FELINE PRACTICE

FELINE PRACTICE

Gary D. Norsworthy, D.V.M.

Acres North Animal Hospital
Fellow, Academy of Feline Medicine
San Antonio, Texas

With 34 contributors

J. B. Lippincott Company
Philadelphia

Acquisitions Editor: Mary K. Smith
Assistant Editor: Anne Geyer
Production Manager: Janet Greenwood
Production: P. M. Gordon Associates, Inc.
Compositor: Achorn Graphics Services, Inc.
Printer/Binder: R. R. Donnelley & Sons

6 5 4 3 2

Library of Congress Cataloging-in-Publication Data

Norsworthy, Gary D.
Feline practice / Gary D. Norsworthy ; with 34 contributors.
p. cm.
Includes bibliographical references (p.) and index.
ISBN 0-397-51204-X
1. Cats—Diseases. 2. Cats—Diseases—Treatment. I. Title.
SF985.N67 1993
636.8′089—dc20 92-41678
CIP

The authors and publisher have exerted every effort to ensure that drug selection and dosage set forth in this text are in accord with current recommendations and practice at the time of publication. However, in view of ongoing research, changes in government regulations, and the constant flow of information relating to drug therapy and drug reactions, the reader is urged to check the package insert for each drug for any change in indications and dosage and for added warnings and precautions. This is particularly important when the recommended agent is a new or infrequently employed drug.

CONTRIBUTORS

Douglas C. Bronstad, DVM
Diplomate, American College of Veterinary Internal Medicine (Internal Medicine)
Animal Diagnostic Clinic
Dallas, Texas

William B. Buck, DVM, MS
Diplomate, American Board of Veterinary Toxicology
Professor of Toxicology
Department of Veterinary Biosciences
Director of Toxicology
National Animal Poison Control Center
College of Veterinary Medicine
University of Illinois
Urbana, Illinois

Robert Crawford Causey, DVM
Section, Comparative Theriogenology
Department of Veterinary Clinical Sciences
School of Veterinary Medicine
Louisiana State University
Baton Rouge, Louisiana

James R. Cook, Jr., DVM, PhD
Diplomate, American College of Veterinary Internal Medicine (Neurology)
Staff Neurologist
Animal Emergency and Referral Center
Fort Pierce, Florida

Rick L. Cowell, DVM, MS
Diplomate, American College of Veterinary Pathologists
Associate Professor of Clinical Pathology
Department of Veterinary Pathology
College of Veterinary Medicine
Oklahoma State University
Stillwater, Oklahoma

Bruce E. Eilts, DVM, MS
Diplomate, American College of Theriogenologists
Associate Professor of Theriogenology
Department of Veterinary Clinical Sciences
School of Veterinary Medicine
Louisiana State University
Baton Rouge, Louisiana

Frances T. Eiserlch, MS, MT (ASCP)
Associate Professor
Program Director
Medical Laboratory Technology
St. Philip's College
San Antonio, Texas

Sharon K. Fooshee, MAG, MS, DVM
Clinical Instructor of Critical Care
Coordinator, Intensive Care Unit
College of Veterinary Medicine
Animal Health Center
Mississippi State University
Mississippi State, Mississippi

Ronald W. Green, DVM, MS
Diplomate, American College of Veterinary Radiology
Associate Professor of Radiology
Veterinary Teaching Hospital
College of Veterinary Medicine
Texas A&M University
College Station, Texas

Richard M. Groff, DVM
Contra Costa Veterinary Emergency Clinic
Concord, California

Jeffery O. Hall, DVM
Diplomate, American Board of Veterinary Toxicology
Teaching Associate, Veterinary Biosciences and Laboratories of Veterinary Diagnostic Medicine
College of Veterinary Medicine
University of Illinois
Urbana, Illinois

Anne M. James, DVM
Acres North Animal Hospital
San Antonio, Texas

Michael W. Knight, DVM
Veterinary Poison Information Specialist
National Animal Poison Control Center
College of Veterinary Medicine
University of Illinois
Urbana, Illinois

Heidi B. Lobprise, DVM
Dallas Dental Service Animal Clinic
Dallas, Texas

Amy R. Marder, DVM
Clinical Assistant Professor
Tufts University School of Veterinary Medicine
Animal Behavior Consultant
Angell Memorial Animal Hospital
Cambridge, Massachusetts

W. Sherman Mathey, DVM
Consulting Veterinarian
Sea World, Inc.
Ultrasound Consulting Practice
San Antonio, Texas

Sandra R. Merchant, DVM
Diplomate, American College of Veterinary Dermatology
Assistant Professor of Dermatology
Department of Veterinary Clinical Sciences
School of Veterinary Medicine
Louisiana State University
Baton Rouge, Louisiana

Joan M. Miller, DVM
Veterinary Poison Information Specialist
National Animal Poison Control Center
College of Veterinary Medicine
University of Illinois
Urbana, Illinois

Gary D. Norsworthy, DVM
Acres North Animal Hospital
Fellow, Academy of Feline Medicine
San Antonio, Texas

L. A. Norsworthy, PhD
Clinical Psychologist
Academic Dean
Northeastern Christian Junior College
Villanova, Pennsylvania

Dale L. Paccamonti, DVM, MS
Diplomate, American College of Theriogenologists
Assistant Professor of Theriogenology
Department of Veterinary Clinical Sciences
School of Veterinary Medicine
Louisiana State University
Baton Rouge, Louisiana

James C. Prueter, DVM
Diplomate, American College of Veterinary Internal Medicine (Internal Medicine)
Head of Medicine
Veterinary Referral Clinic
Cleveland, Ohio

Art J. Quinn, DVM
Diplomate, American College of Veterinary Ophthalmologists
Professor of Ophthalmology
Section Chief, Small Animal Medicine
Boren Veterinary Medical Teaching Hospital
Oklahoma State University
Stillwater, Oklahoma

J. Thomas Ross, DVM
Private Practice, Colonial Veterinary Hospital
Ithaca, New York

Gerard J. Rubin, DVM
Diplomate, American College of Veterinary Internal Medicine (Internal Medicine & Cardiology)
Adjunct Professor
University of Texas Health Science Center
Dallas, Texas
College of Veterinary Medicine
Texas A&M University
College Station, Texas

John E. Saidla, DVM
Director of Continuing Education
College of Veterinary Medicine
Cornell University
Ithaca, New York

Virginia A. Schultz, DVM
Section, Comparative Veterinary Ophthalmology
Boren Veterinary Medical Teaching Hospital
Oklahoma State University
Stillwater, Oklahoma

Fredric W. Scott, DVM, PhD
Diplomate, American College of Veterinary Microbiologists
Honorary First Fellow, Academy of Feline Medicine
Director, Cornell Feline Health Center
Professor of Virology
College of Veterinary Medicine
Cornell University
Ithaca, New York

Eric L. Stair, DVM
Teaching Associate, Veterinary Biosciences and Veterinary Diagnostic Medicine Laboratories
National Animal Poison Control Center
College of Veterinary Medicine
University of Illinois
Urbana, Illinois

Steven Joel Susaneck, DVM
Diplomate, American College of Veterinary Internal Medicine (Internal Medicine & Medical Oncology)
Veterinary Internal Medicine & Oncology Referral Service
Houston, Texas

R. Steve Taylor, DVM
Diplomate, American College of Veterinary Internal Medicine (Internal Medicine)
Staff Internist
Lexington Boulevard Animal Hospital
Sugar Land, Texas

Jane M. Turrel, DVM, MS
Charter Diplomate, American College of Veterinary Internal Medicine (Medical Oncology)
Diplomate, American College of Veterinary Radiology
Radiation Oncologist
Veterinary Oncology Specialties
Pacifica, California

Ronald D. Tyler, DVM, PhD
Diplomate, American College of Veterinary Pathologists
Senior Research Pathologist
Schering Research Institute
Lafayette, New Jersey
Adjunct Professor
Department of Veterinary Pathology
College of Veterinary Medicine
Oklahoma State University
Stillwater, Oklahoma

Robert B. Wiggs, DVM
Diplomate, American Veterinary Dental College
Director, Dallas Dental Service Animal Clinic
Adjunct Assistant Professor
Department of Physiology
Baylor College of Dentistry
Dallas, Texas

Benny J. Woody, DVM, MS
Diplomate, American Board of Veterinary Practitioners (Companion Animals)
Associate Professor
Section Chief, Community Practice
College of Veterinary Medicine
Animal Health Center
Adjunct Professor
Department of Wildlife and Fisheries
Mississippi State University
Mississippi State Mississippi

FOREWORD

Dr. Gary D. Norsworthy is well known and popular on the feline medicine speaking circuit. He was among the first to approach his topics from the perspective of clinical presentation in the way practitioners actually see sick cats, and this point of view is strongly emphasized in *Feline Practice*.

When a small handful of practitioners established "cats only" practices in the early 1970s, success was virtually assured by doing little more than acknowledging the special needs of cats and their owners. Thankfully, such is no longer the case, and feline care has developed into a branch of small animal practice that can take full advantage of the great advances in knowledge about this delightful species.

Drawing on years of practical experience and fine clinical judgment, Dr. Norsworthy has created a book that is specifically directed toward practitioners who accept the challenge of providing excellent primary care under practical circumstances and toward clinical year veterinary students who wish to augment their theoretical knowledge with practical techniques that work.

Many of the chapters that discuss specific syndromes in depth have been written by experts in specialized disciplines and emerging areas of new knowledge. The various authors' individual styles prove advantageous since the book is intended as a reference, and every chapter can stand alone. Each topic is discussed from the perspective that is most clear and useful within the guidelines imposed by the intended audience.

The format of the book is consistent, emphasizing the importance of making definitive diagnoses and including realistic prognoses and alternative treatment approaches. The busy practitioner will find new solutions to old problems and up-to-date, clinically oriented discussions of emerging challenges.

Susan McDonough, V.M.D.
Cat Hospital of Philadelphia

PREFACE

When I graduated from Texas A&M University in 1972, cats were a minor part of most small animal practices. Most small animal practices had a feline caseload that was less than 20% of the practice. When I entered a feline-only practice upon graduation, some of my classmates thought I was slightly crazy; others thought I was wasting my education.

Today, however, there are 57 million cats and 52.5 million dogs in the American veterinary service market, according to a recent AVMA report. The gap between the number of cats and dogs has widened each year since 1987. This shift in pet owners from canine to feline continues to affect veterinary practice. No longer is the cat considered a minor species.

The need for this book is based on the growing importance of the cat in small animal and mixed veterinary practices. It is also based on the practitioner's need for a *practical* reference book. *Feline Practice* is my best effort to create a clinically useful manual for the treatment of feline patients.

My goal has been to create a book for the primary care veterinarian, whether in a feline-only practice or mixed, and also for third- or fourth-year veterinary students. *Feline Practice* provides tools for the handling of feline patients, for client relations, and for diagnostic and therapeutic procedures for common diseases and conditions. Each contributing author has been asked to place emphasis on diagnosis, treatment, and prognosis. Each author also has been asked to organize and present information in a manner that allows the busy practitioner to retrieve clinical information quickly. You, the reader, must be the judge of how effectively we have met this goal.

Gary D. Norsworthy, D.V.M.

ACKNOWLEDGMENTS

I would like to express gratitude to my friends and colleagues who have reviewed parts of this book. Drs. Douglas Bronstad, Kenita Rogers, Connie Guerra, Bill Gibson, Alisa Lane, and Ike Sawyer reviewed most of the chapters. Selected chapters were reviewed by Drs. Don C. Miller, Ronald Green, Claudia Barton, Kohle Herrmann, H. T. Green, and Linda Homco. Their input has helped to ensure scientific accuracy and practicality.

I would like to express gratitude to four of my colleagues who greatly shaped my veterinary career. Dr. David D. White of Dallas employed me as a kennelboy one summer when I was looking for a job. Not only did he give me a job, but his guidance directed me to a career. Dr. Bill Freitag of Seattle was my first boss when I graduated from veterinary college. He set standards of excellence that I have always tried to emulate. Dr. Walter Juliff of Texas A&M University invited me to speak at the first Feline Seminar conducted by the University. His encouragement has given me confidence for my many speaking opportunities. Dr. Don Miller of San Antonio has been my partner for the past 18 years. He has made tolerable a lot of the bumps and bruises of the real world of veterinary practice. To each of these I say "Thank you." You have had more to do with this book than you realize.

Finally, and most importantly, I would like to express gratitude to my wife, Linda, and my children, John and Melissa, for not begrudging me the time needed for this endeavor. I would like to express special thanks to Linda for the hours she put in as my personal secretary and encourager.

CONTENTS

PART I

General Techniques for Feline Practice

1. Breeds of Cats 3
   Anne M. James
2. Addressing and Handling the Cat 28
   Gary D. Norsworthy
3. The History and Physical Examination 31
   Gary D. Norsworthy
4. Kittens 37
   Gary D. Norsworthy and Frances T. Eiserloh
5. Anorexia and Force Feeding 40
   Gary D. Norsworthy
6. Administration of Oral Medications 44
   Gary D. Norsworthy
7. Drug Peculiarities 48
   Gary D. Norsworthy
8. Anesthetics and Anesthesia 56
   Gary D. Norsworthy
9. Blood Collection 62
   Gary D. Norsworthy
10. Blood Transfusions 64
    Gary D. Norsworthy
11. Euthanasia and Grief Management 69
    Gary D. Norsworthy and L. A. Norsworthy

PART II

Diagnostics

12. Laboratory Tests and Testing 81
    Gary D. Norsworthy
13. Cytology 95
    Gary D. Norsworthy
14. Radiology 114
    Ronald W. Green and Gary D. Norsworthy
15. Ultrasonography 144
    W. Sherman Mathey

PART III

Clinical Syndromes

16. Anemia 157
    Gary D. Norsworthy
17. Ataxia/Paresis 164
    James R. Cook Jr.
18. Dyspnea 172
    Gary D. Norsworthy
19. Fever of Unknown Origin 191
    James C. Prueter
20. Icterus 195
    Gary D. Norsworthy
21. Lymphadenopathy 199
    Rick L. Cowell and Ronald D. Tyler
22. Polyuria and Polydipsia 207
    R. Steve Taylor
23. Seizure Disorders 218
    James R. Cook, Jr.
24. Vomiting and Diarrhea 223
    Douglas C. Bronstad and Gary D. Norsworthy

PART IV

Diseases

25. Asthma 231
    Gary D. Norsworthy
26. Behavior Problems 236
    Amy R. Marder
27. Cardiomyopathy and Thromboembolic Disease 244
    Gary D. Norsworthy
28. Cervical Ventroflexion 256
    R. Steve Taylor
29. Cholangitis/Cholangiohepatitis Syndrome 261
    Gary D. Norsworthy
30. Chronic Nasal Discharge 266
    Gary D. Norsworthy

31. Chronic Renal Disease 274
R. Steve Taylor

32. Chylothorax 287
Gary D. Norsworthy

33. Dental Diseases 290
Robert B. Wiggs and Heidi B. Lobprise

34. Diabetes Mellitus 305
Gary D. Norsworthy

35. The Eyes: Extraocular Diseases 317
Art J. Quinn and Virginia A. Schultz

36. The Eyes: Intraocular Diseases 332
Art J. Quinn and Virginia A. Schultz

37. Feline Immunodeficiency Virus Diseases 348
Gary D. Norsworthy

38. Feline Infectious Peritonitis 352
Gary D. Norsworthy

39. Feline Leukemia Virus Diseases 360
Gary D. Norsworthy

40. Feline Urologic Syndrome 369
Gary D. Norsworthy

41. Heartworm Disease 379
Gary D. Norsworthy

42. Heinz Body Hemolytic Anemia and Methemoglobinemia 384
Gary D. Norsworthy

43. Hemobartonellosis 389
Gary D. Norsworthy

44. High-Rise Syndrome 392
J. Thomas Ross

45. Hyperesthesia Syndrome 399
James R. Cook, Jr.

46. Hyperthyroidism 401
Jane M. Turrel and Gary D. Norsworthy

47. Idiopathic Hepatic Lipidosis 408
Gary D. Norsworthy

48. Inflammatory Bowel Disease 413
Douglas C. Bronstad

49. Megacolon 416
Gary D. Norsworthy

50. Multicat Facilities: Disease Control 420
Fredric W. Scott and John E. Saidla

51. Neoplastic Diseases 425
Steven Susaneck

52. Oral Diseases 438
Robert B. Wiggs and Heidi B. Lobprise

53. Pyothorax 454
Gary D. Norsworthy

54. Reproductive Disorders 458
Bruce E. Eilts, Dale L. Paccamonti, and Robert Causey

55. Selected Surgical Procedures 477
Gary D. Norsworthy

56. The Skin: Fungal Diseases 504
Sandra R. Merchant

57. The Skin: Parasitic Diseases 511
Sandra R. Merchant

58. The Skin: Hypersensitivity Diseases 518
Sandra R. Merchant

59. The Skin: Neoplastic Diseases 526
Sandra R. Merchant

60. The Skin: Diseases of Unknown or Multiple Etiology 532
Sandra R. Merchant

61. Systemic Fungal Diseases 540
Sharon K. Fooshee and Benny J. Woody

62. Toxicoses and Toxins 551
Richard M. Groff, Joan M. Miller, Eric L. Stair, Jeffery O. Hall, Michael W. Knight, and William B. Buck

63. Upper Respiratory Infections 570
Gary D. Norsworthy

64. Zoonotic Diseases 577
Gary D. Norsworthy

Appendixes

Appendix A. Drug Formulary: Alphabetical by Generic Name 585

Appendix B. Drug Formulary: Alphabetical by Trade Name 615

Appendix C. Drug Formulary: Alphabetical by Indication 621

Appendix D. Conversion Table: Weight to Body-Surface Area 629

Appendix E. Medication Dosage Charts 631

Appendix F. Differential Overview 635
Gerard Rubin

Index 665

PART I

◇ ◇ ◇

General Techniques for Feline Practice

CHAPTER 1

◇ ◇ ◇

Breeds of Cats

Anne M. James

A breed is a group of animals that a sufficient number of people mutually agree to accept as such; the group must have distinguishing features that set it apart from all others and, therefore, distinctive underlying genetic traits.

It is very difficult to give a rigid definition of a breed. The criteria generally used include unique body conformation, hair color pattern, hair type, and geographic origin of the breed. These are the main criteria covered in this chapter.

The evolution of cat breeds has been influenced over the centuries by several factors:

1. Environmental adaptation
2. Mutations
3. Geographic restrictions
4. Superstitions
5. Human preferences

As cats have spread around the world, they have gradually changed to adapt to their new environments. The two main domestic cat structural types that have been defined—that is, the longhair and shorthair—likely arose as a result of adjustments to cold and warm climates, respectively.

There are many main genes responsible for the genetic variations delineating different breeds. Some of the most recent mutations that have occurred are the Abyssinian ticked tabby pattern, Manx, Rex, hairless Sphynx, wirehair, and curled ear breeds.

Several well-known breeds probably originated as a result of geographic restriction. As an example, cats living in early New England that carried the recessive longhair gene were better able to survive the harsh climate. Through isolation and survival, they became the basis for the Maine Coon breed. The Manx is an example of spontaneous mutation that occurred on an isolated island in the Irish Sea.

Another factor influencing the evolution of cat breeds is cultural differences. In the Orient cats were kept isolated and were bred by monks in monasteries, keeping gene pools separated. This separation helped firmly establish certain breeds. Another example is the Japanese Bobtail breed of cat, which is often given as a gift. This breed is considered to be a sign of good luck or a token of great esteem.

Human preferences for color patterns or unique body types affected migration of many breeds, influencing importation from one country to another. There are a number of breeds that were affected in this way throughout the years.

Cat Shows and the Cat Fanciers' Association

Cat shows serve as a major means of public education about cats in general, and also promote them as a potential member of the American family. Moreover, cat shows allow breeders to assess their breeding programs and improve upon each breed. The first National Cat Show was held in 1871 in London, England. The Maine Coon breed became the first pedigreed American cat breed, and subsequently won best cat at the first large American Cat Show in 1895.

The National Cat Club was established in 1884 in England. The main purpose of early breed registries was to refine and further develop many breeds. The Cat Fanciers' Association (CFA), founded in 1906, had as its original goals the improvement of the general welfare of cats, the promotion of cat shows, and the registration of cats and kittens in America. Currently, the CFA is the largest pedigreed cat registry in the world. There are many other smaller registry groups across the globe.

All of the registry associations have their own set of rules governing the acceptance of new breeds and colors. These rigid rules exist basically to protect the cat fancy from potential decline.

Application for CFA registration requires documentation of 50 specimens and a minimum of 10 breeders working with the new breed. Once registered, the breed may be shown in the noncompetitive "Miscellaneous Class." This allows exposure to the new breed to breeders, judges, and the general public for 5 years. The next step is to achieve "Provisional Breed" status. The breed must have at least 100 specimens and a breed standard proposal, among other requirements. Then the breed must be shown extensively across the country, reports must be made by judges, and in-depth information about the breed must be presented to the CFA board. When 25 different cats have been shown in all 7 regions and a breed standard has been agreed upon, the new breed is then eligible for "Championship" status.

This status confers eligibility for full competition with other breeds.

The number of cats that are family pets has steadily increased, and cats have surpassed dogs as the number one pet in America. It has been estimated that less than 10% of American cats are pedigreed. Almost two thirds of pedigreed cats registered by the CFA in 1988 and 1989 were of the Persian breed.

Specific Breeds

Abyssinian

The Abyssinian (Fig. 1–1) is one of the older cat breeds but has a sketchy history. The Abyssinian has been called the "child of the gods," as it is believed to be descended from the cats of ancient Egypt who lived more than 4,000 years ago.[1] Others believe this cat is related to the small wild cats of North Africa, and originated there. Yet another theory credits British breeders for developing the unique ticking of the Abyssinian from the British Domestic Tabby.[1] Each of these theories has merit, but none has been solidly proven. The name Abyssinian came about because the first Abyssinian cat exhibited at a show in England in the late 1800s came from Abyssinia, now known as Ethiopia.[2]

The Abyssinian breed was first brought to England in 1868, near the end of the Abyssinian War, and was first listed as a separate breed in 1882. By 1900, the name was changed to Ticked or British Ticks. This breed was also sometimes referred to as "Bunny Cats" owing to the coat's similarity to that of wild rabbits. British cross-breeding experimentation produced silver or blue Abyssinians, the first pair of which was exported to the United States in the early 1900s.[1] The first Abyssinian was registered with the CFA in 1917.[3] World War I halted cat breeding in England which, in turn, slowed exportation of Abyssinians to the United States until the late 1930s. The breed has steadily grown in popularity since then.

The Abyssinian is a medium-sized cat with large, brilliant, almond-shaped eyes and alert ears, often with characteristic tufts. Its legs are slim and fine-boned, with small oval paws. The tail is long and tapers to the tip. The Abyssinian gives the overall impression of being alert and athletic.

The characteristic ticking of the Abyssinian's hair is caused by the black or brown tips of each hair. The standard coloring for the Abyssinian is called "normal" in England, but is termed "ruddy" in the United States. It is a rich, burnt sienna color ticked with various shades of dark brown or black, with an orange-brown undercoat. Other colors have occurred in the history of the breed, including red, cinnamon, or sorrel, a lilac or fawn, and blue. The red Abyssinian's coat is coppery-red ticked with a light chocolate brown, with a deep red undercoat. Red Abyssinians received CFA Championship status in 1964 after much debate. In 1984, the blue Abyssinian received CFA Championship status, followed by the fawn in 1990.[2] An Abyssinian of a new color, termed a silver Abyssinian, has recently been seen in Australia, having been developed in New Zealand.

Abyssinians are highly intelligent cats and are easy to train. They love people and have sweet personalities. They are built for agility and are either sleeping or on the go.[1]

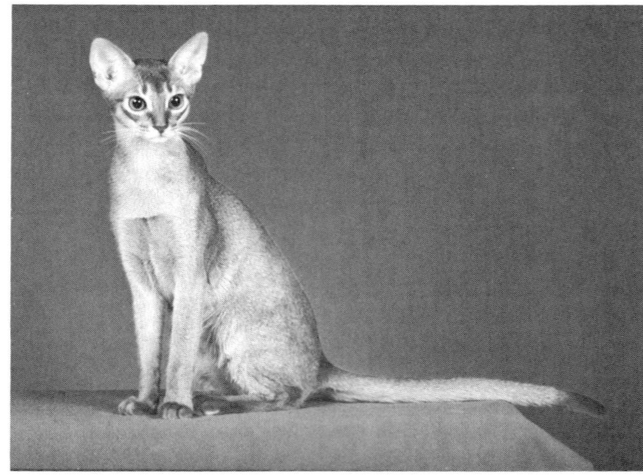

Figure 1–1. Abyssinian. (© Chanan Photography)

They usually prefer not to live in large cat groups, and tend to stay close to their owners. Their voice is considered quiet, even when in heat.

American Bobtail

A breed that has not yet been accepted by the CFA—the American Bobtail—was developed as a result of mating a mixed-breed, short-tailed male to a Siamese female.[2] The dominant Manx tail gene results in cats with tails of varying lengths. The longhair gene has recently been introduced into the breed by mating Himalayan and Maine Coon cats to existing lines.

American Curl (Longhair and Shorthair)

The curled ear of the American Curl breed (Figs. 1–2 and 1–3) is the most recent spontaneous mutation recognized in domestic cats, having occurred in 1981.[2] Grace and Joe Ruga of California noticed that the ears of their long-haired black female cat curled up and back. This female, "Shu-

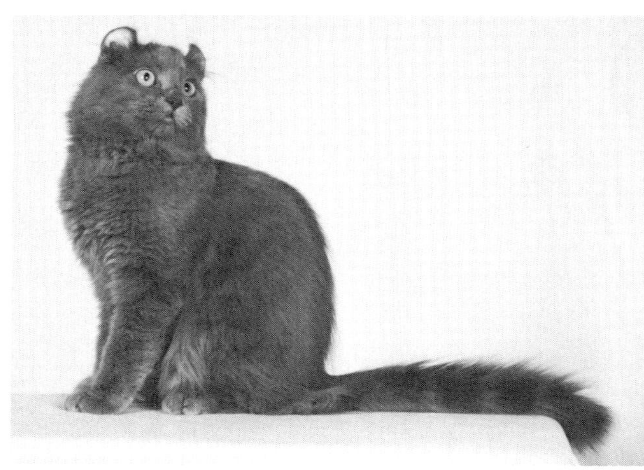

Figure 1–2. American Curl Longhair. (© Chanan Photography)

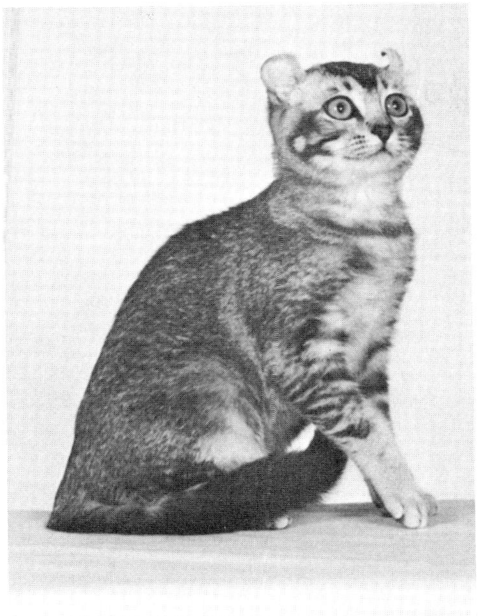

Figure 1–3. American Curl Shorthair. (© Chanan Photography)

lamith," produced kittens with the same uniquely curled ear. She became the foundation cat for the breed. The gene was determined to be a simple dominant gene. Short-haired and long-haired versions have been developed by breeders working to achieve a consistent appearance for both.

The CFA allowed registration of this breed in 1986. Since May of 1991, these cats have been shown in the Provisional class.

The ears of the American Curl have firm cartilage except for the top one third. Toward the center of the back of the head, there is a smooth curving arc. An ear that curls to touch the back of the ear or head is not acceptable.

The most critical factors in defining the uniqueness of this breed are related to the facial expression and ear formation of these cats. The head, eyes, and ears of this breed receive the most attention in the proposed standard.

The head of the American Curl is a modified wedge, with gentle contours. The eyes are large and expressive. This cat is physically well balanced and of medium size, being slightly larger than the Oriental or foreign breeds. The Longhair Curls have a silky, moderately long coat with minimal undercoat. The tail is heavily plumed and full. The Shorthair Curls have a short, soft coat that lies fairly flat. All coat colors and patterns are acceptable, including the Siamese pointed pattern.[2]

A large gene pool has provided a sound foundation for the American Curl. No associated defects have been reported as of yet, and the general public has responded favorably to the breed.[2]

American Shorthair

When domestic shorthairs reportedly first came to North America aboard the Mayflower in 1620, they quickly earned their keep as good hunters and mousers. The tough conditions these hard-working cats survived are still evident in the American Shorthair (Fig. 1–4) today. These cats bred freely for years and kept a fairly consistent look. In 1900, a male shorthair from England named Belle was imported, and subsequently became the first short-haired cat to be registered by the CFA. Belle's owner, Mrs. Jane Cathcart, promoted the shorthair breed in the early 20th century. In 1904, Cathcart registered "Buster Brown," the first American-born Shorthair.[3]

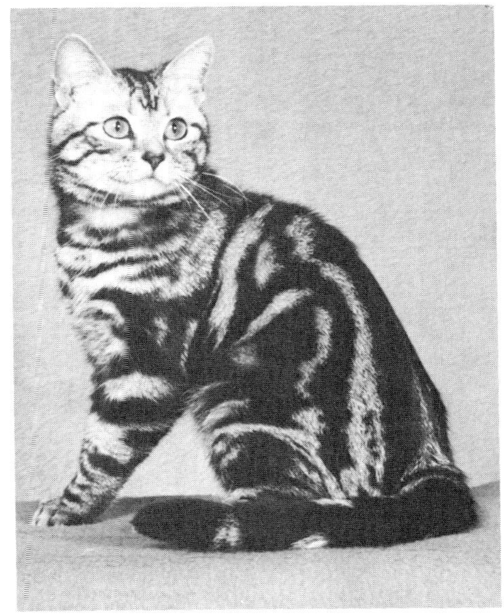

Figure 1–4. American Shorthair. (© Chanan Photography)

Throughout the years, breeders became anxious to distinguish these cats from mixed breed cats. Several hair color patterns were developed that are not seen in modern day mixed breed cats. Originally, the breed was simply known as the Shorthair, but was renamed the American Shorthair in 1966. To retain its roots as a true natural American breed, associations will allow registration of nonpedigreed shorthair cats under certain conditions. In fact, a cat such as this was declared best of breed by the CFA in 1971.[3]

American Shorthairs are generally medium-sized to large cats, with a muscular body and short, hard coat. There are no extremes to this cat, with no part of their anatomy being exaggerated. Their head is large and oblong with full cheeks and strong jaw. Their eyes are wide-set and round. Their legs and tail are medium in length. Over 30 solid colors and patterns are recognized, including calico and tortoiseshell.

These cats are very natural, taking life in stride. They are intelligent, independent, and very loving and gentle with people. Their characteristics as survivors and hunters are evident in their personality and behavior, as they are able to adjust very well.[1] They make good breeders, with an average litter size of four.[3]

American Wirehair

The American Wirehair is one of only a few breeds considered to be truly native to the United States. In 1966, a muta-

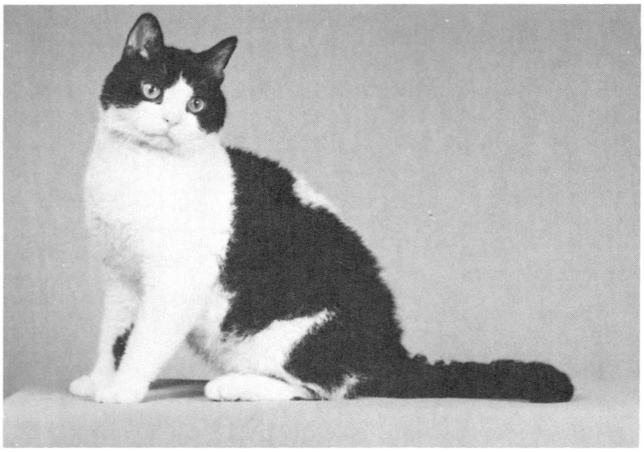

Figure 1–5. American Wirehair. (© Chanan Photography)

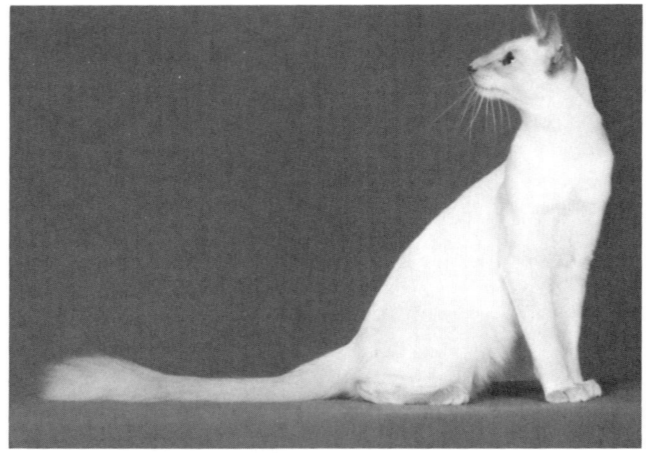

Figure 1–6. Balinese. (© Chanan Photography)

tion occurred among a litter of farm cats near Vernon, New York. One of the kittens had a very wiry coat, which geneticists in England confirmed as a type of coat never seen before in cats. The hairs were crimped and wiry, more so than the Wirehaired Terrier.[3] The breed was then developed and named the American Wirehair (Fig. 1–5).

The first Wirehair, named "Adam," was bred to an unrelated female, which produced wirehaired kittens. This proved that the new gene was dominant. Adam's granddaughter, "Barberry Ellen," was the first homozygous American Wirehair.[3] The breed was granted Championship status by the CFA in 1978.

Breeders today are still working on standardizing the appearance and coat characteristics of this breed, as there is still considerable variation. Breeders want these cats to conform to a standard similar to American Shorthairs, except for the coat description. Adam and his close relatives did not have the ideal appearance, having longer legs, body, and large ears. Many outcrossings have been done to help this breed achieve a uniquely standard appearance. Their body structure and facial features are very similar to American Shorthairs, being well-rounded and medium-sized.

Cats of this breed may be of any color or pattern except Siamese coloring and pattern.[2] The CFA standard for coat states that it must be "very dense, resilient, crimped and coarse."[2] The eyebrows and whiskers are also crimped.

The American Wirehair has a personality that is very similar to that of the American Shorthair except that the former may be slightly more personable to strangers.[2] Like the American Shorthair, they are hearty, sweet-tempered, and very adaptable.

Balinese

The Balinese (Fig. 1–6) acquired its name because its smooth lines and graceful movements, emphasized by its flowing coat, reminded its pioneer breeders of Bali dancers. This cat was developed by breeders in the United States from a mutation that occurred within the Siamese breed, whereby long-haired kittens were among a litter of normal Siamese kittens. These long-haired kittens were considered to be faulty until two breeders in California and New York began to develop this as a separate breed in the 1940s.[1]

Breeders worked to refine the body type and coat quality, and finally gained CFA Championship status in 1970. The appearance of these cats is one of a long-haired Siamese, and they are accepted in the same four colors as the Siamese: seal point, chocolate point, blue point, and lilac point.[2] Balinese cats differ slightly from the Siamese in that their longer coat gives the appearance of a less extreme body type and softer lines, and they have a distinctive plumelike tail.

These cats are lively and affectionate, quick to learn, and want to be a part of the family. They have a softer-toned voice than does the Siamese.[1]

Bengal

The Bengal (Fig. 1–7) breed has not yet been recognized by the CFA. It is the result of cross-mating domestic cats with the native Asian Leopard cat, which is a spotted wild

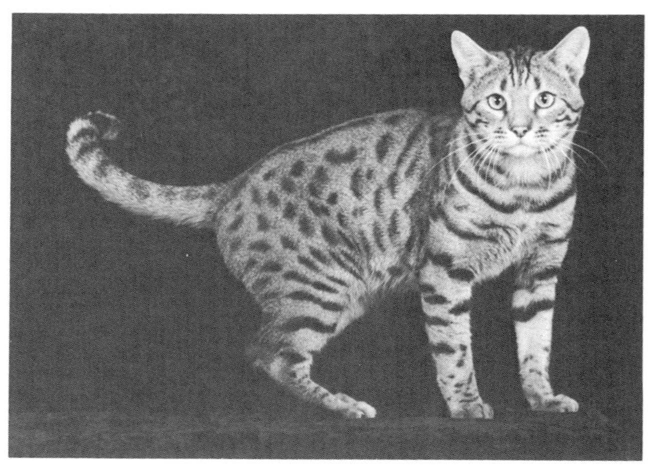

Figure 1–7. Bengal. (© Chanan Photography)

cat with a high degree of pattern contrast.[2] These cats have a wild appearance coupled with a domestic cat temperament.

Birman

The Birman (Fig. 1–8), also known as the "Sacred Cat of Burma," is thought to have originated from sacred cats that were guardians of the temples in Burma. The legend of Birman cats traces back to the time of death of the head monk, Mun-Ha. Sinh, his loyal cat, placed his paws on his master's body at the moment of his death. Sinh then faced the golden goddess of the temple and instantly his white hair turned golden, and his eyes became sapphire blue, as were hers. His paws remained white, denoting purity. Seven days after the head priest died, Sinh died as well, purportedly taking his master's soul to heaven.[1]

In 1919, a Birman pair were sent to France. The male did not survive the trip. The female was pregnant, which led to the development of the breed in France. The first Birmans to enter North America came from France in 1959. A chocolate point male known as "Waddi" came to the Seipels of Fairfax, Virginia.[1] Through extensive breeding, Birmans became well established in the United States and were registered with the CFA in 1966. Champion status was granted in 1967.[2]

The appearance of the Birman is one of robustness; they are a large cat. The head is rounded and the muzzle is large and blunt. The eyes are very expressive, deep, and blue. Other characteristics include short paws, heavy legs, and a large, bushy tail. The hair coat is silky and of medium length, but does not mat easily. The hair on the belly is wavy. The Birman is accepted by the CFA in only the four point colors (seal, chocolate, blue, and lilac).

The four white gloves are unique to the Birman. The front paws should be white up to the second or third joints. Back paws have "gloves" and "laces" extending up the back of the hock, ideally ending in an inverted V.[2]

Birmans are known to adjust well to family living, having lots of charm and personality. They are intelligent and easy to train, possessing a quiet, pleasant voice. They also breed easily and have few problems.

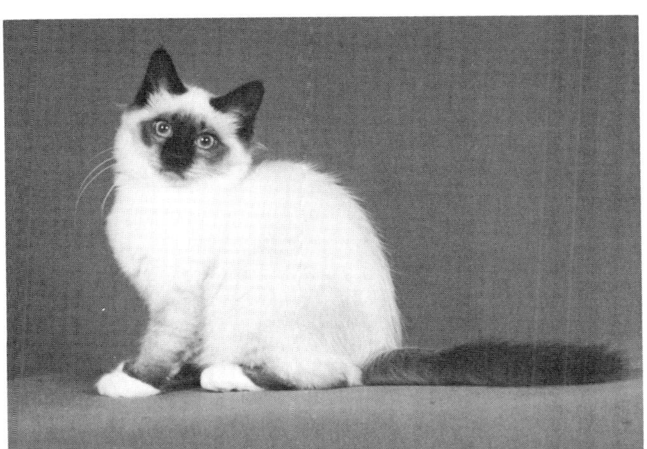

Figure 1–8. Birman. (© Chanan Photography)

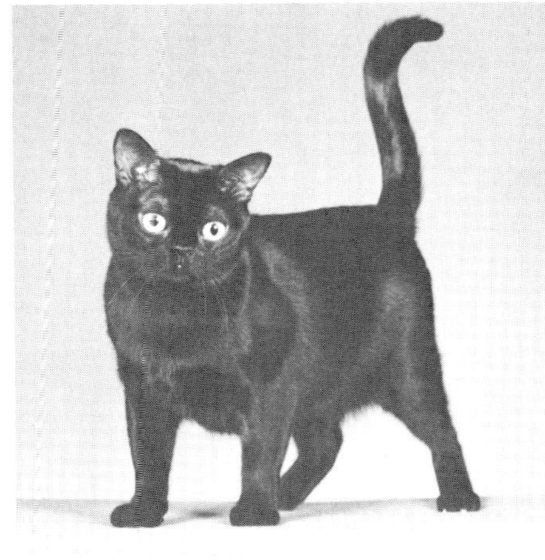

Figure 1–9. Bombay. (© Chanan Photography)

Bombay

The Bombay breed of cat is a man-made, hybrid breed, the product of crossing a black American Shorthair with a Burmese. In 1958, Nikki Horner of Louisville, Kentucky began to develop this new breed with a certain look in mind.[2] Her desire was to produce a copper-eyed short-haired black cat with a sleek coat, a "mini-panther."[1] The name of this breed was inspired by the black leopard of India.[2]

After years of selective breeding, the CFA accepted the Bombay (Fig. 1–9) for Championship status in 1976.[1] Outcrossing to sable Burmese and black American Shorthairs is still allowed.[2]

The Bombay has a round head and full face, with considerable distance between the eyes. The eyes are round and range in color from yellow to deep copper, the latter of which is ideal. The ears are medium in size, broad-based, and rounded at the tips. The body is medium-sized, with a straight tail of average length. The coat is fine, short, and satin-like in texture, and is often said to shimmer like patent leather, black to the roots. Both the nose leather and paw pads must be black to conform to breed standard.[1]

Bombays have an even temperament and are playful, but are not too talkative. They are very hearty and get along well with other cats. They seem to purr constantly, and love attention. The males can be clumsy, but the females are quite graceful.[1]

British Shorthair

In some ways, the British Shorthair breed can be thought of as the British equivalent of the American Shorthair, being first shown in England in the late 1800s.[1] Having been developed from nonpedigreed working cats of Europe, this breed has certain qualities, such as hardiness, stamina, and an ideal temperament, while varying somewhat in appearance. This breed, along with many others, suffered during World War II, and very few pedigreed stud males were left. In the 1950s, many British Shorthairs were outcrossed to larger Persians. This cross-mating successfully restored the stocky body type

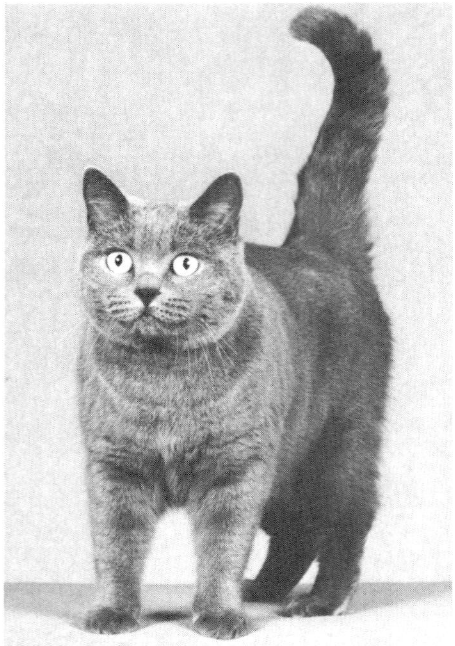

Figure 1–10. British Shorthair. (© Chanan Photography)

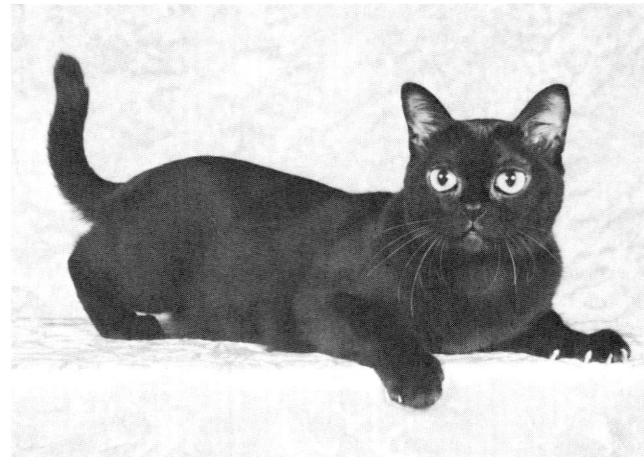

Figure 1–11. Burmese. (© Chanan Photography)

but sacrificed the originally desired short, extremely dense and firm coat. Since then, breeders have worked hard to restore the haircoat to its original type.

The popularity of this breed expanded gradually in the United States during the 1960s and 1970s.[2] Associations in the United States refrained from fully recognizing the British Shorthair (Fig. 1–10) because of the Persian blood in their pedigree. The CFA finally recognized the British Shorthair for Championship status in 1980.

The main distinction between the British Shorthair and other domestic-derived shorthairs is the character of its head,[2] which is round with full cheeks, a firm chin, and a short nose that has a gentle dip. The eyes are large and round, with the color ranging from gold to copper. White cats may have blue eyes or odd eyes (one blue and one gold). The ears are small, rounded, and set well apart. These cats have a compact, powerful body and full chest, with short, strong legs and rounded paws. The tail is short and thick with a rounded tip. The ideal coat is dense and resilient, without woolliness. The coat colors include a variety of solids and a number of patterns. In the earlier days, solid colors were most popular, especially the blue.

British Shorthairs are said to have an even temperament, with lots of intelligence and dignity. Their voice is very quiet, and they can be left alone to entertain themselves. They are exceptionally hardy and resistant to cold weather.

Burmese

The Burmese (Fig. 1–11) was the first pedigreed breed to be developed entirely in the United States.[3] In 1930, Dr. Joseph Thompson imported a walnut-brown female cat named "Wong Mau" from Burma. He was very interested in determining the genetic makeup of these cats from the Orient, which were also known as "copper" cats. Accordingly, Thompson began a controlled breeding program in the hope of establishing a new breed. Wong Mau was mated with a Siamese male, and over several generations, three types of kittens resulted. Of the three types, the cats with the darkest brown body all over (no points) were considered to be the first true Burmese. These breeding experiments led to the establishment of the Burmese gene. All Burmese are homozygous for this gene. (Wong Mau's intermediate coloring indicates she had one Burmese and one Siamese gene. This hybrid of Siamese and Burmese is now known as the Tonkinese breed.)

The Burmese breed was first recognized by the CFA in 1936.[3] With such a small gene pool, however, many outcrossings to Siamese cats continued, and these outcrossings led to a less-than-uniform appearance. The confusion prompted the CFA to suspend registration of the breed in 1947.

Burmese cats were exported to Europe and were recognized as a breed in 1952.[2] Colors other than the original sable brown have been developed. The European Burmese is also a more foreign-looking cat, with a wedge-shaped head and oval eyes, true in appearance to the original cats imported from the United States.

The CFA reinstated registration of Burmese cats in 1953 based upon a new color standard allowing only a "solid coat without markings."[2] The body standard changed several times over the following decade. In the mid-1970s, some breeders began to select for a shorter and shorter muzzle to emphasize the rounded head called for in the standard. These gradual skull changes may have led to a craniofacial lethal deformity in newborn kittens.[2] Breeders are still working to eliminate problems in this breed and to improve the concept of the desirable Burmese appearance.

In 1980, the CFA dealt with the three color variations within the Burmese breed by establishing a separate breed called the Malayan. Two recessive genes remained in Burmese lines, likely as a result of earlier outcrossings with Siamese. The mutant chocolate gene produces a champagne-colored cat. The dilute factor alters the sable to create a blue coat, and the champagne to produce a platinum coat.[2] In 1984, the CFA finally incorporated Malayans into the Burmese breed, but they are classified in a separate Dilute division.[2]

The Burmese cat is surprisingly heavy for its medium size and has good bone structure and muscle development. Its head is round with expressive, wide-set eyes and a full face. The ears are medium-sized and alert, with slightly rounded tips. The tail is straight and of medium length.[1] The eye color should be brilliant gold. The marked feature of all Burmese is their short, dense, glossy coat, which should be satinlike in texture and close-lying. The color of the sable is a rich and warm sable brown, with brown nose leather and paw pads. The champagne coat is a warm honey-beige, with shading to a more pale golden-tan color on the underside. The blue Burmese coat is a medium blue with warm fawn undertones, again shading slightly on the belly. The platinum color is described as a pale dove-grey with slight pinkish shading.[3]

Burmese cats are bundles of energy and are said to remain kittenlike all their lives. They love to be cuddled and are unusually adaptable. They can be jealous, but have nice manners and sweet voices. The Burmese have a characteristic treading movement with their hind legs, termed the Burmese shuffle.[2]

Burmilla

The Burmilla breed came about after a planned crossmating of a British Chinchilla Longhair (Persian) male to a Burmese female in 1982.[2] The results were a shaded silver, short-haired cat of the Burmese type. This breed has been accepted by the Cat Association of Britain as a provisional breed.[2] The largest British association, Governing Council of the Cat Fancy (GCCF), has yet to do so.

California Spangled Cat

The California Spangled Cat breed has been developed by one man over a 15-year period using an assortment of American domestic cat breeds and two foreign cats imported from Africa and Southeast Asia.[2] This short-haired breed has a spotted coat pattern and a "wild look."

Chartreux

The Chartreux breed (Fig. 1–12) was referred to as long ago as 1558 and was supposedly bred by the Carthusian monks in France. These cats were reportedly kept and bred by the monks to keep their monastery, La Grande Chartreuse, free from rats and mice. Throughout history, this cat has been admired by the French for its sturdiness and strong hunting ability. The Chartreux pelt was prized by the Dutch for its thick, wooly texture which is similar to that of an otter.[2]

The first recorded selective breeding began on the small island of Belle-Ill-sur-Mer, off the Northwestern coast of France, around 1928. Free-roaming ancestors of the Chartreux were all of the same type despite cross-breeding with other European cats.[1] After World War II, there were few Chartreux left. To restore the breed, breeders tried out-

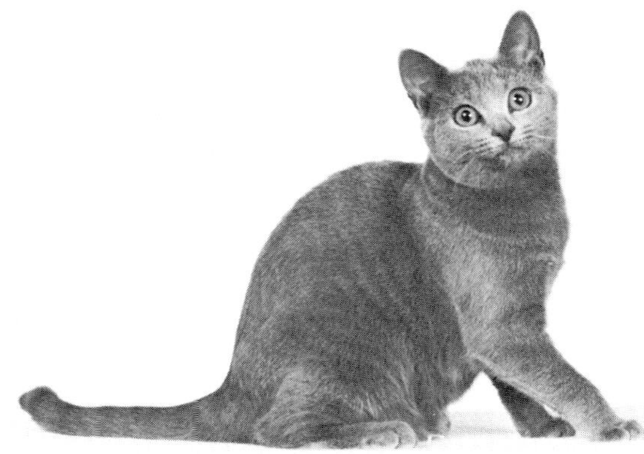

Figure 1–12. Chartreux. (© Chanan Photography)

crossing to Persians and British Blue, but the results were undesirable. Finally, it was decided to use French Blue cats found in the countryside that met the breed standard.

Helen and John Gamon of La Jolla, California went to France in 1970 to find cats of pure lineage to import to the United States. These original imports became one of the foundation breeding stocks for the Chartreux in Canada and the United States. The CFA accepted the breed for registration in 1979, and granted Championship status in 1987.[2]

The Chartreux head and body type set it apart from other blue cats. These cats have a large, broad head, but it is not round. The muzzle is narrow, but not pointed, and its jaws are powerful. Well-developed cheeks and a short, strong, heavy-set neck do not detract from its sweet, smiling expression. The ears are small and set high on the head. The eyes are large and round, and vary in color from pale gold to deep, brilliant orange. The Chartreux's body is robust, with large shoulders and a well-developed chest. The legs seem fairly dainty in comparison to the body. The male is much more massive than the female.

The Chartreux is accepted in the blue color only. The coat is dense and water-repellent, with silver highlights. The nose leather is silver-grey and the paw pads are rose-taupe.[1]

Chartreux cats act in a similar manner to dogs, and sometimes prefer dogs to cats as company. They are energetic and playful, but have a very docile temperament. They tend to be quiet, and are sometimes said to have no voice at all. Legend maintains that these cats took a vow of silence with the monks.[2] Nevertheless, their faint chirping voice is unique to them.

Colorpoint Shorthair

In type, the Colorpoint Shorthair (Fig. 1–13) is identical to the Siamese except for color. This breed resulted from early cross-breeding by cat fanciers in Britain.[2] Their goal was to develop colors other than the traditional four Siamese colors by breeding to Abyssinians and red domestic shorthairs.[2] The early red and seal tortie point cats had poor Siamese body and head type, and the lynx point required great effort to develop perfection in the markings.

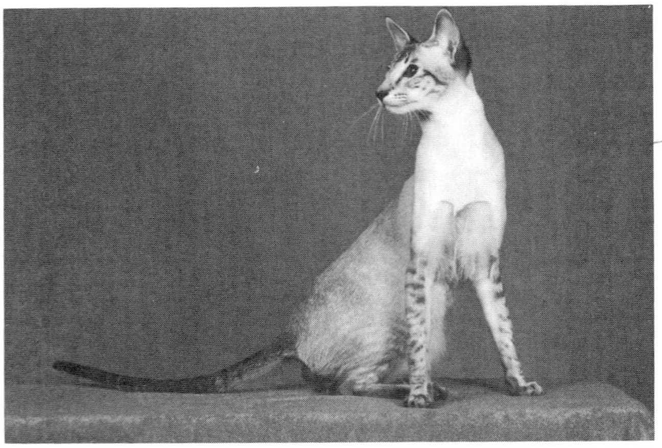

Figure 1–13. Colorpoint Shorthair. (© Chanan Photography)

The CFA does not recognize these cats as Siamese, but did recognize the Colorpoint Shorthair as a breed in 1964.[2] Many other colors have been developed and accepted since their acceptance. Most other associations accept these cats as Siamese.

The standard for Colorpoints is the same as that for Siamese cats except for coat color. There are 10 "lynx point" colors, as well as red point, cream point, blue cream point, seal tortie point, chocolate cream point, lilac cream point, and chocolate tortie point.

The Colorpoint's personality resembles that of the Siamese, as they are intelligent, affectionate, and noisy.

Cornish Rex

The mutation that led to the beginning of the Rex breed occurred in 1950 in Bodmin Moor, Cornwall, England. One male kitten from a litter of farm cats had a distinctive, tightly curled coat, and was subsequently named "Kallibunker." The owner, Mrs. Nina Ennismore, recognized her kitten's uniqueness and consulted Mr. A. C. Jude, a well-known geneticist.[4] The name Rex (Fig. 1–14) was given to this newly developing breed because of the coat similarities to the wavy-haired Rex breed of rabbits.[5]

The first pair of Cornish Rex kittens imported to the United States in 1957 belonged to Fran Blancheri of San Diego, California.[4] The male died before he was able to sire kittens. "La Morna Cove," a blue female, had been bred before leaving England. Two kittens from this litter—"Diamond Lil" and "Marmaduke"—became the main foundation stock in many pedigrees of American Cornish Rex.[2] Marmaduke was outcrossed with other purebred females, thereby helping to develop the wide variety of coat colors of Rex cats.

In Berlin, Germany, in 1951, another Rex mutation was recognized. A doctor working at a hospital discovered a stray black, curly-coated female. When bred to one of her sons, this female produced curly-haired kittens, which became the foundation for the German Rex. Breeding experiments mating Cornish to German Rex cats proved that the varieties were the same mutation.[2] The CFA recognizes the two strains as one breed, and championship status was granted in 1964.[2]

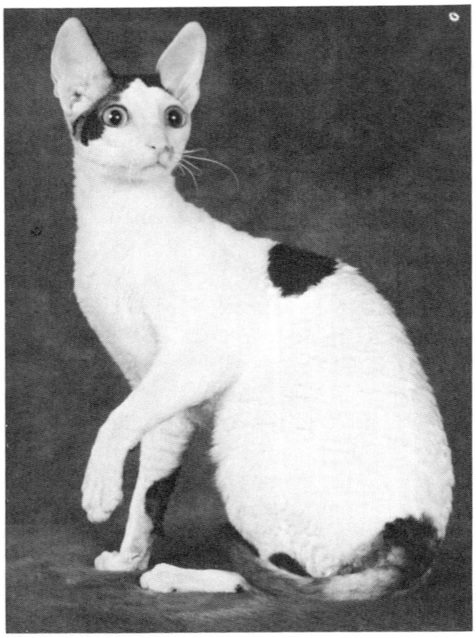

Figure 1–14. Cornish Rex. (© Chanan Photography)

The Cornish Rex is a slender and elegant cat, being described in the CFA standard as having a "racy" body type.[2] They are fine-boned and delicate, with a small to medium-sized body. These cats have a natural arch in their back, with long, well-muscled legs and a slender tail. The head is long and narrow, with oval eyes and large ears. The whiskers are short, curly, and very brittle. The most striking feature is, of course, their unique coat.

Ordinary cat fur normally consists of three hair types: long, coarse guard hairs that act as a protective covering; finer, bristlelike hairs (awn hairs); and a superfine undercoat, the down hair (or wool hair), which provides insulation. The Cornish Rex coat is made up only of the down hair, which accounts for its extreme softness. The marcel-like wave to their coat is the second point of uniqueness to the breed, and they share this quality only with the Devon Rex.[4] Because of a lack of guard hairs, shedding and dander is minimal, which may make this breed acceptable to those who experience allergic problems with cats in general. These cats will feel warm to the touch because of their type of coat, but their body temperature is the same as that of other cats. Cornish Rex cats appear in all colors of the cat world, including solids, tabbies, bi-colors, tortoiseshells, and calicos. Siamese patterns are not accepted by all cat associations.

The Cornish Rex is one of the few breeds that enjoys crowds and excitement; they exhibit a high degree of curiosity and intelligence.[4] It is gentle, yet playful, and a true lap cat and companion. It seldom uses its small voice, and loves all kinds of toys.

Cymric

The longhair variety of the Manx breed is known as the Cymric (Fig. 1–15). In the late 1960s, long-haired kittens began to appear in Manx litters as a result of numerous

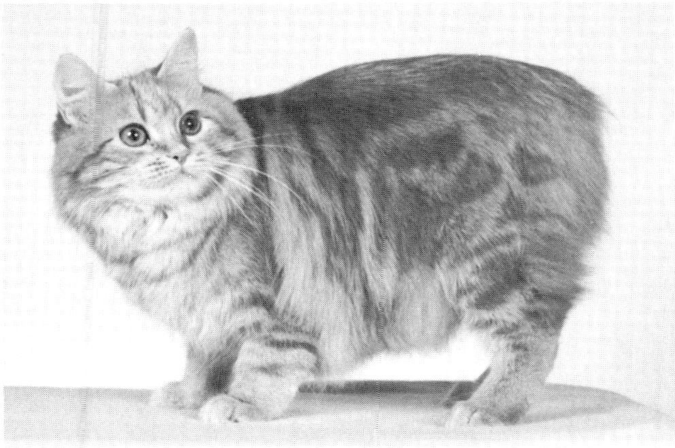

Figure 1–15. Cymric. (© Chanan Photography)

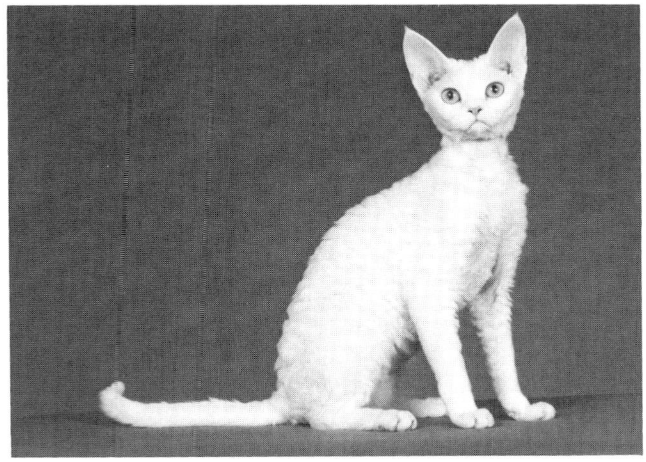

Figure 1–16. Devon Rex. (© Chanan Photography)

outcrossings over the years.[2] The long-haired cats reflected the recessive gene inherited from the outcrosses with tails. Outcrossing is still practiced in England.[2] The Cymric breed gained recognition by numerous associations, and Championship status was granted by the CFA in 1989.[2]

The Cymric standard is very much like that of the Manx, except the coat is of medium length. The coat gradually lengthens from the shoulders to the pelvis. The hair on the breeches, abdomen, and neck ruff is longer than the body hair. Toe and ear tufts are desirable.[2]

Devon Rex

As Rex mutations were discovered, they were tested genetically with the existing Cornish Rex, whose curly-coated gene was known to be autosomal recessive. All were found to be compatible, or were forgotten about, until 1960 when Berl Cox found a curly-coated cat near a tin mine in Buckfastleigh, Devon, England. One of her kittens was a male she named Kirlee, whose father was curly-coated. Being familiar with the Cornish Rex breed, Cox allowed Kirlee to go to Brian Sterling-Webb, a cat breeder. Kirlee was mated to nine Cornish Rex queens, and produced no curly-coated kittens.[2] This newly discovered autosomal recessive gene was acknowledged and named Rex gene II.

In 1968, the R.A.E. Whites of Anglo-Tex Cattery imported a Devon Rex (Fig. 1–16) from England, and the breeding program in the United States began. The CFA did not recognize the Devon Rex for championship status until 1983.[6]

The Devon Rex has an 'elfin look," as described by the CFA standard.[2] This look is created by wide, low-set ears, oversized almond-shaped eyes, a short muzzle, and full, broad cheeks. Topping each ear is a small pointed tuft of hair; sometimes, the hair on the back of the ears is long enough to be seen from the front, in which case the cat is said to have "earmuffs."[6] The Devon Rex is moderate in body size and musculature, with long, fine legs and tail and crinkled whiskers.

The Devon Rex coat is similar to that of the Cornish Rex, except that the Devon Rex does have some thin, irregular, and brittle guard hair. The Devon's fur is more like suede, with the hair curling in many directions or curling tightly in neat rows.[6] Devons are available in a rainbow of shades, identical to the Cornish Rex. The most popular colors are black smoke and white.

The Devon Rex is best described as a playful extrovert, a people-oriented cat.[6] Devons enjoy exploring, and changes and variety in their lives are taken on with great pleasure. They also like to spend time in their owners' laps.

Egyptian Mau

The Egyptian Mau (Fig. 1–17) is a natural breed that is believed to be descended from the ancient cats of Egypt. The name Mau is another name for cat, and is unnecessary in the name. However, all associations that accept this breed use the full name.[1] This cat is considered to be the only naturally domesticated breed of spotted cat. Ancient Egyptian art shows cats with this type of spotting, which are referred to as "fishing and fowling" cats. The ancient ancestor of this breed is thought to be a domesticated spotted subspecies of the African wild cat, *Felis libyca* (ocreata).[2] This cat, which was taken from Ethiopia to Egypt, was important in Egyptian mythology, often being depicted killing rats, mice, and snakes. These cats were so cherished that many were mummified after death, enabling scholars to compare the ancient spotted cats with the Egyptian Mau.[2]

Before World War II, Egyptian Maus were bred and shown in Europe. After the war, an exiled Russian princess named Nathalie Troubetskoy rescued a few surviving Egyptian Maus in Italy. Through her contacts, she was also able to import several cats from the Syrian Embassy to reduce imminent inbreeding.[2]

One of these imported cats was a silver female named "Baba of Fatima." She was one of the three Egyptian Maus brought to the United States from Italy in 1953 by Princess Troubetskoy. Baba of Fatima later became the first Champion in America.[1] The CFA granted Championship status in 1977.

The breed has a unique appearance; its hind legs are longer than the front, and there is a loose flap of skin that extends from the flank to corresponding knee. This is also seen in wild cats, allowing for longer strides when running.[2]

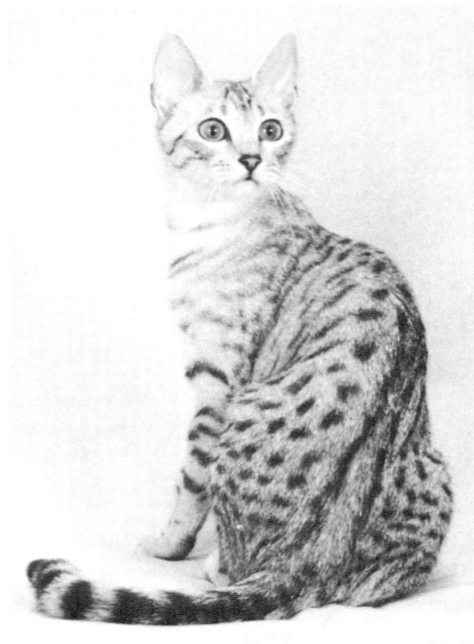

Figure 1–17. Egyptian Mau. (© Chanan Photography)

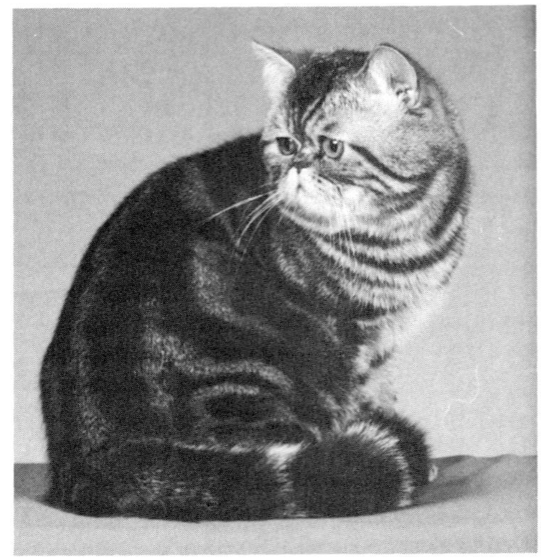

Figure 1–18. Exotic Shorthair. (© Chanan Photography)

Its ears are large, alert, and wide at the base. It is medium in size with well-developed muscle. The head has a slightly rounded, wedge shape. The eyes are large, alert, almond-shaped, and slightly slanted. Eye color is called gooseberry green, but an amber cast is acceptable in terms of the breed standard, but only in young adults up to 1½ years of age. Its feet are small and dainty, and the tail is medium in length.

The hair coat is medium-short, with a lustrous sheen. The color pattern is quite unique, with a characteristic "M" and frown marks on its forehead. These frown marks continue down the back, breaking into spots along the spine. A dorsal stripe continues to the tip of the tail, which is heavily banded and dark at the tip. There are randomly spotted markings on the body that vary in size and shape. The three recognized colors are bronze, silver, and smoke.[1]

This breed of cat, being rather shy, tends to attach itself to one or two people. These cats are loving, and enjoy sleeping in laps. They are built for agility and train easily. Their voice is considered melodious, and they adjust well to children and other pets.[2]

Exotic Shorthair

The Exotic Shorthair breed, like many others, evolved from cross-mating two established breeds. For many years, the Persian was used to restore a certain type or color to British and American Shorthairs. This hybridization also added some undesirable characteristics, such as rounded heads and soft, long coats. The true American Shorthair breeders did not like these new changes. In 1966, Jean Rose, then CFA executive director, along with many others, helped support a new class for this hybrid.[1] Jane Martinke, a prominent CFA judge, convinced the CFA to designate the new breed Exotic Shorthair (Fig. 1–18).[2] This new breed standard was Persian in type but resembled the shorthair in coat length, with a dense, plush coat. By 1967, this new breed was granted Championship status. In the early years of this breed, any shorthair was allowed as an outcross. Now, only Persians are accepted as outcrosses.[2]

Except for the coat, the standards for this breed are identical to those for the Persian. The head is round and massive, with a short nose and full cheeks. The eyes are round and brilliant, and the body size is large to medium. The legs and neck are short, with an overall stocky body type. These cats have been said to have a "teddy bear look."[2]

The coat is medium in length, soft and plush, and it stands out from the cat's body.[2] The coat does not flow, as does that of the Persian, but it is longer than other shorthair coats. The accepted colors and patterns include all of those of the Persian breed. This cat has been shown with other longhairs since 1983.[2]

This cat's dense, soft coat requires less combing and occasional bathing to avoid excessive shedding.[2] These cats love people, children, and other cats, and they enjoy playing. They are sweet, loving, and even-tempered, with no extremes in personality.[1]

Havana Brown

The Havana Brown breed is another one that is not found in a natural state, nor was it created by a spontaneous mutation.[1] In the late 1800s, all-brown cats were imported to England from Thailand. The genetic makeup of these early brown cats was likely not the same.[2] Actual breeding for the Havana Brown did not begin until 1951.[1] Breeders worked intensely to redevelop the self-chocolate brown short-haired cat. The first kitten of this new color, "Bronze Idol," was born in 1954 from the mating of a seal point Siamese to a solid black cat, both of whom were carrying chocolate genes. (This chocolate point gene had to appear in both parents for the Havana to result.[1]) This kitten became the foundation stock of the Chestnut Brown Foreign breed in England.[2] The breed was later renamed Havana, after a rab-

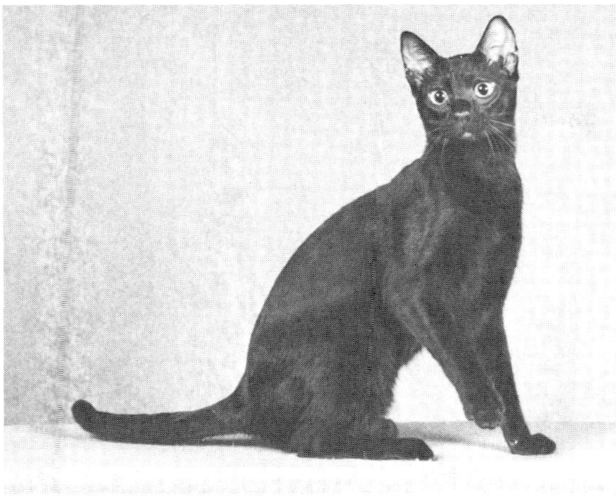

Figure 1–19. Havana Brown. (© Chanan Photography)

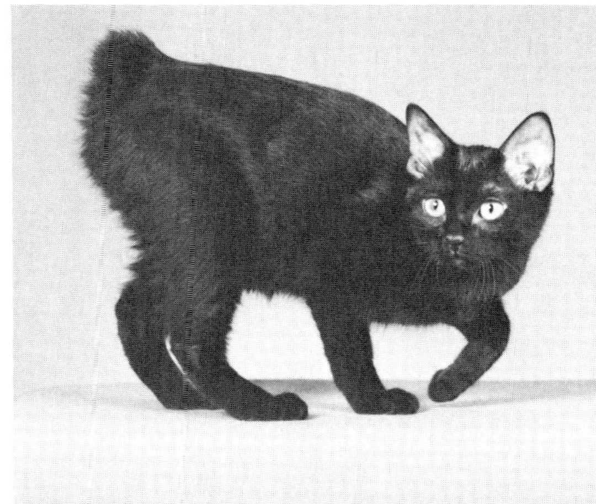

Figure 1–20. Japanese Bobtail. (© Chanan Photography)

bit breed of the same color. The Havanas that remain in England have taken on the appearance of the Siamese, necessitating occasional breedings back to Siamese to maintain type.[1] In fact, by CFA standards, this breed in England would be considered to be a Chestnut Oriental Shorthair.[2]

The first Havanas in the United States were imported from England in the late 1950s. The word "Brown" was added to the name in 1959.[2] American breeders chose not to strive for the foreign-type cat, and the breed gradually emerged with its own unique appearance. In 1964, the CFA granted Championship status to the Havana Brown (Fig. 1–19).

The Havana Brown has a muzzle that has been described to resemble a protrusion on the face, rather than an extension of the head.[2] When viewing its profile, there is a distinct break at the eyes, and the end of the muzzle appears square.[2] There is a slight break or indentation behind the brown whiskers. The ears are large, round-tipped, and wide-set. The eyes are oval and a brilliant, chartreuse green.[1] The body type is graceful and sleek, yet muscular and firm. The legs are long and straight, with a medium-length, slender tail. The coat is medium in length and a warm, mahogany brown color.

The cats are said to have quiet and gentle temperaments.[2] They are highly intelligent and have a great ability to move fast. They are less vocal than the Siamese, and love to play. Affectionate with people and especially other cats, this breed is often called the "feline connoisseur's cat," and is, as yet, surprisingly undiscovered by the general public.[2]

Japanese Bobtail

The Japanese Bobtail (Fig. 1–20) is a natural breed that originated in Japan. This type of cat, often portrayed in ancient Japanese art, is considered to be a symbol of good luck. Statues of these cats are characteristically depicted with one outstretched paw, presumably extended as a sort of greeting to passersby.[1] Accordingly, they are called welcoming cats, or *Maneki-Neko.*[1]

The original cats entering Japan from China and Korea were of a variety of colors, but the calico cats were most cherished.[2] These calico cats were called *mi-ke* (pronounced mee-kay), and were considered by Japanese sailors to be symbols of good luck. The government eventually ordered this cherished breed set free to help save the increasingly important silk and grain industries from mice.[2]

The CFA accepted this breed for registration in 1967, and Championship status was granted in 1976.[1] Appreciation of these cats continues in Japan, and in modern times, many of the pedigreed breeds have been imported.[2] A number of the common street cats have bobbed tails. The bone Structure is often twisted in an S shape, or even a corkscrew shape. Geneticist Dr. Niel Todd proved that the recessive gene responsible for this tail configuration is not the same as the Manx tailless gene, which is dominant.[2] Occasionally, these cats have short, straight tails, but they are never full-length.

The Japanese Bobtail is not related to the Manx. According to the breed standard, its tail, which can be either rigid or flexible, should not extend more than 3 inches.[2] The tail is carried high like a flag, and the hair on the tail is longer and thicker than that on the body. The hair grows in an outward direction, which gives it a pom-pom effect.

The Bobtail's head shape is almost an equilateral triangle, with gently curving lines and high cheekbones.[2] The ears are large and expressive, set wide apart and at right angles to the head. The eyes are large and oval, but alert and wide. The body is medium in size, but shapely and well muscled. The rear legs are longer than the front legs, and all are long and slender. When the cat stands, the rear legs are bent so that its back is level. The coat is medium in length, soft, silky, and without much undercoat.[1] Longhair Bobtails are eligible for AOV (Any Other Variety) registration. The most common colors are bi-colors and tri-colors, along with solid blacks, reds, whites, and tortoiseshells. Other Bobtails may have patterned coats, including any variety of tabby or spotting, with or without white. Vivid colors and dramatic markings seem to be preferred.[2]

The Japanese Bobtail makes a wonderful and loyal house pet. Their quiet, chirping voice adds to their distinctive character. They like to retrieve, love the water, and are great swimmers. They are intelligent, have a great sense of curiosity, and adjust well to their environment.[1]

Javanese and Oriental Longhair

At about the same time the Balinese was becoming well known, breeders were developing long-haired Siamese-style cats with other colorpoints through breedings to American Shorthairs. Cats carrying the recessive gene for long hair were bred to Colorpoint Shorthairs to bring out this gene. These long-haired Colorpoint Shorthairs were designated Javanese (Fig. 1–21), and the CFA granted them Championship status in 1986.[2] In several other associations, this breed is still considered among the Balinese.

In the late 1970s and 1980s, breeders crossed the Balinese with Oriental Shorthairs to achieve a long-haired type. However, breeders found it difficult to maintain ideal body type and to improve upon hair coat quality simultaneously. The Oriental Longhair (Fig. 1–22), the long-haired equivalent of the Oriental Shorthair in terms of color and patterns, was accepted by the CFA for registration in 1988.[2]

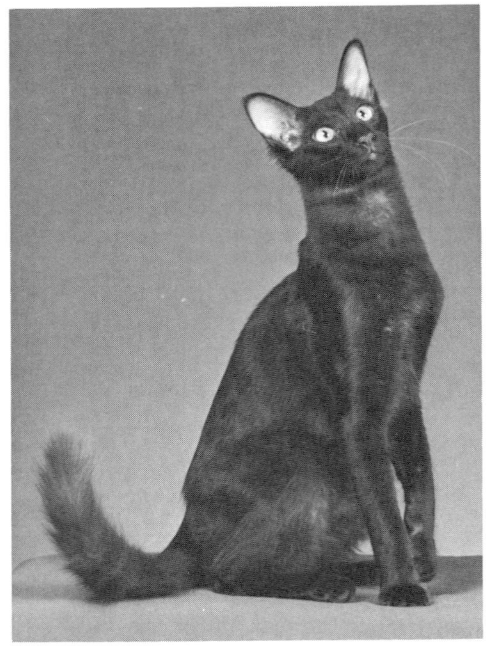

Figure 1–22. Oriental Longhair. (© Chanan Photography)

Korat

This cat is one of three cat breeds depicted in the ancient book *The Cat Book Poems,* which dates back in Thai history from 1350–1767. This cat is known in Thailand as the *Si-Sawat,*[1] and is considered to be one of the oldest and purist breeds. The Korat's (Fig. 1–23) shimmering silver coat signifies wealth to the Thais, and for centuries, this cat has signified good fortune.[2] In early Thailand, they were never sold, but were given as gifts as tokens of honor and esteem.

The Korat was probably first seen at a cat show in England in 1896, where it was entered as a Siamese and was subsequently disqualified. Other breeders often wrongfully claimed this cat as a Russian Blue or Siamese, but there was no record of registry until 1959.

A pair of Korats, "Nara" and "Darra," was sent as a gift to Mrs. Jean Johnson of Oregon in 1959. Her earlier visits to Bangkok sparked her interest in these silver-blue cats, but she was unable to obtain one at that time. This new pair became the first Korats in America.[2] Others were imported during the 1960s, which led to the establishment of the Korat Cat Fanciers' Association in 1965. The Korat was ac-

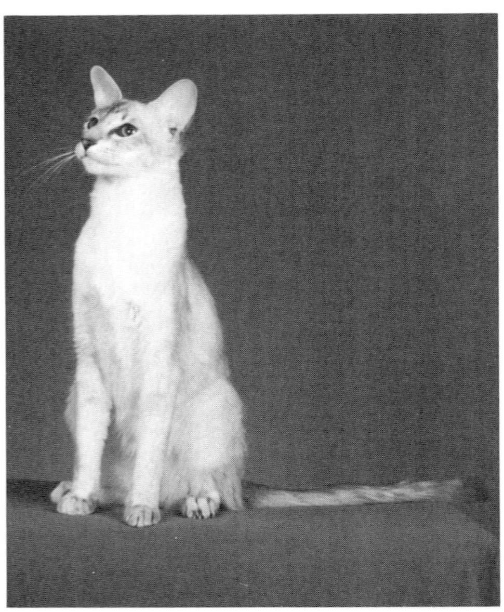

Figure 1–21. Javanese. (© Chanan Photography)

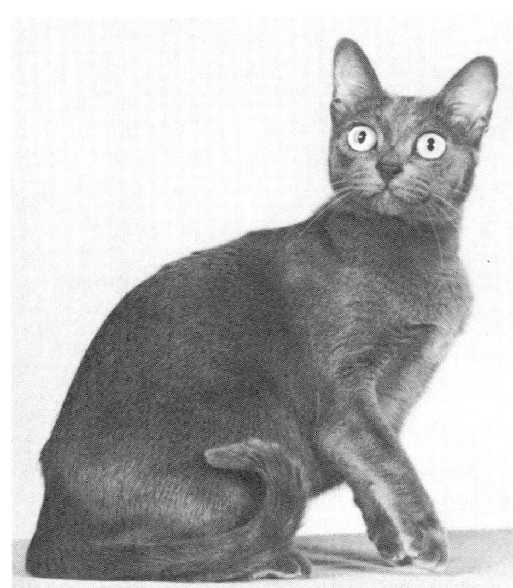

Figure 1–23. Korat. (© Chanan Photography)

cepted for Championship status by the CFA in 1966.[2] The first Korats in Europe were imported into England from the United States in 1972.

The Korat is a unique breed, having a heart-shaped face and large, expressive green eyes. Its ears are large, which gives an alert quality to its expression. The breed is muscular and semi-cobby, with a body that has the "feeling of hard-coiled spring power."[2] The coat is glossy, close-lying, of medium length, and silver blue, with each hair being tipped with silver. This tipping produces a halo-like glow when the light reflects from the tapered hairs. The typical Korat does not acquire its full coat and eye color potential until it is 2 to 4 years of age.[3] Korat breeders insist that no outcrossing occurs, and that all Korats trace back to their ancestors from Thailand.

This breed is known to be very protective of their owners and children.[2] They seem somewhat susceptible to upper respiratory viral infections, so vaccination is imperative.[3] They communicate well with their quiet voices, and love to be petted. They move with caution, and do not like sudden or loud noises.[1]

Longhair Scottish Fold

The Longhair Scottish Fold (Fig. 1–24) has the same appearance as its parent breed, The Scottish Fold, but with a softer, rounded look. The recessive longhair gene evolved within the Scottish Fold litters through approved outcrossing over the years. These cats appear to have no ears at all, as they are folded down and covered by fur.[2] Many early fold breeds were, indeed, long-haired.

Maine Coon

The Maine Coon (Fig. 1–25), as the name implies, originated in its home state of Maine more than 100 years ago. There are many sketchy stories concerning the history of this cat; some have even believed that this cat is part raccoon, although of course, this is genetically impossible.[1] Its bushy tail and raccoon-like dark tabby markings led to the adoption of the name Maine Coon. Also called the "Shag" or "working cat," it is one of the oldest North American breeds.[2]

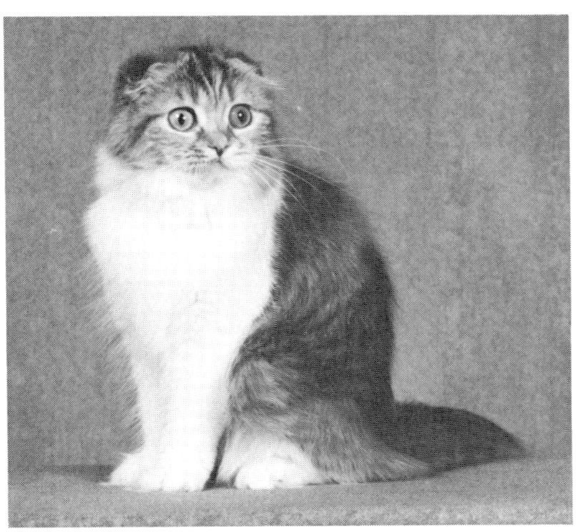

Figure 1–24. Longhair Scottish Fold. (© Chanan Photography)

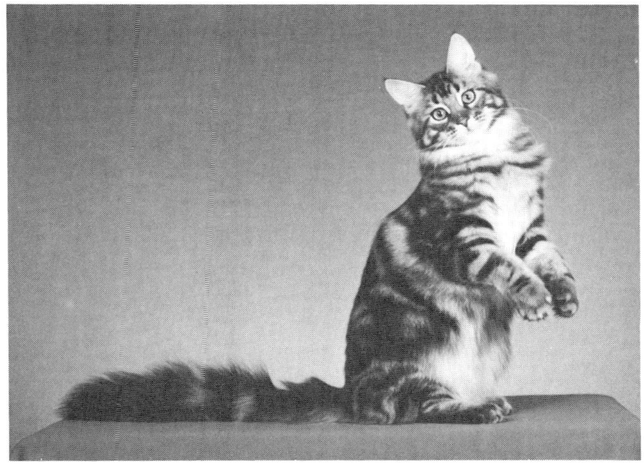

Figure 1–25. Maine Coon. (© Chanan Photography)

Modern-day breeders believe this cat to be the product of crossmating between early long-haired Angoras brought to America by English seamen and domestic short-haired cats from New England.[2] The long-haired cats that resulted from these matings stood the best chance for survival in the harsh winter climate of Maine. Natural selection led to exclusively long-haired cats that were exceptionally hardy and excellent mousers.

Natives of Maine were proud of their big cats, and kept pedigree information for years. These cats were popular at early cat shows in Boston and New York, where a neutered male named "Gosie" won Best Cat at the Madison Square Garden show in 1895.[2] Their popularity as a show cat declined when Persians arrived, but they thrived as household pets.

Because of a small group of persistent breeders, the Maine Coon once again achieved show recognition in the late 1960s. The CFA finally granted Championship status in 1976.

Cats of this breed are large, tall, and long-bodied. Males usually weigh no more than 15 pounds, and females generally weigh less than 12 pounds, despite the myth that describes a 37-pound Maine Coon cat. Its head is medium in length, with a square muzzle and high cheek bones. The ears are well-tufted, wide at the base, and tapered, giving a pointed appearance. The eyes are large and wide set. Eye colors range from green to gold and copper to blue, and odd eyes are allowable. The legs are substantial and wide set, with large, well-tufted paws. The tail is long and wide at the base, with flowing fur. The coat is shaggy and heavy, shorter on the shoulders and longer on the britches.[1] A frontal ruff is desirable. The coat should be silky in texture and should flow with ease. These cats appear to be larger because of their unique coat. Tabby patterns are most common among the breed, but they also come in a variety of other colors, such as tabby and white, bi-color, smoke, shaded, tortoiseshell, and solid.[2] They are slow to develop, and may not reach full size until they are 4 years of age.[3]

Maine Coon breeders believe that no two Coon cats sound alike because of their unique voice.[1] They love to sleep in awkward places and positions. Many consider this cat to be the ideal pet, given its clownlike personality and state of perpetual kittenhood. They are very friendly and outgoing, as well as easy to groom.

Manx

The Manx (Fig. 1–26) breed is a very ancient breed with many legends concerning its origin. One legend states that Irish invaders stole the cats' tails for helmet plumes.[3] Another famous tale maintains that a pair of Manx was the last pair of animals to enter Noah's Ark. In a rush, Noah slammed the door on their tails, rendering them tailless.[2] The best-known story dates back to 1588, when a Spanish ship wrecked near the Isle of Man, and several tailless cats swam ashore and lived to sustain the breed.[2] In addition, for years, the Manx was believed to have evolved from the bobtailed cats that were imported to England from Japan, although it is now well known that Oriental bobtailed cats differ genetically from Manx cats.[2]

Modern science has determined that the Manx's taillessness is a dominant gene, and that the original mutation occurred long ago.[3] There are four basic tail types. A fifth type, the rumpy-riser, is a combination of two basic types and is not widely accepted. The first is the show-quality completely tailless Manx with no complete sacral vertebrae, also called "rumpy."[2] The rump is completely rounded and has a dimple at the base of the spine. By contrast, the so-called "rumpy-riser" has a few flexible tail vertebrae that form a small knob. The CFA allows these cats so long as the rump is rounded. Another variety, known as "riser," has vertebrae that are fused in a vertical position, which is penalized by the CFA standard. A so-called "stumpy" or "stubby" Manx has a short tail with coccygeal vertebrae that are usually movable, but often curved or kinked. A "longy" is a tailed manx that has a normal-looking tail. All of these variations can be registered as Manx, but for show purposes, the "rumpy" is preferred. Many Manx breeders believe it is desirable to dock the tails of the "longy" kittens shortly after birth to increase their acceptance as Manx.

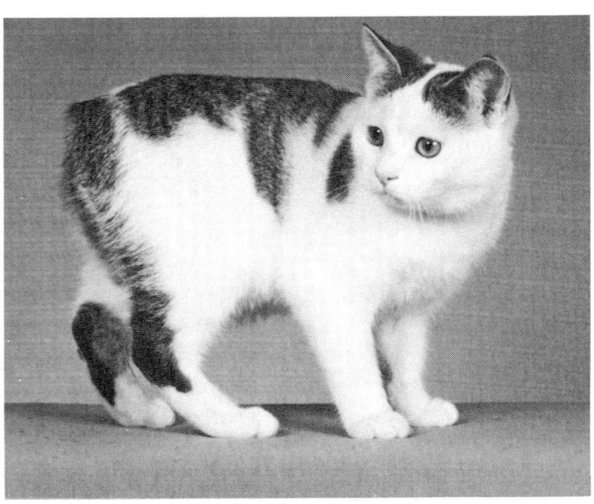

Figure 1–26. Manx. (© Chanan Photography)

Even though it is one of the oldest known breeds, several problems persist with regard to the breeding of Manx cats. First, the Manx gene can cause malformations in portions of the spinal column other than the tail. Spina bifida and vertebral fusions are a few of the many deformities that may occur. (Recently, the prevalence of these problems has been challenged by American breeders who have decreased the incidence of these problems through sound breeding.[2]) Second, the Manx gene is lethal when in the homozygous form, with affected kittens dying in utero. This reduces the average litter size, although it is still considered to be average when compared to that of other breeds.

Manx cats were among the first cats registered in Europe; indeed, a Manx Club existed as early as 1901, in England.[2] The breed was exported to North America in the 1930s.

Breeders aim for the rounded look for the Manx, not only in the rump. The back of the Manx is short, and its cheeks are full. The body is medium-sized and stout, with solid muscling and a sturdy bone structure. Manx cats have round, full eyes and widely spaced, medium-sized ears. The neck is short, and the full chest causes the forelegs to be set well apart.[2] The back legs are much longer than the front, the thighs are heavily muscled, and the pads are small and well rounded. The coat is short and of good texture. It is called a double coat because of the longer, glossy outercoat that overlies the thicker, cottony undercoat.[1] The Manx occurs in a wide variety of colors excepting those showing chocolate, lavender, or Himalayan pattern, or these colors combined with white.

As a pet, the Manx tends to attach itself to one person. It loves children and is easy to train. The Manx's voice is basically quiet. It is affectionate and playful and very intelligent. Most cats of this breed need time to adjust to strangers.

Missouri Rex (Mo Rex)

The Missouri Rex (Fig. 1–27) represents yet another Rex mutation in the cat. The Cornish and Devon Rex both have well-known recessive traits that have established them as distinctive breeds. The American Wirehair and the Wyoming (Selkirk) Rex are examples of autosomal dominant traits resulting in curling of the hair coat. Genetic studies of the relationship between the Missouri Rex and the Wyoming Rex are still in progress.

The present stock originated from a line of unregistered Manx cats, although the tailless gene has been lost from most of the breeding stock. Currently, this breed is being developed with a normal tail, intermediate body type, and a head that does not resemble that of the Manx. The coat is very soft and plush, more like a water-repellent pelt than hair. The hair gently curls and the coat quality is similar throughout life.

At present, the stock is being maintained with the potential for a new breed. Mary DeVeny of Stark City, Missouri is currently working with these cats. Also, a colony has been established in New England to protect the survival of the

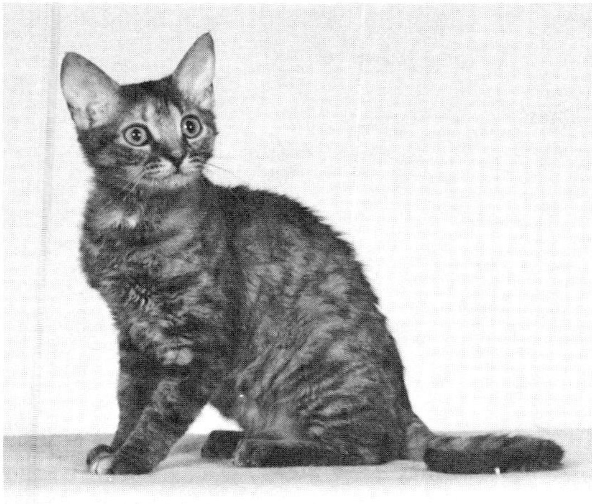

Figure 1–27. Missouri Rex. (© Chanan Photography)

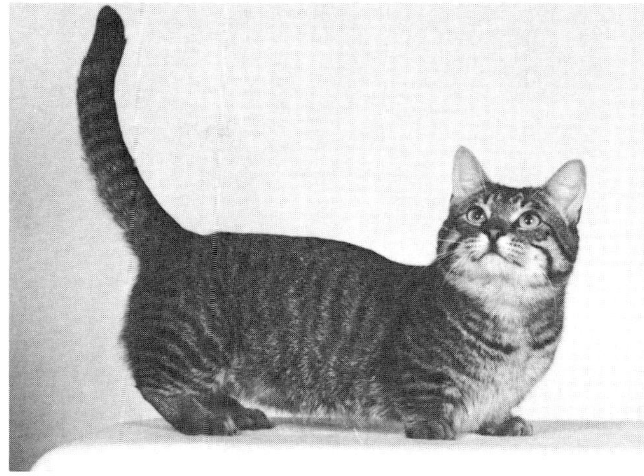

Figure 1–28. Munchkin. (© Chanan Photography)

gene and to conduct further breeding studies to determine whether there is a true relationship to other Rex factors.

The Missouri Rex gene has been determined to be an autosomal recessive trait. Results from crosses with the Devon Rex indicate that this new Rex gene has its own distinct locus. Crosses with the Cornish Rex have not been completed, but phenotypic differences in the hair suggest a genetic difference as well.

Munchkin

Currently, there is a movement to develop a short-limbed breed of cats within the cat fancy. These short-limbed cats have recently been exhibited at cat shows, and the proposed name for the new breed is the Munchkin (Fig. 1–28). The Munchkin is a naturally occurring domestic cat breed. A spontaneous change in genetics introduced a gene similar to that seen in Basset Hounds, Corgis, and dachshunds. Although these cats have only recently been discovered by the cat fancy, previous reports of achondroplastic cats date back to 1944.

The origin of the present stock was a pregnant black female found in Rayville, Louisiana in 1983. Munchkins have also been found in New Hampshire, New York, and Massachusetts. Several colonies were established in Louisiana, and these now span many generations. The available data strongly support an autosomal dominant mode of inheritance that closely resembles human achondroplasia in both phenotype and inheritance pattern. These cats exhibit shortening of the long bones, which is more pronounced in the forelimbs. Marked bowing of the extremities is often present, and is especially prominent in some of the larger males. Also, there is an exaggerated lordosis of the lower thoracic spine, but no other major congenital anomalies. Thus far, the Munchkin has not experienced any particular problems, such as disk disease or joint degeneration, but a complete assessment will take more time to complete.

Munchkin cats run with a gait similar to that of a ferret or squirrel. They turn corners quickly and catch small prey with ease. They do have decreased jumping ability, but climb without difficulty. They have normal reproductive fitness, although an extremely short-limbed, inexperienced male may have difficulty mounting a female initially. The litters average four to five kittens, some of which will be normal and some short-limbed. They come in a variety of coat colors. There is no evidence to suggest that the gene for short legs hampers their quality of life. Extensive studies are in progress to help determine the feasibility of establishing the breed within the cat fancy.

The Munchkin is amusing to watch, and their personality is all cat. They love to play and are very sociable. They get along well with people, as well as other dogs and cats. They also readily accept a harness and leash, and seem to enjoy going for walks.

Nebelung

The look of the Nebelung breed came about as a result of a chance mixed-breed cat mating. The breeder decided to replicate the look of this blue semi–long-haired cat by cross-mating Russian Blues with mixed-breed long-haired cats of similar type.[2]

Norwegian Forest Cat

The history of the Norwegian Forest cat, which sometimes is referred to as the "Skogkatt" or "Wegie," is steeped in mythology. Legend has it that these cats provided the power to pull the chariot of Freya, the Norse goddess of beauty, love, and fertility. In the mid 1800s, this cat was referred to in Norwegian folk tales as the "fairy cat."[2,7] In actuality, this cat is a naturally occurring breed that has lived in Norwegian woods for hundreds of years.

The first efforts to have this breed recognized began in the 1930s. After World War II, the breed neared extinction. Serious breeding programs resumed in the early 1970s. In 1976, the Federation Feline Internationale (FIFe) accepted the breed and granted it Championship status the following year. Modern-day show classes of this breed in Europe are among the largest.[7]

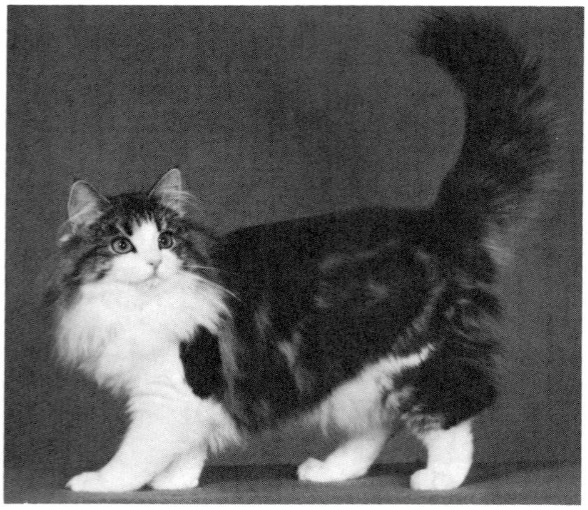

Figure 1–29. Norwegian Forest Cat. (© Chanan Photography)

The Norwegian Forest cat (Fig. 1–29) arrived in the United States about 2 years later. The CFA recognized the breed for registration in 1987; however, it still does not have Championship status, and is instead evaluated in the Miscellaneous class.

The Wegie is a long, heavy-boned cat with a double coat. The outer layer is long and smooth with oily guard hairs, whereas the undercoat is dense and cottony. These cats have a huge ruff, furry hind legs, and a flowing tail. During hot weather, only the outercoat, tail, and ear and toe tufts remain. The head of the Wegie is triangular, with rounded, medium to large ears and almond-shaped eyes. It is thought that the original two colors were brown tabby and black and white, but many other colors are now accepted.

This cat has always been thought of as a sturdy survivor. They are slow to mature and purr constantly.[7] They are friendly and often become very attached to people.

Ocicat

The Ocicat (Fig. 1–30) is the result of cross-breeding Abyssinians to Siamese cats, the first remarkable kitten of which resulted in 1964. A well-known breeder, Virginia Daly of Berkeley, Michigan, had been trying to achieve a ticked tabby-pointed Siamese. The kitten that was born, named "Tonga," had golden spots on an ivory body. The breed was named Ocicat, after a spotted cat of the wild known as the ocelot. This breed is the only spotted domestic breed that has been bred selectively to emulate wild cats in appearance but to retain the gentle temperament of domestic cats.

In addition to the two original breeds, American Shorthairs were added to broaden the genetic base. The Ocicat was recognized by the CFA for registration in 1966; it then achieved Championship status in 1987. Abyssinians are acceptable for outcross breedings until January 1, 1995.[2]

The Ocicat is a medium to large cat of average type. It is well muscled, with a full body and chest. The head is a modified wedge with a gentle rise from the bridge of the nose to the brow. The head is carried gracefully, and the ears are alert and large. Ocicat eyes are large, almond-shaped, and tilted slightly toward the ears. The legs are well muscled, well proportioned, and powerful, and the feet are oval. The tail is long and slim, tapering to the tip.

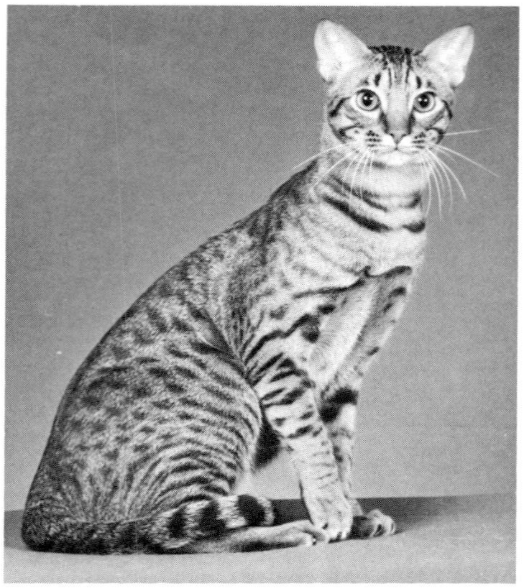

Figure 1–30. Ocicat. (© Chanan Photography)

The coat is close-lying and sleek with large, scattered thumbprint-shaped spots. Each hair has several bands of color except for the hairs of the tip of the tail. The Ocicat is available in most known colors except for the tortoiseshell pattern, which would interfere with the spotting. The 12 colors are as follows: tawny (brown spotted tabby), chocolate, cinnamon, blue, lavender, fawn, silver, chocolate silver, cinnamon silver, blue silver, lavender silver, and fawn silver.

The Ocicat is a hardy, vigorous cat that is outgoing and very devoted to its owner. They are very bright and easy to train, as well as being very social with other people and pets. They make an excellent family companion.[2]

Ojos Azules

The first Ojos Azules (Fig. 1–31) was a blue-eyed red tabby stray seen in San Antonio, Texas, in the late 1970s. The name in the Spanish language means "blue eyes." At one time, blue eyes in a nonwhite self cat were thought to be genetically impossible, but occasionally they would surface in the Southwest portion of the country. The breed originated through spontaneous mutation in the domestic shorthair population. The number of Ojos cats is presently very limited, and outcrossing is encouraged to enlarge the gene pool. There is no particular breed ideal for outcrossing because none is sufficiently close to the Ojos in phenotype. Outcrosses to the unregistered domestic population with similar phenotype is still acceptable until the phenotype is fully set.

The present stock originates from a tortoiseshell female named "Cornflower," that was found in a New Mexico shelter by William Bates in 1984. Bates and Annie Glass, the woman who established the current line, worked to determine the pattern of inheritance starting with "Cornflower." After six generations, it is now clear that the blue-eyed trait is a new autosomal dominant mutation that is distinct from any other in the cat fancy.

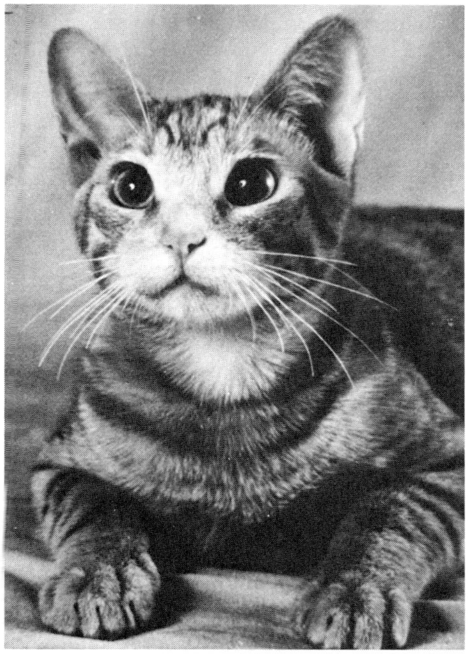

Figure 1–31. Ojos Azules. (Courtesy of Solveig M.V. Pflueger, Ph.D., M.D.)

Cats carrying the trait usually have blue eyes, but can have odd eyes or an eye that is part blue and part gold. The gene can, at times, produce white patches limited to the tail, hip, hind feet, and face. This is distinct from traditional white spotting, and the two traits appear to result from different mechanisms. None of the Ojos produced to date have shown any signs of deafness, a problem seen in other non-pointed blue-eyed cats.

The Ojos Azules is recognized in all categories, and in all colors of all divisions. Pointed and parti-colors must have the characteristic white tail tip, as these colors may have blue eyes unrelated to the Ojos gene. Solid white is discouraged because it is indistinguishable from the usual blue-eyed white. The Ojos is a shorthaired cat of medium build. It has a sweet, appealing expression, with no extremes in type. The word "pretty" should come to mind when looking at a male or female. The eyes should be the dominant feature of the face, being nearly round, slightly almond-shaped, and large. Eye color should be blue or blue-grey, not turquoise or lavender. In odd eyes, the other color may be green, gold, or copper. The coat is short and fine in texture, shiny and silky. White patches are limited to the tip of the tail, the muzzle, and the toes of the hind feet, with lesser degrees being preferred.

Oriental Shorthair

The Oriental Shorthair (Fig. 1–32) conforms to the Siamese type, but is a solid-colored or patterned cat without point color contrast. The original cats imported to England from Thailand were often solid-colored, as well as point-restricted. In the late 1920s, the Siamese Cat Club excluded cats that were neither blue-eyed nor pointed.[2]

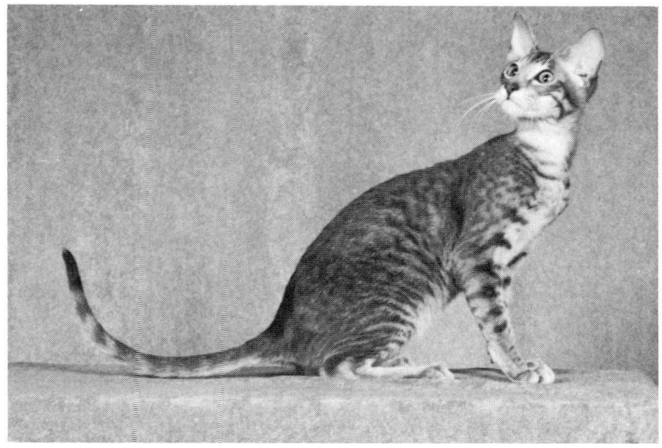

Figure 1–32. Oriental Shorthair. (© Chanan Photography)

After World War II, British breeders began to develop a solid brown cat that carried the Siamese chocolate brown gene. The cat that resulted was recognized in 1958 and called the Chestnut Brown Foreign Shorthair.[2] A British geneticist, Patricia Turner, began a breeding program in 1962 to produce a blue-eyed solid white cat of Siamese type. During her breeding program, many kittens were born with a variety of solid and patterned coloring. These cats were finally accepted in 1977 in England. In 1978, British tabbies of Siamese type were accepted as well.[2] A variety of solid and patterned colors have subsequently been created over the years.

American cat breeders were intrigued by Oriental Shorthairs in England and began to import them in the early 1970s. CFA Championship status was granted in 1977 and the breed was divided into five color groups: solid, shaded, smoke, tabby, and parti-color. All of these cats have green eyes except the whites, which may have either blue or green eyes.[2] Outcrossings to Colorpoint Shorthairs and Siamese are allowed. Pointed cats that result from these outcrossings are not allowed in the Siamese breed. However, CFA rules state that those meeting the Colorpoint Shorthair standard may be shown in their Colorpoint Shorthair class.[2]

The Oriental Shorthair standard is essentially identical to that of the Siamese except for coat color. This breed is accepted in a wide variety of colors and patterns.

As a pet, the Oriental Shorthair is similar to the Siamese in many ways. It is playful and agile, but has a quieter voice that can be raucous. These cats are very outgoing toward other animals and people.

Persian

Bred in a multitude of colors and patterns, Persians (Fig. 1–33) are greatly prized by pet owners all over the world. They have a long and distinguished history, having appeared in cat shows all over the world for more than 100 years. The earliest long-haired cats seen in Europe in the late 16th century came from two locations, Persia and Turkey. These two longhairs of the time were quite different in appearance and were believed to be separate breeds; however, cross-mating often occurred. Eventually, the British came to prefer

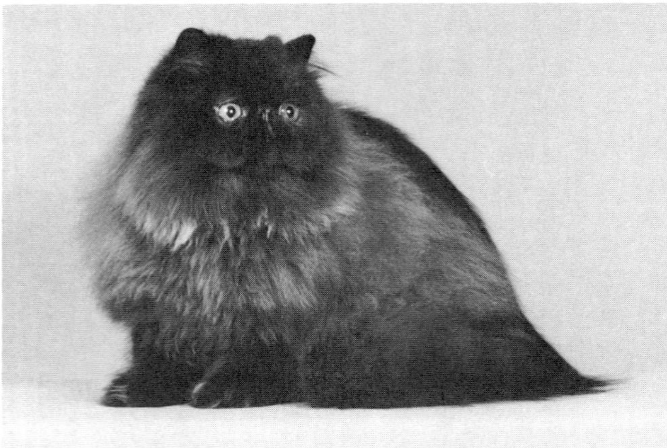

Figure 1–33. Persian. (© Chanan Photography)

the Persian type, primarily to avoid the tendency toward deafness that was characteristic of the blue-eyed white Angoras, as well as the dominance of the white gene, which masks other color genes.[2] By 1901, English show Persians were available in 13 colors.

At the end of the 19th century, Persians were exported to North America and they were soon being bred and shown regularly. The American type of today differs from the British type, each country preferring its own. The American type tends to have a more compact body and luxuriant coat than their British counterparts, as well as a more "extreme" head type. The British believe that the American-style Persian is "overtyped."

Persians may be large to medium in size, with small ears and large, round, brilliant eyes. The head is round, with powerful jaws and a wide skull. Their nose is short and broad with a "break," although the standard is not specific in the degree of nose break.

The standard does call for a "proper bite," as well as symmetry of the face and head.[2] The body of the Persian appears round, and the width across the shoulders and hips should be the same. The bone structure should be heavy and strong, with fairly short legs. The coat is thick, of fine texture, and stands off from the body. The ruff and tail should be full and enormous.[1]

The Persian breed is divided by the CFA into seven categories on the basis of color and pattern. The following is a description of each:

A. ***Solid.*** The coat is even and without markings, and only copper-colored eyes are permitted. White cats compete in separate classes for blue-eyed and odd-eyed (one copper, one blue) cats. The Peke-face red Persian is placed in this category.

B. ***Shaded.*** This division is for cats that have an undercoat of one color, with the tips of the hair being another, darker shade. This includes the so-called cameos, which have a white undercoat and red tips; the silvers, which have a white undercoat with black tips; the tortoiseshells, which have a white undercoat and patched tipping; and the goldens, which have a cream undercoat tipped with black. The "chinchilla" Persian has what is called shell tipping, which is a more subtle color change than the shaded tipping. The cameos and tortoiseshells have copper-colored eyes, whereas the silvers and goldens have green or blue-green eyes that are darkly outlined with black.

C. ***Smoke.*** These cats are very similar genetically to the shaded cats except that the tipping extends more deeply into the coat. The cats appear to be a solid, blue-cream or tortoiseshell on the surface, but have a white undercoat that can be seen when the hair is parted. Solid tipping can be black, blue, red, chocolate, or lilac.

D. ***Tabby.*** Tabby Persians occur in three accepted patterns: classic, mackerel, and patched. The patched tabby has additional red or cream patches, and can be of the mackerel or classic pattern. The Peke-face Red Tabby Persian is also placed in this division. The underlying bone structure of the skull of these cats is different from that of all other Persian types.

E. ***Parti-color.*** This division is for tortoiseshell and blue-cream cats.

F. ***Bi-color.*** This is a new division established by the CFA in 1990. Cats included in this category are of acceptable solid color, but have piebald white spotting. This division also includes tabby cats and whites, calicos, Van calicos, and Van bi-colors. Vans have white bodies with colored legs, tail, head, and ears, and one or two small spots on their bodies.

G. ***Himalayan (Pointed).*** These cats were considered a separate breed until 1984 when the CFA declared that these colorpoint cats constituted a Persian division. This color pattern was developed in the 1920s and 1930s when long-haired and Siamese cats were cross-mated. The Persian look with colorpoint pattern was finally achieved, and these cats eventually became indistinguishable from Persians. Many color points are acceptable, including lynx, blue-cream, solid blue-cream and tortie points. All cats in this division must have vivid blue eyes. Excepted from this class of cats are the solid-colored chocolate and lilac Himalayans, which are shown in the solid Persian class.[2]

Persians are ideal exhibition cats as they have a generally placid, gentle temperament. They are often content merely to sit in the window and look beautiful. Their voices are fairly quiet, and as kittens, they are very playful. The queens have small litters, with two to three kittens being the average.

Ragdoll

The Ragdoll breed (Fig. 1–34) originated in about 1965 when Ann Baker, of Riverside, California, bred a long-haired mixed-breed female to a Birman male.[1] The name for this breed was chosen because of the gentle nature of these cats and their ability to relax when held.[1]

Ragdoll kittens are born white and do not reach full color and maturity until about 3 years of age. Males average about 15 to 20 pounds, and females weigh about 5 pounds less. There are three basic color patterns: bi-color, colorpoint, and mitted. This breed is not yet recognized by the CFA, but has gained acceptance from several other breed registries.

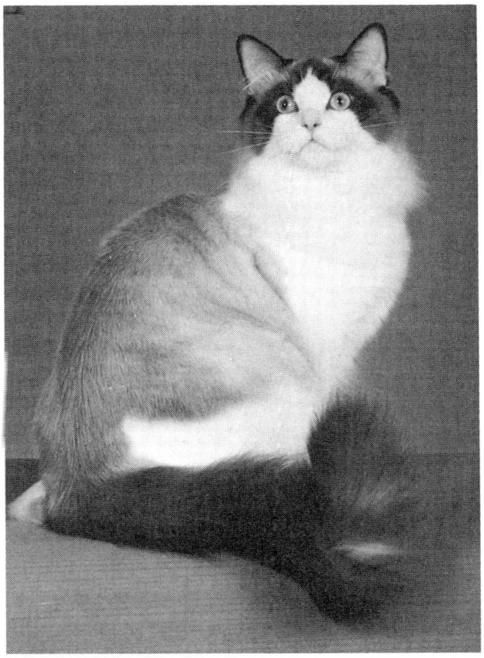

Figure 1–34. Ragdoll. (© Chanan Photography)

The Ragdoll is large in size and long-haired with point-restricted color. The fur is very thick and does not mat easily. The colorpoints are chocolate, seal, lilac, and blue. The head is broad between the eyes and ears, with a rounded chin. The cheeks are well developed with long whiskers. The neck is short and strong and the chest has a full ruff over it. The eyes are large and round. The legs are long and heavy, with the rear legs being longer than the front.[1]

As their name suggests, this breed resembles a ragdoll and will go limp in your arms when picked up. They will walk on a leash, but love to be carried and are very affectionate. They have tiny voices, and when frightened, will hide rather than fight.

Russian Blue

The Russian Blue (Fig. 1–35) is one of many of the older breeds of cats with a somewhat shadowy history. These cats are believed to have originated at the White Sea port of Archangel in Northern Russia, from which sailors took them to western Europe in the 1860s. This cat has been known by several names, including Spanish Blue, Archangel cat, and Maltese Blue.[8]

At the turn of the century, British cat shows included all the short-haired blue cats in the same class, regardless of body type. The British type usually won, and interest in the Russian type dwindled. Indeed, the breed became almost nonexistent during World War II. In the late 1940s and 1950s, Scandinavian breeders began developing the breed. They crossed the Russian Blue with Siamese to produce cats of a more foreign body type. The same outcrossing was being tested by breeders in Britain to the extent that the show standard was rewritten. In 1965, a group of British

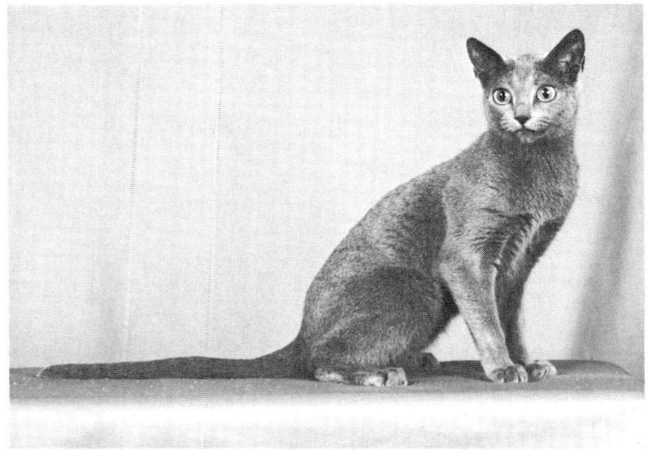

Figure 1–35. Russian Blue. (© Chanan Photography)

breeders attempted to breed away from the Siamese type, and the show standard was changed once again.

Russian Blues existed in the United States as early as 1900, although solid breeding did not begin until 1947, using imported British and, later, Scandinavian cats. These cats were quite varied in type and closely resembled the established blue American Shorthairs, which may have contributed to their lack of popularity. Gradually, the breed was strengthened through increasingly stabilized breeding.[3] Many Russian Blue breeders believe that the British lines are responsible for the light, plush, beautiful coats of these cats, and that their brilliant green eyes are attributable to the Scandinavian lines.

The Russian Blue is a slender, balanced cat, in contrast to domestic-type, stockier cats. The head is a moderate wedge, with wide-set ears. The paw pads are a dusty rose pink, and the nose leather is slate. The tail is wide at the base, long and tapering. Brilliant green eyes set this breed apart from most other breeds; the eye color may range from light apple-green to a deep jade that is almost blue-green.[8] This unique eye color may take up to a year or more to develop. The most striking feature of the Russian Blue, however, is its plush and dense double coat. The outer, longer guard hairs protect and repel water, whereas the short, downy undercoat keeps the cat warm. Each hair is tipped with silver, giving the coat a lustrous sheen.

The Russian Blue is gentle, shy, and refined, but loyal to its owners. They live happily with children and other pets. They use their quiet voices only when they have something to say.[1] They can be affectionate lap sitters, but only at their own choosing. They are also quite obedient, train easily, and are fanatic about cleanliness.[8]

Scottish Fold

In the Perthshire region of Scotland in 1961, a shepherd named William Ross discovered a white female cat with forward-folded ears. Ross and his wife acquired one of this cat's kittens, a white female they named "Snooks." These two cats subsequently became the foundation stock for the breed. The Rosses began to develop this unique breed, ini-

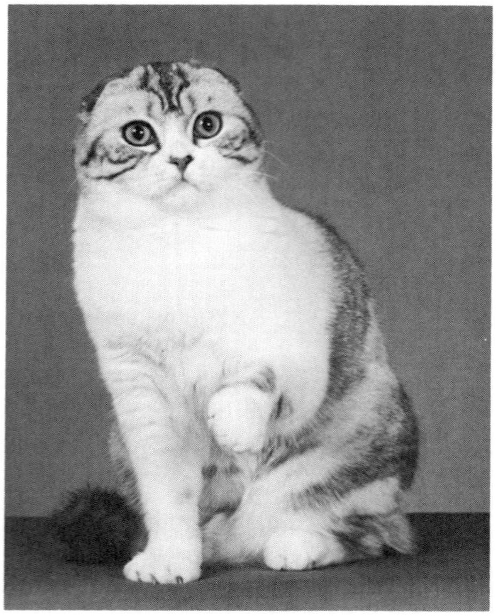

Figure 1–36. Scottish Fold. (© Chanan Photography)

tially cross-breeding to British Shorthairs. It was later discovered that the gene generated by this natural mutation was a simple dominant one.[2]

By 1966, the Scottish Fold (Fig. 1–36) was registered in England. A New England geneticist developed an interest in these cats, and brought three of them to the United States in 1970.[2] The first Scottish Fold was registered in America in 1972, and by the next year, they were accepted by other American associations as well. CFA Championship status was granted in 1978.[2]

In early breedings, outcrossings occurred with a variety of other breeds. The CFA still allows outcrossings to American and British Shorthairs. Several defects related to the folded ear mutation have emerged despite efforts to maintain a large gene pool.

The Scottish Fold was banned in England in 1974 because of ear mite infestation causing deafness. American breeders did not follow suit, believing that the deafness was more likely attributable to genetics, as was the case with blue-eyed whites. Much of the earlier stock of Folds was white. Now Americans are breeding Folds in many other colors and patterns, and the incidence of deafness has been reduced greatly.[2] A more serious condition inherent to the breed is that of skeletal abnormalities—specifically, osteodystrophy. Dr. O.F. Jackson, a British geneticist, first described these abnormalities when cats with folded ears were bred to other cats with folded ears. Affected kittens (usually one out of three folded-ear kittens) have a short, stiff tail and may also have grossly deformed extremities. When one of the affected cats is bred to a straight-eared cat, all the resulting kittens are normal.[2]

A published report of Jackson's discoveries in 1975 stopped Scottish Fold breeding in England. Breeders in the United States took note and began to change their breeding practices. Now it is standard practice to keep straight-eared Folds and to use outcross breeds to produce cats that are not affected with osteodystrophy.[2]

The Scottish Fold has a massive, round head set on a short neck. It has round cheeks, prominent whisker pads, and large, round eyes, all of which contribute to its sweet, expressive smile.[1] There is a considerable distance between the ears, each of which has a definite fold line. The degree of fold will vary from a small and tightly folded ear to a larger, slightly folded ear, but the fold is always forward. These cats have a gently curved profile, and eye color is related to coat color. The body is short, compact, and well balanced. The tail is wide at the base. The coat is thick, short, and very dense, with a soft texture. The Scottish Fold is accepted in a wide variety of colors and patterns.

The Scottish Fold personality is gentle and sweet, which makes them wonderful pets. They are very patient with other pets and children. Like their British domestic ancestors, they are known as very "laid-back" cats.[2]

Selkirk

The Selkirk breed (Fig. 1–37) is the most recent, although unconfirmed, mutation to occur in domestic cats. In 1987, a litter of household cats in Wyoming included a female with an unusually curly coat. This cat was taken to a Persian breeder from the local humane society. The breeder bred her to a black Persian, and three of six resulting kittens had curly coats. Apparently, the curly coat is attributable to a dominant gene, unlike the curly Devon and Cornish Rex genes. The wirehair gene is also dominant, and more genetic work is needed to determine whether this is truly a separate genetic event. The coat is thick, plush, and soft, and falls in loose curls rather than waves.[2] The look is similar to that of the Puli dog.

Siamese

There is much controversy surrounding the early history and origin of the Siamese breed (Fig. 1–38). It is safe to say that this cat is of Eastern origin, with most experts agreeing upon Siam, now known as Thailand, as the country of origin. The oldest known book about cats, *The Cat Book Poems,* which dates back to the 1700s, describes pointed cats with

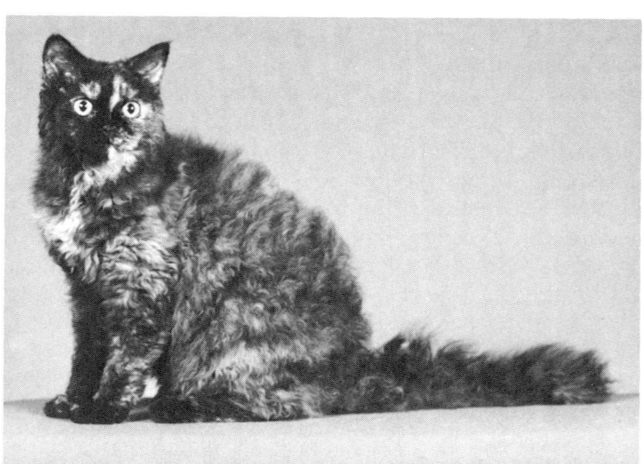

Figure 1–37. Selkirk. (© Chanan Photography)

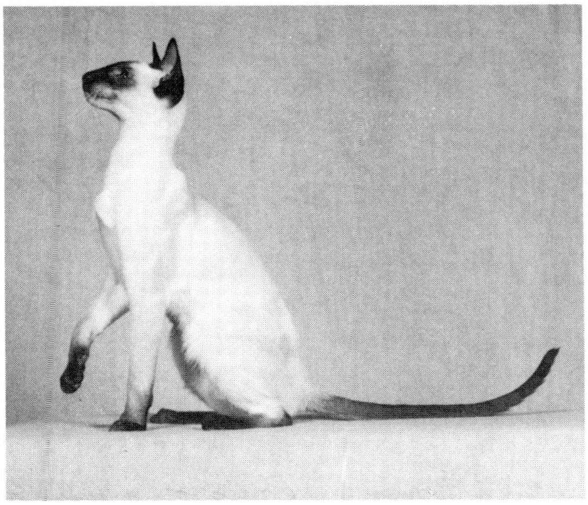

Figure 1–38. Siamese. (© Chanan Photography)

pale coats and dark coloring on the extremities, large ears, and a tapered muzzle. Cherished by the priests and King living in the Royal Palace, the Siamese cat was designated the Royal Cat of Siam.[1,2]

The first official Siamese cats to be imported to the Western world in 1884 were a pair of seal points, given by the King of Siam to the British Consul-General. Earlier imports to England in 1871 were probably not derived from the true temple cats. These Siamese cats caused quite a stir at their first few cat shows in England, and were described as "an unnatural, nightmare kind of cat."[3] The first standards for the Siamese were established in 1892 in England.

Siamese cats began to arrive in the United States in the late 1800s. The first official pair, probably a seal point male and a chocolate point female, belonged to Mrs. Clinton Locke. The American standard for the Siamese breed was drawn up in 1927 by the CFA and was a modified version of the English standard.

The original recognized color was the seal point. Blue points were recognized by the CFA in 1932, but chocolate points did not receive full recognition until 1951. The lilac point, sometimes referred to as the frost point (although some experts recognize the two as having definite differences), was last to be accepted in the United States (1954–55).

Many other point colors have been developed through cross-breeding. The CFA considers only the four classic colors originating from Siam to be true Siamese. Other pointed colors are classified by the CFA as a separate breed, the Colorpoint Shorthair.[2]

The appearance of the Siamese was preceded by centuries of selection. In Siam, crossed eyes and a kinked tail were quite common, but in England, these were considered to be faults and were corrected through selective breeding. The earliest true Siamese cats were small and dainty, with marten-like pointed faces, almond-shaped eyes slanted toward the nose, and large ears. The modern-day Siamese is much the same, with brilliant, piercing blue eyes; sleek, graceful lines; and long, slim legs and tail.

The fur is soft, short, silky to the touch, and lies flat to the body. The ideal body color is uniform, with a definite contrast between body color and point color. The points include the mask, ears, legs, feet, and tail, all of which should be the same shade. The Siamese is accepted in the following colors: seal point, chocolate point, blue point, and lilac point. In countries and organizations that do not recognize the Colorpoint Shorthair as a breed, the colors of the latter may be included in the Siamese breed.[1]

The Siamese is the most popular short-haired breed, based on CFA registration numbers.[2] The Siamese is one of the most playful, intelligent, and affectionate breeds and is highly social. Their best-known traits are their distinct and articulate, noisy voice, and their ability to communicate. Queens are known to have large litters and few reproductive problems. Their gestation length is also unique in that it ranges from 62 to 65 days.[9]

Siberian Cat

The Siberian, a long-haired large cat originating in Russia, has only recently been exported. The first three kittens directly imported to America from Russia by Elizabeth Terrell of Baton Rouge, Louisiana arrived in June of 1990. Siberians (Fig. 1–39) are known for their huge size, with males averaging 17 to 26 lb. Their coat is straight and lustrous, and lacks undercoat. Their ruff is long, with thick curly hair on the belly and breeches. The preferred color pattern is tabby.[2]

Singapura

The Singapura (Fig. 1–40) is a natural breed that was developed from a gene pool native to the Asian island of Singapore. Small cats with a brown-ticked coat pattern have been observed there since 1965. This characteristic coat pattern is thought to be derived from the Abyssinian ticked tabby gene, as modified by the Burmese gene.[2] The black ticking is altered to a deep brown, which results in a softer coat coloring.

Two breeders, Tommy and Hal Meadow, became interested in this breed while living in Singapore. They imported three cats to the United States in 1975 and later acquired

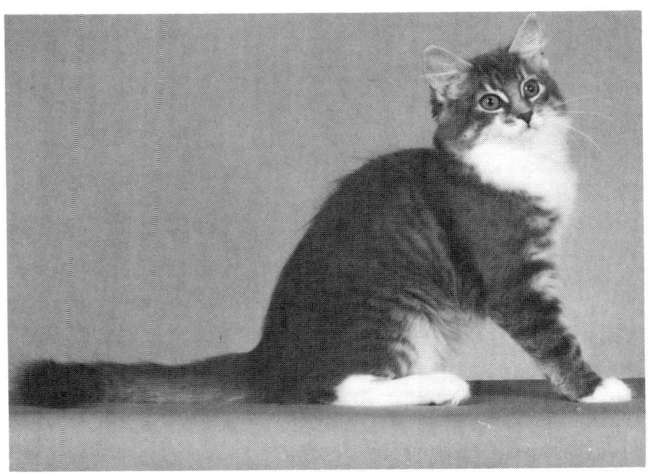

Figure 1–39. Siberian. (© Chanan Photography)

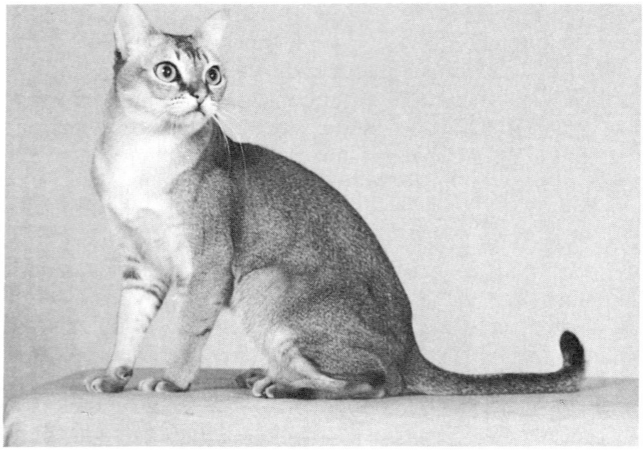

Figure 1–40. Singapura. (© Chanan Photography)

another import from the Society for the Prevention of Cruelty to Animals (SPCA) in 1980. The CFA accepted the breed for registration in 1982 and granted Championship status in 1988. The breed is still fairly rare throughout the United States.

Adult Singapuras are the smallest of the pedigreed breeds, with males averaging about 6 lb and females averaging 4 to 5 lb. This cat has a muscular body and a short, thick neck. The legs are heavily muscled toward the body, with small oval feet. The head is rounded, with a blunt muzzle and well-developed chin. The ears are large and slightly pointed. The eyes are also large, are almond-shaped, and have a slight slant. The eye color may be hazel, green, or yellow. The tail is slender with a blunt tip.

The coat is very short, fine, and close-lying. The ticking effect resembles fine-grained sand.[2] Barring is required on the inner front legs and on the back knee. The color is distinct, with only one color for the breed, known as sepia agouti.

Singapuras are fairly quiet, but are curious and playful. They love to be in the middle of any activity. They are gentle and intelligent, and have excellent mothering instincts. The current demand for the Singapura greatly exceeds their availability.

Snowshoe

The Snowshoe (Fig. 1–41) was developed in the 1960s by cross-mating the Siamese with bi-color American Shorthairs. Since then, breeders have had problems consistently producing the desired white pattern.[2] This breed is short-haired and color-pointed with white on all four feet, and has a moderate, exotic body type.

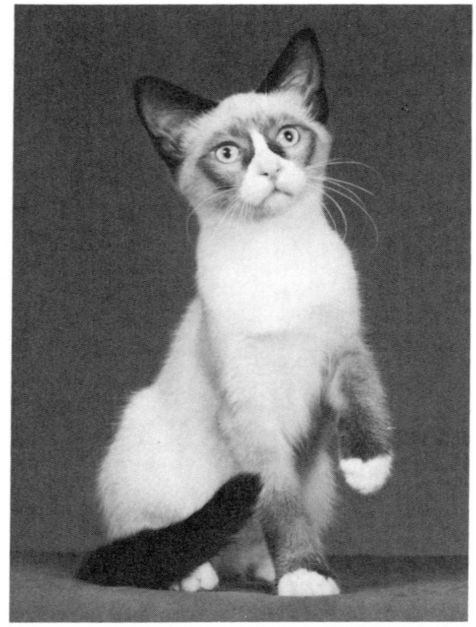

Figure 1–41. Snowshoe. (© Chanan Photography)

Somali

When long-haired kittens first started appearing in purebred Abyssinian litters after World War II, most were quietly sold or kept as pets. The first to be recorded and bred was owned by a Canadian in the 1960s. This male, "Mae-Ling Tutseita of Dunedin," founded the oldest Canadian line.[2] About the same time, an Abyssinian breeder in the United States named Evelyn Mague, of Gillette, New Jersey, began to develop and breed her long-haired Abyssinians. Other Abyssinian breeders were very reluctant to accept these cats as long-haired Abyssinians. Mague chose the name Somali (Fig. 1–42) because Somalia forms two borders of Ethiopia, which used to be called Abyssinia.[10] Gradually, other Abyssinian breeders with long-haired cats surfaced, and in 1972, Mague founded the Somali Cat Club of America. The CFA granted Championship status to the Somali in 1979.

The appearance of the Somali has been compared to that of a wild animal or of a striking red fox. They are medium to large in size with a slightly rounded, wedge-shaped head. The chin is rounded, and their ears are large

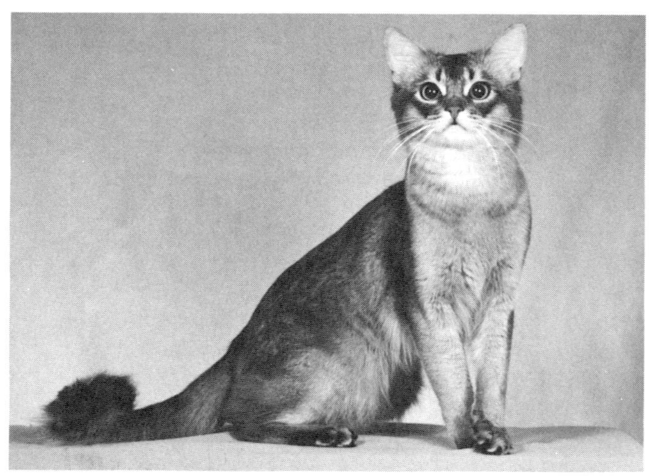

Figure 1–42. Somali. (© Chanan Photography)

and alert. The eyes are almond-shaped, large, and expressive. Gold or green eye color is acceptable. One exceptional feature of this cat is its foxlike appearance owing to its bushy tail, ticking, and full breeches and ruff. These cats are very athletic and agile.

The Somali has a double coat that is medium in length, as well as fine and soft. The ticking of the coat is similar to that of the Abyssinian, with contrasting bands of light and dark. The colors are red, ruddy, blue, and fawn—just as with the Abyssinian.

The Somali is very alert and affectionate, but is fairly quiet and rarely uses its voice. They are profoundly curious and intelligent. When playtime is over, they will seek a warm lap to serve as a nap site. They adapt to changes well and train easily.

Sphynx

The Sphynx (Fig. 1–43) breed resulted from a spontaneous mutation that occurred in Canada in 1966. One kitten from a litter was entirely hairless. The hairless gene is simple recessive. Several breeders took an interest, but found this cat to be difficult to breed. The CFA accepted the Sphynx for registration and with provisional status, only to revoke both later.

The kittens are born nude and later gradually grow a little hair. Their body conformation is striking, with wrinkled skin that sweats. Their head is longer than it is wide, and the neck is very slender. The body is hard and muscular with medium bone structure. The paws are long and dainty, with slender toes. The cat is not really hairless, but is covered with very short down that is barely visible to the eye and touch. The ears, tail, muzzle, feet, and scrotum have short, soft hair. There are no whiskers or eyebrows. This cat came from domestic lines, which allows for a great variety of coat and eye color.

The Sphynx as a pet is a very loving but independent cat. They are people-oriented but do not like other cats.[1] They do not like to be held, but are content to stand in your lap and purr. They have a characteristic stance, with one foreleg lifted. They prefer to lie on warm surfaces.

Tonkinese

The Tonkinese (Fig. 1–44) is a hybrid offspring that evolved from mating Siamese and Burmese cats. The Burmese gene is partially dominant to the Siamese gene, which results in a pointed cat with much deeper body color. Most first generation Tonkinese were produced from a seal-point Siamese and a sable Burmese, although other Siamese colors have been produced experimentally. The first cross produces all Tonkinese. Tonkinese are bred only to Tonkinese to maintain the 50:50 ratio of the two breeds. These Tonkinese matings produce solid Burmese and pointed Siamese as well as Tonkinese, and can never be eliminated from the breed. These offspring are called "variants" and are very valuable in breeding programs.[2]

It is believed that Tonkinese cats have existed for many years, but were never officially recognized. In fact, a cat named "Wong Mau," the foundation stock for the Burmese breed, would, by today's standards, probably be considered a Tonkinese. Modern breeding experiments involving Tonkinese began in the 1960s in the United States and Canada. The breed finally acquired its name in 1967. The CFA granted Championship status in 1984.[2]

The Tonkinese breed not only has a blend of coat colors, but also has a varied body type as well. It is a medium-sized, well-muscled cat. The head is a modified wedge with a somewhat blunted muzzle. The ears are medium in size and alert. The eyes are nearly almond-shaped and wide set. The eye color is uniquely aqua. Its paws are dainty and oval and its legs are fairly slim. The coat is medium-short, close-lying, soft, and lustrous. The coat should be rich and evenly shaded, with a slightly lighter hue on the underside. The four accepted coat colors for Tonkinese are: natural mink with dark brown points and medium brown body, champagne mink with medium brown points, blue mink, and platinum mink.[2] A fifth color—honey mink—is no longer recognized by the CFA.

Tonkinese cats are friendly and affectionate, and love to be around people. They are intelligent and playful, yet only slightly vocal. They are easy to groom and a hardy breed.

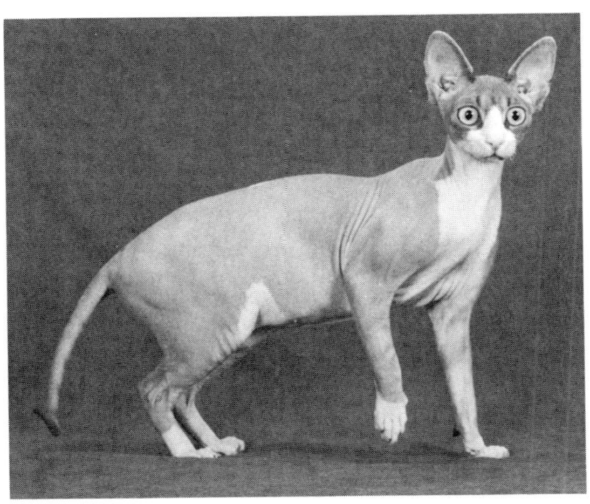

Figure 1–43. Sphynx. (© Chanan Photography)

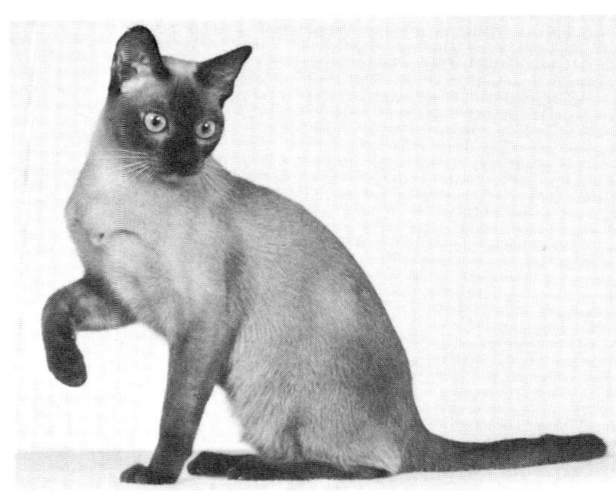

Figure 1–44. Tonkinese. (© Chanan Photography)

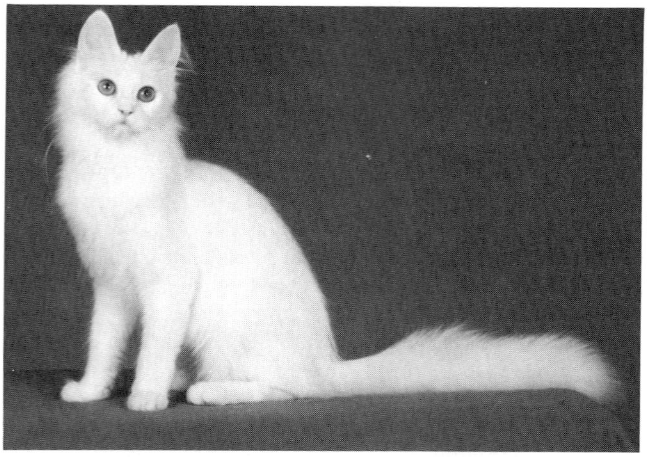

Figure 1–45. Turkish Angora. (© Chanan Photography)

Turkish Angora

The Turkish Angora (Fig. 1–45) is believed to have originated in Ankara, Turkey. This breed, which dates back to the 1600s, is one of many with a speculative past. For centuries, Europeans used the word Angora to denote a long-haired cat. Long-haired cats from Turkey and Persia were introduced into Europe in the 17th century. Sea traders probably brought these cats to America from Europe during the same time period. A letter written in 1856 describes a beautiful long-haired variety of cat that predominated in the eastern part of Turkey.

In the late 1800s, the British began to notice major differences between two specific popular longhairs. The Persian had a rounded face, short nose, and a woolly coat that was of equal length over the entire body. The Angora was a longer cat with a pointed nose and fine, soft, flowing hair. Also, the Angora's hair was longer on the tail, britches, ruff, and around the neck than on the rest of the body.[1] Gradually, the Persian became the preferred breed, and Angoras became scarce except in Turkey.

The Turkish government began a breeding program at the Ankara Zoo in the early 20th century. Their goal was to preserve the pure white Angoras with blue eyes, amber eyes, or a combination of these two eye colors. In the 1960s, several American breeders began to import Angoras from the Ankara Zoo. These breeders founded The Original Turkish Angora Society in the late 1960s to help promote the breed.[2] The CFA granted Championship status in 1973, accepting only a white coat color. Other recessive colors appeared periodically, and were later acknowledged by the CFA in 1978. In England, cats known as "Angoras" and "Turkish" cats are not the same as the Turkish Angora.

The Turkish Angora is medium in size with a definite wedge-shaped head and tapering chin. The ears are wide-based, long, and tufted, and are set high on the head. The eyes are large and almond-shaped. These cats are light-boned with long legs. The hind legs are longer than the front, and the paws are small and dainty. The tail, which is wide at the base and full, and which tapers to the end, is carried lower than the body, but without dragging. When the cat is happy, the tail is carried as a flag over the body. The Angora's coat is silky, slightly wavy, and of medium length. Any color or color pattern is acceptable except those exhibiting Siamese hybridization.[2]

It has been said that this cat loves water. They are very alert and intelligent with great adaptability. The Angora is not very talkative, but it is a polite cat, and easy to train. As with many breeds of cats, some blue-eyed whites may be partially or totally deaf. These cats still make wonderful pets.[2]

Turkish Van

It is believed that a true breeding variety within the Turkish Angora breed—the Turkish Van—developed in the area of the great Lake Van in Turkey. These cats are known for their red or auburn coloring, which is restricted to the head and ears; the rest of the body is white. (This has come to be known in all breeds as the Van pattern.) Like the Turkish Angora, they have a love for water. In Britain, this new variety is known as the Turkish cat. Two Britons imported a pair to England and began a breeding program. This breed has now been recognized by several breed registries in Europe and America.

The auburn and white Van cats imported to England were the original preferred color, although black and white cats are more common in the Lake Van area. These cats also carry a dilution factor that allows cream and white combinations, as well as blue and white.[2] Occasionally, calicos and tortoiseshells are produced as well.

A British breeder brought some of these cats to the United States in 1982. Within a few years, interest escalated and more Vans have continued to be imported. The breed was recognized by the CFA for registration in 1988.[2]

The Turkish Van (Fig. 1–46) is considered to be one of the largest domestic cats.[2] They have broad shoulders and hips, and wide-set, long legs. Males average 12 to 18 lb, whereas generally females weigh 7 to 12 lb. The head is a

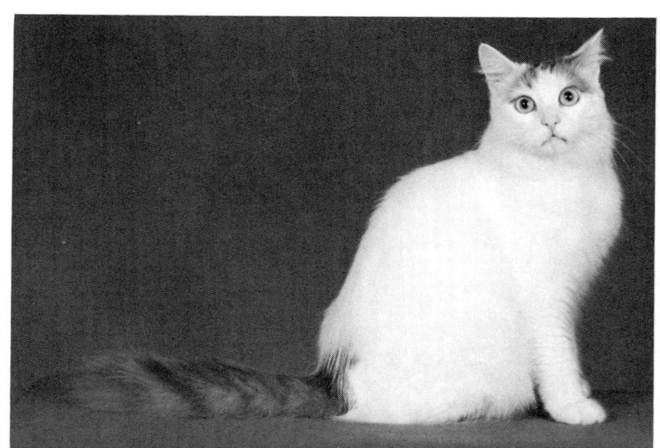

Figure 1–46. Turkish Van. (© Chanan Photography)

modified wedge that is fairly broad, to match their body size. The tail is very full and is constantly in motion.

The coat is soft, silky, and semilong; in fact, it feels similar to cashmere, but lacks an undercoat. This minimizes the tendency for the hair to tangle or knot. The coat takes time to develop and varies in length according to the time of the year.

The Turkish Van has a gentle disposition, but these cats need their space to help them to adapt to household living. Not all of them like to swim, although they are more likely to do this than most cats. They are very athletic and playful.

Acknowledgments. The author would like to thank Mr. Richard Katris of Chanan Photography, Mira Loma, California for the superior quality photographs for this chapter.

The author would also like to thank Solveig M.V. Pflueger, Ph.D., M.D., of Baystate Medical Center, Springfield, Massachusetts, for the extensive information provided on the Missouri Rex, Munchkin, and Ojos Azules breeds, which are very new to the cat fancy.

REFERENCES

1. Wilson M. Encyclopedia of American Cat Breeds. Neptune, NJ: TFH Publications, Inc., 1978.
2. Wastlhuber J. History of Domestic Cats and Cat Breeds. In: Pedersen N, ed. Feline Husbandry, Goleta, CA: American Veterinary Publications. Inc., 1991:1.
3. Wright M, Walters S. The Book of the Cat. New York: Summit Books, 1980:20.
4. Urcia I. All About Rex Cats. Neptune, NJ: TFH Publications, Inc., 1982:5.
5. Carr W. The New Basic Book of the Cat. New York: Charles Scribner's Sons, 1978:57.
6. Pare C. The Devon Rex. Cat Fancy 1991;34(5):44.
7. Maggitti P. The Norwegian Forest Cat. Cats Magazine 1991; 48(3):5.
8. Urcia I. This Is The Russian Blue. Neptune City, NJ: TFH Publications, Inc., 1983:5.
9. Dunnill M. The Siamese Cat Owner's Encyclopedia. New York: Howell Book House, Inc., 1974:12.
10. Maggitti P. The Somali. Cats Magazine 1991;48(7):5.

CHAPTER 2

◇ ◇ ◇

Addressing and Handling the Cat

Gary D. Norsworthy

It has always been a frustration to me the way clients have assessed my professional competence. I have performed commendable diagnostic feats and heroic therapeutic deeds, only to be deserted for a colleague because the cat jumped and cried when I gave an injection. I have heard colleagues described as "good veterinarians" because they talked to and understood their patients, even though their professional skills left much to be desired. The hard-learned lesson for all of us is that the mechanics of handling the feline patient are often more important to the client than the fact that we spent half of our lives in school studying anatomy, physiology, pathology, and so on. This chapter offers some techniques, some of which have been hard-learned, which may help your client to view you as a "good veterinarian."

I also recommend to you an article published in the September 1990 issue of *Cat Fancy Magazine* and written by Margaret Reister, DVM. This article, entitled "Cats and Their Vets," is a summary of a recent survey of readers of that magazine. Among other things, she found that 50% of the respondents in the survey had changed veterinarians as a result of dissatisfaction.

Demonstrate a Liking for Cats

Some veterinarians do not particularly care to treat cats. Amazingly, many of these are in small animal practices in which cats constitute a significant percentage of their patient load. When cat lovers detect this ambivalence or downright dislike, they often seek another veterinarian who is not so inclined.

The best way to demonstrate that you like cats and enjoy working with them is to keep a resident "hospital cat" that feels at home with your clientele. This cannot be just any cat; rather, it must be one that has an outgoing personality and that seeks attention from strangers. This cat should spend quite a bit of time roaming the reception area looking for people to charm. If your practice is not exclusively feline, your hospital cat should not be afraid of dogs.

Such a cat is not easy to find. We are fortunate to have one that meets these criteria and more. Jokingly, we tell our clients that this cat is in charge of public relations; however, there is more truth than fiction in that statement. He strongly conveys the message that our staff and our veterinarians like cats.

Cats Are Not Small Dogs

In the past, the cat has been treated as if it were the medical equivalent of a Chihuahua or a Toy Fox Terrier. However, the cat and the dog are separate species manifesting significant differences. Some of these differences are biological; however, many of the features that distinguish the feline species relate to their basic psychological makeup. The cat is a very independent and private creature. It is unusual for a cat to be gregarious enough to approach an unknown human. Rather, cats accept humans only on their terms, and often not at all.

The following are suggestions, based on 20 years of clinical experience with cats, for dealing successfully with the feline patient:

- Suggest to owners that their cat(s) always travel in a carrier or a cage. Because some cats become very agitated when traveling by car, driving may be very dangerous if they are left unrestrained. Following a hospital visit, a cat may become even more agitated, making the return trip potentially more dangerous.
- As cats are generally fearful of dogs, try to provide a separate space in your reception room for cats and their owners. If separate reception rooms or areas are not feasible, the feline patient and its owner should be ushered into an empty examination room as soon as possible. Most cat owners would prefer to wait in the isolation of an examination room than in a larger room in the company of barking dogs.
- Upon entering the examination room, close the door, move slowly, and greet the client softly. Address the owner while ignoring the cat. A cat will be less apprehensive if it, rather than the veterinarian, is the first to explore and initiate contact.
- If the cat is in a carrier, open the carrier door to give the cat an opportunity to exit. Most will not do so, but enough will to make the effort worthwhile.
  - If the cat does not exit the carrier, have the owner reach in the carrier for the cat. The cat will be much

less apprehensive when handled by familiar hands accompanied by a familiar voice.
  - If the cat does not exit the carrier and the owner has difficulty extracting it, *slowly* turn the carrier on end with the door positioned downward. Leave the carrier in this position until the cat rests its two front or two rear feet on the table. This may take a few seconds to a couple of minutes. When this occurs, lift the carrier upward, and the cat will remain on the table. Do not try to shake the cat out of the carrier, as the cat will only resist and the owner will often be uncomfortable with this approach.
  - As soon as the cat is out of the carrier, close the carrier door. If given the chance, most cats will return to the safety of the carrier, in which case the entire process must begin again.
- When the cat is out of the carrier, stroke it and talk to it, but do not pick it up initially. After the cat has had an opportunity to examine you and the surroundings, you may then pick it up affectionately. Most cat owners will be impressed by your attempts to befriend their cat.
- At each visit, make a point to say something complimentary about the cat, within the limits of sincerity. Most clients relish positive statements made about their prized pet and companion, and most are looking for a veterinarian who genuinely likes their cat. Any statement that is detrimental to their cat will quickly alienate the client, effectively negating all of your years of schooling and experience.
- Your value and competence as a veterinarian are also being tested when you administer injections to a cat in the presence of its owner If the cat reacts negatively, you may be instantly labeled a "cat hater" or a "bad veterinarian." To minimize such negative reactions, consider adopting the following practices:
  - Use a sharp 22- or 25-gauge needle. Bargain brand needles are often not as sharp as first-quality needles, and the loss of a client can quickly negate any initial savings.
  - When drug bioavailability permits, administer injections by the subcutaneous (SC) route instead of intramuscularly (IM). The area of loose skin on the dorsal midline between the scapulae is the preferred site of injection.
  - Ask the owner to help restrain the cat while the needle is being inserted if he or she is willing. Lightly pinch the skin at the injection site just prior to inserting the needle.
  - After inserting the needle, ask the owner to turn the cat loose. Then, grasping the cat by the nape, slide it along the examination table, preferably toward the end of the table, while simultaneously administering the injection (Fig. 2–1). The cat will be sufficiently distracted by the motion, and especially by the threat of being pulled off the end of the table, that it will not react to the injection. The cat will remain untraumatized, the owner will be happy, and you will be considered a "good veterinarian."
  - If an intramuscular injection is necessary, the injection should be made in the semimembranosus or semitendinosus muscle, about midway between the hip joint and the knee. The injection site should be on the caudalmost aspect of the leg. This location avoids the sciatic nerve and is less painful than many IM injection sites.
  - Administer IM injections slowly, as rapid infusion is more painful.

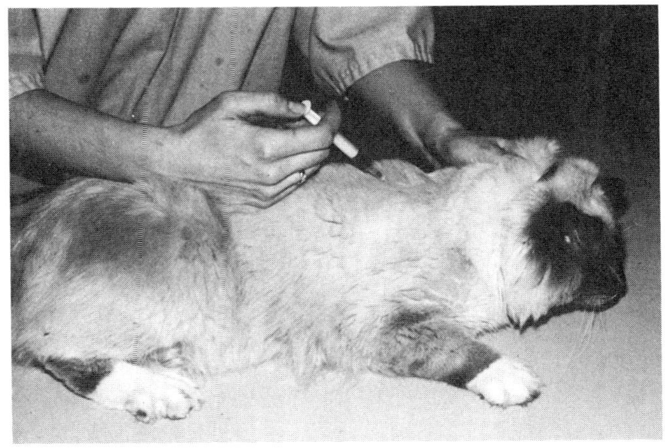

Figure 2–1. **To make a "painless" subcutaneous injection, insert the needle between the scapulae. Administer the injection while pulling the cat along the examination table. The cat will become distracted by the movement and will be unaware of the injection.**

- The fractious cat offers unique challenges to the veterinarian. Whereas a fractious dog can generally be restrained with force, a fractious cat will almost always be the victor in a cat:doctor encounter. The following are suggestions for managing the fractious cat:
  - Appreciate the consequences of a cat bite—for you, your technician, and the owner. Consider the fact that approximately 50% of cat bites to human hands become infected,[1] and that an infected cat bite can result in septicemia and hospitalization of the victim. If the owner is bitten, legal action against the veterinarian is possible.
  - If you or the owner are not able to coax a fractious cat from its carrier, disassemble the carrier and lift off the top. As soon as the top is removed, cover the entire body of the cat with a heavy bath towel. If possible, perform the examination and treat the animal while the cat is in the bottom half of the carrier; then quickly reassemble the carrier.
  - If the cat is out of its carrier, cover it with a heavy bath towel. Covering the cat's head will help to calm the cat and will prevent it from knowing where to strike
  - Some clinicians advocate the use of a "cat bag" for restraint. Although I appreciate their views, I do not share their enthusiasm for this type of restraint for several reasons. First, cats that truly need that degree of restraint can rarely be placed in a cat bag. Second, most owners find such "feline straitjackets" to be objectionable, considering them to be demeaning to their pet.

- Many practitioners find a fish net to be useful in handling fractious cats. These nets may be used to retrieve fractious cats from cages or to catch those that escape within the hospital. They are especially useful in administering injections, as they provide easy access to the injection site.
- Using heavy gloves to restrain fractious cats is usually not a successful approach, as cats can bite through even very thick leather gloves. Moreover, those gloves that are truly cat-proof are usually too bulky to use effectively. The use of radiographic gloves is discouraged because they do not offer any real protection against bites, and because the damage done to the gloves renders them unsafe for radiographic protection.
- When hospitalizing a fractious cat, separate it from as much dog noise and visual intimidation as possible. Do not allow hospital personnel to taunt or further aggravate this cat. A towel covering the front of the cage helps to calm many cats.
- Use extreme caution in choosing anesthetics and tranquilizers for the fractious cat. (This subject will be discussed in more detail in Chapter 8.)
- Keep in mind that a number of physiologic changes occur in the excited cat that will affect blood chemistry parameters, including the glucose level, and white blood cell, neutrophil, eosinophil, and lymphocyte counts. These influences must be considered when interpreting blood profile results. Some excited cats will also experience a rise of 1° to 2°F in body temperature.
- Following a visit to the hospital, suggest that the client keep the cat indoors for several hours. Cats that are not confined have been known to leave home and not return. This is especially true of cats that have undergone surgery (ovariohysterectomy, neutering, etc.).

REFERENCE

1. Elliot DL, Tolle SW, Goldberg L, Miller JB. Pet-associated illness. J Am Anim Hosp Assoc 1986;22:387.

CHAPTER 3

◇ ◇ ◇

The History and Physical Examination

Gary D. Norsworthy

Despite the advanced technology now available, the patient's history and physical examination remain the two most important components of diagnosing disease. When diagnostic testing commences before the history and physical examination are performed, many questions will remain unanswered, and unnecessary expense may be incurred by the client.

The History

The principles underlying a systematic and complete approach to history taking include the following:

- Ask the client to discuss or list the primary clinical complaints, then take control of the conversation with a list of specific questions. If the client remains in control of the conversation, the discussion may wander aimlessly, focusing on trivia rather than on important points.
- Ask the client about the cat's diet, concentrating on the percentage of table food that is fed.
- Ask whether this cat is indoors only, outdoors only, or both indoors and outdoors.
- Establish whether there are other pets in the household and whether they are well.
- Inquire whether other pets or neighborhood animals have died or been sick recently. If so, ask the client about their diagnosis.
- Ask whether the cat has a history of engaging in cat fights, especially if abscesses or cellulitis are evident.
- Phrase questions objectively so as not to prejudice the client's answer.

  Example

  "Has there been any change in your cat's water consumption?"

  versus

  "He is drinking a lot of water, isn't he?"
- If more than one family member is present, allow each to offer an answer. The answers will often differ; you must weigh each answer and make a judgment as to which, if any, are valid. In my experience, school-aged children often provide more reliable information than do their parents, presumably because they have more frequent contact with the cat on a daily basis.
- Establish the duration of the various events and abnormalities described.
- Be alert for evasive answers that may reflect the owner's unwillingness to admit a failure to observe the animal closely or to admit that the condition has been present for several days or weeks.

  Example

  Q: "Is your cat eating?"

  A: "The bowl is empty each day after the cats finish eating." (Since there are several cats in the household, the answer given is actually an evasion.)
- If a cat is presented for trauma that is unrelated to a collision with an automobile or a fight with another animal, be aware that owner abuse may be involved. This is especially true if the client reports that the cat has sustained multiple falls. Such clients are likely to answer questions evasively, and will often offer contradictory explanations of the events preceding the injury or illness
- Do not limit the list of differential diagnoses too quickly. By so doing, you may fail to ask important questions.
- Be aware that the cat may be manifesting more than one disease process at any one time. Continue to probe the cat's history even if you are sure of a diagnosis. Concentrate on any elements of the history that contradict diagnoses that are being considered.
- Be sure to assess accurately the cat's appetite for the last few days and for the last several weeks. Some diseases, such as hyperthyroidism and diabetes mellitus, are initially characterized by polyphagia but subsequently result in anorexia.
- If weight loss has occurred, establish how rapidly the weight was lost, as well as what percentage of body weight was lost.
- If the condition is chronic, ask about seasonality, especially if pruritus is a component.
- The scope of this text does not permit the listing of every question pertaining to every body system for each

patient. However, you may find it useful to develop a list of specific questions based on key words or clinical signs that arise in the course of history taking. The following is an example of such a list relating to a history of vomiting.

Is the cat vomiting, or merely regurgitating its food?

What is being vomited?

What is the duration of the vomiting?

How many times has vomiting occurred within the last 24 hours? Within the last 48 hours?

Does the cat have a history of anorexia, decreased appetite, increased appetite, or normal appetite?

Does vomiting occur immediately after eating?

Is diarrhea present?

What has the cat's pattern of water consumption been over the last 24 hours? Over the last 30 days?

Are any other pets in the household vomiting?

- When examining a well cat, such as during the annual vaccination visit, concentrate on taking an especially good history and performing a thorough physical examination. Certain key questions should be asked, including:

  How long have you owned this cat?

  Has there been a weight change? If so, what percentage of body weight has been lost or gained? What is the total number of pounds involved?

  What is the cat's diet? Is it fed dry or canned food? What percentage of the cat's diet is table food or treats? Does the cat eat a generic food, or dog food?

  How much water does the cat drink? Has there been a change in the amount consumed?

  Is there a history of recent or recurrent episodes of vomiting or diarrhea?

  Does the cat have a history of fight wounds or abscesses?

  Have any cats in the household or in the immediate neighborhood died recently? Have any been seriously ill or been diagnosed as having feline leukemia virus (FeLV) or feline immunodeficiency virus (FIV) in the last year?

  When did the cat last receive its vaccinations (if a new patient)? (Note: This question will reveal the type of care the cat routinely receives.) Has the cat previously been vaccinated for FeLV or feline infectious peritonitis (FIP) (if a new patient)?

  Is this cat presently taking any medication?

- Be alert to clinical complaints whose diagnosis may require additional clarification or careful wording of questions to avoid misunderstanding or misinterpretation. Common examples include the following:[1]

  Not Eating. Is the cat interested in food? Does the cat have difficulty chewing or swallowing?

  Not Walking Normally. Is the cat reluctant to move? Is there weakness, or is it lameness? Is pain elicited when touching or moving a leg or joint?

  Not Urinating Normally. Does straining or vocalization occur during urination? Is the urine any color other than pale yellow? Has there been any change in water intake? Does the cat urinate any place except the litter box or outside?

  Not Defecating Normally. What is the consistency of the stool? Does vocalization occur when the cat attempts to defecate? Is there a history of urinary blockage or difficulty urinating? When the cat strains, does any stool (or urine) pass?

  Unusual Behavior. Is the cat's behavior continual or episodic? Is the cat an unspayed female? If it is a tom cat, is there an unspayed female cat nearby that might be in heat?

  Vomiting. What is the consistency and content of the vomitus? How often does vomiting occur and when does it occur in relation to eating? Does coughing precede the vomiting?

The Physical Examination

As with the history-taking process, it is customary for the clinician to examine every body system in every patient. However, certain situations make this unnecessary or impractical, including time constraints (five clients waiting), "red flag" statements made by the client (constipation), and pathognomonic findings (a urinary bladder the size of a baseball). When circumstances permit, however, the following assessments should be made during the physical examination.

General Assessment

The cat's weight should be assessed and the cat categorized subjectively as emaciated, thin, normal, heavy, or obese. If the cat has a long hair coat, palpation is generally necessary to make a correct assessment. Palpation of the dorsal spines of the vertebrae, the ilium, and the greater trochanters will allow a correct assessment of the degree of fleshing. As the cat moves around the examination room, its activity level should be evaluated as hyperactive, normal, or lethargic. However, it is important to solicit the owner's input in this regard, as the cat's activity during the examination may not be representative of its usual pattern of activity. The cat's attitude—aggressive, shy, or attention-seeking—is also important to note.

Skin and Hair Coat

The condition of the skin and hair coat reflect the general condition of the cat. Areas of focal alopecia and bilateral truncal alopecia should be identified (Fig. 3–1). Excessive dandruff and an unkempt hair coat often indicate that the cat is not grooming itself properly. Some cats are fastidious groomers and others are not; however, sick cats usually become lax about grooming, resulting in an unkempt appearance and an oily hair coat. Areas of dermatitis and ulcer-

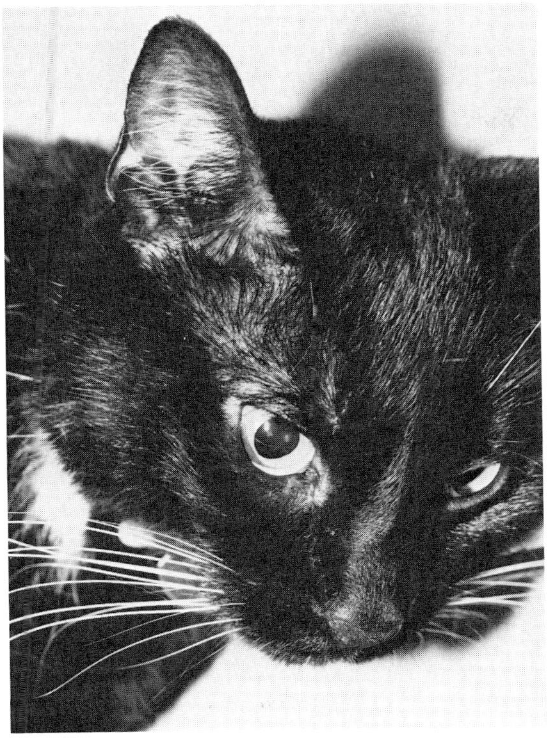

Figure 3–1. **Preauricular alopecia is a normal finding that is especially noticeable in cats with black hair coats. The hair is often thin between the eyes and the pinnas.**

ation should be sought. Seemingly innocent areas of ulceration on the ear tips of white cats may be the initial manifestation of squamous cell carcinoma. One should examine the cat and palpate for dermal/epidermal masses. Hair that epilates easily is generally a sign of disease. The chin should be examined for comedones or swelling.

Eyes

Hyperemia and swelling of the conjunctivae are not normal. Icterus may be visible on the sclera. The corneas should be clear. There should be no evidence of hyphema or hypopyon in the anterior chambers. The irides should be homogeneous and similar in color to each other (except in odd-eyed cats). The irides often become mottled in appearance in cats older than 10 to 12 years of age. A change in iris color occurs in some FeLV-infected cats and in blue-eyed cats with anterior uveitis. The pupils should be responsive to light. Blindness of any etiology will cause the pupils to become persistently dilated (Fig. 3–2). The third eyelids should not be visible in the healthy cat. If they are prolapsed, several disease states or conditions may be present, including tapeworms, diarrhea (of any cause), weight loss, general debilitation, and Horner's syndrome. Some tranquilizers will also cause third eyelid prolapse. The lenses should not be visible. Cloudiness of the lens usually indicates cataract formation (see Fig. 3–2). Epiphora is common in brachycephalic cats, such as Persians, or in any cat with

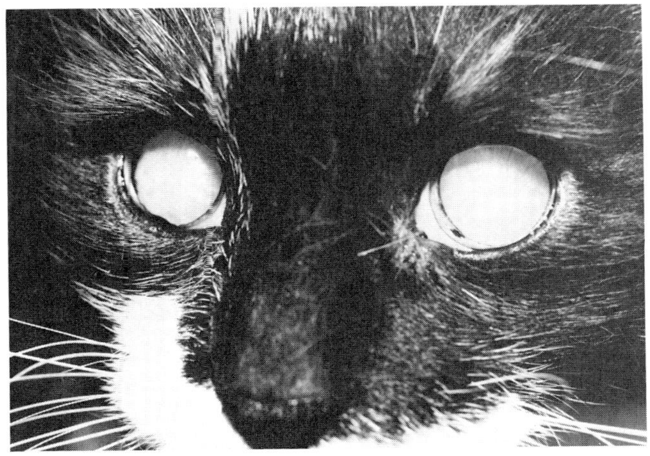

Figure 3–2. **This cat's persistent pupillary dilation indicates blindness. The densely white lenses indicate cataract formation.**

nonfunctional or poorly functioning nasolacrimal ducts. Cats with orange hair coats usually develop black pigment depositions on the lid margins (Fig. 3–3*A*). This increases with age and is not related to a malignant process. The retinas should be examined for lesions typical of several systemic diseases, including FIP, toxoplasmosis, and FeLV infections.

Nose

A nasal discharge is never a normal sign. The nature of the discharge and its duration should be assessed. Ulceration of the nasal planum may occur secondary to some respiratory viruses, immune-mediated diseases, and squamous cell carcinoma. Cats with orange hair coats usually develop black pigment depositions on the nasal planum (see Fig. 3–3*A*). As with the pigmentation that involves the eyelid margins, this pigment deposition increases with age and is unrelated to malignancy.

Ears

The ears should be examined for any odor or signs of discharge. If either is present, the cause should be investigated. The ear canals should be visualized for masses or deep wax plugs. Abnormal carriage of the pinna may be the result of fighting, untreated aural hematomas (Fig. 3–4), or tumor(s).

Mouth

Before opening the mouth, the cat should be observed for drooling, and the upper lips should be lifted on each side to observe for masses, missing or broken teeth, tartar formation, ulcerations of the gingiva or labia, and gingival color. The periodontal area should be examined for gingival hyperemia and hyperplasia. When the mouth is opened, the odor of the breath should be noted. One should look for

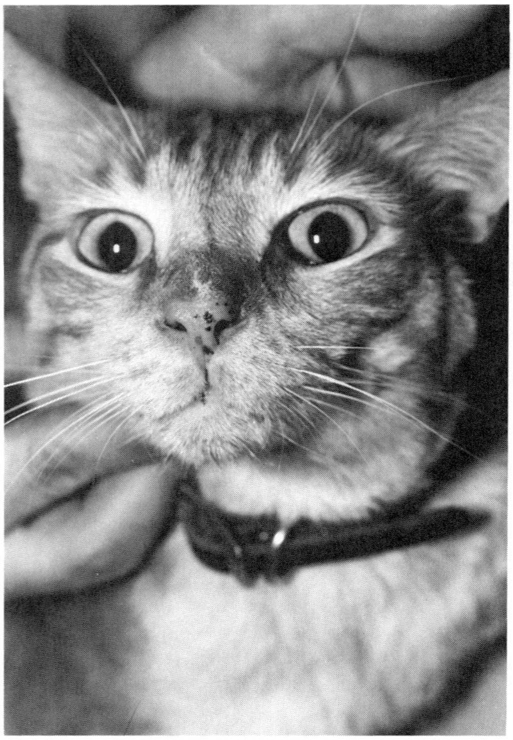

A

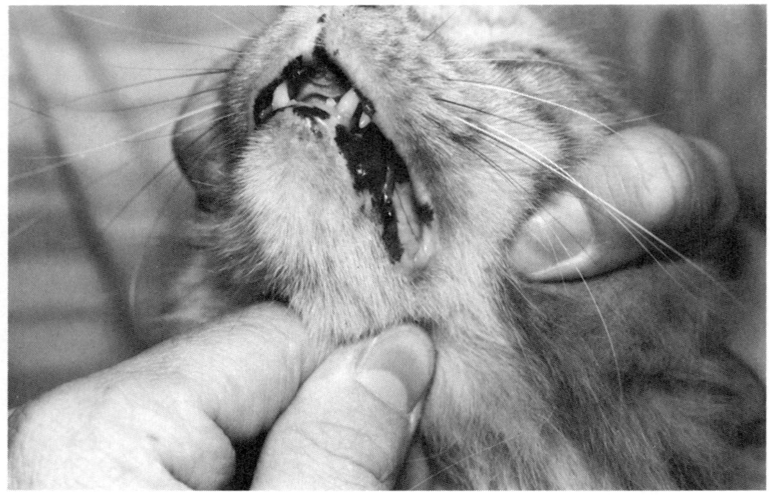

B

Figure 3–3. Cats with orange hair coats exhibit deposition of black pigment on the upper and lower eye lid margins (*A*), the nasal planum (*A*), and the lips (*B*). This pigment deposition is age-related but is not associated with malignancy.

signs of icterus on the soft palate, as well as for masses and ulceration anywhere in the mouth. The tongue should be lifted with a blunt instrument to facilitate the search for foreign bodies (especially string) or masses. The pharynx and tonsils should be examined. Cats with orange hair coats usually develop black pigment depositions on the lips (see Fig. 3–3*B*). As when it involves the eyelid margins and the nasal planum, this pigmentation increases with age and is unrelated to malignancy.

The teeth may be helpful in determining age, especially in kittens (Fig. 3–5). The permanent upper central incisors erupt at about 4 months of age, whereas the corresponding permanent canine teeth erupt at about 6 months of age. These are the most reliable dental indicators of age. Although tartar formation is dependent on a number of factors, including diet and individual variations, it is unusual for a cat to have significant tartar formation prior to 2 years of age.

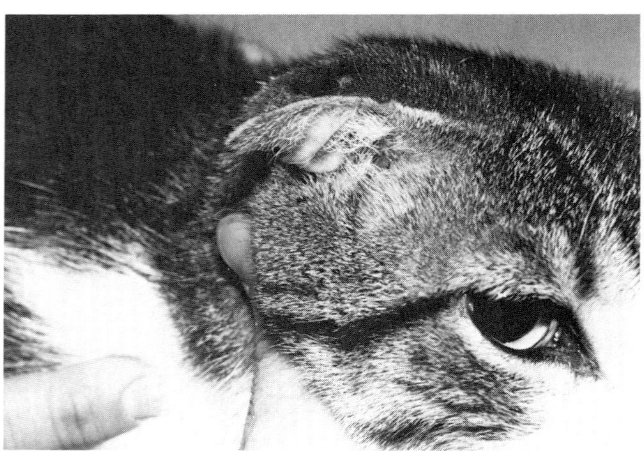

Figure 3–4. Abnormal pinna carriage may be attributable to fighting, untreated aural hematomas (as in this cat), or a tumor.

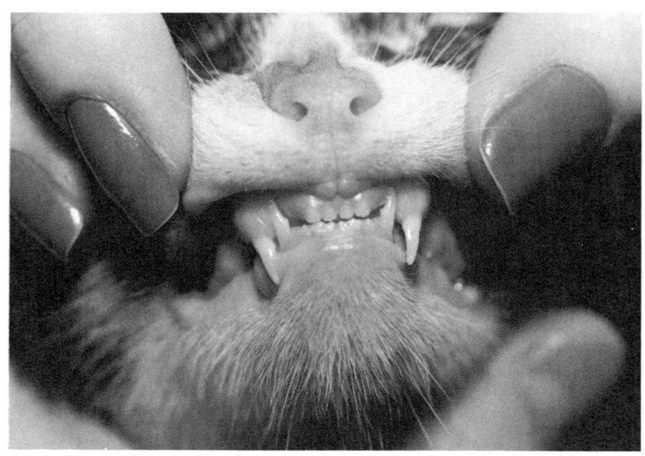

Figure 3–5. A cat's age can be assessed accurately as deciduous teeth are shed and the adult teeth erupt. Because the first four incisors—the first adult teeth—have erupted in this cat, its age is just over 4 months.

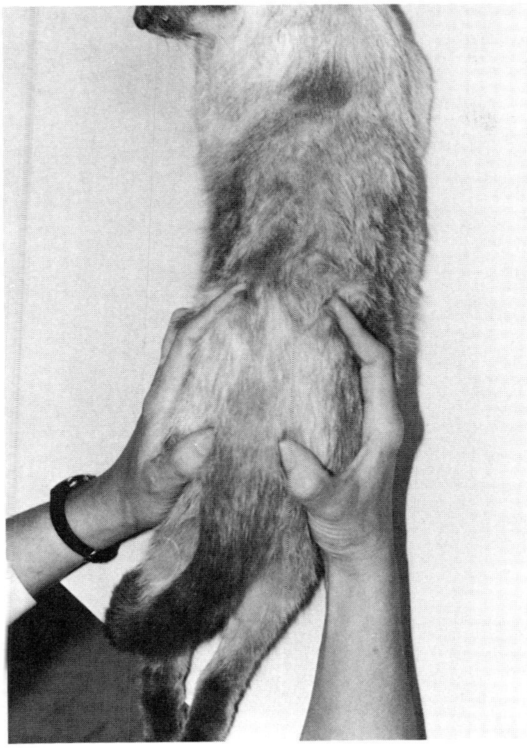

Figure 3–6. The presence of a luxated coxofemoral joint or a fractured femoral head or neck may be suspected by palpating the greater trochanter of the femur in relation to the wing of the ilium (index fingers) and the point of the ischium (thumbs). This assessment is most effective when the knees of the cat are in extension.

Neurologic Parameters

Some neurologic tests are difficult to perform in an examination room setting. However, testing for proprioceptive deficits and placing reflexes can be done in this setting. The cranial nerves can also be tested. The cat should be observed for any evidence of head tilt or anisocoria. If the cat will walk, it can be evaluated for ataxia; however, this condition is more likely to be observed and reported by the owner.

Cervical Area

The cervical area should be palpated to detect enlargement of or pain involving the thyroid gland, lymph nodes, or salivary glands.

Musculoskeletal System

Major muscle groups should be palpated for atrophy. Persistent ventroflexion of the neck is pathologic. If lameness is present, each joint of the affected leg should be palpated for evidence of pain or crepitus. Palpation of the feet can be misleading. Cats may falsely withdraw as if in pain because their feet are somewhat sensitive, or because of the way in which they have been restrained. If palpation does elicit pain, the other feet should be palpated for comparison; then the presumably painful one should be palpated again to determine whether the sensitivity is reproducible. The coxofemoral joints are often luxated, and femoral head or neck fractures are common. If either occurs, the femur will displace dorsally. The relationship of the wing of the ilium, the ischial tuberosity, and the greater trochanter should be determined by palpation (Fig. 3–6). Assessing the relationship of the first two of these is also helpful when a pelvic fracture is suspected. The toenails of older cats should be inspected for lack of nail shedding and to determine whether they have grown into the toe pads owing to inadequate sharpening (Fig. 3–7). If a traumatic injury is suspected, the toenails should be examined, as frayed nails are often present in such cats (Fig. 3–8).

Peripheral Lymph Nodes

The peripheral lymph nodes (submandibular, prescapular, superficial inguinal, and popliteal) should be palpated for swelling. If they are normal, they are generally only barely palpable.

Mammary Glands

The mammary glands should be palpated for evidence of pain, enlargement, or the presence of a mass.

Chest

The cat's heart should be auscultated to determine the heart rate and rhythm, and to rule out the presence of a murmur. The lungs should be auscultated for evidence of crackles, wheezes, and dullness. The ribs of the anterior chest should be gently compressed. In young cats, a lack of compressibil-

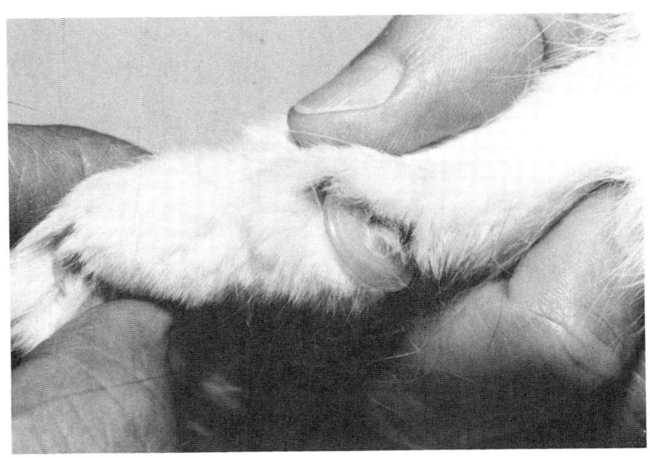

Figure 3–7 This 14-year-old-cat discontinued proper sharpening of its toenails, as evidenced by nail thickening secondary to the buildup of dead nail tissue. Because the nails were allowed to grow unchecked, they curled into the toe pad.

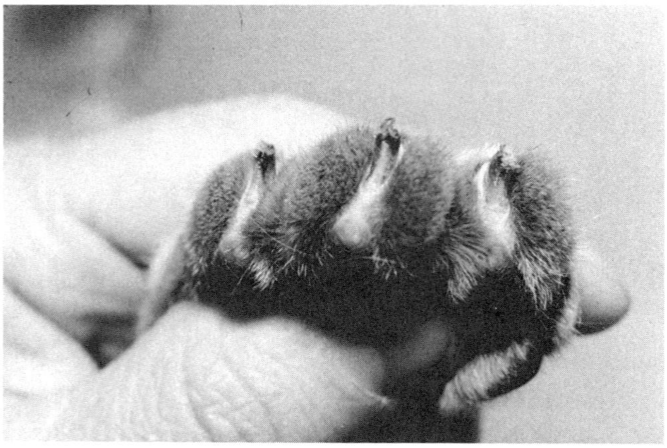

Figure 3–8. In cases of possible traumatic injury, the cat should be examined for frayed toenails. The nails may become frayed in the process of dashing from in front of a motor vehicle or in sliding down a roof or tree prior to a fall.

ity often indicates a mediastinal mass. This is more difficult to interpret in adult cats.

Abdomen

The abdomen should be assessed by palpation. A doughy feeling to the abdomen may indicate the presence of ascites. Splinting in response to abdominal palpation, or attempts to evade palpation generally indicate pain, which may be a sign of pancreatitis, gastrointestinal distress, a urinary obstruction, urocystoliths, or peritonitis. Most of the cat's major organs (liver, kidneys, stomach, small and large intestines, spleen, and urinary bladder) are palpable, and each should be assessed for size, shape, location, and pain. The intestines should be evaluated for the presence of excessive intraluminal gas or increased thickness of the intestinal walls. Abnormal masses or foreign bodies should be identified. If the mesenteric lymph nodes are palpable, they are abnormal. Any evidence of uterine enlargement or fetuses should be noted.

Perianal Area

The perianal area should be examined for evidence of tapeworm segments, which are usually found at the anus or stuck to the perianal hair (Fig. 3–9). Inflammation of the anus may be the only clue to the presence of diarrhea. If the anal sacs are palpable, they are probably abnormally full. One should observe the vulvar opening for any evidence of a vaginal discharge. Because of the fastidious nature of most cats, an actual flow of purulent material is rarely observed, even if open-cervix pyometra is present.

Characteristics of Male Cats

The testicles of the male cat should be descended and palpable by 4 months of age. Male cats are fertile and capable of

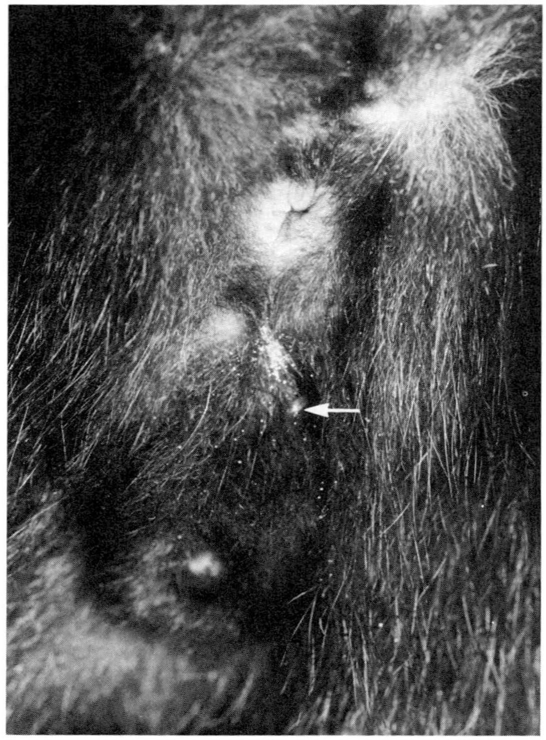

Figure 3–9. The examination should include an inspection of the perineal area. Tapeworm segments (*arrow*) or their fragments may be seen attached to the hair just below the anus. Because these fragments may not pass daily, the owner should also be instructed to observe for them.

breeding by 7 to 9 months of age, even though most of the secondary sexual characteristics do not develop that early. The cheeks of the male cat enlarge and the neck thickens by 2 to 3 years of age. Spraying of urine may be observed as early as 8 to 9 months of age, but generally begins at 1 to 2 years of age. Territorial influences have a bearing on the initiation of that behavior. A strong urine odor becomes prominent by 1.5 to 2.5 years of age.

Characteristics of Female Cats

There are no obvious secondary sexual characteristics that develop in female cats. However, the onset of estrus may occur as early as 4 months of age, or as late as 10 to 12 months of age. A number of external factors affect the timing of this, such as temperature, number of hours of light per day, and the presence of other cycling queens in the area.

REFERENCE

1. Schaer M. The Medical History, Physical Examination, and Physical Restraint. In: Sherding RG, ed. The Cat: Disease and Clinical Management. New York: Churchill Livingstone, 1989:7.

CHAPTER 4

◇ ◇ ◇

Kittens

Gary D. Norsworthy and Frances T. Eiserloh

Veterinarians are frequently consulted for information on breeding cats and raising kittens. If handled properly, this affords the practitioner an opportunity to acquire several new patients and clients. When newly acquired kittens are presented for examination and/or vaccination, the veterinarian has an opportunity to cultivate or recultivate a positive, long-term doctor-client relationship.

Breeding Cats and Raising Kittens

There is a sizable volume of information that the novice cat breeder needs to know. However, busy practitioners generally do not take the time to address the many possible scenarios that may develop. Rather, these situations are usually handled on an as-needed basis. Owners requesting more explicit instructions about gestation, labor, and delivery should be referred to the many excellent texts on cat care that are available to the lay public.

Estrus

The female cat comes into estrus many times each year. The estrus lasts about 2 to 3 weeks. If she is not bred, she will return to estrus in 1 to 2 weeks. This cycle will continue until she is bred or for several estrus cycles. The interestral period varies, depending on geographic and environmental factors (e.g., temperature and length of light).

Most female cats require 3 or 4 breedings within a 24-hour period for ovulation to occur. Once ovulation has occurred, the female cat will go out of heat within a day or two.

Gestation Period

The gestation period for cats ranges from 60 to 67 days and averages 65 days; most cats deliver between Days 63 and 65. The only way to accurately determine the stage of pregnancy is to count days from the time of breeding. It is mandatory to record the breeding date(s) so this is possible. The queen should be examined 3 weeks after breeding to determine pregnancy by palpation.

Difficult Delivery (Dystocia)

Although most cats deliver without need for assistance, problems do arise that require the attention of a veterinarian. Owners should be informed that professional assistance should be sought if any of the following occur:

1. Intense labor ≥20 min without a kitten being delivered.
2. Intense labor ≥10 min while a kitten or a fluid-filled bubble is visible in the birth canal.
3. The queen experiences acute depression or marked lethargy.
4. The body temperature exceeds 103°F (via a rectal thermometer).
5. Fresh blood discharges from the vagina for more than 5 minutes.

Dystocia may be managed with or without surgery. The condition of the queen, size of the litter, and size of the kittens are factors used in making that decision.

Instructions for Owners of a New Kitten

When a client presents a new kitten for its first examination and series of vaccinations, the veterinarian should be prepared to instruct the client in proper kitten care. This discussion should include information concerning vaccinations, intestinal parasites, diet and feeding, neutering/spaying, breeding, and declawing. Time should also be allowed to answer the client's questions.

Because these consultations can be quite lengthy, it is often helpful to provide the client with a written set of instructions. This material, which can be presented to the client at the beginning of the consultation, can serve as the basis of one's presentation. The contents of the document should be quickly scanned so that the client will know what information is presented. Only the important points should be covered; the details are best left for the client to read at home. Once the material has been reviewed briefly, the practitioner can then answer any questions the client may have. This approach is more efficient than a typical question-and-answer format, and it is more likely to impart the information needed.

Raising Orphaned Kittens

An orphaned kitten is one that is unable to eat from a bowl and whose mother has been lost or killed; alternatively, such a kitten may have been rejected by the mother. Many rejected kittens are sick and will not survive, even with intensive care. However, many orphaned kittens can be raised very successfully.

As with basic kitten care, a handout devoted to orphan care may be helpful to the client. It is important that the client understand the proper steps for feeding the kitten, keeping it warm, and stimulating the kitten's urination and defecation. The client must also have the proper equipment and food for feeding the kitten. If tube feeding is chosen, the technique should be demonstrated. Most clients are initially fearful of orogastric tube feeding, so a demonstration of its ease and safety is essential.

Early Kittenhood

For the first month of life kittens require a minimal amount of care because their mothers will feed and care for them. To some degree, the length of time before the eyes open varies with the breed. Siamese frequently have their eyes open within 5 to 7 days; other breeds average about 9 days. Some Persian kittens may not open their eyes for 11 days. If swelling or bulging is noted under the eyelids, open them gently, using a cotton ball dampened with warm water. If the swelling is due to infection, pus will exit the open eyelids and should be treated. If the eyes have not opened within 11 days of age, they should be opened as described.

Vaccinations

Kittens are provided some immunity to many feline diseases by their queen, whose antibodies cross the placenta and enter the kittens' circulation. Some antibodies also are provided in the queen's milk. These "maternal antibodies" protect the kittens against the diseases to which the queen is immune, which explains why it is desirable to booster the queen's vaccinations within a few months prior to breeding.

Although very protective, maternal antibodies last for only a few weeks, after which the kitten becomes susceptible to disease. The vaccination program should be started at about 6 to 8 weeks of age. Kittens should be vaccinated against feline parvovirus (enteritis), respiratory viruses, and rabies. If the kitten will be allowed to go outdoors or to be in contact with cats that go outdoors, leukemia and feline infectious peritonitis vaccine should also be considered.

Intestinal Parasites

Intestinal parasites are common in kittens. Symptoms include general poor condition, chronic soft or bloody stools, loss of appetite, loss of luster of the haircoat, and weight loss. Some parasites are transmitted from the queen to her kittens and others are carried by fleas. Some are transmitted through the stool of an infected cat.

A microscopic examination of the feces will reveal the eggs of most of these parasites. Generally this test should be performed at the time of the first vaccinations; however, it may be performed as early as 3 weeks of age if a parasite problem is suspected. Treatment is based on the type of parasites found, although some elect to treat all kittens because they know that some fecal tests can be falsely negative.

Deworming

Some broad-spectrum anthelminthics are suitable for use in kittens at 3 and 6 weeks of age. This approach has the advantage of treating parasites that are not consistently diagnosable with fecal examinations. Coccidia and giardia are not affected by these products, however, so kittens, particularly those with diarrhea, should have stools examined microscopically.

Normal Kitten Development

Knowing what is normal or abnormal for the newborn, 2-week-old, or 4-week-old kitten can be confusing. The reflexes that one expects to see in a 6-month-old kitten or in an adult cat may or may not apply to very young kittens. An excellent review of normal kitten development from birth to 8 weeks of age has recently been published.[1] The information included in this publication is summarized in the following list.

Birth Through Day 6

Closed eyelids

Poorly developed visual system[2]

Light-induced blink reflex present in most

Closed external ear canals

Heart rate: > 200 beats/min

Respiratory rate: 15–35 breaths/minute (through week 4)[3]

Considerable motor activity during sleep (through week 1)

Strong rooting response[4]

Righting response

Sucking reflex

Seal postural reflex

Panniculus reflex

Anogenital reflex

Tonic neck reflex

Magnus neck reflex

Front legs supportive of weight from 3–4 days of age

Scratch reflex from 2–4 days of age[4]

Nonvisual placing response in forelimbs beginning at 2–3 days of age

Days 7 Through 13

Light-induced blink reflex present up to 13 days of age

Eyelids separated at 5–14 days of age

Corneal and palpebral reflexes[4]

Mild corneal cloudiness for up to 2–3 weeks

Divergent strabismus until 8 weeks of age

Disappearance of seal postural reflex[4]

Days 14 Through 20

Open external ear canals at 6 to 14 days of age[4]

Development of thermoregulatory system

Hindlimbs supportive of weight

Ability to elevate body completely off table (range of 5–25 days of age)

Extensor postural thrust response[4]

Disappearance of rooting response[4]

Days 21 Through 27

Disappearance of light-induced blink reflex

Strong menace reflex

Pupillary light reflexes[4]

Change from blue-gray irides to adult coloration

Functional hearing[4]

Ability to sit; unsteady walking ensues 1–2 days later

Ability to retract claws[4]

Disappearance of tonic neck and magnus neck reflexes[5]

Adultlike vestibular nystagmus[6]

Disappearance of sucking reflex[7]

Days 28 Through 34

External ear canals large enough for otoscopic examination

Possible climbing ability (range of 23–40 days of age)

Air righting response (when dropped from a height)[8]

Hemiwalking (range of 3–6 weeks of age)

Disappearance of anogenital and scratch reflexes[4]

Onset of raking of soft dirt or litter in litter box

5 Weeks of Age

All postural reactions (range of 6–8 weeks)

Definition of Terms

Anogenital reflex: Controls elimination behavior up to 3 weeks of age at a time when the kitten cannot voluntarily urinate or defecate

Corneal reflex: Blinking of the eyelids in response to touching of the cornea

Extensor postural thrust: Extension of a kitten's hind limbs to touch a table or other hard surface in response to being held, with hands around its chest, in a vertical position

Magnus neck reflex: A reflex elicited by rotation of the kitten's neck to one side while the kitten is in dorsal recumbency; there is extension of the limbs on the side to which the head is turned, and flexion of the opposite limbs.

Menace reflex: A reflex elicited by first covering one of the kitten's eyes and then gesturing menacingly with a hand directed at the other eye. The kitten should flinch or withdraw.

Nonvisual placing response: Touching of the dorsum of the kitten's front paws to a hard surface or table while being suspended off the table by the rear legs

Palpebral reflex: Immediate closure of the kitten's eyelid in response to touching of the eyelid

Panniculus reflex: Twitching of the skin in response to cutaneous stimulation (such as pin pricking) along the thoracolumbar region

Righting response: The ability of the newborn kitten to move from lateral to sternal recumbency

Rooting response: Burrowing into warm objects

Scratch reflex: Scratching movements made with the ipsilateral hindlimb in response to repetitive scratching of the kitten's side

Seal postural reflex (Landau reflex): Extension of all four of a kitten's legs in response to being suspended by the ventral midline in a normal dorsoventral position

Slow blink reflex: Slow blinking of the eyelids in response to a light shone through kitten's closed eyelids

Sucking reflex: Turning of a kitten's head toward a stimulus, followed by sucking movements; this reflex is strongest immediately after awakening.

Tonic neck reflex: Extension of the forelimbs and simultaneous flexion of the hindlimbs in response to dorsal extension of the neck. This response is reversed when the neck is flexed.

REFERENCES

1. Hoskins JD. Clinical Evaluation of the Kitten: From Birth to Eight Weeks of Age. Compend Contin Ed Pract Vet 1990;12:1215.
2. Thorn F, Gollender M, Erikson P. The development of the kitten's visual optics. Vision Res 1976;16:1145.
3. Finley JP, Kelly C. Heart rate and respiratory patterns in mild hypoxia in unanesthetized newborn mammals. Can J Physiol Pharmacol 1986;64:122.
4. Beaver BV. Veterinary Aspects of Feline Behavior. St. Louis: CV Mosby Co, 1980:1.
5. Kornegay JN. The nervous system. In: Hoskins JD, ed. Veterinary Pediatrics: Dogs and Cats from Birth to Six Months. Philadelphia: WB Saunders Co, 1990:95.
6. Fish MW, Windle WF. The effect of rotary stimulation on the movements of the head and eyes in newborn and young kittens. J Comp Neurol 1932;54:103.
7. Kovach JK, Kling A. Mechanisms of neonate sucking behavior in the kitten. Anim Behav 1967;15:91.
8. Warkentin J, Carmichael L. A study of the development of the air-righting reflex in cats and rabbits. J Genet Psychol 1939;55:67.

CHAPTER 5

◇ ◇ ◇

Anorexia and Force Feeding

Gary D. Norsworthy

Anorexia is a component of many feline diseases. Because it is easily observed by owners, it is often the reason the sick cat is presented for veterinary care. As the causes of anorexia are so diverse[1] (Table 5–1), the practitioner is often presented with a diagnostic dilemma that may require several days to resolve. If anorexia continues during the diagnostic period, a number of secondary disorders may begin, some of which may be more life-threatening than the primary cause of anorexia. These include glycogen depletion, decreased plasma fibronectin levels, decreased immune function, decreased strength and muscle mass, decreased albumin levels, delayed healing, hepatic and gastrointestinal involution, idiopathic hepatic lipidosis (IHL), and "nitrogen death."[2] Therefore, it is important for the practitioner to simultaneously treat the anorexia and pursue diagnosis and treatment of the underlying primary disease.

Chemotherapeutic Methods

Certain drugs may have a direct stimulatory effect on the appetite and can be used to great advantage in cases of anorexia of short duration. Unfortunately, all of these drugs are inconsistent in their effect; they may work well in some cats, but not at all in others. Despite this, their use is warranted because of the profound effects that one or more of these drugs may have in certain cats. It should be emphasized that trial and error is the only method available for testing the effects of these drugs on appetite in any given cat. Table 5–2 lists some drugs that the author has found to be effective in selected anorectic cats.[3] However, their use should not delay the practitioner from aggressively pursuing a diagnosis for the cause of anorexia.

Physical Methods

Because chemical appetite stimulants are inconsistently effective, the practitioner must be prepared with alternative modes of treatment. Food can be administered successfully to a nonvomiting, anorectic cat if the correct food is chosen to meet the cat's nutritional needs and if the correct mode of administration is used.

Nutritional Needs

In order to formulate a proper diet for the anorectic cat, one must consider the higher caloric intake required by the ill, stressed cat compared to that suitable for a healthy, nonstressed cat. The basal energy requirement (BER) is increased 25% in cats with acute medical illnesses without sepsis, 50% in those with diseases requiring major surgery, and 75% in those with acute diseases or injuries involving serious infection or sepsis.[2] On average, an ill, hospitalized 9-lb cat has a BER of approximately 250 to 300 kcal per 24 hours.

The first objective of force feeding, then, is to ensure adequate energy intake. The second objective is to choose a diet with a sufficiently high caloric density so that two (or possibly three) daily feedings can be used to meet the cat's energy needs without causing vomiting. Finally, the third objective is to use a delivery system that is tolerated by the cat and that can be used rapidly by the busy practitioner or by the owner.

Selection of Diet

The author's diet of choice for anorectic cats consists of Prescription Diet Feline p/d (Hill's Pet Products, Topeka, KS), water, and Wesson Oil (Beatrice/Hunt-Wesson, Inc., Fullerton, CA). A can of Feline p/d contains 675 kcal. If a sick cat were to consume half a can in 24 hours, its energy requirements would be met. However, water must be added to liquefy the diet so that it will pass through a 16- to 18-French feeding tube. Adding enough water to liquefy this diet results in a caloric density of about 1 kcal/mL. Thus, a 9-lb cat would need about 250–300 mL of the mixture every 24 hours. Because only about 100 mL of food or fluid can be placed in a 9-lb cat's stomach without causing vomiting, three feedings at 6–8 hr intervals would be needed per day. This is not a workable schedule for the average practitioner. To solve this problem, the food's caloric density can be increased by adding vegetable oil to the Feline p/d and water mixture. Wesson Oil has a caloric density of 9.4 kcal/mL. By adding a small amount to the Feline p/d and water mixture, the caloric density can be raised to 1.35 kcal/mL,

Table 5–1. Causes of Anorexia in Cats[1]

Primary Anorexia
Neurologic causes
Cerebral edema
Intracranial pain
Hypothalamic neoplasia, infection, or trauma
Psychological causes
Diet with objectionable taste, odor, or texture
Stress
Altered routine or environment
Loss of smell
Secondary Anorexia
Pain from any source
Abdominal organ disorders
Abdominal enlargement or serosal distention
Inflammation
Neoplasia
Toxic agents
Exogenous drugs or poisons
Endogenous metabolic wastes, endotoxins, or pyrogens
Endocrine conditions
Adrenal insufficiency
Hypercalcemia
Neoplasia (any site)
Infectious diseases
Miscellaneous causes
Cardiac failure, motion sickness, high ambient temperatures, gastritis (nausea), intestinal cramping
Pseudoanorexia
Oral cavity disorders
Dental disease, foreign bodies, stomatitis
Paralysis of the hypoglossal nerve or muscles of mastication
Fractures or luxations of the mandible or maxilla
Retrobulbar abscess or neoplasia
Blindness
Esophagitis

Adapted, with permission, from Lorenz MD. Disturbances of Food Intake: Anorexia and Polyphagia. In Lorenz MD, Cornelius LM, eds. Small Animal Medical Diagnosis. Philadelphia: JB Lippincott, 1987:27.

while still maintaining a well-balanced diet for the cat. The author recommends the following:

PWW* Diet = 1 15-oz can of Feline p/d®
+
10 oz. of water
+
2 oz of Wesson Oil

The mixture is blenderized at the fastest (i.e., liquefy) setting so that it will pass through a 16- to 18-French feeding tube. Twice-daily administration of 100 mL of this mixture is sufficient to meet the energy requirements of a 9-lb, stressed cat. Unused portions can be stored in a refrigerator for several days. It should be warmed to body temperature in a microwave oven before each use.

*PWW = Feline p/d, water, and Wesson Oil

Deficiencies of the PWW Diet

The PWW diet has two disadvantages. First, it is somewhat low in protein. The stressed 9-lb cat needs about 25 g of protein per day; the PWW mixture supplies only about 19 g. If the cat requires special feeding for 2 weeks or less, this deficiency is usually not significant. However, if the anorectic cat must be fed this mixture for longer than 2 weeks, protein supplementation will be required. This can be accomplished by adding 5½ packed tablespoons of Casec Powder (Mead Johnson Nutritionals, Evansville, IN), a supplement that is 88% protein, to the PWW formula, thereby boosting the daily protein level to 25 g. Other protein supplements are available in pharmacies and health food stores. As long as the quantity of protein in these supplements is comparable to that of Casec, they can be substituted at an equal volume.

Second, the PWW diet is deficient in terms of fluid volume. If an anorectic cat is not drinking on its own, about 90 mL of fluid should be administered per day, either by stomach tube, intravenously (IV), or subcutaneously (SC).

Administration Methods

Various methods have been used to administer blenderized diets to anorectic cats. The PWW diet will easily pass through a 16 French or larger feeding tube. If a smaller tube is used, the PWW diet can be strained with a kitchen strainer without affecting the diet's nutritional value.[4] The strained diet will pass through an 8 French or larger feeding tube or a standard syringe. Feeding the entire prescribed amount the first day may result in vomiting owing to a reduced gastric capacity or diarrhea secondary to decreased intestinal function. Therefore, the following schedule is recommended:

Day 1. Feed ⅓ of the total amount required

Day 2. Feed ⅔ of the total amount required

Day 3. Administer a full feeding

Orogastric Tube Feeding

Feeding by orogastric tube is the author's most frequent approach to the *hospitalized* anorectic cat. A 16- or 18-French feeding tube can be used comfortably in most 9-lb cats. The author's preference is an 18-French 16-inch Feeding Tube and Urethral Catheter (Monoject, Division of Sherwood Medical, St. Louis, MO). In order to prevent obstructions of the tube, the side ports in the distal end of the tube should be enlarged to about double their normal size.

The 60-cc Monoject Catheter-Tipped Syringe (Monoject, Division of Sherwood Medical, St. Louis, MO) and the Feline Mouth Speculum (Jorgensen Laboratories, Inc., Loveland, CO) complete the equipment requirements. Two persons are needed for feeding most cats. One person restrains the cat by holding both front legs in one hand and both rear legs in the other. The second person holds the cat's head in one hand and inserts the mouth speculum with the other. When the speculum is in place, the tube is inserted and the food is passed through it by syringe (Fig. 5–1). It should not be administered so rapidly that vomiting is induced. The

Table 5–2. Appetite-stimulating Drugs*

Drug	Recommended Dose	How Supplied
Diazepam (Valium)†	1–2 mg orally or 0.5 mg IV	2-mg tablets or 5 mg/mL injectable solution
Oxazepam (Serax)†	0.3–0.4 mg/kg orally	15-mg 5-sided tablets
Flurazepam (Dalmane)†	0.1–0.2 mg/kg orally	15-mg capsules
Chlordiazepoxide (Librium)†	1.25–2.5 mg orally	5-mg capsules
Cyanocobalamin (Vitamin B_{12} Injectable)	1,000 μg SC	1,000-μg/mL injectable solution
Boldenone undecylenate (Equipoise)	5 mg IM or SC	50 mg/mL injectable solution

*None of these drugs are consistently effective. Only trial-and-error usage will determine whether a particular drug will be effective in any given cat.

†If sedation occurs, reduce the dosage.

Adapted, with permission, from Norsworthy GD. Providing nutritional support for anorectic cats. Vet Med 1991;86:589.

operator is encouraged to hold the syringe-tube junction to prevent the tube from dislodging.

The only serious complication—passage of the food into the lungs, which is always fatal—occurs among cats that aggressively fight passage of the tube. Therefore, if a cat arduously resists this procedure, 1 to 2 mg of diazepam should be administered intramuscularly (IM) or SC. This may stimulate the cat's appetite so that eating occurs, or it may sedate the cat adequately so that the orogastric tube may then be passed. If neither occurs, do not continue to force the cat to swallow the tube; otherwise, disastrous results may follow.

A 16- or 18-French feeding tube is not appropriate for small cats or kittens. Rather, an 8- or 12-French feeding tube should be used for these patients. The PWW diet will pass through these tubes if the food is strained and if the distal end of the tube is removed.

After the cat has been fed, the mouth speculum and feeding tube should be soaked in a cold sterilization solution. This is especially important after use in cats with respiratory or feline leukemia virus (FeLV) infections, but is also recommended after use in other cats, as well, as so many anorectic cats are infected with contagious microorganisms.

The feeding syringe is designed to be disposable, but it can be used for multiple feedings. With repeated use, the rubber part of the plunger will swell, ultimately making it unusable. However, if the rubber is first lubricated with a water-soluble lubricant or some of the liquefied food prior to use, it will continue to perform adequately for several weeks or months.

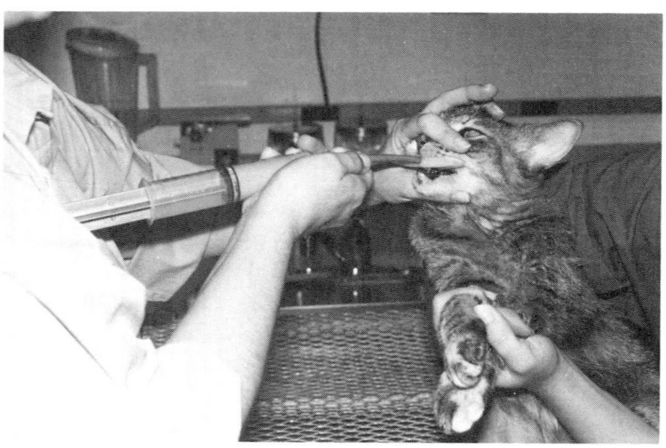

Figure 5–1. **Orogastric tube feeding generally requires two persons—one to restrain the cat, holding its front legs in one hand and its rear legs in the other; and the other to place the mouth speculum, restrain the head, insert the tube, and administer the food.**

Syringe Feeding

For home feedings, the PWW diet can be strained through a kitchen strainer and then administered through a standard syringe. This method requires a cooperative patient and a dedicated owner. If a 12-cc syringe is used to feed a 9-lb cat, about 17 syringefulls must be administered within 24 hours. Daily feedings should be divided into at least 2 feeding sessions.

Although syringe feeding is a very laborious method of feeding an anorectic cat, it may be the method of choice in some situations, especially if the cat is one that does poorly away from home or if the owner's financial resources prohibit the expense of hospitalization.

Surgically Implanted Feeding Tubes

Various surgical techniques have been used to implant feeding tubes in anorectic cats. It is beyond the scope of this chapter to describe all of these. Some require specialized equipment for placement; some do not permit the use of foods as thick as the strained PWW diet. Each has advantages and disadvantages.

The Esophagostomy Tube. The author's preferred technique is the esophagostomy tube. No specialized equipment is needed for placement, a very brief period of anesthesia is needed, and the tube is generally well tolerated by the patient.[5] This method is appropriate for long-term home feeding. Its placement is described in Chapter 55.

The esophagostomy tube allows for the administration of PWW diet—strained with a kitchen strainer—as often as necessary to meet the cat's nutritional requirements. The tube does not interfere with the cat's ability to swallow, so when the cat's appetite returns, it will commence eating.

The Pharyngostomy Tube. Another approach to feeding is the placement of a pharyngostomy tube, which is inserted through the skin of the neck, through the pharynx, and then into the esophagus. This procedure requires no specialized equipment for placement and requires only a few minutes of anesthesia. Although pharyngostomy tubes have been used extensively for many years, they have two disadvantages as compared to esophagostomy tubes. If they are not properly placed, the hyoid apparatus may be permanently damaged. Also, when such a tube is in place, swallowing becomes difficult in some cats, making it difficult or impossible to determine when the cat's appetite has returned.

The Nasogastric Tube. The nasogastric (or nasoesophageal) tube is a 3.5- to 5-French tube that is passed through the nasal meatus into the stomach (or esophagus). It is well tolerated by some cats, but not by others. Some cats will tolerate it only if an Elizabethan collar is worn. The main disadvantage of this tube is its diameter. Blenderized diets will not pass through tubes this small, necessitating the use of expensive liquid diets.

The Gastrostomy Tube. The gastrostomy tube passes through the skin and abdominal wall directly into the stomach. It is held in place by an inflated balloon around the distal end of the catheter. It is positioned either by laparotomy and gastrotomy or by endoscopy. Both methods require general anesthesia.

The gastrostomy tube is generally well tolerated by the cat and has a diameter that is sufficiently large to permit use of blenderized foods. Moreover, its removal does not require further surgery.

One disadvantage of the gastrotomy tube is the need for major surgery (laparotomy and gastrostomy) for placement or for specialized equipment (endoscope) not found in most veterinary practices. Certain cats, such as those with IHL, are generally not good candidates for major surgery. Another disadvantage is the likelihood of bacterial peritonitis should the tube's insertion point into the stomach not seal properly or should the cat dislodge the tube. In one study,[6] 2 of 11 (18%) cats with a gastrostomy tube died as a result of complications related to the tube. Its use should be reserved for practitioners who use it frequently.

Conclusion

Anorexia in the cat is a common condition which, left untreated, can transform a curable, minor disease into a major illness. Aggressive treatment of affected cats, either with the aid of appetite-stimulating drugs or with various force-feeding methods, can hasten their recovery and may even be life-saving.

REFERENCES

1. Lorenz MD. Disturbances of Food Intake: Anorexia and Polyphagia. In: Lorenz MD, Cornelius LM, eds. Small Animal Medical Diagnosis. Philadelphia: JB Lippincott, 1987:27.
2. Crowe D. Understanding the nutritional needs of critically ill or injured patients. Vet Med 1988; 83:1242.
3. Norsworthy, GD. Providing nutritional support for anorectic cats. Vet Med 1991; 86:589.
4. Lewis L, Morris ML, Hand MS. Anorexia, Inanition, and Critical Care Nutrition. In: Lewis L, Morris ML, Hand MS, eds. Small Animal Clinical Nutrition III, 3rd ed. Topeka, KS: Mark Morris Associates, 1987:5.
5. Crowe DT. Nutritional Support for the Hospitalized Patient: An Introduction to Tube Feeding. Compend Contin Ed Pract Vet 1990; 12:1711.
6. Jacobs G, Cornelius L, Allen S, Greene C. Treatment of idiopathic hepatic lipidosis in cats: 11 cases (1986–1987). J Am Vet Med Assoc 1989; 195:635.

CHAPTER 6

◇ ◇ ◇

Administration of Oral Medications

Gary D. Norsworthy

Surveys of human patients taking oral medications have consistently shown that less than 50% do so exactly as directed, even if a life-threatening disease exists.[1] If these same people are asked to administer oral medication to a patient who is uncooperative, we can expect the compliance level to be even less. Moreover, if medications are not administered in a timely fashion, the therapeutic results are jeopardized.

It is important for the veterinarian to prescribe the correct medication, the correct dose, and the correct dosage interval. However, it must be realized that the average cat owner has no concept of how to get the medication into the cat's stomach. One of the most effective means of increasing owner compliance is to issue specific instructions.[2] Conversely, if specific instructions are not given to the client, results will be poor. The following suggestions have proven helpful to the author. Note that some of these approaches differ considerably from those that are appropriate for dogs.

Forms of Medication and Administration Methods

The following are guidelines for administering oral medications. These recommendations may be presented to cat owners in order to increase compliance with the prescribed medication regimen.

Liquid Medications

Many cats will swallow liquid medications more readily than tablets or capsules. However, this is not true of all cats, so a blanket recommendation for liquids is not appropriate. When liquid medications are prescribed, the following guidelines may be helpful:

- The liquid prescribed must have a taste that is desirable (or at least not objectionable) to the cat. Just because a taste is desirable to humans does not make it desirable to the cat. Even though most humans like cherry-flavored medications, most cats do not because they do not typically like sweet tastes.
- The liquid must be in a concentration that allows a dosage of no more than 2 mL at a time. This can be a problem when prescribing liquid medications formulated for children.
- Liquids are especially useful for cats or kittens weighing less than 5 lb, as it is generally easier to dose medications with accuracy in this weight range.
- Liquids are useful when a cat is being force-fed by the syringe method or via an esophagostomy tube (See Chapter 5). The medication can generally be added to the food without detection by the cat.

Nonliquid Medications

Several strategies may be used to facilitate the administration of nonliquid medications. Some of the elements to consider are as follows.

Pill Size. Because of the small size of a cat's mouth, any pill that is prescribed must be of a size that permits it to be swallowed without difficulty. Some common antibiotics that meet this small size requirement include Amoxi-Tabs and Clavamox, Cefa-Tabs, and Baytril.

Tablets versus Capsules. As a rule, capsules are larger than tablets of an equivalent drug dose. They also have a long axis, which makes them more difficult to swallow than tablets. Therefore, when given the choice, the tablet form of a drug is preferred over a capsule.

Hiding Medications in Food ("Trojan Horse" Method). The hiding of medications in food is a common and generally successful strategy for medication administration in dogs. However, the relative size or quantity of tablets and liquids makes this technique less successful in cats. Also, cats seem to be more sensitive to unfamiliar tastes than dogs, which also contributes to the failure of this method. In order to improve the chances of success of this method, the following strategy may be helpful:

- Use a very small tablet, if available.
- Place the small tablet in a ball of food measuring approximately 0.5 cubic inches.
- Select a food with a strong aroma, such as fish or liver.

- Commercial cat treats, such as Bonkers (Martha White Foods, Nashville, TN) also seem to work well.
- Three balls of food or three cat treats should be given to the cat before regular feeding (i.e., when the cat is hungry). Only one of the three should contain the tablet. The tablet-laden ball of food or treat should be given third, after the cat has begun to believe that these "goodies" have no strings attached.

Masking the Taste of and Lubricating Tablets or Capsules. Capsules become sticky when the least amount of moisture touches them, making them difficult to swallow. Moreover, tablets that are not coated or that have been broken in half often impart an objectionable taste to the cat. To solve these problems, the capsule or broken surface of the tablet should be covered with a substance that provides lubrication and masks the taste of the medication. Such a substance should be one that is commonly available to owners, such as butter or margarine.

Administering a Tablet or Capsule. The following are guidelines for administering tablets or capsules to a cat. If the medication is to be given at home as well, the client should be allowed to participate fully in the pilling process.

- Place the cat on a countertop, a table, or a bar stool without a back. The latter option is a powerful distraction to the cat, as it usually becomes so concerned about falling off the small stool top that minimal attention is paid to the pilling process (Fig. 6–1). Do not place the cat on the floor or in someone's lap, as the cat considers these areas to be personal territory and thus will tend to struggle more.
- Have an assistant stand behind the cat, placing his or her forearms parallel and next to the cat's long axis. The cat is thus cradled between the forearms in such a fashion that dorsal recumbency must be retained. The assistant then grasps the cat's front legs to prevent the cat from clawing the person administering the tablet or capsule.
- Instruct the client to grasp the cat's head firmly, using the following grip (for the right-handed person):

  The little finger of the left hand is placed behind the cat's right ear and the ring finger is placed behind the cat's left ear (Figure 6–2*A*).

  The first finger and thumb of the same hand are placed under the ridge of bone below the cat's left and right eyes, respectively. This puts the palm of the hand above the cat's head, but not touching it (Fig. 6–2*B*).

  The client then raises the cat's head so that the nose is at a 45° angle to the horizon; the cat's mouth will open slightly (see Fig. 6–2*B*). The owner should be shown the "pill slot" on the caudal aspect of the tongue (Fig. 6–2*C*).
- The client then administers the tablet or capsule in the following manner:

  The client holds the tablet or capsule in the right hand between the first finger and the thumb.

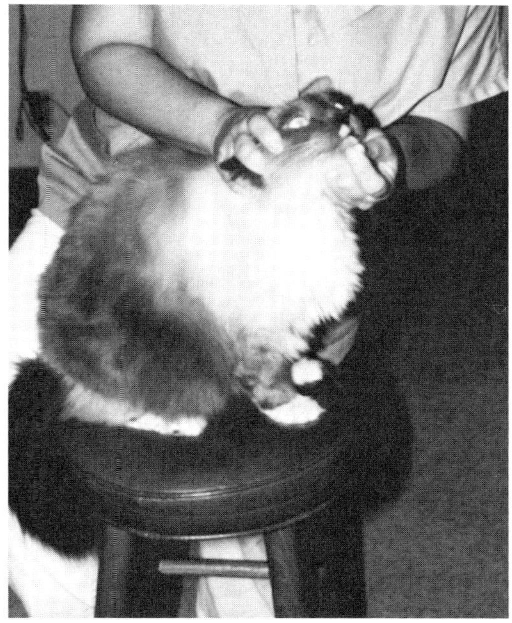

Figure 6–1. **Administering oral medication can be facilitated by placing the cat on a stool without a back. The cat will be distracted by the small surface and will be less intent on resisting the pill.**

  Using the right ring finger, the client then opens the cat's mouth by pushing downward on the lower incisor teeth.

  The tablet or capsule is then dropped into the so-called "pill slot" (Fig. 6–2*D*).

  The lower jaw is released but the head is not.

  The head is held at a 45° angle to the table and the mandible is gently pushed upward until the cat swallows. During swallowing, the cat will extend its tongue from the mouth so the client will know when the cat's head may safely be released (Fig. 6–2*E*). Stroking the cat's throat will not facilitate swallowing and so should be avoided.
- If the cat is reluctant to swallow the pill, 1 to 2 mL of water may be flushed into the cat's mouth using a 3-cc syringe. This forces the cat to swallow and also serves to lubricate the pill.
- Some cats are prone to excessive salivation, especially if the pill has an objectionable taste or if the patient is a Siamese or Siamese crossbreed. This may also be a conditioned reflex in some cats that is manifested when they hear the rattle of the pills in the pill vial. As it is very difficult to administer a pill to a salivating cat, the best approach is to allow the cat to rest for 10 to 30 minutes and to try again.
- As an alternative to this method, pilling devices are sold commercially. These are miniature forms of the balling guns that are used on cattle and horses. They work well in some cats, but not so well in others. Likewise, some

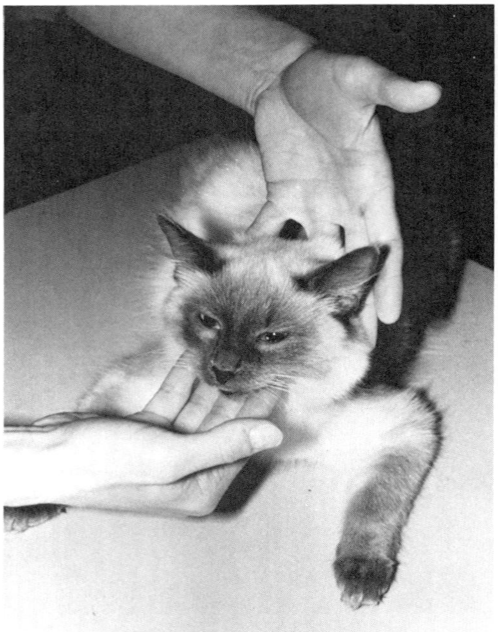

A

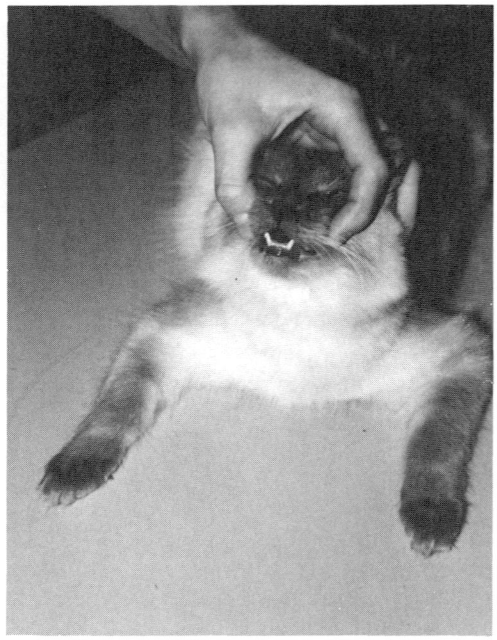

B

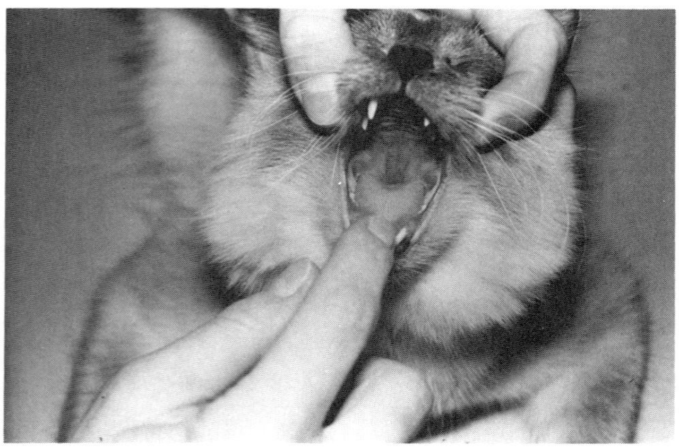

C

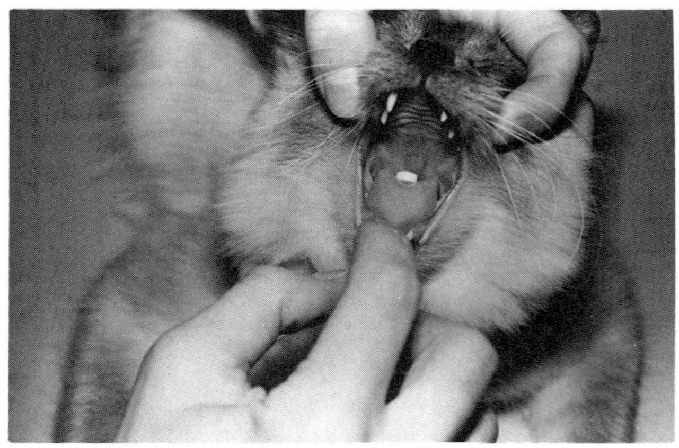

D

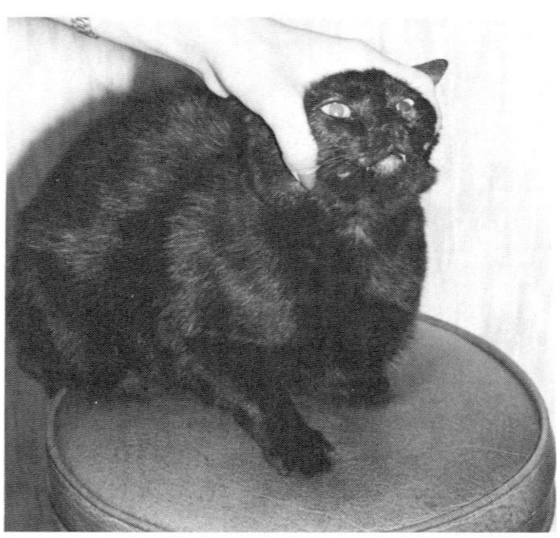

E

Figure 6–2. Holding the cat's head properly greatly facilitates the administration of a capsule or tablet. (*A*) For a right-handed person, the 4th and 5th fingers of the left hand are placed behind the cat's ears at the base of the skull. (*B*) The index finger and the thumb are then placed below the cat's eyes. (*C*) The "pill slot" in the center and caudal aspect of the cat's tongue will be visible. (*D*) The tablet or capsule is dropped into the "pill slot," as far back into the mouth as possible. (*E*) The cat will extend its tongue when swallowing occurs. The nose should be elevated by gently pushing up on the mandible until this occurs or the cat will be able to expel the pill from the mouth.

owners have good success with them and others find them awkward to use.

Dissolving Medications in Liquids

When direct administration of pills or the hiding of medications in food is not successful, one may try dissolving the medication in a liquid. This method is also useful if a tablet or capsule that was formulated for humans is used and the quantity prescribed makes pill division inaccurate.

- Crush the tablet, or part thereof, into a powder. If the tablet is enteric-coated, the enteric coating must be removed because it will usually not dissolve in the solvent that is used.
- Pour the crushed tablet or capsule's contents into a tasty liquid, such as Vitamino 4× (TechAmerica Veterinary Products, Kansas City, MO) after determining the correct concentration and dosing quantity.*
- Administer the medication with a dropper or syringe directly into the cat's mouth, or mix it into the cat's food.

REFERENCES

1. Hayes RB, Taylor DW, Sackett DL, eds. Compliance in Health Care. Baltimore: Johns Hopkins University Press, 1979:25.
2. Straw B. What veterinarians should know about client compliance. Topics Vet Med 1991;2(2):14.

*Adequate testing has not been performed to determine whether the efficacy of various drugs is altered when mixed with liquids, such as Vitamino 4×. If a lack of response or unusual side effects occur, another means of administering the drug should be used.

CHAPTER 7

◇ ◇ ◇

Drug Peculiarities

Gary D. Norsworthy

Franz Inglefinger, the late and widely respected editor of the *New England Journal of Medicine,* stated:

> Eighty-five percent of all people who bring complaints and symptoms to their physicians are suffering from self-limiting disorders. That is, more than four times out of five, what ails you is well within the reach of the body's own healing mechanisms.

If this observation is extrapolated to the feline patient, it is clear that caution must be exercised in treating the cat so as not to compromise its immune system or inadvertently induce another disease process, especially one that is not self-limiting, through the choice of treatment modalities. Rather, the clinician should strive to help the 15% of patients with non–self-limiting disorders while not hurting the 85% that will recover regardless of whether they receive medical care. It should also be remembered that, because of the cat's unique ability (or inability) to metabolize some of the common drugs that are used, drug toxicity is more prevalent in the cat than in the dog.

The goal of drug metabolism is to convert lipid-soluble drugs to a water-soluble form that can be excreted via the urinary system. This process is generally described as consisting of two phases.[1] Phase I results in the breakdown of the drug. Unfortunately, this breakdown may result in the production of toxic metabolites. In other words, the drug may not be toxic, but its breakdown products may be. Phase II consists of the conjugation process. The liver is responsible for conjugating the drug's metabolites to large molecules that may be removed from the body. Glucuronide and glutathione are integral agents in this process. Unfortunately, the cat is deficient in stores of glucuronyltransferase, the enzyme necessary for glucuronide to process the metabolites. Moreover, cats store only minimal amounts of glutathione. Because these two agents are present in limited quantities, the excretion of toxic metabolites is prolonged, which permits them to accumulate in the body. For example, the cat's excretion rate of aspirin is approximately 3 days.[2] Because the safe dosage interval for aspirin in the cat is 3–4 days, it is given twice weekly.

The reader is referred to Appendices A through C in this text for a listing of drugs suitable for the cat, with appropriate dosages given for specific uses. In addition, the following sections present some general guidelines for drug selection, dosage, and administration.

Drugs to Be Avoided in the Feline Patient

Some drugs should not be used in treating cats, including the following:

Acetaminophen. This is an over-the-counter (OTC) drug that is available in tablet or oral liquid form. One 325-mg tablet can be fatal to an adult cat. Acetaminophen causes methemoglobinemia[3] (see Chapter 42).

Benzocaine. This is a prescription drug available as a topical spray (Cetacaine). It has been used to anesthetize the larynx to aid intubation and in the urethra to aid catheterization of cats with a urethral obstruction. If administered during inspiration, it may be inadvertently sprayed into the trachea, which results in absorption by the lungs. Moreover, there is concern that, when used in cats with a urethral obstruction, benzocaine may be absorbed from the bladder mucosa owing to the highly inflamed state of the bladder at that time.[4] Benzocaine is also available as an OTC topical cream with a trade name of Lanacaine. If this is applied to ulcerated skin, it is absorbed readily.[5] Benzocaine causes methemoglobinemia (see Chapter 42).

Benzyl Alcohol. This preservative has been used in lactated Ringer's solution and is approved for use in large animals. However, when administered to cats, it results in ataxia, hyperesthesia, muscle fasciculations, and death. This preservative is no longer found in fluids available today, but it may still be present in older, stored fluids.[6]

Chlorinated Hydrocarbons. A number of drugs are included in the category of chlorinated hydrocarbons (lindane, chlordane, etc.). All are extremely toxic to the cat when applied as a parasiticidal dip[7] (see Chapter 62).

Hexachlorophene. This antibacterial soap (pHiso-Hex) can cause irreversible brain damage if it is absorbed through the skin. It is particularly dangerous if used in its undiluted form on the skin of kittens.[8]

Methylene Blue. This drug is often a component of combination drugs used to treat urinary infections. In the past, it was used rather extensively in treating the symptoms of the feline urologic syndrome (FUS), generally without toxic effects. However, some cats have been known to develop severe methemoglobinemia after just a few doses of this substance. Because its efficacy has not been confirmed, and because it is impossible to predict which cats will suffer severe toxic effects, it is not recommended for use in the cat[9] (see Chapter 42).

Phenazopyridine. This drug is combined with sulfa drugs (Azo Gantrisin) and is commonly used in humans to treat urinary tract infections. Cat owners may have it in their home medicine cabinet. It causes methemoglobinemia in cats[10] (see Chapter 42).

Phenytoin. This drug, marketed as Dilantin, is commonly used as an anticonvulsant in the dog. Its excretion in the cat may take as long as 4–5 days. Moreover, its anticonvulsant activity is far less than that of phenobarbital in most cases. Therefore, it is not efficacious at safe intervals and is not safe at efficacious intervals.[11]

Phosphate Enemas. These products, including Fleet Enema, are sold as OTC preparations. When used in cats with severe constipation, such as in those with megacolon, such products may be retained in the colon long enough to allow absorption of excessive quantities of the phosphate ion. This leads to potentially fatal hyperphosphatemia, hypocalcemia, and hypernatremia.[12]

Drugs to Be Used with Certain Restrictions in the Feline Patient

The following drugs may safely be used in the treatment of cats provided certain restrictions are observed:

Aspirin. This is an OTC drug that is often given to cats by their owners to relieve pain or fever. Its plasma half-life is 9 hours in the dog, but 38 hours in the cat.[13,14] Therefore, it should only be given to cats every 3–4 days. A dose of 1.25 gr (¼ of a regular-strength adult aspirin, or one baby aspirin) is appropriate for relief of fever or pain in a 10-lb cat. However, the client must be warned not to repeat the dose within 3 days. The same dose is used as an anticoagulant in cats with cardiomyopathy.[15]

Chloramphenicol. High doses of this antibiotic (i.e., 250 mg or more b.i.d.) can cause marked appetite depression, to the point of anorexia, as well as a nonregenerative anemia.[16] However, it is generally safe to use at a dosage of 50 to 100 mg b.i.d. (5–10 mg/lb).

Griseofulvin. Marketed as Fulvicin, this drug has been used for many years in treating dermatophytosis in the cat. Pancytopenia has been associated with its use in some cats,[17] and cerebellar damage has been reported in one kitten receiving the drug.[18] However, these occurrences are considered to be idiosyncratic and uncommon. Severe neutropenia has been reported in 6 of 7 cats infected with feline immunodeficiency virus (FIV) that were treated with griseofulvin.[19] Because of these findings, one should be alert to the hematologic and neurologic status of any cat receiving griseofulvin. Despite these potential drawbacks, it is still the drug of choice for dermatophytosis in cats except for those with an FIV (see Chapter 56).

Lidocaine. This drug is available as an injectable agent. It can be toxic to the cat when given intravenously (IV) at standard canine doses. It should be used to treat life-threatening cardiac arrhythmias only after treatment with digoxin and propranolol has failed. When administered subcutaneously, as for local anesthesia, it is considered to be safe. It is also available as a topical spray and is safe to use on a cat's larynx to facilitate intubation.[20]

Megestrol Acetate. Marketed as Ovaban and Megace, this drug is used to treat a variety of ailments in the cat. It has profound anti-inflammatory and antiemetic effects. However, it may cause behavioral changes, polyphagia, weight gain, polydipsia, polyuria, mammary gland hyperplasia or carcinoma, pyometra, or diabetes mellitus.[21] For an extensive discussion of this drug, see the section entitled "Clinical Use of Megestrol Acetate" later in this chapter.

Nonsteroidal Anti-inflammatory agents. As in humans and dogs, these drugs may cause gastrointestinal ulceration to the point of perforation. Except for aspirin, the only drug in this category that the author uses is flumixin meglumine (Banamine), as it is often effective in the treatment of cats with lumbar spondylosis and arthritis.

Pepto-Bismol. This OTC preparation is commonly used for diarrhea. It is an excellent intestinal protectant and can be very efficacious. However, it contains salicylates (i.e., aspirin) and can be toxic if the dose is excessive. For a 10-lb cat, a safe dose of regular-strength Pepto-Bismol would be 1 tablespoon (15 mL) or less per 24 hours.[22] (One tablespoon is equivalent to 3/4 of a Pepto-Bismol tablet.)

Smooth Muscle Relaxants. Antispasmodic drugs used for diarrhea, such as Lomotil, or for urethral spasm may result in bizarre behavior in some cats. Behavioral signs include pawing at the mouth, hiding in dark places, and withdrawal. Moreover, in some cats, excretion of this drug is prolonged. Because these drugs dilate the pupils, their duration of action can be monitored by the owner. If the pupils are dilated when another dose is scheduled, the drug should not be administered. It should only be resumed when the pupils are normally responsive to light. (The author frequently uses Lomotil, at a dosage of ½ tablet (0.008 mg) b.i.d., for a 10-lb cat.)

Tetracycline. This antibiotic is particularly good for treating hemobartonellosis and some respiratory viruses. It has been used in the past for mixed or unknown infections. However, many antibiotics are now available that surpass it in efficacy. This drug commonly causes a marked fever of up to 105°F. Less commonly, it may cause depression, vomiting, and/or diarrhea. In the author's opinion, its only indication in the cat is for treatment of hemobartonellosis.

Thiacetarsamide. Marketed as Caparsolate, this drug is used to treat heartworms. At a dosage of 1 mg/lb b.i.d. for 2 consecutive days (for a total of 4 doses), it has been shown to have a 21% mortality rate in healthy cats owing to an acute, fulminating respiratory distress syndrome (RDS).[23] However, other clinicians have used it in cats without similar toxic results[24] (see Chapter 41). This drug has also been used to treat hemobartonellosis at a dosage of 0.5 mg/lb s.i.d. IV for 2 doses 48 hours apart. Used at this dosage, extensive trials of this drug have not demonstrated problems with toxicity[25] (see Chapter 43).

Thiamylal sodium. Manufactured under the trade name of Biotal, this ultra–short-acting barbiturate is commonly used for anesthetic induction or for brief surgical procedures. Animals develop a decreased tolerance to this agent after multiple exposures. If this occurs, the dosage must be reduced by as much as 50% to prevent adverse cardiac and respiratory effects.

Urinary acidifiers. As a cat's urine will become alkaline following each meal (*postprandial alkaline tide*), an acidifier must be given with each meal if it is to be effective. Because cats generally prefer to eat very small amounts of food 12 to 20 times per day, often taking only one mouthful at a time, acidification of the urine is best accomplished by adding an acidifier to the food. As many commercial cat foods are now formulated in this fashion, there are few indications for the use of urinary acidifers (one being the cat that refuses to eat an acidified cat food). Ammonium chloride and dl-methionine are the only such products with proven efficacy that are currently on the market. Both are available in a chewable fashion—Methioform and UroEze. The clinician should be aware that methionine has been shown to produce a Heinz body hemolytic anemia if administered at a dose of 250 mg/lb or more.[26]

Clinical Use of Megestrol Acetate

Megestrol acetate is marketed as a veterinary prescription drug known as Ovaban, available in 5- and 20-mg chewable tablets, and as a human prescription drug known as Megace, available in 20- and 40-mg tablets. The Food and Drug Administration (FDA) has approved it for veterinary use only for the postponement of estrus and the alleviation of false pregnancy in the dog. However, it has been shown to be an effective drug for a variety of diseases in the cat. One disadvantage of megestrol acetate is that, with repeated use, a number of mild to serious adverse effects may occur. As discussions with a number of newly graduated veterinarians from many states has led the author to the realization that this drug's use is being strongly discouraged under any circumstances, another look at this drug's relevance to clinical practice is appropriate.

Physiologic Effects

Megestrol acetate is known to cause a variety of physiological effects, including the following:[27]

- Antigonadotropic effects (estrus suppression)[28]
- Antiandrogenic effects (spermatogenesis suppression)[28]
- Induction of growth hormone release (potential for diabetes mellitus and acromegaly)[29]
- Glucocorticoid properties (adrenal response suppression and adrenal atrophy induction)[30]
- Effects on the behavioral centers (behavior, sleep patterns, thirst, and appetite effects)[28,31]
- Anti-inflammatory effects (in a wide spectrum of tissues)[28,31]
- Effects on the hair growth cycle and melanocytes (alopecia and hyperpigmentation)[32]
- Immunosuppression of T-lymphocytes (immune response suppression)[32]

Indications

Given the documented physiological effects of megestrol acetate, it should not be used indiscriminately. However, it has been used successfully in the treatment of a number of feline diseases, as shown in Table 7–1.

Adverse Effects

The preceding list of physiological effects is the basis for understanding the extensive adverse side effects that may

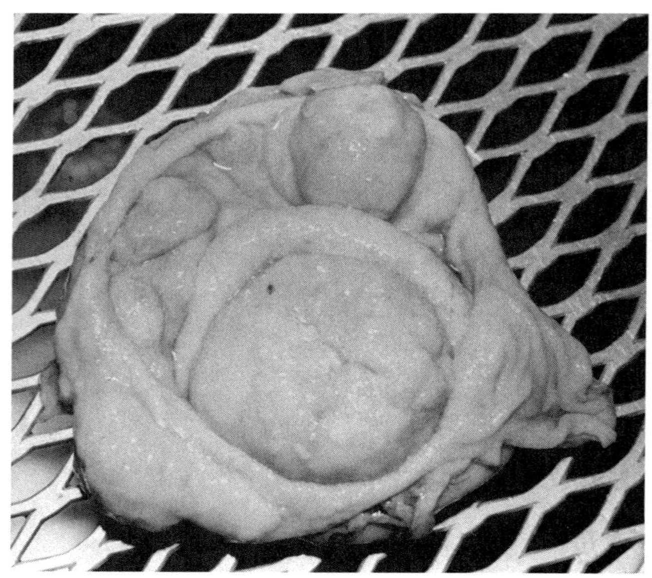

Figure 7–1. This gastric adenocarcinoma was present in a cat whose vomiting was controlled with megestrol acetate (5 mg every 7 days) for all but the last 2 weeks of the last 6 months of its life.

Table 7–1. Indications for and Recommended Dosage of Megestrol Acetate in the Cat

System/Behavior	Dosage	Indication(s)
Integumentary	Allergies to fleas, food, and inhalant allergens[27] Miliary dermatitis complex[27] Eosinophilic granuloma complex[27] Feline acne (chin) "Stud tail"[27] Psychogenic alopecia[27] Feline endocrine alopecia[27]	2.5–5 mg s.i.d. for 5–7 days; then 2.5–5 mg q 5–10 days
Urinary	Dysuria secondary to feline urologic syndrome (FUS)[27]	5 mg s.i.d. for 5–7 days
Reproductive[27]	Estrus suppression	5 mg s.i.d. for 3 days; then 2.5–5 mg q 7 days
	Estrus termination	5 mg s.i.d. for 3 days
Ophthalmologic	Eosinophilic keratitis*	5 mg s.i.d. for 5–10 days (to response); then 1.25–2.5 mg q 3–4 days
Behavioral changes[33]	Spraying Aggression Male roaming	5 mg s.i.d. for 7 days; then 2.5–5 mg q 5–10 days
Digestive	Vomiting (see Figure 7–1)	5 mg s.i.d. for 5–7 days; then 5 mg q 5–10 days
	Gingivitis/stomatitis	5 mg s.i.d. for 5–10 days (to response); then 5 mg q 5–10 days

*Megestrol acetate is the drug of choice for this disease.[34]

be caused by megestrol acetate. The following side effects have been well documented.

- Weight gain
- Polydipsia and polyuria
- Behavioral changes (aggression or passivity)
- Skin changes (alopecia, seborrhea, and atrophy[28,31,35])
- Iatrogenic hyperadrenocorticism[30,36]
- Suppression of spermatogenesis
- Benign mammary hypertrophy (fibroadenomatosis)[28] (Fig. 7–2)
- Mammary adenocarcinoma[31]
- Pyometra and endometritis[27]
- Diabetes mellitus[31]

Recommendations for the Practitioner

One of the basic principles of good medical practice is to establish a firm diagnosis so that a specific therapeutic approach may be devised. Because of megestrol acetate's powerful anti-inflammatory and antiemetic actions, the use of this drug as the primary treatment for pruritus or vomiting is very tempting. However, when this drug is chosen without first aggressively pursuing a definitive diagnosis and without considering alternative drugs, serious ethical and/or legal questions are raised. Nonetheless, following proper diagnosis, there are some situations in which this drug's use is justified (keeping in mind, however, that this drug is not

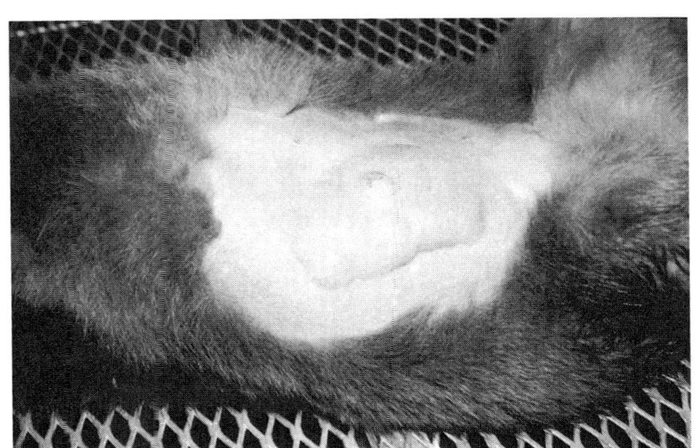

Figure 7–2 Benign mammary hypertrophy (fibroadenomatosis) was caused by megestrol acetate in this male cat. He was treated with a dosage of 5 mg every 7 days for more than 2 years before this occurred.

Table 7–2. Common Drug Interactions in Humans

Initially Prescribed Drug	Additional Drug(s)	Interaction Effect
Acidifying agents (ammonium chloride, methenamine, etc.)	Weak acid drugs	↑ Response
	Weak base drugs	↓ Response
Alkalizing agents (sodium bicarbonate, Na_2HPO_4, etc.)	Weak acid drugs	↓ Response
	Weak base drugs	↑ Response
Aminoglycoside antibiotics (streptomycin, dihydrostreptomycin, neomycin, kanamycin, paromomycin, gentamicin, amikacin, sisomicin, etc.)	Other aminoglycoside antibiotics	↑ Neuromuscular blockade
		↑ Nephrotoxicity
	Ethacrynic acid	↑ Ototoxicity
	Methoxyflurane	↑ Nephrotoxicity
	Tubocurarine	↑ Neuromuscular block
	General anesthetics	↑ Neuromuscular block
	Polymixins	↑ Nephrotoxicity and neuromuscular blockade
Ammonium chloride	Sulfonamides	Crystalluria
Amphotericin B	0.9% NaCl	Precipitation of amphotericin
	Corticosteroids	↑ K^+ depletion
	Digitalis	↑ Digitalis toxicity
Antacids (Aluminum hydroxide, magnesium compounds, $NaHCO_3$, Calcium carbonate, etc.)	Nitrofurantoin	↓ Absorption of nitrofurantoin
	Oxacillin	↓ Absorption of oxacillin
	Penicillin	↓ Absorption of penicillin
	Sulfonamides	↓ Absorption of sulfonamides
	Tetracyclines	↓ Absorption of tetracyclines
	Iron	↓ Absorption of iron
Aspirin	Heparin	↑ Bleeding
Barbiturates	Acidifying agents	↑ Barbiturate potentiation
	Central nervous system (CNS) depressants	↑ Additive effect
Calcium salts	Digitalis glycosides	↑ Cardiac arrhythmias
	Tetracyclines	↓ Absorption and activity
	Aminoglycosides	↓ Neuromuscular blockade
Cephalosporins	Gentamicin	↑ Nephrotoxicity
	Lactated Ringer's solution	↓ Cephalothin sodium
Chloramphenicol	Iron	↓ Response to iron
	Cyanocobalamine	↓ Response to cyanocobalamine
	Dicumarol	↑ Clotting time
	Penicillins	Chloramphenicol may interfere with penicillin activity
	Barbiturate	Prolongs anesthesia (enzyme inhibition)
Corticosteroids	Amphotericin B	↑ K^+ depletion
Cyanocobalamine	Neomycin	↓ Absorption of cyanocobalamine
	Chloramphenicol	↓ Response to cyanocobalamine
Digitalis glycosides	Neomycin	↓ Absorption of digitalis
	Amphotericin B	↑ K^+ depletions; digitalis toxicity
	Calcium products	↑ Cardiac arrythmias
	Furosemide	Digitalis toxicity
	Phenylbutazone	↑ Metabolism of digitalis
Erythromycin	Halothane	Possible hepatotoxicity
	Lincomycin	Possible antagonism
	Penicillin	Possible antagonism

Table 7–2 (*Continued*)

Initially Prescribed Drug	Additional Drug(s)	Interaction Effect
Estrogens	Phenobarbital	↑ Metabolism of estrogens
Furosemide	Digitalis glycosides	Digitalis toxicity
Gentamicin	Carbenicillin	In vitro inactivation when mixed in same bottle or syringe
	Cephalosporins	↑ Nephrotoxicity
Griseofulvin	Phenobarbital	↓ Absorption of griseofulvin; potentiation of barbiturate
Iron products	Chloramphenicol	↓ Response to iron
	Tetracycline	↓ Absorption of tetracycline
Kaolin-Pectin	Lincomycin	↓ Absorption of lincomycin and other drugs
Lincomycin	Erythromycin	Possible antagonism
Metheramine	Sulfonamides	↑ Crystalluria
Methoxyflurane	Tetracycline	↑ Nephrotoxicity
	Aminoglycosides	↑ Nephrotoxicity
Neomycin	Digitalis glycosides	↓ Absorption of digitalis
	Penicillin-V	↓ Absorption of penicillin V
	Cyanocobalamine	↓ Absorption of cyanocobalamine
	Alkalizers	↑ Activity
Nitrofurantoin	Antacids	↓ Absorption of nitrofurantoin
	Acidifiers	↑ Activity
Penicillins	Neomycin	↓ Absorption of penicillin
	Chloramphenicol	Chloramphenicol may interfere with penicillin activity
	Dextrose solutions (pH ≥ 8.0)	Penicillin inactivation
	Erythromycin	Possible antagonism
	Tetracycline	Possible antagonism
	Antacids	↓ Absorption of penicillin
Phenobarbital	Estrogens	↑ Metabolism of estrogens
	Griseofulvin	↓ Absorption of griseofulvin
Phenylbutazone	Digitalis glycosides	↑ Metabolism of digitalis
Procaine and related local anesthetics	Sulfonamides	Antagonism
Salicylates	Ammonium chloride	↑ Blood level of salicylates
Sulfonamides	Antacids	↓ Absorption of sulfonamides
Tetracyclines (chlortetracycline, oxytetracycline, Demethylchlortetracycline, doxycline, Minocycline, etc.)	Penicillin	Possible antagonism
	Iron products	↓ Absorption of tetracycline
	Methoxyflurane	↑ Nephrotoxicity
Thyroid hormone	Ketamine	Hypertension; tachycardia
Trimethoprim	Furosemide	↑ Incidence of thrombocytopenia
Vitamin B complex with Vitamin C	Chloramphenicol	↓ Antibiotic activity
	Erythromycin	↓ Antibiotic activity
	Nitrofurantoin	↓ Antibiotic activity
	Potassium penicillin-G	↓ Antibiotic activity

Key: ↑ Increased or enhanced; ↓ decreased or inhibited

Adapted from Talbot RB. Appendix 1: Drug Interactions. In Talbot RB. Veterinary Pharmaceuticals and Biologicals, 7th ed. Lenexa: Veterinary Medicine Publishing Co., 1991:887.

FDA-approved for any use in the cat). These situations include the following:

- Diseases for which it is the drug of choice, such as eosinophilic keratitis
- Conditions that respond best when megestrol acetate is used only to achieve control. Once control is achieved, the cat may be switched to another drug, such as a corticosteroid, for maintenance therapy. Idiopathic vomiting, some cases of gingivitis/stomatitis, and diseases of the eosinophilic granuloma complex are examples of such conditions.
- Diseases that are initially controlled by treatment with megestrol acetate, but that do not lend themselves to alternative maintenance therapy (e.g., some cases of gingivitis/stomatitis).

The second principle that must be followed in administering megestrol acetate is using the lowest effective dose at the widest effective interval. The doses given in Table 7–1 include a daily loading dose to achieve control, followed by a maintenance dose. The maintenance dose should be begun as soon as possible and the least dosage and widest interval should be chosen. If a dose greater than 5 mg once weekly is required for maintenance, the risk of adverse side effects increases.

The last principle of megestrol acetate therapy is client education. The client should be informed of the possible side effects of the drug and of the early signs of possible problems. These include polydipsia and polyuria (diabetes mellitus and hyperadrenocorticism), weight gain, mammary masses (even in males), and aggressive behavior.

Drug Interactions[37]

It is a common practice to administer several drugs simultaneously. This generally produces additive or synergistic results. However, such a practice can also produce adverse consequences. The interaction of two or more drugs may occur as a result of (1) mixing solutions outside the animal body, or (2) reactions occurring within the body after the administration of two or more drugs by the same or different routes. The drug interactions that may occur include the following:

1. Direct chemical and physical interactions
2. Altered absorption following administration by the oral or parenteral routes
3. Effects on protein binding
4. Changed rate of drug metabolism
5. An increase or decrease in body clearance by renal, hepatic, or other routes
6. Interaction of drugs at the receptor site
7. Interactions related to changes in the acid–base balance of body fluids

Any of the preceding can result in a variety of unexpected responses, including no response, a reduced response, or an increased response, some of which may be associated with toxic reactions that range in severity from minimal to severe, including death.

The drug interactions listed in Table 7–2 are based on the human species, and so there may be exceptions for the feline species. However, this list should serve as a general guideline for administering multiple drugs to cats.

REFERENCES

1. Booth DM. Drug therapy in cats: Recommended dosing regimens. J Am Vet Med Assoc 1990;196:1845.
2. Davis LE, Westfall BA. Species differences in biotransformation and excretion of salicylate. Am J Vet Res 1972;33:1253.
3. Finco DR, Duncan JR, Schall WD. Acetaminophen toxicosis in the cat. J Am Vet Med Assoc 1975;166:469.
4. Krake AC, Arendt TD, Teachout DJ, et al. Cetacaine-induced methemoglobinemia in domestic cats. J Am Anim Hosp Assoc 1985;21:527.
5. Wilkie DA, Kirby R. Methemoglobinemia associated with dermal application of benzocaine cream in a cat. J Am Vet Med Assoc 1988;192:85.
6. Cullison RF. Toxicosis in cats from use of benzyl alcohol in lactated Ringer's solution. J Am Vet Med Assoc 1983;182:61.
7. McDonald JM, Miller TA. Parasiticide Therapy in Small Animal Dermatology. In: Kirk RW, ed. Current Veterinary Therapy IX. Philadelphia: WB Saunders, 1986:571.
8. Thompson JP, Senior DF, Pinson DM, Moriello KA. Neurotoxicosis associated with the use of hexachlorophene in the cat. J Am Vet Med Assoc 1987;190:1311.
9. Schechter RD, Schalm OW, Kanek JJ. Heinz-body hemolytic anemia associated with the use of urinary antiseptics in the cat. J Am Vet Med Assoc 1973;162:37.
10. Harvey JW, Kornik HP. Phenazopyridine toxicosis in the cat. J Am Vet Med Assoc 1976;169:327.
11. Shell L. Antiepileptic drugs. Compend Contin Educ Pract Vet 1984;6:432.
12. Atkins CE, Tyler R, Greenlee P. Clinical, biochemical, acid-base, and electrolyte abnormalities in cats after hypertonic sodium phosphate enema administration. Am J Vet Res 1985;46:980.
13. Conlon PD. Nonsteroidal drugs used in the treatment of inflammation. Vet Clin North Am (Small Anim Pract) 1988;18:1115.
14. Davis LE, Westfall BA. Species differences in biotransformation and excretion of salicylate. Am J Vet Res 1972;33:1253.
15. Atkins CE, Snyder PS. Cardiomyopathy. In: Allen DG, ed. Small Animal Medicine. Philadelphia: JB Lippincott, 1991:269.
16. Watson ADJ, Middleton DJ. Chloramphenicol toxicosis in cats. Am J Vet Res 1978;39:1199.
17. Kunkle GA, Meyer DJ. Toxicity of high doses of griseofulvin in cats. J Am Vet Med Assoc 1987;191:322.
18. Levy JK. Ataxia in a kitten treated with griseofulvin. J Am Vet Med Assoc 1991;198:105.
19. Shelton GH, Grant CK, Lindenberger ML, Abkowitz JL. Severe neutropenia associated with griseofulvin therapy in cats with feline immunodeficiency virus infection. J Vet Intern Med 1990;4:317.
20. Booth DM. Drug therapy in cats: A systems approach. J Am Vet Med Assoc 1990;196:1502.
21. Romatowski J. Use of megestrol acetate in cats. J Am Vet Med Assoc 1989;194:700.
22. Papich MG, Cavis CA, Davis LE. Absorption of salicylate from an antidiarrheal preparation in dogs and cats. J Am Anim Hosp Assoc 1987;23:221.
23. Turner JL, Lees GE, Brown SA, et al. Thiacetarsamide in healthy cats: Clinical and pathological observations. J Am Anim Hosp Assoc 1991;27(3):275.

24. Dillon R. Feline dirofilariasis. Vet Clin North Am (Small Anim Pract) 1984;14:1185.
25. Fishler JJ, Birzele FD. Feline Infectious Anemia. In: Kirk RW, ed. Current Veterinary Therapy V. Philadelphia: WB Saunders, 1974:358.
26. Maede Y, Hoshino T, Inaba M, Namioka S. Methionine toxicosis in cats. Am J Vet Res 1987;48:289.
27. White SD. Megestrol Acetate: Indications and Effects. In: August JR, ed. Consultations in Feline Internal Medicine. Philadelphia: WB Saunders, 1991:263.
28. Kunkle GA. Feline dermatosis. Vet Clin North Am (Small Anim Pract) 1984;14:1065.
29. Eigenman JE. Disorders Associated with Growth Hormone Oversecretion: Diabetes Mellitus and Acromegaly. In: Kirk RW, ed. Current Veterinary Therapy IX. Philadelphia: WB Saunders, 1986:1006.
30. Chastain CB, Graham CL, Nichols CE. Adrenocortical suppression in cats given megestrol acetate. Am J Vet Res 1981;42:2029.
31. Scott DW. Feline dermatology 1900–1978: A monograph. J Am Anim Hosp Assoc 1980;16:440.
32. Muller GH, Kirk RW, Scott DW. Dermatologic Therapy. In: Muller GH, Kirk RW, Scott DW, eds. Small Animal Dermatology, 3rd ed. Philadelphia: WB Saunders, 1983:174.
33. Borchelt PL, Voith VL. Diagnosis and treatment of elimination behavior problems in cats. Vet Clin North Am (Small Anim Pract) 1982;12:676.
34. Brightman AH, Vestre WA, Helper LC. Chronic eosinophilic keratitis in the cat. Feline Pract 1979;9(3):21.
35. Chastain CB, Ganjam VK. Clinical Endocrinology of Companion Animals. Philadelphia: WB Saunders 1986:460, 540.
36. Scott DW. Feline dermatology 1979–1982. J Am Anim Hosp Assoc 1984;20:537.
37. Talbot RB. Appendix 1: Drug Interactions. In Talbot RB. Veterinary Pharmaceuticals and Biologicals, 7th ed. Lenexa, KS: Veterinary Medicine Publishing Co., 1991:887.

CHAPTER 8

◇ ◇ ◇

Anesthetics and Anesthesia

Gary D. Norsworthy

Anesthesia: Science and Art

In the last 10 to 15 years, a great deal of scientific progress has been made in the field of veterinary anesthesia. A significant number of new anesthetic agents have become available. The American College of Veterinary Anesthesiologists has led the way in promoting research. However, the typical primary care veterinarian does not have the on-site services of a veterinary anesthesiologist. In the average practice, monitoring of the patient's anesthetic status is often performed by an on-the-job–trained technician or by the surgeon. Because of this situation, successful monitoring of the patient requires a distinct familiarity with the animal and its responses during the various planes of anesthesia. This is somewhat of an objective assessment, but it is also somewhat subjective. The experienced practitioner learns to get the "feel" of the effects of various anesthetics on the patient, which is what the author terms "the art of veterinary anesthesia."

To promote this "art of veterinary anesthesia," it is recommended that the surgeon follow two principles:

1. Become familiar with a few anesthetics or anesthetic combinations and use them frequently enough to get a feel for how the properly regulated patient should appear during surgery and recovery and what the signs of impending difficulty are.
2. Do not use a new or infrequently used anesthetic or anesthetic combination in critical or crisis situations. Consider, for example, the use of isoflurane. Because this anesthetic is quite expensive, it may seem wasteful to use it for routine cases. Rather, a more judicious use would be to reserve it for cats with cardiac compromise, such as those with hyperthyroidism. If one does not have the "feel" for this anesthetic, one may misinterpret, or miss entirely, the early signs of difficulty.

Anesthetic Options

If one existed, the "perfect" anesthetic would have the following characteristics:[1]

It would rapidly induce loss of consciousness.

It would have a controllable duration of action.

It would be technically easy to administer.

It would produce easily identifiable levels of anesthetic depth.

It would allow rapid alteration of the levels of anesthetic depth.

It would have a wide margin of safety.

It would produce no toxic metabolites.

It would be predictably and spontaneously eliminated, regardless of renal or hepatic function.

It would be receptor-specific, making its actions reversible with specific antagonists.

It would be unaffected by variations in patient age or disease.

It would be economical to use.

There are many anesthetics and anesthetic combinations that offer a good surgical plane of anesthesia and a wide margin of patient safety. However, there is no anesthetic that has all of the qualities just listed; rather, each has certain advantages and disadvantages. The following is not an exhaustive list of anesthetics, but it does include those anesthetic agents and combinations of agents that have been used routinely by the author. (For a more complete list, see Table 8–1.[2])

Ultra–short-acting barbiturates, such as thiamylal (Bio-Tal) or sodium thiopental (Pentothal)

Dose. When diluted to 3% to 4%, a dose of approximately 2 mL per 10 lb is given to effect. Atropine or glycopyrrolate is appropriate, and can be mixed in the same syringe.

Advantages and Indications. These agents produce short-acting effects that allow full recovery within 4 to 6 hours. They are appropriate for use in neutering, abscess drainage, intubation, and other procedures of a similar length.

Disadvantages. These agents must be given intravenously (IV). Some cats will experience a brief period of excitation during recovery. Repeated use within several days may result in cumulative effects, thus necessitating lower subsequent doses. They are controlled substances.

Table 8–1. Anesthetics and Anesthetic Combinations

Anesthetic Agent(s)	Recommended Dose(s)*	Concentration(s)	Dose(s) for 10-lb Cat	Antagonist
Pentobarbital (Pentobarbital USP)	11 mg/lb IV	65 mg/mL	1.7 mL IV (to effect)	Yohimbine
Sodium thiopental (Pentothal)	2.3–4.5 mg/lb IV	2% (20 mg/mL); may be 2%–5%	1.15–2.3 mL IV (to effect)	
Thiamylal (Bio-Tal)	2.3–4.5 mg/lb IV	2% (20 mg/mL); may be 0.5%–4%	1.15–2.3 mL IV (to effect)	
Ketamine (Ketaset, Vetalar)				
IV	0.2–0.9 mg/lb	100 mg/mL	0.02–0.09 mL	Yohimbine
IM	4.5–9 mg/lb	100 mg/mL	0.4–0.9 mL	Yohimbine
Ketamine (Ketaset, Vetalar) + diazepam (Valium)				
IV	2.3 mg/lb of ketamine + 0.3 mg/lb of diazepam	Ketamine: 100 mg/mL Diazepam: 5 mg/mL	0.23 mL of ketamine + 0.6 mL of diazepam	Yohimbine (for ketamine only)
IM	4.5–9 mg/lb of ketamine + 0.23 mg/lb of diazepam	Ketamine: 100 mg/mL Diazepam: 5 mg/mL	0.4–0.9 mL of ketamine + 0.5 mL of diazepam	Yohimbine (for ketamine only)
Ketamine (Ketaset, Vetalar) + Acepromazine (PromAce)	4.5–9 mg/lb of ketamine + 0.2 mg/lb of acepromazine IM	Ketamine: 100 mg/mL Acepromazine: 10 mg/mL	0.4–0.9 mL of ketamine + 0.2 mL of acepromazine	
Ketamine (Ketaset, Vetalar) + xylazine (Rompum)	4.5–9 mg/lb of ketamine + 0.13–0.23 mg/lb of xylazine IM	Ketamine: 100 mg/mL Xylazine: 20 mg/mL	0.4–0.9 mL of ketamine + 0.07–0.12 mL of xylazine IM	
Tiletamine-zolazepam (Telazol)				
IV	0.45–1.4 mg/lb	100 mg/mL	0.05–0.14 mL	
IM	3.6–6.8 mg/lb	100 mg/mL	0.35–0.68 mL	
Yohimbine (Yobine)	0.11 mg/lb IV	2 mg/mL	0.55 mL	

*The doses listed are averages. However, individual patient variation demands that each be given to effect.

Used by permission from Muir WW, Swanson CR. Principles, Techniques, and Complications of Feline Anesthesia and Chemical Restraint. In: Sherding RG, ed. The Cat: Disease and Clinical Management. New York: Churchill Livingstone, 1989:81.

A combination of ketamine and diazepam

Dose (for a 10-lb cat). A dose of 0.5 mL of ketamine (50 mg) plus 0.5 mL of diazepam (2.5 mg) is given IV. The two are mixed together in a syringe and then 1/2 of the dose is administered as a bolus; the remainder is then administered, if needed, to effect. Atropine (Atropine Injectable, S.A., Fort Dodge Laboratories, Fort Dodge, IA) or glycopyrrolate is appropriate and can be mixed in the same syringe.

Advantages and Indications. This combination of anesthetics produces medium-acting effects, allowing procedures lasting up to 30 minutes but still permitting full recovery within 6 to 8 hours. This combination is appropriate for dematting, teeth cleaning, intubation, suturing of lacerations, and the like. Compared to barbiturates, this combination of agents produces better laryngeal relaxation, thus facilitating intubation.

Disadvantages. Although IV administration is preferred, intramuscular (IM) or subcutaneous (SC) administration is possible, albeit with slower onset of action and slightly increased dosage requirements. These drugs are more expensive than the barbiturates, and diazepam is a controlled substance.

A combination of ketamine and acepromazine

Dose (for a 10-lb cat). A combination dose of 1.0 to 1.5 mL (100 to 150 mg) of Ketamine plus 0.25 mL (2.5 mg) of acepromazine (Acepromazine Maleate Injection, TechAmerica Veterinary Products, Kansas City, MO) is mixed together in a syringe and given as an IM bolus. Atropine or glycopyrrolate is appropriate and can be mixed in the same syringe.

Advantages and Indications. This combination produces long-lasting effects, allowing adequate relaxation for brief intra-abdominal procedures, such as ovariohysterectomies or cryptorchid surgery.

These anesthetics should be given IM, but SC dosing is acceptable. The latter results in a slower onset of action and the need for a slightly increased dosage.

Disadvantages. This combination of anesthetics does not allow adequate muscle relaxation for prolonged intra-abdominal procedures or for orthopedic procedures. A prolonged recovery time (12 to 18 hours) requires hospitalization overnight. Indeed, some cats do not fully recover for up to 48 hours.

Anesthetic gases, such as methoxyflurane (Metophane), halothane (Fluothane), and isoflurane (AErrane).

Dose. These anesthetic gases are given via endotracheal tube to effect. Dosage percentages vary somewhat according to the agent used, the condition of the patient, and the procedure performed. Administration of atropine or glycopyrrolate is appropriate.

Advantages and Indications. These anesthetic agents produce long-lasting effects for major abdominal, thoracic, spinal, cranial, and orthopedic procedures. Halothane and isoflurane may be administered by face mask or induction chamber. In addition, these anesthetics are excellent for performing caesarean sections because only minimal amounts cross the placenta.

Intubation

The cat is considerably more difficult to intubate than the dog because the cat's laryngeal reflex is easily evoked. In fact, the cat's larynx can remain tightly closed for an incredibly long period of time, even to the point of causing cyanosis. In order to simplify the intubation process, the following suggestions are offered:

- Tie a 1- to 2-inch wide, 15-inch long piece of gauze around the endotracheal tube before passing the tube. This will be used later to secure the tube to the cat's head.
- Choose an endotracheal tube with a diameter no larger than 5 mm.
- In particularly difficult cats, use a Cole-style tube (Portex Cole-style Endotracheal Tube, Jorgensen Laboratories, Inc., Loveland, CO). The distal end of this tube is tapered, facilitating insertion. However, this tube is not cuffed.
- Use a stylet made from a stiff piece of wire (i.e., a coat hanger) or a stiff canine urinary catheter. Distally, it should be placed just at the end of the endotracheal tube. Proximally, it should exit the tube and be bent in such a way that the stylet can be held and used to direct the tube. If a metal stylet extends past the end of the endotracheal tube, there is a risk of injuring the larynx.
- Have an assistant hold the cat's head in such a way as to avoid placing the fingers in the cat's mouth. If the cat's soft palate is touched, a strong reflex will occur that will often result in the cat firmly closing its mouth.
- For the right-handed operator, grasp the cat's tongue with the left index finger and thumb. Use of a gauze sponge will make holding the tongue much easier. Firmly extend the tongue from the cat's mouth so as to expose the pharynx fully.
- Apply 4% lidocaine (Xylocaine) to the larynx, either as an aerosol spray or as a liquid that is painted on with a cotton-tipped applicator, until the larynx is no longer stimulated by the applicator. (This step is optional.)
- Pass the endotracheal tube to a point just short of the larynx. (If the larynx is touched, it will close tightly.)
- While holding the endotracheal tube near the larynx, wait for the cat to open the larynx (i.e., during inhalation).
- Using the little finger of your left hand, lift the larynx by pressing on the ventral surface of the cat's trachea.
- When the larynx opens, quickly and smoothly pass the tip of the tube into the laryngeal opening. If the tip of the tube is tapered, rotate the tube to align the point into a vertical plane because the cat's larynx opens in a vertical plane first.
- Pass the tube to the desired depth and secure it to the cat's head by tying the gauze behind the cat's head.
- Inflate the cuff and attach the endotracheal tube to the anesthetic machine.

Non-Rebreathing System

Because of the small capacity of the cat's respiratory system as compared to the hoses and bag of an anesthetic machine, careful anesthetic management may be difficult. Therefore, a non-rebreathing anesthetic system, such as the Mini Bain Anesthesia Circuit (Jorgensen Laboratories, Inc., Loveland, CO) or the Ayres T (Fraser-Harlake, Orchard Park, NY), should be used in cats to overcome this problem. These items attach to an anesthetic machine in place of the normal hoses and bag.

Monitoring

Because the typical primary care veterinary practice does not have a trained anesthesiologist in attendance for surgical procedures, some form of monitor must be utilized. In the author's opinion, anesthetic monitoring equipment should meet the following criteria:

1. The monitor must be reasonably priced. The importance of this criterion will vary somewhat from one practice to another, but price will always be a factor.
2. The monitor must be easy to connect to the patient.
3. The monitor must function without the need for continual adjustments.
4. The monitor should have the ability to detect patient difficulties before a crisis level is reached. In the author's experience, cardiac arrest has never occurred in an anesthetized animal prior to apnea. Therefore, if apnea can be detected at its onset, the patient will still have reasonably normal cardiac function and can usually be revived by discontinuing anesthesia or by initiating forced ventilation.
5. The monitor should alert the surgeon at the onset of apnea. A loud audible tone is preferable.

Table 8–2. Anesthetic Monitors

Parameter(s) Monitored	Type of Monitor	Manufacturer
Respiratory rate	Vet Alarm Respiratory Monitor	Jorgensen Laboratories, Loveland, CO
Respiratory rate	The Beeper	Spencer Instrumentation, Irvine, CA
Respiratory rate, tidal and minute volume	Respirometer	Fraser-Harlake, Orchard Park, NY
Rate, end tidal PCO_2, anatomic deadspace	Capnograph	Biochem Intern, Inc., Waukesha, WI
PaO_2, $PaCO_2$, pH	Blood gas machine	Instrumentation Labs, Inc., Lexington, MA
Heart sounds and temperature	Esophageal stethoscope and temperature monitor	Portex, Wilmington, MA
Amplified heart sounds	Heart sound amplifier and audio monitor	Bickford, Inc., Wales Center, NY
Arterial pressure monitor (direct or indirect)	Blood pressure monitor	Datascope Corp., Paramus, NJ
Arterial pressure monitor (direct or indirect)	Blood pressure monitor	Critikon, Inc., Tampa, FL
Core body temperature	Temperature monitor	Sunbeam Corp., Shubuta, MS

Adapted from Muir WW, Swanson CR. Principles, Techniques, and Complications of Feline Anesthesia and Chemical Restraint. In: Sherding RG, ed. The Cat: Disease and Clinical Management. New York: Churchill Livingstone, 1989:81.

6. The monitor should be dependable and should be able to perform for many months or years without maintenance.

There are several monitors available that fulfill these criteria. The following have been used by the author:

> Vet Alarm Respiratory Monitor (formerly marketed as apALERT), Jorgensen Laboratories Inc., 1450 N. Van Buren Ave, Loveland, CO 80538 (303–669–2500)
>
> The Beeper and The Beeper Plus, Spencer Instrumentation, 17286 Citron, Irvine CA 92175 (714–786–4011)

These monitors connect easily into the breathing circuit, monitor apnea (with variable settings, measured in seconds, for an acceptable duration of apnea), sound a loud audible tone when the acceptable length of apnea is exceeded, and are reasonably priced for the average veterinary practice. In addition to these features, The Beeper Plus has a heart rate monitor with an alarm for both tachycardia and bradycardia.

For a more complete listing of anesthetic monitors, see Table 8–2.

The Fractious Cat

The fractious cat is a challenge in many ways. The handling and restraint of this type of patient were discussed in Chapter 2, as were the physiologic effects of such behavior on blood parameters.

Such cats are also a unique challenge when anesthesia is administered. When excited, the cat releases large amounts of endogenous catecholamines. This is part of the cat's well-developed "fight-or-flight" reflex that results in tachycardia, myocardial hypoxia, peripheral vasoconstriction with rebound vasodilation, and respiratory alkalosis.[3] If an anesthetic is administered in conjunction with these events, the results may be cardiac fibrillation and arrest, especially if cardiac depressants, hypotensive agents, or both, are used.

The author has witnessed these effects on three occasions. On each occasion, the cat was very agitated and aggressive and was given a rather painful IM injection that included a cardiac depressant and a hypotensive agent. Death of the patient ensued within a few minutes. To avoid this situation, the following suggestions are offered:

- Minimize aggravation to fractious cats prior to anesthetic induction by keeping them away from the sight and sound of dogs. If you do not have a separate ward for cats, leave the cat in a carrier in an examining room or other quiet place.
- Do not allow any of your staff to antagonize these cats further.
- Consider using an induction chamber, either a fish tank or any of the commercially available chambers (Induction Chamber, Veterinary Concepts, Inc., Spring Valley, WI) (Fig. 8–1). You will, however, need to weigh the time and expense involved in induction using these chambers.
- Remove the cat from the hospital cage with a device that minimizes struggling. The Snappy Snare (Campbell Enterprises, Brush Prairie, WA) may facilitate this task, but it should be used with extreme caution to avoid choking or panicking a patient.
- Use a squeeze-type cage to handle the cat. Cages that permit SC injections are preferred. Commercially avail-

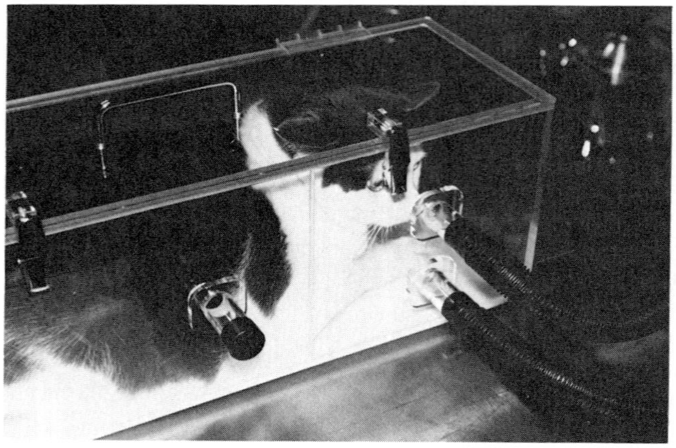

Figure 8–1. The Induction Chamber (Veterinary Concepts, Inc., Spring Valley, WI) permits anesthetic induction of a fractious cat with halothane or isoflurane. A removable partition allows the chamber to accommodate three sizes of cats.

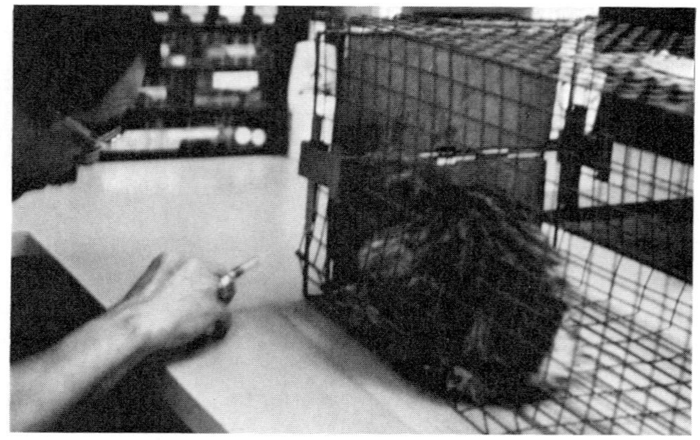

Figure 8–3. Ketamine can be administered orally through an open-end feline urinary catheter. A 2-mL dose is injected into the cat's mouth. It will be absorbed through the oral or respiratory mucosa to produce sedation within about 10 minutes. Care should be taken not to get it in the cat's eyes.

able cages include the Wild Child (Veterinary Concepts, Inc., Spring Valley, WI) (Fig. 8–2) and the Portable Omnicage (Campbell Enterprises, Brush Prairie, WA).

- Administer anesthetic combinations SC. Although the SC route prolongs the time it takes for the anesthetic to take effect (compared to IV or IM administration), it is definitely less stressful to the cat. If this method is used, an increased dose is usually required, or additional anesthetic may need to be administered after the cat relaxes.
- Avoid the IV administration of cardiac depressants, such as barbiturates and xylazine, or vasodilators, such as acepromazine.
- Use anesthetic regimens that are minimally damaging to cardiac output and blood pressure. The following are recommended (for the 10-lb cat):[2]

  Ketamine (0.5 mL) + diazepam (0.5 mL), administered IM or SC. When the cat is calm, administer more ketamine (0.25 mL) and diazepam (0.25 mL) IV, if needed.

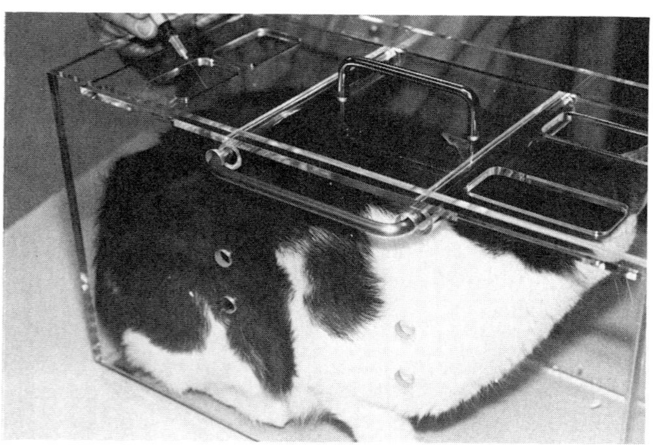

Figure 8–2. The Wild Child (Veterinary Concepts, Inc., Spring Valley, WI) is a squeeze cage that permits injections to be made without risk to the patient or the veterinarian.

  Ketamine, administered orally (the author's preferred regimen). Begin with 2 mL of ketamine in a 3-mL syringe to which is attached an open-end feline urinary catheter (Sovereign 3½-French Tom Cat Catheter, Sherwood Medical, St. Louis, MO). When the cat hisses, inject the entire amount into the cat's mouth (Fig. 8–3). (The excited cat is generally preoccupied by watching you, and usually does not see the clear catheter that can be slipped into or near the mouth.) Whether the Ketamine is absorbed from the oral mucosa or goes into the trachea and is absorbed from the lungs, the results are the same. The actual dose is 1.0 mL (10 mg/

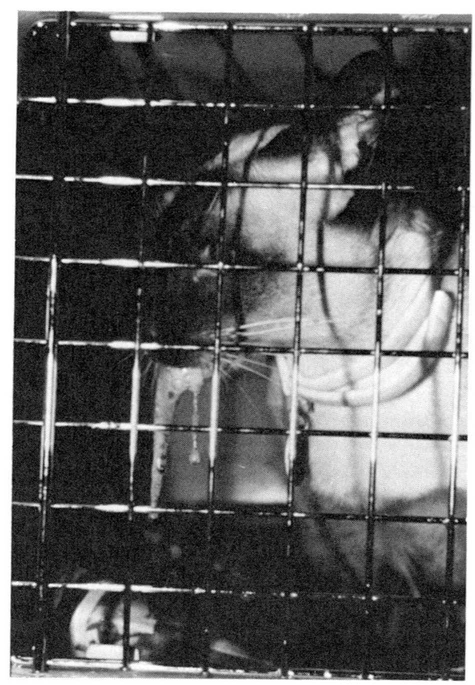

Figure 8–4. Ketamine causes the transient side effect of drooling.

lb), but generally, administration of 2 mL is necessary for 1.0 mL to be absorbed.[4]

The sedative effects of the drug will be evident within about 10 minutes and will last only about 10 to 15 minutes. When the cat is calm, an additional dose of Ketamine and diazepam is administered IV to effect, followed by intubation if desired.

The only undesirable side effect is salivation (Fig. 8–4). Oral ketamine causes severe drooling, presumably because of its taste. However, this is a transient effect.

REFERENCES

1. Tranquilli W. Veterinary anesthesia: Present day and future methodologies. Vet Messenger 1988;1:4.
2. Muir WW, Swanson CR. Principles, Techniques, and Complications of Feline Anesthesia and Chemical Restraint. In: Sherding RG, ed. The Cat: Diseases and Clinical Management. New York: Churchill Livingstone, 1989:81.
3. Mandelker L. Anesthetic trivia, pitfalls and solutions. Vet Forum 1985;8:8.
4. Macy DW, Siwe ST. The use of ketamine as an oral anesthetic in cats. Feline Pract 1977;7(1):44.

CHAPTER 9

◇ ◇ ◇

Blood Collection

Gary D. Norsworthy

Because the cat has smaller peripheral veins than the average dog, blood collection can be somewhat more difficult. Blood can be easily collected from only two peripheral veins—the cephalic vein and the jugular vein. The former is quite small and its use requires a great deal of patience on the part of the practitioner or technician. Blood may also be collected in small quantities from a cut toe nail, from a nicked marginal ear vein, or from the medial saphenous vein.

The Cephalic Vein

The equipment needed for blood collection from the cephalic vein includes a 3-, 6-, or 12-cc syringe, a 20- or 22-gauge needle, and a tourniquet. A ¼-inch wide rubber band that is secured by a small hemostat can serve as a tourniquet for this vein. Unless contraindicated for the blood test in question, the syringe should be heparinized. Because blood collection from this vein is quite slow, the blood is likely to clot in the syringe or needle if an anticoagulant is not used.

To collect blood from the cephalic vein, the tourniquet is applied just above the elbow. Its application is critical to success because if it is applied too tightly, the cephalic vein as well as the radial artery will be occluded. In this instance, after the small amount of blood that is available is removed from the vein, the vein will not refill, so blood collection will stop. If this occurs, the total yield will be 0.1 to 0.2 mL of blood in the syringe and no more. Loosening the tourniquet so the radial artery is no longer occluded will resolve the problem.

Once the tourniquet is applied, the cephalic vein will fill and become quite prominent just below the elbow. The application of isopropyl alcohol to the area will make the vein even more visible. Only rarely should one have to shave the hair from the area; indeed, most owners prefer that the hair not be shaved.

Because this is a small vein, successful blood collection requires patience. Talking to or stroking of the cat may be helpful in keeping the animal calm and still. The use of a 20-gauge needle may also be helpful. (Note: Laboratory technicians are taught not to draw blood through a needle smaller than 20 gauge owing to the risk of vacuum-induced hemolysis. However, a 22-gauge needle is acceptable if patience is used and a good entry into the vein is achieved.)

Most cats will permit 5 to 10 mL of blood to be drawn from the cephalic vein, which amount is generally adequate for blood profiles. When blood collection is completed, pressure should be applied to the venipuncture site to prevent hematoma formation. This is especially true if repeated venipunctures are necessary. Many practitioners use adhesive tape for this purpose; however, the difficulty in removing this kind of tape can be very frustrating to cat owners. Masking tape is an excellent alternative. It has adequate adhesion to be effective, is removed much easier, and is considerably less expensive than adhesive tape.

Some tests, such as a blood glucose or hematocrit determinations, can be performed using only a few drops of blood. A blood smear requires only one drop of blood. In these situations, a 25-gauge needle is appropriate. This size needle is especially desirable when multiple samples must be taken in one day, as is the case when performing a glucose curve. A capillary tube can be filled by inserting it into the hub of the needle (Fig. 9–1). Enough blood can be collected in this manner to perform several important tests, including a hematocrit or glucose level, or to make a blood smear.

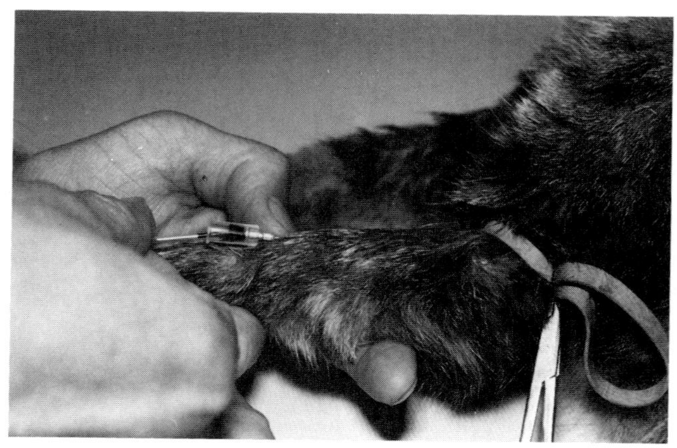

Figure 9–1. **A 25-gauge needle is inserted into the cephalic vein, after which a capillary tube can be filled and the blood used to perform several vital tests. Note the hemostat-rubber band tourniquet.**

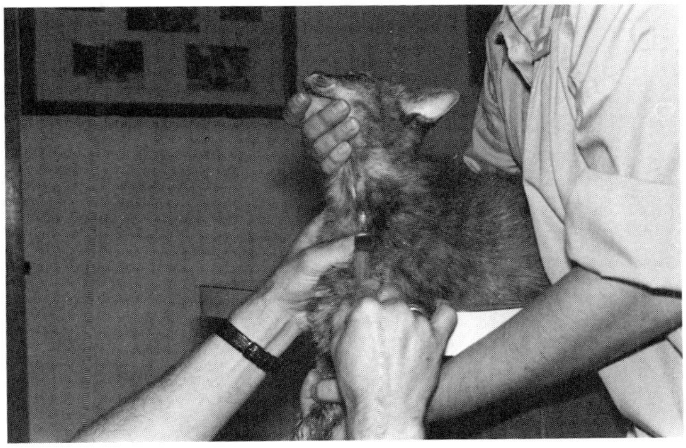

Figure 9–2. To collect blood from the jugular vein, have an assistant elevate the cat's chin, directing the head slightly away from the side selected. The front legs should be held over the edge of a table. The jugular vein is then occluded with the left thumb while the syringe and needle are directed with the right hand.

The Jugular Vein

The jugular vein is considerably larger than the cephalic vein, but its use for blood collection requires a considerable degree of cooperation from the cat. If a clean entry is made into this vein, 12 mL of blood can be collected without an anticoagulant and the sample can be placed in an anticoagulated tube in adequate time. However, if the cat is uncooperative, this vein may be difficult or impossible to use.

To collect blood from the jugular vein, the cat's head should be elevated upward to expose the cervical area and it should be turned slightly away from the side of the venipuncture. The hair should be clipped from the area in most cats, but this is often unnecessary if the cat has a thin to medium body build and if isopropyl alcohol is applied. Although some cats do well with minimal restraint, such as occurs with raising the head, other cats require additional restraint. For the latter, restraint is achieved by extending the front legs of the cat downward, over the edge of a table. This form of restraint requires the help of one assistant in most cases, but a second assistant may need to hold the back legs if the cat resists (Fig. 9–2).

The venipuncture is made into the vein with the needle directed cranially. Blood is drawn rapidly through a 20-gauge needle into a 6- or 12-cc syringe. When an adequate sample is obtained, the cat's head is allowed to return to a normal position and pressure is applied at the venipuncture site to prevent hematoma formation.

Toenails and the Marginal Ear Vein

Small samples of blood can be collected by cutting a toenail into its vein or by nicking a lateral ear vein. In either case, a few drops of blood are collected in a hematocrit tube and a white blood cell pipette (Unopette, Becton-Dickinson, Rutherford, NJ) Another drop is placed on a microscope slide and a blood smear is made immediately. These methods of blood collection usually do not meet with the approval of the owner, so they should not be performed in the owner's presence. In cats with poor circulation or in very small cats, these methods may be the only successful means of blood collection.

CHAPTER 10

◇ ◇ ◇

Blood Transfusions

Gary D. Norsworthy

A blood transfusion can be a life-saving treatment in the severely anemic cat. More often, because most severely anemic cats are suffering from incurable diseases, it is a treatment that maintains life long enough for a diagnosis to be made.

Indications for Blood Transfusion

Because of the expense involved in transfusions, the clinician should be sure that the owner understands that many severe anemias are the result of incurable diseases. Because anemias secondary to the feline leukemia virus (FeLV) are so common, this virus should be part of the differential diagnosis in almost all anemic cats. Anemic cats should undergo three tests initially, all of which can be performed in a hospital laboratory using minimal equipment. The purpose of these tests is to determine the likelihood of the cat having an incurable disease.

1. An FeLV test should be performed to determine whether the FeLV is likely to be the cause of the anemia.

   A positive FeLV test means that the short-term prognosis is guarded and the long-term prognosis is grave. Many owners elect euthanasia for an FeLV-positive cat, despite the fact that many of these cats, if treated, can survive for many months. The owner should be fully informed of the options and prognosis, and should be allowed to make the final decision.
2. A blood smear should be obtained, stained with Diff-Quik (AHS Caribe, Inc., Aguada, Puerto Rico), and observed to determine whether the anemia is regenerative or nonregenerative (Fig. 10–1) (see Chapter 16). Cats with regenerative anemias can survive with a lower packed cell volume (PCV) than can those with nonregenerative anemias.

   The presence of macrocytes is the best indicator of bone marrow activity. Macrocytes are the transitional cells between a nucleated red blood cell (RBC) (the metarubricyte) and a mature erythrocyte. They are also called reticulocytes; however, the reticulum cannot be visualized unless a reticulocyte prep is performed using new methylene blue stain. Macrocytes are characteristically larger than mature erythrocytes, and have a bluish-colored cytoplasm. They are released from the bone marrow in response to anemia.

   Another indicator of bone marrow activity is the presence of Howell-Jolly bodies. These are dense, dark bodies found in the cytoplasm of the mature erythrocyte. They are generally seen in less than 10% of the erythrocytes, and only if the bone marrow response is marked. Thus, their absence does not rule out bone marrow activity.

   If the stained blood smear indicates bone marrow activity, the erythrocytes should be observed for the presence of *Hemobartonella felis*. As with Howell-Jolly bodies, their absence on a blood smear does not exclude their presence in the cat, and their presence on a blood smear is very meaningful (see Chapter 43).

   After examining a stained blood smear, there may still be some uncertainty concerning bone marrow response. A better understanding is possible with a reticulocyte stain. (For more information about this technique and its interpretation, see Chapters 12 and 16.)
3. If the cat is not visibly icteric, 0.5 mL of blood or more should be centrifuged to determine whether icterus is present in the serum.

   If the cat has a nonregenerative anemia and is icteric, the likelihood of a nontreatable disease is heightened. The owner should be so advised before a decision on a blood transfusion is made.

The cat possesses a tremendous ability to compensate for severe disease processes. Indeed, it is not uncommon for a cat with a hematocrit of 4% to be in fairly stable condition. Therefore, decisions regarding blood transfusion should be made with that fact in mind.

Another factor that determines the urgency of a blood transfusion is the stress under which the cat will be for the next 24 hours (or until further laboratory testing can be completed). If the cat is to be hospitalized, then there is less urgency for blood transfusion than if the cat were to be allowed outdoors in very cold or hot weather, or in situations that might require defense from another cat or a dog.

Other factors that should be considered are the cat's general clinical condition, the owner's financial limitations and desires, the availability of suitable feline blood, and the

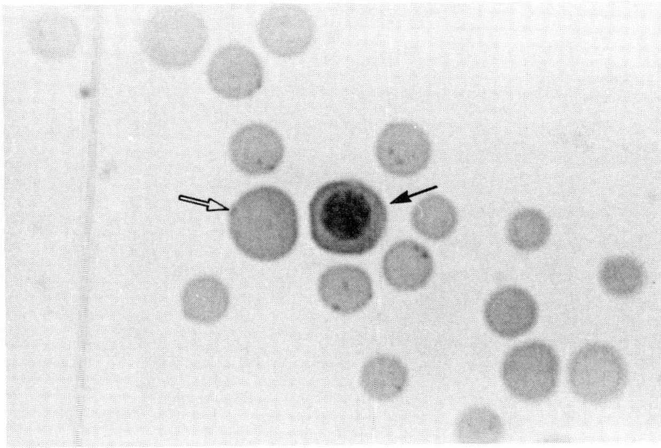

Figure 10–1. **Several indicators of bone marrow response can be seen in this photomicrograph. The nucleated cell in the center of the field (*solid arrow*) is a metarubricyte, or nucleated red blood cell (RBC). The large cell to the left of the metarubricyte is a macrocyte (*open arrow*). If this cell were stained with new methylene blue, its reticulum would be visible. The other cells are mature erythrocytes. Many of the mature RBCs contain *Hemobartonella felis* on their surface.**

availability of appropriate equipment for blood collection and administration.

In summary, the major determinants for a blood transfusion are the hematocrit level, the type of anemia (regenerative versus nonregenerative), and the stress factors that will be present over the next 24 hours. Certain other factors that have been mentioned must also be considered. As a general rule, a transfusion is indicated if (1) the hematocrit is less than 15% and the anemia is nonregenerative; or (2) the hematocrit is less than 10% and the anemia is regenerative.

Blood Collection, Storage, and Administration

Blood can be freshly collected from a donor for immediate use. The donor should not be anemic and should be free of FeLV, the feline immunodeficiency virus (FIV), and *Hemobartonella felis.* In most cases, it is best to sedate or anesthetize the donor to ensure proper restraint. A combination of ketamine (50 mg) (Ketaset), diazepam (2.5 mg) (Valium), and atropine (0.2 mg) (Atropine Sulfate), given intravenously (IV), may be used for sedation of a 10-lb cat. Acepromazine (PromAce Injectable) should be avoided because it interferes with platelet function and lowers the blood pressure.[1]

No more than 6 mL of blood per pound of body weight should be taken from a donor, and an equal volume of replacement fluids should be administered. Most healthy adult cats can safely donate 50 mL of blood every 2 weeks. If the donor is used more often than every 30 days, the PCV should be assessed before any more blood is donated.[1] Replacement fluids are best administered IV immediately upon removal of the blood, but the administration of fluids intraperitoneally or even subcutaneously is often sufficient.

If the blood is to be used immediately, heparin is a suitable anticoagulant. Approximately 750 U (0.75 mL) of heparin should be drawn into a 60-mL syringe before blood collection. Although suitable for this purpose, heparin does have the disadvantage of activating platelets. Although active platelets will not be given the blood recipient, microthrombi may be. For this reason, acid-citrate-dextrose (ACD) and citrate-phosphate-dextrose-adenine (CPDA-1) are preferred over heparin for anticoagulation. CPDA-1 has the additional advantage of a prolonged storage life.[2] If either ACD or CPDA-1 is used, 8 mL of the anticoagulant solution should be placed in a 60-cc syringe before collecting the donor's blood.[1] An 18- or 19-gauge needle inserted into the jugular vein is the preferred collection method, but cardiopuncture has also been used successfully, albeit with an attendant risk of myocardial damage.

If the blood is to be stored for more than 24 hr, ACD solution or CPDA-1 is preferred. Both are more expensive than heparin, but use of ACD or CPDA-1 allows storage of blood at 40° F (i.e., refrigerator temperature) for 3 to 4 weeks and 6 weeks, respectively.[3] Blood collection bags are somewhat preferable to glass bottles because the latter may activate some clotting factors, and they do not preserve platelet function.[2] The Animal Blood Bank (PO Box 1118, Dixon, CA, 916–678–3009) is one source of cat-sized donor bags, CPDA-1, and cat-sized blood administration filters that minimize loss of blood when giving a transfusion.

In most situations, whole blood is administered IV. A 20-gauge butterfly catheter is inserted into one of the cephalic veins and attached to the filter-containing blood administration set. The cat's leg is attached to the end of a table or counter with a cord around the foot to keep the leg extended. When properly secured, one person can restrain the cat and administer the blood transfusion. The butterfly catheter allows for some movement of the recipient and for gentle mixing of the blood during administration (Fig. 10–2).

Blood may also be administered into the medullary cavity of the proximal femur. An 18- or 20-gauge needle is

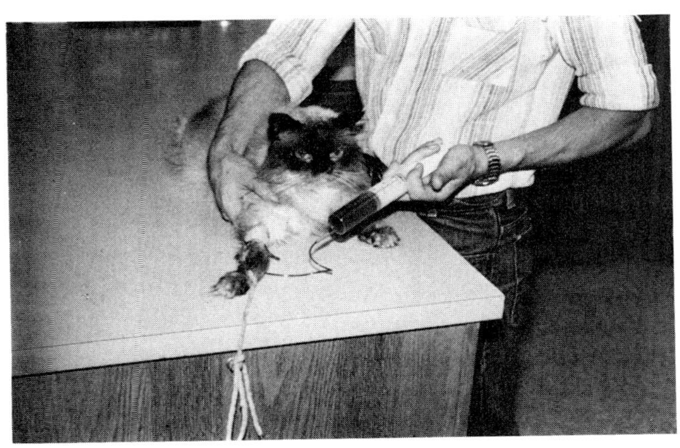

Figure 10–2. **A simple method of administering a blood transfusion begins by securing the cat's foot to the end of a table. Most cats will pull against the tie, thereby keeping the leg extended. A 19- or 20-gauge butterfly catheter is then placed in the cephalic vein; this allows the operator to restrain the cat and administer the blood simultaneously.**

inserted into the trochanteric fossa after administration of a local anesthetic. The blood is absorbed at the rate of approximately 1 drop per second.[4] The intraperitoneal route is not recommended because absorption is slow and incomplete.[1] Regardless of the mode of administration, blood should not be administered through a needle or catheter smaller than 20-gauge in order to minimize erythrocyte destruction.

The recommended administration rate is 4 to 5 mL per minute.[5] Rapid administration of blood may cause nausea and vomiting. If either of these occurs, the rate of administration should be reduced. During administration, the cat should be observed for facial edema or dyspnea, which would indicate a transfusion reaction. If either of these occurs, the transfusion should be discontinued and rapid-acting corticosteroids should be administered at shock dosage levels.

Crossmatching

Transfusion reactions can be life-threatening, or they may result in the destruction of the transfused erythrocytes. To avoid such a reaction, every effort should be made to crossmatch the blood types of the donor and recipient precisely.

The following procedure can be used to crossmatch blood types:

1. Collect small amounts of blood from the donor and the recipient in heparinized syringes or other containers. Separate the RBCs from the plasma by centrifugation for 10 minutes at 3,000 rpm.
2. Prepare the following for the test:
   - Donor plasma
   - Recipient plasma
   - Donor 4% RBC suspension*
   - Recipient 4% RBC suspension*
3. Set up four slides for the following tests:
   - ***Slide 1.*** 1 drop of donor plasma and 1 drop of donor 4% RBC suspension (donor control test: no reaction should be noted)
   - ***Slide 2.*** 1 drop of recipient plasma and 1 drop of recipient 4% RBC suspension (recipient control test: no reaction should be noted)
   - ***Slide 3.*** 1 drop of donor plasma and 1 drop of recipient 4% RBC suspension (minor crossmatch)
   - ***Slide 4.*** 1 drop of recipient plasma and 1 drop of donor 4% RBC suspension (major crossmatch)
4. Gently rock the slides from side to side.
5. Observe Slides 3 and 4 for agglutination reactions within 5 to 15 minutes (at room temperature).
6. Interpretation
   - Anti-A and Group A cells produce strong agglutination when mixed together.
   - Anti-B and Group B cells produce weak agglutination, which is generally not visible to the naked eye.
   - A Group-B recipient and a Group A donor:
     Slide 3—no reaction (negative)
     Slide 4—agglutination (positive)
   - A Group-A recipient and a Group B donor:
     Slide 3—agglutination (positive)
     Slide 4—no reaction (negative)[6]

*0.2 mL of packed RBCs and 4.8 mL of 0.9% saline

Frequency of Blood Types

If Type A or Type B blood is transfused into a *matched* recipient, the erythrocytic half-life (the maximum survival time of 50% of the erythrocytes) will be 33 days. If Type B blood is transfused into a Type A cat, the erythrocytic half-life will be 2.3 days and there will be a mild systemic reaction. If Type A blood is transfused into a Type B cat, the erythrocytic half-life will be 1.4 hours, and moderate to severe systemic signs of a reaction will be noted.[7] Thus, it would seem logical that crossmatching be performed prior to any transfusion.

However, the reality is that crossmatching is not routinely performed in most veterinary practices. For years, cats have been transfused without the benefit of crossmatching and with only rare transfusion reactions. Recent studies now explain why. In three studies conducted in the United States, the blood type of more than 1,000 cats was determined. In these studies, less than 1% of the cats tested were Type B.[8–10]

However, subsequent studies have found that certain lines of purebred cats have a significantly higher incidence of Type B blood than that found in domestic shorthair and longhair cats. In some breeds, as many as 59% of the cats tested had Type B blood. For a complete listing of breed incidence, see Table 10–1.[9–12] Therefore, before transfusing purebred cats, it is advisable to perform a crossmatch first. If incompatibility with the normal hospital donor is established, it will be necessary to find a Type B donor or to abort the transfusion.

The existence of Type AB blood has also been documented as a rare occurrence in cats in the United States.[13] It has been found in a few Scottish Fold, Birman, British Shorthair, and Domestic Shorthair (DSH) cats. Type AB cats can be safely transfused with either Type A or Type B blood.

Blood typing may be indicated for more than just blood transfusions. It is also useful when breeding purebred cats. Neonatal isoerythrolysis (NI) has been documented in cats and is one of the causes of the "fading kitten syndrome." If kittens receive antibodies to their RBCs from their queen

Table 10–1. Frequency of Blood Types in Cats in the United States

Breed	Number of cats	Type A (%)	Type B (%)
Domestic Shorthair (DSH)/Domestic Longhair (DLH)*	1,072	99.7	0.3
Abyssinian	194	79.8	20.1
Birman	216	82.4	17.6
British Shorthair	85	41.2	58.8
Devon Rex	100	57.0	43.0
Himalayan	35	80.0	20.0
Persian	170	75.9	24.1
Scottish Fold	27	85.2	14.8
Somali	27	77.8	22.2
Miscellaneous others†	41	80.5	19.5

*Of these, 964 were DSH and 108 were DLH; 82% were from the Philadelphia area.

†Less than 6 per breed.

Adapted from Giger U, Bucheler J, Patterson DF. Frequency and inheritance of A and B blood types in feline breeds of the United States. J Heredity 1991;82:15.

via the colostrum, NI will occur. This condition occurs most commonly when Type B queens are mated with Type A toms.[2] It can also occur in Type AB kittens born to Type B queens.[13] First or subsequent litters may be affected, and it may occur in one kitten or in the entire litter. To prevent NI, Type B queens should only be bred with Type B toms.[2]

Blood typing is available from many veterinary commercial laboratories or from the following:

Dr. Urs Giger
University of Pennsylvania
School of Veterinary Medicine
Section of Medical Genetics
3850 Spruce Street
Philadelphia, PA 19104–6010

Stormont Laboratories
1237 E. Beamer St.
Woodland, CA 95695

One half milliliter of EDTA blood is required.

Other Complications Associated with Transfusions[5]

Bacterial Contamination

Extreme care should be taken during collection and administration to prevent blood contamination. Dark brown or black supernatant plasma indicates digested hemoglobin from bacterial growth. If this blood is administered, the recipient will show a febrile response within 15 to 20 minutes.

Hemorrhage

If a large quantity of blood that is deficient in clotting factors (platelets, fibrinogen, Factors V and VIII) is administered, the recipient may experience bleeding. This can also occur if blood is stored in glass bottles; this is because the glass surface activates the platelets and Factor XII, resulting in their consumption.

Circulatory Overload

If the recipient has a normal blood volume and an increased venous return, vascular overload can occur if blood is transfused at a rapid rate. Cats with chronic anemia and impaired kidneys are most prone to this condition. Signs include vomiting, urticaria, and pulmonary edema. It is best not to exceed a rate of 10 mL of transfused blood per pound of body weight per 24 hours.[3]

Other Reactions

Pulmonary microembolization and respiratory insufficiency can occur if microaggregates develop in stored blood. If blood is stored for more than 5 days, it should be filtered. Most blood administration sets contain a filter. If too little blood is placed in an ACD bottle, citrate toxicity, in the form of hypocalcemia, can occur. When blood cells become hemolyzed, potassium is released. This can cause hyperkalemia, resulting in heart failure. Cardiac failure can also occur if cold, refrigerated blood is transfused. Stored blood should be warmed to body temperature before being used for a transfusion.

Quantity of Blood Transfused

The goal of a transfusion should be to elevate the PCV to a level that is high enough to get the cat out of danger, but not so high as to send negative feedback to the bone marrow, thereby causing it to decrease erythrocyte production. A PCV of 18% will satisfy both of these criteria.

Various formulas have been proposed to determine how much blood is appropriate for a transfusion. In order to be accurate, a formula must consider three factors:

1. The hematocrit or PCV of the recipient
2. The weight of the recipient
3. The hematocrit or PCV of the donor

Table 10–2 can be used to make this determination. This formula will result in the recipient's PCV rising to 18%.

Table 10–2. Volume of Blood (mL) Needed per Pound of Body Weight of Recipient Cat*

PCV of Recipient	PCV of Donated Blood (including anticoagulant)										
	30%	32%	34%	36%	38%	40%	42%	44%	46%	48%	50%
4%	16.3	15.3	14.4	13.6	12.9	12.3	11.7	11.1	10.6	10.2	9.8
6%	14.1	13.1	12.4	11.7	11.2	10.5	10.1	9.5	9.1	8.8	8.4
8%	11.7	10.9	10.3	9.7	9.2	8.8	8.3	8.1	7.6	7.3	7.1
10%	9.3	8.8	8.2	7.8	7.4	7.1	6.7	6.4	6.1	5.8	5.6
12%	7.1	6.6	6.2	5.8	5.5	5.3	5.1	4.8	4.6	4.4	4.2
14%	4.7	4.3	4.1	3.9	3.7	3.5	3.3	3.2	3.1	2.9	2.8

Example:	
PCV of recipient	6%
PCV of donated blood	46%
Weight of recipient	7 lb
Volume of blood needed per pound	9.1 mL (from table)
Mutiplied by weight of recipient	× 7 lb
Total volume of blood needed	63.7 mL*

*Based on posttransfusion PCV of 18%

Key: PCV, packed cell volume

Used by permission from Norsworthy GD. Blood transfusions in the cat. Feline Pract 1977;7:29.

Because of fluid compartment equilibrations, this predetermined PCV will not occur until about 12 to 24 hours following the transfusion. Therefore, in order to verify the results, a PCV should be performed on the recipient about 24 hours posttransfusion.

A note of precaution. Table 10–2 is based on the collective PCV of both the donated blood and the anticoagulant.[14] If heparin is used as the anticoagulant, its volume is so small that the PCV of the donated blood will not be affected by its addition. However, if ACD solution is used, its volume will cause considerable dilution of the donated blood, thus reducing the PCV. To allow for this, the PCV of the donated blood should be determined on the basis of the blood in the ACD bottle, not the blood taken directly from the donor cat.

REFERENCES

1. Rentko VT, Cotter SM. The procedure for treating anemic cats. Vet Med 1990;85:605.
2. Smith CA. Transfusion medicine: The challenge of practical use. J Am Vet Med Assoc 1991;198:747.
3. Green CE. Practical considerations of blood transfusion therapy. Proceedings, AAHA 47th Annual Meeting, San Francisco, CA, 1980:187.
4. Otto C. Intraosseous infusion of fluids and therapeutics. Compend Contin Educ Pract Vet 1989;11:421.
5. Blue J. Basic principles of feline blood transfusion. Feline Health Topics (Cornell University) 1990;1:4.
6. Auer LA, Bell K. Feline Blood Transfusion Reactions. In: Kirk RW, ed. Current Veterinary Therapy IX. Philadelphia: WB Saunders Co., 1985:515.
7. Bucheler J, Giger U. Transfusion of Type A and B blood in cats. Proceedings, 8th Annual American Colege of Veterinary Internal Medicine Forum, 1989.
8. Bird MS, Cotter SM, Gibbons G, Harris S. Blood groups in cats. Companion Anim Pract 1988;2:31.
9. Giger U, Kilrain CG, Filippich LJ, Bell K. Frequencies of feline blood groups in the United States. J Am Vet Med Assoc 1989;195:130.
10. Giger U, Bucheler J, Patterson DF. Frequency and inheritance of A and B blood types in feline breeds of the United States. J Heredity 1991;82:15.
11. Giger U. Frequency of feline A and B blood types in purebred cats and their clinical importance [Abstract]. Proc Am Soc Vet Clin Pathol 1989;40:7.
12. Giger U. Feline blood groups and incompatibility reactions. Proc Am Coll Vet Intern Med 1990;12:319.
13. Griot-Wenk M, Giger U. Cats with Type AB blood in the United States [Abstract]. J Vet Intern Med 1991;5:139.
14. Norsworthy GD. Blood transfusions in the cat. Feline Pract 1977;7:29.

CHAPTER 11

◇ ◇ ◇

Euthanasia and Grief Management

Gary D. Norsworthy and L. A. Norsworthy

Although the death of a patient is the veterinarian's ultimate failure, it is also ultimately inevitable. Death may occur in the young or the old; it may be anticipated or unexpected. But regardless of when or how, it will have effects on the pet owner and on the owner's relationship with the veterinarian. If the euthanasia procedure is handled well and appropriate respect is given the owner, the doctor/client relationship will be strengthened. However, if it is managed poorly, or if insensitivity is perceived by the owner, the client/doctor relationship will likely be permanently severed.

This chapter addresses the factors relating to euthanasia and how the veterinarian may assist the pet owner in dealing with the loss of a cherished pet.

Euthanasia

Indications

Euthanasia of a pet may be contemplated by the owner because of intense pain or suffering, terminal illness, poor quality of life, or owner convenience. Most owners consider euthanasia to be a viable option when the pet experiences persistent pain or suffering. If pain or suffering cannot be relieved with reasonable medical therapy, the owner may seek to protect the pet from continued discomfort by choosing euthanasia.

Progressive terminal illness becomes distressing to the cat and owner alike. When it becomes obvious that a disease cannot be controlled and/or the costs (both emotional and financial) are too great, euthanasia becomes a likely option. Euthanasia is also frequently chosen when the pet can no longer enjoy quality life. Although loss of "quality life" may have several definitions, it is generally defined as an inability of the cat to participate in the routine functions of being a family member and companion. However, in the case of a barn cat, it may be defined as no longer being able to chase mice, climb into the loft of the barn, or participate in other such activities.

Another reason for considering euthanasia is convenience. For example, the family may be moving into an apartment that will not allow pets, and a new home for the cat cannot be found. Another example would be the owner's desire to get rid of a cat that is not a desirable pet. This decision may be the result of a lack of affectionate behavior on the part of the cat, or of behavior that is objectionable, such as inappropriate elimination. This presents an ethical dilemma for both the owner and the veterinarian because a healthy cat is being considered for euthanasia. Each practitioner must carefully consider all aspects of this issue and make a decision that is acceptable to his or her value system. In doing this, the practitioner must realistically consider what is likely to happen to the cat if the request is denied. The alternative chosen by some owners may be less desirable than properly performed euthanasia.

Terms to Use and Terms to Avoid

Certain words related to death are rather harsh. These include "kill" and "expired." Words or phrases, such as "passed away," "passed on," "slipped away," or even "died" convey the same meaning without negative connotations.

Certain words related to what is done with the body are also harsh. These include "disposal," "dumpster," "landfill," and "city dump." It is far better to say that the cat was "buried," even if that burial occurred in a landfill. The term "euthanasia and disposal" is rather commonly used, but may be offensive to most owners.

Terms that can be misunderstood include "put down" and "put to sleep." The former term is commonly used by breeders to mean euthanasia. However, if a nonbreeder uses that term, always ask questions to be sure euthanasia is what is intended. "Put to sleep" can imply euthanasia or anesthesia. That, too, needs clarification before either is performed.

Who Should Make the Decision?

The cat is the legal and moral responsibility of the pet owner, and the ultimate decision for euthanasia rests with the owner. However, some owners are reluctant to make that irreversible decision. Some will defer to your expert knowledge and experience because they respect your judgment. Others simply do not want to feel responsible so they will thrust the decision on the veterinarian. They may verbalize, 'I cannot bring myself to do this." The concepts that need to be understood in this instance are sharing information, giving advice, and making a decision.

Sharing information is supplying the client with the facts in a neutral way. It involves conveying the results of a professional assessment of the medical situation of the cat to the owner in an objective manner. By contrast, giving advice is considering the facts and formulating an opinion of what actions are appropriate, based on one's own value system and understanding of the situation. Both of these approaches should prove beneficial to the client who makes the final decision. However, encouraging or leading the client into a decision may be perceived by the client as taking responsibility for the decision. This may seem expeditious at the time, but may result in difficulties later. If the client later regrets the decision or experiences cognizant dissonance (i.e., inner conflict) in the form of guilt, the practitioner will likely be held responsible.

On the other hand, if the veterinarian is asked to make the decision concerning euthanasia—"If this were your cat, what would you do, doctor?"—it is prudent to remind clients that only they know the value of the cat in the context of their relationship with that cat. However, if the owner persists, an honest opinion should be given.

In summary, sharing information should be done freely, giving advice should be done cautiously, and, except for exceptional situations, decision making should be left to the client.

Filling the Void

Sometimes euthanasia can be predicted several weeks or months in advance because of advancing age or a progressive disease. If so, the owner may wish to obtain another cat well in advance of the departure of the dying cat. If another cat is obtained in that manner, the void left by the dead cat will be "prefilled," so the sense of loss may not be as great.

However, if terminal illness or injury occurs suddenly, the void left in the family may be significant. If the emotional attachment to the dead cat is minimal or moderate, a replacement may be obtained immediately without adverse emotional consequences. However, if the emotional attachment to the dead cat is great, a cat that is quickly obtained may be viewed as a second-class replacement, or even resented by certain family members. In addition, this cat may be compared to the dead cat, never being perceived as an individual. If the replacement cat does not have most of the same qualities that endeared the dead one to the owner, it will become a disappointment to the owner, and may ultimately be rejected. Therefore, if terminal illness occurs suddenly, it is best to advise the owner to wait a few weeks or months to get another cat.

Timing

Euthanasia can cement the bonds between you and your client or it can destroy those bonds, depending upon how it is handled. Timing is one of the most important determinants of this outcome, and timing involves the cat and the owner(s).

The timing must be correct for the cat. The health of the cat must be such that euthanasia is truly indicated. This determination is generally based on pain or suffering and/or quality of life. Sometimes this determination is easily arrived at; other times, it may be equivocal. When the conclusion must be made on the basis of subjective criteria, clinicians must rely on their training and experience to make this judgment, and should convey this to the owner.

The timing must also be correct for the client. The client (and preferably all family members) must be convinced that euthanasia is in the best interest of the cat. This often requires that all family members be consulted, even children. It also may take several days of discussions within the family, with or without the veterinarian's input. However, if the decision is made prematurely, one or more family members may harbor resentments that may persist for many years.

Some diseases and trauma situations progress or occur so rapidly that it may be difficult for the owners to accept euthanasia readily. This is more likely to occur in feline patients than in other species because of the cat's secretive nature. Many very ill cats will conceal severe disease until the crisis level is reached. When such a cat is presented to the veterinarian, the owner may not have even remotely considered the possibility of euthanasia. In this situation, the owner's first impulse may be to reject that assessment and to request, or even demand, a second opinion. The clinician should not be offended by such a request, and should agree to it. In reality, the owner is not rejecting the veterinarian's clinical expertise, but rather is rejecting euthanasia because the timing is not correct. The owner is in a state of denial and has not had time to accept the finality of the situation. Fortunately, this state of denial may only last a few minutes to hours, and the client will generally become more rational and accepting of the outcome.

In summary, euthanasia should not be recommended until the owner(s) and preferably, all family members, are convinced that it is justified and necessary for the cat.

Supporting the Decision

Many owners will go through an agonizing process of deciding in favor of euthanasia. This is especially true if the cat does not have a terminal disease but is simply old, has multiple incurable but not fatal diseases, or has a history of recurrent illness. Such situations frequently produce feelings of guilt which the owner must address. These owners frequently verbally review the cat's medical history, often in great detail, as if preparing a case for the decision. This process occurs partially because of their respect for the veterinarian and partially because of their guilt feelings. Even though this is a time-consuming process, the client should be allowed to vent these feelings and pursue this course. The veterinarian should agree with the thought process and the decision. Otherwise, feelings of guilt may continue for many years and the client may no longer feel comfortable in the veterinarian's presence, seeking another veterinarian in the future.

Even when the cat's physical condition makes euthanasia clearly appropriate, many owners will still have doubts about whether or not the decision was correct. Once the decision is made, always verbally agree with it, even to the point of making statements that reinforce it. Realizing that this is an irreversible decision, statements such as, "This is really the right thing to do" will greatly help to remove doubts and guilt feelings that many owners will have. Commending the client's courage in making the right decision on behalf of the cat is also helpful.

A euthanasia release form is recommended. It should state that the cat has not bitten anyone recently and that the owner approves of the euthanasia. This is one method of documenting that euthanasia is what has been decided upon and ensuring that terms, such as "put down" or "put to sleep," have not been misinterpreted.

The Owner's Presence

Some owners wish to be present at the time of euthanasia. There are several possible motivations for such a request. The owner may simply wish to be with the cat "to the end." Other owners feel as if they are deserting the cat if they just leave their pet to be euthanized. Another possible motivation is a desire to be sure that the cat is actually dead. By observing the euthanasia, the client knows that the cat has not been the victim of experiments nor sold for research purposes. A third possible motivation is that the client needs to be assured that euthanasia was performed in a painless, humane manner.

If children are present, the clinician should briefly explain that the cat's death is final, that the pet is not suffering, and that everything possible was done to restore the cat to a state of health, but that it was not possible. After giving the child(ren) time to say goodbye to the pet, the veterinarian should ask if there are any questions. Even if they do not have any questions at that point, remember that it may take some time to formulate and express questions. Indeed, they may not ask questions until 2 or 3 weeks later.

The owner's presence can be important to the owner, but it can also increase the stress level. Therefore, if the owner asks for advice on this matter, the practitioner may choose to discourage him or her from observing the euthanasia on the basis that it may be more difficult for the owner in the long run. However, if the owner wishes to be present, this request should not be denied.

The location for euthanasia is important. The client(s), patient, and clinician should be alone in a quiet room. An examination room is often quite suitable; however, lasting negative memories may be associated with that particular room. On subsequent visits with other pets, some clients may request not to be put in that particular room again. Therefore, the use of the least-used examination room for euthanasia purposes should be considered.

The clinician should ensure that other events occurring in the hospital do not become distractions. Interruptions from incoming phone calls, another client, or nonemergency events should not be permitted. The client deserves the veterinarian's complete and undivided attention at that moment. An effort should also be made to ensure that conversations and laughter from other parts of the hospital are not audible, as these can be very distressing to clients.

Facial tissue should be provided for the client's convenience. Clients, especially men, frequently do not anticipate the need for such and are often unprepared. Your thoughtfulness will be appreciated.

When performing euthanasia in the presence of the owner, it is very important that the procedure go smoothly. Stroking the cat and talking to it are reassuring to the owner and are calming to the cat. These actions also allow the clinician to be remembered as a caring person, even in the face of a difficult task. If repeated attempts at venipuncture must be made, or if the cat struggles or cries in pain, the owner will be left with an indelibly negative impression. If the cat is fractious, pretreatment with a tranquilizer (acepromazine or xylazine) will usually be effective. If the cat has poor peripheral veins, advance placement of an intravenous (IV) catheter may be helpful, if possible. Cardiopunctures are distressing to most clients and should be reserved for desperate situations. A generous dose of euthanasia solution should be used to increase the rapidity of its action. If the cat gasps following the injection, this response should be explained as a reflex, and the owner should be assured that there was no pain or awareness on the part of the cat.

Following the injection, the heart should be auscultated with a stethoscope so that an official pronouncement of death can be made. This is something that the owner needs to hear. At that point, some clients wish to spend a few minutes alone with the pet's body. Others wish it to be removed immediately. The clinician should try to ascertain from the client's body language which is preferred. In either case, the client should be allowed to stay in the room for a few minutes to gather composure before facing other staff members or clients.

If the client has not already paid for the services and is visibly upset, it may be best to state that a bill will be sent in the mail rather than to request payment at this time. Most clients greatly appreciate this gesture, and collection problems rarely occur if the euthanasia and billing are handled in a professional manner. However, other clients may wish to clear their account before leaving as part of the closure process. Be sure that the needed information is relayed to the receptionist quickly so that the transaction is not prolonged.

Explaining What to Expect

When owners ask for a description of what euthanasia involves, they want to hear that it is quick and painless. It should be described as a procedure in which a drug, which is essentially an anesthetic, is injected IV. The owner should be told that the cat will go to sleep, as for surgery, but will not awaken.

It is alarming to many clients that the eyelids of the animal do not close at the time of death. Because of this, some may even question whether the cat is, in fact, dead. It may also be alarming to them that urination and defecation may occur with death. An explanation of these events prior to euthanasia is encouraged.

Technique

Two aspects of euthanasia must occur correctly: the choice of drug and its administration. The only nonscheduled, currently available drug approved by the Food and Drug Administration (FDA) for euthanasia is Beuthanasia-D Solution. However, its effects are not always as smooth and rapid as might be desired. By adding one part of ketamine to four parts of Beuthanasia-D Solution, the results are much smoother and more pleasing to the observing client. (The drugs will appear to precipitate when they are mixed, but the cloudiness in the syringe will disappear within 1 to 2 minutes.)

Smooth drug administration is critical if the client elects to observe the procedure. A clean cephalic venipuncture with a 22-gauge needle is the preferred approach. (Beuthanasia-D Solution does not pass through a 25-gauge needle very well.) However, if the veins have been punctured repeatedly, or if they do not distend fully, difficulty may be encountered. The medial saphenous vein is an alternative if the cephalic vein is not usable. If the cat is fractious, the procedure may be very difficult. If the situation permits, sedation of a fractious cat with acepromazine or xylazine prior to the euthanasia injection may be very helpful.

Disposition of the Body

Most veterinary practices offer several options for final disposition of the cat's body. Burial by the owner at home or on rural property, burial by a municipal agency, cremation, or burial in a pet cemetery are common examples. The clinician should understand the details and cost of each and be prepared to share this information with the owner. If euthanasia occurs unexpectedly, the owner may not be prepared to make a decision on this matter; in such cases, the practitioner should offer to store the cat's body, usually by freezing, until such a decision is possible. If burial on the owner's property or other available property is selected, the owner's child(ren) should be permitted to be present.

Sympathy Card

An expression of sympathy is both appropriate and appreciated in many situations. There are exceptions, but most clients will go through a grieving process and will appreciate the clinician's expression of concern and support (Fig. 11–1). The use of a sympathy card that is inscribed with a message, handwritten by the veterinarian and mailed in a hand-addressed envelope, is perceived as being both thoughtful and sincere. An appropriate inscription may follow these lines:

> Dear Mary,
>
> Fluffy was one of my very special patients. I will share in your loss.
>
> Thanks to your excellent care, she had many years of quality life. However, the decision you (or we) made was the correct one for Fluffy.
>
> Thanks for letting me be a part of her care.
>
> Personally Signed

The choice of the card is important. Several companies make cards with an inscription and picture that are very appropriate.* The sympathy card should be mailed the day of or day after euthanasia. If the client did not pay at the time of euthanasia, the bill for the services should be sent a day or two *after* the sympathy card is mailed. A record should be made of the specific card and personal inscription because if another cat belonging to the same owner is euthanized within a few weeks or months, the client is likely to recognize a duplicate card or inscription. Another solution is to buy sympathy cards in small quantities and change the card selected with each subsequent order.

Charges

Euthanasia is a legitimate professional service. The veterinarian incurs some direct costs, such as the drug used and, in some cases, the costs for burial of the body. However, some clients believe that this procedure should be performed at no charge in certain circumstances. The results of a survey conducted by Margaret Reister, DVM for *Cat Fancy Magazine* were published in the September, 1990 issue of this periodical. Dr. Reister cited one respondent whose feelings toward her veterinarian were very positive because two of her older cats that had required constant care were euthanized at no charge. Another respondent who paid for euthanasia of her cat was impressed that her veterinarian had made a contribution in honor of her cat to a local veterinary college. This is an issue that each practitioner must decide, but one that should be considered carefully.

Grief of Other Pets

Many cats or dogs that have lived in close association with a euthanized cat will also go through a grieving process. It is not unusual for the surviving pets to search the house for the missing pet for several days. They may refuse to eat, or they may only eat when coaxed or fed by hand. Some become very withdrawn, as if depressed. These pets should be given an extra amount of care and attention. Most go through their grieving process in 5 to 10 days, then return to normal.

By contrast, some surviving pets will actually become increasingly extroverted and affectionate. Generally, these pets were submissive to the deceased animal and now feel free to become dominant. If the owner obtains another pet, the surviving pet may again become the submissive one, or it may become even more determined to be the dominant pet in the household.

Grief Management

No matter what the cause of death, the owner is likely to experience a sense of loss. The veterinarian is in a unique position to help during this time. There is extensive literature in the area of grief, loss, and bereavement. Although

*Some companies that make cards of sympathy designed for veterinary clients include: Woodgeard Graphics, Inc., Rte. 5–12–765-Rte 34, Bryan, OH 43506; Straight Status, Inc., PO Box 445, New Castle, IN 47362; Pet Lover, Inc., PO Box 295, Shawnee Mission, KS 66201–0295; and SmartPractice, 3400 East McDowell, Phoenix, AZ 85008–7899.

June 10, 1992

Dr. Gary D. Norsworthy
Acres North Animal Hospital
16302 San Pedro
San Antonio, TX 78232

Dear Dr. Norsworthy,

We received your sympathy card today recognizing our loss of Whiskers, our pet and family member. Thank you so very much for your thoughtfulness and the concern which you exhibited toward Whiskers while he was under your care.

As a Doctor of Veterinary Medicine, and possibly a pet owner yourself, I am sure you recognize and appreciate the love, affection and loyalty that one develops for a pet, especially after so many years (15 years). My wife, Judy, and my daughter, Beth, were deeply touched by your card and were very grateful when I told them of your considerate and generous treatment of Whiskers and me at our last visit to your hospital.

Needless to say, I will be delighted to recommend you to anyone needing your professional services in the future. From one Aggie to another, again, thank you so much for your professionalism, TLC, and personal concern for Whiskers and his family.

Sincerely,

The LaVoy Family
(Bob, Judy, and Beth)

Figure 11–1. Euthanasia, if handled properly, can result in the owner having strong positive feelings toward the veterinarian. The sympathy card can be an important means of demonstrating your sensitivity to the situation, and it is usually very appreciated by the client.

most of the research has focused on the loss of a spouse, child, or other human loved one, much can be gained by reviewing and adapting this information to the loss of a pet.

Terminology

Many terms related to grief, loss, and bereavement have emerged from the literature of medicine, psychology, theology, philosophy, and literature. Consequently, many of the terms have been used interchangeably or ambiguously within varying contexts. Therefore, a few of the significant terms in this area need to be briefly defined.

Bereavement refers to a separation or loss through death.

Bereavement reactions consist of physiological, psychological, or behavioral responses to the death of another.

Grief is an intense feeling of emotional suffering caused by a loss through death. *Grief process* refers to the change of feeling states over time.

Grief work is the term applied to the concept that it requires energy or effort to "work through" a loss.

Factors Affecting the Grief Process

When a person loses a pet as a result of death, reactions may include a host of emotional responses ranging from depression to relief. In addition to the unique personalities of the owners, there are some factors that can be identified that can help explain and predict the reaction of the person to the loss of his or her pet. Burnell and Burnell have identified eight factors that are most important to clinicians when dealing with people working through the grief process.[1] These are:

1. The nature of the person's relationship to the deceased
2. The individual's coping behaviors and mental health
3. The individual's basic beliefs and attitudes toward death
4. The person's level of intelligence and maturity
5. The individual's past history of losses
6. The individual's ethical, cultural, and religious background
7. Any "unfinished business" with the deceased
8. The person's social support system

In trying to predict how a client might be affected by the loss of a pet, it is particularly important to consider the nature of the relationship with the pet or the needs that were met by the pet. If the pet was the individual's sole companion, a significant source of security, or a source of great emotional comfort, the person is likely to suffer a great sense of loss that will require a considerable time to complete the grief work, if it can be successfully done. The more knowledgeable the veterinarian is of the type of relationship the client had with the pet, the more effective he or she will be in intervening.

Categories of Grief Manifestation

Knowing the importance assigned to the pet by the owner can help the veterinarian predict the intensity of loss that is likely to follow the death of the pet. The clinician's sensitivity to the reactions of the owner may be increased by an awareness of the ways in which grief reactions may be manifested. The manifestations of grief in an adult can be classified into four categories:[1]

1. Physical symptoms
2. Mental symptoms
3. Emotional symptoms
4. Behavioral manifestations

Physical Symptoms. Researchers[2-4] have identified several physical symptoms that may be attributed to the grieving process. These include:

- Sensations of somatic distress
- A feeling of tightness in the throat
- Choking, with shortness of breath
- The need to sigh
- An empty feeling in the abdomen
- Muscle weakness
- Sobbing and crying
- Sensitivity to noise
- Tightness in the chest
- Lack of coordination
- Dry mouth
- Gastrointestinal disturbances
- Insomnia
- Marked irritability

Mental Symptoms. A variety of mental symptoms may be associated with the grief process, including:[1]

- Confusion and disbelief, especially in the initial stage
- Experiences of hearing and/or seeing the dead; this causes some people to retreat in silence, whereas others seek comfort in sharing these recent experiences with trusted friends, including their veterinarian
- An inability to concentrate, which may be manifested as:
  - Being absent-minded
  - Getting lost on the way to familiar places
  - Misplacing personal items
  - Missing appointments

Emotional Symptoms. Common emotional reactions are likely to include the following:[5-7]

- Denial
- Sadness
- Depression
- Guilt
- Anger
- Relief

Behavioral Manifestations. There are a host of behavioral changes that may result from the grieving process. These include:

- Self-damaging behaviors, including starting or increasing smoking, drinking, or drug abuse
- Withdrawal or avoidance of social occasions
- Aimless activities
- Avoidance of any reminder of the deceased or, conversely, a fascination with objects associated with the dead pet

Stages in the Grief Process

Averill[8] described three stages of grieving: shock, despair, and recovery. Several other theoreticians have modeled the grief process according to the stages of the dying process described by Kübler-Ross.[9] These stages are denial, bargaining, anger, depression, and acceptance. It should be kept in mind that the theories that conceptualize grief stages are not delineated by rigid boundaries; indeed, it would be misleading to do so. Instead, a person is likely to have characteristics of more than one stage at a time.

Likewise, the bereavement process has no sharp end point; rather, there are new levels of adaptation. Adaptation is probably best described as a process of replacing the dead pet with other involvements on both emotional and temporal levels. However, even when adaption is complete, it is not uncommon for the owner to experience a recurrence of grief during special times, such as the birthday of the deceased pet. Finally, even though there may not be any calendar or yardstick that can predict or measure how long the bereavement process will last, there are some significant factors that can be used as indicators. These include:

- The amount of time invested
- The significance of the pet
- The needs met by the pet
- The lack of other sources to meet the needs previously met by the pet
- The degree of attachment to the pet
- The cognitive development of the bereaved

Bereavement Reactions in Children

Age, or more specifically, cognitive development, is a salient factor that affects the grief reaction of a person. Several significant differences between children and adults have been noted in terms of their reactions to loss. The grief process of children varies in duration and intensity according to their age and cognitive development. A child's ability to conceptualize death has been explained by several sources. In a study by Burnell and Burnell,[1] children who had been classified according to age exhibited some important distinguishing characteristics with regard to their reactions to loss.

Two- and Three-Year-Olds

Children who are 2 or 3 years of age typically have no idea of what death means. They are likely to confuse death with sleep. By the age of 3, the concept of death may cause some anxiety, although this occurs more commonly at ages 5 to 6. Children younger than 3 years of age may manifest grief through the loss of speech and generalized distress. Children who are 2 or 3 years of age should be told that their pet has died and that the pet will not return. To allay any guilt feelings, the child should be told that the reason the pet will not return is unrelated to any rejection of the child or to anything the child may have said or done. Generally, children in this age group have no difficulty replacing the lost pet with another.

Four-, Five- and Six-Year-Olds

Children ages 4 through 6 are likely to have some understanding of death, albeit in a limited capacity. Frequently, children in this age group associate death with life and consciousness. From the child's perspective, the pet may be thought to live in the ground while continuing to eat, breathe, and play. Alternatively, the child may assume that the pet has gone somewhere else and is asleep, though still alive. During this time span, the child is likely to believe that death is reversible and not final. Thus, they might expect the pet to return.

Children of these ages tend to conceptualize death as an unnatural event. Thus, they may need reassurance that it is a natural and inevitable occurrence. They may suspect that angry feelings can assure death. Therefore, they need to know that any anger they may have had toward the pet was not responsible for the death of their pet. It is also very important for a child to know that their anger, or that of others, will not cause their own death. The death of their pet may cause the frightening realization that they, too, may die, causing them to think that it is only by being lucky and careful that they can avoid it. They should be reassured that they will not die because of the death of their pet. In other words, let them know that death is not contagious.

Children in this age group may manifest their grief by disturbances in bladder and bowel control, eating, and sleeping. If any of these behaviors occur, the child should be encouraged to talk about the loss of their pet and should be given help in identifying and expressing their concerns and feelings. It should be remembered that children's expressions of intense emotions are not continuous. Therefore, they are more likely to benefit from several brief discussions about death, rather than one or a few prolonged discussions.

Seven-, Eight-, and Nine-Year-Olds

Children in this age group begin to understand the irreversibility of death. Generally, such children believe that death only occurs to others. Thus, their personal security may not be threatened by death unless they begin to direct their concern about death to their parents. This worry might be expressed in a question such as "Who will take care of me if . . . ?" Children of these ages tend to be very curious about death. Therefore, it is particularly important to give them time to ask questions. Parents should listen to their statements and answer their questions as clearly as possible.

Children in this age group might exhibit their grief through the development of school problems, learning problems antisocial behavior, hypochondriacal concerns, or aggression. Other manifestations of grief may include withdrawal, overattentiveness, or clinging behavior.[10] Cain, Fast, and Erickson,[11] in writing about the effects of the loss of a sibling, stated that troublesome emotions and behaviors may appear months or even years after the loss. Although this has not specifically been documented in the case of the loss of a pet, one should be sensitive to the possibility that the symptoms of grief might not occur immediately following the death of a pet.

Ten- and Eleven-Year-Olds

Children ages 10 and 11 years generally come to understand death as a process that is natural, inevitable, and universal. Death is understood as final, and the reactions of children older than 11 years of age tend to be the same as those of adults. However, variations do occur, depending on the child's emotional and intellectual development.[12]

Adolescents

Much of the information presented thus far in this text has focused on the adult pet owner. Using the chronological ages of 12 through 18 years as the period of adolescence, very few differences have been identified between adolescents and adults in terms of their reactions to losses. However, one predominant reaction that is associated with adolescence is denial. It would be invalid to assume that a lack of emotional display of grief means that the adolescent is not grieving. It is also likely that acting out behaviors, such as the use of alcohol, drugs, or tobacco, or sexual promiscuity, may be manifested as displaced grief.

Recommendations for the Veterinarian

As a way of summarizing these findings, the following list of "do's and don'ts" in dealing with survivors, adapted from Burnell and Burnell, may be applied to the pet owner.[1] Because there is great variation in the degree of an owner's attachment to a pet, the clinician must use good judgment in determining which of these suggestions are appropriate.

- Always be truthful. Do not attempt to shield the pet owner by withholding information. Tell the pet owner everything you honestly know.
- When telling the pet owner about the cat's death, be available for a short period of time. If the owner is notified by telephone, remain on the line long enough

to allow the person to begin to accept the reality of the death, and be available to answer questions. If you tell the owner in person about the pet's death, remain available long enough for them to begin to accept the reality of the death, and be available to answer questions. Be supportive and reassure owners that you understand that the death of their pet can cause an intense sense of loss and pain.

- Be prepared for denial to be an initial response to the news. It may be necessary to repeat information about the loss several times. Denial is a process of protecting oneself from the pain of the loss. Therefore, let the pet owner set the pace for acceptance of the loss.
- Use terminology that can be easily understood. When someone is upset, they may have little desire or energy to ask for clarifications.
- Prepare the pet owner for what they will see. Explain that the eyelids of the cat will not be closed. If trauma was the cause of death, prepare them for the fact that certain parts of the body may be missing or abnormal. If surgical equipment is present (including an endotracheal tube), explain its use before it is seen. The general appearance of the room should be neat and clean.
- Reassure the pet owner that all reasonable measures were taken to preserve life. Even if it seems obvious, it is important to explain that everything within the realm of current technology was utilized.
- Always refer to the pet by name after death. This shows appropriate respect for the significance of the pet.
- Answer questions about suffering. Reassure them that everything possible was done to avoid suffering. In the case of euthanasia, explain that the pet did not suffer during the procedure.
- Allow time for the owners to be with their pet after death. Allowing adequate time to be alone with the pet after death may be an important component of the healing process in response to grief.
- Be prepared for expressions of anger. This is not a time to be defensive, or to change the subject. The focus should be on the owner's pain, with demonstration of empathetic understanding and support. The more you show appropriate sensitivity to their feelings, the more likely pet owners will associate pleasant memories, rather than negative ones, with you and the clinic. This increases the likelihood that they will continue to return to your clinic for the care of other or future pets.
- Validate the pet owner's grief. Pet owners may think that their feelings are inappropriate or not understood. Your acknowledgment and acceptance of their feelings can be very reassuring and comforting to them.
- Avoid such phrases as "You'll get over it," as these statements may convey the message that you do not believe that the owner's pet was very important, or that the owner's feelings are appropriate. The phrase, "Time will ease the pain," is more likely to be perceived as being supportive. Refrain from saying "I understand how you feel," because people react differently to similar situations. Rather, the phrase, "It must be hard for you," is more likely to be well-received by the owner as an acknowledgment of his or her pain.
- Send a sympathy card or other expression of your understanding and concern.
- Consider making a donation in the pet's name to a veterinary foundation* or to a veterinary school.
- Recommend the Pet Loss Support Hotline, University of California at Davis, 1–916–752–4200. This line is operational from 6:30 to 9:30 PM (Pacific Time), Monday through Friday.
- Make the following suggestions to parents concerning their children's reactions.†

1. The news of the cat's death should never be withheld from a child. To avoid guilt, frightening fantasies, and fears, the truth should be explained in simple terms and questions should be encouraged.
2. The child should be reassured that everything was done to provide quality life as long as possible.
3. If the cat's death occurs unexpectedly, any misinterpretations by the child should be quickly corrected.
4. Children should be reassured that they cannot die in connection with the death of their pet. Explain that death is not contagious.
5. The child may have a tendency to feel responsible for the death because of past anger toward the pet or lack of care for the pet (i.e., not feeding, etc.). Reassure them that they are not responsible for the death of the cat.
6. Have the child repeat what is understood about the cat's death as though they were speaking to a friend. This provides an opportunity to clarify misconceptions and to check their understanding.

REFERENCES

1. Burnell GM, Burnell AL. Clinical Management of Bereavement: A Handbook for Health Care Professionals. New York: Human Services Press, 1989:35.
2. Parkes CM, Brown RJ. Health after bereavement: A controlled study of young Boston widows and widowers. Psychosomatic Med 1972;34:449.
3. Warden JW. Grief Counseling and Grief Therapy. New York: Springer, 1982.
4. Holmes TH, Rabe RH. The social readjustment rating scale. J Psychosomatic Res 1967:11:213.
5. Kalish RA. Death, Grief and Caring Relationship. Monterey, CA: Brooks Cole, 1985.
6. Parks CM, Weiss RS. Recovery From Bereavement. New York: Basic Books, 1983.
7. Engel GL. A life setting conducive to illness: The giving-up-given-up complex. Ann Intern Med 1968;69(2):294.
8. Averill JR. Grief: Its nature and significance. Psychological Bull 1968;70:721.
9. Kübler-Ross E. On Death and Dying. New York: Macmillan, 1983.

*One such foundation is the American Animal Hospital Association Foundation, PO Box 150899, Denver, CO 80215–0899; 303–279–2500.

†Adapted from Burnell GM, Burnell AL. Clinical Management of Bereavement: A Handbook for Health Care Professionals. New York: Human Services Press, 1989:35.

10. Raphael B. The Anatomy of Bereavement. New York: Basic Books, 1983.
11. Cain A, Fast I, Erickson M. Children's disturbed reactions to the death of a sibling. Am J Orthopsychiatry 1964;34:741.
12. Gartley W, Bernasconi M. The concept of death in children. J Genet Psychol 1967;110:71.

SUPPLEMENTAL REFERENCES

For Adults

1. Anderson MK. Coping With Sorrow on the Loss of Your Pet. Riverside, NJ: Peregrine Press, 1987.
2. Church JA. Joy in a Woolly Coat. New York: H. J. Kramer, Inc., 1987
3. Jewett CL. Helping Children Cope with Separation and Loss. Boston: The Harvard Common Press, 1982.
4. Mooney S. A Snowflake in My Hand. New York: Dell Publishing, 1983.
5. Nieburg HA, Fisher A. Pet Loss: A Thoughtful Guide for Adults and Children. New York: Harper & Row, 1982.
6. Quackenbush J, Graveline D. When Your Pet Dies: How to Cope with Your Feelings. (New York: Simon & Schuster, 1985.
7. Tatlebaum J. You Don't Have to Suffer: A Handbook for Moving Beyond Life's Crises. New York: Harper & Row, 1989.

For Children

1. Balter L. A Funeral for Whiskers. New York: Barron's Educational Series, 1991.
2. Eatrick C. The Accident. Boston: Clarion Books, 1976.
3. Mellonie B, Ingpen R. Lifetimes. New York: Bantam Books, 1983.
4. Rogers F. When a Pet Dies. New York: G. P. Putnam & Sons, 1988.
5. Viorst J. The Tenth Good Thing About Barney. Philadelphia: Atheneum, 1975.
6. Wilhelm H. I'll Always Love You. Glendale, CA: Crown Publishing Group, 1985.

PART II

◇ ◇ ◇

Diagnostics

CHAPTER 12

◇ ◇ ◇

Laboratory Tests and Testing

Gary D. Norsworthy

In the last 20 years, there has been a tremendous increase in the number of laboratory tests available to the veterinary practitioner. The tests that are now available at a reasonable cost allow the practitioner to diagnose many diseases that, only a few years ago, could be diagnosed only by histopathologic studies or necropsy. The purpose of this chapter is to discuss relevant facts concerning feline laboratory testing and to present the techniques for and interpretation of some of these tests.

Important Concepts

Sensitivity versus Specificity

The sensitivity and specificity of various laboratory tests allow us to determine their accuracy and reliability.

Sensitivity refers to the amount of antigen, antibody, or other substance that is detectable by a given test. If the test has a high sensitivity, only a minute quantity of the substance need be present to be detected. Tests with high sensitivity are unlikely to yield false-negative results. Conversely, if the test has a low sensitivity, the likelihood of false-negative results increases.

Specificity refers to the ability of a test to demonstrate a positive reaction only to the substance in question. If a test has a high specificity, it will be unlikely to test positive for any other substance; thus, false-positive results are unlikely. Conversely, if the test has a low specificity, false-positive results are more likely to occur.

Some examples of feline tests can be used to illustrate these concepts. For instance, one of the early tests for feline leukemia virus (FeLV) antigens was also found to react to murine leukemia virus antigens, so a positive result could mean infection with either virus. Therefore, that test was said to have a low specificity. However, because false-negative results were unlikely, it was considered to be a highly sensitive test. By contrast, some tests for heartworm antigens have been found to have a low sensitivity, as demonstrated by one study in which fewer than 75% of the cats that had heartworms at necropsy had previously tested positive for heartworm antigens. Thus a low sensitivity meant a significant number of false-negative results.

Antigen versus Antibody Tests

Some of the tests for feline diseases detect the presence of antigens and some detect antibodies. There are important differences between the two that impact on test results.

Testing for the presence of antigen is a direct test for the presence of the pathogen in question. If an antigen test with a high sensitivity and high specificity yields a positive result, one can be assured that the pathogen is present. Examples of feline antigen tests currently in use include the FeLV test (indirect fluorescent antibody [IFA], blood enzyme-linked immunosorbent assay [ELISA], and tears/saliva ELISA) and some of the tests for heartworm. (Heartworm antibody tests are also available.) If these tests are positive, one can be assured that the pathogen is present because the test detects antigen released from the pathogen.

Testing for antibodies is not as straightforward, as there are several potential problems that may interfere with accurate test results. Because antibodies are produced by the host and not the pathogen, an effective immune response must be present. If this does not occur, false-negative results will be reported. It may take several days to several months for cats to develop antibodies after the initial exposure to a virus. This time period varies with the specific virus involved. Cats that are infected with the feline immunodeficiency virus (FIV) take at least 2 weeks, and up to 2 years, to develop enough antibodies to react to the test. During that prepatent period, the test will be negative even though the virus has infected the cat. During the terminal stages of an FIV infection or feline infectious peritonitis (FIP), antibody depletion may occur. As more and more virus (antigen) is produced, antigen:antibody complexing occurs at an increased rate until there are no longer any free antibodies in the serum. With no antibodies present, the antibody test will be negative. This is one of the greatest frustrations of veterinary practice.

Normal Values

The following reference values are listed for the reader's convenience. Because commercial veterinary laboratories may use different normal values as a result of regional or technical variations, the reader is encouraged to consult the specific laboratory for possible adjustments to the values listed.

*Biochemical Profile**

Test	Normal Value	Unit
Hematologic Values		
White blood cells (WBC)	5.5–19.5	$\times 10^3/mm^3$
Red blood cells (RBC)	5.5–10.0	$\times 10^6/mm^3$
Hemoglobin (Hb)	8–15	g/dL
Hematocrit (Hct)	25–45	%
Mean corpuscular volume (MCV)	39–55	μm^3
Mean corpuscular hemoglobin (MCH)	13–17	μg
Mean corpuscular hemoglobin concentration (MCHC)	30–36	%
Monocytes	3–10	%
Lymphocytes	12–30	%
Segmented neutrophils	60–70	%
Prothrombin time (PT)	5–13	sec
Activated partial thrombo-plastin time (APTT)	10–20	sec
Fibrinogen	100–400	mg/dL
Platelets	200–800	$\times 10^3$
Biochemical Values		
Glucose	70–115	mg/dL
Blood urea nitrogen (BUN)	15–35	mg/dL
Creatinine	1.0–2.0	mg/dL
Cholesterol	75–150	mg/dL
Total bilirubin	0.0–0.8	mg/dL
Direct bilirubin	0.0–0.6	mg/dL
Total protein	5.2–7.9	g/dL
Albumin	2.1–4.0	g/dL
Globulin	3.9–6.5	g/dL
Albumin/globulin (A/G) ratio	0.5–1.3	Ratio
Alkaline phosphatase	10–200	μ/L
Aspartate aminotransferase (AST [SGOT])	5–100	μ/L
Alanine aminotransferase (ALT [SGPT])	10–150	μ/L
Lactate dehydrogenase (LDH)	10–400	μ/L
Creatinine phosphokinase (CPK)	10–500	μ/L
Amylase	0–2600	μ/dL
Lipase	0–700	μ/L
Calcium	7.2–12.2	mg/dL
Phosphorus	3.0–5.5	mg/dL
Sodium	145–155	mEq/L
Potassium	4.3–5.2	mEq/L
Chloride	111–126	mEq/L
Total Carbon dioxide (CO_2)	17–28	mEq/L
Anion gap	12–30	mEq/L
Serum osmolality	280–325	mOsm/kg
Sodium/potassium (Na/K) ratio	29–41	
Protein/creatine ratio	0–0.25	
Protein, quantitative	0–5	mg/kg/24 h
Bile acids	0–15	mmol/L
Gamma-glutamyl transpeptidase (GGTP)	1–20	μ/L

(continued)

*Used by permission of Dr. Robert Bartsch, Southwest Veterinary Diagnostic Laboratory, Phoenix, AZ.

Hemostatic Values

Test	Normal Value	Unit
Activated clotting time	<65	sec[1]
Bleeding time	1–5	min[2]
Whole blood coagulation time (glass)	8	min[2]
Whole blood coagulation time (cap tube)	5.0–5.4	min[3]
Activated coagulation time of whole blood at room temperature	60–125	sec[4]
PT	8.1–9.1	sec[3]
Russell's viper venom time	9	sec[5]
Prothrombin consumption	20	sec[5]

*Blood Values at Different Ages**

Age	RBC (millions/ µL)	Hb (g/dL)	Packed Cell Volume (PCV) (%)	WBC (µL)	Neutrophils (per µL)	Lymphocytes (per µL)
Birth	4.95	12.2	44.7	7,500		
2 weeks	4.76	9.7	31.1	8,080		
5 weeks	5.84	8.4	29.9	8,550		
Average	4.80	7.5	26.2	11,770	4,600	6,970
Range	3.90–5.70	6.6–8.4	21.0–33.5	7,500–14,500		4,500–9,400
6 weeks	6.75	9.0	35.4	8,420		
8 weeks	7.10	9.4	35.6	8,420		4,900
Average	5.90	7.5	26.2	12,400	7,500	1,925–10,100
Range	3.30–7.30	7.5–15.0	22–38	6,900–23,100		

*Modified from Jain NC, Hematologic Values. In: Jain NC, Schalm's Veterinary Hematology, 4th ed. Philadelphia: Lea & Febiger, 1986.

*Endocrine Tests**

Test	Normal Value	Unit
Triiodothyronine (T_3)	60–140	ng/dL
Thyroxine (T_4)	0.6–2.5	µg/dL
Free T_4	3.0–9.0	pmol/L
Pre–thyroid-stimulating hormone (TSH)	0.6–3.5	µg/dL
Post-TSH	2–3 × normal resting value	µg/dL
Cortisol	2.5–6.0	µg/dL
Pre-adrenocorticotropic hormone (ACTH)	2.5–6.0	µg/dL
Post-ACTH	3–4 × normal resting non-stressed value	µg/dL
Pre-dexamethasone	2.5–6.0	µg/dL
Post-dexamethasone	½ of baseline value (low dose)	µg/dL
Post-dexamethasone, 6–8 h	<1.0 (high dose)	µg/dL
Progesterone	18+: pregnancy or corpus luteum phase (PG Dx only to Day 40)	ng/mL
Progesterone	0–14: Cyclic or follicular phase	ng/dL

*Used by permission of Dr. Robert Bartsch, Southwest Veterinary Diagnostic Laboratory, Phoenix, AZ.

*Protein Electrophoresis**

Test	Normal Value	Unit
Total protein	5.2–7.9	g/dL
Albumin	2.1–3.3	g/dL
Globulin		
Alpha 1	0.2–1.1	g/dL
Alpha 2	0.4–0.9	g/dL
Beta	0.9–1.9	g/dL
Gamma	1.7–4.4	g/dL

*Used by permission of Dr. Robert Bartsch, Southwest Veterinary Diagnostic Laboratory, Phoenix, AZ.

Bone Marrow[7]

Test	Normal Value	Unit
Erythrocytic cells	26	%
Granulocytic cells	59	%
Myeloid:erythroid ratio (average)	2.47:1	
Myeloid:erythroid ratio (range)	0.60–3.90:1	
Other cells	15	%

Urine[7]

Test	Normal Value	Unit
Color	Light yellow	
Turbidity	Clear	
pH	5.0–7.0	
Specific gravity		
Minimum	1.001	
Maximum	1.080	
Usual limits (normal food & water intake)	1.018–1.050	
Volume	22–30	mg/kg/day
Osmolality		
Usual range	500–1200	mOsm/kg
Maximal limits	2,000–2,400	mOsm/kg
Osmolality plasma	300	mOsm/kg
Creatinine	110–280	mg/dL
Urea	1.0–3.0	g/dL
Protein	0–20	mg/dL
Amylase	30–120	Somogyi units
Protein sulfosalicylic acid	0–trace	
Protein Multistix (Miles Laboratories)	0–1+	
Glucose	0	
Ketones	0	
Bilirubin	0	
Cats with high specific gravity (5%)	1+	
Urobilinogen	0–1	Ehrlich unit
Urobilinogen	< 1:32	Wallace-Diamond

Cerebrospinal Fluid[7]

Test	Normal Value	Unit
Color	Clear; colorless	
Pressure	<100	mm H_2O
Cells	<5	% lymphocytes per µL
Protein	<20	mL/dL
Glucose	85	mg/dL

*Electrocardiographic Values in Lead II**

Test	Normal Value
Heart Rate (beats per minute)	140–240
Rhythm	Sinus rhythm, infrequent sinus arrhythmia
P wave	0.2 mV, 0.04 sec; positive in leads II & aV1; may be isoelectric or positive in lead I
PR interval	0.05–0.09 sec (inversely related to heart rate)
QRS complex	0.9 mV, 0.04 sec; more variable than in the dog; the mean electric axis in the frontal plane is often insignificant. Often, the QRS complex is nearly isoelectric in all frontal plane limb leads (horizontal heart).
QT interval	0.16–0.18 sec
ST segment	No significant depression, elevation, or coving
T wave	0.3 mV; should be free of repolarization charges and marked depression or elevation
Electrical axis	0–160°

*From Allen DG. Special Techniques. In: Allen, DG, ed. Small Animal Medicine. Philadelphia: JB Lippincott, 1991:1035; and Ettinger SJ. Cardiac Arrhythmias. In: Ettinger SJ, ed. Textbook of Veterinary Internal Medicine. Philadelphia: WB Saunders, 1989:1055. Used by permission.

Diseases Affecting Common Feline Tests

The following charts are intended to be used as quick references when interpreting various tests. These are not exhaustive lists, but represent the most common disease conditions that should be considered. The reader is referred to Appendix F for a similar approach to diseases based on predominant clinical signs. The combination of these two sources can be very helpful in the diagnostic process.

Diseases Affecting the Complete Blood Count (CBC)[10–15]

Packed Cell Volume, Red Blood Cells and Hemoglobin

Decreased

Hemorrhage

Trauma
Surgery
Clotting Disorders
Hookworm
Fleas

Hemolysis

Hemobartonellosis
Autoimmune disease
Cytauxzoonosis
Propylthiouracil
Drugs causing Heinz body anemias (see Chapter 42)
FeLV (rare)

Bone marrow suppression

FeLV
FIV
Chronic inflammatory diseases
Bone marrow neoplasia, including LSA
Drugs (CHPC, etc.)
Deficiencies (B_{12}, folic acid, iron, etc.)
Chronic renal failure

Increased

Dehydration
Hyperthyroidism
Hypoxemia (cardiopulmonary disease)
Splenic contraction

Total White Blood Cells

Decreased

FeLV
Panleukopenia
Overwhelming sepsis
FIV
Bone marrow neoplasia, including LSA
Bone marrow exhaustion or arrest

Increased

Physiologic causes (epinephrine)
Stress (glucocorticoids)
Chronic inflammation
Chronic infection
Leukemias (FeLV)

Neutrophils

Decreased

FeLV
Panleukopenia
Drugs (chloramphenicol, etc.)
Overwhelming sepsis, including bacterial peritonitis
Acute viral infections
FIV

Increased

Physiologic causes (epinephrine)
Stress/excitement (glucocorticoids)
Acute or chronic inflammation
Acute or chronic infection
Granulocytic leukemia (FeLV) (rare)

Lymphocytes

Decreased

Glucocorticoids (exogenous or hyperadrenocorticism, ACTH therapy)
Chronic infections/debilitating disease
Surgery/trauma/shock
Renal failure
Chylothorax with repeated chest drainage
Chemotherapy/irradiation

Increased

Physiologic stress/excitement
Chronic inflammation
Lymphocytic leukemia (FeLV)
Lymphosarcoma (FeLV)
Temporary increase following some vaccinations

Eosinophils

Decreased

Glucocorticoids (exogenous or hyperadrenocorticism, ACTH therapy)
Inflammation with stress

Increased[1,11,12,15,16]

Parasitism (hookworms, roundworms, tapeworms, lungworms, heartworms, fleas, mosquito bites)
Ear mites
Toxoplasma species
Giardia species
Cutrebra species
Allergic bronchitis/asthma
Eosinophilic gastroenteritis (chronic inflammatory bowel disease)
Dermatitis (allergic, eosinophilic granuloma complex, pemphigus foliaceus, systemic lupus erythematosus [SLE])
Masteocytoma (mast cell tumor)
Eosinophilic leukemia (FeLV)
Hypereosinophilic syndrome
Mast cell leukemia (FeLV)
Hypersensitivity/anaphylaxis
Hypoadrenocorticism (not a consistent finding)
Infections (chronic sinusitis/rhinitis, panleukopenia)
Enteric lymphosarcoma
Chronic feline urologic syndrome
Chronic renal disease
Cardiomyopathy
Immune-mediated hemolytic anemia
Hyperthyroidism
Soft tissue trauma (chronic inflammation)

Basophils

Increased

Concurrent with eosinophilia in hypersensitivity (heartworm disease)
Masteocytoma (Mast cell tumor)
Chronic inflammation of skin and mucous membranes
Hyperadrenocorticism

Monocytes

Increased

Chronic inflammation/necrosis
Internal hemorrhage
Hemolytic diseases

Suppuration in body cavity (FIP, pyothorax, etc.)
Monocytic leukemia (FeLV) (rare)

Thrombocytes

Decreased

FeLV diseases
Autoimmune thrombocytopenia
Splenomegaly
Disseminated intravascular coagulation (DIC)
Drugs
Bone marrow neoplasia, including LSA
Bone marrow exhaustion or arrest

Increased

Drugs (vincristine)
Splenectomy
Acute hemorrhage
Chronic infections
Trauma
Iron deficiency secondary to chronic hemorrhage

Diseases Affecting the Biochemical Profile[11,13,14]

Alanine Aminotransferase (ALT, Formerly SGPT)

Increased

Cholangiohepatitis
LSA (FeLV)
Hepatic lipidosis
FIP hepatopathy
Liver toxins (acetaminophen, etc.)
Liver trauma

Albumin

Decreased

Chronic hepatic insufficiency
Chronic starvation
Hemorrhage
Renal insufficiency (with proteinuria)
Ascites
Pleural effusion
Intravenous (IV) fluids
Hypoadrenocorticism
Protein-losing enteropathy

Increased

Dehydration

Alkaline Phosphatase

Increased

Cholangiohepatitis
Hepatic LSA (FeLV)
Hepatic lipidosis
FIP hepatopathy
Cholestasis
Bone growth in young kittens
Corticosteroids (endogenous or exogenous)

Amylase/Lipase

Increased

Pancreatic inflammation, necrosis, or neoplasia
Renal disease
Intra-abdominal diseases
Diabetic ketoacidosis
Neoplasia of the liver

Anion Gap

Decreased

Decreased albumin levels
Hypercalcemia
Hypermagnesemia
Multiple myeloma

Increased

Diabetes mellitus (ketoacidosis)
Azotemia
Dehydration
Drugs (penicillin, carbenicillin, salicylate)
Dehydration
Hypocalcemia
Hypomagnesemia

Bicarbonate (HCO_3)

Decreased

Diarrhea
Renal failure
Diabetes mellitus (ketoacidosis)
Drugs (ammonium chloride, ethylene glycol)

Increased

Vomiting of gastric contents
Drugs (sodium bicarbonate, lactate, citrate)

Bilirubin

Increased*

Hepatocellular disease (>50% direct bilirubin)
Biliary obstruction (>75% direct bilirubin)
Hemolysis (>50% indirect bilirubin)

Calcium

Decreased

Renal failure
Necrotizing pancreatitis
Ethylene glycol toxicity (antifreeze)
Dietary deficiency
Hypoparathyroidism (secondary to thyroidectomy, all-meat diets)
Hypovitaminosis D
Phosphate-containing enema
Hypoalbuminemia
Hyperadrenocorticism
Artifactual (chelation by ethylenediamine tetraacetic acid [EDTA])

*These percentages are less reliable in the cat than in the dog, but are useful generalities, especially in the first few days of disease.

Increased

Young, growing kittens
Neoplasia, especially lymphosarcoma
Hypervitaminosis D (dietary)
Hypoadrenocorticism
Artifactual (lipemia)

Globulin

Decreased

Chronic hepatic insufficiency
Chronic starvation
IV fluids

Increased

Chronic inflammation (FIP, systemic fungal diseases, chronic gingivitis, etc.)
Neoplasia (LSA, plasma cell myeloma, etc.)

Glucose

Decreased

Starvation
Chronic malabsorption
Hepatic insufficiency
Hypoadrenocorticism
Chronic sepsis
Islet cell tumor of the pancreas (rare)
Sample held on erythrocytes
Overdose of insulin

Increased

Diabetes mellitus
Physiologic (epinephrine)
Drugs (glucocorticoids; progesterones, including megestrol acetate [Ovaban], glucose-containing fluids; ACTH therapy)
Hyperadrenocorticism
Postprandial testing
Acute pancreatitis
Overdose of insulin (Somogyi overswing)

Phosphorus

Decreased

Inadequate dietary intake
Hypercalcemia of neoplasia (pseudohyperparathyroidism)
Excess insulin (iatrogenic or insulinoma-induced)
Diabetes mellitus
Hypovitaminosis D
Glucose-containing fluids (intracellular shift)
Alkalosis (intracellular shift)

Increased

Artifactual (sample held on erythrocytes or hemolysis)
Young cats
Decreased renal function
Hypervitaminosis D
Hypoparathyroidism (secondary to thyroidectomy, all-meat diet)
Tissue trauma or necrosis

Potassium

Decreased

Vomiting
Diarrhea
Excessive HCO_3 or lactate therapy
Hyperpnea/metabolic alkalosis (pleural effusion, pneumonia, etc.)
Insulin therapy
Chronic anorexia
Chronic hepatic insufficiency
Drugs (furosemide, mannitol, 5% dextrose, corticosteroids, etc.)
Chronic renal failure
Postobstructive diuresis
Hyperadrenocorticism

Increased

Urethral obstruction
Ruptured ureter, bladder, or urethra
Hypoadrenocorticism
Massive crush injuries
Acidosis (diabetes mellitus, etc.)
Severe or acute renal failure
Artifactual (thrombocytosis)

Sodium

Decreased

Increased glucose or protein
Vomiting
Severe diarrhea
Hypoadrenocorticism
Diuretics
Renal failure
Congestive heart failure
IV fluids with low sodium content (especially 5% dextrose)
Hypervolemia
Compulsive water drinking
Metabolic acidosis
Hypothyroidism

Increased

Vomiting
Diarrhea
Renal water loss (diabetes insipidus, renal insufficiency, hyperadrenocorticism, pyometra, etc.)
Water deprivation
Increased sodium intake (dietary, IV fluids, $NaHCO_3$, etc.)
Diabetes mellitus (nonketotic)

Blood Urea Nitrogen (BUN)

Decreased

Protein-restricted diet
Urea loss secondary to polyuria/polydipsia
Urea loss secondary to IV fluids
Hepatic shunt

Increased

Prerenal (dehydration, decreased cardiac output, shock, high-protein diet [BUN only])
Renal insufficiency
Postrenal (urethral obstruction; ruptured ureter, bladder, or urethra)

Laboratory Tests

There are a number of important tests that are performed on feline patients on an infrequent basis. Some of these are discussed because their infrequent use means that the technique and interpretation must be researched each time they are used.

Most blood analysis is done by commercial veterinary laboratories. However, there are some situations in which rapid answers are needed. Some of the tests presented in this chapter are included because they may be performed while the results of more sophisticated laboratory tests are pending.

ACTH Level (Endogenous)

Purpose/Indication: To differentiate cats with pituitary-dependent hyperadrenocorticism (PDH) from those with functioning adrenocortical tumors

Technique: Submit plasma for ACTH level.

Interpretation:
1. >40 pg/mL: PDH
2. <20 pg/mL: Adrenocortical tumor

ACTH Stimulation Test

Purpose/Indication: To determine whether the adrenal cortex has the ability to be stimulated or overstimulated by ACTH; used in cats that are thought to have hyperadrenocorticism

Materials:
ACTH gel
2 Heparinized syringes

Technique:
1. The cat should fast for at least 12 hours.
2. Collect a preinjection, heparinized blood sample.
3. Inject ACTH gel at the rate of 1 U/lb intramuscularly (IM).
4. Collect a 30-minute postinjection, heparinized blood sample.

Interpretation:
1. Normal[17]
   - Baseline: 1.0–4.4 μg/dL (mean: 2.9 μg/dL)
   - 30-minute: 6.8–12.1 μg/dL (mean: 11.1 μg/dL)
2. Likely abnormalities
   - Hyperadrenocorticism*[17]
     a. Baseline: 1.2–11.5 μg/dL (mean: 5.6 μg/dL)
     b. 30-minute: 12.1–25.7 μg/dL (mean: 16.7 μg/dL)
   - Hypoadrenocorticism: Little change over baseline value.

*Note: There is some overlap in terms of test results between normal and hyperadrenocorticoid cats.

Activated Clotting Time[18]

Purpose/Indication: To test the cat's intrinsic blood clotting system; used to diagnose bleeding disorders

Materials: Glass tube containing diatomaceous earth (Becton-Dickinson, tube No. 6522).

Technique:
1. Place 2 mL of whole blood in the tube.
2. Incubate the sample at 37°C for 60 seconds and then evaluate it every 5 seconds until clotting occurs.

Interpretation:
1. Normal: <65 seconds[19]
2. Likely abnormalities: The clotting time will be prolonged if the intrinsic blood clotting system is defective. However, more than 95% of the coagulation proteins must be absent for the time to be prolonged.

Baermann Technique

Purpose/Indication: To recover parasite eggs (especially those of lungworms) that are heavier than the standard solutions used for fecal flotation; indicated for cats with a cough

Materials:
Funnel or beaker with an exit port at the bottom
Rubber hose attached to the exit port
Clamp to occlude the rubber hose
Fecal flotation solution
Microscope slide
Microscope

Technique:
1. Place the fecal sample and a standard fecal flotation solution in the funnel or beaker
2. Macerate the fecal sample to release the eggs.
3. Allow the material to stand in the funnel or beaker for 5 to 10 minutes.
4. Collect a sample from the rubber tube, exiting the bottom of the apparatus, for microscopic examination.

Interpretation: Likely abnormalities: The eggs of *Capillaria aerophila* or *Aelurostrongylus abstrussus* will be recovered from most cats with lungworms.

Bile Acid Concentrations[19]

Purpose/Indication: To test for the level of bile acids in serum following a meal (as bile acids are produced and cleared by the liver, this is a test of liver function); used in cases in which liver failure or biliary obstruction is suspected.

Materials: Can of cat food

Technique:
1. After a 12-hour fast, collect a serum sample.
2. After feeding the cat, collect a 2-hour postprandial serum sample.

Interpretation:
1. Normal: Fasting sample: <2 μmol/L, postprandial sample: <10 μmol/L

2. Likely abnormalities: In hepatic disease, either or both samples will be >20 μmol/L, which is an indication for a liver biopsy.

Bone Marrow Aspiration

Purpose/Indication: To collect cells from the bone marrow for examination; used to detect diseases of the hematopoietic system when a CBC is not diagnostic.

*Materials:**

16- or 18-gauge biopsy needle (Jorvet Bone Marrow Needle, Jorgensen Laboratories, Loveland, Co., or Rosenthal or Osgood Needle, Becton-Dickinson Co., Rutherford, NJ)
12-mL syringe
Scalpel with pointed blade (optional)
Surgical drape
Watch glass
Microhematocrit tubes
Microscope
Microscopic slides
Stain

Technique:

1. Administer general anesthetic to or heavily sedate the cat.
2. Surgically prep a 2- to 3-cm in diameter area of the skin over the greater trochanter of one femur. (The bone marrow may also be aspirated from the proximal humerus and the ilium.)
3. Cover the area with a surgical drape.
4. Make a nick incision in the skin over the greater trochanter (optional).
5. While palpating the greater trochanter, insert the biopsy needle through the skin and soft tissue until it comes into contact with the greater trochanter.
6. Advance the biopsy needle medially until it falls into the trochanteric fossa (Fig. 12–1 *A, B*). Be careful not to pierce the sciatic nerve. If the sciatic nerve is encountered, the leg will twitch.
7. With a twisting motion, force the biopsy needle through the cortex and into the marrow cavity (Fig. 12–1*C*). Remove the stylet from the biopsy needle.
8. Using the 12-mL syringe, aspirate material until a blood-like substance enters the syringe. A sample of 0.5 to 1.0 mL is sufficient.
9. Spray the marrow aspirate onto a watch glass. Tilt the watch glass so that the liquid runs away from the particles of bone (Fig. 12–2).
10. Using a microhematocrit tube or pipette, pick up 2 or 3 particles of bone (Fig. 12–3), then place them on a microscopic slide.
11. Lightly crush the particles of bone with another microscopic slide, then pull the slides apart.
12. Allow the slide to air-dry, then stain it. If it is to be sent to a laboratory for interpretation, it should be air-dried or fixed in methanol, but not stained. Sev-

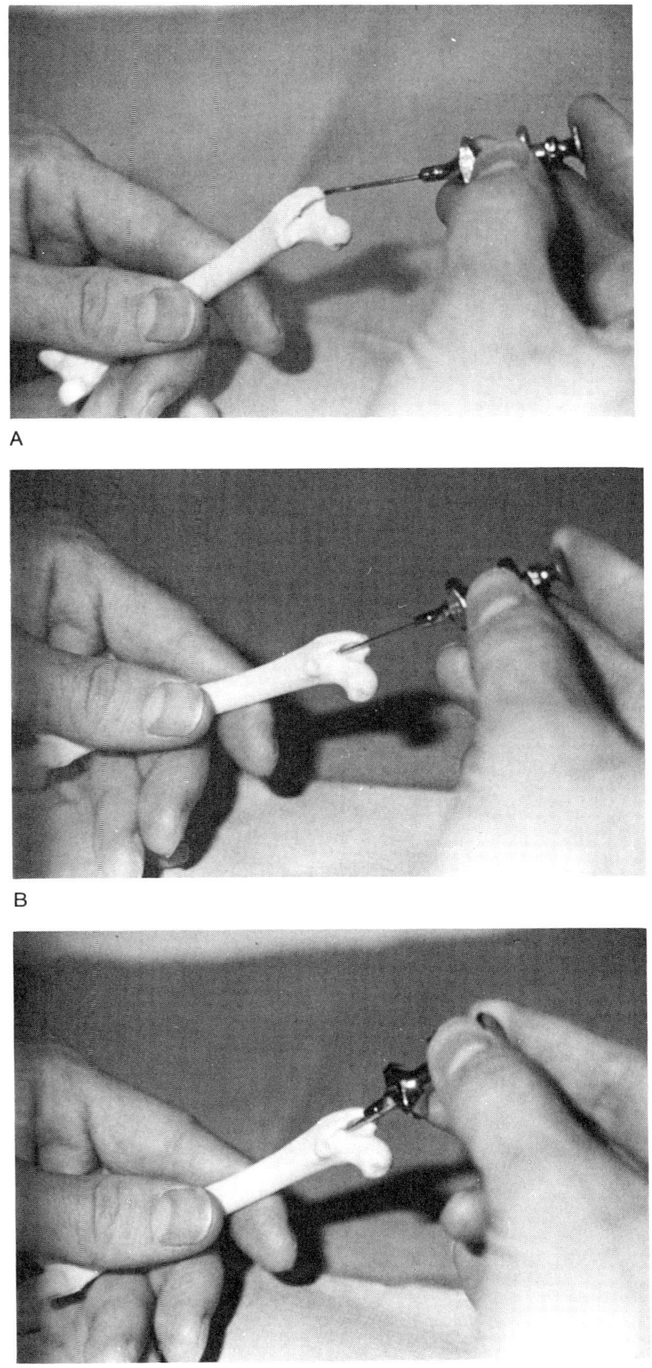

A

B

C

Figure 12–1. Bone marrow aspiration. (*A*) The tip of the needle is placed on the greater trochanter. (*B*) The tip of the needle is "walked off" the greater trochanter into the trochanteric fossa. (*C*) With a twisting motion, the needle is forced into the marrow cavity.

*Note: The use of an anticoagulant is discouraged because of the possible adverse effects on cell morphology. However, it is preferred by many clinicians.

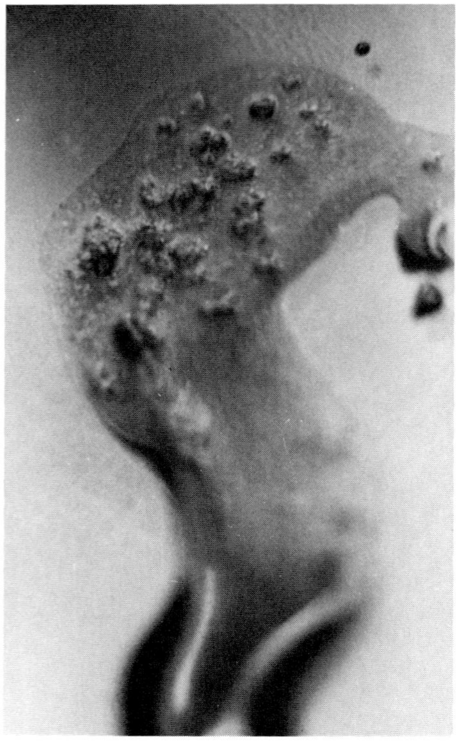

Figure 12–2. **The watch glass is tipped so that the blood runs away from the particles of bone.**

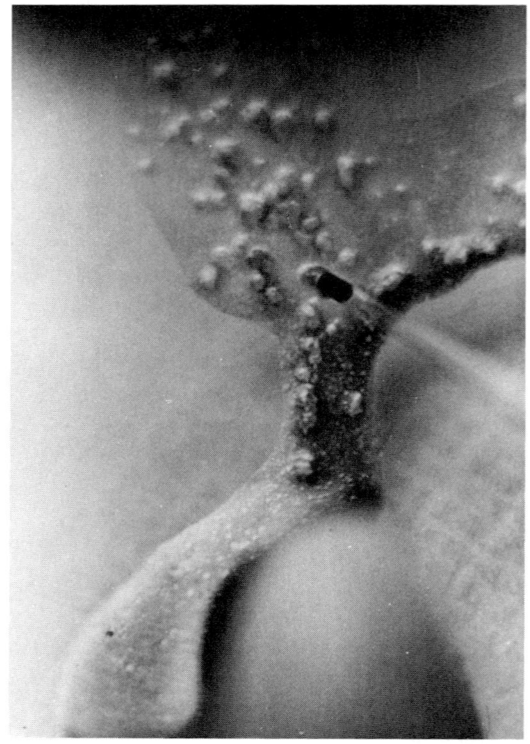

Figure 12–3. **The particles of bone obtained by bone marrow aspiration are picked up using a hematocrit tube or a pipette.**

eral slides should be submitted so special stains can be performed if needed.

13. Examine the slide under magnification (100× and 1,000×).

Interpretation:

1. Normal: The normal feline myeloid-erythroid ratio is reported to be 1.6:1.0.[20]
2. Likely abnormalities: An overwhelming increase of one cell line may indicate a leukemia or a physiologic need for certain cells. For example, an acute bacterial infection will stimulate myeloid cell production, and anemia will stimulate erythroid cell production. Marrow exhaustion is typified by a lack of cellularity of the specimen. Poor technique will also produce a scantily cellular sample.

Buffy Coat Prep

Purpose/Indication: To assemble a concentration of white blood cells; used to facilitate examination of large numbers of WBCs, most notably to detect mast cells when a mast cell tumor has been diagnosed

Materials:

1 to 3 mL of whole blood with anticoagulant
Centrifuge
Centrifuge tube
Microscope
Microscopic slide
Blood stain
Microhematocrit tube

Technique:

1. Centrifuge blood for 5 minutes at 3,500 rpm.
2. Cover the top end of the microhematocrit tube with one finger.
3. Lower the bottom end of the microhematocrit tube through the plasma layer of the blood to the buffy coat layer (between the plasma and the RBCs).
4. Remove the finger from the top of the microhematocrit tube to allow the buffy coat layer to enter the tube.
5. Reposition the finger on top of the microhematocrit tube.
6. Remove the microhematocrit tube from the centrifuge tube.
7. Blow the cells in the microhematocrit tube onto the microscopic slide.
8. Smear the cells onto the slide, as for a routine blood smear.
9. Stain the slide and examine it under magnification (1,000×).

Interpretation: Likely abnormalities: If the mast cell tumor has metastasized to the bone marrow, spleen, or liver, mast cells (and large numbers of eosinophils) will be present.

Cholinesterase[21]

Purpose/Indication: To confirm or exclude organophosphate toxicity

Likely Abnormality: Toxicity is confirmed if the cholinesterase level is less than 500 U/L.

Creatinine Clearance Test (Endogenous)[22]

Purpose/Indication: To measure reduced glomerular filtration rate (GFR) in an effort to detect abnormalities before BUN and serum creatinine levels are elevated; used in animals with polydipsia and polyuria that have normal BUN and creatinine levels.

Technique:

1. Weigh the cat (kg).
2. Determine the collection time interval. This may range from 20 minutes to 24 hours. The longer the time, the more accurate the results.
3. Empty the cat's bladder by manual expression or catheterization. If the collection time is to span less than 2 hours, the bladder should be rinsed with saline to remove any creatinine that might be adherent.
4. At the midpoint of the collection time, draw blood for serum creatinine testing.
5. Collect urine periodically so that all of the urine is obtained during the collection period. If the bladder was rinsed initially, rinse it again and add the saline wash solution to the collected urine.
6. Record the amount of time in the collection period and the amount of urine collected.
7. Mix all of the urine (and any saline wash solution) collected. Remove one aliquot.
8. Determine the creatinine concentration in the aliquot of urine.
9. Calculate the creatinine (CR) clearance by applying the following formula:

   $$\text{Creatinine clearance} = [(U\ Cr)\ (U\ V)] / [(S\ Cr)\ (T)\ (Wt)]$$

   where U Cr is urine creatinine (mg/dL), U V is urine volume (mL), S Cr is serum creatinine (mg/dL), T is time (minutes), and Wt is weight (kg).

Interpretation: Normal: 1.6–3.8 mL/min/kg

Ether Clearance Test[23]

Purpose/Indication: To determine whether a fluid is chyle or pseudochyle; used when milky colored fluid is removed from the chest cavity

Materials:

2 test tubes
10% Potassium hydroxide
Diethyl ether

Technique:

1. Place one part of the suspect fluid in each of two test tubes.
2. Add 2 drops of 10% potassium hydroxide to each tube.
3. Add one part water to one tube and one part diethyl ether to the other.
4. Mix both tubes by inverting them.

Interpretation:

1. Chyle: The fluid in the diethyl ether tube will become transparent. (The tube containing water is a control. It will remain milky.)
2. Pseudochyle: The fluid in the diethyl ether tube will remain milky. (The tube containing water is a control. It will also remain milky.)

Fat Absorption Test

Purpose/Indication: To determine whether fat is being absorbed from the gastrointestinal tract; used when maldigestion or malabsorption is suspected

Materials:

Corn oil
Several heparinized blood samples

Technique:

1. Administer corn oil to the cat via a stomach tube at a rate of 5 mL/kg.
2. Collect 1 mL of heparinized blood at 0, 1, 2, 3, and 4 hours.
3. Centrifuge each sample to observe for the presence of lipemia.
4. If lipemia does not occur, repeat the test as described, except add 1 tablespoon of Viokase Powder to the corn oil prior to administration.

Interpretation:

1. Normal: Lipemia will occur in at least one of the samples when corn oil is administered without Viokase.
2. Likely Abnormalities:
   - Malabsorption: No lipemia will occur with administration of corn oil alone.
   - Maldigestion: No lipemia will occur with administration of corn oil and Viokase.

Heinz Body Stain*

To identify Heinz bodies on RBCs

Purpose/Indication: When Heinz body anemia (methemoglobinemia) is suspected

Materials:

1 mL of anticoagulated blood
Microhematocrit tube
2 microscopic slides
New methylene blue stain

Technique:

1. Place one drop of anticoagulated blood and one drop of new methylene blue stain on a microscopic slide.
2. Using the microhematocrit tube, mix the two together.
3. Fill the microhematocrit tube with the mixture.
4. Allow the mixture to incubate at room temperature for 15 minutes.
5. Blow one drop of the mixture onto the second mi-

*This is the same procedure as a reticulocyte stain. Heinz bodies can also be seen with a modified Wright's stain; however, they will not be stained a different color than the rest of the RBCs.

croscopic slide and smear it as for a routine blood smear.

6. Allow the slide to dry; then examine it under magnification (1,000 ×).

Interpretation:

1. Normal: Less than 2% of RBCs should contain Heinz bodies. Cats eating foods containing propylene glycol (semi-moist foods) are likely to have an increased number of Heinz bodies despite being clinically normal.
2. Likely Abnormality: If more than 10% of the RBCs contain Heinz bodies, methemoglobinemia of any cause (i.e., acetaminophen, methylene blue, etc.) is present. (See Chapter 42.)

Platelet Estimation

Purpose/Indication: To make a rapid platelet estimation

Technique:

1. Formula 1: Platelet count/μL = (number of platelets/number of WBCs) × WBC/μL[24]
2. Formula 2: Platelet count/μL = (number of platelets per oil immersion field × 20,000)[19]

Reticulocyte Count

Purpose/Indication: To quantify the percentage of reticulocytes in the peripheral RBC population; used to determine whether an anemia is regenerative or nonregenerative (i.e., whether the bone marrow is responsive). (See Chapter 16.)

Materials:

1 mL of anticoagulated blood
Microhematocrit tube
2 Microscopic slides
New methylene blue stain

Technique:

1. Place one drop of anticoagulated blood and one drop of new methylene blue stain on a microscopic slide.
2. Using the microhematocrit tube, mix the two together.
3. Fill the microhematocrit tube with the mixture.
4. Allow the mixture to incubate at room temperature for 15 minutes.
5. Blow one drop of the mixture onto the second microscopic slide and smear it as for a routine blood smear.
6. Allow the slide to dry, then examine it under magnification (1,000 ×).

Interpretation:

1. Normal: Feline reticulocytes have two forms—punctate and reticulated. The small punctate forms are not counted. The large reticulated ones are counted as a percentage of the total number of RBCs. A regenerative anemia will have a corrected (aggregate) reticulocyte count of 4% or greater.
2. Likely Abnormality: A nonregenerative anemia will have a corrected (aggregate) reticulocyte count of less than 2%.

Reticulocyte Count (Corrected)

Purpose/Indication: To correct the reticulocyte count for determining the PCV* of the patient.

Technique: Corrected reticulocytes = Actual PCV/Normal PCV × % reticulocytes

T_3 Suppression Test[25]

Purpose/Indication: To determine thyroid function; appropriate for cats with clinical signs of hyperthyroidism but with a normal or marginally elevated T_4 level.

Materials: Liothyronine (Cytomel or Cytobin)

Technique:

1. Collect blood to determine T_3 and T_4 levels. Separate serum and freeze or refrigerate.
2. Administer liothyronine (25–30 μg) q8h for 7 doses.
3. Two to four hours after the seventh dose, collect blood for the second T_3 and T_4 level determinations.
4. Submit the pre-pill and post-pill blood samples for T_3 and T_4 determinations at the same time to the same laboratory.

Interpretation:†

1. Normal: A post-pill T_4 level of less than 1.5 μg/dL, and a T_4 level that is 50% or less of the pre-pill T_4 level.
2. Likely abnormalities: In cats with hyperthyroidism, the post-pill T_4 level will be greater than 1.5 μg/dL.

Transtracheal Wash[8]

Purpose/Indication: To collect material for analysis from the trachea, bronchi, and possibly, the bronchioles; useful in diagnosing respiratory diseases when radiographs and other tests are not diagnostic.‡

Materials:

12- to 18-inch, 14- to 16-gauge IV catheter
20 mL of nonbacteriostatic, sterile saline
6- or 12-mL syringe

Technique:

1. Heavily sedate or anesthetize the cat.
2. Clip and prep the skin of the ventral cervical area just caudal to the larynx.
3. Pass the catheter through the skin, between two tracheal rings, and down the trachea to the level of the primary or secondary bronchi.
4. Inject 3 to 5 mL of saline through the catheter. As soon as a cough occurs, as much of the saline as possible should be aspirated into the syringe. (The yield is unlikely to exceed 20%.)

*Note: The normal PCV of the cat should be designated as 35%.

†Note: If the post-pill T_3 level is not greater than the pre-pill T_3 level, the liothyronine was not administered or absorbed properly and the test should be repeated.

‡A lung aspirate is often more meaningful, as the sample is taken directly from the lung parenchyma. That procedure should be performed first in most cases. (See Chapter 13.)

5. Repeat the procedure up to three times until a visibly productive sample is obtained.
6. Perform bacterial culture and cytology.

Interpretation:

1. Normal: A few inflammatory cells, including some eosinophils, may be recovered.
2. Likely abnormalities:
   - Bronchopneumonia: Recovery of an excessive number of inflammatory cells and/or bacteria
   - Asthma or heartworms: A large number of eosinophils
   - Neoplasia: Rarely, recovery of neoplastic cells

Tracheal Wash*[8]

Purpose/Indication: To collect material for analysis from the trachea, bronchi, and possibly, the bronchioles; useful in diagnosing respiratory diseases when radiographs and other tests are not diagnostic.†

Materials:

12- to 18-inch, 14- to 16-gauge sterile urinary catheter
Sterile endotracheal tube
20 mL of nonbacteriostatic, sterile saline
6- or 12-mL syringe

Technique:

1. Anesthetize the cat.
2. Pass the endotracheal tube into the trachea so that it does not become contaminated with oral cavity substances.
3. Pass the catheter through the endotracheal tube and down the trachea to the level of the primary or secondary bronchi.
4. Inject 3 to 5 mL of saline through the catheter. As soon as a cough occurs, as much of the saline as possible should be aspirated into the syringe. (The yield is unlikely to exceed 20%.)
5. Repeat the procedure up to three times until a visibly productive sample is obtained.
6. Perform bacterial culture and cytology.

Interpretation:

1. Normal: Recovery of a few inflammatory cells, including some eosinophils
2. Likely abnormalities:
   - Bronchopneumonia: Recovery of an excessive number of inflammatory cells and/or bacteria
   - Asthma or heartworms: A large number of eosinophils
   - Neoplasia: Rarely, recovery of neoplastic cells

Trichogram[26]

Purpose/Indication: To determine whether or not a cat's hair loss is attributable to self-trauma (chewing, scratching, licking)

Materials:

1 Microscope slide
Microscope
A few drops of mineral oil
Serrated thumb forceps or small hemostats

Technique:

1. Using the thumb forceps or hemostats, pluck a tuft of hair from the periphery of the area of hair loss.
2. Place the hair in a drop of mineral oil on the microscopic slide.
3. Examine under magnification (100 ×) and (1000 ×), concentrating on the distal ends of the hair shafts.*

Interpretation:

1. Normal: In cats with nontraumatic hair loss, the distal ends of the hair shafts will be tapered to a point.
2. Likely abnormality: In traumatic hair loss, the distal end of the hair shafts will be blunted and ragged.

WBC Count (Corrected)[24]

Purpose/Indication: To correct the WBC count for the presence of circulating nucleated RBCs (NRBC) in cats with suspected regenerative anemia

Technique:

$$\text{Corrected WBC} = (\text{initial WBC} \times 100) / (100 + \text{NRBC})$$

WBC Estimation from Blood Smear[24]

Purpose/Indication: To rapidly estimate the WBC count

Technique:

$$\text{WBC} = (\text{average number of WBC/HPF}\dagger \times \text{patient's PCV}) / 33\% \text{ (mean normal PCV for species)}$$

WBC Estimation from Hct Tube[24]

Purpose/Indication: To rapidly estimate the WBC count

Technique: The first percent of the buffy coat equals 20,000 WBC/μL. Each subsequent percent equals 10,000 WBC/μL.

REFERENCES

1. Bartsch R. Personal communication. Southwest Veterinary Diagnostic Laboratory, Phoenix, AZ.
2. Seager SW, Fletcher WS. Collection, storage, and insemination of canine semen. Lab Anim Sci 1972;22:177.
3. Osbaldiston GW, Stowe EC, Griffith PR. Blood coagulation: Comparative studies in dogs, cats, horses, and cattle. Br Vet J 1970;126:512.
4. Byars TD, Ling GV, Ferris NA, Keeton KS. Activated coagulation time (ACT) of whole blood in normal dogs. Am J Vet Res 1976;37:1359.
5. Rowsell HC. Blood Coagulation and Hemorrhage Disorders. In: Medway W, Prier JE, Wilkinson JS, eds. Textbook of Veterinary Clinical Pathology. Baltimore: Williams and Wilkins, 1969:247.

*This is basically the same procedure as a transtracheal wash, but the catheter and the method of passing the catheter into the lungs are different.

†A lung aspirate is often more meaningful, as the sample is taken from the lung parenchyma. That procedure should be performed first in most cases.

*The examination will be easier if the distal ends of the hair shafts are placed together on the slide.

†HPF = high-power field.

6. Jain NC. Hematologic Values. In: Jain NC. Schalm's Veterinary Hematology, 4th ed. Philadelphia: Lea & Febiger, 1986.
7. Bentinck-Smith J, French TW. A Roster of Normal Values for Dogs and Cats. In: Kirk RW, ed. Current Veterinary Therapy X 1989:1335.
8. Allen DG. Special Techniques. In: Allen DG, ed. Small Animal Medicine. Philadelphia: JB Lippincott, 1991:1035.
9. Ettinger SJ. Cardiac Arrhythmias. In: Ettinger SJ, ed. Textbook of Veterinary Internal Medicine. Philadelphia: WB Saunders, 1989:1055.
10. Green CE. Hematologic Problems. In: Lorenz MD, Cornelius LM, eds. Small Animal Medical Diagnosis. Philadelphia: JB Lippincott, 1987:527.
11. Rich LJ, Coles EH. Tables of Abnormal Blood Values as a Guide to Disease Syndromes. In: Ettinger SJ, ed. Textbook of Veterinary Internal Medicine, 3rd ed. Philadelphia: WB Saunders, 1989:11.
12. Center SA, Randolph JF. Eosinophilia. In: August JR, ed. Consultations in Feline Internal Medicine. Philadelphia: WB Saunders Co, 1991:349.
13. Cornelius LM. Abnormalities of the Standard Biochemical Profile. In: Lorenz MD, Cornelius LM, eds. Small Animal Medical Diagnosis. Philadelphia: JB Lippincott, 1987:539.
14. Cornelius LM. Abnormal Blood Gases, pH, and Anion Gap. In: Lorenz MD, Cornelius LM, eds. Small Animal Medical Diagnosis. Philadelphia: JB Lippincott, 1987:604.
15. Mason KV, Evans AG. Mosquito bite-caused eosinophilic dermatitis in cats. J Am Vet Med Assoc 1991;198:2086.
16. Neer TM. Hypereosinophilic syndrome in cats. Compend Contin Educ Pract Vet 1991;13:549.
17. Feldman EC, Nelson RW. Hyperadrenocorticism: Feline Cushing's Syndrome. In: Feldman EC, Nelson RW, eds. Canine and Feline Endocrinology and Reproduction. Philadelphia: WB Saunders, 1987:186.
18. Hammer AS, Couto CG. Disorders of Hemostasis and Principles of Transfusion Therapy. In: Allen DS, ed. Small Animal Medicine. Philadelphia: JB Lippincott, 1991:173.
19. Forrester SD, Rogers KS, Willard MD. Diagnosis and Management of Primary and Secondary Feline Hepatic Disease. Fel Pract 1990;18(2):15.
20. Gilmore CE. Bone Marrow and Peripheral Blood in Cats: Technique and Normal Values. J Vet Pathol 1964;1:18.
21. Christman C. Organophosphate toxicity. Friskies Res Dig 1989;25(3):4.
22. McCaw DL, Fleming EJ, Mikiciuk MG. Selecting the right diagnostic tests for renal disease. Vet Med 1989;84:266.
23. Fossum TW, Birchard SJ. Chylothorax. In: Kirk RW, ed. Current Veterinary Therapy X. Philadelphia: WB Saunders, 1989:393.
24. Feldman BF, Thomason KJ. Useful Indexes, Formulas, and Ratios in Veterinary Laboratory Diagnostics. Compend Contin Educ Pract Vet 1989;11:169.
25. Peterson ME, Graves TK, Gamble DA. Triiodothyronine (T_3) Suppression Test: An Aid in the Diagnosis of Mild Hyperthyroidism in Cats. J Vet Intern Med 1990;5:233.
26. Miller, WH. Symmetrical truncal hair loss in cats. Compend Contin Educ Pract Vet 1990;12:461.

CHAPTER 13

◇ ◇ ◇

Cytology

Gary D. Norsworthy

Cytology is a relatively new diagnostic modality for the veterinary practitioner. It has been taught on a widespread basis since about 1985, and is now a standard discipline in all American veterinary schools.

The author has presented lectures on cytology to practitioners since 1983. The feedback theme that is consistently repeated in these seminars is, "I was taught cytology, but I do not use it in my practice. I am not a pathologist and do not have any desire to be one." This attitude is widespread because, when cytologic diagnosis is taught, emphasis is generally placed on its use in diagnosing neoplasia, with considerable stress placed on the identification of many tumor types.

Cytology is a tremendous tool for the primary care veterinarian; its use is certainly not limited to pathologists. This chapter will demonstrate that the primary care veterinarian can use cytology to understand nonneoplastic, as well as neoplastic, processes. In fact, the clinician may find that its use in nonneoplastic processes is more valuable than in neoplastic processes.

In addition to its diagnostic usefulness, cytology is also extremely cost-effective. In many situations, a cytologic preparation will contain as much information as a histologic preparation. When cytologic examination is compared to histopathology, its ease of sample acquisition, the time lapse until results are available, and the cost to the client make it clearly superior as an initial test.

Cytology: What It Is and How to Do It

The Lump Dilemma

Almost every day the practitioner is presented with a cat with a dermal or epidermal mass. This presents a dilemma, as the owner must be told that one of three treatment alternatives is appropriate:

- Cut it out (i.e., surgical removal).
- Wait it out (i.e., do nothing and hope the immune system resolves it).
- Rub it out (i.e., dispense a topical medication for the owner to apply).

Without cytologic examination, a recommendation is largely an educated guess. The safest choice is to remove all masses surgically, but this is a form of medical overkill. The use of cytology allows one to classify the mass so that a rational recommendation can be made.

Cytology versus Histopathology

Cytology is not synonymous with histopathology. The difference may be illustrated with this example:

> You are a forest ranger. A large number of trees in your district are dying, and it is your job to diagnose the problem. You know that you must sample some of the dead or dying trees. You may randomly sample trees in several areas of the forest, or you may take an acre of trees and study them as a group.

The first method—random sampling of several trees—is analogous to cytology. With cytology, relatively small numbers of cells are collected from various locations in the lesions or organ. The second method—studying an entire acre of trees—is analogous to histopathology. With histopathology, one is studying a larger number of cells and studying them as they are related to one another.

Some diseases can be reliably identified with cytologic methods. For instance, the identification of *Histoplasma capsulatum* in a liver aspirate is adequate evidence for a diagnosis of histoplasmosis. However, there are also some diseases that require histopathologic examination. Examination of aspirated material from a granuloma caused by feline infectious peritonitis (FIP) will reveal a sterile inflammatory pattern, which is typical of many diseases. Histopathologic examination of such a lesion, however, will reveal the granuloma and the vasculitis that are consistent with FIP.

Equipment

A cytologic specimen is not the same as a biopsy specimen. For a biopsy specimen, a wedge or core of tissue is removed from the lesion with a scalpel or a large-gauge biopsy needle. For a cytologic specimen, a small number of clusters of cells or individual cells are removed from the lesion, generally through a small-gauge hypodermic needle.

Making a cytologic preparation can generally be accomplished with the equipment found in a veterinary hospital.

The following are needed:

- 3-, 6-, or 12-cc syringes
- 25-, 22-, and 20-gauge needles
- Microscopic slides
- A modified Wright's stain (Diff-Quik)
- A centrifuge with tubes
- A microscope with 1,000× magnification capability

There are several modified Wright's stains on the market. However, Diff-Quik Stain (AHS del Caribe, Inc., Aguada, Puerto Rico) requires less than 1 minute for specimen staining and gives consistently uniform results.

There are two things one should know about Diff-Quik stain. First, the initial solution is primarily methyl alcohol. If the lid is left off of the staining jar, it will evaporate quickly. To help compensate for the evaporative loss, one need not change this solution. Rather, when the level gets low, more solution can be added to the existing amount in the staining jar. Second, the third solution (the blue dye) tends to become exhausted much sooner than the second solution (the red dye). As this becomes evident on cytologic preparations, one may increase the number of dips of the slide in the solution (or the length of time for each dip). If increasing the contact time still results in pale blue staining, the solution should be discarded, the staining jar cleaned (with alcohol, not water), and replacement solution added. At the same time, the red solution should also be replaced.

A high-quality microscope must be used for reading cytologic preparations or frustration will result and cytology will often be abandoned. Even if the sample is properly collected, mounted, and stained, without a high-quality microscope, it is worthless. The financial returns from cytology will pay for a new microscope in a few months. The purchase of a binocular microscope is well worth the difference in cost.

One addition to a microscope that is very helpful is a pair of wide-field, 15× eyepieces. These increase magnification by 50% and permit visualization of structures that might otherwise be missed.

Other Stains

There are several other stains that are used for special situations. Each has advantages and disadvantages. Diff-Quik is desirable because of its ease and versatility. A few situations make new methylene blue (NMB) stain advantageous. Because Diff-Quik is alcohol-based, crystals, fat, and mucin may be dissolved by it. NMB is water-based so it will not dissolve these substances. By contrast, thus, NMB should be used when looking for urine crystals and when examining a suspected salivary mucocele.

Cell Collection Techniques

Collection of cells may be accomplished by four methods: tissue aspiration, tissue impression, tissue scraping, and fluid aspiration.

Tissue Aspiration

The following equipment is needed for tissue aspiration.

- 3-, 6-, or 12-cc syringe
- 25-gauge needle
- Microscope slide
- Diff-Quik stain

The technique for performing a tissue aspiration involves the following steps:

1. Entrap the mass with the fingers of one hand.
2. Insert the needle into the center of the mass (Fig. 13–1*A*) using the other hand.
3. Produce a vacuum in the syringe by pulling back on the plunger (Fig. 13–1*B*).
4. While maintaining the vacuum within the syringe, redirect the needle within the mass several times to collect cells from several areas of the mass (Fig. 13–1*C*).*
5. Release the vacuum in the syringe (Fig. 13–1*D*).
6. Withdraw the needle from the mass.
7. Remove the needle from the syringe. Fill the syringe with air and reattach it to the needle (Fig. 13–1*E*).
8. Spray the cells onto a microscope slide (Fig. 13–1*F*).
9. Spread the cells into a thin layer on the microscope slide. There are several ways of doing this. The needle can be touched into the center of the cells and used to drag "fingers" of cells outward (Fig. 13–2). Alternatively, another microscope slide may be used to apply gentle pressure to the mass of cells; when the two slides are pulled apart, the specimen will be ready for staining. Regardless of which method is chosen, the cells should be treated as if they were very fragile. This is because, in many diseases, the cells are very easily lysed, and overvigorous handling of the cells will result in the creation of cellular debris that is not readable.
10. Stain the slide with Diff-Quik.
11. Examine the slide under magnification, first at 100×, then at 1,000×. (*Note:* If the cells are not first examined under the lower [100×] magnification, one will not gain a perspective of the relative numbers of normal and abnormal cells.) This perspective is important in order to clearly assess the situation.

Tissue Impression

The following equipment is needed for performing a tissue impression:

- Microscope slide
- Diff-Quik stain

A tissue impression may be performed on a lesion on the skin surface, on the surface of a surgically exposed organ or tissue, or on the cut surface of an organ. To perform a tissue impression, the following steps should be followed:

1. Blot the tissue with a paper towel to remove as much fluid as possible from the surface.

*The amount of tissue collected is generally so small that it will not enter the syringe. However, there will be hundreds of cells that remain within the needle only.

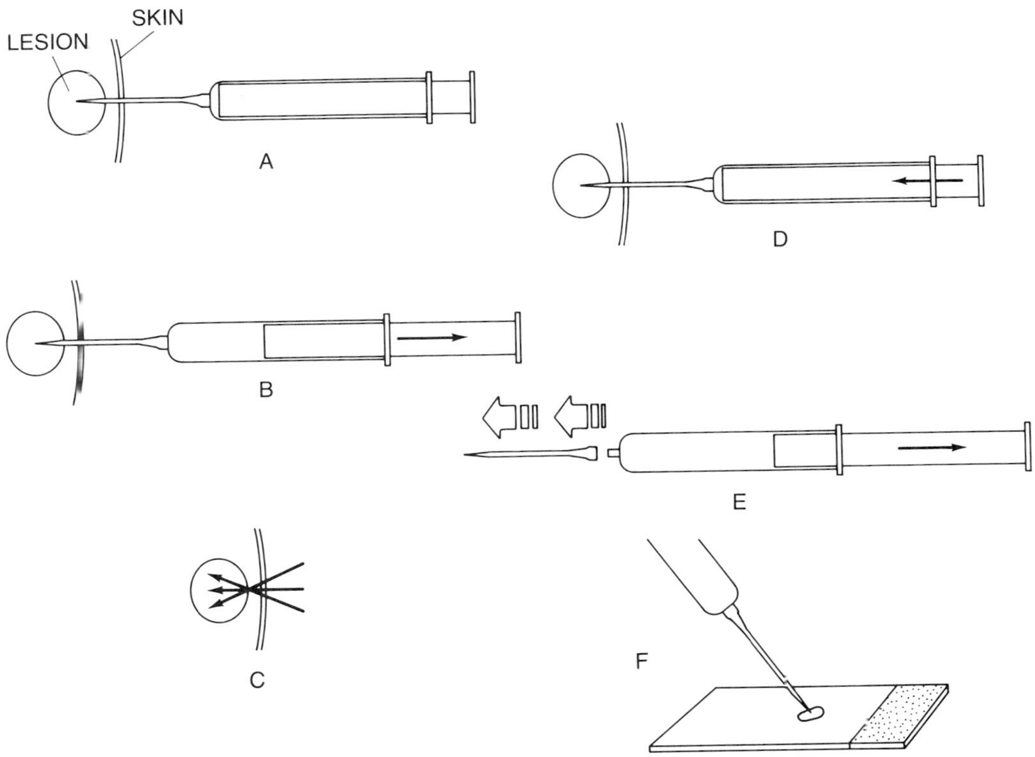

Figure 13–1. (*A*) Aspiration of a mass begins with the insertion of a needle into the mass. (*B*) Full suction is then applied with the syringe. (*C*) The needle is redirected within the mass while the suction is maintained with the syringe. (*D*) The negative pressure is released before the needle is withdrawn from the mass. (*E*) The needle is detached from the syringe, the syringe is filled with air, and then the needle is reattached. (*F*) The aspirated cells are sprayed onto a microscope slide, spread, and stained. (Used by permission of Heinz K. Grohs, M.D.)

2. Press the microscope slide directly onto the tissue.
3. Stain the slide with Diff-Quik stain.
4. Examine the slide under magnification, first at 100×, then at 1,000×.

Tissue Scraping

The following equipment is necessary for a tissue scraping:

An instrument for scraping, such as that which would be used for a skin scraping (the author's preference is a dental spatula)

Microscope slide

Tissue scraping is indicated for dense tumors, such as squamous cell carcinoma, which do not exfoliate cells easily. If a tissue impression is made and very few cells are recovered, a tissue scraping should be performed. The following is the procedure for a tissue scraping:

1. Blot the tissue with a paper towel to remove as much fluid as possible from the surface.
2. Scrape the surface of the mass to collect cellular material.
3. Transfer the cellular material to a microscope slide.
4. Stain the slide with Diff-Quik.
5. Examine the slide under magnification, first at 100×, then at 1,000×.

Fluid Aspiration

The following equipment is needed to aspirate fluid for cytologic examination:

3-, 6-, or 12-cc syringe

22- or 20-gauge needle

Microscope slide

Centrifuge

Diff-Quik stain

Fluid aspiration may be performed on fluid from a body cavity, such as the chest or abdomen, or from a cystic lesion. The technique for fluid aspiration involves the following steps:

1. Insert the needle into the fluid and aspirate at least 1 mL of fluid (if possible) into the syringe.
2. Centrifuge the fluid and pour off the supernatent.*
3. Resuspend the sediment with the remaining fluid in the centrifuge tube.
4. Pour the cell-rich fluid from the centrifuge tube into a microscope slide.
5. Make a smear of the fluid, as for a blood smear.

*If less than 1 mL of fluid is obtained, omit centrifugation and place the fluid direcly on the microscope slide.

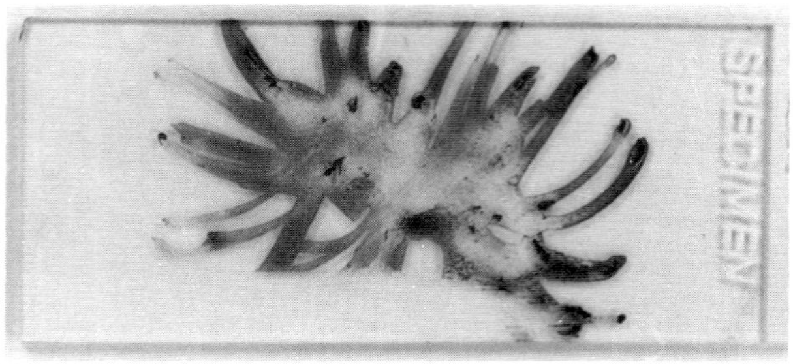

Figure 13–2. One method of spreading the cells on the slide is to touch the needle into the drop of cellular material, repeatedly dragging it outward to produce "fingers" of cellular material.

6. Stain with Diff-Quik stain.
7. Examine the slide under magnification, first at 100× then at 1,000×.

Cytologic Interpretation

Basic Cellular Patterns

There are several full-color books available that illustrate cell and organ patterns. Some of these are listed at the end of this chapter.

It is essential to learn the characteristics of the basic cell to be able to read a cytologic preparation (Table 13–1). The references cited in Table 13–1 refer to one of three inexpensive cytology or hematology manuals with photomicrographs that clearly demonstrate the essential cells. Because the stain used in these manuals is Diff-Quik stain, positive identification of cells requires that the appearance of the cells on microscopic examination be identical to that depicted in the manuals.

Although cytology is often viewed as a complex subject, it can be simplified to the understanding of four distinct cellular patterns, only three of which apply to pathologic processes.

1. *Normal Organ Pattern.* This pattern includes the normal cells found in each body organ. Each organ and its cells are different from the others. For instance, liver cells are distinctly different from kidney cells. Likewise, blood cells are distinctly different from lung cells, although the former may be found in aspirates of nearly all organs (Fig. 13–3).

   When aspirating sample material from an organ, one should identify the normal organ cells first, to confirm that the desired organ has been sampled. Only then should the other cellular patterns be sought. Blood and fat are commonly found because they can be found in nearly any organ.
2. *Inflammatory Pattern.* This pattern indicates that the body is responding immunologically to an insult. It is the first of the three pathologic cellular patterns. If neutrophils, lymphocytes, macrophages, plasma cells, eosinophils, and/or plasma cells are present, the pattern is termed inflammatory (Fig. 13–4*A*,*B*).

   Most inflammatory cells are found in the blood, and blood cells are found in most organs and lesions. Therefore, classifying a lesion as inflammatory must allow for the presence of blood.

   The cellular response may be described as purulent, pyogranulomatous, or granulomatous. Likewise, inflammation is also further characterized in terms that attempt to quantify its duration—that is, acute, subacute (or chronic active), or chronic. The presence or ab-

Table 13–1. Cells the Veterinary Practitioner Should Be Able to Identify

Cell	Reference	Page/Figure No.
Erythrocyte	a	23/12.1–12.3
Neutrophil	b	23/3.1,3.2
Lymphocyte	b	35/4.26
Lymphoblast	b	35/4.24
Eosinophil	a	15/6.8; 17/7.6
Macrophage (monocyte)	b	31/4.5–4.7
Mitotic figure	b	42/5.16
Bacteria		
Rods	c	33/3
Cocci	c	31/7; 33/8
Pityrosporon/Malassezia	c	49/1–3
Simonsiella/Caryophanon	c	49/1–3
Histoplasma	c	47/7,8
Mast cells	b	41/5.12,5.13
Melanoma cells	c	103/1,2
Epithelial cells	c	137/5,6
Sarcoma cells	c	93/1–4
Adenocarcinoma cells	c	111/3.6

[a] Rich LJ. Morphology of Canine and Feline Blood Cells. St. Louis, MO: Ralston Purina Co., 1974.
[b] Rebar AH. Handbook of Veterinary Cytology. St. Louis, MO: Ralston Purina Co., 1980.
[c] Perman V, Alsaker RD, Riis RC. Cytology of the Dog and Cat. South Bend, IN: American Animal Hospital Association, 1979.

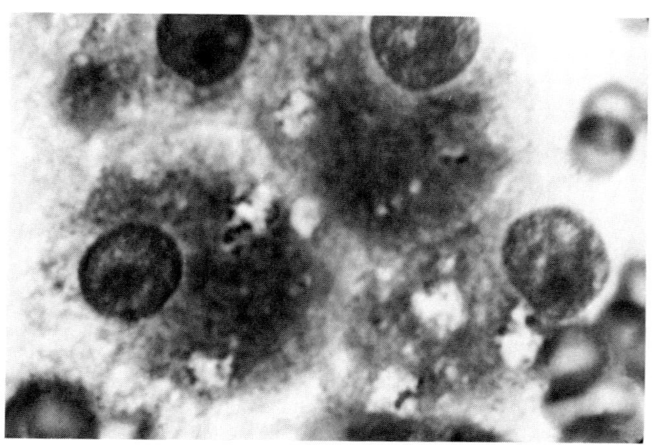

Figure 13–3. Aspiration of any organ should yield some normal organ cells. The four large cells shown are normal liver cells (hepatocytes) from a liver aspirate.

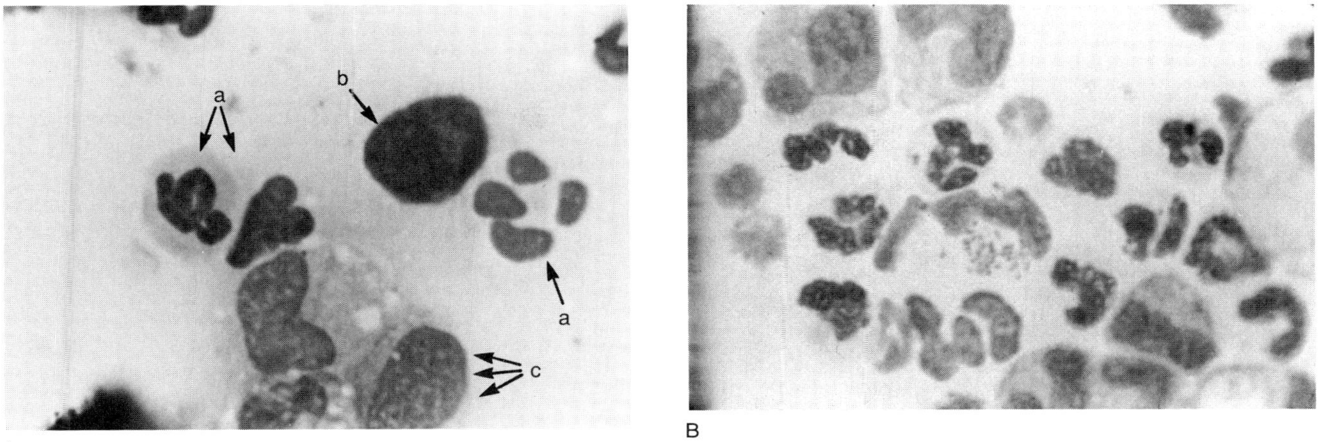

A B

Figure 13–4. (*A*) The aseptic inflammatory pattern is characterized by the presence of neutrophils, lymphocytes, monocytes, and occasionally, eosinophils or plasma cells without microorganisms. Three neutrophils (*a*), a plasma cell (*b*), and three monocytes (*c*) are seen in this field. (*B*) The septic inflammatory pattern is characterized by the presence of neutrophils, lymphocytes, monocytes, and sometimes eosinophils accompanied by microorganisms. This photomicrograph shows bacteria that has been phagocytized by the neutrophil in the center of the field (*arrow*).

sence of bacteria or other microorganisms differentiates between septic and aseptic inflammation.

3. *Neoplastic Pattern.* This pattern, which is the second of the three pathologic cellular patterns, is characterized by the presence of neoplastic cells (Fig. 13–5). (The characteristics of neoplasia are listed in a later section in this chapter.) Identification of the specific type of tumor is not necessary for a cytologic specimen to be definitively identified as neoplastic. Once the diagnosis of neoplasia is made, appropriate recommendations, such as biopsy, cryosurgery, or surgical excision, can be formulated. Histopathologic examination is appropriate for confirmation of the diagnosis.
4. *Mixed Pattern.* This pattern represents a combination of inflammatory and neoplastic patterns. It is the third of the three pathologic cellular patterns. Many types of neoplasia will evoke an inflammatory reaction in the nearby tissues. For example, if the neoplasia is on the body surface, the cat will often lick or chew at it, which results in an inflammatory response. Therefore, both inflammation and neoplasia can exist simultaneously (Fig. 13–6).

   If a mixed pattern is present, the neoplastic cells are considered to be the predominant finding, and rec-

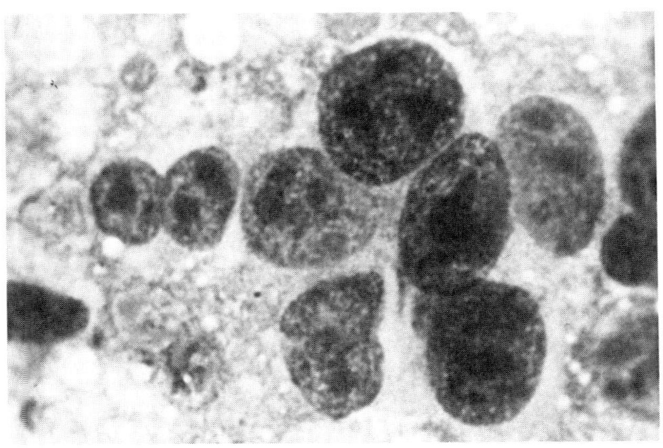

Figure 13–5. The neoplastic pattern is typified by the presence of at least three, and preferably four of the typical characteristics of malignant cells listed on page 100. These cells demonstrate nuclear enlargement, an increased nuclear/cytoplasmic ratio, multinucleation and marked indention of the nuclei secondary to abnormal mitosis, and variations in nuclear size and shape.

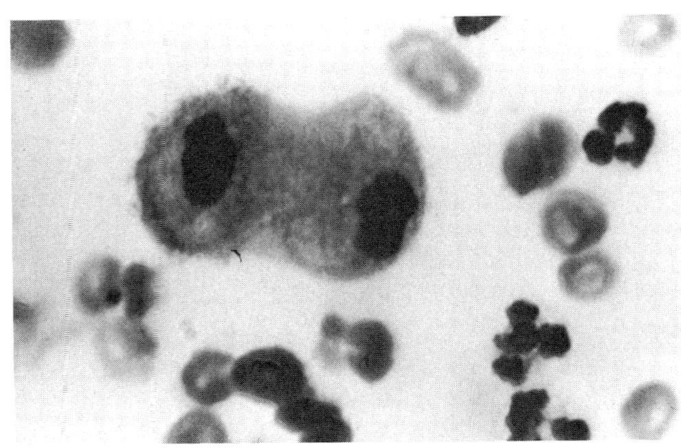

Figure 13–6. The mixed cellular pattern exhibits characteristics of both inflammation and neoplasia. This occurs most often when a malignant tumor involves the skin surface. In this photomicrograph, a mitotic figure is surrounded by inflammatory cells.

ommendations for treatment should be made as if they were the only finding.

Inflammatory Cellular Subpatterns

The inflammatory pattern may be further classified as follows:[1]

Septic versus Aseptic

Aseptic inflammatory patterns are characterized by inflammatory cells without the presence of microorganisms (see Fig. 13–4*A*). Foreign body reactions and vaccine reactions are examples. Conversely, the presence of bacteria or fungal elements is the typical finding in *septic* inflammatory patterns (see Fig. 13–4*B*).

Bacteria may be classified as rod-shaped or coccal. Examples of fungi that may be identified are *Histoplasma capsulatum* and *Cryptococcus neoformans*.

Purulent versus Granulomatous versus Pyogranulomatous versus Eosinophilic

These subclassifications are based on the types of cells present in the exudate. The inflammatory response may be described as *purulent* (or *suppurative*) if greater than 85% of the inflammatory cells are neutrophils. The response is termed *granulomatous* if inflammatory giant cells or numerous epithelioid macrophages, or both, are present. A combination of these two responses is termed *pyogranulomatous*. If numerous eosinophils are present, the reaction is termed *eosinophilic or allergic*.

Acute versus Subacute versus Chronic

This subclassification is an attempt to quantify the duration of the disease process. The *acute* pattern is one in which more than 70% of the inflammatory cells are neutrophils. The *subacute* (or *chronic active*) pattern is characterized by a ratio of neutrophils to macrophages of approximately 50:50. The *chronic* pattern is one in which greater than 50% of the inflammatory cells are macrophages.

Characteristics of Neoplasia

Cells undergoing neoplastic transformation exhibit several specific characteristics. For the sake of contrast, the characteristics of normal cells are listed first, followed by the characteristics of neoplastic cells.

1. Characteristics of normal cells
   - Homogeneous appearance of cells when examined by low-power magnification
   - Nuclear:cytoplasmic ratio of 1:3 or 1:4
   - Uniform size and number of nuclei per cell
   - Uniform size and number of nucleoli per cell
   - No (or very rare) mitotic figures
2. Characteristics of malignant cells (see Fig. 13–5)
   - Enlargement of the nucleus. Cells with nuclei larger than 10 μm in diameter* are suspected to be malignant. This nuclear enlargement is attributable to polyploidy, or doubling of DNA without subsequent nuclear division.
   - Increased nuclear:cytoplasmic ratio (sometimes to 1:1). It must be remembered that lymphocytes normally have a 1:1 ratio.
   - Multinucleation and marked indention of the nuclei as the result of abnormal mitosis. It must be remembered, however, that multinucleation also occurs in certain types of benign cells, such as transitional cells of the urinary tract, osteoclasts, mesothelial cells, macrophages, and giant cells. Occasionally, binucleate hepatocytes may be found as a normal variation. In general, isokaryosis in a multinucleated cell suggests a benign or reactive process. Multinucleated tumor cells should show at least mild (and sometimes marked) anisokaryosis.
   - Abnormal or frequent mitosis. Mitotic figures are occasionally seen in normal mesothelial cells or macrophages, and are not uncommon in reactive lymph nodes.
   - Variations in the size and shape of the nuclei
   - An increase in the size and number of nucleoli. Enlargement of the nucleolus by more than 5 μm in diameter is strongly suggestive of a malignant process.
   - Increased basophilia of the cytoplasm. This implies an increased RNA content of the cell, which results in rapid cell growth. Some cells may have such blue cytoplasm that distinction of the nuclear/cytoplasmic borders is difficult.

At least three, and preferably four, of these criteria should be met to justify diagnosis of a malignant lesion. Nuclear criteria are more reliable than cytoplasmic criteria. Finding only a small number of abnormal cells may indicate a malignant lesion; on the other hand, it may mean a reactive or dysplastic process. This is especially true if chronic inflammation is superimposed on normal tissue. Continually finding abnormal cells warrants appropriate radiographic studies, endoscopic examinations, exploratory surgery, or other diagnostic tests.

A tumor that has numerous characteristics of a malignant lesion may be interpreted as being malignant. On the other hand, aspirates that have only one or no malignant characteristics should not be interpreted as indicating benignity. Benignity is a histopathologic diagnosis only, as many Grade I carcinomas are so well differentiated that the cytologic characteristics of malignancy are absent. In these cases, the diagnosis of a malignant lesion can only be made on the basis of abnormal arrangements of cells on histopathologic examinations. Tumors that often are extremely well differentiated and yet are malignant include thyroid carcinoma, perianal adenocarcinoma, ovarian carcinoma, and many low-grade mammary carcinomas.[2]

The information included in Figure 13–7[3] can be used to determine the specific type of tumor found upon aspiration and cytologic examination of a specimen.

*The average diameter of a red blood cell in cats is 6 μm.

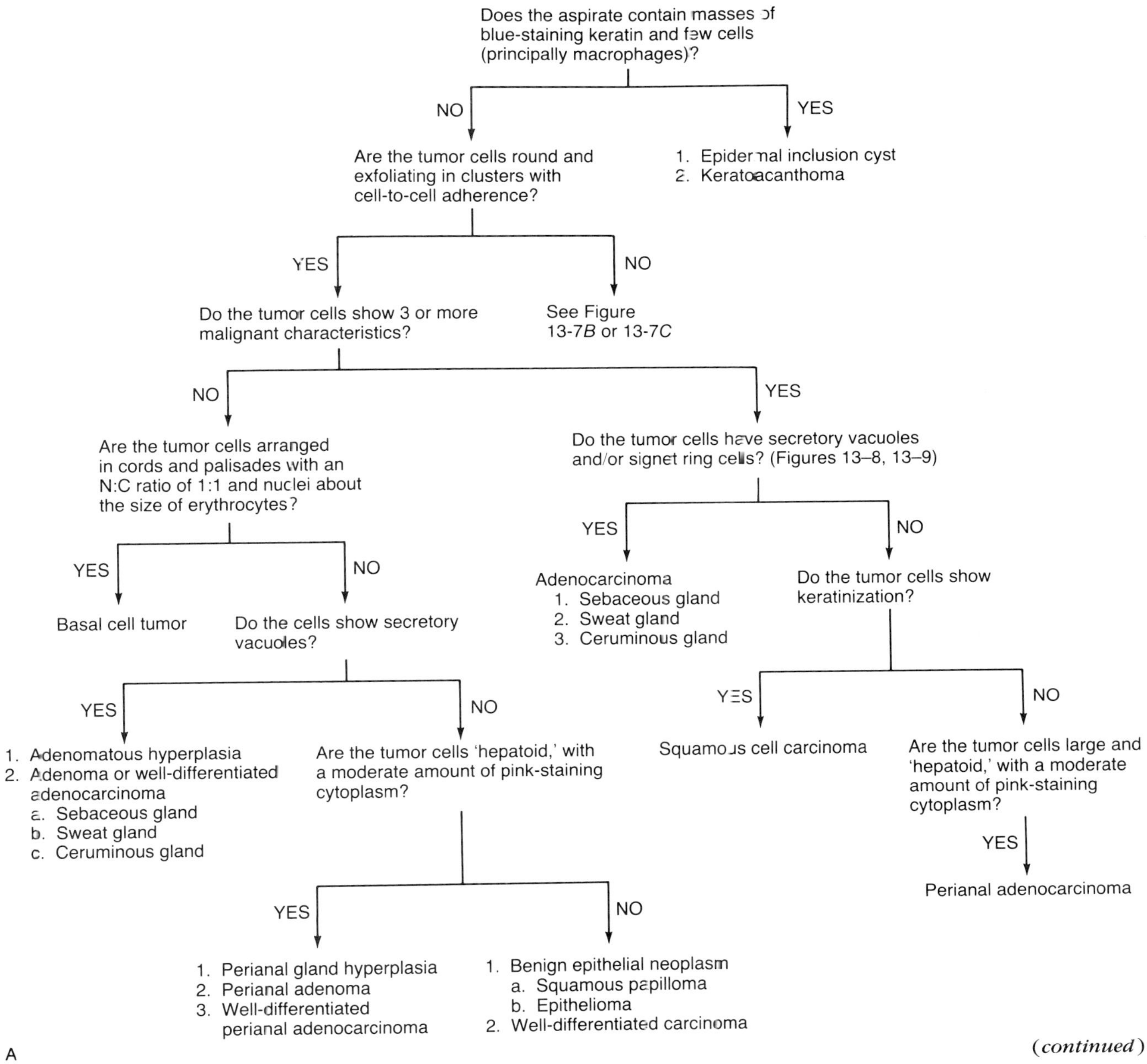

(*continued*)

Figure 13–7. Algorithms can be used to differentiate (*A*) nodules of epithelial origin, (*B*) nodules of nonepithelial origin, and (*C*) round cell tumors.[3] (Used by permission of Veterinary Learning Systems Co., 425 Phillips Boulevard, Suite 100, Trenton, NJ 08618.)

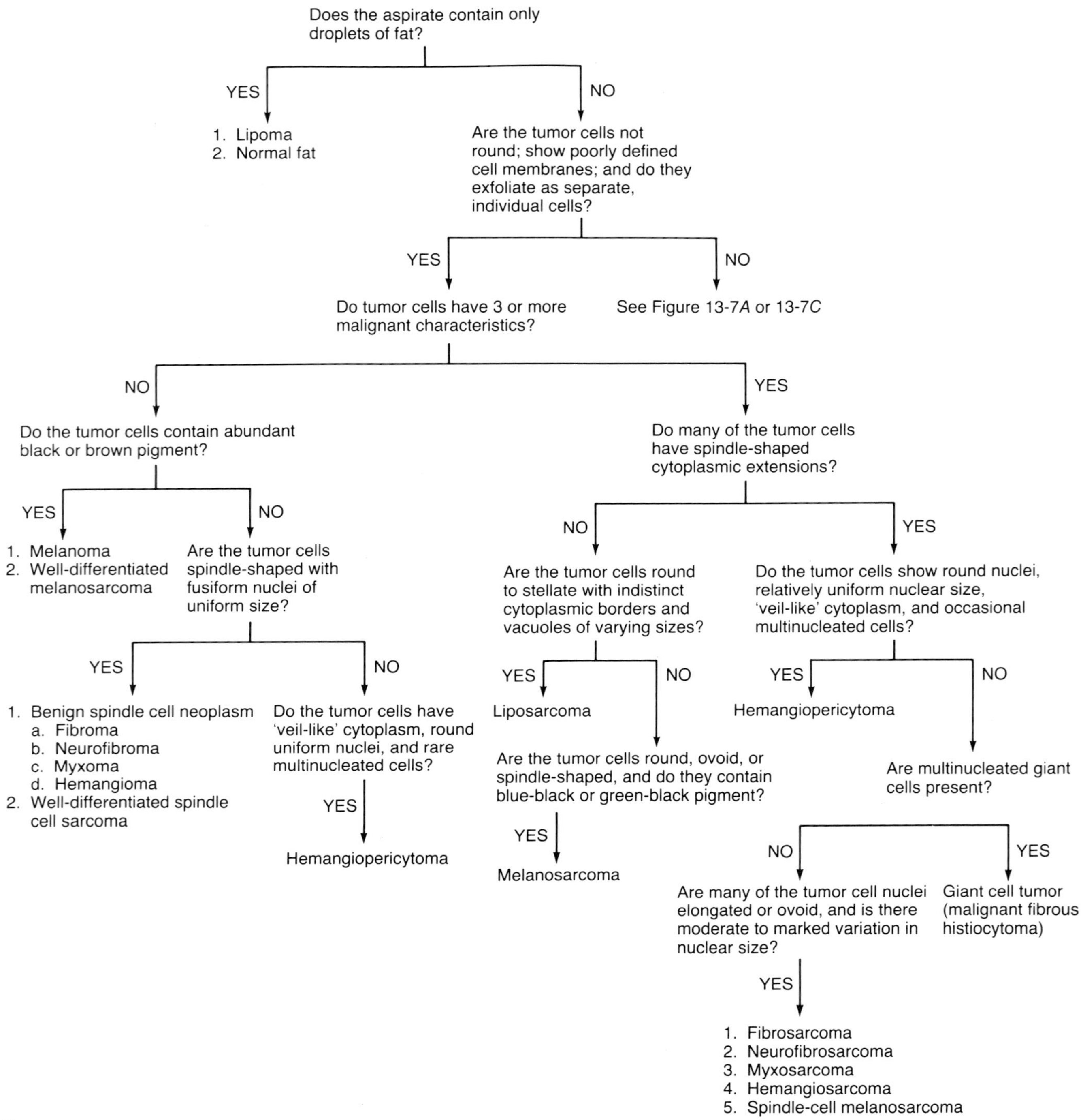

B

Figure 13–7 (continued)

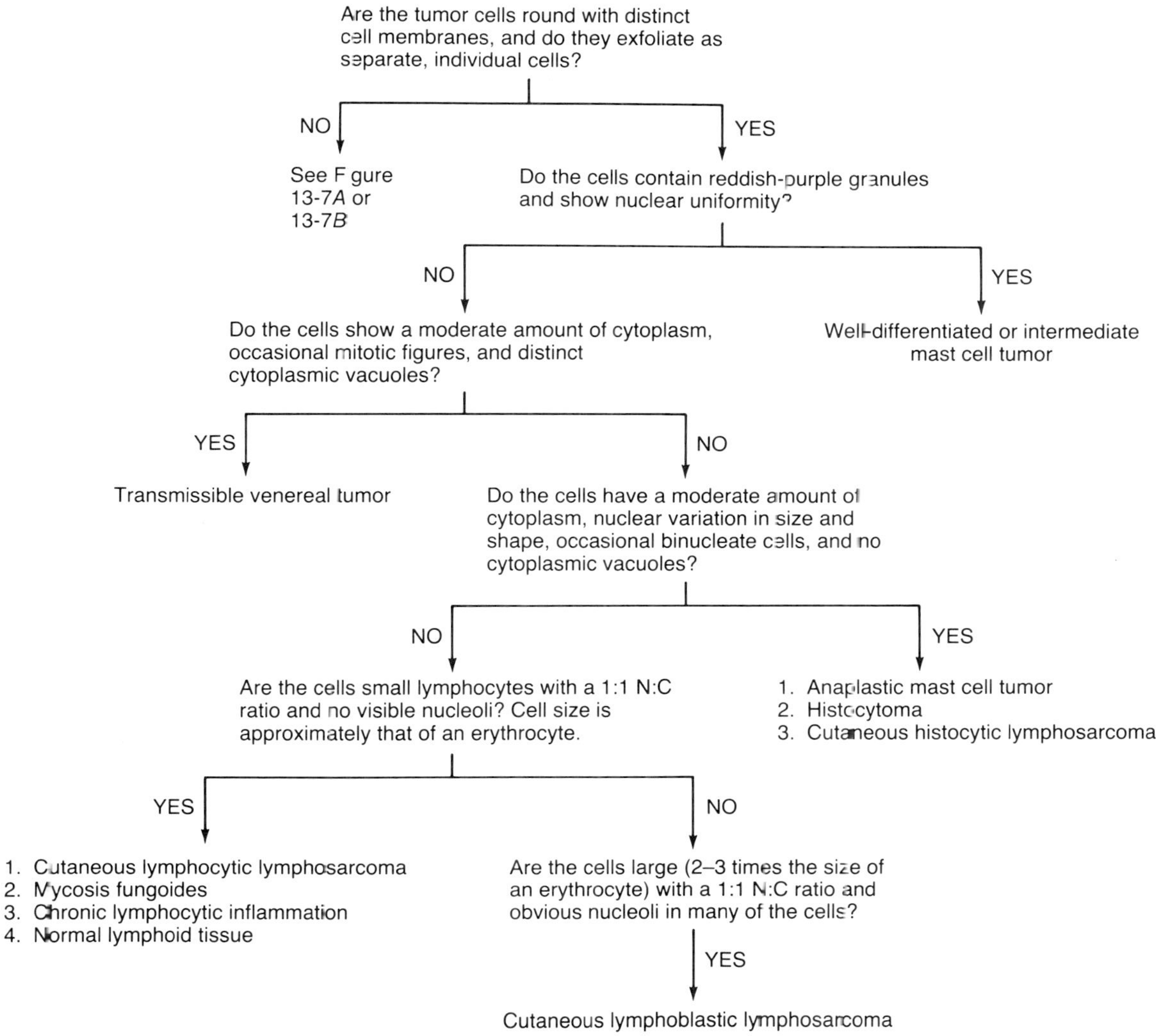

C

Figure 13–7 (continued)

Tissue Aspirates

Technique

The fine-needle aspiration of a cytologic sample from various body organs is generally a simple process involving palpation and immobilization of the organ in question, with subsequent aspiration of material. Some organs better lend themselves to this technique than others. For instance, the cat's kidneys are much easier to palpate and immobilize than is the spleen because the kidneys are relatively fixed in their position. Some organs, such as the adrenal glands, are so small that they are not candidates for aspiration. Other organs, such as the lungs, must be aspirated with utmost care because of their vascularity, their friability, and their proximity to other vital organs.

General anesthesia or tranquilization may facilitate the aspiration process. However, sedation is generally not needed because of two factors. First, the cat is generally somewhat oblivious to a puncture with a 25- or 22-gauge needle. Second, most cats undergoing organ tissue aspiration are so sick that this procedure elicits no reaction.

The procedure for tissue aspiration is as follows:

1. The skin is surgically prepped; usually, an area that is 1 to 2 cm in diameter is sufficient.
2. A technician restrains the cat for the aspiration procedure.
3. When the patient's skin has been prepped, the clinician entraps the target organ with one hand and performs the aspiration procedure with the other. The chances of obtaining a sample of diagnostic quality are increased if two organ tissue aspirations are performed.
4. When the tissue sample is collected, the cells are smeared on a microscope slide so that a layer of tissue that is one cell in thickness is present. (If the cells are smeared too vigorously, they may rupture, resulting in a meaningless sample.)
5. The cells are then stained with Diff-Quik Stain.

Hemorrhage is generally not a significant complication of organ tissue aspiration if care is taken in performing the aspiration, and if a 25-gauge needle is used. Even tissue from the spleen can be aspirated successfully without the likelihood of hemorrhage.[4] However, if the cat is icteric or anemic, and if tissue is to be aspirated from a vascular organ it is advisable to obtain either a clotting profile or at least a clotting time prior to tissue aspiration.

Organ-Specific Considerations

Liver

The liver is one of the most frequently aspirated organs in cats because of the high incidence of liver disease in this species. Indeed, a liver aspiration should be considered to be a routine diagnostic procedure for icteric cats.

The liver is an organ that yields a high diagnostic success rate from cytologic sampling. However, it is helpful to precede a liver aspiration with abdominal radiographs in order to determine the best site for needle entry. The size of the liver can vary considerably with various disease processes, as can the size of the falciform ligament. The size of the latter greatly influences the location of the liver, another reason that radiographs are valuable adjuncts to proper site selection. However, if a radiograph is not available, the liver of most cats can be aspirated by inserting the needle between the 8th and 9th or 9th and 10th ribs at the level of the costochondral junction (Fig. 13–8). Liver tissue should be aspirated from each side of the abdominal wall.

If the gallbladder is greatly distended, as in the case of a biliary obstruction, bile and/or cells are likely to be aspirated from it, as well as from the liver. However, this is not likely to be a problem in terms of gallbladder function.

The liver lies adjacent to the body wall. It is neither necessary nor desirable to insert the needle deeply into the liver. A needle insertion depth of 1/4 to 3/8 inches is generally adequate to obtain a representative sample without the likelihood of lacerating the liver. Therefore, a 25-gauge, ⅝-inch needle is ideal.

When examining a liver aspirate, the presence of liver cells should be verified (see Fig. 13–3). If liver cells are not found, the procedure should be repeated. If liver cells are present, the search for inflammatory or neoplastic cells can begin. Because the liver is such a vascular organ, a large number of blood cells, including neutrophils, will be present in the aspirate. Before a liver aspirate is interpreted as having an inflammatory pattern, one must consider the neutrophil count in the blood. If the peripheral neutrophil count is elevated, there will be a large number of neutrophils in the liver aspirate, which may or may not indicate hepatitis.

The common feline diseases diagnosed by liver aspiration include the following:

1. Hepatic lipidosis (Fig. 13–9*A*,*B*)

   Findings: A large number of round fat droplets, either within the cytoplasm of the hepatocytes or extracellularly, or both. An inflammatory pattern, consisting of neutrophils and macrophages, is often present (see Chapter 47).

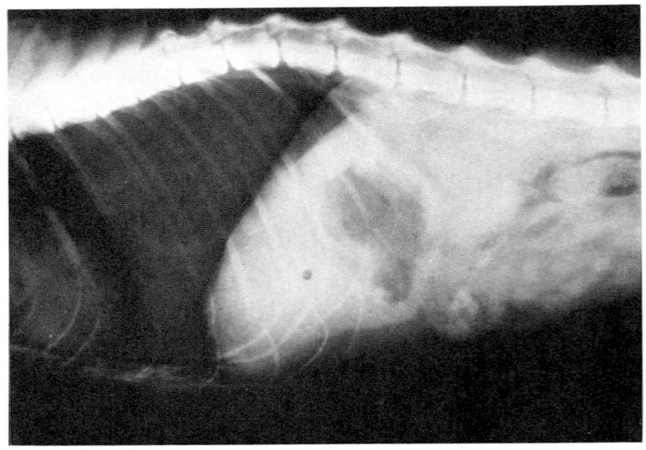

Figure 13–8. **In performing a liver aspiration, the site of needle insertion is best determined by a lateral radiograph. However, if one is not available, success is usually achieved by inserting the needle in the 8th or 9th intercostal space at the level of the costochondral junction. The dot on this radiograph indicating the proper location is in the 9th intercostal space.**

2. Lymphosarcoma (Fig. 13–10)

   Findings: Large numbers of lymphoblasts and several mitotic figures (see Chapter 39)

3. Histoplasmosis (Fig. 13–11)

   Findings: A subacute, septic inflammatory pattern consisting of neutrophils, macrophages, plasma cells, and *H. capsulatum* organisms (see Chapter 61)

4. Cholangiohepatitis, FIP, blunt trauma, or toxicosis (see Fig. 13–4*A*)

   Findings: A sterile inflammatory pattern consisting of neutrophils and macrophages. Even though these diseases have identical cytologic patterns, their prognoses are vastly different. This is one cytologic pattern that warrants a biopsy and histopathologic studies in order to establish a final diagnosis.

5. Bacterial hepatitis

   Findings: A septic inflammatory pattern consisting of neutrophils, macrophages, and cocci or rod-shaped bacteria. If this pattern is found, another aspirate should be performed. The second sample should be used for culture and sensitivity (aerobic and anaerobic).

Spleen

The spleen can be aspirated with a 25-gauge needle without significant likelihood of hemorrhage, even in thrombocytopenic cats.[4] When enlarged, localization, immobilization, and aspiration of the spleen are relatively simple, unless the cat is obese.

The common diseases diagnosed by spleen aspiration are:

1. Mast cell tumor or mastocytosis (Fig. 13–12*A*,*B*)

   Findings: Copious numbers of mast cells. These cells are so distinctive that their recognition is almost en-

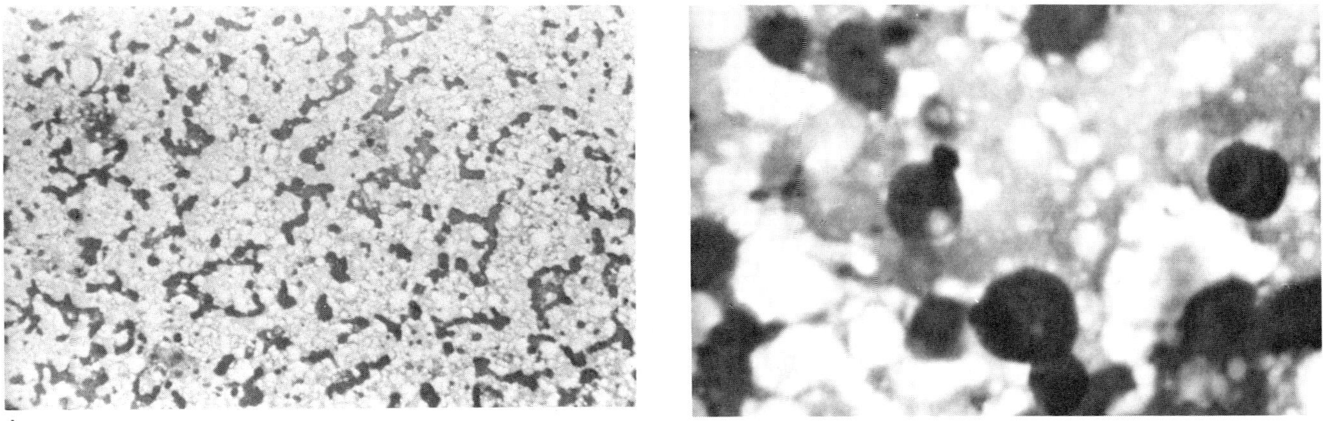

A B

Figure 13–9. (*A*) Hepatic lipidosis is characterized by the presence of a large amount of fat in the liver aspirate. The round white vacuoles in this field (magnification 100×) are fat droplets. (*B*) The fat droplets typical of hepatic lipidosis are readily visible between, and usually within, the hepatocytes (magnification 1000×).

sured, even for the inexperienced cytologist. The basophilic granules will fill the cytoplasm; they will also be free in the intracellular space because of the rupture of the fragile cells (see Chapter 51).

If this diagnosis is made, the cat should immediately receive an antihistamine to counteract the effects of the histamine release that will occur.

2. Lymphosarcoma (see Fig. 13–10)

   Findings: Lymphoblasts and mitotic figures. The cytologic pattern of lymphosarcoma in the spleen is the same as in any other organ (see Chapter 39).

3. Erythremic myelosis

   Findings: Erythrocytic precursors, as would normally be found in the bone marrow. This is a disease induced by the feline leukemia virus (FeLV) that may be difficult to differentiate from extramedullary hematopoiesis.

4. Hemangiosarcoma

   Findings: Typically, only normal blood cells are found, suggesting a normal aspirate. Hemangiosarcomatous cells do not exfoliate well unless a tissue scraping is performed. If they are found, they are plump, spindle-shaped cells (see Chapter 51).

5. Feline hypereosinophilic syndrome/eosinophilic leukemia*

   Findings: Copious numbers of eosinophils. Feline hypereosinophilic syndrome is a poorly understood, nonneoplastic disease that may be confused with eosinophilic leukemia. The former is characterized by band and segmented eosinophils, whereas the latter is char-

*This is not a common finding, but it is so unique that it is worth mentioning.

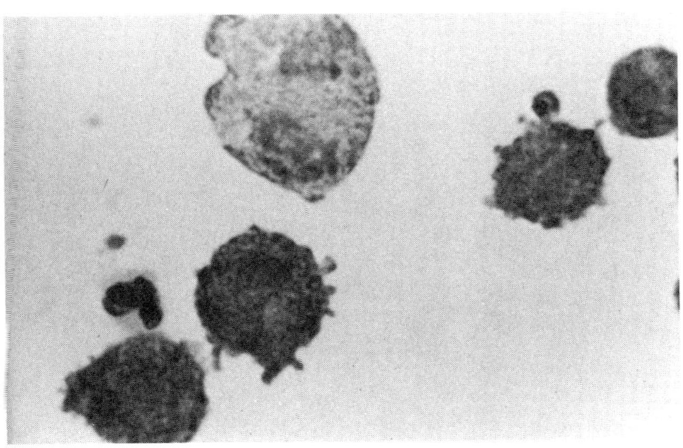

Figure 13–10. Lymphosarcoma is characterized by the presence of lymphoblasts and mitotic figures. The cytologic findings will be the same for lymphosarcoma detected in masses or in effusions. These cells were recovered from a pleural effusion.

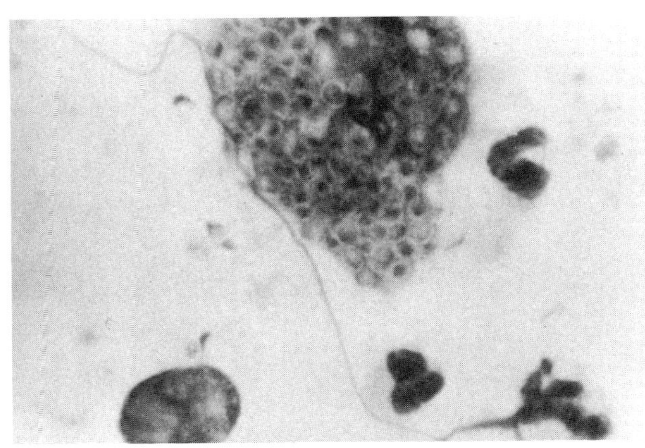

Figure 13–11. The macrophage at the top of this field engulfed *Histoplasma capsulatum* organisms. This finding is diagnostic for this organism, whether obtained from lymph nodes, lung, liver, or other organs.

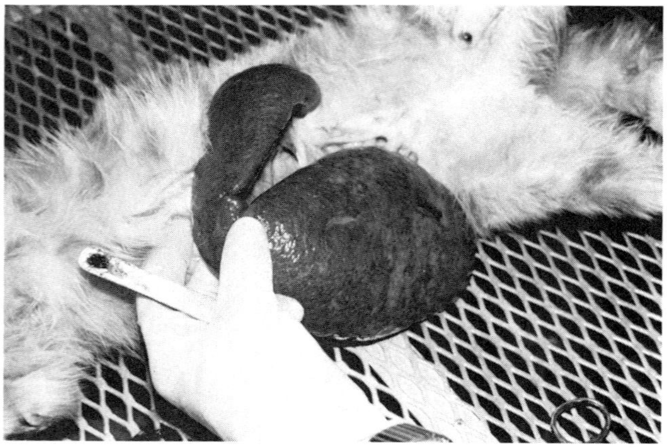

A

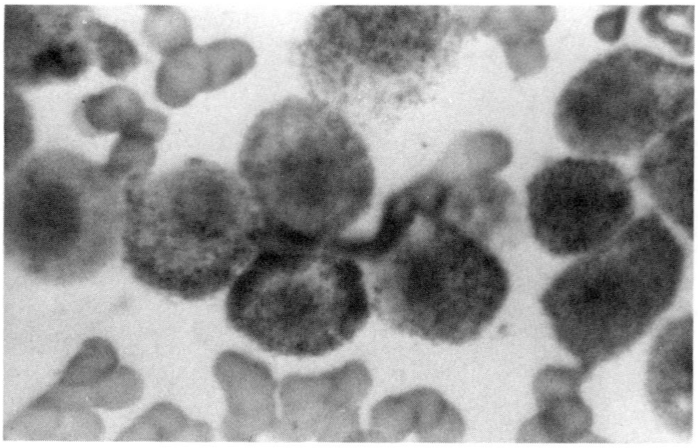

B

Figure 13–12. (*A*) The spleen of this cat was massively enlarged, a typical finding in splenic mastocytosis. (*B*) The aspirate obtained from the spleen of the cat in Figure 13–12*A* contains copious mast cells. The cytoplasm of these cells is filled with purple granules. Because these cells are very friable, it is common to find extracellular granules throughout the field. Mast cell tumors in other locations have the same appearance.

acterized by both band and segmented eosinophils and less differentiated cell forms.[5]

Other Abdominal Masses/Enlarged Organs

Abdominal masses are generally discovered by palpation. Radiographic studies may facilitate their localization, but rarely provide a definitive diagnosis. In palpating a mass, it is helpful to note whether or not the mass can be moved freely within the abdomen. Those that are movable are usually within the small intestine or uterus.

Common abdominal masses and their locations include the following:

1. Stomach wall masses (Fig. 13–13)

   Findings: Usually, neoplastic cells. As in the intestinal tract, the most common tumors are lymphosarcoma and adenocarcinoma. Because of the acidity in the stomach, bacteria are usually not found in the aspirate.

2. Intraluminal gastric masses (Fig. 13–14)

   Findings: Amorphous debris. The most common masses within the cat's stomach are hairballs and cellophane (or other) wrappings from meat or other foods. Bacteria and cells are generally absent. This represents a nonspecific finding that warrants endoscopy or gastrotomy.

3. Neoplastic intestinal masses

   Findings: Neoplastic cells, most commonly, lymphosarcoma and adenocarcinoma. Intestinal lymphosarcoma is found in cats of all ages and is usually not associated with a positive FeLV test. Adenocarcinoma is typically

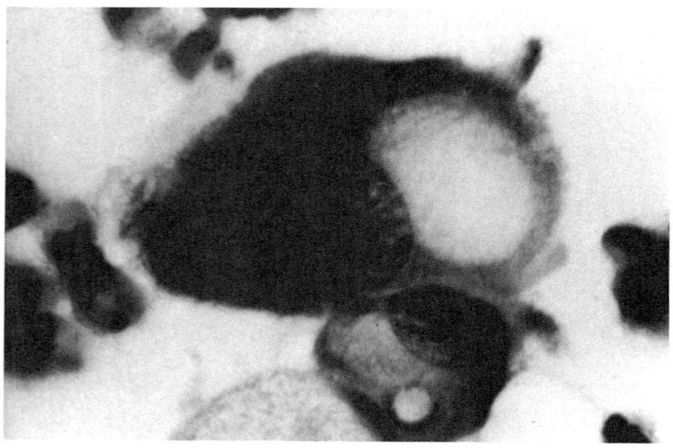

Figure 13–13. Signet ring cells are often found in adenocarcinomas. The large cell in the center of the field has a large singular vacuole that is typical of this cell. Such a cell may be found in adenocarcinoma involving the mammary glands or intestinal walls, or any other location.

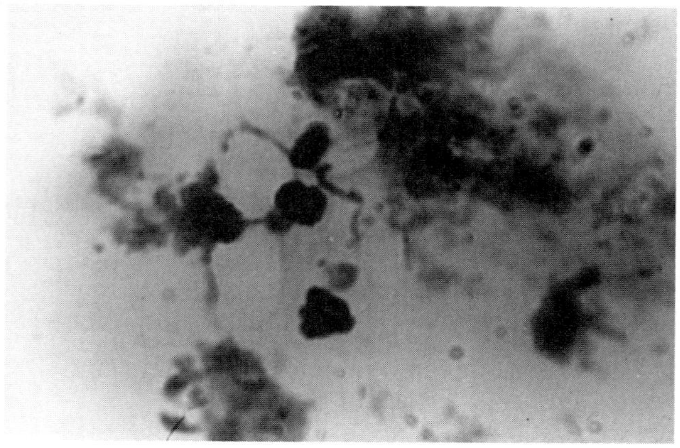

Figure 13–14. The amorphous debris depicted, which is typical for normal gastric contents, was aspirated from the stomach of a cat with a palpable intraluminal stomach mass. This cat had swallowed a cellophane meat wrapper. Note the absence of bacteria.

found in cats older than 10 years of age. Both of these diseases are usually accompanied by enlargement of the mesenteric lymph nodes. These masses are freely movable, and aspirates may contain bacteria from within the intestinal tract (see Chapters 39 and 51).

4. Kidney enlargement

   Findings: Neoplastic cells or a sterile inflammatory pattern. The most common diseases causing renal enlargement are lymphosarcoma and FIP. Lymphosarcomatous kidneys are usually smooth, and aspirates generally yield lymphoblasts and mitotic figures. Kidneys of cats with FIP generally have granulomas that extend above the normal renal contour (i.e., so-called "lumpy-bumpy" kidneys). The cytologic pattern is a sterile, inflammatory one. Other neoplasms may also be found in the kidneys, and will yield other types of neoplastic cells.

   Polycystic and hydronephrotic kidneys are also found in the cat. Renal aspiration in affected cats will yield a significant amount of fluid, a finding that is not typical for lymphosarcoma or FIP.

   Structural damage to the kidneys may occur if the aspiration is performed within the renal pelvis. Therefore, it is suggested that aspirations be directed at the renal poles.

5. Mesenteric lymph node enlargement

   Findings: Neoplastic cells or lymphoid hyperplasia. The most common cause of enlargement of the mesenteric lymph node is lymphosarcoma, which may occur as a primary disease or secondary to lymphosarcoma of the intestinal tract. Adenocarcinoma of the intestinal tract may also cause mesenteric lymph node enlargement. Infectious processes, including FIP and fungal diseases, will produce lymphoid hyperplasia or an inflammatory pattern that is either sterile or septic (see Chapter 21).

Lung

Cats are affected by a number of diffuse lung disorders, making lung aspiration appropriate in many cases. It is essential that thoracic radiographs be obtained prior to lung aspiration in order to differentiate between focal and diffuse disease. Without the aid of ultrasonography or image intensification, it is very difficult and unsafe to aspirate a focal lesion, such as a mass, within the lung parenchyma.

Except when pneumothorax is present, the lung is immediately adjacent to the thoracic wall. Therefore, the depth of needle penetration into the thoracic cavity need only be ⅛ to ¼ inches to yield an adequate sample of the lung parenchyma. The use of a 25-gauge, ⅝-inch needle is recommended.

Because needle penetration into the lung parenchyma is very superficial, the site of entry is not too critical. Generally, needle insertion at the level of the 9th to 11th ribs and midway between the dorsal and ventral midlines is acceptable. The procedure should also be repeated on the contralateral side.

Because the lungs are almost constantly in motion owing to inspiration and expiration, there is significant risk for laceration of the lung parenchyma. If this happens, the resulting hemorrhage or pneumothorax may be fatal. To avoid this situation, the following strategies may be helpful. First, respiratory movements may be arrested temporarily by having an assistant hold the cat's mouth closed while occluding the nasal openings as the aspiration is being performed. (Doing this for more than a few seconds, however, will cause the cat to struggle.) Second, needle penetration and withdrawal should be accomplished in one rapid motion and should be completed within no more than 2 seconds.

The common diseases diagnosed by lung aspiration include the following:

1. Feline asthma

   Findings: A sterile, inflammatory pattern consisting of neutrophils, eosinophils, and a few mast cells. A significant number of eosinophils may be found in the normal feline lung. The cat with asthma usually has more eosinophils than neutrophils (see Chapter 25).

2. Systemic fungal pneumonias

   Findings: An inflammatory pattern with fungal organisms present. Figure 13–11 provides a good example of *H. capsulatum.* (See also Chapter 61.)

3. Bacterial pneumonia/lung abscess

   Findings: An inflammatory pattern with rod-shaped or coccoid bacteria. These are not common findings in the cat.

4. FIP

   Findings: A sterile, inflammatory pattern with neutrophils and macrophages (see Fig. 13–4*A*). As this pattern is not specific for FIP, a definitive diagnosis of FIP requires further hematologic and clinical studies (see Chapter 38).

Thoracic Masses

Thoracic masses are generally detected by radiographic studies. In many of these cases, aspiration cytology is a noninvasive means of confirming such a diagnosis. Often, the alternative for obtaining a tissue sample is thoracotomy.

Most feline thoracic masses are located in the anterior mediastinum or in the lung parenchyma. The former are candidates for aspiration cytology, but the latter are usually too small to be aspirated safely.

The site of aspiration should be determined by radiography. As anterior mediastinal masses enlarge, they displace the adjacent lung tissue, so that there is generally little risk of damaging the lung parenchyma. There is a risk of penetrating the anterior vena cava, but this is unlikely if the needle is inserted through the lateral thoracic wall near the sternum.

The common diseases diagnosed include the following:

1. Lymphosarcoma (see Fig. 13–10)

   Findings: Lymphoblasts and mitotic figures. This is the most common disease causing a mass in the anterior mediastinum (see Chapter 39). Cytologic studies are usually diagnostic.

2. Thymoma (Fig. 13–15)

   Findings: Mature lymphocytes, sometimes accompanied by epithelial cells. This is an uncommon condition,

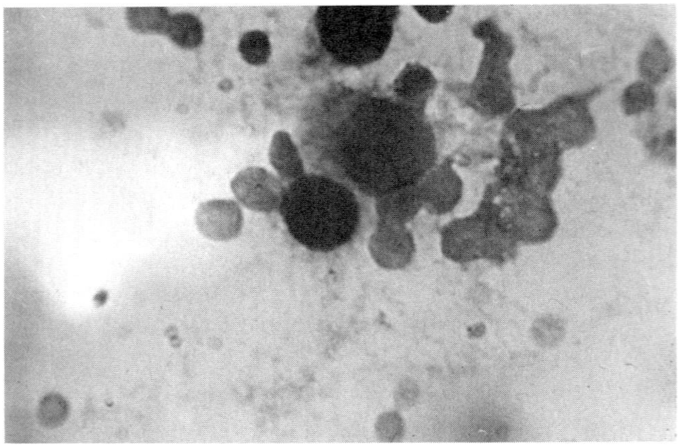

Figure 13–15. **When normal lymphocytes are aspirated from an anterior thoracic mass, it is likely to be a thymoma, although some thymic lymphosarcomas will have similar cells. Thymomas have both epithelial cells and lymphocytes, and have a much better prognosis than does anterior thoracic lymphosarcoma.**

but it has a much more favorable prognosis than does lymphosarcoma.

Dermal/Epidermal Masses and Ulcerations

Masses that occur within the dermis or epidermis can be classified just as those that occur within the body cavities. One should try to determine whether the mass is inflammatory or neoplastic. Once that decision is made, an appropriate therapeutic regimen can be formulated.

Inflammatory Lesions. Inflammatory masses and ulcerations are characterized by the presence of neutrophils, macrophages, lymphocytes, plasma cells, eosinophils, and/or microorganisms, and by the absence of neoplastic cells. The common inflammatory masses and ulcerations found in the cat include the following:

1. Vaccine reaction granulomas (see Fig. 13–4*A*)

   Findings: Neutrophils, macrophages, and occasionally, eosinophils or plasma cells. These granulomas may occur up to 3 weeks postinjection. If no bacteria are present, as in most cases, antibiotics are not indicated. Local heat will enhance resolution, but the lesion will resolve even if no treatment is given.
2. Foreign body granulomas (see Fig. 13–4*A*)

   Findings: Neutrophils, macrophages, and occasionally, eosinophils or plasma cells. The cytologic findings are identical to those associated with vaccine reaction granulomas. Resolution can occur without treatment, but these granulomas may require surgical removal. Most foreign bodies are radiolucent.
3. Abscesses/cellulitis secondary to cat fights (see Fig. 13–4*B*)

   Findings: Neutrophils, macrophages, and bacteria. Surgical drainage should be performed in cats with abscesses, but it is not indicated for cellulitis. Systemic antibiotics are indicated for both.
4. Fungal granulomas (see Figs. 13–11 and 13–16)

   Findings: Neutrophils, macrophages, and fungal organisms. Systemic fungal granulomas, especially those secondary to *H. capsulatum,* may occur on any part of the body. Confirmation of the presence of fungal organisms is diagnostic. (See Chapter 61.)
5. Eosinophilic granuloma complex (Fig. 13–17*A,B*). (See Chapter 60.)

Neoplastic Masses. Neoplastic masses are characterized by the presence of neoplastic cells. There are many neoplastic masses that occur on or within the dermis or epidermis. They should be removed surgically. The exact diagnosis can be left to the histopathologist. The common ones include the following:

1. Mast cell tumors (see Fig. 13–12*B*)

   Findings: Copious numbers of mast cells, often accompanied by eosinophils. Before surgical removal is attempted, the cat should be medicated with antihistamines. Cryosurgery is contraindicated. This is potentially a fatal disease in the cat. (See Chapter 51.)
2. Squamous cell carcinoma (Fig. 13–18)

   Findings: Cytologic studies are often nondiagnostic in these cases. This is one of the dense tumors whose cells do not exfoliate easily. Tissue impression or aspiration often will not reveal neoplastic cells. A tissue scraping of the surface of a squamous cell carcinoma is more likely to result in exfoliation of cells that will provide a meaningful cytologic preparation. (See Chapter 51.)
3. Lipoma (Fig. 13–19)

   Findings: "Skeleton" cells accompanied by fat droplets from ruptured cells. This is a benign tumor that is generally not surgically removed unless it causes discomfort to the cat (or the owner). Some mast cell tumors have a similar appearance to lipomas on gross examina-

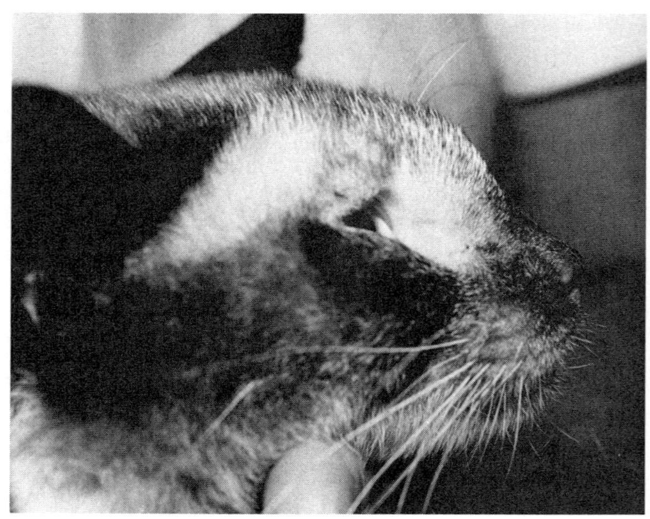

Figure 13–16. **The area of swelling between this cat's eyes was aspirated. *Histoplasma capsulatum* was recovered, as seen in Figure 13–11.**

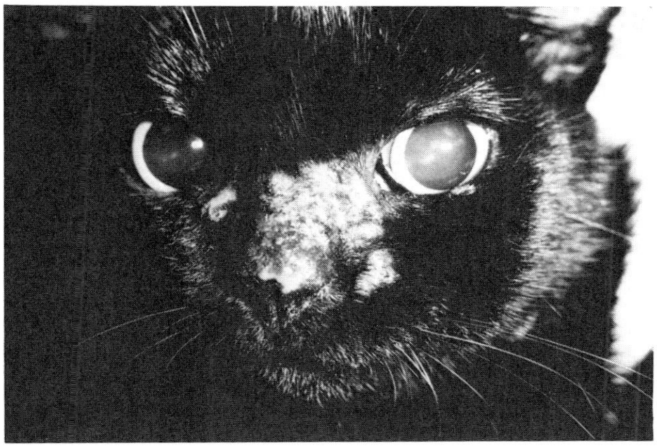

A

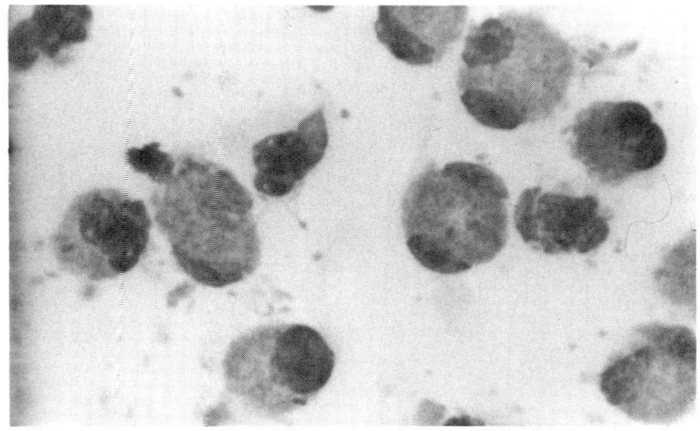

B

Figure 13–17. (*A*) A tissue scraping was performed to recover cells from the ulcerated lesion on the skin of this cat's nose. (*B*) The cells from the skin of the cat in Figure 13–17*A* were predominantly eosinophils. This is typical of eosinophilic granuloma complex dermatitis.

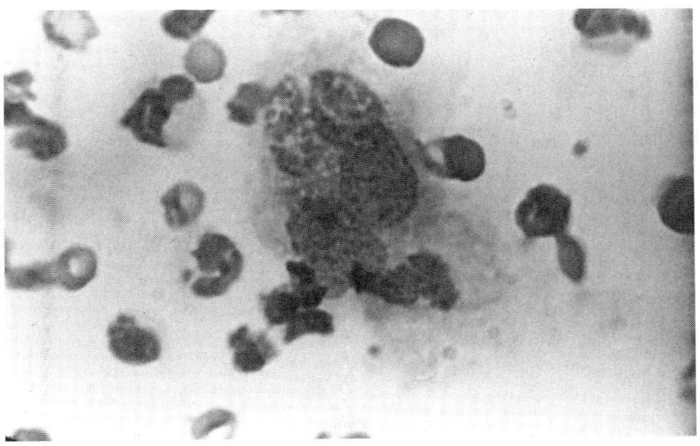

Figure 13–18. The cells of a squamous cell carcinoma may be recovered by scraping the lesion. Because this is a dense tumor, a tissue impression may not recover the neoplastic cells.

tion, so all soft masses should be aspirated and identified.

4. Mammary adenocarcinoma (see Fig. 13–13)

   Findings: Neoplastic cells that sometimes include signet ring cells. Cytologic specimens may be aspirated from mammary masses or taken from fluids expressed from adjacent nipples. This is a very aggressive tumor in the cat, as it metastasizes much earlier than in the dog. It should always be treated with liberal, aggressive surgical excision, including excision of local lymph nodes. (See Chapter 51.)

5. Melanoma (Fig. 13–20)

   Findings: Neoplastic cells containing amorphous inclusions of black pigment. The finding of the black pigment is diagnostic; however, the amelanotic melanoma, which can be just as serious, cannot be diagnosed by

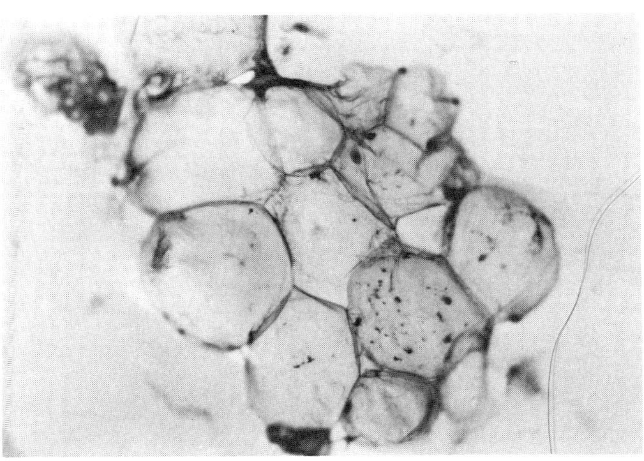

Figure 13–19. Large lipid-filled lipocytes are characteristic of lipoma.

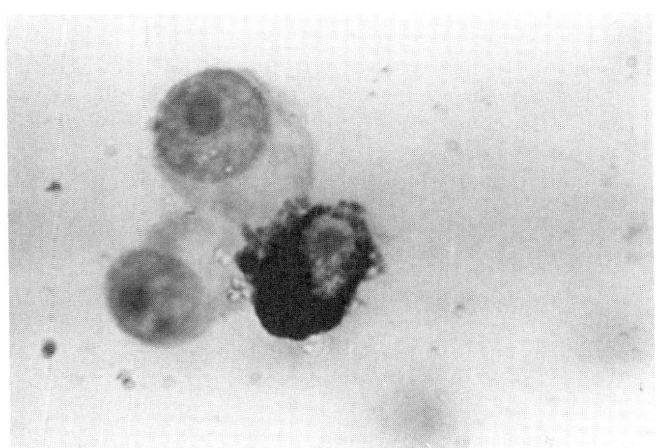

Figure 13–20. The black granules that fill the cytoplasm of the cell in the center of the field are typical of a melanoma.

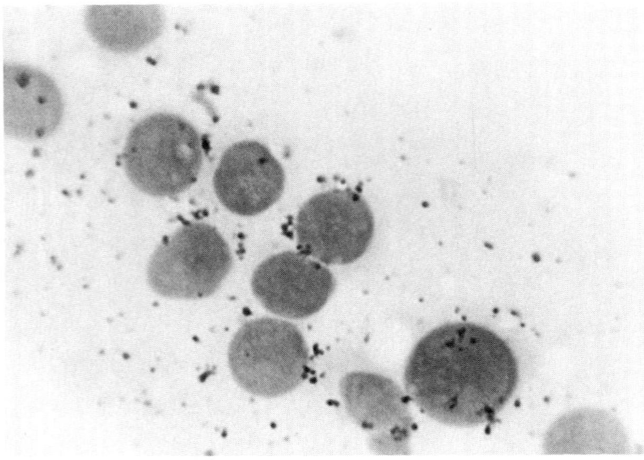

Figure 13–21. **The basal cell tumor is characterized by cells that align themselves in rows or ribbons. If this cellular pattern is not present, this tumor may be confused with a histiocytoma.**

cytologic means. Aggressive therapy is indicated if long-term survival is to occur (see Chapter 51).

6. Basal cell tumor (Fig. 13–21)

   Findings: Neoplastic cells with large nuclei and large amounts of cytoplasm. These cells may occur in groups or individually and frequently align themselves in a characteristic row or ribbon of cells. If the cells are not arranged in a ribbon, they may easily be confused with a histiocytoma.

Lymph Nodes

Lymph node cytology is discussed in Chapter 21.

Body Fluid Aspirates

The fine-needle aspiration of fluids from various body cavities is generally a simple process. The cavity is identified and aspirated, as discussed previously.

The body cavities from which aspirates are most commonly obtained are the thoracic and abdominal cavities. Other structures subject to aspiration include the subcutaneous tissues, the urinary bladder, bony cavities (such as the frontal sinuses), and the ventricles of the brain, all of which may be affected by cystic lesions. In addition, a spinal tap is a form of aspiration cytology.

Fluid in the thoracic cavity is identified by radiography. The typical radiographic signs include a reduction in the gas-filled lung parenchyma and, on the lateral view, the appearance of "leafing" of the lungs owing to their flotation in fluid (see Chapter 18).

Fluid in the abdominal cavity may be identified visually, radiographically, or by palpation. If there is a significant amount of fluid present, the abdomen will be grossly distended. This may also occur if a large intra-abdominal mass is present, or if the cat is in an advanced stage of pregnancy. Radiographically, fluid has the same density as most soft tissue organs. When fluid is present, the abdomen has a homogeneous appearance. The only contrasting densities would be gas or osseous densities. On palpation, a fluid-filled abdomen has a "doughy" feeling. Experience will allow one to identify this feel.

Technique

General anesthesia or tranquilization may facilitate the aspiration process, but they are generally not needed. This is because of two factors. First, the cat is generally somewhat oblivious to a puncture with a 22- or 20-gauge needle. Second, most patients needing fluid aspiration are ill enough so that this procedure elicits no reaction.

The only preparation needed is a surgical prep of the skin. Usually, an area 1 to 2 cm in diameter is all that needs to be prepped.

A technician is needed to restrain the cat during the fluid aspiration. When the patient's skin has been prepped, the target cavity is secured with one hand and the aspiration procedure is performed with the other. The cat should be positioned so that gravity helps to put the fluid in contact with the needle. For thoracic and abdominal aspirations, the cat is generally positioned in sternal recumbency or in a standing position.

If 1 mL or more of fluid is collected, the sample is centrifuged and the sediment is smeared on a microscope slide. If less than 1 mL of fluid is collected, a direct smear is made, as with a drop of blood. The microscope slide is stained with Diff-Quik Stain.

Other Tests

Some feline diseases producing body fluids can be diagnosed by cytologic studies alone. Other diseases require additional tests in order to make a definitive diagnosis. Although there will be some variation from case to case, the other appropriate tests generally include the following:

- White blood cell (WBC) count
- Specific gravity
- Total protein
- Bacterial culture and sensitivity (aerobic and anaerobic)
- Electrophoresis
- Cholesterol:triglyceride ratio

Pleural Effusions

Any fluid in the pleural space is abnormal. Radiography is the most common method used to diagnose pleural effusion. (The typical radiographic appearance has already been described.)

Any disease producing pleural effusion is serious; however, not all such conditions are fatal. A rapid, accurate diagnosis is imperative if therapy is to be successful.

Once a fluid sample is collected, the most valuable initial tests that should be performed are cytologic studies (relative cell numbers and specific cell types) and a specific gravity determination. The latter is actually an indirect measurement of the total protein level or, more accurately, the total solid level. Based on this information, the common diseases involving the pleural space may be differentiated as follows:

1. Lymphosarcoma (see Fig. 13–10)

   Findings: Lymphoblasts and mitotic figures. There are generally copious numbers of lymphoid cells, many of which are mature lymphocytes. The specific gravity is typically less than 1.018. On radiographic examination, the trachea is elevated owing to the presence of an anterior mediastinal mass (see Chapter 39).
2. FIP (see Fig. 13–4*A*)

   Findings: Sterile, inflammatory pattern with neutrophils and mature lymphocytes. Because of the large amount of protein in the fluid, the slide will have a homogeneous pink background. Typically, there is a relatively small number of these cells, but exceptions occur. The specific gravity is greater than 1.018, indicative of the high protein level (see Chapter 38).
3. Pyothorax (see Fig. 13–4*B*)

   Findings: Large numbers of band and segmented neutrophils with large numbers of bacteria. The specific gravity is greater than 1.018 owing to the presence of thick, purulent fluid. An anaerobic culture should be performed because of the high incidence of anaerobic bacteria. This is the only common disease of the cat causing bacteria-laden pleural effusion (see Chapter 53).
4. Cardiomyopathy

   Findings: Small numbers of mononuclear cells. The specific gravity is less than 1.018. Pulmonary edema is likely because of the typical left-sided heart failure that is present. However, if right-sided or biventricular failure occurs, pleural effusion may result (see Chapter 27).
5. Chylothorax (Fig. 13–22)

   Findings: Numerous, very small lymphocytes. The very small size of the lymphocytes, which are the same diameter as red blood cells, is the key finding in this condition. Although primary chylothorax does occur, this disease is usually secondary to another disease, such as lymphosarcoma, cardiomyopathy, heartworms, or trauma. The primary disease typically determines the specific gravity of the fluid (see Chapter 32).

A summary of diagnostic criteria for pleural effusions is presented in Table 13–2.

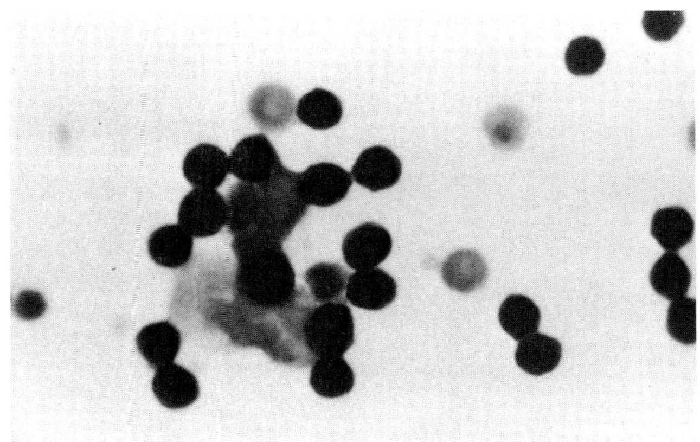

Figure 13–22. **Chylous pleural effusion is typified by moderate to large numbers of small lymphocytes that are approximately the same diameter as erythrocytes. The dark cells shown are lymphocytes, whereas the light cells are red blood cells.**

Abdominal Effusions

Fluid collection within the abdominal cavity is not a common occurrence in the cat. When such a fluid collection is present, however, the most valuable initial tests that should be performed are cytology (relative cell numbers and specific cell types), a specific gravity determination, and bacterial culture and sensitivity.

Recovery of fluid may be difficult if less than 150 mL of fluid is present in the abdomen. If this is the case, 100 to 200 mL of a warm, sterile isotonic fluid can be infused into the abdomen and recovery attempted again. If this procedure is necessary, the specific gravity of the recovered fluid will be different from that of the undiluted fluid within the abdomen.

1. FIP (see Fig. 13–4*A*)

   Findings: Sterile, inflammatory pattern with neutrophils and mature lymphocytes. Because of the large amount of protein in the fluid, the slide will have a homogeneous pink background. Typically, there is a relatively small number of these cells, but exceptions do occur. The specific gravity level is greater than 1.018, which is indicative of the high protein level. This is by far the most common cause of abdominal effusion in the cat (see Chapter 38).
2. Septic peritonitis

   Findings: Large numbers of band and segmented neutrophils, macrophages, and bacteria (often a mixed population). If this pattern is found, the most likely causes are a ruptured intestinal tract, usually secondary to neoplasia (Fig. 13–23) or a foreign body; a ruptured urinary bladder with bacterial cystitis; a ruptured intra-abdominal abscess (involving the liver, spleen, kidney, etc.); a ruptured uterus (pyometra) (Fig. 13–24); trauma; or bite wounds.
3. Aseptic peritonitis (see Fig. 13–4)

   Findings: Large numbers of band and segmented neutrophils and macrophages. If this pattern is found, the most likely causes are a ruptured urinary bladder secondary to trauma, a ruptured gallbladder, or irritant peritonitis (secondary to gloving powder, surgical sponges, etc.)
4. Hemorrhage

   Findings: Normal blood cells. This condition is usually caused by trauma, surgical hemorrhage, or ruptured hemangiosarcoma.

Table 13–2. Summary of Findings in Conditions Associated with Feline Pleural Effusion

Condition	Radiographic Findings	Cytologic Findings	Specific Gravity*	No. of Cells
Lymphosarcoma	Fluid and mass	Lymphoblasts, mitotic figures; no bacteria	<1.018	Large
Feline infectious peritonitis	Fluid	Neutrophils, lymphocytes, macrocytes; no bacteria	>1.018	Small
Pyothorax	Fluid	Neutrophils, lymphocytes, macrocytes; copious bacteria	>1.018	Large
Cardiomyopathy	Abnormal heart shape; pulmonary edema/effusion	Few cells; no bacteria	<1.018	Small
Chylothorax	Fluid	Very small lymphocytes; no bacteria	Variable†	Large

*This is actually a measurement of the total serum protein (solids) level. A specific gravity of 1.018 equals a total protein level of 2.5 mg/dL.
†This condition is generally the result of another disease process. The primary disease will determine the specific gravity. (See Chapter 32.)

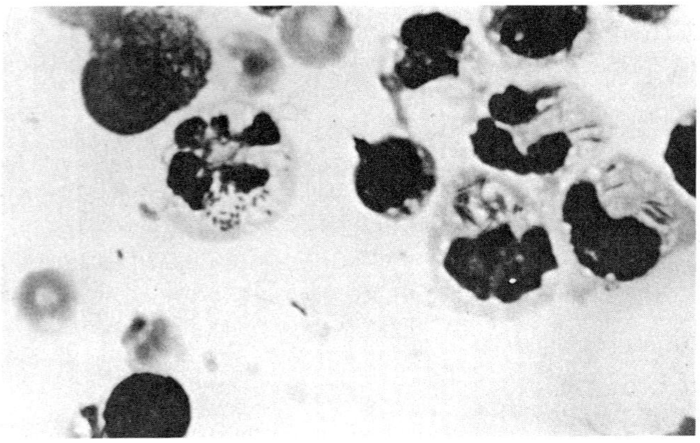

Figure 13–23. Fluid recovered from a cat's abdomen is seen to have a septic inflammatory pattern. The cat had a ruptured ileum secondary to an adenocarcinoma.

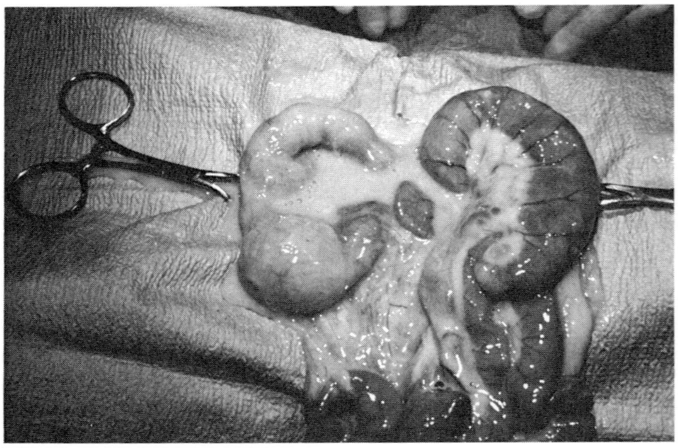

Figure 13–24. The fluid recovered from this cat's abdomen exhibited a septic inflammatory pattern. The cat had a ruptured uterus secondary to pyometra.

5. Ascites

   Findings: Low cell numbers in a fluid with a specific gravity of less than 1.018. This is the typical fluid of congestive heart failure; however, this is not common in the cat.

Other Fluids

Nasal discharges, vaginal discharges, external ear discharges, draining tracts, and urine are examples of other fluids that may be examined cytologically. The staining and evaluation process is the same as for any other fluid. Likewise, each fluid should be classified as either inflammatory, neoplastic, or mixed.

REFERENCES

1. Tyler RD, Cowell RL, Baldwin CJ, Morton RJ. Introduction. In: Cowell RL, Tyler RD, eds. Diagnostic Cytology of the Dog and Cat. Goleta, CA: American Veterinary Publications, 1989:1.
2. Barton CJ. Cytologic diagnosis of neoplastic diseases. J TX Vet Med Assoc 1983;45:41.
3. Barton, CL. Cytologic diagnosis of cutaneous neoplasms: An algorithmic approach. Compend Contin Educ Pract Vet 1987;9:18.
4. O'Keefe DA, Cuoto CG. Fine needle aspiration of the spleen as an aid in the diagnosis of splenomegaly. J Vet Intern Med 1987;1:102.
5. Latimer KS, Meyer DJ. Leukocytes in Health and Disease. In: Ettinger SJ, ed. Textbook of Veterinary Internal Medicine, 3rd ed. Philadelphia: WB Saunders, 1989:2181.

SUPPLEMENTAL REFERENCES

1. Rebar AH. Handbook of Veterinary Cytology. St. Louis, MO: Ralston Purina Co., 1980.*
2. Rich LJ. Morphology of Canine and Feline Blood Cells. St. Louis, MO: Ralston Purina Co., 1974.*
3. Perman V, Alsaker RD, Riis RC. Cytology of the Dog and Cat. South Bend, IN American Animal Hospital Association, 1979.
4. Cowell RL, Tyler RD. Diagnostic Cytology of the Dog and Cat. Goleta CA. American Veterinary Publications, Inc., 1989.

*The Purina books are available from PMG Veterinary Marketing, 6 RPL, Ralston Purina Co., Checkerboard Square, St. Louis, MO 63164.

CHAPTER 14

◇ ◇ ◇

Radiology

Ronald W. Green and Gary D. Norsworthy

The purpose of this chapter is to illustrate some of the radiographic findings in common diseases of the cat and to describe some of the special procedures that the private practitioner should find suitable for use in feline patients.

Digestive System

Esophagogram

Goal(s)

- To demonstrate the size, shape, and location of the esophagus. If fluoroscopy is available, the motility of the esophagus may also be studied.

Clinical Indications

- Regurgitation or vomiting

Materials

1. Barium sulfate
   - Paste form: Esophatrast or E-Z Paste
   - Liquid form (30% W/V): Colibar-V *or* Organic iodine: Gastrografin
2. 60-cc syringe

Technique

1. Obtain survey radiographs of the cervical and thoracic regions.
2. Administer 10 to 15 mL of barium sulfate per os.
3. Increase the X-ray exposure 5 to 10 kVp as compared to the survey radiographs. Make lateral and ventrodorsal radiographs. Oblique views are optional.

Normal Findings

- The barium sulfate paste should afford excellent detail for viewing the esophageal mucosa. The proximal two thirds of the esophagus has longitudinal folds. The caudal one third has an irregular mucosal pattern that produces a herringbone pattern (Fig. 14–1).
- It is not uncommon to record a bolus of contrast material in the esophagus. If there is a question as to whether this is a normal peristaltic wave, another radiograph should be obtained. If the dilated area is attributable to a normal peristaltic wave, subsequent radiographs will fail to demonstrate the bolus in the same location.

Common Lesions

- Megaesophagus will appear as a dilated esophagus filled with contrast medium (Fig. 14–2, *A* and *B*). There is usually no evidence to suggest peristalsis.
- Strictures of the esophagus will show narrowing of the esophagus at the level of the stricture, with a dilatation or diverticulum cranial to the stricture.
- Mediastinal masses will displace the esophagus dorsally (Fig. 14–3).
- Hiatal hernias may displace the cardiac portion of the stomach into the caudal thorax.
- An irregular mucosal pattern in the distal esophagus suggests gastric reflux esophagitis.
- A gastroesophageal intussusception displaces the stomach into the esophagus. When an orogastric tube is passed, the tube appears to double back within the esophagus (Fig. 14–4, *A* and *B*).
- Inflammation of the esophagus appears as an irregular mucosal pattern.
- Radiolucent foreign bodies may be coated by the contrast medium. There may be dilation of the esophagus cranial to the foreign body.
- Thickening of the wall, or a mass originating from the wall of the esophagus, may be a result of neoplasia or mycosis.
- Extraesophageal tumors may displace the esophagus.
- Contrast medium outside the esophagus may be a result of perforation.

Miscellaneous

- If tranquilization is needed, acepromazine is the tranquilizer of choice. It should be administered at a rate of 0.5 to 1.0 mg/lb intramuscularly (IM) or intravenously (IV).
- General anesthetics should be avoided.
- Gastrografin has a bitter taste which may cause excessive salivation in the cat.
- Aspiration of Gastrografin will result in pulmonary edema.

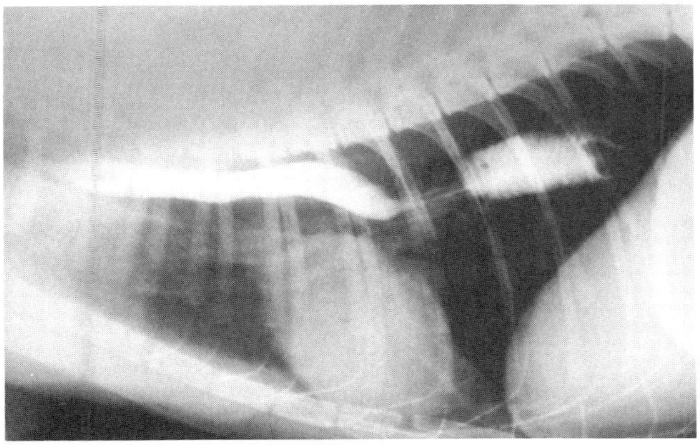

Figure 14–1. On this normal esophagogram, the cranial two thirds of the esophagus is seen to have linear striations. The caudal one third has a herringbone pattern.

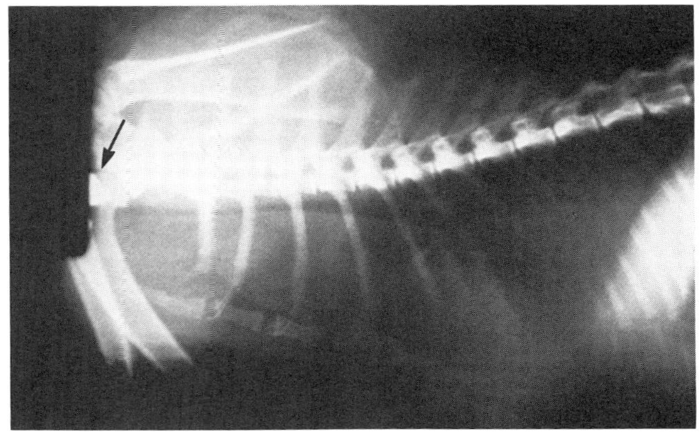

Figure 14–3. An anterior thoracic mass, such as lymphosarcoma, will compress the esophagus, preventing barium from entering at the level of the thoracic inlet (*arrow*).

Upper and Lower Gastrointestinal Series

Goals

- To determine the size, shape, and location of the stomach, small bowel, and large bowel
- To determine patency of the stomach and bowel

Clinical Indications

- Vomiting
- Regurgitation
- Diarrhea
- History of trauma, with a possible diaphragmatic hernia

Materials

1. Barium sulfate (30% W/V)
   or
   Iohexol (Omnipaque 240) diluted 1:2 or 1:3 with tap water
   or
   Organic iodine (Gastrografin)
2. 60-cc Syringe
3. 12- or 18-French orogastric tube (Feeding Tube and Urethral Catheter, Monoject, Division of Sherwood Medical, St. Louis, MO)

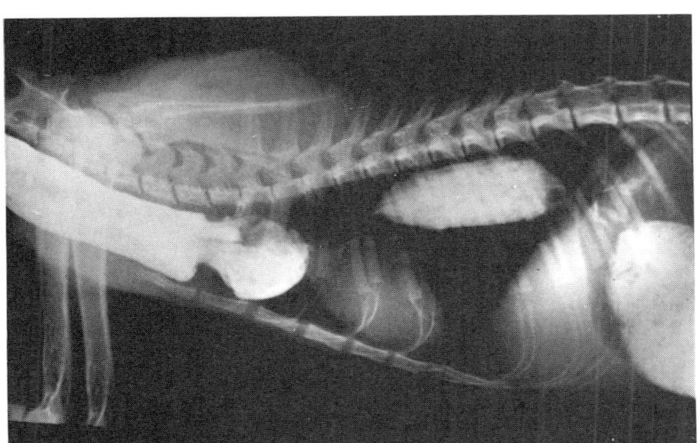

A

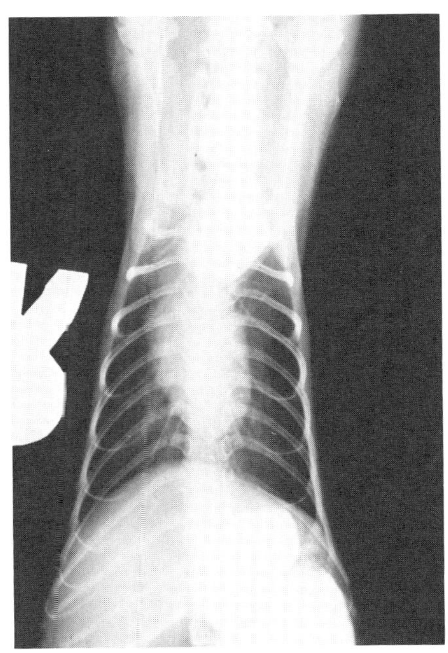

B

Figure 14–2. (*A*) Megaesophagus is easily visualized when the barium reaches the esophagus. The contrast material fills the greatly distended organ. (*B*) A ventrodorsal view of the same cat as in Figure 14–2A.

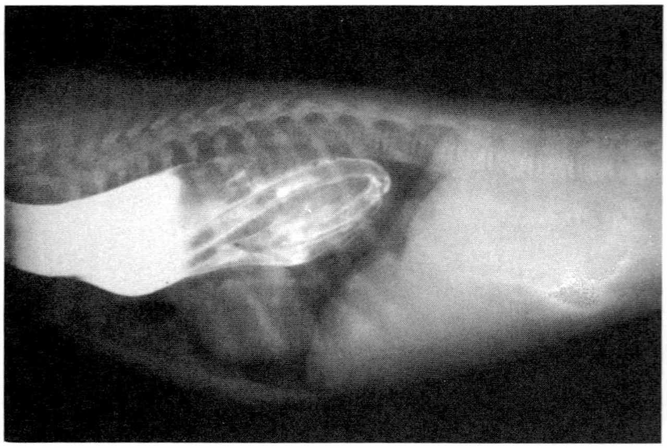

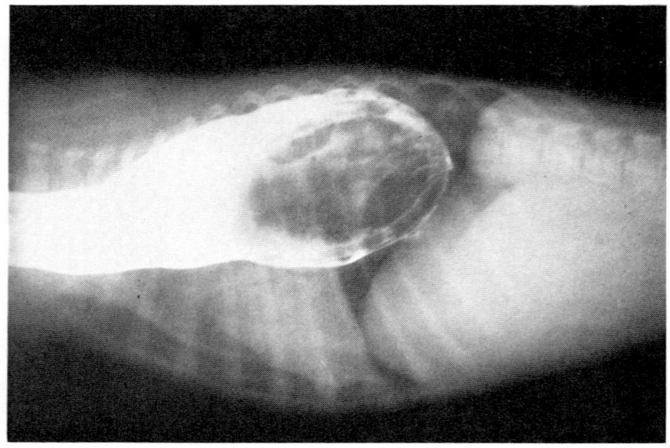

A B

Figure 14–4. (*A*) The esophageal dilation and filling defect seen in this radiograph is typical for a gastroesophageal intussusception. The tube is in the stomach, and the stomach is within the esophagus. (*B*) Another view of the same cat as in Figure 14–4A.

4. Mouth speculum (Feline Mouth Speculum, Jorgensen Laboratories, Loveland, CO)

Technique

1. Allow the cat nothing by mouth for 12 to 24 hours prior to the procedure.
2. Administer a soapy water enema 3–4 hours prior.
3. Obtain survey lateral and dorsoventral radiographs of the abdomen.
4. Administer 30% barium sulfate or iohexol through the orogastric tube at a rate of 5 mL/lb of body weight.
5. If an esophagogram has not been performed and vomiting or regurgitation is present, the final 10 mL of contrast should be administered as a swallow to allow visualization of the esophagus.
6. Increase the radiographic exposure 5 to 10 kVp as compared to the survey radiographs.
7. Obtain right lateral and dorsoventral abdominal radiographs.
   - If a barium swallow is administered, obtain lateral and dorsoventral radiographs of the thorax and cranial abdomen *immediately*.
   - If the lesion is thought to be in the stomach, four views of the stomach should be obtained—right lateral, left lateral, ventrodorsal, and dorsoventral.
   - Right lateral and dorsoventral views should be made at 5, 15, 30, and 60 minutes, or until the contrast material fills the large bowel.
   - Based on clinical judgment and transient time, more or fewer radiographs may be made during the study. A questionable lesion should be re-radiographed for confirmation even if a second dose of contrast must be administered.

Normal Findings

- The transit time from the stomach to the large bowel is approximately 60 minutes when barium is utilized.
- If a rupture of the stomach or bowel is suspected, iohexol should be used. Using Gastrografin, transit time from the stomach to the large bowel is approximately 1–2 hours.
- The pyloric outflow tract is near the midline on the dorsoventral view (Fig. 14–5).
- The duodenum (only) may exhibit multiple peristaltic waves which are sometimes referred to as the "string of pearls" sign (Fig. 14–5). This should not be confused with a linear foreign body or with ulceration.

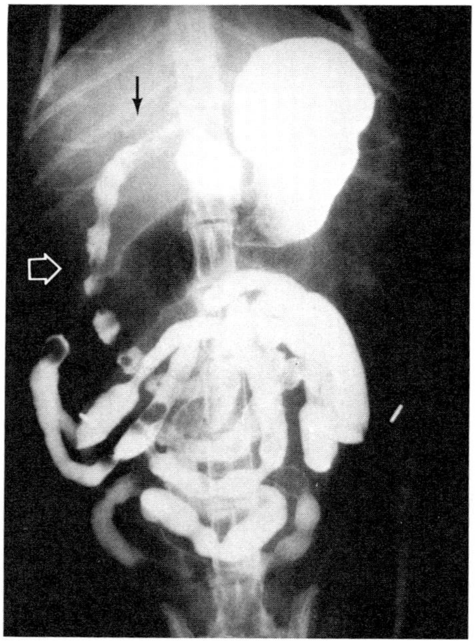

Figure 14–5. A normal upper gastrointestinal study. The pylorus is located near the midline on the ventrodorsal view (*solid arrow*). The pattern in the duodenum is attributable to peristalsis and is often called the "string of pearls" sign (*open arrow*). It should not be confused with a linear foreign body.

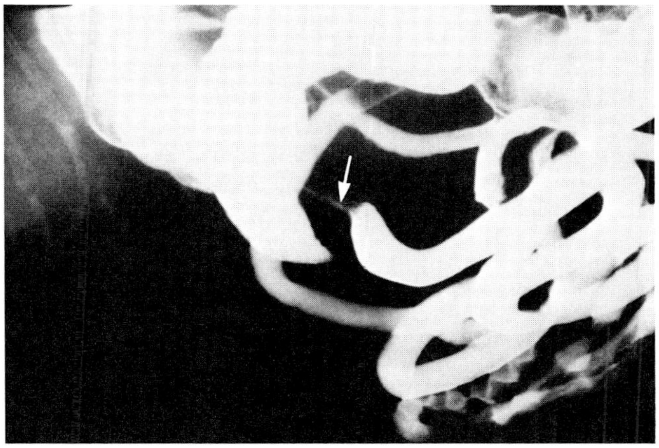

A

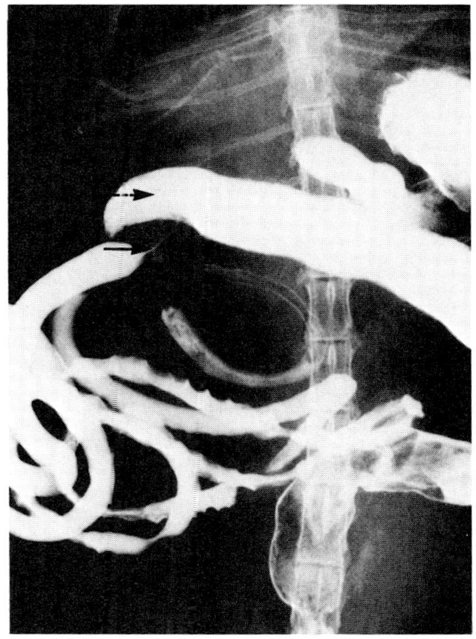

B

Figure 14–6. (*A*) Lateral view of the abdomen. The narrowed segment of ileum (*arrow*) just proximal to entering the colon is normal. (*B*) A ventrodorsal view of the same cat shows a narrowing of the ileum (*solid arrow*) just proximal to its entry into the colon. The barium then enters the cecum (*dashed arrow*).

- As the contrast material leaves the stomach, the rugal folds should be well delineated.
- The cecum of the cat is a blind pouch that is much smaller than that of the dog.
- The ileocolic valve is often seen as a narrowing of the ileum (Fig. 14–6, *A* and *B*).

Common Lesions

- Inflammatory changes of the stomach and small bowel (gastroenteritis) will cause irregular margination of the contrast within the mucosal wall. There may be "smudging" of the gastric mucosa, with poor visualization of the rugal folds. If there is mucus or blood in the stomach or bowel, barium may clump or flocculate. Mucosal margination is ill-defined with Gastrografin.
- Ulcers in the stomach or bowel will fill with contrast material. These irregular fillings may persist after the contrast material has left the area.
- A perforated gastric (Fig. 14–7, *A* and *B*) or intestinal (Fig. 14–8) ulcer is indicated by contrast material exiting the gastrointestinal tract.

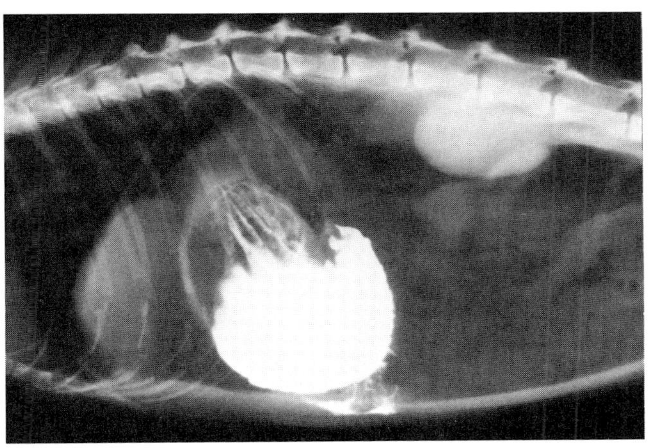

A

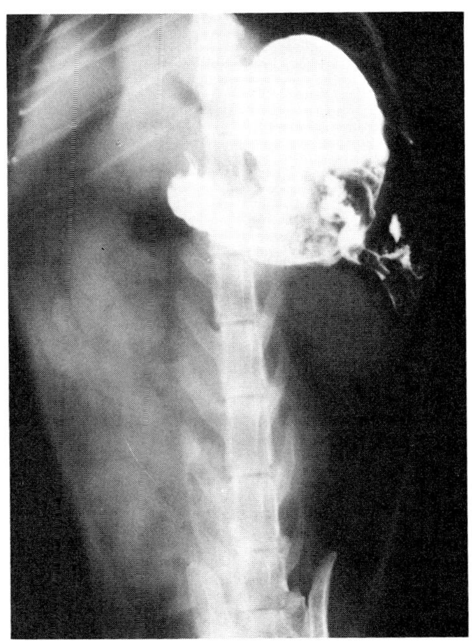

B

Figure 14–7. (*A*) A perforating gastric ulcer allows the contrast medium to escape into the peritoneal cavity. (*B*) A ventrodorsal view of the same cat as in Figure 14–7A.

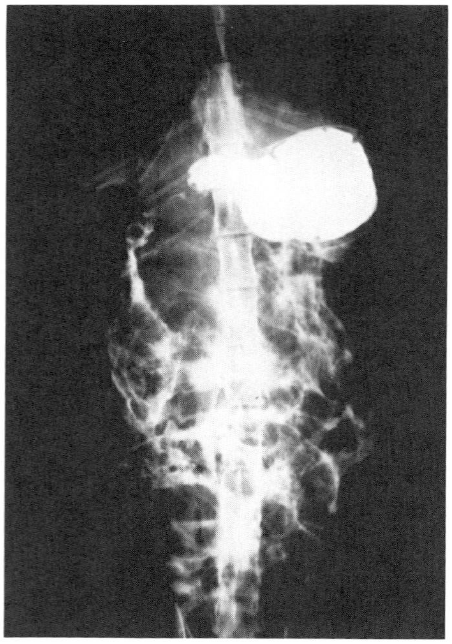

Figure 14–8. Barium was administered to a cat with a perforating duodenal ulcer. Free barium can be seen in the abdomen. If perforation is suspected, iohexol is the contrast medium of choice, as barium is very irritating to the peritoneum.

- Linear foreign bodies will cause the bowel to gather on itself (Fig. 14–9, *A* and *B*). This radiographic finding is sometimes referred to as "accordion pleating" or "gathering." The small bowel may not be evenly distributed throughout the abdomen, but may be displaced into one small quadrant of the abdominal cavity. Linear foreign bodies may cause complete occlusion of the small bowel.
- Retained barium in absorptive foreign bodies, such as cloth or hairballs, may be visualized after the rest of the barium passes (Fig. 14–10).
- Radiolucent foreign bodies may cause complete or incomplete obstruction of the stomach or bowel. With complete obstruction, there is generally dilation of the stomach or bowel proximal to the obstruction (Fig. 14–11, *A–C*). There may be coating of the radiolucent foreign body or an interface with the contrast material and the foreign body.
- Intussusception may cause the small bowel to assume a "coiled spring" appearance. It may also be represented as a very small, thin line of contrast material coursing through the intussuscepted bowel, or as a portion of dilated bowel proximal to the obstruction (Fig. 14–12, *A–C*).
- Neoplasia and fungal lesions are represented as infiltrative bowel diseases. Infiltration of the bowel wall will cause an irregular pattern (Fig. 14–13, *A* and *B*). Short, constrictive lesions are sometimes thought to have an "apple core" appearance. Fungal diseases tend to be seen most often in the duodenum. Neoplasia, especially lymphosarcoma, may be generalized in the wall of the bowel.

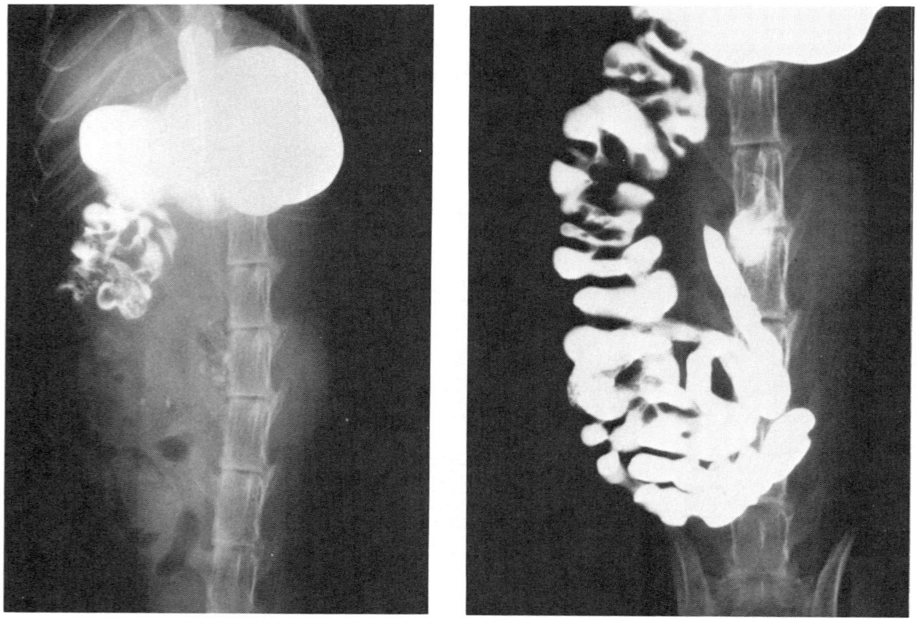

A B

Figure 14–9. (*A*) The convoluted appearance of this proximal duodenum is a classic indication of a linear foreign body, such as string. (*B*) Another linear foreign body has caused an obstruction in the jejunum, resulting in convolution of the duodenum and proximal jejunum.

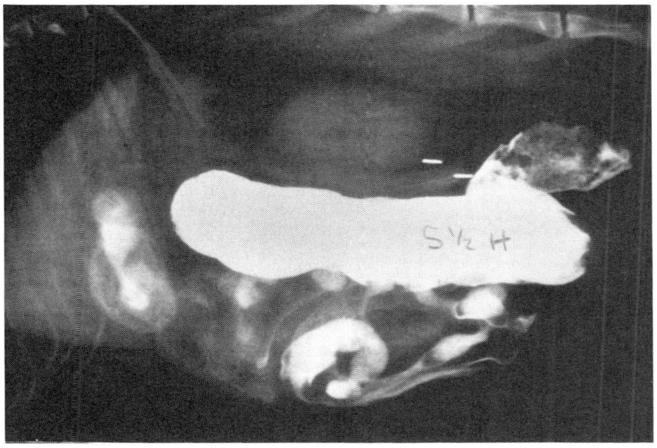

Figure 14–10. Hair balls are not visible unless they retain barium. The majority of the barium has passed from the stomach, but the barium in the hair ball is still prominent, even after 5.5 hours.

Miscellaneous

- If a tranquilizer is required, acepromazine is the drug of choice.
- If Gastrografin is used, it is not uncommon for some of the contrast medium to be absorbed and excreted by the kidneys. Therefore, a gastrointestinal series and excretory urogram may be obtained simultaneously.
- If the patient is dehydrated or has an electrolyte imbalance, Gastrografin should not be used.
- Powdered barium (Barium USP) will often flocculate as it passes through the gastrointestinal tract. This artifact may be misdiagnosed as inflammation.

Barium Enema

Goals

- To determine the size, shape, and location of the colon and rectum
- To determine the patency of the colon and rectum

Clinical Indications

- Rectal bleeding
- Hematochezia (bright red blood)
- Dyschezia

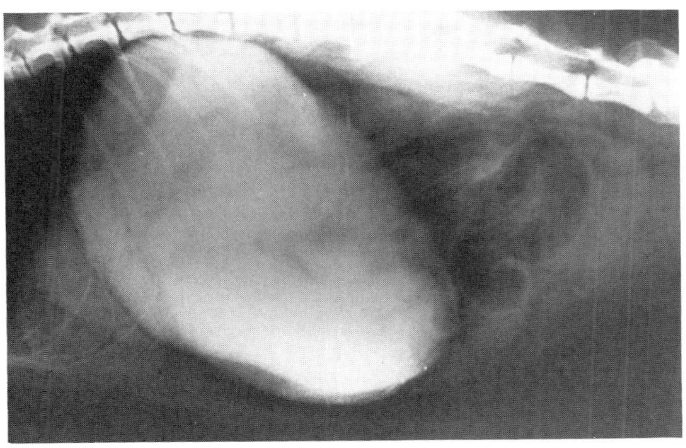

A

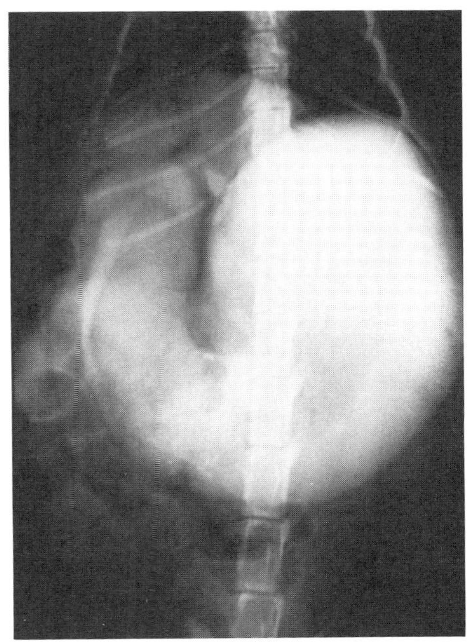

B

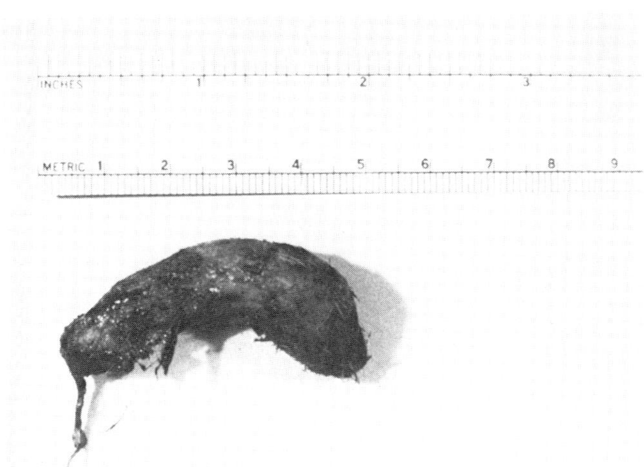

C

Figure 14–11. (*A*) Lateral view of a distended stomach. This degree of gastric distention is characteristic of intestinal obstruction. (*B*) Ventrodorsal view of the same cat as in Figure 14–11*A*. (*C*) A hair ball was found to be the cause of duodenal obstruction which resulted in the gastric distention seen in Figures 14–11, *A* and *B*. The hair ball was not visible radiographically.

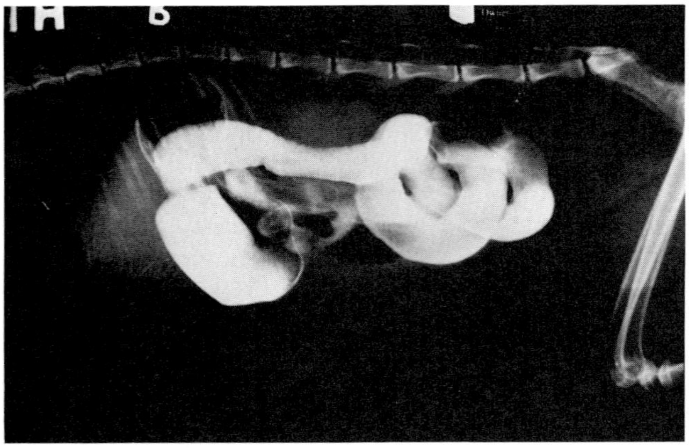

A

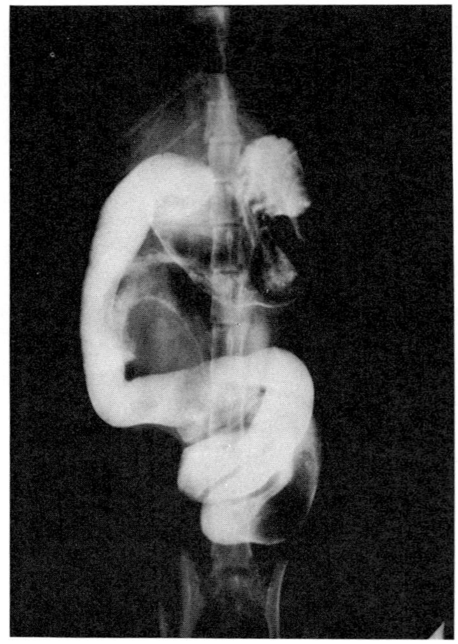

B

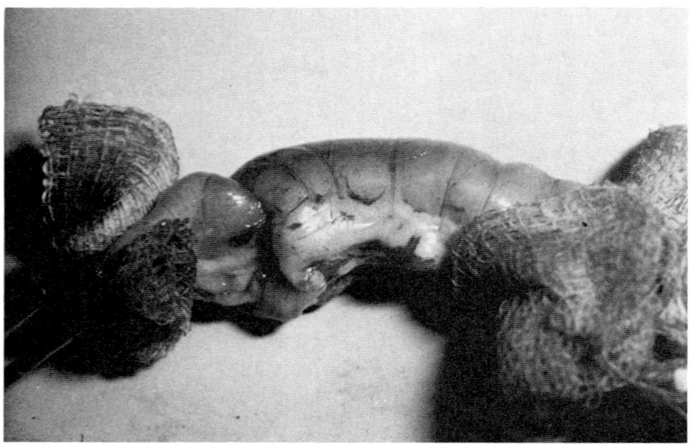

C

Figure 14–12. Intestinal obstruction results in dilation of the bowel proximal to the lesion. Barium is seen to fill this dilated jejunum. (*B*) A ventrodorsal view of the same cat as in Figure 14–12*A*. (*C*) An intussusception was found in the distal jejunum of this cat.

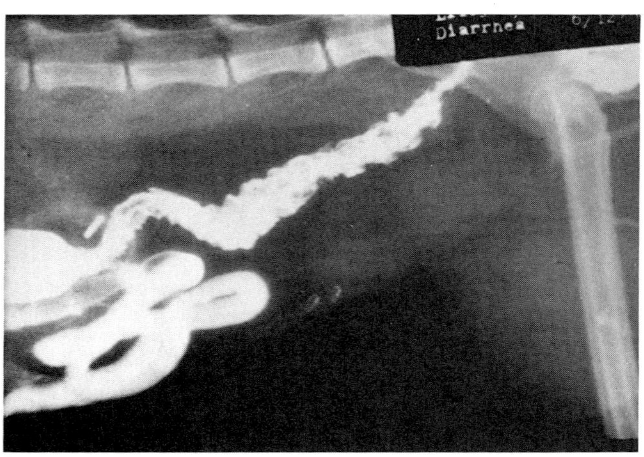

A

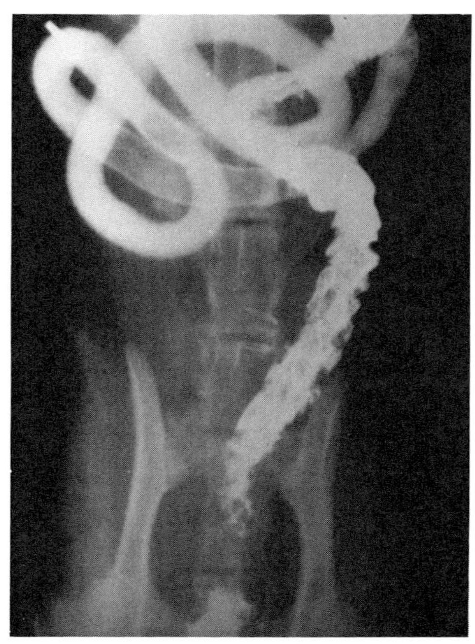

B

Figure 14–13. (*A*) Infiltrative bowel diseases, such as lymphosarcoma and histoplasmosis, change the shape of the bowel wall from smooth to ragged, as is the case with this colon. (*B*) A ventrodorsal view of the same cat as in Figure 14–13*A*.

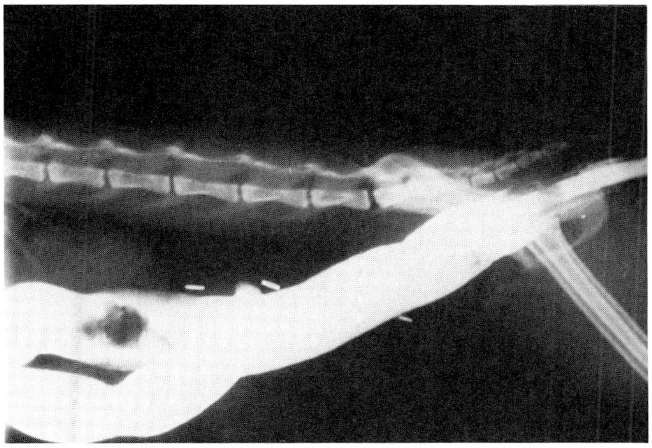

A

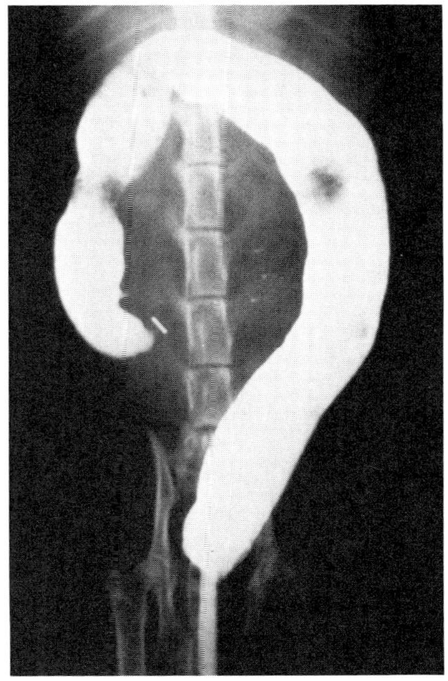

B

Figure 14–14. (*A*) A normal barium-filled colon has a smooth wall. (*B*) On the ventrodorsal view, the colon has the shape of a question mark.

Materials

1. Barium sulfate: 30% W/V
2. 16-French Foley catheter (Rusch Gold Foley Catheter, Willy Rusch, Stuttgart, Germany)
3. 60-cc Syringe

Technique*†

1. Allow the cat nothing by mouth for 12 to 24 hours prior to the procedure.
2. Administer a general anesthesia.
3. Perform a soapy warm water enema 3–4 hours prior.
4. Obtain survey radiographs of the abdomen.
5. Place the distal end of a Foley catheter in the rectum and inflate the cuff.
6. Administer barium at a dose of 5 mL/lb of body weight.
7. Increase the radiographic exposure 5 to 10 kVp as compared to the survey radiographs.
8. Obtain right lateral and ventrodorsal radiographs of the caudal abdomen.

Normal Findings

- The colon will have the appearance of a question mark on the ventrodorsal view (Fig. 14–14, *A* and *B*). The colon and rectum should be distended so that the mucosal surface is smooth.

*An examination of the colon may be included in an upper and lower gastrointestinal series if radiographs are made with barium in the colon and rectum. A barium enema dilates and more completely fills the colon, permitting better visualization. It is indicated if the findings of the upper and lower gastrointestinal series are equivocal.

†A negative contrast study may be performed prior to the barium study by distending the colon with room air.

Common Lesions

- Strictures and masses will be visualized easily. These may be attributable to scar tissue or fungal or neoplastic diseases.
- Infiltrative bowel diseases, especially neoplastic diseases will create an irregular mucosal surface (see Fig. 14–13, *A* and *B*).
- Megacolon causes the colon to dilate abnormally. Its size is generally equal to or greater than two times the length of the body of L7 (Fig. 14–15).

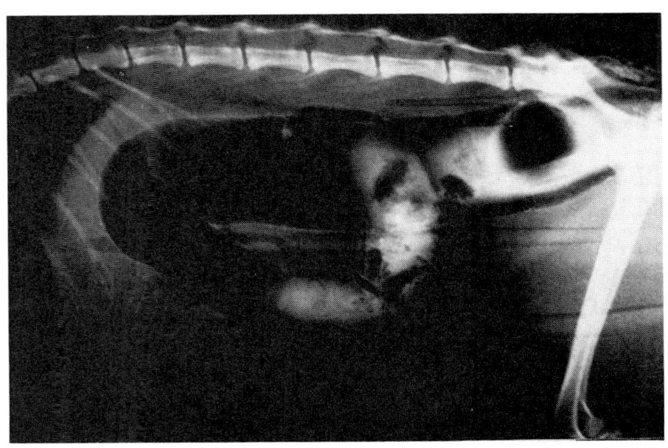

Figure 14–15. Megacolon is characterized by a colonic diameter that is equal to or greater than two times the length of the body of L7. For this radiographic view, air has been used to distend the colon to demonstrate its diameter.

Urinary System

Excretory Urogram (Intravenous Pyelogram)

Goal

- To determine the size, shape, and location of the kidneys, ureters, and urinary bladder

Clinical Indications

- Hematuria
- Pyuria
- Fever of unknown origin
- Abdominal masses
- Poor visualization or nonvisualization of the kidneys on plain radiographs
- Incontinence
- Urine in the peritoneal cavity and/or retroperitoneal space.

Materials

1. Water-soluble organic iodine contrast agent for intravenous use (Renografin-76)
2. 22-Gauge needle and 12-cc syringe*

Technique

1. Allow the cat nothing by mouth for 12 to 24 hours prior to the procedure.
2. Administer a soapy warm water enema.
3. Perform scout radiographs of the abdomen.
4. Inject Renografin-76 IV at a rate of 1 mL/lb (400 mg of iodine/lb).
5. Increase the radiographic exposure by 5 to 10 kVp as compared to the scout radiographs.
6. Obtain lateral and ventrodorsal abdominal radiographs once the injection is complete.
7. Obtain lateral and ventrodorsal abdominal radiographs at 5, 15, and 30 minutes after the injection. Fewer or more radiographs may be indicated, depending on the rate of renal filtration of the contrast material.

Normal Findings

- The radiographs made at the conclusion of the injection will demonstrate the nephrogram stage of the excretory urogram. There will be an increased opacity of the renal parenchyma (Fig. 14–16, *A* and *B*). The size, shape, and location of the kidneys can be determined from this phase of the examination.
- The pyelogram phase of the study will be seen on subsequent radiographs. The pelves and collecting system, as well as the ureters and urinary bladder, will be imaged on the 5-, 15-, and/or 30-minute radiographs (Fig. 14–16*C*). Filling defects in the ureters may be seen and/or expected owing to normal peristalsis.

Common Lesions

- Nonvisualization of a kidney may be the result of renal agenesis or poor renal function (Fig. 14–17, *A* and *B*). If the blood urea nitrogen (BUN) level is greater than 100 mg/dL, the kidneys will not be able to concentrate the contrast medium.
- Neoplasia, such as lymphosarcoma, and feline infectious peritonitis (FIP) may cause unilateral or bilateral enlargement of the kidney (Fig. 14–18, *A* and *B*). Additionally, hydronephrosis and polycystic renal disease can cause enlargement of the renal silhouettes on the excretory urogram (Fig. 14–19).
- End-stage kidneys may be seen as small, irregularly marginated kidneys.
- A tear of the renal capsule or of a ureter will cause contrast medium to leak into the retroperitoneal space or peritoneal cavity, or both.
- Ectopic ureters, which are often enlarged (hydroureter), will empty into the urethra or vagina.
- Pyelonephritis may be seen as an enlarged and irregular filling of the pelvis of the kidney. Hydroureter of the proximal ureter may also be visualized.
- A subcapsular cyst may be seen as an opacified kidney surrounded by a fluid-filled sac.
- Cystic kidneys will exhibit irregular filling of the cortex and medulla of the kidney. There may be isolated areas where the contrast material concentrates (Fig. 14–20, *A–E*).
- Renal calculi may cause filling defects in the kidneys or ureters, or both (Fig. 14–21, *A* and *B*).

Miscellaneous

- Injection of the IV contrast media used for urography will sometimes cause retching or regurgitation, or both. This usually occurs immediately after the start of the injection, but is not a contraindication for completing the injection or the procedure.

Urinary Cystogram

Goals

- To determine the size, shape, and location of the urinary bladder
- To demonstrate the thickness and margination of the bladder wall
- To visualize masses or uroliths within the urinary bladder

Clinical Indications

- Hematuria
- Stranguria
- Polyuria
- Incontinence
- Crystalluria

Contraindication

- Pyuria

Materials

1. 3.5 French urinary catheter (Tomcat Catheter, Sherwood Medical, St. Louis, MO)
2. Water-soluble organic iodine contrast media (Renografin-76
3. Gas source: Carbon dioxide (CO_2), nitrous oxide (N_2O), or room air

*Some clinicians prefer to substitute a 22-gauge butterfly catheter for the 22-gauge needle.

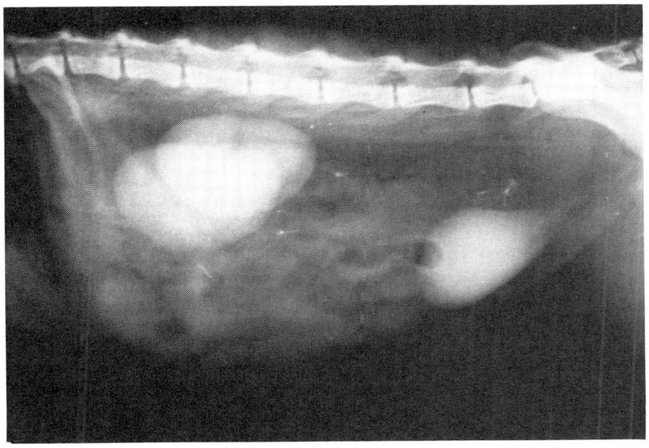

A

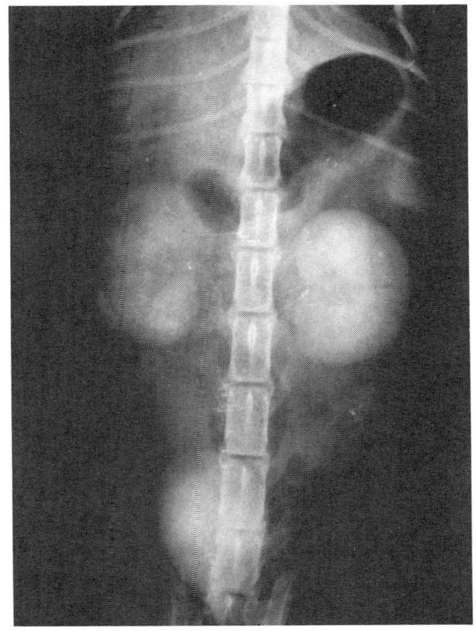

B

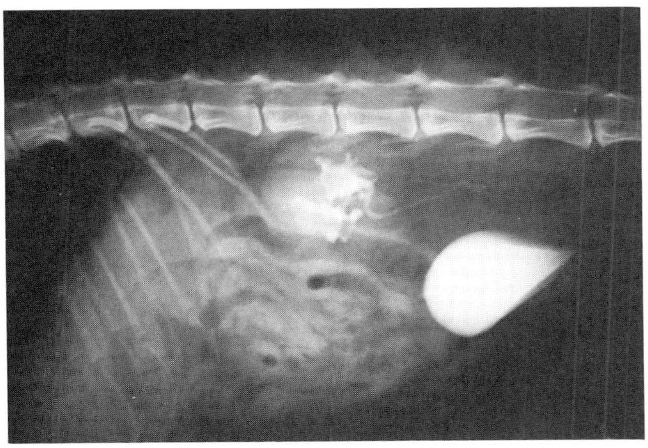

C

Figure 14–16. (*A*) When an excretory urogram is performed on a normal cat, contrast material may be seen in the renal cortex from *T* = 0 (the end of the injection) to *T* = 10 minutes. (*B*) A ventrodorsal view obtained during the excretory urogram performed on the same cat as in Figure 14–16*A*. (*C*) At *T* = 10–20 minutes, contrast material can be seen in the renal pelves, the ureters, and the urinary bladder.

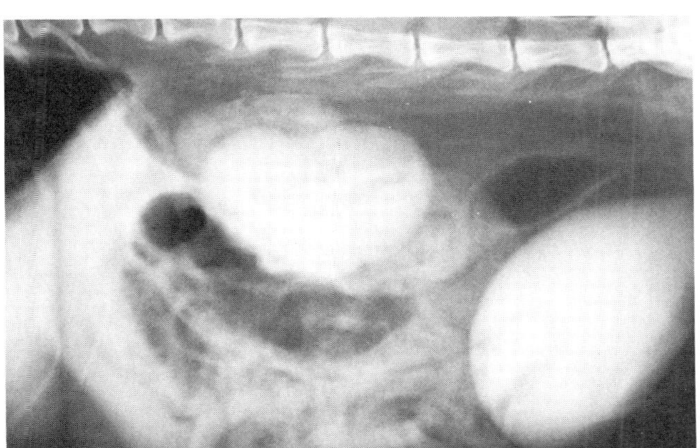

A

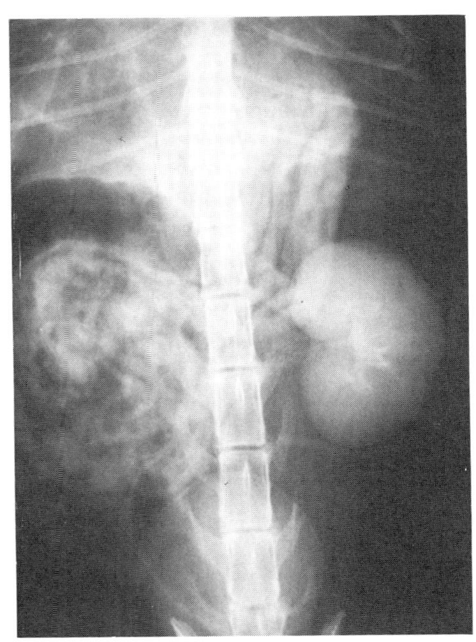

B

Figure 14–17. (*A*) This excretory urogram demonstrates that the size of the right (cranial) kidney is decreased. Because the excretion of the contrast material is delayed, it can be seen in the visceral vasculature. (*B*) A ventrodorsal view of the same cat as in Figure 14–17*A*. The contrast material in the visceral vasculature obscures the right kidney.

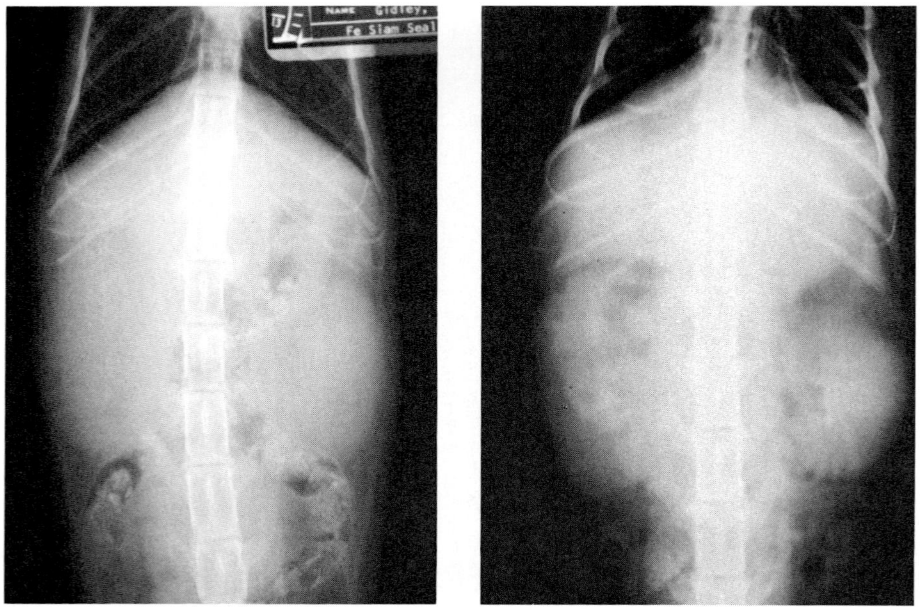

A B

Figure 14–18. (*A*) A ventrodorsal view of a cat with bilateral renal enlargement that is typical of lymphosarcoma or feline infectious peritonitis (FIP). (*B*) A ventrodorsal view obtained during an excretory urogram in a cat with lymphosarcoma of the right kidney. The right kidney contains minimal contrast material, whereas the normal left kidney has a small amount of contrast material in the renal pelvis.

General Technique

1. Allow the cat nothing by mouth for 12 to 24 hours prior to the procedure.
2. Administer general anesthesia.
3. Administer a soapy warm water enema.
4. Obtain scout radiographs of the caudal abdomen.
5. Insert a catheter into the urinary bladder. Male cats can be catheterized easily using a 3.5-French catheter. Female cats can be catheterized with a 3.5-French catheter using an otoscope and a vaginal speculum (Fig. 14–22). To accomplish this, the female cat is placed in ventral recumbency. Her rear legs are positioned over the edge of the table, and her rear quarters are lifted slightly from the table by her tail. Because the urethral opening is on the ventral midline of the vagina, it is essential that the cat be positioned in true ventral recumbency and not allowed to roll to either side. The lighted vaginal speculum is slowly passed cranially into the vagina until the slit-shaped opening of the urethra is visualized. The urethral opening is just cranial to the clitoral fossa. The catheter is passed through the speculum into the urethra. If the speculum is large enough, it can be removed from the operating field by sliding it over the catheter. If not, it must remain in place; this is not desirable, however, because the speculum will restrict ease of operation. If difficulty is encountered using this method of catheterization, the cat should be placed in dorsal recumbency with her legs pulled cranially. By passing the catheter along the midline of the floor of the vagina, the urethra can often be catheterized easily.
6. Evacuate the urine from the urinary bladder.
7. Inject contrast medium.
8. Increase the radiographic exposure by 5 kVp as compared to the scout radiograph.
9. Obtain lateral and ventrodorsal radiographs of the caudal abdomen.

Technique for a Positive Contrast Cystogram

1. After evacuating the urinary bladder, fill the bladder with Renografin-76, diluted 1:1 or 1:2 with sterile saline, until it is taut. Generally, 40 to 60 mL of diluted Renografin are needed. The urethra/vagina can be occluded

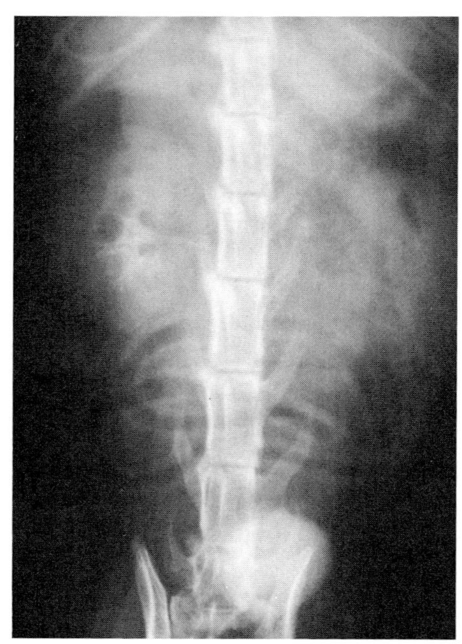

Figure 14–19. The right kidney of this cat with hydronephrosis is enlarged. The enlarged renal pelvis contains contrast material.

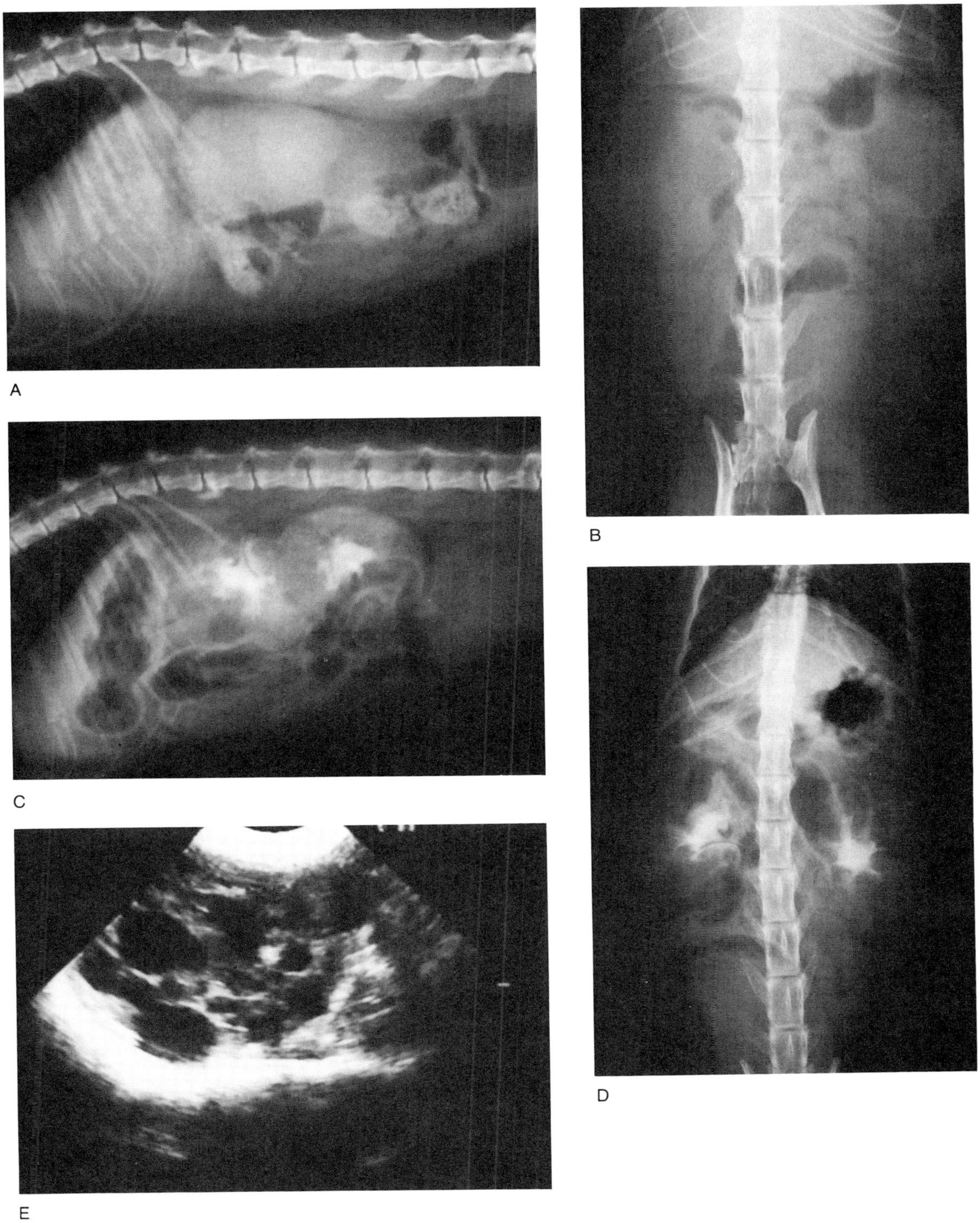

Figure 14–20. (*A*) These enlarged kidneys are typical of polycystic renal disease. (*B*) A ventrodorsal view of the same cat as in Figure 14–20*A*. (*C*) When an excretory urogram is performed, the irregularly shaped renal pelves can be seen. (*D*) A ventrodorsal view of the same cat as in Figure 14–20*C*. (*E*) A sonogram of a cat with polycystic kidneys clearly reveals multiple cysts within the renal parenchyma.

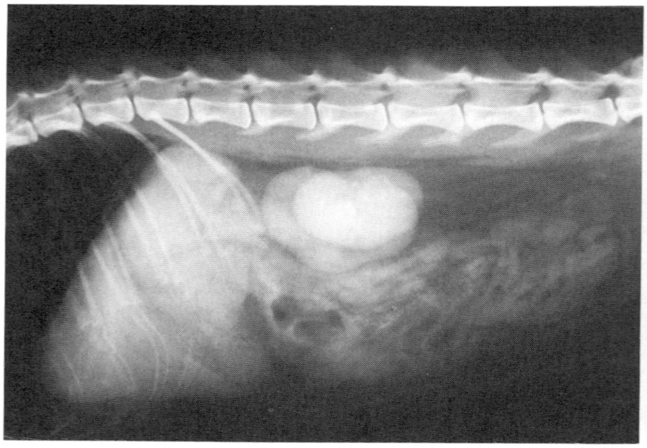

A

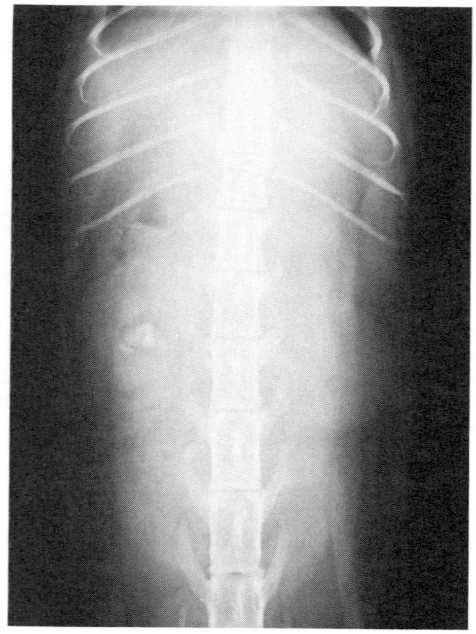

B

Figure 14–21. (*A*) A calculus can be seen in the right kidney. (*B*) A ventrodorsal view of the same cat as in Figure 14–21A.

with digital pressure to prevent backflow of the contrast material.

2. Obtain lateral and ventrodorsal radiographs, increasing the radiation exposure by 5 kVp over that of the scout radiographs. An oblique ventrodorsal view is optional.

Technique for a Double Contrast Cystogram

1. Evacuate the positive contrast material from the bladder, leaving a "puddle" of positive contrast material in the bladder.
2. Inject negative contrast material (gas) into the urinary bladder until the bladder is taut.
3. Obtain lateral and ventrodorsal radiographs, reducing the radiograpic exposure by 5 kVp compared to that of the scout radiographs. An oblique ventrodorsal radiograph is optional.

Technique for a Negative Contrast Cystogram (Pneumocystography)

1. Inflate the urinary bladder with negative contrast material (gas) until the urinary bladder is taut.
2. Obtain lateral and ventrodorsal radiographs using the same level of radiographic exposure as for scout radiographs, or reducing it by 5 kVp.

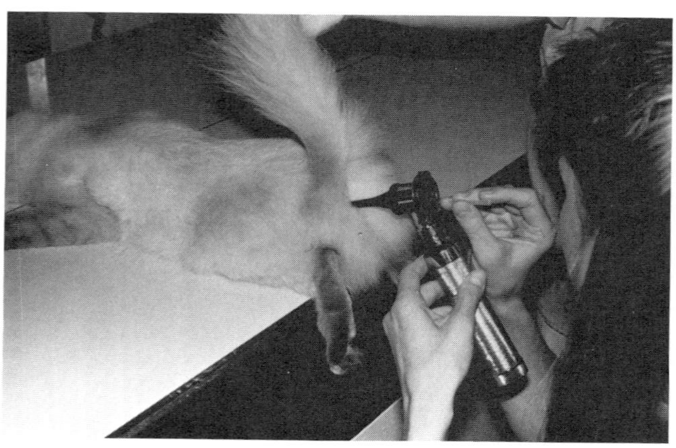

Figure 14–22. The female cat can be catheterized with a 3.5-French tom cat catheter, using an otoscope as a vaginal speculum. If possible, one should use an otoscope cone that is large enough to allow the large end of the catheter to pass through it.

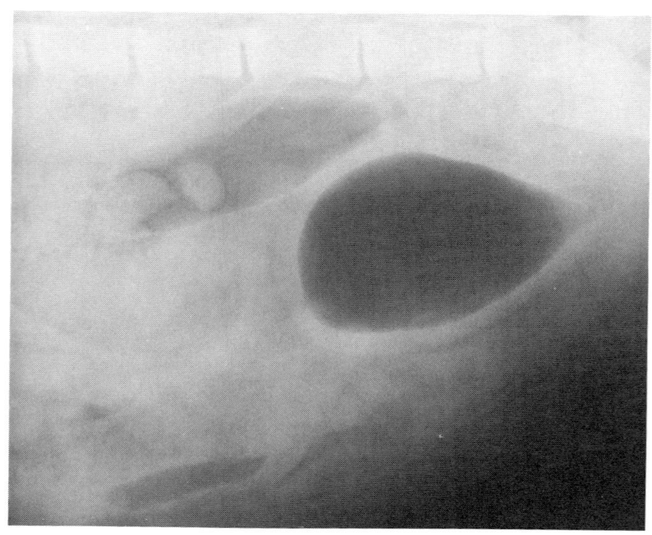

Figure 14–23. A negative contrast cystogram is performed by injecting air into the bladder. Although the lumen is smooth, the thickened bladder wall can be visualized.

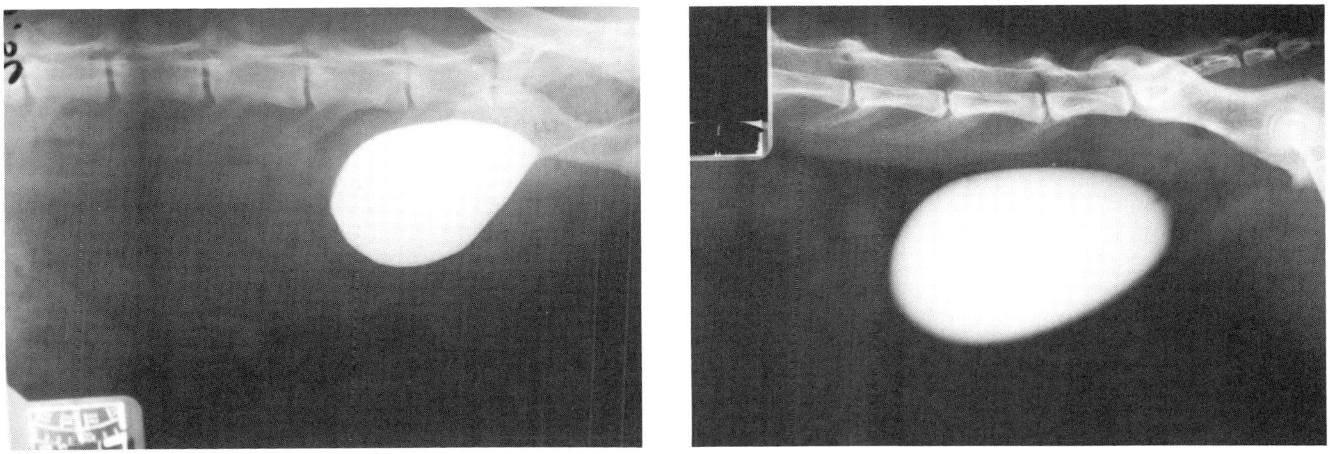

A B

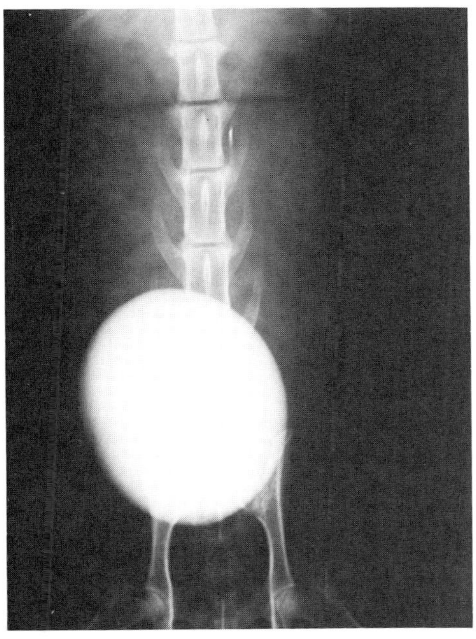

C

Figure 14–24. (*A*) A positive contrast cystogram is performed by injecting Renografin-76 into the bladder. The thickened bladder wall is not as visible as in Figure 14–23 because the radiographic exposure is increased by 5–10 kVp. (*B*) A positive contrast cystogram of a normal bladder with a smooth lumen. (*C*) A ventrodorsal view of the bladder of the same cat as in Figure 14–24*B*.

Normal Findings

- A negative contrast cystogram (pneumocystogram) provides good detail of the bladder wall (Fig. 14–23). The mucosal surface should be smooth, and the bladder wall should be uniform and approximately 1 mm thick. The urinary bladder should be circular or ovoid.
- The positive contrast cystogram will reveal findings similar to those derived from the pneumocystogram (Fig. 14–24, *A–C*). The shape of the urinary bladder can easily be determined by this technique. Bladder wall thickness will not be as apparent as with the negative contrast study owing to the increased radiographic exposure.
- The double contrast cystogram affords good mucosal visualization, as the mucosal surface is coated with the positive contrast medium. A small amount of contrast medium should be seen in the dependent central portion of the urinary bladder (Fig. 14–25, *A–C*).

Common Lesions

- A thickened bladder wall and irregular margination of the mucosal surface are common findings in cats with chronic cystitis (Fig. 14–26, *A–D*).
- Radiopaque uroliths may be visualized on double contrast and negative contrast cystograms, but are usually invisible on positive contrast cystograms (Fig. 14–27).
- Radiolucent uroliths are best visualized on double contrast cystograms appearing as filling defects within the pooled contrast medium. They may also appear to be radiopaque on some negative contrast studies (Fig. 14–28, *A* and *B*).
- A ruptured bladder or urethra is best visualized by positive contrast cystography. If there is a possibility that the urinary bladder is ruptured, the positive contrast cystogram is the procedure of choice. The positive contrast material will be seen to leak into the abdominal cavity (Figs. 14–29, *A* and *B* and 14–30, *A–C*).

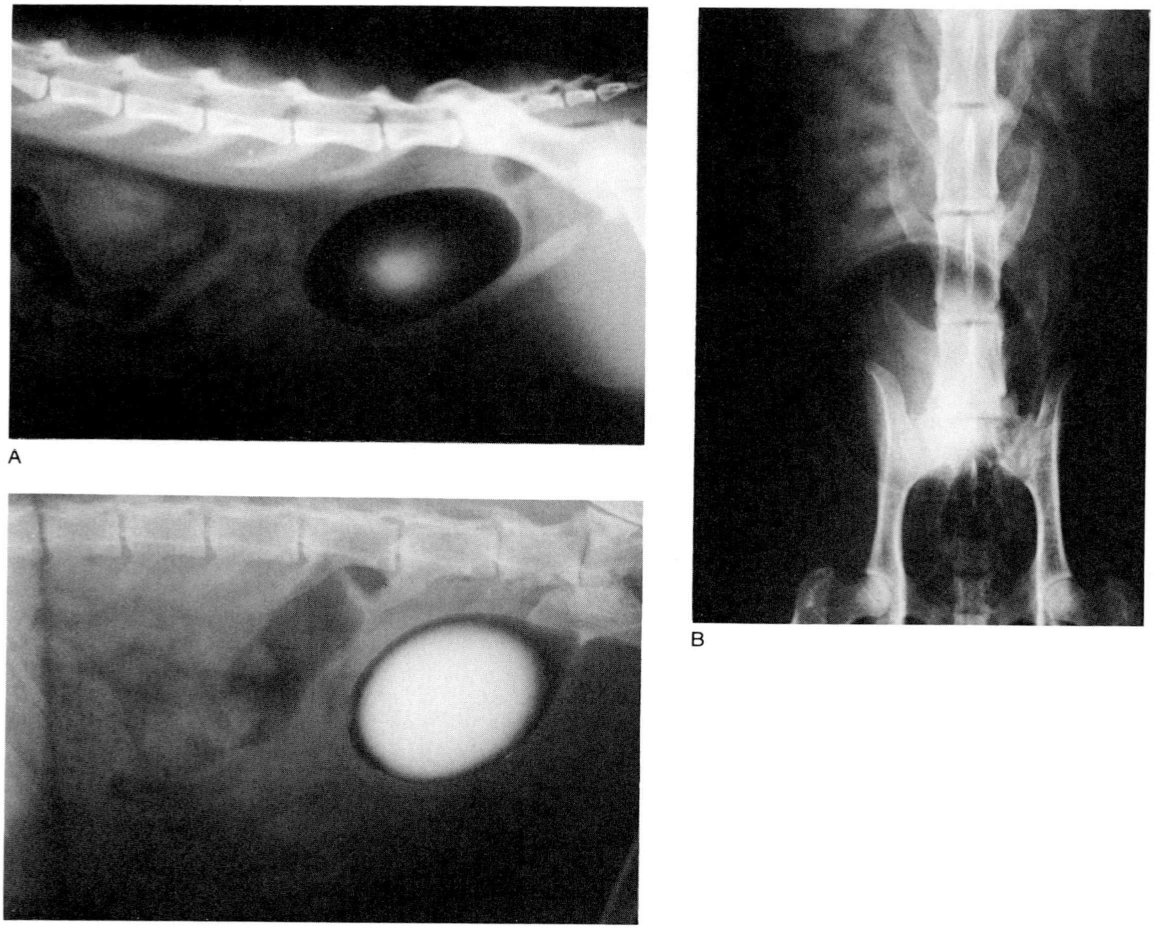

A

B

C

Figure 14–25. (*A*) A double contrast cystogram is performed on a bladder that contains a small amount of contrast material (from the positive contrast cystogram) and that has been distended with air. (*B*) A ventrodorsal view of the bladder of the same cat as in Figure 14–25*A*. Visualization of the bladder is obstructed by the superimposed pelvis. (*C*) An oblique view of the same cat as in Figure 14–25*A* (as evidenced by the position of the lumbar vertebrae). This view allows visualization of parts of the bladder not seen on the lateral view because of superimposition of the pelvis.

- Both neoplasia and polyps will cause filling defects and irregular margination of the bladder mucosal surface. Tumors have a tendency to be seen in the caudal aspect of the bladder or at the neck (Fig. 14–31, *A* and *B*), whereas polyps and bladder wall thickening secondary to chronic cystitis will often be seen in the cranial aspect.
- Urachal diverticula are seen in the cranial aspect of the urinary bladder, often only when the bladder is completely distended (Fig. 14–32, *A–D*).

Miscellaneous

- Reflux of contrast medium into the ureters is not uncommon.
- Fatal air embolism secondary to pneumocystography has been reported in the cat. For this reason, CO_2 and N_2O are suggested for pneumocystography and double contrast cystography, although room air has been used very successfully by many clinicians for many years.
- Ruptured bladders are often difficult to detect with pneumocystography.
- The bubble formation that results from a failure to evacuate all of the urine from the bladder will have a honeycomb type of appearance (Fig. 14–33).
- Some clinicians prefer to perform a pneumocystogram prior to the positive contrast and double contrast procedures.
- On the double contrast cystogram, gas bubbles tend to cause circular radiolucent filling defects at the junction of the contrast material and the gas; uroliths tend to congregate in the dependent central portion of the contrast material.
- Hematomas usually have smooth borders and cause filling defects, which may be centralized or located at the periphery of the contrast medium (Fig. 14–34).

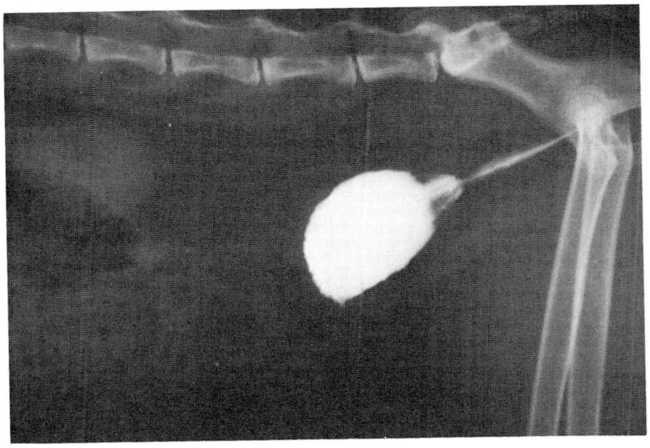

A

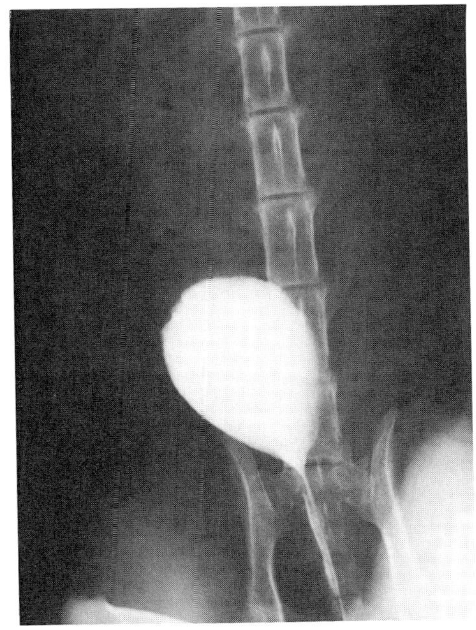

B

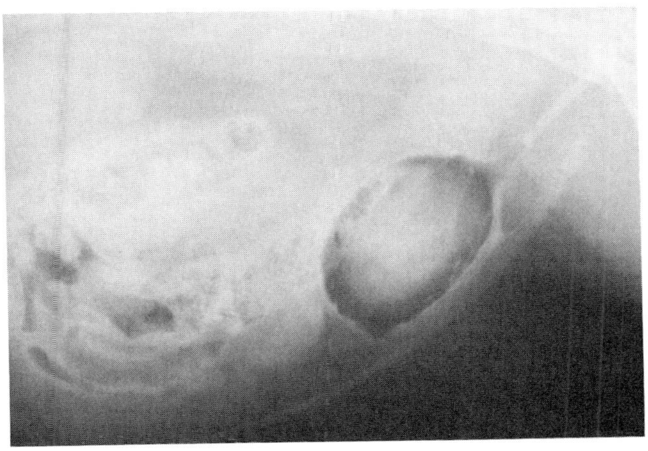

C

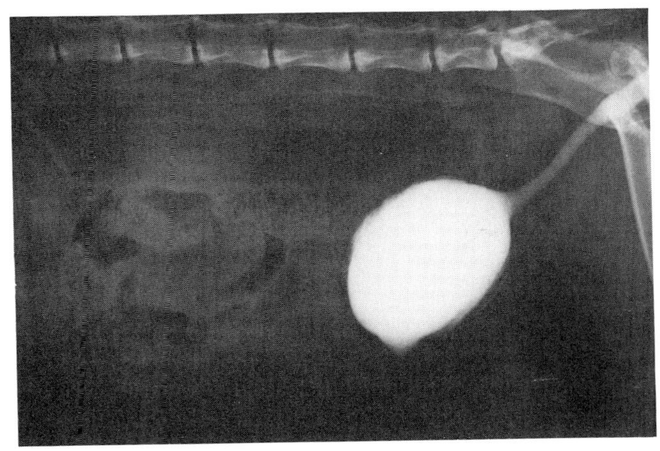

D

Figure 14–26. (*A*) An irregular bladder wall can be seen on this positive cystogram in a cat with chronic cystitis. (*B*) A ventrodorsal view of the same cat as in Figure 14–26*A*. (*C*) An irregular bladder wall, secondary to chronic cystitis, can be seen in this negative cystogram. (*D*) A positive contrast cystogram performed on the same cat as in Figure 14–26*C*. Note that contrast material has infiltrated the bladder wall.

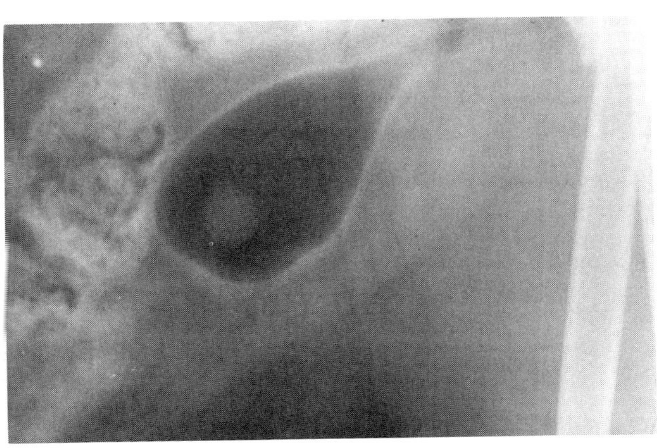

Figure 14–27. A radiopaque stone may be seen on a scout radiograph or on a negative contrast urogram, as shown here.

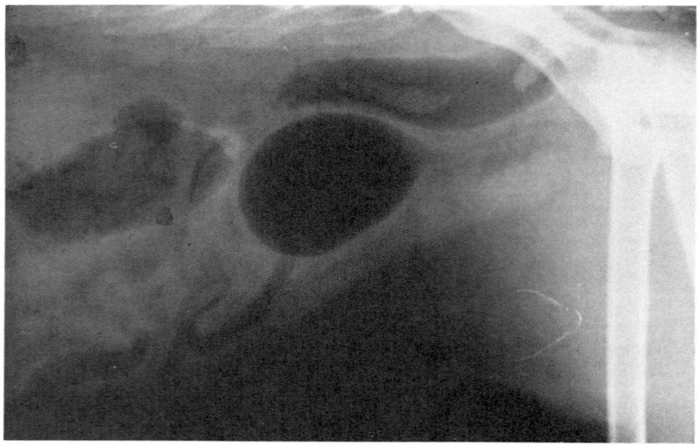

A

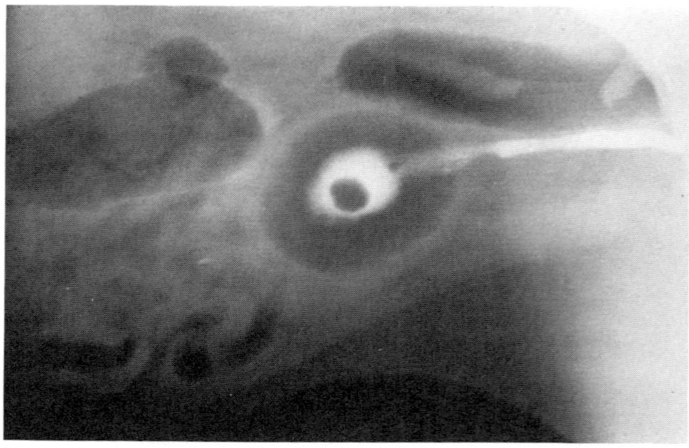

B

Figure 14–28. (*A*) Radiolucent stones are not visible on scout radiographs or on positive contrast urograms. (*B*) Radiolucent stones are best visualized as filling defects in a pool of positive contrast material, as in this double contrast cystogram.

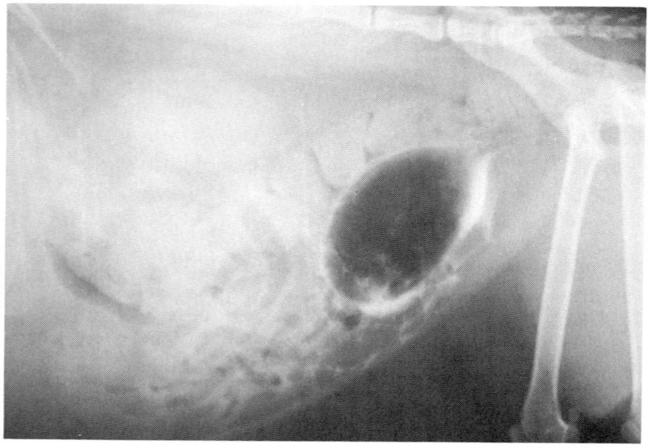

A

Figure 14–29. (*A*) A double contrast cystogram demonstrates positive contrast material that is free in the abdominal cavity. This has occurred as a result of a ruptured bladder. (*B*) A ventrodorsal view of the same cat as in Figure 14–29A.

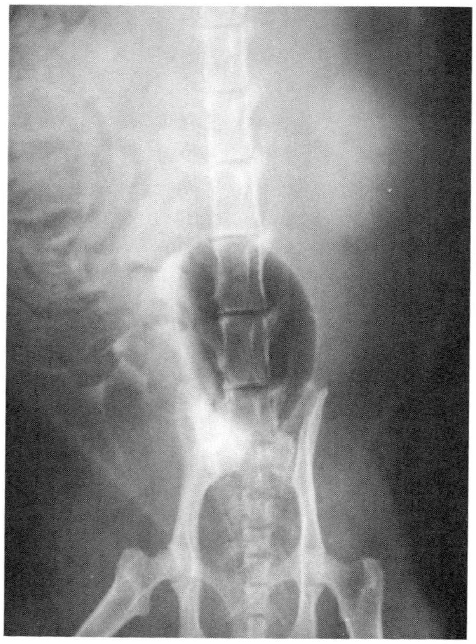

B

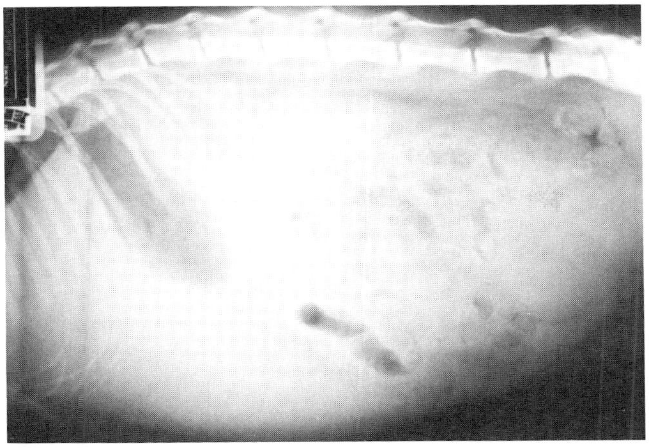

A

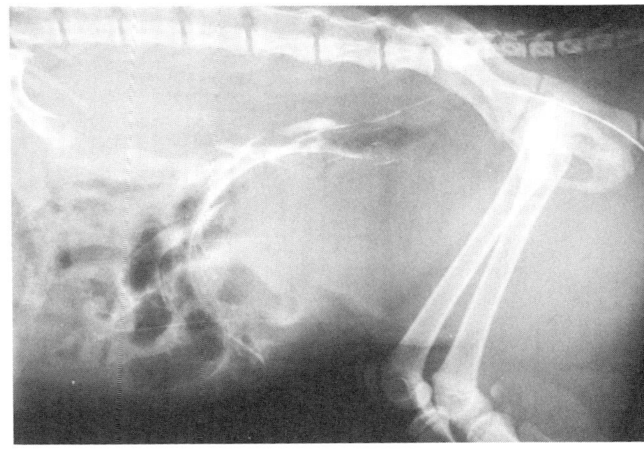

B

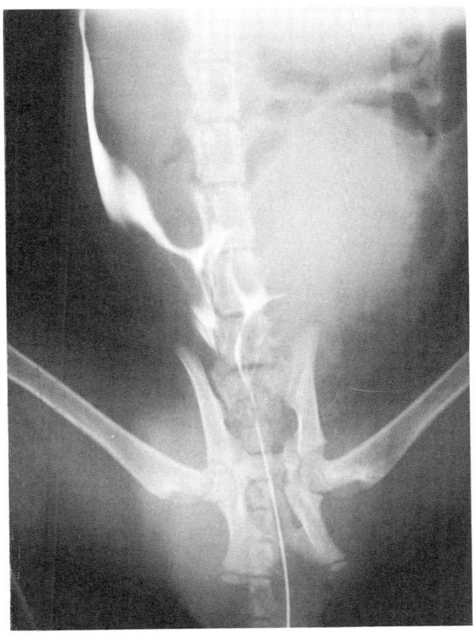

C

Figure 14–30. (*A*) The only hint of a ruptured urinary tract in this cat is a homogeneous water density throughout the abdomen. However, this could be attributable to any abdominal fluid. (*B*) When positive contrast material is injected into the urethra and bladder of the same cat as in Figure 14–30*A*, it can be seen to diffuse throughout the abdominal cavity. This cat had a ruptured urethra secondary to a pelvic fracture. (*C*) A ventrodorsal view of the same cat as in Figure 14–30*B*.

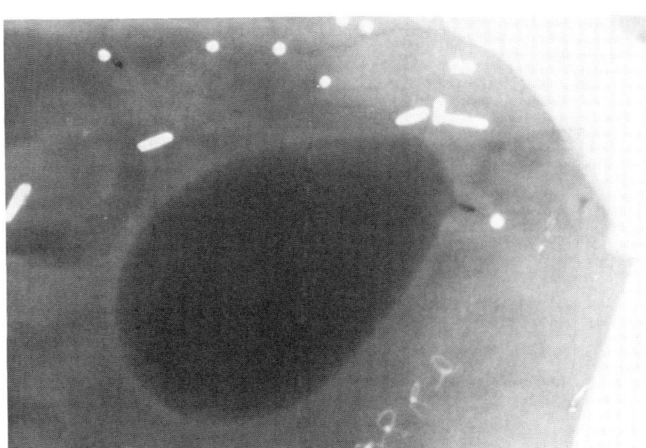

A

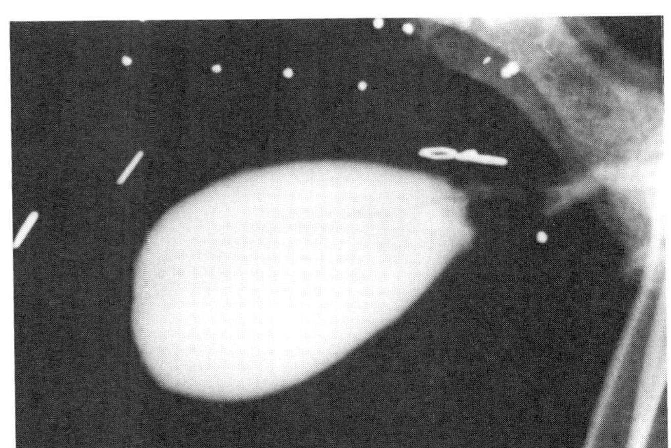

B

Figure 14–31. (*A*) This pneumocystogram reveals a filling defect in the neck of the urinary bladder. (*B*) The filling defect seen in Figure 14–31*A* is even more obvious in this positive contrast cystogram. A transitional cell carcinoma was found at surgery.

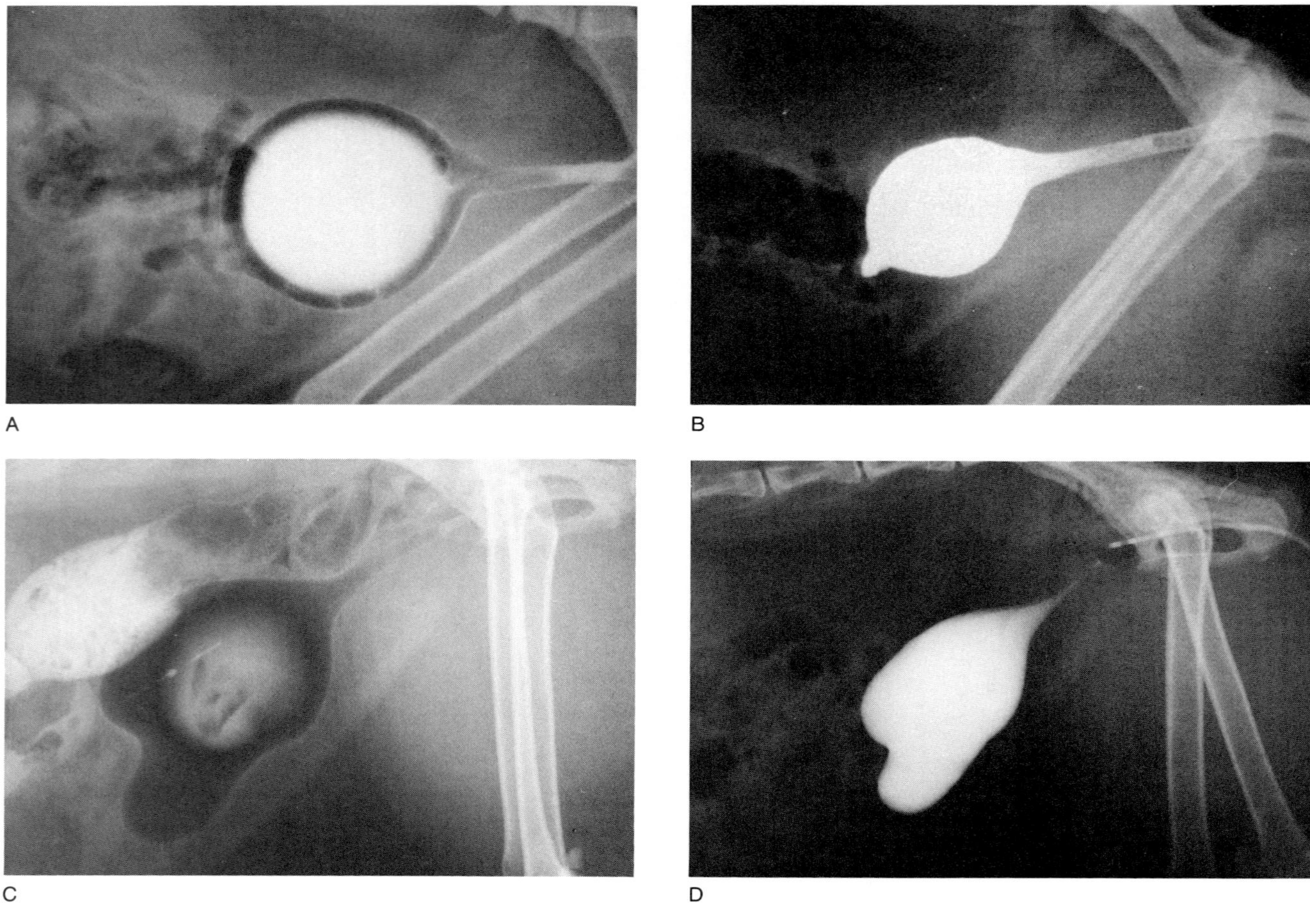

Figure 14–32. (*A*) A small vesicourachal diverticulum is barely visible on a negative or double contrast cystogram. (*B*) The small vesicourachal diverticulum seen in Figure 14–32*A* is better visualized on a positive contrast cystogram. (*C*) This unusually large vesicourachal diverticulum is clearly visible on a negative contrast cystogram. (*D*) The same large vesicourachal diverticulum as seen in Figure 14–32*C* is clearly visible on a positive contrast cystogram.

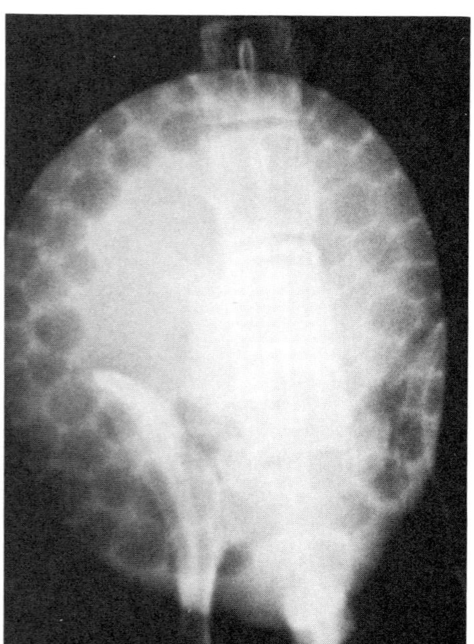

Figure 14–33. A honeycomb appearance is typical of bubbles within the bladder. This may occur when gas is injected into a bladder that has not been completely emptied of urine.

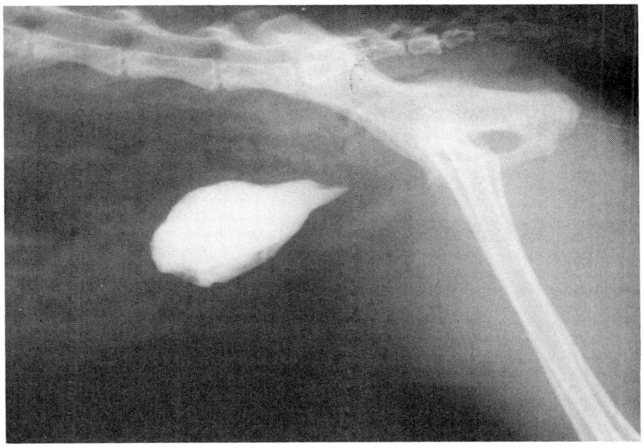

Figure 14–34. **Filling defects found on a positive cystogram indicate masses. These masses are blood clots, which may be radiographically indistinguishable from tumors.**

Urethrogram (Male)[1]

Goals

- To determine the size, shape, and location of the urethra
- To determine the patency of the urethra

Clinical Indications

- Stranguria
- Anuria
- Stranguria despite being able to pass a urinary catheter easily

Materials

1. Water-soluble organic contrast agent (Renografin-76)
2. 12-cc Syringe
3. 3.5-French catheter
4. Radiolucent (wooden) spoon

Technique

1. Administer a soapy warm water enema (desired, but not mandatory).
2. Administer general anesthesia.
3. Obtain survey lateral radiographs of the caudal abdomen.
4. Fill the urinary bladder with sterile saline until it is moderately taut.
5. Pass a catheter 1 cm into the penile urethra and occlude the urethra around the catheter with digital pressure. A lead shield should be used to protect one's fingers from the radiographic beam.
6. Inject 5 to 10 mL of contrast material into the urethra while an assistant applies pressure to the urinary bladder with the radiolucent spoon. Pressure is applied to the bladder to create a pressure gradient within the bladder that encourages retention of the contrast material within the urethra. Care should be taken not to cause bladder rupture.
7. A lateral radiograph is obtained while the contrast material is being injected.

Normal Findings

- The radiographs should show the mucosa of the urethra to be smooth.
- The distal one half of the urethra will be somewhat S-shaped unless it is artificially straightened by applying caudal tension on the penis.
- The cranial half of the urethral lumen will be about 1 to 2 mm in diameter.
- Beginning at the level of the bulbourethral glands and proceeding caudally, the urethral lumen will taper until the penile urethra is about 0.5 mm in diameter (Fig. 14–35).

Common Lesions

- Strictures may occur at any point in the urethra, but they are most likely to occur at the level of or just cranial to the bulbourethral glands. On a lateral radiograph, this will be at about the level of the coxofemoral joints.
- A stricture will cause dilation of the urethra caudal to it because the pressure gradient is from caudal to cranial (Fig. 14–36, *A–C*).

Miscellaneous

- An alternative technique has been described in which contrast material is placed in the bladder, and a radiograph is obtained during induced voiding.[2]

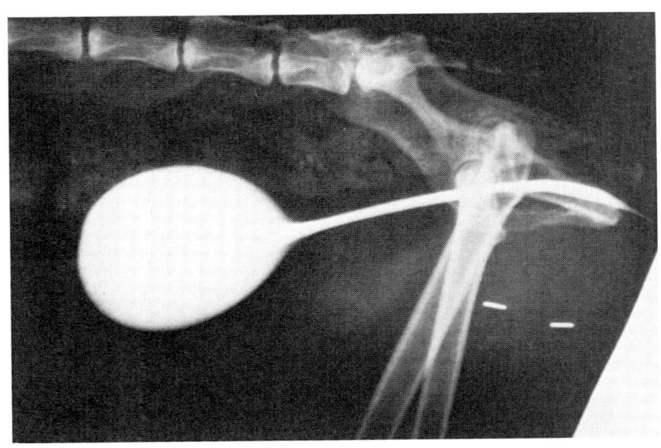

Figure 14–35. **A normal urethrogram demonstrates a urethra that is narrowed distally. The distal end of the urethra is artificially straightened by caudal traction on the cat's penis. (Used by permission of Veterinary Medicine Publishing Co.)**

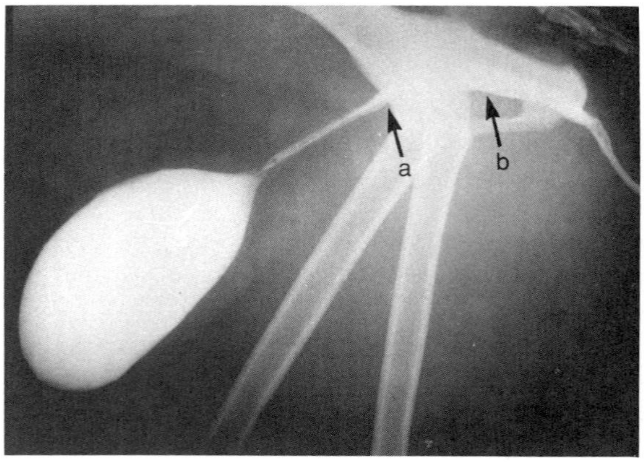

A

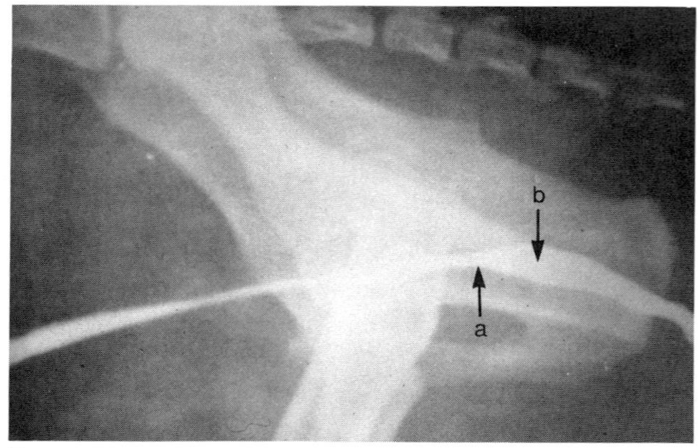

B

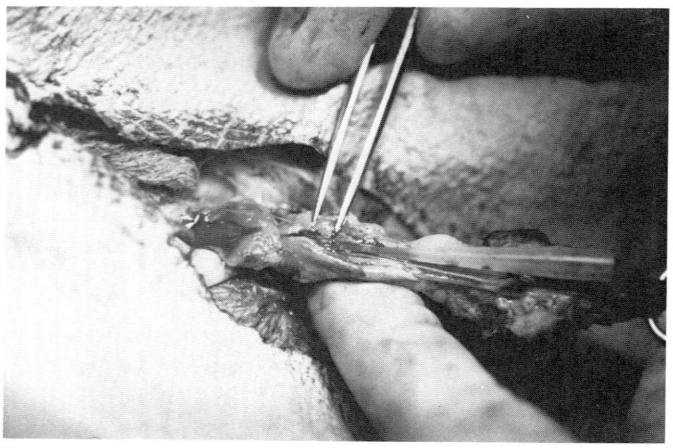

C

Figure 14–36. (*A*) A stricture (*a*) is present at the level of the bulbourethral glands, as evidenced by the dilated urethra (*b*) caudal to it. The coxofemoral joints are superimposed over the strictured area. (Used by permission of Veterinary Medicine Publishing Co.) (*B*) Another view of the strictured urethra showing the dilated urethra (*b*) caudal to the stricture (*a*). (Used by permission of Veterinary Medicine Publishing Co.) (*C*) When a perineal urethrostomy was performed on the same cat as in Figures 36*A* and *B*, a urethral urolith was found to be the cause of the stricture. (Used by permission of Veterinary Medicine Publishing Co.)

Nervous System

Myelogram

Goal

- To visualize the size and shape of the spinal cord

Clinical Indications

- Ataxia
- Paresis
- Paralysis

Materials

1. Iohexol (Omnipaque 240)
2. 22-Gauge spinal needle, 1.5 or 3.0 inches long, with stylet (Sherwood Medical, St. Louis, MO or Becton-Dickinson, Rutherford, NJ)

Technique

1. Administer general anesthesia.
2. Surgically prepare the injection site (either the cisterna magna or L5–6 or L6–7).
3. Place the needle into the subarachnoid space.
   - *Cisterna magna.* The landmarks for this injection site are the occipital protuberance and the wings of the

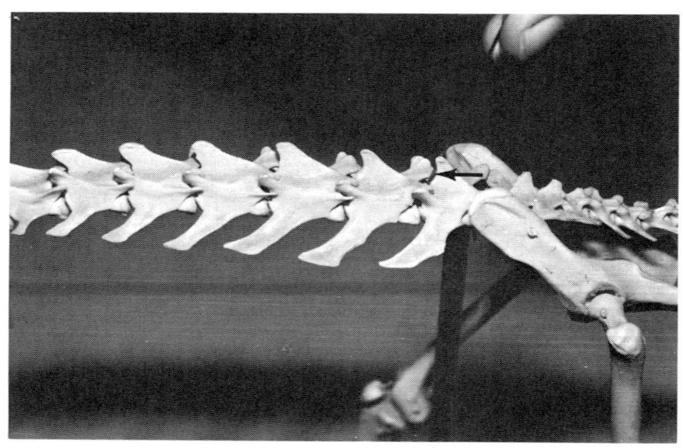

Figure 14–37. The preferred sites for a subarachnoid injection of contrast material are the cisterna magna, L5–6, and L6–7. To make an injection at L6–7, the spinal needle (arrow) is directed ventrally and slightly cranially, just cranial to the dorsal process of L7, while the cat's spine is flexed. (See text for more details.)

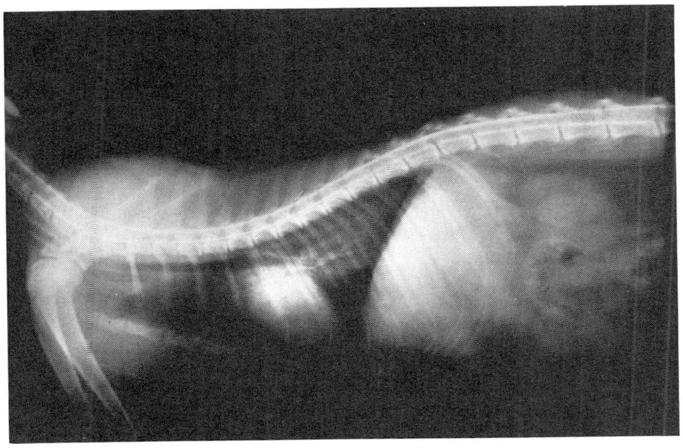

A

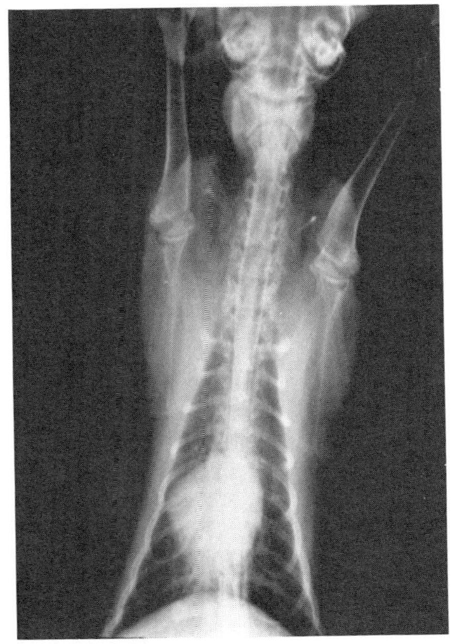

B

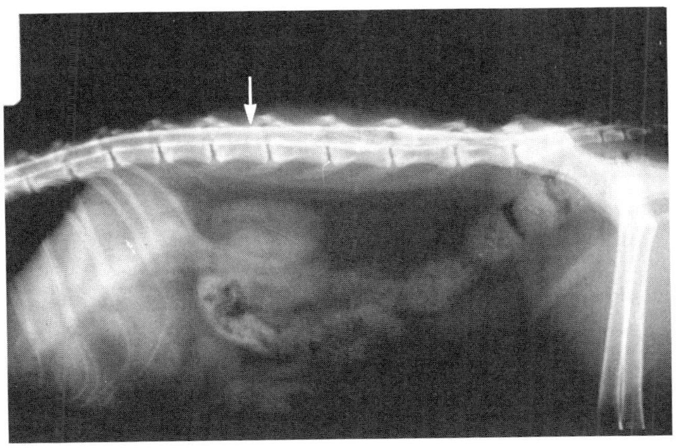

C

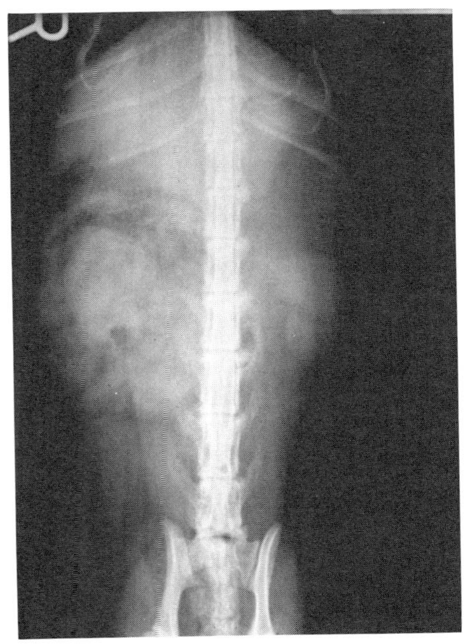

D

Figure 14–38. (*A*) A lateral view obtained during a cervical and thoracic myelography. A smooth, regular column of dye is seen in a normal cat. (*B*) A ventrodorsal view of the same cat as in Figure 15–38*A* shows a widened spinal cord at C4–7. (*C*) A lateral view of a lumbar myelogram. A smooth, regular column of dye is seen in a normal cat. (*D*) A ventrodorsal view of the same cat as in Figure 14–38*C* reveals a widened spinal cord at L4–6.

atlas. The needle should be placed at the intersection of imaginary lines from the occipital protuberance to the dorsal process of the atlas and a line perpendicular to the first line, just cranial to the wings of the atlas. Sometimes, a small depression may be palpated at this site. The needle is carefully placed into the cisterna magna. A slight "pop" is usually felt as the needle passes through the dura mater. When the stylet is removed from the needle, clear cerebrospinal fluid (CSF) should flow from the needle; however aspiration may be required to obtain CSF. Approximately 50% of the calculated volume of contrast material should be removed from the subarachnoid space. For example, if the calculated volume of contrast material is 2.0 mL, approximately 1.0 mL of CSF should be removed. The calculated dose is

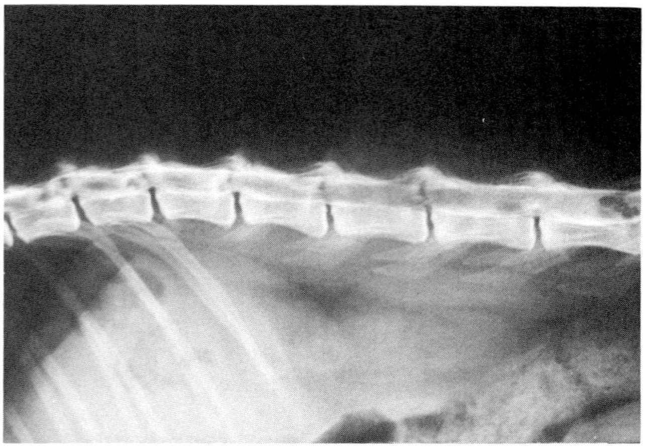

Figure 14–39. A break in the dorsal dye column at L3–4 (*arrow*) in a cat with posterior paresis indicated the need for exploratory surgery. Lymphosarcoma was found.

0.2 mL/lb. Needle placement may be accomplished with the patient in sternal recumbency or in lateral recumbency.

If difficulty is encountered such that the needle strikes bone instead of entering the subarachnoid space, the needle should be moved 1 to 2 mm caudally for another attempt.

- *L5–6 or L6–7.* The landmark for this injection site is the dorsal spinous process of L6 or L7. The needle is placed on the midline at the level of the dorsal spinous process and is directed slightly cranially (Fig. 14–37). The needle is passed through the joint between L5–6 or L6 and L7 and through the spinal cord until the ventral surface of the spinal canal is encountered. A twitch generally occurs in the rear legs as the needle passes through the spinal cord. The needle is backed out very slightly until CSF can be aspirated to confirm the needle's presence in the subarachnoid space.

4. Inject the contrast medium. The bevel of the needle is directed caudally for an injection into the cisterna magna, and the contrast medium is injected slowly. One of the authors (RWG) prefers to direct the bevel of the needle cranially during a lumbar injection; the other author (GDN) prefers to direct the bevel of the needle caudally. Too rapid an injection at the lumbar site is likely to place dye extradurally or within the central canal of the spinal cord.

Normal Findings

- The contrast medium should appear as parallel radiopaque lines that outline the spinal cord.
- On the ventrodorsal view, the dye column should be widest at C4–7 and L4–6 (Fig. 14–38, *A–D*).

Common Lesions

- Spinal cord lesions are uncommon in the cat.
- Lymphosarcoma in the spinal canal (Fig. 14–39) and ruptured intervertebral disks (Fig. 14–40, *A* and *B*) are the two most common spinal lesions found.

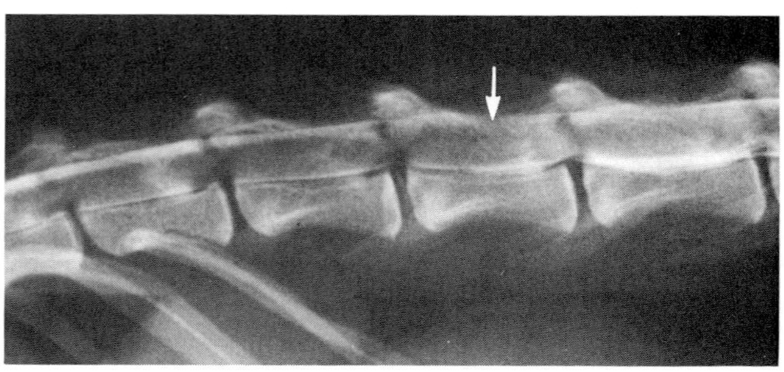

A

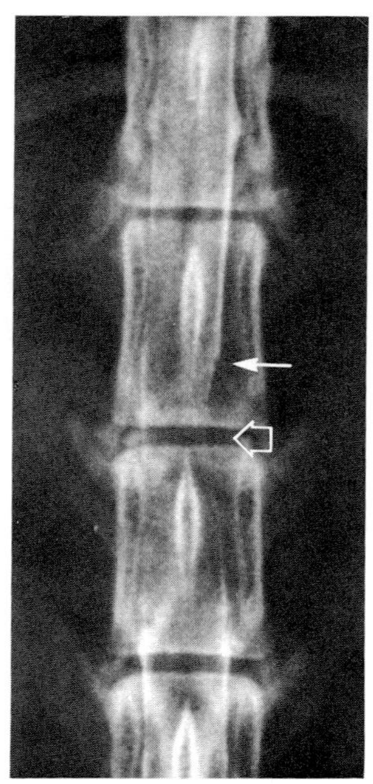

B

Figure 14–40. (*A*) A break in the dorsal dye column at L2–3 (*arrow*) in a cat with posterior paralysis indicated the need for exploratory surgery. A ruptured disk was found. (*B*) A ventrodorsal view of the same cat as in Figure 14–40*A*. The left dye column deviates toward the midline (*solid arrow*) and then disappears at L2–3 (*open arrow*).

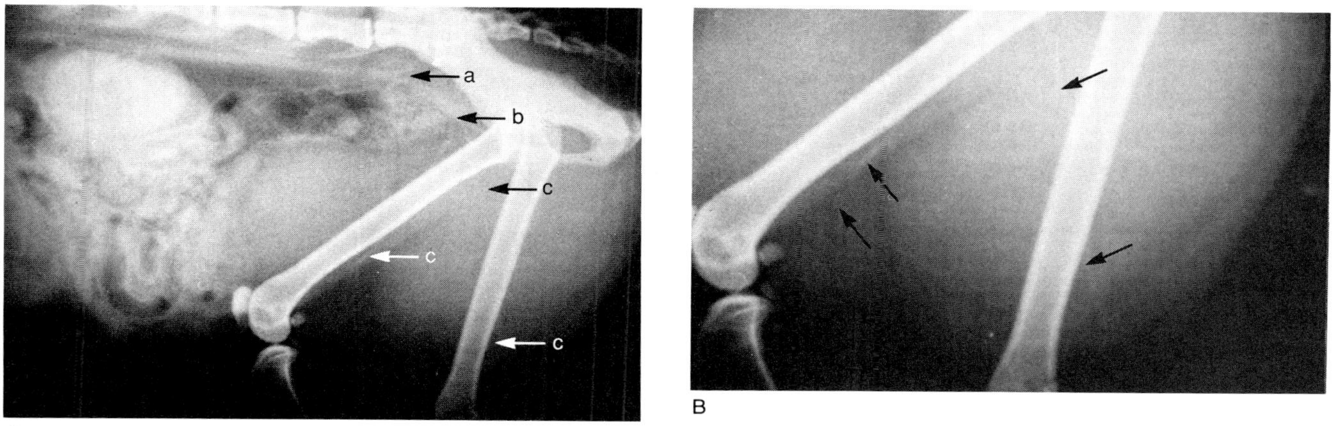

B

A

Figure 14–41. (*A*) When a nonselective angiogram is performed on a cat with normal aortic and femoral circulation, the contrast material can be seen in the aorta (*a*), at the aortic trifrucation (*b*), and in the femoral arteries (*c*). (*B*) A close-up of Figure 14–40*A* reveals the contrast material in the femoral arteries (*arrows*), demonstrating that aortic and femoral circulation is normal.

Cardiovascular System

Nonselective Angiogram of the Aorta

Goal

- To determine patency of the aorta and its major branches

Clinical Indications

- Paresis
- Paralysis (especially if its onset is peracute)

Contraindication

- Dilated cardiomyopathy with pleural effusion

Materials

1. 20-Gauge IV catheter (Saftiwing Scalp Vein Set, Cutter Medical, Berkeley, CA)
2. 12-cc Syringe
3. Water-soluble contrast medium for IV use (Renografin-76)

Technique

1. Obtain lateral survey radiographs of the abdomen and lateral and ventrodorsal radiographs of the thorax (for evidence of cardiomyopathy and pleural effusion).
2. Sedate the cat by administering 0.1 mL (10 mg) of ketamine intravenously.
3. Position the cat in lateral recumbency without the rear legs being superimposed upon one another (i.e., scissored). The procedure is facilitated if the cat is secured to the radiographic table with masking or adhesive tape.
4. Rapidly inject the IV contrast medium at a rate of 1.0 mL/lb into the cephalic or jugular vein. Preplacement of an IV catheter minimizes technical problems with the injection. The injection should be rapid so that the contrast medium is administered as a bolus.
5. Obtain a radiograph 1 to 3 seconds after the conclusion of the injection.
6. If the first radiograph is not of diagnostic quality, the procedure may be repeated.

Normal Findings

- The aorta and cranial mesenteric, renal, internal iliac, and femoral arteries may be visualized (Fig. 14–41, *A* and *B*).

Common Lesions

- Thromboembolic disease, usually secondary to cardiomyopathy, will obstruct the flow of the contrast media. This is most commonly seen at the level of the internal iliac arteries (Fig. 14–42). However, obstruction may also be seen at the level of the renal arteries to the level of the femoral arteries. (For further discussion, see Chapter 27.)

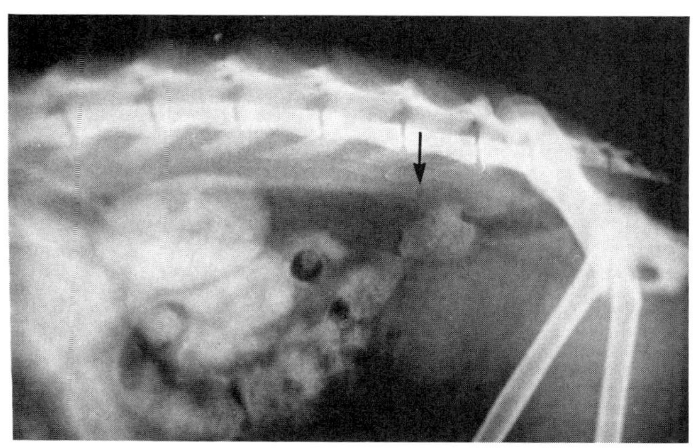

Figure 14–42. When a nonselective angiogram is performed on a cat with an aortic embolus, the contrast material will end abruptly at the point of the obstruction (*arrow*).

Nonselective Angiogram of the Heart

Goal

- To visualize the size of the ventricular chambers and the thickness of the ventricular walls

Clinical Indication

- Cardiomyopathy (for differentiation of the various forms)

Contraindication

- Dilated cardiomyopathy with pleural effusion

Materials

1. 20-Gauge IV catheter (Saftiwing Scalp Vein Set, Cutter Medical, Berkeley, CA)
2. 12-cc Syringe
3. Water-soluble contrast medium for IV use (Renografin-76)
4. Rapid cassette changer*

Technique

1. Obtain lateral and ventrodorsal survey radiographs of the thorax (for evidence of cardiomyopathy and pleural effusion).
2. Sedate the cat by administering 0.1 mL (10 mg) of ketamine intravenously.
3. Position the cat in lateral recumbency. The procedure is facilitated if the cat is secured to the radiographic table or film changer with masking or adhesive tape.
4. Rapidly inject IV contrast medium at the rate of 1.0 mL/lb into the cephalic or jugular vein. Preplacement of an IV catheter minimizes technical problems with the injection. The injection should be rapid so that the contrast medium is given as a bolus.
5. Obtain the first radiograph when 80% of the injection is completed; two additional radiographs should be obtained as quickly as the cassettes can be changed and the radiograph machine recycled. These films should be taken about 3 to 5 seconds apart.*
6. If the first radiographic series is not of diagnostic quality, the procedure may be repeated.

Normal Findings

- On the first exposure, contrast material will be present in the right side of the heart and in the pulmonary arteries; some may be seen in the lungs as well (Fig. 14–43).
- On the second or third exposure, contrast material will be seen in the pulmonary veins, in the left side of the heart, and in the aorta (Fig. 14–44).
- If large enough cassettes are used, the aortic trifurcation can also be seen.

Common Lesions

- If the cat has congestive cardiomyopathy, the left ventricular walls will be thinner than normal, and the left ventricular chamber will be larger than normal (Fig. 14–44).
- If the cat has hypertrophic cardiomyopathy, the left ventricular walls will be thicker than normal, and the left ventricular chamber will be smaller than normal. (For further discussion, see Chapter 27.)

*A cassette changer is contructed so that three cassettes are placed in a movable tray. The cat is positioned on a radiolucent (wooden) platform above the cassette tray so that the cat does not move when the cassette tray does. For best results, a grid is placed between the cat and the cassettes.

*The X-ray beam is centered just caudal to the heart. If 11 × 14 inch cassettes are used, the heart and aortic trifurcation may be seen on the same exposure. If that is possible, the rear legs should be scissored to prevent superimposition. If that is not possible, the X-ray beam should be centered on the heart. If an aortic study is needed, it may be done immediately following this one.

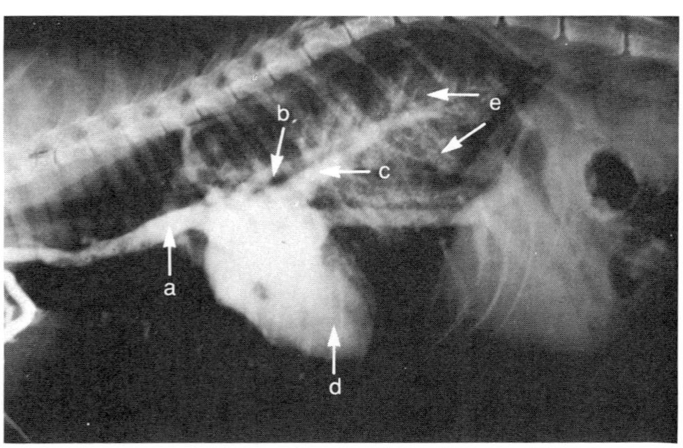

Figure 14–43. A nonselective angiogram demonstrates the structures of the heart and adjacent vessels. The anterior vena cava (*a*), main pulmonary artery (*b*), pulmonary vein (*c*), and left ventricle (*d*) are visible. Contrast material can be seen in the lung parenchyma (*e*).

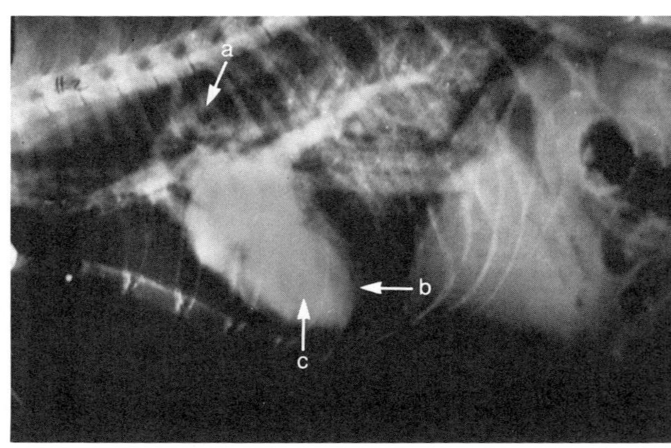

Figure 14–44. A radiograph obtained 5 seconds after that pictured in Figure 14–42 demonstrates the structures previously noted, plus the aorta (*a*). The left ventricular free wall (*b*) is of normal thickness, but the left ventricle (*c*) is dilated. These findings are diagnostic for congestive cardiomyopathy.

Respiratory System

For a discussion of the radiographic findings in the common feline diseases affecting the respiratory system, see Chapter 18.

The Skull

Routine ventrodorsal and lateral views of the skull will not allow adequate visualization of certain structures of the skull. Special positioning is needed to be able to image the tympanic bullae, the temporomandibular joints (TMJs), the frontal sinuses, and the nasal cavity.

Tympanic Bullae

The tympanic bullae are best viewed with a slightly oblique lateral view. Right and left lateral oblique views allow each bulla to be evaluated without superimposition of other structures (Fig. 14–45). The ventrodorsal view of the skull will demonstrate the bullae; however, there will be superimposition of other bones, which may make evaluation difficult. It is important for the skull to be positioned so that the tympanic bullae are symmetrical with each other. Such precise positioning requires that the patient receive general anesthesia. A well-positioned skull will allow for comparison of one tympanic bulla to the other.

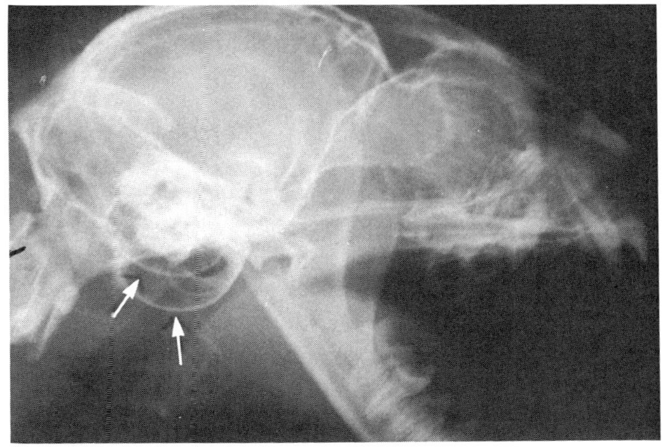

Figure 14–45. The tympanic bullae are best visualized with an oblique view of the skull (*arrows*). These bullae are of normal thickness.

Common Lesions

Inner and middle ear infections may cause an increased opacity of the tympanic bullae (Fig. 14–46). Lysis of bone, as well as soft tissue swelling, may be signs of osteomyelitis and tumors of the bullae.

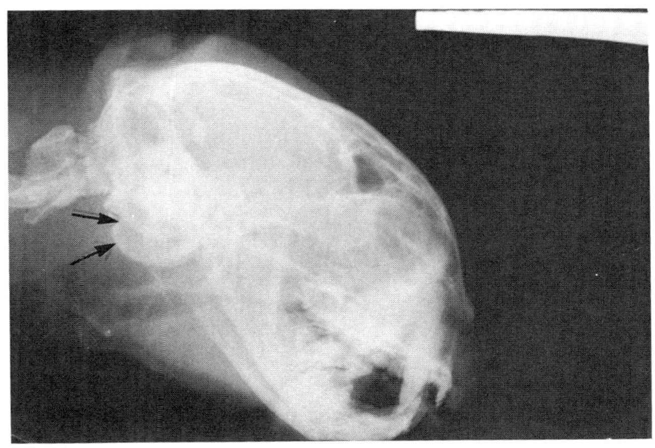

Figure 14–46. Abnormally thickened tympanic bullae (*arrows*) are seen in this cat with otitis interna and media.

Temporomandibular Joints

The TMJs are best visualized with lateral oblique views and a ventrodorsal view. The lateral oblique views allow the TMJs to be seen without superimposition of other structures (Fig. 14–47). The ventrodorsal view allows one TMJ to be compared to the other. Positioning is critical for proper radiographic evaluation; therefore, the patient should receive general anesthesia.

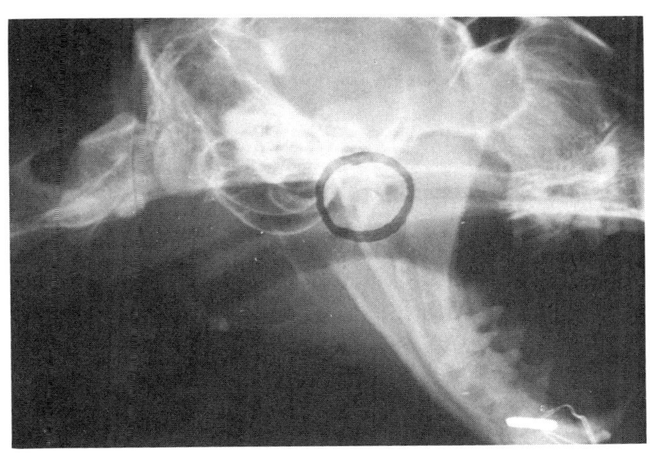

Figure 14–47. A normal temporomandibular joint (*circle*).

Common Lesions

Fractures and luxations are common findings in patients sustaining traumatic injuries (Fig. 14–48). Luxations of the TMJs and fractures of the mandibles can be confirmed radiographically. Improper alignment of the teeth is a strong indicator of TMJ luxation or mandibular fracture.

Frontal Sinuses

The air-filled frontal sinuses can easily be identified on a lateral radiograph (Fig. 14–49). The ventrodorsal view is helpful, but may be more difficult to evaluate because there is superimposition of other structures. The rostral caudal view of the frontal sinuses—sometimes called the skyline view—allows optimal visualization (Fig. 14–50*A*). General anesthesia is required to achieve proper positioning. Poor

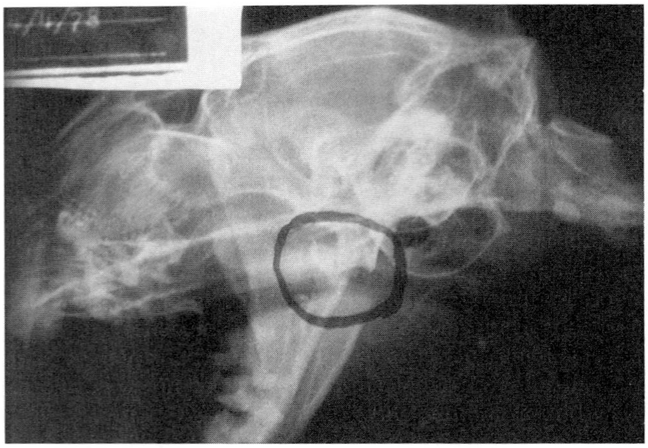

Figure 14–48. A luxated temporomandibular joint (*circle*).

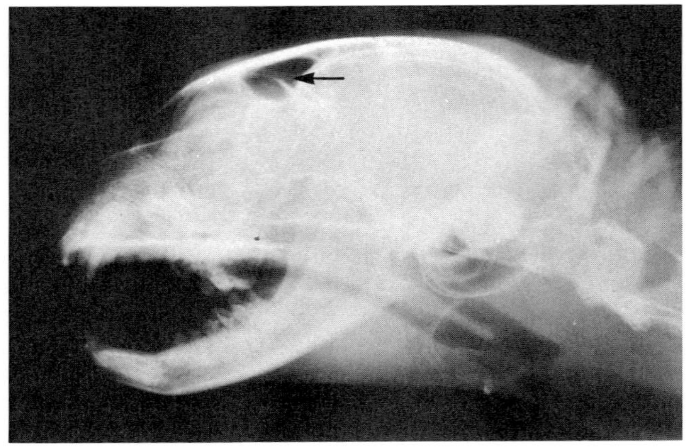

Figure 14–49. A lateral view of the skull will demonstrate the frontal sinuses (*arrow*). If they are normal, they will be seen to contain a gas density.

positioning may result in an erroneous or inconclusive evaluation (Fig 14–50*B*).

Common Lesions

Sinus infections, tumors, and foreign bodies may cause osseous lysis and/or increased opacity of the frontal sinuses and surrounding structures (Fig. 14–50*A* and 14–51). (For further discussion, see Chapter 30.)

Nasal Cavity

The nasal cavity can be visualized with a ventrodorsal view of the skull; however, superimposition of the mandibles restricts the view of the cranial one third to one half of the nasal cavity (Fig. 14–52). An open-mouth ventrodorsal view avoids the superimposition of the mandibles (Fig. 14–53, *A* and *B*). This view requires the patient to receive general anesthesia. The patient must be positioned so that the right and left nasal cavities are symmetrical. Even brachycephalic breeds can be evaluated when proper positioning is utilized.

Common Lesions

Infections, tumors, and foreign bodies may cause lysis of the nasal turbinates and the vomer. Increased opacity of the nasal cavity is also common with infections, tumors, and foreign bodies. (For further discussion, see Chapter 30.)

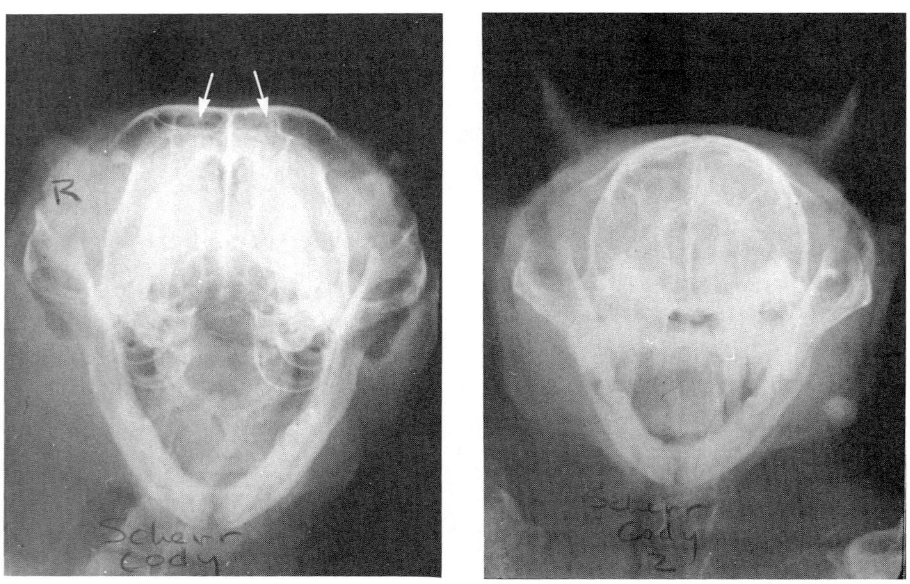

A B

Figure 14–50. (*A*) The frontal sinuses (*arrows*) can be viewed individually with a "skyline" (rostral caudal) view of the skull. (*B*) If the skull is slightly malaligned, the frontal sinuses will not be visible. (This is the same cat as in Figure 14–50*A*.)

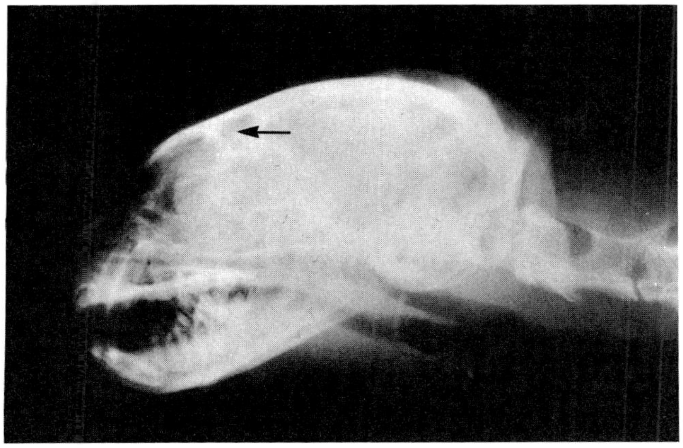

Figure 14–51. When the frontal sinuses are infected, they are filled with a water density (*arrow*).

Celiogram

Goal

- To document communication between the abdominal and thoracic cavities

Clinical Indication

- Suspected diaphragmatic hernia

Materials

1. 12-cc Syringe
2. 22-Gauge needle
3. Water-soluble organic iodine contrast agent (Renografin-76)

Technique

1. Inject Renografin-76 at a dose of 1 mL/lb into the abdominal cavity. Sedation is generally not required and is discouraged if the cat is dyspneic. The injection should not be made into the falciform ligament; rather the recommended injection site is in the flank, midway between the kidneys and urinary bladder.
2. Make a lateral and ventrodorsal radiograph that includes the thoracic and abdominal cavity.

Findings

- If the diaphragm is intact, the contrast material will be confined to the abdominal cavity.
- If a diaphragmatic hernia is present, contrast material will be seen in the thoracic cavity as well as the abdominal cavity (Fig. 14–54, *A* and B).

Pneumoperitoneogram

Goal

- To better visualize the abdominal organs

Clinical Indication

- To evaluate the size, shape, and location of the stomach, liver, kidney, urinary bladder, uterus, and distal colon

Contraindications

- Ascites
- Peritonitis
- Diaphragmatic hernia

Materials

1. 60-cc Syringe
2. 3-Way valve
3. 20- or 22-Gauge needle with stylet, or a plastic IV catheter with stylet
4. CO_2, N_2O

Technique[3]

1. Allow the cat nothing by mouth for 12 hours prior to the procedure.
2. Administer a soapy warm water enema.
3. Administer a sedative or general anesthetic.
4. Aseptically prepare the injection site, which is halfway between the umbilicus and the pubis.
5. Place the needle or catheter through the abdominal wall into the peritoneal cavity.
6. Remove the stylet and aspirate. If blood, urine, or intestinal contents are aspirated, remove the needle and reposition it.
7. Inject the contrast medium (gas) into the peritoneal cavity to achieve moderate abdominal distention.
8. Obtain radiographs in the dorsoventral, ventrodorsal, right lateral, and left lateral positions.

Normal Findings

- The various abdominal organs will be outlined by the gas, facilitating their delineation (Fig. 14–55).

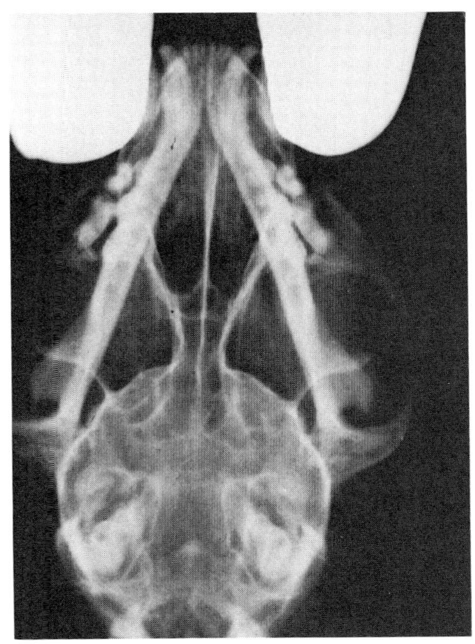

Figure 14–52. A ventrodorsal view of the skull superimposes the mandible on the cranial one third to one half of the nasal cavity.

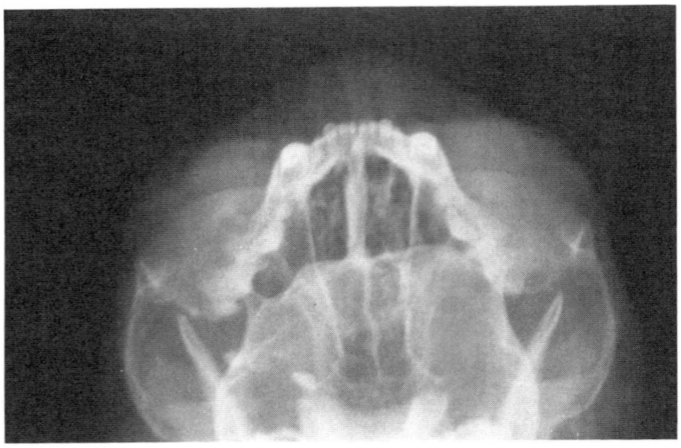

A

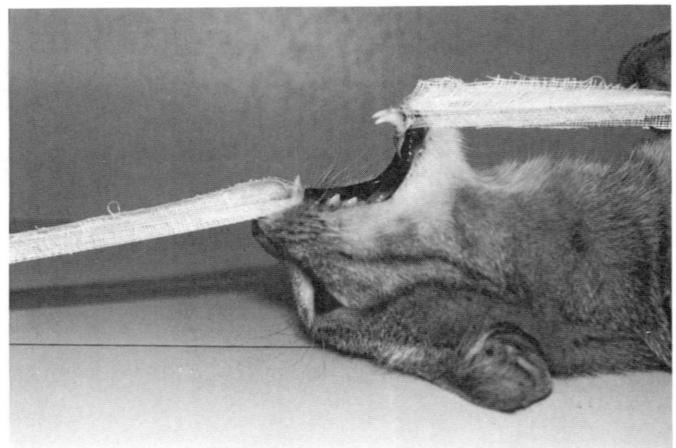

B

Figure 14–53. An open-mouthed ventrodorsal radiograph allows visualization of the nasal cavity, even in brachycephalic breeds. The mandible is retracted caudal to the nasal cavity. (*B*) The cat's mouth can be opened at a 90 degree angle so that the nasal cavity can be viewed without mandibular superimposition. The use of gauze strips to position the mouth prevents exposure of the operator's fingers.

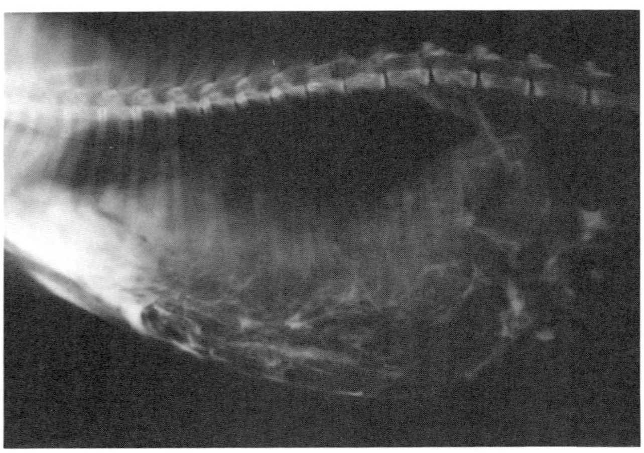

A

Figure 14–54. (*A*) A celiogram was performed on this cat by injecting Renografin-76 into the abdominal cavity. The contrast material can be seen in the thoracic and abdominal cavities, confirming the presence of a diaphragmatic hernia. (Courtesy of Dr. Lewis Hanks, Austin, TX) (*B*) A ventrodorsal view of the same cat as in Figure 14–54*A*.

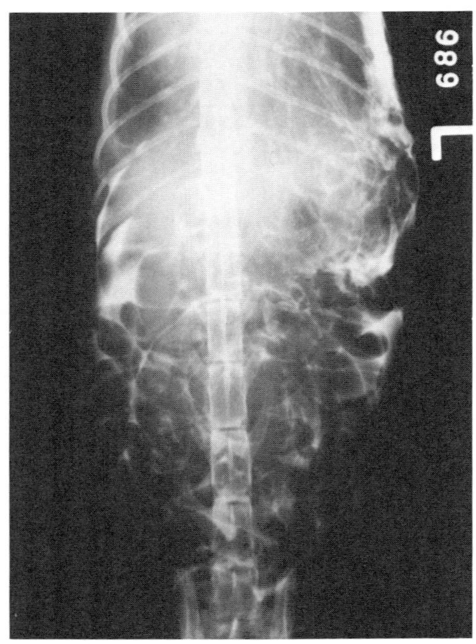

B

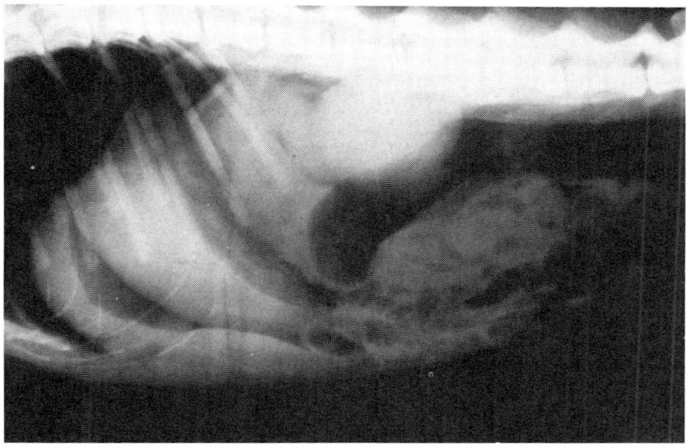

Figure 14–55. A pneumoperitoneogram was performed on this cat by injecting air into the abdominal cavity. Air dissects between the organs, allowing improved visualization of the viscera. Note the individual lobes of the liver and the spleen.

Miscellaneous

- Ultrasonographic examination may provide the same information without invasion of the peritoneal cavity (see Chapter 15).
- Too much gas in the abdomen may exert pressure on the diaphragm, causing dyspnea.
- Intravascular air embolization may occur, resulting in dyspnea and cardiovascular abnormalities. If this occurs, the patient should be placed in left lateral recumbency (left side down) so that intravascular air will accumulate on the right side of the heart and be disseminated to the lungs rather than to the systemic circulation.
- A pneumoperitoneogram that is performed in a patient with a diaphragmatic hernia may result in pneumothorax and may be fatal.
- This technique may be particularly helpful in cats with minimal intra-abdominal fat (i.e., young or emaciated cats).

REFERENCES

1. Norsworthy, GD. The steps in performing a urethrogram in male cats. Vet Med 1991;86:110.
2. Johnston GR, Feeney DA. Localization of feline urethral obstruction. Vet Clin North Am 1984;14:555.
3. Ticer JW. The Abdomen. In: Ticer JW, ed. Radiographic Technique in Small Animal Practice. Philadelphia: WB Saunders Co, 1975:335.

CHAPTER 15

◇ ◇ ◇

Ultrasonography

W. Sherman Mathey

Ultrasound is a noninvasive imaging modality that poses no radiation danger to the patient or operator. Ultrasonography uses very high frequency sound waves directed into soft tissues. Following interaction with body tissues, a portion of the sound waves is reflected toward the sound source. These reflected sounds (echos) are analyzed, then transmitted to and displayed on a screen as a visible image for diagnostic interpretation. Unlike radiology, ultrasonography is a non-ionizing technique that reveals insight into the texture as well as the anatomy and internal architecture of the tissues.

The hand-held transducer is the heart of the ultrasound machine. It contains one or more crystals with piezoelectric (pressure–electric) properties. When piezoelectric crystals are deformed by pressure, electricity results. The piezoelectric effect enables the crystal to convert electrical energy into mechanical sound or energy. Pulsated electrical deformation of the crystal produces small sound waves that impart kinetic energy to tissue molecules. When these sound waves are reflected and return to the transducer, the crystal is again deformed, generating an electric current that is then displayed on an oscilloscope. Amazingly, the transducer receives sound 99% of the time, while sending sound waves less than 1% of the time during imaging. The frequencies employed in diagnostic sonography range from 3 to 10 MHz (megahertz) compared with the highest frequency audible to the human ear, which is only about 20 KHz.

Facts and Artifacts

Although this chapter does not contain a detailed discussion on the physics of applied ultrasound, there are several excellent references available.[1-5] Some basic facts and artifacts must be understood, however, in order to avoid misinterpretation of the displayed image.[6,7]

Fact 1: Properties of Sound. The three important properties of a sound wave are its velocity, frequency, and wavelength. Frequency is measured in hertz (Hz) and diagnostic ultrasound frequencies range from 3 to 10 MHz.

The wavelengths of ultrasound are less than 1.0 mm, and the average velocity of sound in soft tissue in 1540 m/sec. The relationship between velocity (V) and frequency (f) and wavelength (λ) of sound can be expressed as $V = (f)(\lambda)$.

Since the velocity of sound in any given medium is constant, the wavelength of the sound wave is inversely proportional to its frequency. Therefore, when frequency is increased, wavelength must decrease. This concept is important when understanding transducer frequency and its effects on resolution and penetration.

Fact 2: Acoustic Impedance. A traveling ultrasound wave crosses many interfaces of tissue that differ in density or compressibility (the change in tissue volume due to pressure). The velocity of ultrasound in tissue is constant, even over a wide range of frequencies. Acoustic impedance is defined as the product of the density and the propagating velocity. Any difference in acoustic impedance can be employed to distinguish one soft tissue from another or to identify pathology within an organ.

Fact 3: Attenuation. Attenuation is the removal of energy or intensity from the sound beam as it passes through tissues. A combination of absorption and scattering of the sound waves accounts for most of the energy lost. The decibel (dB) is the unit used to compare changes in intensity. Attenuation equals 1 dB/cm/MHz in soft tissues. For example, a 3.0 MHz sound beam would be attenuated at a rate of 3.0 dB/cm, and a 5.0 MHz beam is attenuated at a rate of 5.0 dB/cm. Therefore, lower frequency sound beams provide greater tissue penetration than higher frequency beams.

Artifact 1: Acoustic Shadowing. As a strong reflector, such as gas or bone, blocks the passage of the sound beam, a dark band appears in the distant field beyond the reflector. This artifact tends to be more pronounced with a higher frequency transducer, and is a beneficial artifact that may aid in the detection of small calculi in the kidney, urinary bladder, or gallbladder. Refraction of the sound beam distal to the margins of a rounded fluid-filled structure (gallbladder or cyst) is another form of acoustic shadowing termed "edge shadowing."[8]

Artifact 2: Reverberation. This artifact occurs at highly reflective interfaces. Strong returning echoes cause the formation of another echo at the transducer face, and this new echo is reflected back into the examined tissue. The result is a second echo (and possibly several more) displayed twice as far from the original acoustic interface. Reverberation is commonly seen at soft tissue or fluid interfaces with gas. A classic example is the highly reflective interface between the lungs and the diaphragm.[9]

Artifact 3: Distant Enhancement. Sound waves pass unimpeded through a homogeneous tissue, which has low acoustic impedance, resulting in a brighter area immediately beneath the fluid. This artifact is useful in confirming that an echo-free region is indeed fluid filled.[10]

Artifact 4: Mirror Image. A mirror image artifact occurs at highly reflective interfaces and is caused by multiple internal reverberations between the tissues creating the interface, such as the diaphragm/lung interface. Some echoes are delayed in returning to the transducer and are displayed as if they originated beyond the original interface. This artifact can produce a liver image on the thoracic side of the diaphragm or the appearance of a second heart beyond the pericardium/lung interface.

Image Display Modes

Ultrasound information is displayed in three basic forms.[11]

1. ***A-Mode (Amplitude Mode).*** This is the simplest form of image display consisting of vertical peaks along a horizontal axis where the height of each peak corresponds to the amplitude or strength of the echo. This display mode measures only the depth of interfaces and is not useful for visualizing anatomy or organ motion.
2. ***M-Mode (Motion Mode).*** A single ultrasound beam is directed into a body part, and the returning echoes are displayed as a series of dots along a vertical line. The position of each dot represents depth and the strength of the echo, and a moving tracing of the dots results in a pattern representing the motion of the tissue interface. M-Mode is used in echocardiography to determine the action of the heart and its valves, chamber size and wall thickness, and degree of motion.
3. ***B-Mode (Brightness Mode).*** This mode displays amplitude as a function of dot brightness. Strong echoes have bright dots, while weaker echoes are displayed in variable shades of gray. A two-dimensional anatomic image is obtained by displaying the summation of dots from several scans. In real time B-mode scan imaging, many sound beams are continually emitted in a pulse sequence, either by an array of many crystals or the movement of a single crystal. Real time imaging is the most commonly used display mode in medical sonography.

Transducers

The most important component of the transducer, or scan head, is the piezoelectric crystal. The thickness of each crystal determines the frequency of the sound it generates. The most commonly used piezoelectric crystals are manufactured from quartz, tourmaline, and man-made ceramics. The higher the frequency of sound produced, the finer the resolution, but the trade-off is greater attenuation of the beam in tissue. The characteristic crystal frequencies used in veterinary ultrasonography range from 3 to 10 MHz. In feline practice, the high frequency 7.5 MHz is good for cardiac and ocular examinations. This choice is based on the demand for higher resolution with little need for deep penetration. The lower frequency 5-MHz transducer is more practical for the examination of feline abdomens in which deeper penetration at the loss of some resolution is wise.[8]

Transducer Configurations

A linear array scanner forms the sound beam by electronically firing individual crystals in a defined sequence. These crystals, which vary in number from 60 to 256, give a rectangular field of view. The advantage of this type of transducer is a larger field of view without loss of resolution. The disadvantage is the necessity for a large amount of contact area, or "footprint," on the body surface, which is of little practical use in feline ultrasound. Transducers with a smaller convex scanning surface have recently been designed for the veterinary market.

Sector transducers produce a fan-shaped field of view. This sector configuration is produced mechanically by wobbling a single crystal or by rotating multiple crystals within the transducer across the scan window. A newer technology, termed "phased array," uses a fixed array of many crystals that are sequentially pulsed to produce a fan-shaped beam. The advantage of sector scanners is a smaller scan surface area, and therefore, a smaller area of skin contact. This feature is important when the imaging window is restricted by ribs, lungs, or abdominal gas. The disadvantage is the potential difficulty in identifying and relating structures because of the smaller field of view.

Image Interpretation

Soft tissue organs have characteristic echo patterns based on variation in cellularity and stromal composition. Fluid-filled structures, solid tissue masses, and calculi can be identified by observing some general ultrasonographic characteristics:

1. ***Hyperechoic (Echogenic):*** very bright or white echoes representing highly reflective interfaces (i.e., bone, gas, collagen)
2. ***Hypoechoic:*** fewer echoes appearing as different shades of gray (i.e., soft tissues, fat)
3. ***Anechoic:*** lacking echoes, appearing black as a result of complete transmission of sound (i.e., fluid)

The ability to differentiate between solid and cystic lesions is fundamental to ultrasonography. The edges of a cyst are well defined with strong acoustic enhancement of the far wall, and internally a cyst is echo free. Cystic structures with a cellular component (abscesses or hematomas) appear hypoechoic internally. The borders may be irregular, and the acoustic enhancement is not easily observed. Complex lesions appear both hyperechoic and hypoechoic. The best example of this pattern is neoplasia. The normal parenchymal order for intraabdominal organs from least echogenic (hypoechoic) to most echogenic (hyperechoic) is kidney, liver, spleen, and then prostate.

Clinical Application

Liver

The liver normally lies within the costal arch. The size and shape of the liver is variable, and the normal liver is composed of several types of tissue. Ultrasound provides an insight into liver parenchyma, which is uniform in echo pattern.[12] The uniqueness of hepatic texture is due to the interspersing of collagen, fat, and blood vessels. Landmarks include the diaphragm, which is seen as a thin echogenic line that moves in synchrony with respiration. Another characteristic landmark in feline liver ultrasound is falciform fat. The streaked linear pattern of fat is in contrast to the coarse but more uniform pattern of the liver. In the cat, the quantity of falciform fat can be extensive compared with the amount of normal liver (Fig. 15–1).[13]

Imaging Technique

There is no single correct position of the patient for imaging. Circumstances and temperament often dictate the imaging position. Dorsal or lateral recumbency facilitates nearly all examinations of the liver and other abdominal organs. It is important that the organ be evaluated from the right, left, and ventral scan planes. Scanning in two planes with longitudinal and transverse orientation of the transducer will ensure a thorough examination. In order to fully assess the liver parenchyma, it is necessary to compare it with the parenchyma of other organs (i.e., spleen, kidney). Therefore, the entire abdomen should always be imaged. Some patients are best scanned while standing. This may require clipping hair over the ribs to permit intercostal examination.

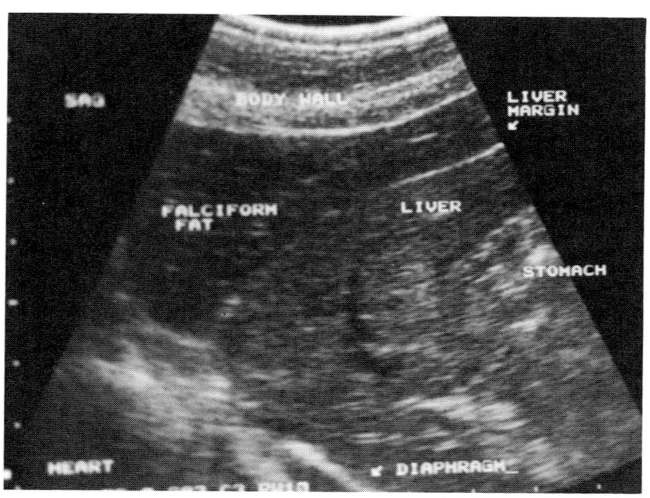

Figure 15–1. **Normal liver. Note the different ultrasonographic texture of falciform fat. (Courtesy of Corometrics Medical Systems, Inc., Wallingford, CT.)**

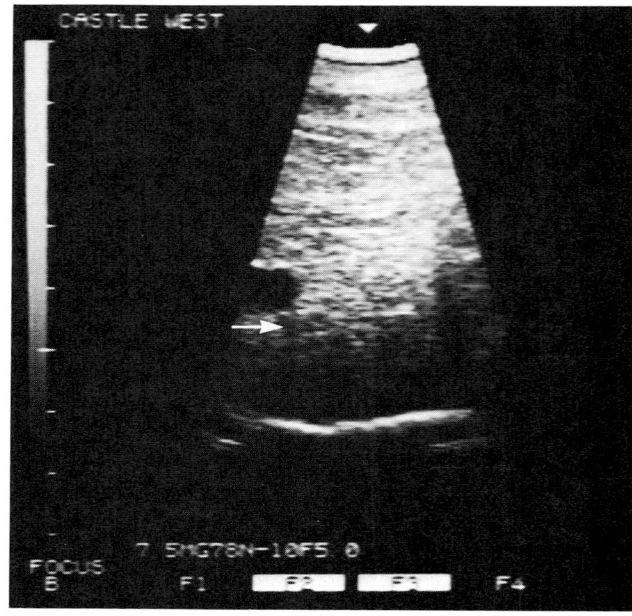

Figure 15–2. **Transverse ultrasound image showing a hyperechoic liver. In addition, acoustic shadows are seen originating from the edges of the gallbladder (*arrow*).**

Liver Disease

Hepatic disease is classified as diffuse or focal, depending on the ultrasound appearance. Present technology does not allow histologic diagnosis.[14]

Diffuse. Diseases of the hepatic parenchyma are characteristically either hypoechoic or hyperechoic. It is important to compare the liver echogenicity with that of other organs to avoid misinterpretation. Machine gain and intensity settings are variables that also can affect the interpretation of the overall echogenicity. Examples of diseases that cause a diffuse hypogenic liver include lymphosarcoma and congestion. A more common finding is a hyperechoic liver, which is often due to hepatic lipidosis or fibrosis (Fig. 15–2).

Focal. Focal liver disease is much easier to recognize. Ultrasound allows differentiation between solid and cystic focal lesions (Fig. 15–3). Focal lesions fall into one of the following three categories (Table 15–1).

Gallbladder

The normal gallbladder has a thin, smooth wall and anechoic content. Bile stasis causes bile to become echogenic, making it more difficult to distinguish the gallbladder from surrounding liver parenchyma (Figs. 15–4 to 15–6). Sludge and choleliths are often incidental findings. Cholecystic calculi are not common in cats but are easily detected due to mineralization and acoustic shadowing (Fig. 15–7). If suppurative cholangitis/cholangiohepatitis is suspected, evaluation of the gallbladder wall for thickness and irregularity,

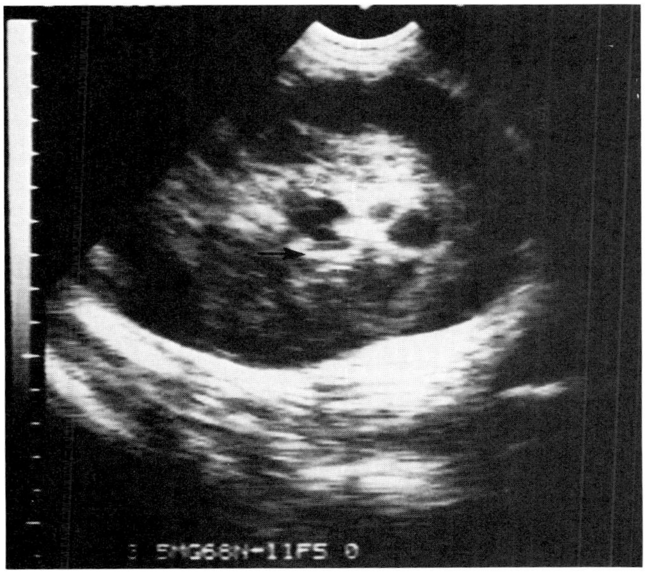

Figure 15–3. Longitudinal liver scan with an increase in uniform echogenicity. Two focal hypoechoic lesions are present. The *arrow* shows an example of distant enhancement. The diagnosis was lymphosarcoma.

along with dilated intrahepatic bile ducts, can aid in the diagnosis.

Pancreas

The normal pancreas is not visible with ultrasound because it is isoechoic (the same echogenicity) as the surrounding tissues. This organ is slender with no discrete borders and is usually surrounded by fat. An important landmark for pancreatic identification is the right kidney, which is located just behind the right costal arch. The right branch of the pancreas lies ventral to the right kidney. Additional landmarks are the aorta, caudal vena cava, and portal vein. Stomach and duodenal gas result in acoustic shadowing, making imaging difficult. Several ways to handle the gas problem include positioning the cat in right lateral recumbency and imaging from beneath the right side, adding water by a stomach tube to outline the gastric fundus, which can then

Table 15–1. Types of Focal Lesions

Category	Examples
1. Anechoic	Hepatic cyst (uncommon)*
2. Hypoechoic	Abscess, hematoma, or cystic neoplasia
3. Mixed (progression of necrosis and liquefaction)	Noncystic neoplasia or benign nodular hyperplasia

*The gallbladder should be identified before making a diagnosis of a cyst.

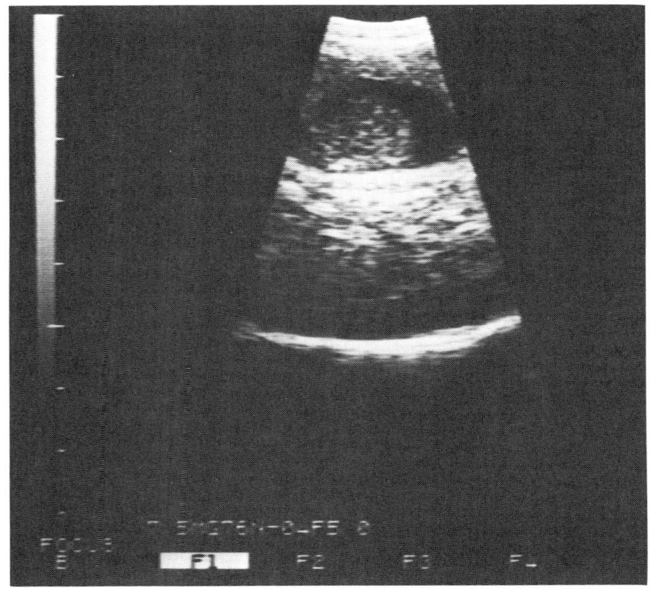

Figure 15–4. Transverse gallbladder scan. Bile within the gallbladder contains echos reflecting bile stasis. Note the distant enhancement.

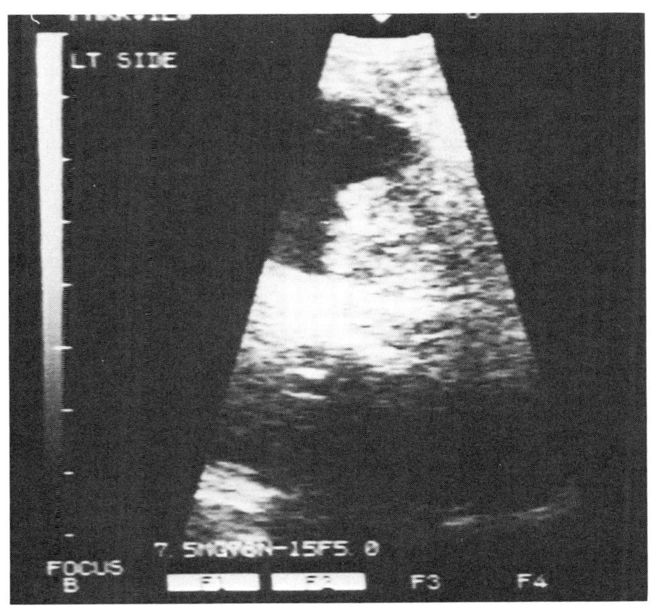

Figure 15–5. Transverse gallbladder scan with a different echodensity than in Figure 15–4. Bile stasis obscures the neck of the bladder. Neoplasia would be a differential.

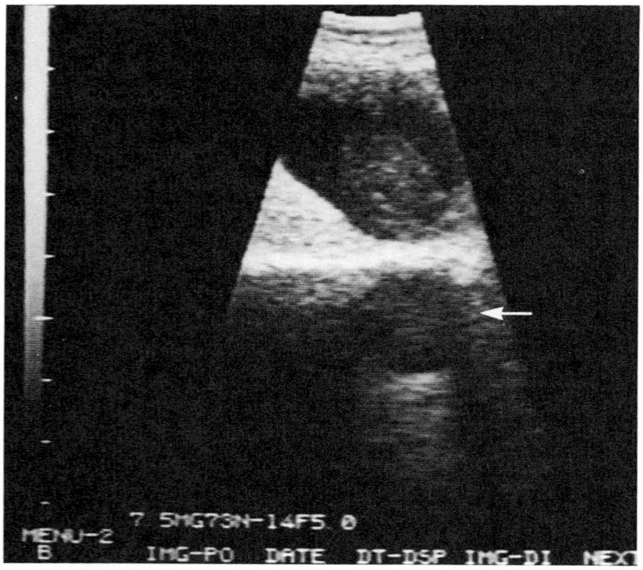

Figure 15–6. Transverse gallbladder scan with bile stasis. The *arrow* denotes a mirror-image artifact.

be used as an imaging "window," and injecting sterile saline into the abdomen to produce a clearer image of the right upper quadrant.

Pancreatic disorders in cats are not well documented. Those that directly or indirectly affect the pancreas include trauma (Fig. 15-8), neoplasia, cholangiohepatitis, inspissated bile syndrome, and pancreatitis. The typical sonographic signs of pancreatitis are as follows:[15]

1. Decrease in echogenicity relative to the surrounding mesentery as a result of edema, hemorrhage, or necrosis
2. Increase in adjacent mesenteric echogenicity due to cellular infiltrates associated with inflammation and fat saponification
3. Thickening of the wall of the descending duodenum accompanied by hypomotility
4. Focal pain response to transducer pressure (inconsistent)

Kidney

The normal kidney appears as an ovoid structure on longitudinal scans and is more rounded on transverse projections.[16,17] A thin echogenic line representing the capsule may be visualized but often only when the capsule is perpendicular to the sound beam. The renal cortex is hyperechoic as compared with the medulla. The corticomedullary junction is well demarcated by a thin echo and populated by bright echoes that represent arcuate arteries.[18] The cavity of the renal pelvis is not seen but is surrounded by varying amounts of fat, which may cause acoustic shadowing.[19] It is not normal to see evidence of fluid accumulation within the

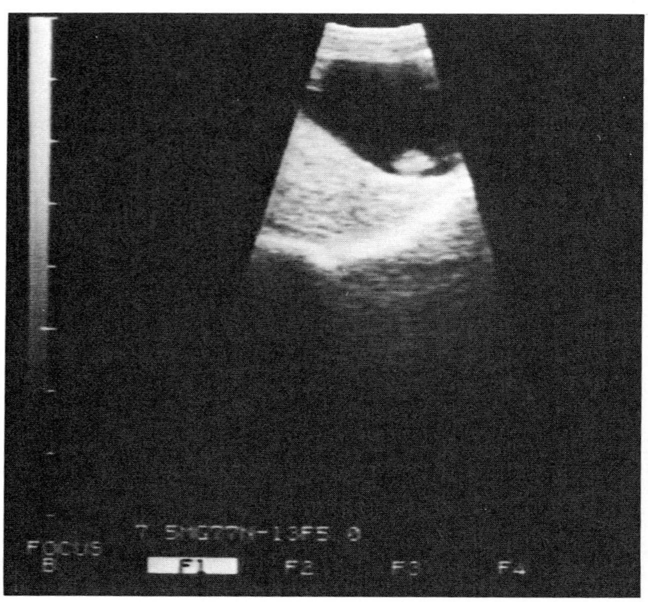

Figure 15–7. Transverse gallbladder scan with a discrete mass free within the lumen. Because no acoustic shadowing is present, this is most likely bile sludging or a polyp. Choleliths generally create acoustic shadowing.

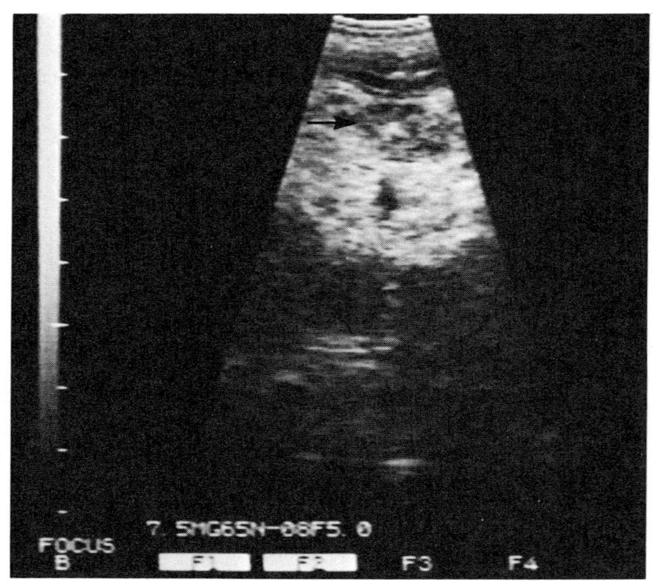

Figure 15–8. Longitudinal scan of the pancreas. Hyperechoic mesentery surrounds the pancreas (*arrow*). This is not to be confused with distant enhancement.

renal pelvis, and the normal proximal ureter is not visualized with ultrasound.

Imaging Techniques

The extreme mobility of the feline kidneys must be considered. The slightest abdominal pressure by the transducer can displace the kidney or change its orientation. The right kidney lies in the renal impression of the liver. When the patient is placed in dorsal recumbency, the cranial pole of the right kidney lies within the costal arch. The proximity of the descending duodenum and the ascending colon further complicates renal scanning. Both traverse the ventral surface of the kidney. Therefore, the best images of the right kidney are achieved by scanning the eleventh or twelfth intercostal spaces. The left kidney is easier to image because it is located laterally with the spleen, which may be used as an imaging window.

Diffuse Renal Parenchymal Disease

Hyperechoic kidneys are often associated with diffuse infiltrative diseases primarily involving the renal cortex (Fig. 15–9). Many infiltrative diseases of the renal parenchyma appear sonographically similar. Therefore, a biopsy sample is needed to determine the cause.[20] Examples of hyperechoic change include glomerulonephritis, chronic interstitial nephritis, amyloidosis, and nephrocalcinosis. End-stage kidney disease results in increased echogenicity due to fibrosis as well as a small, shrunken appearance with irregular margins and decreased cortical thickness.

Occasionally, a hyperechoic ring is seen at the corticomedullary junction, which is often associated with renal tubular necrosis. Ethylene glycol toxicity is also characterized by a hyperechogenic cortex. The cause of this increased echo pattern is thought to be crystal deposition within the renal tubules.

Hypoechoic kidneys are less frequently encountered. Lymphosarcoma is a disease that may result in decreased renal echogenicity. Low power setting, improper gain setting, attenuation due to retroperitoneal fat, and different transducer frequencies can mimic hypoechoic kidneys. Therefore, the kidney echo-texture should be compared with other organs prior to judging renal echogenicity.

Focal Renal Parenchymal Disease

Although it is not possible to distinguish different cell types in focal renal disease, ultrasound can identify solid versus cystic lesions. Solid lesions, if benign, are characterized by smooth margination and minimal disruption of the normal renal architecture. Malignant lesions tend to be invasive and cause gross disruption. In cats, most renal neoplasms have been characterized by multifocal sonolucent nodules, the majority of which were lymphosarcomas.

Cystic lesions are fluid filled and often encapsulated. Ultrasonographically, cysts appear as well-demarcated, cavitated anechoic to hypoechoic areas within soft tissue. A cyst generally contains anechoic tissue fluid, although in the presence of cellular debris the fluid will appear hypoechoic. Differentiation between a cyst and a hypoechoic nodule can be based on the fact that a true solid nodule that is hypoechoic will lack the far enhancement characteristic of a cyst. Cystic disease can be solitary or multifocal. Solitary renal cysts are usually benign and infrequently result in clinical signs. Polycystic disease is often accompanied by progressive renal failure.[21] If severe, the renal architecture may be disrupted (Fig. 15–10).

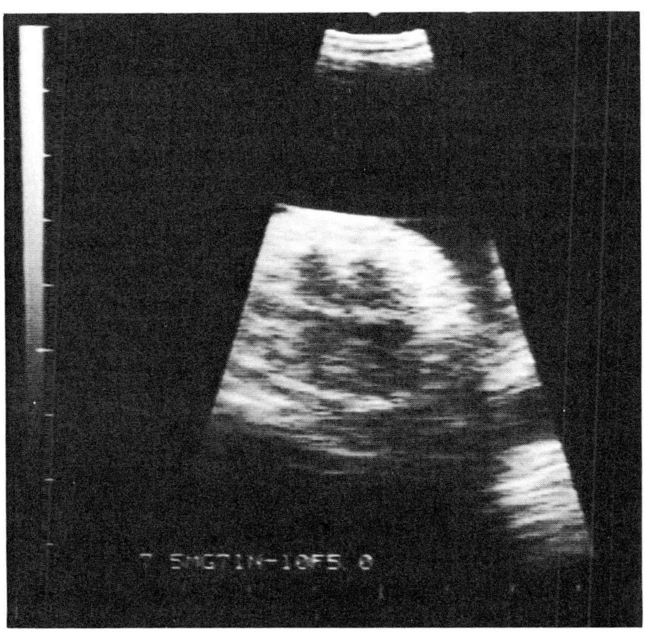

Figure 15–9. Longitudinal renal scan. The hyperechogenic cortex is the result of ethylene glycol toxicity.

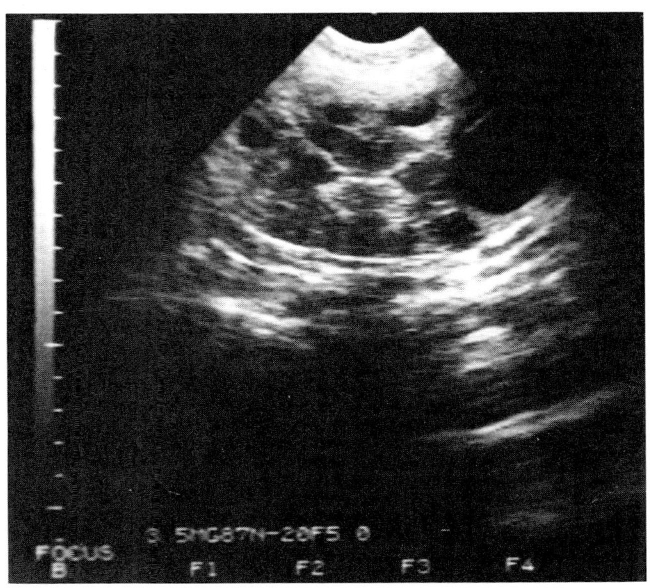

Figure 15–10. Longitudinal renal scan of polycystic kidneys.

Urinary Bladder

The urinary bladder is most easily recognized and most accurately examined when it is full. If the bladder contains only a small amount of urine, the wall will appear artifactually thickened, which may be confused with inflammatory wall disease. The descending colon may also lead to misinterpretations. When it is full it may impinge on the bladder wall; the distortion created can mimic a mural or intraluminal mass. Mineral fragments in the colon may cast shadows that can be mistaken for cystic calculi. Two important findings in bladder ultrasonography are sediment and calculi.[22] Although sediment can be a normal finding, it can suggest urolithiasis. Cystic calculi are easily detected. Irrespective of their mineral composition, calculi are strongly echogenic and cast clear acoustic shadows (Figs. 15–11 and 15–12).

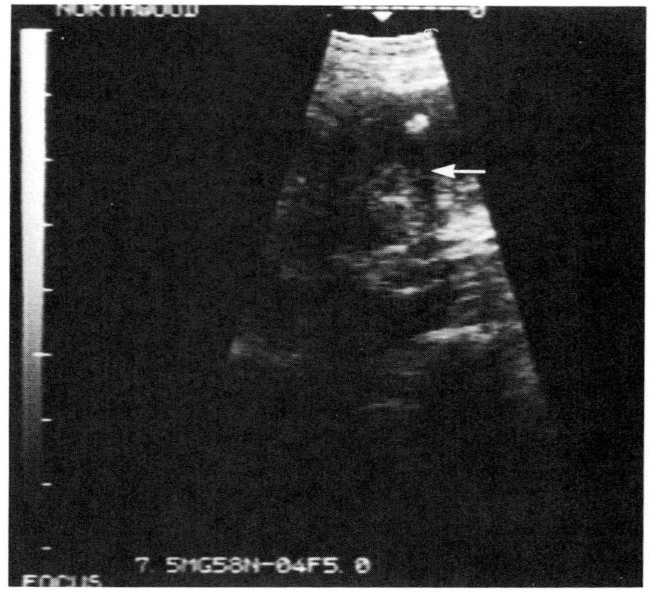

Figure 15–11. Longitudinal bladder scan. The calculi shows acoustic shadowing (*arrow*). Note that the calculi is not adherent to the wall.

Pregnancy

Ultrasound is the preferred method of noninvasive imaging for pregnancy with detection as early as 14 days postovulation (Fig. 15–13).[23] The most common error in obstetrical sonography is failure to detect pregnancy due to a small litter size or examination too early in gestation.[24] Ultrasonography demonstrates fetal viability from the time the gestational sacs are first visualized. Monitoring of fetal movement and heart rate can assess fetal distress.[25] Estimation of the number of fetuses based on ultrasonography is not totally reliable, especially with larger litters. Ultrasonography can differentiate between other causes of uterine enlargement including pyometra, pseudopregnancy, and neoplasia.

Gastrointestinal Tract

When used in conjunction with survey abdominal radiography, ultrasonographic evaluation of the gastrointestinal (GI) tract is most sensitive for focal disease and mesenteric lymph node involvement.[26,27] Because of the length of the GI tract and its variable location within the abdominal cavity, systematic scanning of the entire abdomen is necessary to detect focal lesions. Localization of the lesion by palpation will decrease scanning time and increase detection sensitivity. Once a lesion has been identified, careful evaluation of the proximal and distal contiguous bowel loops in both cross-section and long-axis scan planes will assist interpretation. Usually only three of the five anatomic layers of small bowel can be identified, yielding a characteristic target, or bull's eye, appearance in cross section. The layers that can be seen are the thick hyperechoic serosa, the thick hypoechoic mucosa, and the thin hyperechoic mucosal surface.

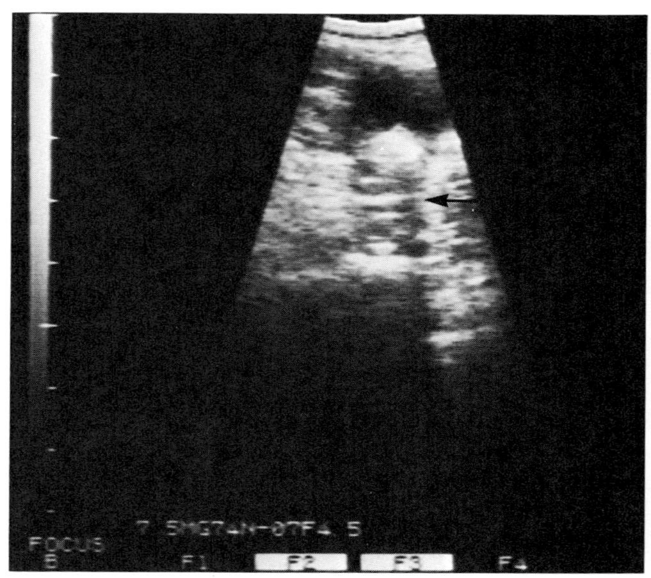

Figure 15–12. Longitudinal bladder scan. The bladder is not distended, but the calculi shadows (*arrow*).

Intussusception

The ultrasonographic appearance of intussusception can best be described as a tube within a tube. The outermost layers represent the doubled bowel loop known as the intussuscipiens or receiving segment. The lumen of the intussuscipiens contains additional bowel wall layers representing the intussusceptum or invaginated segment of the intussusception.[29] The central hyperechoic band within the intussusceptum represents trapped luminal contents (Fig. 15–14).

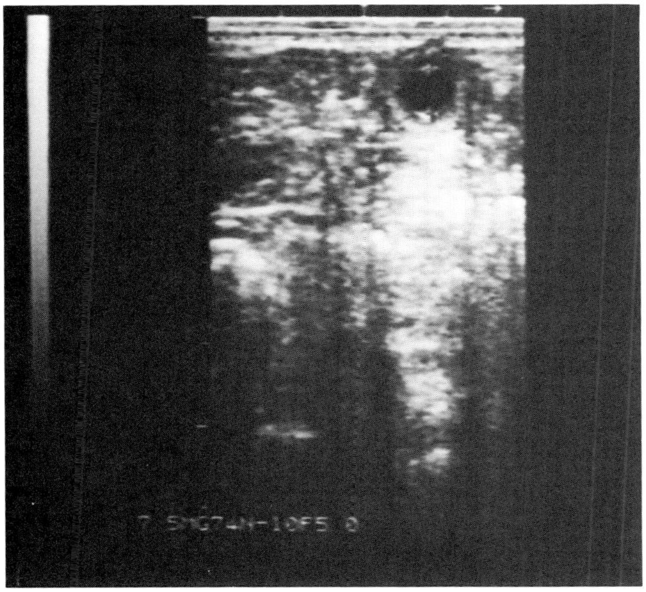

Figure 15–13. Longitudinal abdominal scan showing an 18-day pregnancy. Note the distant enhancement.

Mural Thickening

In transverse section, mural thickening will maximize the target appearance. Longitudinal scanning should confirm the thickening, which will exceed the 2 to 4 mm that is normal for the small bowel and descending colon. Neoplasia, muscular hypertrophy of the pylorus, acute or chronic inflammation, granuloma, hemorrhage, or edema of the wall should be included in the differential diagnosis. Asymmetrical bowel-wall thickening is more typical of neoplasia.

Ascites

Ascites due to a transudate is hypoechoic and can readily be seen in the abdominal cavity. Peritoneal fluid transmits sound well, resulting in parenchymal organs being more prominent and relatively more echogenic owing to distant enhancement (Fig. 15–15).

The nature of the peritoneal effusion can be assessed by comparing it with urine in the bladder. Normal urine is sonographically defined as anechoic because it is a uniform medium without echoes. Relatively echogenic peritoneal effusion, referred to as complex fluid, indicates the presence of cellular or particulate (i.e., fibrinous) debris. The latter is characteristic of peritonitis, which is also often accompanied by apparent increased thickness of the peritoneal surfaces. Adhesions between bowel loops can be demonstrated by applying external abdominal pressure with the transducer resulting in a gathered movement of all the involved loops. When effusion is associated with neoplastic disease of the peritoneum, masses may be seen in the mesentery or on the peritoneal surface.

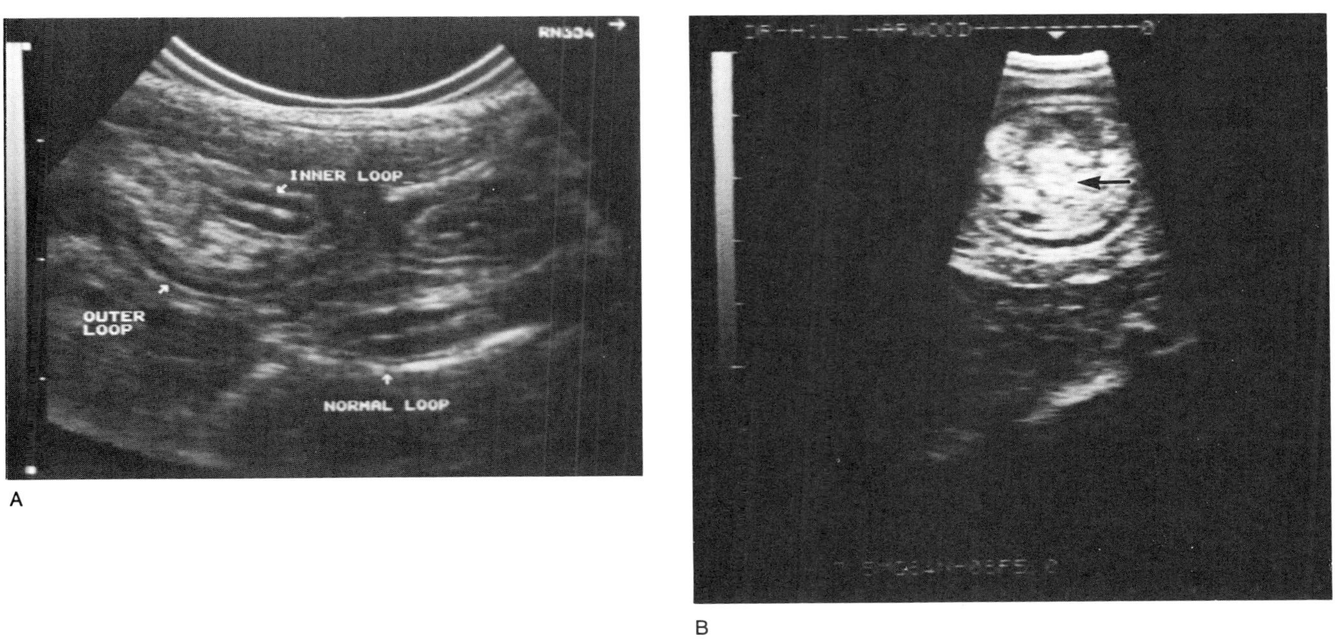

Figure 15–14. (*A*) Normal longitudinal sectional ultrasound of the intestinal tract (*normal loop*) and cross sectional ultrasound of an intussusception (*inner loop* and *outer loop*). (Courtesy of Corometrics Medical Systems, Inc., Wallingford, CT.) (*B*) Cross sectional ultrasound of the small intestine. The *arrow* is the site of an intussusception.

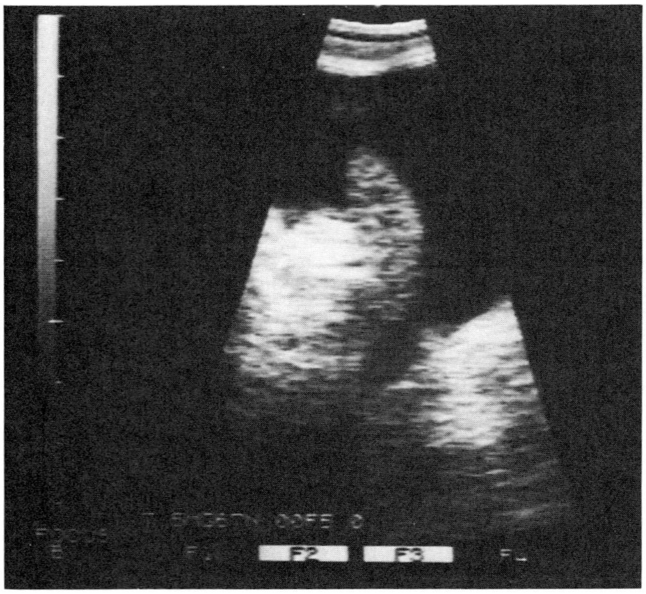

Figure 15–15. **Longitudinal abdominal scan with a large volume of ascites. The organs are hyperechoic.**

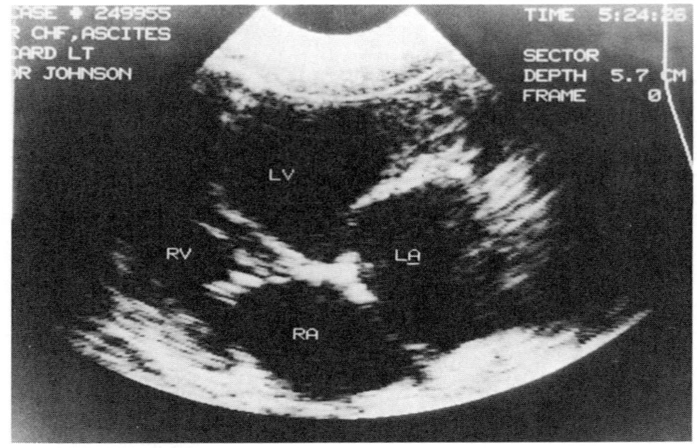

Figure 15–16. **Apical four-chamber view with dilatation of all four chambers due to congestive (dilated) cardiomyopathy. (Courtesy of Dr. R. W. Green, College Station, TX.)**

Heart

Although radiographic impressions of cardiac enlargements are reliable, they often do not discriminate among dilation, hypertrophy, and pericardial fluid accumulations. Cardiac examination with real-time scanning systems can assess the motion, thickness, and function of the heart wall; the motion, structure, and function of the valves; the size of chambers and outflow tracts; the presence of masses associated with the heart, and pericardial and pleural fluid accumulations.[30,31,32] The best acoustic windows to assess the heart are the right and left ventral intercostal spaces. The locations vary from the third to the fifth intercostal space and from 1 to 8 cm lateral (dorsal) to the sternum. Assessment is best dorsal to the sternum and ventral to the lung. In cats, the entire heart can be examined from the right side. The left side is the best window for an apical four-chamber view. This position is important in a Doppler or color-flow study.[33] The transducer of choice should have a small contact surface to allow easy access between the ribs. A 7.5-MHz transducer with close focusing is necessary to achieve resolution of anatomic structures. Positioning of the cat is critical. The quality and size of images obtained from the dependent side of the thorax in lateral recumbency are often superior to those obtained standing. The dependent side for imaging can be created by laying the cat on a table that contains a hole for the transducer. If this position is not feasible, the cat should be placed in a standing or sternal position with the thoracic spine flexed laterally to increase the size of the intercostal window. The structures of the left side of the heart are easier to image than those of the right side.[34] In most cases, the left atrium, mitral valve, left ventricle, aortic valve, and ascending aorta can be visualized. Short axis images of the left ventricle should be made at multiple levels. Clear images of the right atrium, tricuspid valve, pulmonary valve, and pulmonary outflow tract are more difficult to obtain because of lung interference over these thinner structures. The aim of the cardiac examination is to evaluate the four chambers of the heart, note the cardiac rate and rhythm, and evaluate the motion of the ventricular walls and the interventricular system. It is important to establish a scanning protocol that fulfills all of these aims. Both long axis (parasagittal) and short axis (transverse) views should be performed during the study.[35]

Cardiomyopathy

Cardiomyopathy is the most common form of acquired heart disease.[36] Dilated and hypertrophic forms occur, and some cases seem to have features of both forms. Ultrasound allows differentiation between the two major types, which is of utmost therapeutic importance.[37] Dilated cardiomyopathy is characterized by eventual dilation of all four cardiac chambers (Fig. 15–16).[38] The left ventricular wall has a decreased end-systolic thickness, and contractility is reduced.

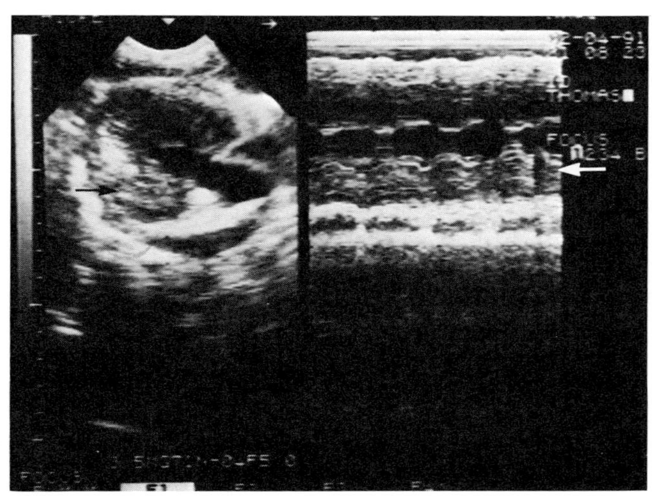

Figure 15–17. **Parasternal long-axis view of hypertrophic cardiomyopathy. On the right is M-mode. The *arrows* denote a thickened left ventricle.**

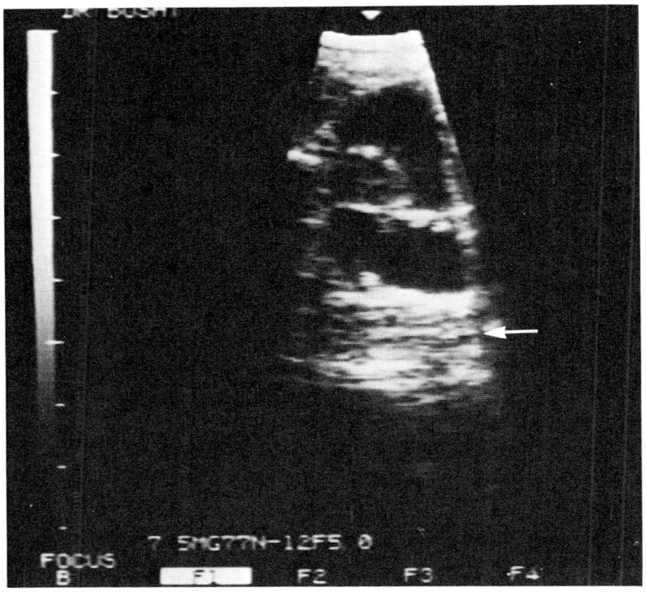

Figure 15–18. Parasternal long-axis scan of the thorax. A small lymphosarcoma was imaged. Mediastinal fat is distal to the mass. Reverberation (*arrow*) is present due to the small thorax.

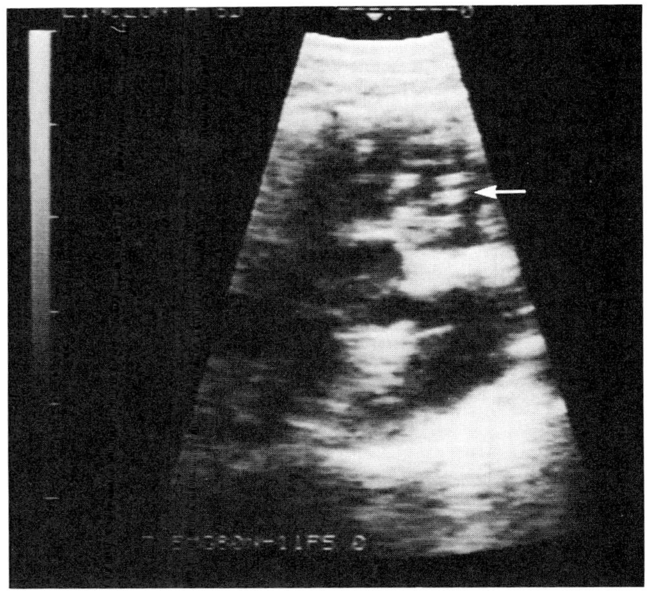

Figure 15–20. Parasternal short-axis scan. The *arrow* shows adult heartworms in the right ventricle as parallel lines.

The aortic outflow may be narrowed. In hypertrophic cardiomyopathy, the ventricular free walls and septum are thickened, resulting in a reduced left ventricular chamber volume (Fig. 15–17). Hypertrophic cardiomyopathy may be a sequel to hyperthyroidism.[39]

Pleural Space

The pleural space, like the lung, cannot be imaged when it is normal.[40] However, pleural fluid can be imaged and may be associated with cardiovascular disease, infection, masses in or near the pleural space, trauma, and lymphatic disease. Ultrasound imaging can differentiate many of these conditions (Figs. 15–18 to 15–20).

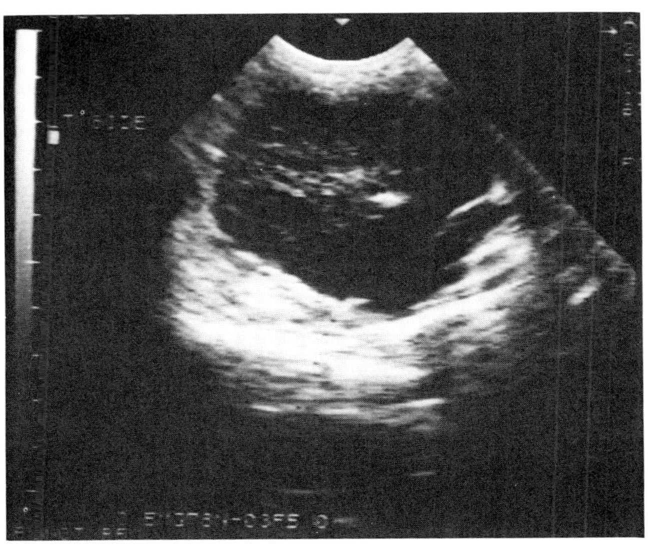

Figure 15–19. Parasternal long-axis view of the thorax. A large hypoechoic mass is present. The ventral thoracic wall is the hyperechoic area under the tumor.

REFERENCES

1. Herring DS, Bjornton G. Physics, facts and artifacts of diagnostic ultrasound. Vet Clin North Amer [Sm Anim Pract] 1985;16:1107.
2. Kremkau FW Physical Principles. In: Kremkau FW, ed. Diagnostic Ultrasound Physical Principles and Exercises. New York: Grune & Stratton, 1980:1.
3. Feeney DA, Fletcher TF, Hardy RM. Basics of Diagnostic Ultrasonography. In: Feeney DA, Fletcher TF, Hardy RM, eds. Atlas of Correlative Imaging Anatomy of the Normal Dog. Philadelphia: WB Saunders, 1991:353.
4. Bartrum RJ, Crow HC. Practical Physics. In: Bartrum RJ, Crow HC eds. Realtime Ultrasound: A Manual for Physicians and Technical Personnel, 2nd ed. Philadelphia: WB Saunders, 1983:1.
5. Powis RL. Ultrasound science for the veterinarian. Vet Clin North Amer [Equine Pract] 1986;2:3.
6. Wortman JA, Rantanen NW. Alternate Imaging. In: Thrall DE, ed. Textbook of Diagnostic Radiology. Philadelphia: WB Saunders, 1986:541.
7. Miles KG. Basic Principles and Clinical Applications of Diagnostic Ultrasonography. Compend Contin Ed Pract Vet 1989;11:609.
8. Barr F. Common Imaging Artifacts. In: Barr F, ed. Diagnostic Ultrasound in the Dog and Cat. London: Blackwell Scientific, 1990:12.9.
9. Stone LR. Diagnostic Ultrasound in Marine Mammals. In: Dierauf LA, ed. Handbook of Marine Mammal Medicine. Boca Raton: CRC Press 1990:235.
10. Park DP, Nyland TG, Lattimer JC, et al. B-Mode gray scale ultrasound: Imaging artifacts and interpretation principles. Vet Radiol 1981;22:204.

11. Colby J. Artifacts and image quality in ultrasound. Equine Vet Sci 1988;5:295.
12. Feeney DA, Johnston GR, Hardy RM. Two-dimensional, gray scale ultrasonography for assessment of hepatic and splenic neoplasia in the dog and cat. J Am Vet Med Assoc 1984;184:68.
13. Schelling CG, Saunders HM, Wortman, JA. Normal Abdomen. In: Schelling CG, ed. Veterinary Ultrasound Atlas. Wallingford: Corometrics, 1990:1.
14. Nyland TG, Hager DA, Herring DS. Sonography of the Liver, Gallbladder, and Spleen. Semin Vet Med Surgery 1989;4:13.
15. Smith FWK, Jr. Feline pancreatitis: A review. Compend Anim Pract 1987;1:4.
16. Cartee RE, Seber BA, Patton CS. Ultrasonographic diagnosis of renal disease in small animals. J Am Vet Med Assoc 1980;176: 426.
17. Konde LJ, Wrigley RH, Park RD. Ultrasonographic anatomy of the normal canine kidney. Vet Radiol 1984;25:173.
18. Walter PA, Feeney DA, Johnston GR, Fletcher TF. Feline renal ultrasonography: Quantitative analyses of imaged anatomy. Am J Vet Res 1987;48:596.
19. Walter PA, Johnston GR, Feeney DA, O'Brien TD. Renal ultrasonography in healthy cats. Am J Vet Res 1987;48:600.
20. Konde LJ, Park RD, Wrigley RH. Comparison of radiography and ultrasonography in the evaluation of renal lesions in the dog. J Am Vet Med Assoc 1986;188:1420.
21. Biller DS, Chew DJ, DiBartola SP. Polycystic kidney disease in a family of persian cats. J Am Vet Med Assoc 1990;196:1288.
22. Biller DS, Kantrowitz B, Partington BP, Miyabayashi T. Diagnostic ultrasound of the urinary bladder. J Am Anim Hosp Assoc 1990;26:397.
23. Shille WM, Gontarck J. The case of ultrasonography for pregnancy diagnosis in the bitch. J Am Vet Med Assoc 1985;187:1021.
24. Poffenbarger EM, Feeney DA. Use of gray scale ultrasonography in the diagnosis of reproductive disease in the bitch: 18 cases (1981–1984). J Am Vet Med Assoc 1986;189:90.
25. Johnston SD, Raksil S. Fetal loss in the dog and cat. Vet Clin North Amer [Sm Anim Pract] 1987;17:535.
26. Nyland TG, Bernard WV. Application of abdominal ultrasound. Calif Vet 1982;36:21.30.
27. O'Brien TR. Radiographic Diagnosis of Abdominal Disorders in the Dog and Cat: Radiographic Interpretation, Clinical Signs, Pathophysiology. Philadelphia: WB Saunders 1981;1.
28. Pennick DG, Nyland TG, Fisher PE, Kerr LY. Ultrasonography of the normal canine gastrointestinal tract. Vet Radiol 1989;30:272.
29. Pennick DG, Nyland TG, Kerr LY, Fisher PE. Ultrasonographic evaluation of gastrointestinal disease in small animals. Vet Radiol 1990;31:134.
30. Pipers FS, Hamlin RL. Clinical use of echocardiography in the domestic cat. J Am Vet Med Assoc 1980;176:57.
31. Thomas WP, Sisson D, Bauer TG. Detection of cardiac masses in dogs by two dimensional echocardiography. Vet Radiol 1984;25:65.
32. Lusk RH, Jr, Ettinger SI, Barr EA. Ultrasound diagnosis of a feline heart tumor. Cardiac carcinomatosis in a cat. Calif Vet 1987;41:9.
33. Nelson TR, Pretorius DH. The Doppler signal: where does it come from and what does it do? Amer J Roent 1988;151:439.
34. Thomas WP. Two dimensional, real-time echocardiography in the dog. Vet Radiol 1984;25:50.
35. Boon J, Wingfield WE, Miller CW. Echocardiographic indices in the normal dog. Vet Radiol 1983:24;214.
36. Bonagura JD, Herring DS. Echocardiography: Acquired heart disease. Vet Clin North Amer [Sm Anim Pract] 1985:15;1209.
37. Pion PD, Kittleson MD, Rogers Q, Morris JG. Myocardial failure in cats associated with low plasma taurine: A reversible cardiomyopathy. Science 1987;237:764.
38. Soderberg SF, Boon JA, Wingfield WE, Miller CW. M-Mode echocardiography as a diagnostic aid for feline cardiomyopathy. Vet Radiol 1983:24;66.
39. Bond BR, Fox PR, Peterson ME, Skavaril RV. Echocardiographic findings in 103 cats with hyperthyroidism. J Am Vet Med Assoc 1988;192:1546.
40. Forrester SD. The categories and causes of pleural effusion in cats. Vet Med 1988;83:894.

PART III

◇ ◇ ◇

Clinical Syndromes

CHAPTER 16

◇ ◇ ◇

Anemia

Gary D. Norsworthy

Anemia is defined as a deficiency of red blood cells (RBCs). It is generally accepted that anemia is present in the cat if the packed cell volume (PCV) is less than 25%; however, the normal values of some commercial veterinary laboratories may differ slightly. Anemia is a common disorder in the cat, but it is much less common now than it was 15 to 20 years ago. (See Appendix F for a comprehensive list of causes of anemia in cats.)

Historical Perspective

Prior to our understanding of the feline leukemia virus (FeLV), most regenerative anemias were diagnosed as acute feline infectious anemia (FIA), whereas most nonregenerative anemias were designated as bone marrow exhaustion secondary to chronic FIA.

Although FeLV was discovered in 1964, serologic testing for this disease did not become available to the veterinary practitioner until 1973. At that time, Dr. William D. Hardy, Jr. developed the indirect fluorescent antibody (IFA) test. With that tool, the veterinary practitioner was able to diagnose FeLV-induced anemias that previously had been misdiagnosed. Because FeLV-induced anemia was the most common type of anemia at that time, the practitioner's handling of the anemic cat was greatly enhanced by this diagnostic test.

Diagnosis

It is the nature of the sick feline patient to appear relatively healthy until a disease reaches a crisis level. Thus, it is not uncommon for a cat with anorexia and lethargy, described as being of a few days' duration, to be presented only after the PCV has dropped to 4%. Usually, an anemia of that magnitude will have developed over a period of several weeks, but the owner may not become aware of the disease state until the crisis stage is reached.

The clinical signs of anemia will vary greatly according to the degree of anemia present. To the owner, an anemic cat may appear to be normal. However, physical examination will often reveal pallor of the mucous membranes. Care should be exercised in interpreting the color of the nasal planum, especially of white cats, as it may appear to be nearly white at a given time, changing to rosy pink within a few hours as a result of cardiovascular fluctuations and other factors. Severe anemia may be accompanied by a rapid respiratory rate, dyspnea, an increased heart rate, and/or a systolic murmur. Physical examination may reveal splenomegaly and icterus of the skin and mucous membranes. Icterus is often first visible on the cat's soft palate, so the physical examination should include inspection of the oral cavity.

A minimum of three tests must be performed to evaluate the anemic cat properly: (1) an RBC count or a PCV level, (2) an RBC evaluation based on a blood smear, and (3) a reticulocyte count. If blood is submitted to a commercial laboratory, the first two tests are routinely performed as part of the complete blood count (CBC). The third—the reticulocyte count—must specifically be requested. If a nonveterinary laboratory is utilized, it is essential that the technician realize that feline reticulocytes are counted differently than are those of humans or dogs.

In some situations, it is necessary for these tests to be performed in-house. Compared to an RBC count, the PCV level is simpler to determine, less expensive, and less likely to be subject to technical errors, and it can be performed within about 5 minutes. It is essential that a high-speed centrifuge specific for microhematocrits be used.

A blood smear evaluation should note the following (see Chapter 12):

- Percentage of polychromatophilic erythrocytes (Figs. 16–1 and 16–2)
- Percentage of nucleated RBCs (see Fig. 16–1)
- Presence of RBC inclusions, such as Heinz bodies (see Fig. 16–2)
- Presence of Howell-Jolly bodies (Fig. 16–3)
- Presence of RBC parasites, such as *Hemobartonella felis* (see Fig. 16–1) and *Cytauxzoon* species (Fig. 16–4)
- Presence of spherocytes
- Presence of fragmented RBCs
- Relative number and types of leukocytes
- Relative number of platelets

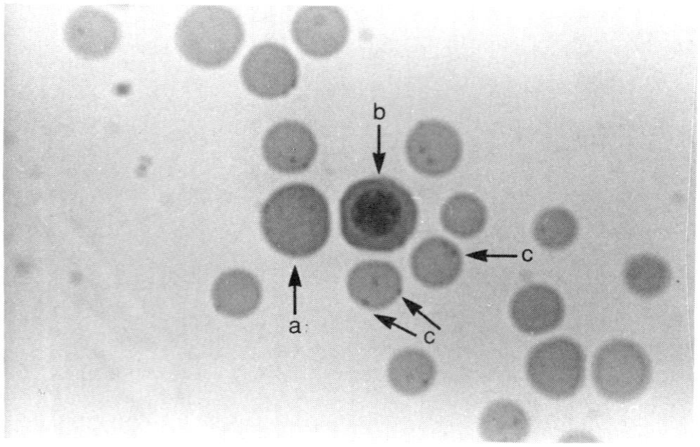

Figure 16–1. The large cell to the left of center (*a*) is a reticulocyte, also known as a macrocyte because of its increased diameter as compared to mature erythrocytes. The large cell next to it (*b*) is a metarubricyte, one of the nucleated red blood cells. *Hemobartonella felis* is an epicellular parasite that can be seen on several of the mature erythrocytes (*c*). (Diff-Quik stain)

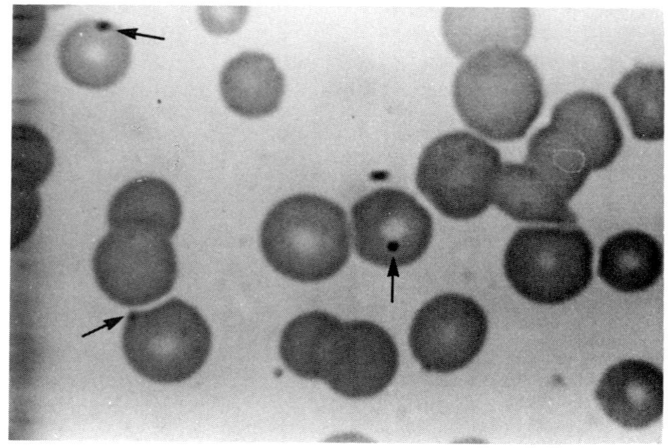

Figure 16–3. Three cells in this field contain a prominent, dense spot known as a Howell-Jolly body (*arrows*). This generally indicates increased bone marrow activity. (Diff-Quik stain)

Reticulocytes are identified by the precipitation of residual RNA that is visible when stained with a supravital dye, such as new methylene blue. The reticulocyte count allows measurement of bone marrow activity. The cat has two types of reticulocytes: the smaller punctate form and the larger aggregate form (Fig. 16–5). Following acute blood loss, the number of punctate reticulocytes peaks at 10 to 20 days, then gradually declines over the next 4 weeks. By contrast, the number of aggregate reticulocytes peaks at 4 to 7 days. Therefore, aggregate reticulocytes reflect bone marrow responses occurring within the previous week, whereas punctate reticulocytes generally reflect the bone marrow activity occurring several weeks prior to the examination. For this reason, a feline reticulocyte count should include only the aggregate forms. If both types are counted, the percentage for each must be noted (see Chapter 12). The reticulocyte count should be corrected to account for the size of the peripheral RBC pool in which the reticulocytes are diluted. The formula for this calculation is as follows:

% Reticulocytes (corrected)
= (% reticulocytes) × (PCV of patient/normal PCV*)

*For the sake of this formula the normal PCV in cats is 35%.

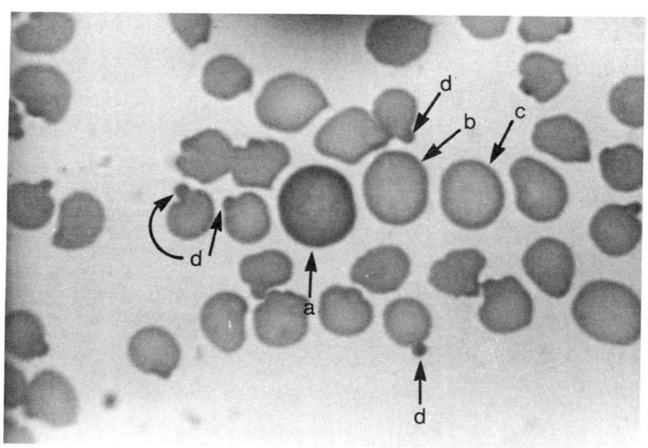

Figure 16–2. The large cell in the center of the field (*a*) and the two cells to its right (*b* and *c*) are reticulocytes or macrocytes. Several of the surrounding mature erythrocytes have protrusions known as Heinz bodies (*d*). (Diff-Quik stain)

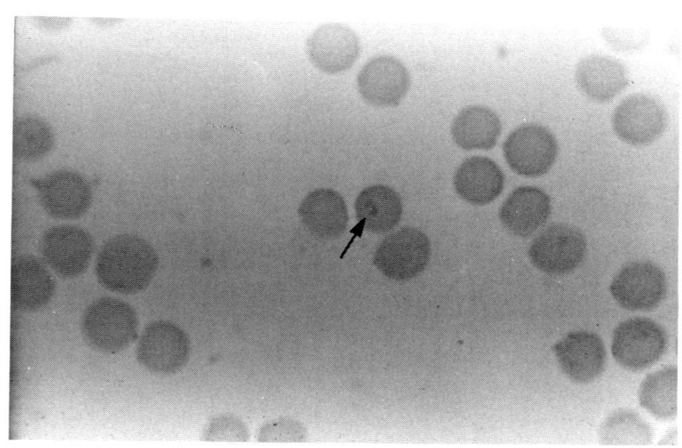

Figure 16–4. One of the three cells in the center of this field contains a ring-form piroplasm, *Cytauxzoon felis* (*arrow*). (Diff-Quik stain)

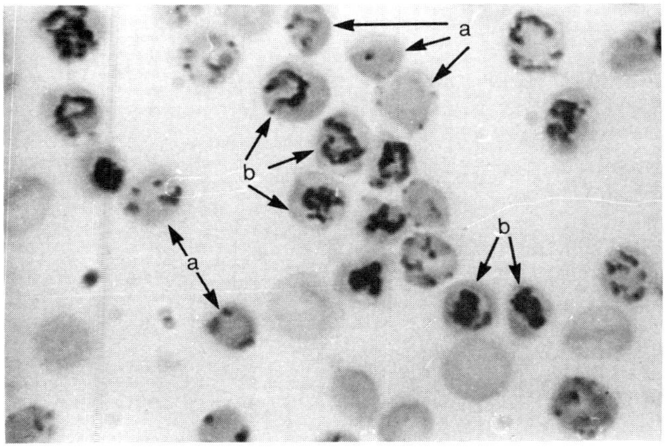

Figure 16–5. **Punctate and aggregate reticulocytes are prominently displayed when stained with new methylene blue stain. The smaller cells containing only a few dark spots are of the punctate form (*a*). Aggregate reticulocytes contain multiple dark spots (*b*); these cells generally have a larger diameter than do the punctate cells.**

Recognizing that many anemias cannot be diagnosed merely on the basis of the three tests just discussed, Table 16–1 lists the other tests that are appropriate for differentiating the various causes of anemia.

Underlying Mechanisms

Anemia may be caused by one or more of three mechanisms—hemolysis, blood loss, or bone marrow suppression. The first two do not affect the bone marrow adversely, so RBC production is accelerated by positive feedback in an attempt to correct the peripheral deficiency. These are termed regenerative or responsive anemias. By contrast, bone marrow suppression results in reduced or arrested red blood cell production. Anemias induced in this manner are considered to be nonregenerative or nonresponsive anemias. Because the average peripheral RBC survival time in the cat is 75 days, a cat will become clinically anemic in a few weeks once RBC production ceases or is significantly impaired.

Anemia can also be caused by more than one disease or mechanism acting simultaneously. Indeed, a lack of bone marrow response does not always mean that blood loss or hemolysis has not contributed to the anemic state. In cats with FeLV-induced bone marrow suppression and hemobartonellosis, for example, *H. felis* destroys RBCs by hemolysis, but the bone marrow cannot regenerate because of FeLV suppression. As a general rule, nonregenerative anemias have a poorer prognosis than do regenerative anemias, as a large percentage of the nonregenerative cases are FeLV-related.

Bone Marrow Response

A number of complex pathways must be intact for the bone marrow to produce RBCs. Interruption of this process along any of these pathways will result in ineffective erythropoiesis.

The steps involved in erythrocyte maturation are listed in Table 16–2. The first four cells listed—rubriblasts, prorubricytes, rubricytes, and metarubricytes—are found in the bone marrow of cats that are not anemic. Aggregate reticulocytes are also found primarily in the bone marrow, and may also constitute up to 1% of the peripheral RBC population in normal cats. A small number of punctate reticulocytes (1% to 10%) may be found in the peripheral circulation.

Table 16–1. Diagnostic Considerations in Anemic* Cats

Reticulocytes: Increased

Blood smear examination: Heinz bodies (acetaminophen, etc.)
Hemobartonella felis (feline infectious anemia)
Cytauxzoon felis (cytauxzoonosis)
Microcytic, hypochromic red blood cells (iron deficiency)

History: Recent surgery or trauma (hemorrhagic anemia)

Physical examination: Fleas, ticks (hemorrhagic anemia)

Fecal examination: Hookworms (hemorrhagic anemia)
Occult or gross blood (gastrointestinal bleeding)

Urinalysis: Hematuria (hemorrhagic anemia)

Platelet count: Thrombocytopenia (hemorrhagic anemia)

Reticulocytes: Decreased

Feline leukemia virus (FeLV) test: Positive (FeLV marrow suppression)

Feline immunodeficiency virus (FIV) test: Positive (FIV marrow suppression)

Blood urea nitrogen level: Increased (chronic renal failure)

Clinical signs: Fever, weight loss, poor appetite (chronic inflammatory diseases, chronic neoplasia, chronic infections)

History: Drugs, toxins

*Packed cell volume of less than 25%

Table 16–2. Progressive Stages of Red Blood Cell Production

1. Rubriblast
2. Prorubricyte
3. Rubricyte
4. Metarubricyte
5. Aggregate reticulocyte
6. Punctate reticulocyte
7. Erythrocyte

Erythrocytes are limited to the peripheral circulation, although bone marrow aspiration may reveal some circulating through the bone marrow as peripheral cells.

In anemic cats, erythropoiesis is greatly accelerated if the bone marrow is normal. Immature erythrocytic forms will be released into the peripheral circulation in an attempt to compensate for the erythrocytic deficiency. The degree of anemia will determine which immature forms are released. In cats with mild anemia (those with a PCV of 20% to 25%), 1% to 2% of the peripheral RBCs may be aggregate reticulocytes, and more than 10% may be punctate forms. In cats with severe anemia (those with a PCV of less than 12%), the aggregate reticulocytes may account for 4% to 6% of the peripheral RBCs, the punctate reticulocytes may represent 20%, and RBC forms as immature as rubricytes and metarubricytes may occur peripherally.

The degree of activity of the bone marrow can be determined by a peripheral blood smear. Generally, the greater the percentage of immature RBCs present, the greater the bone marrow response, as long as an orderly progression of cells occurs. However, there is one situation in which an orderly progression of cells does not occur. Erythremic myelosis is an FeLV-induced leukemia of the red cell line. Tremendous bone marrow activity is typical of this disease; however, the PCV does not rise because erythropoiesis progresses only through the metarubricyte stage. The peripheral blood smear will be saturated with immature RBCs, yet the cat will remain anemic.

There are other indicators of bone marrow activity as well. Because aggregate reticulocytes are larger and bluer than mature erythrocytes, anisocytosis (diversity of size) and polychromasia (diversity of color) will be noted. These larger cells will also increase the mean corpuscular volume (MCV). Howell-Jolly bodies are frequently seen on many of the mature RBCs.

Care should be exercised in judging bone marrow activity on the basis of the presence of nucleated RBCs, as they are only significant if the number of reticulocytes is greater than the number of nucleated RBCs and if the release of cells from the bone marrow is orderly. In severe acute anemias, nucleated RBCs may be released from the bone marrow in an attempt to rectify an RBC deficit quickly. Bone marrow response may or may not follow. Erythremic myelosis causes large numbers of nucleated RBCs to appear in the peripheral circulation without a resultant rise in the PCV. In some myeloproliferative disorders, extramedullary hematopoiesis may occur in the liver and spleen. The cells produced in these locations are not subject to the same release mechanisms as are cells produced by bone marrow; therefore, immature RBCs may be released prematurely.[1]

Once a cat's bone marrow response has been evaluated, the practitioner is in a position to further classify the anemic process. As a diagnostic reference, Figure 16–6 presents a flow chart that includes many of the conditions discussed in the following section.[2]

Diagnosis Based on Bone Marrow Response

Regenerative Anemias

As mentioned previously, regenerative anemias may be caused by hemolysis or blood loss. In most hemolytic anemias, plasma protein concentrations are normal, whereas they are decreased in most hemorrhagic anemias. Other methods used to differentiate between hemolytic and hemorrhagic anemias include an examination of body cavities and excretions (e.g., urine, vomitus, and stool) for the presence of blood, and a fecal examination for intestinal parasites, especially hookworms. Icterus, bilirubinuria, and hemoglobinuria are indicative of a hemolytic disorder, as are Heinz bodies, stomatocytes, spherocytes, and blood parasites.

Once hemolysis has been diagnosed, further testing should include an FeLV test and a test for the feline immunodeficiency virus (FIV). A Coombs' test is optional, as it is of limited value in differentiating feline diseases. If hemorrhage is suspected, tests to confirm or deny hemostatic disorders are indicated.

Regenerative Anemias Secondary to Hemolysis

Hemolysis may be caused by several feline diseases. The hemolytic process is recognized by Heinz bodies, spherocytes, fragmented erythrocytes, and blood parasites.

The two most common hemolytic anemias in the cat are the Heinz-body anemias and FIA caused by *H. felis*. Less likely causes include the intracellular parasite of the *Cytauxzoon* species and autoimmune hemolytic anemia (AHA).

Heinz-body anemias are characterized by the presence of Heinz bodies within the RBCs. These Heinz bodies are aggregates of precipitated hemoglobin that occur as a result of exposure to oxidants. Oxidants that have been implicated in the cat include methylene blue, acetaminophen, benzocaine, and phenazopyridine. Propylene glucol, which is an additive contained in many semimoist cat foods, may induce this process or, more likely, it may sensitize the cells to other oxidants.

Heinz bodies may be visualized using a Wright's stain, such as Diff-Quik (AHS del Caribe, Inc., Aguada, Puerto Rico) (see Fig. 16–2), or they may be more dramatically demonstrated using new methylene blue stain (Fig. 16–7). Many affected cats will recover once the source of the oxidant is identified and eliminated. However, those with severe anemias may require a blood transfusion and supportive care, including the administration of oxygen and intravenous (IV) fluids (see Chapter 42).

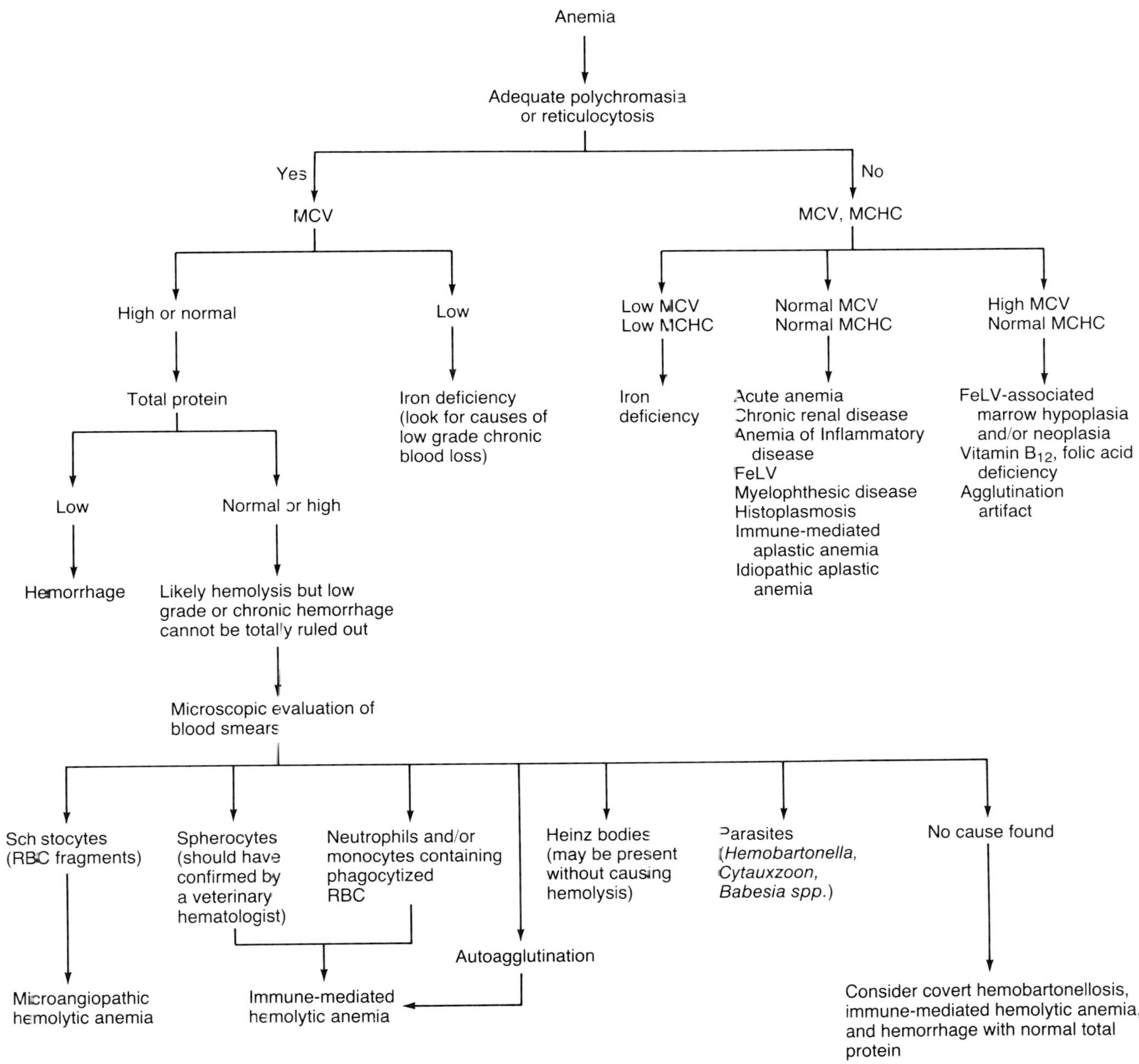

Figure 16–6. Flow chart for evaluating anemic cats.[2] (Courtesy of Rick L. Cowell and Ronald D Tyler, Oklahoma State University, Clinical Pathology Teaching File.)

H. felis is an epicellular parasite that causes RBC destruction. It may be visualized, either as cocci or rods in chains, in RBCs that are stained with several stains, including a Wright's stain (see Fig. 16–1). However, because of the cyclic nature of this parasitemia, multiple blood samples may be required to confirm the presence of this parasite. Many cats with FIA will test positive to the Coombs' test.[3] Because of the low incidence of regenerative anemias secondary to other diseases, one should suspect hemobartonellosis as the cause of non–Heinz-body regenerative anemias even if *H. felis* cannot readily be identified (see Chapter 43).

Feline cytauxzoonosis is a rare hemolytic anemia caused by the intracellular parasite *Cytauxzoon felis.* The organism appears as a ring-form piroplasm within RBCs that have been stained with a Wright's stain (see Fig. 16–4). It is most likely transmitted by ticks. The prognosis is grave, as no effective treatment has been discovered to date.[4]

AHA is a rare disease of cats that causes hemolysis. This disease is controversial, as it may be confused with hemo-

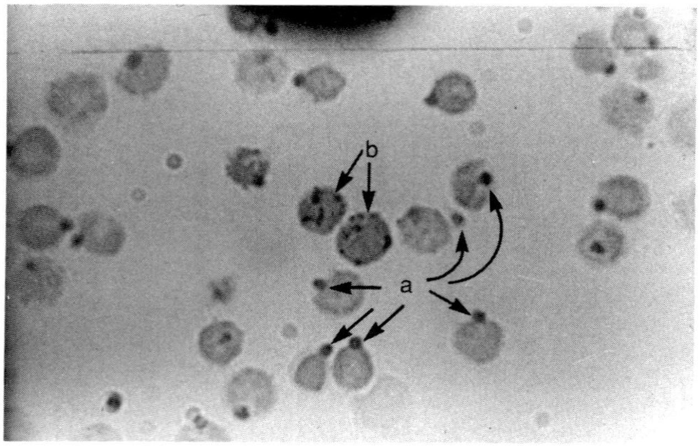

Figure 16–7. **Heinz bodies (*a*) are readily evident when stained with new methylene blue stain. Two punctate reticulocytes can be seen in the center of the field (*b*).**

bartonellosis without parasitemia; cats with either disease may test positive to the Coombs' test, but the latter is responsive to tetracycline. AHA is usually associated with FeLV.

Propylthiouracil, a drug occasionally used to treat hyperthyroidism, can cause an immune-mediated hemolysis.[5] Because this is not the drug of choice for hyperthyroidism, it is not commonly used. However, cats that are receiving long-term medical therapy only and that have experienced side effects with methimazole may be treated with propylthiouracil. The latter may also be used in cats when methimazole is not available.

Regenerative Anemias Secondary to Blood Loss

Anemias secondary to blood loss are not common in cats. Moreover, hookworms and ticks, which are major causes of hemorrhagic anemias in dogs, only occasionally affect cats severely enough to cause anemia. Cats commonly have fleas, but rarely do they cause sufficient blood loss to induce anemia except in otherwise debilitated cats or in kittens.

An acute loss of a large volume of blood is generally the result of trauma or surgery. Such cases are generally easily diagnosed based on the cat's history and the clinical findings.

Chronic blood loss is more likely than an acute loss to cause clinical anemias, but such a cause is still uncommon. Chronic blood loss may result from occult gastrointestinal bleeding, chronic immune-mediated thrombocytopenia, or chronic hematuria.

Iron deficiency anemia is rare except in kittens. Kittens normally go through a stage of iron deficiency between 1 and 10 weeks of age. At its peak, the anemia may produce a PCV of less than 15%; however, it will return to normal adult values by 12 to 15 weeks of age. This is the stage when kittens are most susceptible to the effects of fleas and other blood-sucking parasites. Iron supplementation is warranted if parasites are present; however, iron overload can occur if a deficit is not present. Oral ferrous sulfate may be administered at a daily dose of 10 to 25 mg.[6]

Nonregenerative Anemias

Cats with a suppressed bone marrow will become anemic over a period of several weeks. Because of the slow onset, the cat may be profoundly anemic at the time of diagnosis, with a PCV as low as 4%.

The most common nonregenerative anemia in the cat is caused by FeLV, which accounts for about 70% of the cases. One unique feature of FeLV-induced anemias of this type is macrocytosis. These cats often have an MCV of greater than 50 fl.[1] Another virus that can cause a nonregenerative anemia is FIV. Therefore, an FIV test and an FeLV test should be among the initial tests performed.

The next most common cause of feline nonregenerative anemia is chronic disease. A wide variety of inflammatory diseases, such as systemic fungal infections, feline infectious peritonitis (FIP), and neoplastic diseases, may be responsible. These diseases generally cause a normocytic, normochromic anemia that will self-correct if the primary disease is eliminated. Anemia can also result from chronic renal disease, in which there is decreased production of erythropoietin by the diseased kidneys. This type of anemia is generally mild and of minor clinical significance. It will self-correct if renal function improves.

In addition, some drugs may cause a nonregenerative anemia in cats. For instance, chloramphenicol may suppress bone marrow function as a result of direct injury to precursor cells. It is a reversible anemia once the drug is withdrawn.

A pancytopenia will result from an aplastic anemia, as all three cell lines are damaged. FeLV is the most likely etiologic agent, but drug or chemical exposures should be considered if the results of an FeLV test are negative.

Finally, the bone marrow may be infiltrated by tumors or fungal infections. Either of these conditions may also cause a nonregenerative anemia.

Concurrent Causes of Anemia

A cat may have more than one anemia-producing disease concurrently. The most notable is hemolysis-producing hemobartonellosis that is a stress-related disease occurring secondary to another disease. If a large number of *H. felis* are found on the red blood cells, but a bone marrow response is not evident, another disease may be affecting the bone marrow (such as those mentioned in the previous section on nonregenerative anemias).

Bone Marrow Examination

If the aforementioned tests are not diagnostic, a bone marrow aspiration should be performed. This procedure is detailed in Chapter 12. A bone marrow aspirate can be very helpful in the diagnosis of cytotoxic damage, myelophthisis, and abnormal erythroid maturation.[7] Occasionally, FeLV can be detected by performing an IFA test on a bone marrow sample in a cat that has FeLV-negative peripheral blood. For this reason, unstained bone marrow slides should be saved for this test.

REFERENCES

1. Kociba GJ. Feline Anemia. In: Kirk RW, ed. Current Veterinary Therapy X. Philadelphia: WB Saunders, 1989:425.
2. Cowell RL, Tyler RD. Diagnosis of Anemia. In: August JR, ed. Consultations in Feline Internal Medicine, 1st ed. Philadelphia: WB Saunders, 1991:336.
3. Zulty JC, Kociba GJ. Cold agglutinins in cats with hemobartonellosis. J Am Vet Med Assoc 1990;196:907.
4. Hribernik TN, Barr SC. Parasitic Blood Diseases of Dogs and Cats. In: Kirk RW, ed. Current Veterinary Therapy X. Philadelphia: WB Saunders, 1989:419.
5. Peterson ME, Ferguson DC. Thyroid Diseases. In: Ettinger SJ, ed. Textbook of Veterinary Internal Medicine, 3rd ed. Philadelphia: WB Saunders, 1989 1632.
6. Blue JT. Anemia in cats. Feline Health Topics 1990;5:3.
7. Greene CE. Hematologic Problems. In: Lorenz DM, Cornelius LM, eds. Small Animal Medical Diagnosis. Philadelphia: JB Lippincott, 1987:527.

CHAPTER 17

◇ ◇ ◇

Ataxia/Paresis

James R. Cook, Jr.

Ataxia and paresis are common presenting complaints from cat owners. Because these are nonspecific signs, the primary clinician must carefully correlate all available information, including signalment, history, and physical and neurologic examination findings, in order to develop a logical differential diagnosis list and diagnostic plan. Ataxia and paresis imply nervous system disease; however, the clinician should be alert for multisystemic problems that may cause neurologic signs secondarily. This is especially important in view of the need for anesthesia for many diagnostic procedures of the nervous system.

This discussion is limited to diseases of the central or peripheral nervous system (CNS or PNS). However, thromboembolic disease may cause an acute onset of paresis or paralysis of a foreleg or of one or both hindlegs. This disease, including its differentiation from CNS disease, is discussed in Chapter 27.

Signalment

The age, breed, and sex of the patient are helpful in establishing the general category of disease causing clinical abnormalities. Hard and fast rules do not always apply to age and sex predispositions, but certain generalizations can be made with some degree of confidence. For example, storage diseases are typically seen in juvenile to young adult animals, while non-feline leukemia virus (FeLV) related neoplasia is found in older animals. Bacterial infections and septicemia with nervous system effects are more common in adult intact males who live outdoors and fight with other cats. The clinician should use common sense and practicality in evaluating this information.

The breed of the patient is of extreme importance, since many diseases have a breed predilection or may even be limited to a specific breed of cat. Table 17–1 contains a partial listing of CNS/PNS diseases and breed predispositions. For a more complete list, reference textbooks should be consulted.[1,2]

History

The history should be as complete as reasonably possible. Any information concerning the patient's past health and environment, including travel, diet, vaccinations, and other pets in the household, may be important in the case evaluation. A humorous but distressingly true statement is that the most important historical information is that which the clinician has not yet obtained. This axiom can be applied to diagnostic tests and radiographic views as well. Again, common sense will point out the value of some historical information; e.g., multiple animals affected would indicate an infectious or environmental (dietary deficiency, toxin exposure) etiology.

An extremely important aspect of the history is determining the progression of signs over time. Major disease categories in the DAMNIT scheme (see Table 17–2) can be grouped according to whether they are acute or chronic, progressive or nonprogressive, or variable (see Table 17–3). With complete signalment and history information, the clinician can begin developing some ideas as to the general disease category before moving on to lesion localization and a diagnostic plan.

Physical Examination

The physical examination is important in detecting signs of polysystemic disease that could cause secondary neurologic signs or complicate anesthetic episodes. Fever, respiratory abnormalities, cardiac arrhythmias, abdominal enlargement/organomegaly, pallor, ocular disease, skin and haircoat problems, and excessive weight gain or loss are all indicative of multiple organ system involvement. In patients whose disease process is confined entirely to the central nervous system, or in cases of primary neuromuscular disease, the general physical examination may be normal and the only detectable abnormalities may be those associated with the neurologic examination.

Lesion Localization

The neurologic examination (NE), a form of physical examination with special emphasis on nervous system function, is used to localize a lesion or lesions within the nervous system. The NE does not diagnose diseases but is used in conjunction with historical data to localize the lesion to a particular level of the nervous system and to formulate a

Table 17–1. Breed Predilections for CNS/PNS Disorders

Manx	Neural tube anomalies with myelodysplasia
Siamese	GM1 gangliosidosis, sphingomyelin lipidosis, ceroid lipofuschinosis, mucopolysaccharidosis, hydrocephalus, congenital vestibular disease
Abyssinian	Glucocerebrosidosis
Burmese	Congenital vestibular disease, encephalocele
Korat	GM1 gangliosidosis
Egyptian Mau	Spongiform degeneration
Persian	Mannosidosis
Domestic	GM1 and GM2 gangliosidosis, sphingomyelin lipidosis, glycogenesis, mucopolysaccharidosis VI, mannosidosis, neuroaxonal dystrophy, neurofilament accumulation, globoid cell leukodystrophy, metachromatic leukodystrophy

diagnostic plan. The NE is also used to aid in determining prognosis and in monitoring response to therapy by serial examinations.

The NE is a series of general observations (mental state, gait, abnormalities noted from the general physical) and hands-on manipulations of the patient (cranial nerve responses and reflexes, thorough ophthalmic examination, postural reactions, spinal reflexes, and sensory examination). The different portions of the NE can be performed in whatever order the clinician finds comfortable so long as the NE is performed consistently and results are recorded as the NE progresses. The author prefers the order listed above because it allows a step-by-step progression through the various portions of the nervous system, providing a sound base for the thought processes necessary to localize the lesion. It also completes the most sensitive and critical portions of the NE before the subject's patience and cooperative spirit are exhausted and saves the more noxious sensory tests for the end of the exam (after those portions requiring working around the teeth and jaws are completed). An exhaustive review of the interpretation of NE abnormalities is beyond the scope and intent of this chapter; readers requiring review on NE interpretation should consult a reference textbook.[3] Extreme precision in localizing lesions is not essential for good case management, but the reader should be able to recognize lesions of the forebrain, hindbrain, cerebellum, major sections of the spinal cord, and individual peripheral nerves, as well as diffuse neuromuscular disease. The difference between central and peripheral vestibular disease should also be appreciated.

Table 17–2. DAMNIT Scheme of Disease Classification

Degenerative
Anomalies (congenital)
Metabolic
Neoplastic/**N**utritional
Infectious/**I**nflammatory/**I**schemic
Toxins/**T**raumatic

Table 17–3. Time/Sign Progression

Acute, nonprogressive
 Anomalies, ischemic injury, trauma
Acute, progressive
 Infectious diseases, inflammatory diseases
Chronic, progressive
 Degenerative diseases, neoplasia
Variable or episodic
 Metabolic disease, nutritional deficiencies, toxins

Clinical Presentation

This section presents a brief description of a representative clinical patient for each of the major disease categories as listed in the DAMNIT scheme. Some general correlations will be made among history, physical and NE findings, and basic clinical pathology. In many cases there is the potential for diffuse or multifocal lesions that can result in signs other than ataxia or paresis, e.g., seizures if the forebrain is affected.

Degenerative/Storage Diseases

The patient with degenerative or storage disease is typically a juvenile or young adult and, in many instances, may be a purebred animal. While the nervous system signs are most pronounced, these are whole-body diseases, and there may be obvious skeletal or ocular abnormalities as well. The entire nervous system may be affected, causing multifocal or diffuse deficits. The onset and progression of signs will be chronic and progressive, often over several weeks to a few months. Routine laboratory tests (complete blood count [CBC], serum biochemistries, and urinalysis) are usually noncontributory. The diagnosis should be suspected from the history and clinical signs. Specialized assays of enzyme activity (usually available only from research laboratories) from serum and blood cells or biopsies of nervous or other representative tissues are necessary for absolute confirmation. These diseases are rare and invariably progressive and unresponsive to treatment. Death or euthanasia is the usual outcome.

Anomalies

The affected patient is usually a neonate or juvenile. The signs are present at birth or become noticeable when the kitten becomes ambulatory and are nonprogressive. Skeletal deformities may be found on physical examination, with neurologic deficits referable to the level of the nervous system affected. Routine laboratory tests are not likely to provide valuable information. While the diagnosis is usually obvious from the physical exam and NE, confirmation and determination of the degree of malformation can be evaluated by survey and contrast radiography or nuclear imaging. Treatment is usually limited to decompression or stabilization of spinal lesions, if feasible.

Metabolic Disease

The signalment of these patients can be highly variable; their problems can be both congenital (portosystemic shunt) and acquired (chronic renal failure). The history can also vary considerably; organ failure may be an insidious process until a certain critical level is reached, and then a precipitous change in clinical signs occurs. There is, however, frequently a history of waxing/waning symptoms that gradually worsen with time. Frequently there is a history of episodic signs with a time-dependent relationship with meals. The physical examination usually provides evidence of a systemic disorder such as poor body condition or hair coat, pallor, weakness, etc. The NE may reflect encephalopathy in acute phases. In more chronic compensated states, neurologic deficits may be very minor (mild loss of strength) to absent. Routine laboratory tests frequently reflect organ dysfunction. Specific tests of major organ and endocrine function and biopsies confirm the diagnosis. Many of these conditions can be treated successfully or even cured.

Neoplastic Disease

Non-FeLV neoplasia is normally a disease of older cats, with chronic, progressive signs over weeks to months. Occasionally acute signs may be seen from hemorrhage within a large neoplasm. FeLV-related neoplasia may be present in any age patient, and signs may be both acute and multisystemic. There may be marked physical abnormalities if the primary neoplasm is in the vertebral column or skull or if the nervous system effects are due to metastasis from a distant primary tumor in the skeleton or another major organ system. With primary nervous tissue tumors, physical abnormalities are usually minor, and the NE reflects a solitary focal lesion. Routine laboratory values are normal. Survey and contrast radiography, cerebrospinal fluid analysis, and nuclear imaging studies confirm the diagnosis and help determine the feasibility of surgical therapy or chemotherapy.

Nutritional Deficiency

These patients may have a variable signalment, but the history will almost always include an inappropriate or severely unbalanced diet or loss of appetite with little food intake at all. Progression of signs will be different, depending on the deficient nutrient and how the deficiency is manifested. Physical examination may reflect nutritional imbalance by poor body condition, weight loss, and poor hair coat. Neurologic deficits may range from skeletal pain and reluctance to walk to profound ataxia/paresis. Routine laboratory tests may be relatively normal or may show abnormalities of calcium, phosphorus, or renal function in cases of secondary hyperparathyroidism.

Inflammatory/Infectious Disease

The signalment of cats with inflammatory/infectious disease will not be consistent, but the history will usually describe an acute onset of signs with fairly rapid progression over hours to days. Fever, ocular involvement, pain, and other evidence of systemic illness may be present during physical examination. The NE frequently shows diffuse or multifocal abnormalities, including hyperesthesia during palpation. The CBC will typically show inflammatory changes; serum biochemistries and urinalysis will not show significant changes unless a major organ system is also involved in the disease process. Serum levels of muscle enzymes, infectious disease titers, microbial cultures and antibiotic sensitivity, immune function tests, cerebrospinal fluid analysis, or appropriate tissue biopsies and histology may be needed for definitive diagnosis.

Ischemia/Infarction

Cats with ischemic nervous system injury are usually mature adults. The clinical signs are peracute in onset (minutes to a few hours) and typically are nonprogressive. Some limited improvement may occasionally be seen after the acute phase. In rare cases, signs will be progressive and cause considerable worsening of the cat's clinical condition or even death within 24 hours. Physical examination is usually unremarkable (excepting those cases of cardiomyopathy with saddle thrombus formation) and neurologic deficits will be referable to the level of nervous system that has been infarcted. Routine laboratory data are not significantly altered in most cases. Cardiac evaluation, survey and contrast radiography, and nuclear imaging will define the lesion further and aid in the final diagnosis. In the case of infarction within the central nervous system, the diagnosis may not be confirmed except by elimination of other potential causes unless tissue samples are available for histology.

Trauma

Trauma may occur in cats of any age. The onset of signs is peracute (usually instantaneously) with minimal progression. Improvement may occur following the acute injury depending on the severity of the initial lesion. Rarely, signs may progress or worsen following trauma due to edema, persistent hemorrhage, or myelomalacia. The physical findings generally include abrasions, contusions, laceration, hemorrhage, and other manifestations of trauma. The NE deficits will be consistent with the level of the nervous system injured. Routine laboratory tests are unlikely to show significant changes. The diagnosis can usually be made by the history and the physical appearance of the patient. Survey and contrast radiography and nuclear imaging studies may further define the extent and severity of the injury and provide more prognostic information.

Toxin Exposure

Deliberate toxin ingestion by cats is rare due to their selective dietary habits. Except in cases of very palatable substances such as antifreeze/ethylene glycol, toxicosis is usually from self-grooming following accidental contact or iatrogenic from products applied by owners, groomers, or veterinarians. For this reason, affected animals may be of any age or breed. Signs are typically acute and progressive within minutes to hours of exposure. Slowly progressive signs from chronic low-level exposure to organophosphates is described but is rarely seen clinically. Systemic signs (vomiting, diarrhea, dyspnea, hypersalivation, abnormal behavior) may be reported. The physical examination will be unremarkable in most acute cases unless there is still a detectable odor or foreign substance present. Neurologic deficits may be profound and frequently more abnormalities than just ataxia or paresis are seen. Routine laboratory values should be normal unless a major organ failure has also occurred from the toxicosis. The specific diagnosis is normally made from clinical signs and a compatible exposure history. Specific toxin assays are also available from many commercial labs.

Differential Diagnosis

With the information presented in the previous sections and accurate lesion localization, the practitioner should be able to formulate a reasonable list of differential diagnoses. Table 17–4 lists common differential diagnoses for ataxia/paresis divided by general neuroanatomic location and the progression of signs over time. References are cited for those readers wishing more information on a particular disease.

Diagnostic Plan

The approach to diagnosis must be individually tailored to each patient; however, certain general principles will always apply. As previously mentioned, signalment and history are of paramount importance in determining the general type of disease; the NE localizes the primary lesion so that appropriate tests may be focused on the affected area of the nervous system. A minimum data base (MDB) consisting of a CBC, serum biochemical panel, and urinalysis should be performed on every patient. This accomplishes two tasks. First, if there is a metabolic or systemic illness that may be causing or complicating the clinical condition, MDB abnormalities will help the clinician determine the organ system involved and select further laboratory tests. Ancillary tests may include specific organ function tests, endocrine function, immune studies, infectious disease titers, and microbial culture and antibiotic sensitivity. Cardiac evaluation and specific toxin assays might be indicated as well by the history and physical examination. Secondly, as most patients with neurologic disease will eventually undergo at least one

Table 17–4. Differential Diagnoses

Cranial

Forebrain

Acute, nonprogressive
Hydrocephalus,[4] feline ischemic encephalopathy,[5] encephalocele,[6] head trauma

Acute, progressive
FIP,[7] toxoplasmosis,[8] FeLV/FIV syndromes,[9] cryptococcosis,[10] bacterial encephalitis,[11] feline polioencephalomyelitis,[12] parasite migration[13]

Chronic, progressive
Meningioma,[14] other primary neural tissue tumors (rare), metastatic neoplasia, GM1 gangliosidosis,[15] GM2 gangliosidosis,[16] mannosidosis,[17,18] glycogenosis,[19] sphingomyelinosis,[20] ceroid lipofuschinosis,[21] globoid cell leukodystrophy,[22] glucocerebrosidosis,[23] spongiform degeneration,[24] metachromatic leukodystrophy[25]

Variable or episodic
Hepatic encephalopathy,[26] lead toxicosis, organophosphate toxicosis

Hindbrain/Cerebellum/Vestibular System

Acute, nonprogressive
Trauma, feline ischemic encephalopathy, cerebellar hypoplasia,[27] idiopathic vestibular syndrome[28,29]

Acute, progressive
Same as for forebrain, otitis media with vestibular signs (may also cause facial paralysis)

Chronic, progressive
Same as for forebrain; neuroaxonal dystrophy[30]

Variable or episodic
Thiamine deficiency[31]

Spinal Cord

Acute, nonprogressive
Trauma, intervertebral disk herniation,[32] fibrocartilaginous embolism,[33] sacrocaudal deformities in Manx cats

Acute, progressive
Myelomalacia following injury,[32] tetanus,[34] others as listed for acute, progressive forebrain diseases

Chronic, progressive
Same as listed for chronic, progressive forebrain disease; hypervitaminosis A,[35] mucopolysaccharidosis,[36] degenerative myelopathy[37]

Neuromuscular Disease (Diffuse)

Acute, nonprogressive
Rarely if ever reported

Acute, progressive
Tick paralysis,[38] botulism,[39] polyradiculoneuritis,[40] acute polymyositis[41]

Chronic, progressive
Neurofilament accumulation,[42] "dying-back" syndromes,[43] chronic polyneuropathy/polymyopathy,[44] diabetic neuropathy[45]

Episodic or variable
Myasthenia gravis,[46] polymyopathy syndrome,[47] organophosphate toxicosis, various other toxins, hypoadrenocorticism,[48] hypothyroid neuropathy,[49] steroid-induced myopathy[50]

Neuromuscular Disease (Focal)

Acute, nonprogressive
Focal nerve lesions are almost invariably traumatic, e.g., brachial plexus avulsion, sciatic nerve injection injury, radial paralysis. May see monoparesis rarely secondary to focal spinal cord infarction[33]

Acute, progressive
Ischemic neuromyopathy secondary to hypertrophic cardiomyopathy and saddle thrombus formation,[51] others rarely described

Chronic, progressive
Peripheral nerve or nerve root tumor (rarely described)

anesthetic procedure, the MDB will help determine the patient's anesthetic risk and alert the clinician to any unsuspected metabolic conditions that might complicate anesthesia.

Following the establishment of a MDB, the clinician can then outline a more complete plan to eliminate or confirm the differential diagnoses. Survey and contrast radiography, cerebrospinal fluid (CSF) analysis, electrodiagnostic tests, nuclear imaging techniques, and biopsies for histology are all applicable diagnostic tools. Performance of infectious disease testing may be indicated again at this time, if not already suggested by physical examination and MDB results. The analysis of CSF is a valuable part of the vast majority of neurology work-ups, except for some very specific exceptions, and can be performed by most practitioners if they wish to learn collection and analysis methods.[52] Many other diagnostic procedures in neurology may eventually require referral to a specialty clinic or university veterinary teaching hospital. Table 17–5 lists the general diagnostic procedures typically followed in evaluating the different parts of the nervous system or of metabolic diseases that may cause secondary neurologic deficits. Some leeway should be allowed in evaluating the individual patient; not every patient will require all tests listed, while others may need other tests not normally used in that part of the nervous system. In most cases, however, a diagnosis should be obtained by following the procedures below. If a review of electrodiagnostics is desired, a textbook should be consulted.[53]

Table 17–5. Diagnostic Procedures: Minimum Data Base

Cranial

Blood lead, bile acid assay, cholinesterase levels if indicated by history or MDB abnormalities
Infectious disease testing (FeLV/FIP/FIV/cryptococcus titer/toxoplasma titer) if indicated by history, MDB, or physical examination
Deep otoscopic exam (for vestibular signs)
Skull radiographs (including tympanic bullae views)
CSF analysis
Electroencephalogram (forebrain)
Brainstem evoked potentials (hindbrain)
Nuclear imaging studies (CT and MRI)
Intracranial angiography if CT/MRI unavailable
Infectious disease testing, microbial culture and antibiotic sensitivity, immune studies (antinuclear antibody, Coombs' test) if indicated by CSF results
Biopsy (cerebral cortex, cerebellum)

Spinal Cord

Infectious disease testing if indicated by history or physical examination
Survey radiographs CSF
Myelography
Infectious disease testing, microbial culture and antibiotic sensitivity, immune studies if indicated by CSF results
Somatosensory-, spinal-, and motor-evoked potentials
Biopsies (terminal patients or necropsy only)

Neuromuscular Disease

Electromyography/nerve conduction/repetitive stimulation
Serum muscle enzyme levels
Toxoplasma titer
Botulism toxin bioassay
Myasthenia antibody
Thyroid stimulation testing
Adrenal function
Nerve and muscle biopsies
Blood lead, cholinesterase levels

Therapy

The goal of therapy is to remove or cure the inciting cause of the problem. If cure or removal is not possible, then symptomatic therapy is applied. Because of the blood–brain barrier, treatment of central nervous system disease poses some difficulties and medications must be selected carefully for maximum efficacy.

Antimicrobial Therapy

Antimicrobial medication should be selected based on the results of culture and antibiotic sensitivity of organisms from CSF or other appropriate tissues. Pending these results, or if for some reason they cannot be obtained, broad-spectrum agents should be used. Antibacterial drugs that penetrate the nervous system readily include chloramphenicol and trimethoprim-sulfa combinations. If the blood–brain barrier is damaged by inflammation, penicillins and cephalosporins may cross in therapeutic amounts. Aminoglycosides will not enter the nervous system in therapeutic amounts even when severe blood–brain barrier damage has occurred. Little is known currently about the efficacy of quinolone derivatives in nervous system infection. Ideally, the drug selected should be bacteriocidal and be available in intravenous form so that initial parenteral treatment can provide rapid therapeutic levels. The author prefers ampicillin (10 mg/kg TID to QID) or trimethoprim-sulfa (15 mg/kg BID). While chloramphenicol penetrates the nervous system very readily, it is bacteriostatic and clinical results are usually poorer than with bacteriocidal drugs. In addition, it tends to cause anorexia and depression in cats at higher doses—an undesirable effect in an animal already ill.

Treatment of toxoplasmosis requires more specific antimicrobial medication. Pyrimethamine (0.5 to 1 mg/kg/day) with sulfadiazine or triple sulfas (60 mg/kg/day) is recommended. Clindamycin (30 to 40 mg/kg/day divided TID or QID) has fewer side effects but may not enter the nervous system as well.[54] Antifungal therapy is limited primarily to amphotericin B, ketoconazole, and flucytosine. Flucytosine must be used carefully because it can be toxic to cats. Dosages and frequency of antifungal drugs will vary with the mycotic agent being treated[55] (see Chapter 61).

There are currently no specific agents to treat the viruses commonly associated with nervous system disease in cats (FeLV/feline infectious peritonitis [FIP]/feline immunodeficiency virus [FIV]). A symptomatic treatment scheme has been suggested for FIP,[56] but treated animals still decline rapidly and continue to be a source of contagion for other cats. Therefore, the author recommends that affected cats be humanely euthanatized until more effective therapy is available. Patients with FeLV and FIV may live several years with supportive care and treatment of secondary illnesses associated with these viruses, but they should be isolated from other cats at all times. Vaccines for FIP and FeLV have recently been introduced for general use, but their long-term efficacy in preventing natural infection remains to be proven.

Neoplasia Therapy

The best treatment for neoplasia is surgical removal, if possible. Of the feline nervous system tumors, meningiomas are the most common and are usually benign. If the tumor is located in an accessible area, surgical removal may be curative; this tumor also responds to radiation therapy. Treatment of other nervous system tumors (gliomas, astrocytomas, lymphosarcoma) should rely on chemotherapy or radiation. Several protocols exist for the treatment of lymphosarcoma and related lymphoid neoplasia that affect the nervous system,[57,58] but treatment of feline gliomas and astrocytomas has not been particularly successful. Treatment of metastatic neoplasia in the nervous system is not practical or likely to result in significant improvement in the length or quality of the patient's life.

Trauma Therapy

Traumatic injury to nervous tissue can be treated both surgically and medically. Surgery is for those instances in which removal of disk material, bone fragments, or hematomas is required for decompression or when stabilization of fractures or luxations is necessary.[59–61] Medical therapy is intended to control edema and other potentially harmful biochemical changes within the neural parenchyma following injury. Treatment of edema has classically been with osmotic agents, particularly mannitol (2 gm/kg, IV drip over 30 to 60 minutes). Mannitol is indicated for intracranial injuries but probably has little benefit in spinal cord injury.[62] Controlled studies indicate that the most effective and readily available chemical therapy for spinal cord injury is methylprednisolone sodium succinate (30 mg/kg IV). To be effective, this drug needs to be administered within 45 to 60 minutes following the injury. These studies also demonstrated that other agents recommended for acute nervous system trauma (dexamethasone, thyroid-releasing hormone, naloxone, mannitol, and DMSO) had no more effect than intravenous saline used in the control group animals.[62]

Toxins

If a particular toxin is detected, a specific antidote should be administered. In veterinary medicine, one of the most common poisonings is organophosphates or related insecticide compounds. In the early stages, atropine and/or 2-PAM are indicated. The specific active ingredient should be determined if possible before treatment is begun.[63] Dying-back neuropathies are suspected to occur with chronic exposure; there is no known effective therapy.[43] (A dying-back neuropathy is a delayed neurotoxicity that is characterized by axonal death followed by retrograde motor nerve degeneration to the level of the spinal cord.) Lead poisoning is also occasionally diagnosed in cats. Treatment is by removal of the source and chelation therapy.[64] Other intoxications may occur sporadically; there are now poison control centers that can provide information for veterinarians on an emergency basis. If a specific antidote is not available or if toxicosis cannot be confirmed, supportive care is the only option available.

Nutritional Therapy

In most instances, correction of dietary imbalances will result in rapid resolution of the clinical disease. In cats with thiamine deficiency, parenteral administration of 50 to 100 mg daily during the first few days of treatment may be necessary. There have been many anecdotal accounts of vague or nonspecific neurologic signs that have responded to administration of taurine. Although no controlled studies have been performed, these accounts are impossible to ignore in the face of current knowledge of the importance of taurine in feline metabolism and homeostasis. Therefore, taurine supplementation (500 mg daily) might be considered as an adjunct treatment in cases where a specific diagnosis cannot be reached or if conventional therapy is ineffective.

Antivertigo Therapy

Acute vestibular disease produces dramatic clinical signs that make home management difficult in the early phases. Any inciting causes such as otitis media should be treated (see *Antimicrobial Therapy* above).[7] The treatment of vertiginous signs is primarily by sedation with phenobarbital (1/8 to 1/4 gr BID) or diazepam (2 to 3 mg TID to QID) and restraint if needed to prevent injury from uncontrolled ataxia and rolling. Antihistamines with antivertigo properties have not been particularly effective in the author's experience. Many cases undergo spontaneous resolution.

Anticonvulsant Therapy

See Chapter 23

REFERENCES

1. Oliver JE, Hoerlein BF, Mayhew IG. Appendix II. Species and Breed Predisposition for Noninfectious Disease. In: Oliver JE, Hoerlein BF, Mayhew IG, eds. Veterinary Neurology. Philadelphia: WB Saunders, 1987:525.
2. Fenner WR. Neurologic Disorders. In: Sherding RG, ed. The Cat: Diseases and Clinical Management. New York: Churchill Livingstone, 1989:1163.
3. Oliver JE, Lorenz MD. Neurologic Examination. In: Oliver JE, Lorenz MD, eds. Handbook of Veterinary Neurologic Diagnosis. Philadelphia: WB Saunders, 1983:19.
4. Silson M, Robinson R. Hereditary hydrocephalus in the cat. Vet Rec 1969;84:477.
5. Zaki FA, Nafe LA. Ischemic encephalopathy and focal granulomatous meningoencephalitis in the cat. J Small Anim Pract 1980;21:429.
6. Zook B, Sostaric BR, Draper DJ, Graf-Webster E. Encephalocele and other congenital craniofacial anomalies in Burmese cats. Vet Med Small Anim Clin 1983;78:695.
7. Kornegay JN. Feline infectious peritonitis: The central nervous system form. J Am Anim Hosp Assoc 1978;14:580.

8. Kyle RJ. Toxoplasma encephalitis in a cat. NZ Vet J 1975;23:13.
9. Pedersen NC. Feline Leukemia Virus Infection. In: Pedersen NC, ed. Feline Infectious Diseases. Goleta, CA: American Veterinary Publications, 1988:83.
10. Wilkinson GT. Feline cryptococcosis: A review and seven case reports. J Small Anim Pract 1979;20:749.
11. Fenner WR. Bacterial Infections of the Central Nervous System. In: Greene CE, ed. Infectious Diseases of the Dog and Cat. Philadelphia: WB Saunders, 1990:184.
12. Vandevelde M, Braund KG. Polioencephalomyelitis in cats. Vet Pathol 1979;16:420.
13. Cook JR, Levesque DC, Nuehring LP. Intracranial cuterebral myiasis causing acute lateralizing meningoencephalitis in two cats. J Am Anim Hosp Assoc 1985;21:279.
14. Nafe LA. Meningiomas in cats: A retrospective clinical study of 36 cases. J Am Vet Med Assoc 1979;174:1224.
15. Blakemore WF. GM1 gangliosidosis in a cat. J Comp Pathol 1972;82:179.
16. Cork LC, Munnell JF, Lorenz MD et al. GM2 ganglioside lysosomal storage disease in cats with B-hexosaminidase deficiency. Science 1977;196:1014.
17. Vandevelde M, Fankhauser R, Bichsel P et al. Hereditary neurovisceral mannosidosis in a family of Persian cats. Acta Neuropathol 1982;58:64.
18. Walkley SU, Blakemore WF, Purpura DP. Alterations in neuron morphology in feline mannosidosis. Acta Neuropathol 1981; 53:75.
19. Sandstrom B, Westman J, Ockerman PA. Glycogenosis of the central nervous system in the cat. Acta Neuropathol 1969; 14:194.
20. Snyder S, Kingston R, Wenger D. Animal model of human disease: Neimann-Pick disease. Sphingomyelinosis of Siamese cats. Am J Pathol 1982;108:252.
21. Greene PD, Little PB. Neuronal ceroid-lipofuscin storage in Siamese cats. Can J Comp Med 1974;38:207.
22. Johnson KH. Globoid leukodystrophy in the cat. J Am Vet Med Assoc 1970;157:2057.
23. Van Den Berg P, Baker M, Lange A. A suspected lysosomal storage disease in Abyssinian cats. Part I: Genetic, clinical, and clinical pathological aspects. J South Afr Vet Assoc 1983;48:195.
24. Kelly DF, Gaskell CJ. Spongy degeneration of the central nervous system in kittens. Acta Neuropathol 1976;35:151.
25. Hegreberg GA, Thuline HC, Francis BH. Morphologic changes in feline leukodystrophy. Fed Proc 1971;30:341.
26. Levesque DC, Oliver JE, Cornelius LM et al. Congenital portocaval shunts in two cats: Diagnosis and surgical correction. J Am Vet Med Assoc 1982;181:143.
27. Shepherd DE, deLahunta A. Central nervous system disease in the cat. Compend Contin Ed Pract Vet 1980;2:306.
28. Burke EE, Moise NS, deLahunta A, Erb HN. Review of idiopathic vestibular syndrome in 75 cats. J Am Vet Med Assoc 1985; 187:941.
29. deLahunta A. Vestibular System—Special Proprioception. In: deLahunta A, ed. Veterinary Neuroanatomy and Clinical Neurology, 2d ed. Philadelphia: WB Saunders, 1983:238.
30. Woodard JC, Collins GH, Hessler JR. Feline hereditary neuroaxonal dystrophy. Am J Pathol 1974;74:551.
31. Martin CL. Thiamine Deficiency in the Dog and Cat. In: Kirk RW, ed. Current Veterinary Therapy IV. Philadelphia: WB Saunders, 1971:69.
32. Seim HB, Nafe LA. Spontaneous intervertebral disk protrusion with associated myelopathy in a cat. J Amer Anim Hosp Assoc 1981;17:201.
33. Cook JR. Fibrocartilaginous embolism. In: Luttgen PL, ed. Vet Clin North Amer [Small Anim Pract] 1988;18:581.
34. Baker JL, Waters DJ, deLahunta A. Tetanus in two cats. J Am Anim Hosp Assoc 1988;24:159.
35. Hayes KC. Nutritional problems in cats: Taurine deficiency and Vitamin A excess. Can Vet J 1982;23:2.
36. Haskins ME, Jezyk PF, Desnick RJ et al. Mucopolysaccharidosis in a domestic short-haired cat—A disease distinct from that seen in the Siamese cat. J Am Vet Med Assoc 1979;175:384.
37. Mesfin GM, Kusewitt D, Parker A. Degenerative myelopathy in a cat. J Am Vet Med Assoc 1980;176:62.
38. Barsanti JA. Botulism, Tick Paralysis, and Polyradiculoneuritis (Coonhound Paralysis). In: Kirk RW, ed. Current Veterinary Therapy VII. Philadelphia: WB Saunders 1980:773.
39. deLahunta A. Lower Motor Neuron-General Somatic Efferent. In: deLahunta A, ed. Veterinary Neuroanatomy and Clinical Neurology, 2nd ed. Philadelphia: WB Saunders, 1983:53.
40. Lane JR, deLahunta A. Polyneuritis in a cat. J Am Anim Hosp Assoc 1984;20:1006.
41. Schunk KL. Feline Polymyopathy. In: Proceedings of the 2nd Annual Forum of the American College of Veterinary Internal Medicine 1984:1970.
42. Vandevelde M, Greene CE, Hoff E. Lower motor neuron disease with accumulation of neurofilaments in a cat. Vet Pathol 1976; 13:428.
43. Braund KG. Organophosphate/Carbamate Toxicity. In: Braund KG, ed. Clinical Syndromes in Veterinary Neurology. Baltimore: Williams & Wilkins, 1986:149.
44. Braund KG. Diseases of Peripheral Nerves, Cranial Nerves, and Muscles. In: Oliver JE, Hoerlein BF, Mayhew IG, eds. Veterinary Neurology. Philadelphia: WB Saunders, 1987:353.
45. Kramek BA, Moise NS, Cooper B, Raffe MR. Neuropathy associated with diabetes mellitus in the cat. J Am Vet Med Assoc 1984;184:42.
46. Scott-Moncrieff JC, Cook JR, Lantz GC. Acquired myasthenia gravis in a cat with thymoma. J Am Vet Med Assoc 1990; 196:1291.
47. Averill DR. The Nervous System. In: Holzworth J, ed. Diseases of the Cat. Philadelphia: WB Saunders, 1986:873.
48. Peterson ME, Johnessee J, Gilbertson SR. Spontaneous Feline Hypoadrenocorticism (Addison's Disease). In: Scientific Proceedings of the American College of Veterinary Internal Medicine 1982:92.
49. Feldman EC, Nelson RW. Hypothyroidism. In: Feldman EC, Nelson RW, eds. Canine and Feline Endocrinology and Reproduction. Philadelphia: WB Saunders, 1987:55.
50. Feldman EC, Nelson RW. Hyperadrenocorticism. In: Feldman EC, Nelson RW, eds. Canine and Feline Endocrinology and Reproduction. Philadelphia: WB Saunders, 1987:137.
51. Tilley LP, Lord PF, Wood A. Acquired Heart Disease and Aortic Thromboembolism in the Cat. In: Kirk RW, ed. Current Veterinary Therapy V. Philadelphia: WB Saunders, 1974:305.
52. Cook JR, DeNicola DB. Cerebrospinal fluid. In: Luttgen PL, ed. Vet Clin North Amer [Small Animal Pract] 1988;18:475.
53. Redding RW, Bowen JM, Myers LJ, Coulter DD, Oliver JE. Electrophysiologic Diagnosis. In: Oliver JE, Hoerlein BF, Mayhew IG, eds. Veterinary Neurology. Philadelphia: WB Saunders, 1987:111.
54. Lappin MR, Greene CE, Winston S, Toll SL, Epstein ME. Clinical feline toxoplasmosis: Serologic diagnosis and therapeutic management of 15 cases. J Vet Int Med 1989;3:139.
55. Greene CE, O'Neal KG, Barsanti JA. Antimicrobial Therapy. In: Greene CE, ed. Clinical Microbiology and Infectious Diseases of the Dog and Cat. Philadelphia: WB Saunders, 1984;144.
56. Weiss RC. Feline Infectious Peritonitis and Other Coronaviruses. In: Sherding RG, ed. The Cat: Diseases and Clinical Management. New York: Churchill Livingstone, 1989:333.
57. Matus RE. Chemotherapy of Lymphoma and Leukemia. In: Kirk RW, ed. Current Veterinary Therapy X. Philadelphia: WB Saunders, 1989:482.
58. Hardy WD, MacEwen EG. Hematopoietic Tumors. In: Withrow

SJ, MacEwen EG, eds. Clinical Veterinary Oncology. Philadelphia: JB Lippincott, 1989:362.

59. Swaim SF. Small Animal Thoracolumbar, Lumbosacral, and Sacrocaudal Surgery. In: Oliver JE, Hoerlein BF, Mayhew IG, eds. Veterinary Neurology. Philadelphia: WB Saunders, 1987:416.
60. Sorjonen DC. Small Animal Cervical Surgery. In: Oliver JE, Hoerlein BF, Mayhew IG, eds. Veterinary Neurology. Philadelphia: WB Saunders, 1987:442.
61. Oliver JE. Cranial Surgery. In: Oliver JE, Hoerlein BF, Mayhew IG, eds. Veterinary Neurology. Philadelphia: WB Saunders, 1987:470.
62. Hoerlein BF, Redding RW, Hoff EJ et al. Evaluation of naloxone, crocetin, thyrotropin releasing hormone, methylprednisolone, partial myelotomy, and hemilaminectomy in the treatment of acute spinal cord trauma. J Am Anim Hosp Assoc 1985;21:67.
63. Meerdink GL. Organophosphorus and Carbamate Insecticide Poisoning. In: Kirk RW, ed. Current Veterinary Therapy X. Philadelphia: WB Saunders, 1989:131.
64. Bratton GR, Kowalczyk DF. Lead Poisoning. In: Kirk RW, ed. Current Veterinary Therapy X. Philadelphia: WB Saunders, 1989:152.

CHAPTER 18

◇ ◇ ◇

Dyspnea

Gary D. Norsworthy

Terminology and Clinical Findings

Dyspnea, defined as labored, difficult, or painful breathing, is the result of a variety of complex physiological processes. Dyspnea is present in a variety of diseases affecting the respiratory or cardiovascular systems. A comprehensive list of the causes of dyspnea in the cat is found in Appendix F.

An understanding of the mechanisms of dyspnea requires knowledge of a number of terms that describe various sounds and functions of the respiratory system. Some of these are listed in Table 18–1. By strict definition, true *dyspnea* is labored, difficult, or painful breathing, as mentioned previously. *Polypnea* and *tachypnea* are virtually synonymous with dyspnea and are used to describe a respiratory rate that is greater than normal. Many cats seen in veterinary practices are diagnosed as being "dyspneic" when, in reality, only the respiratory rate is notably abnormal. In this chapter, the term *dyspnea* will be applied to cats that may only have an increased respiratory rate, with the understanding that this increased rate will progress to true dyspnea if the underlying disease goes unchecked.

Coughing is a common finding in respiratory diseases of dogs and most other species; however, it does not occur frequently in cats, even in the presence of pulmonary edema. When coughing is present, the clinician should consider the differential diagnoses of feline asthma, lungworm infection, heartworm disease, chylothorax, and larval migration.

Dyspnea may be manifested by several clinical signs, of which open-mouth breathing is the most obvious. However, by the time dyspnea progresses to that point, the cat is often in critical condition. Ideally, dyspnea should be noted at the stage of rapid, shallow breathing. Although the cat's respiratory rate may range from 20 to 60 breaths per minute, a resting respiratory rate of greater than 50 breaths per minute is highly indicative of early dyspnea. At the beginning of a physical examination, the cat's respirations should be observed carefully, with particular attention to both the rate and depth of respiration. Dyspneic cats may also be observed to lie only in sternal recumbency (orthopnea) (Fig. 18–1). The owner should be questioned as to whether the cat rests, or even sleeps, exclusively in this position.

Many cats are reported to have had an acute onset of dyspnea. When a definitive diagnosis is established, however, it will be obvious to the clinician that the condition did not occur acutely. This discrepancy rarely indicates inattention on the part of the client. Rather, it reflects the nature of cats. At the onset of respiratory compromise, affected cats will compensate by reducing their level of activity. Because most cats spend a great deal of time sleeping or resting, this reduction of activity may go unnoticed. When the degree of compromise becomes severe, or when the cat is stressed, the dyspnea will be noticed by the owner and reported as being of acute onset.

A number of diseases that cause dyspnea in the cat are discussed in this chapter; however, special attention should be paid to the most common ones:

- Diaphragmatic hernia
- Pneumothorax
- Lymphosarcoma
- Feline infectious peritonitis (FIP)
- Pyothorax
- Chylothorax
- Feline asthma
- Cardiomyopathy

Physical Examination

Dyspneic cats should be examined and handled with a great deal of caution, as even minor amounts of stress may result in respiratory insufficiency and death. The following guidelines may be helpful in dealing with cats in critical condition:

- The cat should be placed in an oxygen cage for a few minutes before any examination procedures are performed.
- The cat should not be placed in dorsal recumbency, even for radiographs. A dorsoventral (DV) view of the chest is much less stressful than a ventrodorsal view (VD). The lateral view can also be stressful, so initially, it may be best to obtain only a DV view.
- Because pleural effusion accompanies dyspnea in so many cases, thoracocentesis of both sides of the chest may be attempted if an initial DV radiograph is not feasible. If 50 to 100 mL of fluid can be removed from the chest, respirations will improve. If the cat has pneu-

Table 18–1. Definition of Terms Relating to Respiratory Sounds and Patterns

Term	Definition
Crackles	Short, explosive, nonmusical respiratory sounds
Dyspnea	Labored, difficult, or painful breathing
Orthopnea	Difficulty breathing while in a recumbent position
Polypnea	Increased rate of breathing (not necessarily associated with distress)
Rales	Abnormal respiratory sounds classified as dry or moist
Rhonchus	A dry, course rale in the bronchial tubes that is caused by partial obstruction
Stridor	A shrill, harsh sound made during inspiration that originates from the upper airways; a loud wheeze
Tachypnea	Excessively rapid and usually shallow respirations
Wheezes	Continuous, musical respiratory sounds of varying pitch

mothorax, thoracocentesis will result in the beneficial removal of air from the pleural space.

- Intravenous (IV) administration of one 25-mg dose of furosemide (Lasix) may be very helpful in many cats, and is only strictly contraindicated if dehydration is present.
- IV administration of one 5-mg dose of dexamethasone (Dexamethasone Sodium Phosphate Injection) or one 100-mg dose of prednisolone sodium succinate (Solu-Delta Cortef) may have beneficial effects in many cats.[2] There are no diseases that cause feline dyspnea for which this procedure is strictly contraindicated. A dramatic response to such treatment is a good indicator that the cat has feline asthma or heartworm disease with pulmonary eosinophilic infiltrate.

The cat should be examined for the clinical signs or findings listed in Table 18–2. A different diagnosis may then be established.[1]

Diagnosis

Thoracic Radiography

The single most important diagnostic test for dyspnea is a good-quality thoracic radiograph. As mentioned previously, the DV view is the least stressful for the cat, and may be the only view feasible in some cats. The radiographs should be examined for the following:[1]

Radiographic technique and positioning—If either is poor, interpretation will be compromised.

Phase of respiration—Inspiration causes the diaphragm to be flattened, whereas expiration causes it to be dome-shaped.

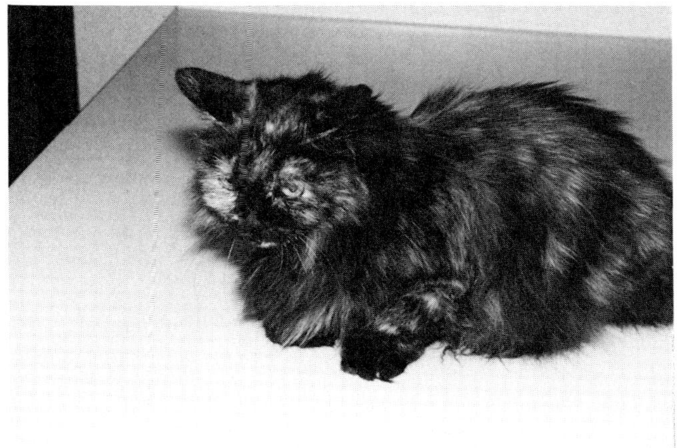

Figure 18–1. The dyspneic cat is most comfortable in sternal recumbency and will consistently assume this position when lying down and even when sleeping.

Lung pattern—It should be classified as interstitial, alveolar, or mixed.

Free air in the pleural space, mediastinum, esophagus, or stomach

Pulmonary vascular changes—Any overcirculation or blunting of the pulmonary arteries should be noted.

Pleural effusion

Cardiac size and shape

Cranial mediastinal mass

Intact diaphragm

Tracheal position and compression or flattening

Intratracheal/intrabronchial densities

Aerophagia—Its presence may be the only radiographic indicator of dyspnea in some cats (Fig. 18–2).

It is essential that pleural effusion, which accompanies many of the common diseases that cause dyspnea, be recognized. The fluid should be removed from the chest to improve pulmonary function and should be analyzed as part of the diagnostic work-up. The radiographic signs of pleural effusion (Fig. 18–3) include the following:

Fissure lines between the lung lobes

Rounding of the lung borders at the costophrenic angles

Mediastinal widening

Ventral scalloping of the lung borders (lateral view)

Obscured cardiac and diaphragmatic silhouettes

Separation of the lung margins from the thoracic wall

Pneumothorax is air in the pleural space. The radiographic signs of pneumothorax (Fig. 18–4) include the following:[3,4]

Underinflated lungs that appear to be more dense than normal and that are displaced from the thoracic wall

Hyperlucent pleural space adjacent to the lungs

Table 18–2. Differential Diagnosis of Dyspnea

Clinical Examination Findings	Likely Differential Diagnoses
Signs of trauma (scrapes, lacerations, bite wounds, multiple frayed toenails)	Diaphragmatic hernia Pneumothorax Lung lobe torsion
Mucous membrane color	
Pallor	Anemia Shock
Cyanotic or bluish	Shock Right-to-left cardiac shunts Pleural effusion Methemoglobinemia
Bright red	Carbon monoxide toxicity Smoke inhalation
Deep red (injected)	Sepsis Polycythemia Excitement
Ulcerative oral lesions	Lesions secondary to biting of an electrical cord
Pink, frothy discharge from nose or mouth	Pulmonary edema
Jugular pulse/distention	Right-sided cardiac failure (cardiomyopathy, heartworm disease, etc.)
Reduced compressibility of anterior thoracic wall*	Anterior thoracic mass (e.g., lymphosarcoma)
Absence of femoral pulse	Aortic thromboembolism
Abdominal palpation	
"Empty" feeling	Diaphragmatic hernia
Mass	Tumor, with metastatis to lungs, or anemia
Ascites	Feline infectious peritonitis (FIP), which may also affect the chest findings†
Mammary palpation	
Mass	Tumor, with metastasis to lungs, or anemia
Pulmonary auscultation	
Muffled lung sounds	Obesity Pleural effusion Pneumothorax Emphysema
Crackles	Pulmonary edema Pulmonary infiltrative diseases Bronchitis with secretions
Wheezes	Feline asthma Intraluminal masses, exudates, or foreign bodies
Cardiac auscultation	
Systolic murmur	Cardiomyopathy Bacterial endocarditis Mitral insufficiency Physiologic causes (anemia, fever)
Gallop rhythm	Cardiomyopathy Stress (transient)
Chest wall percussion	
Hyperresonance	Pneumothorax
Hyporesonance	Pleural effusion Diaphragmatic hernia Lung consolidation

*More meaningful in young cats.
†Any fluid may cause dyspnea as a result of diaphragmatic pressure.

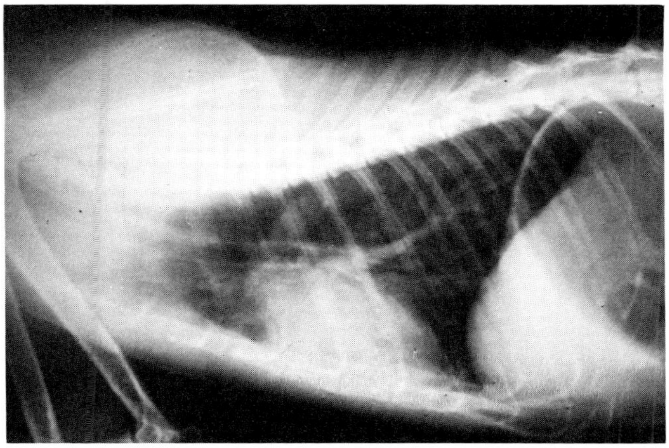

A

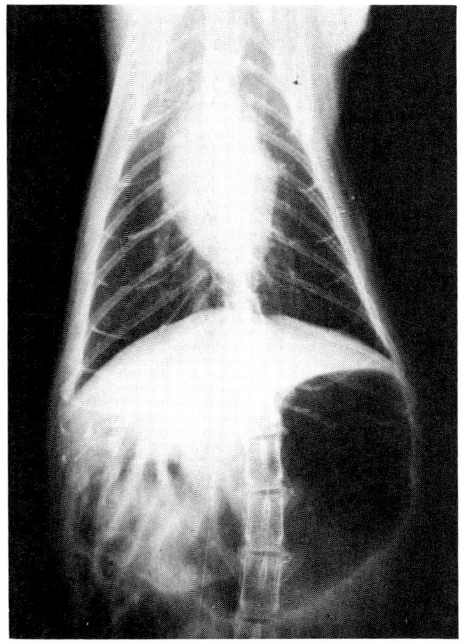

B

Figure 18–2. (*A*) This cat had a history of open-mouth breathing. Although the chest was normal on radiographic examination, the large amount of gas in the stomach indicated aerophagia and substantiated the owner's observations of dyspnea. (*B*) A ventrodorsal view of the same cat as in Figure 18–2*A* reveals gas in the stomach and intestines.

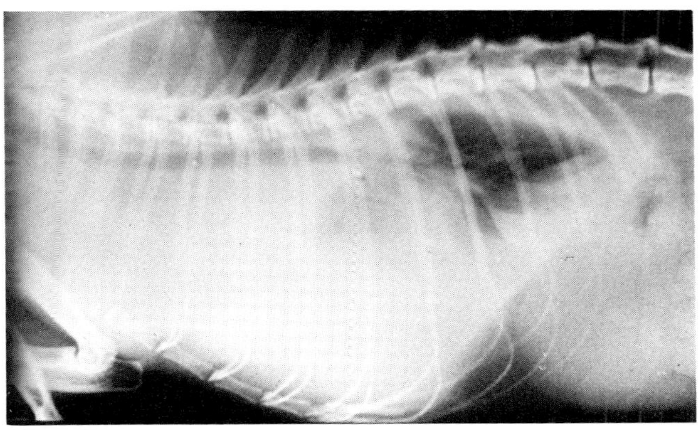

A

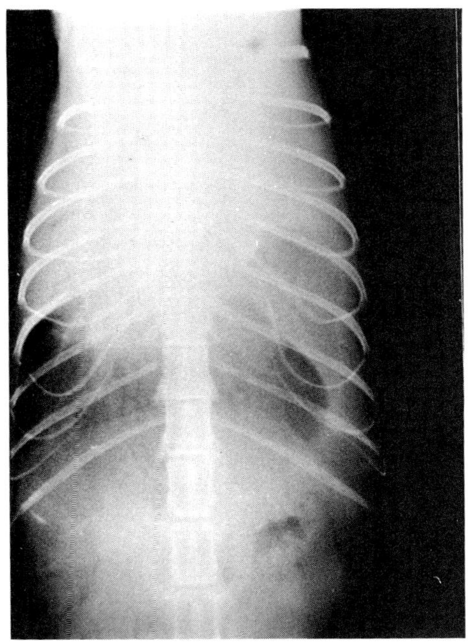

B

Figure 18–3. (*A*) Pleural effusion compresses the pulmonary parenchyma, resulting in dyspnea. The radiographic signs of pleural effusion, regardless of its disease of origin, include fissure lines between the lung lobes, rounding of the lung borders at the costophrenic angles, mediastinal widening, ventral scalloping of the lung borders, and obscured cardiac and diaphragmatic silhouettes. The tracheal elevation is a typical finding in cats with an anterior mediastinal mass. (*B*) A ventrodorsal view of the same cat as in Figure 18–3*A* shows rounding of the lung borders, mediastinal widening, obscured cardiac and diaphragmatic silhouettes, and separation of the lung margins from the thoracic wall.

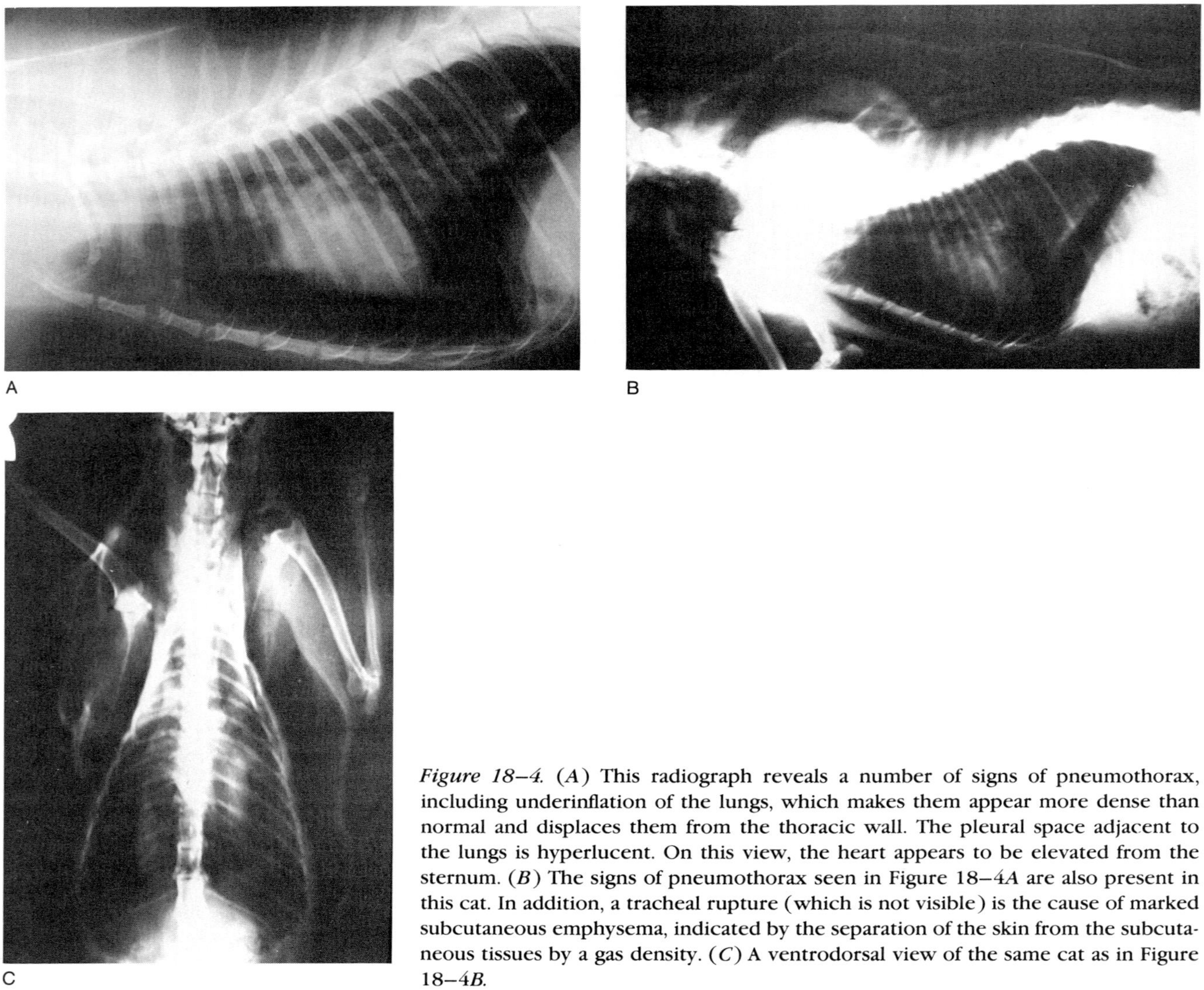

Figure 18–4. (*A*) This radiograph reveals a number of signs of pneumothorax, including underinflation of the lungs, which makes them appear more dense than normal and displaces them from the thoracic wall. The pleural space adjacent to the lungs is hyperlucent. On this view, the heart appears to be elevated from the sternum. (*B*) The signs of pneumothorax seen in Figure 18–4*A* are also present in this cat. In addition, a tracheal rupture (which is not visible) is the cause of marked subcutaneous emphysema, indicated by the separation of the skin from the subcutaneous tissues by a gas density. (*C*) A ventrodorsal view of the same cat as in Figure 18–4*B*.

No evidence of bronchial or vascular markings

Apparent elevation of the heart from the sternum on the lateral view

Increased visibility of the cranial vena cava and esophagus in cases of pneumomediastinum; visualization of the serosal surface of the trachea

Pleural Fluid Analysis

If pleural effusion is present, the fluid should be removed by thoracocentesis to improve respiration and to facilitate diagnosis. The minimum tests that should be performed are a specific gravity level and a cytologic examination of the sediment. Other tests that may be indicated include a bacteriologic culture, both aerobic and anaerobic; a white blood cell (WBC) count, and determination of the triglyceride:cholesterol ratio. See Table 18–3 for a summary of the findings in the five most common causes of pleural effusion based on radiographs and pleural fluid analysis.

Other Diagnostic Tests

Because dyspnea can be caused by such a wide array of diseases, a number of other diagnostic tests may be appropriate in selected situations, including the following:

Fine needle aspiration of the lungs or mediastinal masses can be performed without sedation in most cats. (See Chapter 13 for details concerning the technique.)

Tracheal wash can provide tracheal and bronchial samples suitable for cytologic study and culture. (See Chapter 12 for details concerning the technique.)

Bronchoalveolar lavage can provide alveolar-level samples suitable for cytologic examination and culture.[5,6]

Endoscopy of the trachea and its bifurcation may be useful in diagnosing tracheal masses or a collapsed trachea.

Exploratory thoracotomy with lung biopsy can provide a definitive diagnosis in cats with certain types of tumors.

Table 18–3. Differentiation of Diseases Associated with Pleural Effusion*

Condition	Radiographic Findings	Cytologic Findings	Specific Gravity†	Cell No.
Lymphosarcoma	Fluid and mass	Lymphoblasts, mitotic figures; no bacteria	<1.018	Many
Feline infectious peritonitis	Fluid	Neutrophils, lymphocytes, macrocytes; no bacteria	>1.018	Few
Pyothorax	Fluid	Neutrophils, lymphocytes, macrocytes; copious bacteria	>1.018	Many
Cardiomyopathy	Abnormal heart shape; pulmonary edema/effusion	Few cells; no bacteria	<1.018	Few
Chylothorax	Fluid	Very small lymphocytes; no bacteria	Variable‡	Many

*See chapters specific to each disease cited for more complete information on diagnosis.
†This is actually a measurement of the total serum protein (solids) level. A specific gravity of 1.018 equals a total protein level of 2.5 mg/dL.
‡This disease is usually caused by another disease, althoughh it may occur as a primary idiopathic condition. The primary disease generally determines the specific gravity. The most common primary diseases causing chylothorax include anterior mediastinal masses (usually lymphosarcoma), cardiomyopathy, heartworm disease, and trauma.

Echocardiography and *nonselective cardiac angiography* are useful in diagnosing cardiac diseases, including cardiomyopathy and heartworm disease.

Retinal examination can be helpful in cases of FIP, lymphosarcoma, histoplasmosis, and toxoplasmosis.

Gastrointestinal barium series or *celiogram* can confirm the presence of a diaphragmatic hernia. (See Chapter 14 for details concerning these techniques.)

Fecal Baermann technique is indicated if lungworms are suspected. (See Chapter 12 for details concerning the technique.)

Serologic and hematologic tests that may be helpful include a complete blood count (CBC), total serum protein, albumin:globulin (A:G) ratio, serum electrophoresis, modified Knott's and antigen heartworm tests, titers for systemic fungi and toxoplasmosis, antibody test for feline coronavirus, antibody test for the feline immunodeficiency virus (FIV), and antigen test for the feline leukemia virus (FeLV).

Classification of Diseases Causing Dyspnea

Many different classifications have been proposed to characterize dyspnea. One logical means of grouping these diseases and disorders is to differentiate them according to anatomic location.

Airway Diseases and Disorders

When *tracheal rupture* occurs (usually secondary to trauma), inspiration will not be effective in carrying oxygen-containing air to the lungs. Rather, inspiration and expiration will force air through the rupture into the adjacent tissues, resulting in subcutaneous emphysema (see Fig. 18–4. Pneumothorax may or may not be present, depending on the location of the tracheal rupture.

Tracheal collapse is most commonly caused by pressure from an extraluminal mass (Fig. 18–5). Although lymphosarcoma is the most common cause, other benign and malignant tumors of the anterior thorax may also compress the trachea (Fig. 18–6). A few cases of idiopathic collapsed trachea have been reported in cats, similar to the same phenomenon that occurs in small breeds of dogs (Fig. 18–7).

Tracheal obstruction may occur as the result of a foreign body or an intraluminal mass (Fig. 18–8).

Tracheal strictures may result from endotracheal tube accidents, as may occur with overinflation of the cuff or tracheal damage inflicted by the metal stylet used to place the tube. In addition, other traumatic injuries may cause scar tissue formation which, in turn, may result in stricture.

Bronchial obstruction may be attributable to foreign bodies, benign or malignant masses, thick secretions, or bronchiectasis

Extrapulmonary Diseases and Disorders

Pulmonary compression by extrapulmonary, intrathoracic masses is often a cause of dyspnea in the cat. Anterior mediastinal lymphosarcoma is the most common mass causing lung compression in the cat (see Fig. 18–5). Aspiration cytology of large cell lymphosarcoma will reveal both lymphoblasts and mitotic figures. Thymomas may also be a cause of dyspnea in the cat (see Fig. 18–6). Aspiration cytology in these cases will reveal normal, mature lymphocytes, which are also found in small cell lymphosarcoma. Other malignant or benign tumors, although uncommon, may also cause pulmonary compression.

Pleural effusion is one of the most common causes of dyspnea. It is present in most of the common diseases that cause dyspnea (lymphosarcoma, FIP, pyothorax, chylothorax, and cardiomyopathy). It may also be present in cats with long-standing diaphragmatic hernias. Fluid in the pleural space physically compresses the lungs. If an anterior mediastinal mass is also present, the trachea is often elevated (see Fig. 18–3*A*).

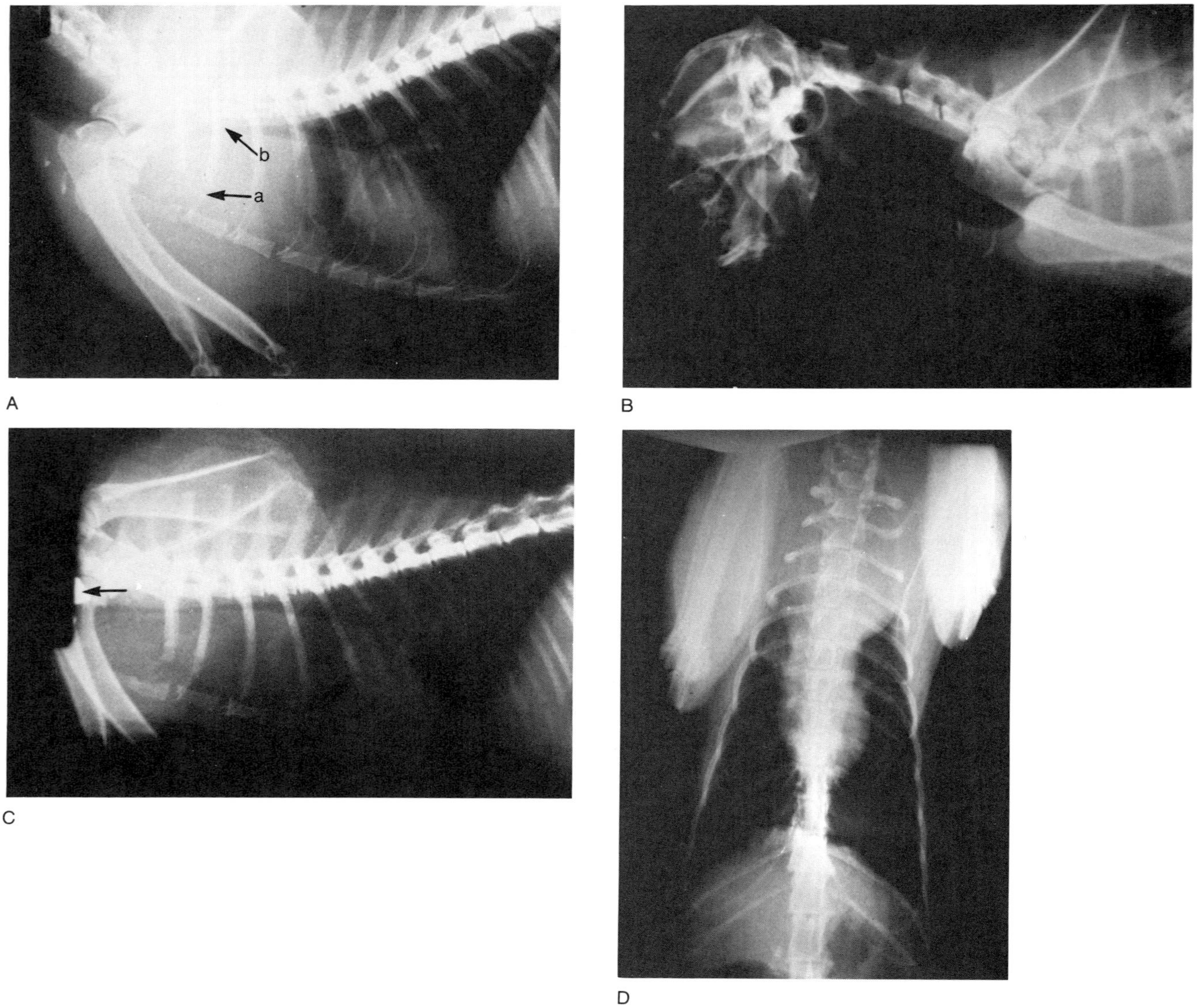

Figure 18–5. (*A*) A large anterior mediastinal lymphosarcoma (*a*) is causing dyspnea secondary to collapse of the trachea (*b*) and the adjacent lung parenchyma. This cat had no pleural effusion. (*B*) Another cat with an anterior mediastinal lymphosarcoma that is compressing the trachea and esophagus. A gas-filled, dilated esophagus is seen in the cervical area. (*C*) When a barium swallow was performed in the same cat as in Figure 18–5*B*, the barium stopped abruptly at the thoracic inlet (*arrow*). (*D*) A ventrodorsal view of the same cat as in Figure 18–5*A* demonstrates a large anterior mediastinal mass (lymphosarcoma) without the presence of pleural effusion.

Compression secondary to ectopic or enlarged organs will result in reduced pulmonary capacity. There are several examples of such compression-producing conditions. Diaphragmatic hernias (Fig. 18–9, *A* and *B*), which are generally traumatically induced, may be unilateral or bilateral. Affected cats may require immediate surgery; others may survive for long periods merely by limiting their activity and minimizing stress. Barium-enhanced radiographs and sonography may help to confirm a suspected diaphragmatic hernia (Fig. 18–9, *C* and *D*). Pericardial diaphragmatic hernias, which are generally congenital, are openings in the diaphragm that allow communication between the pericardial sac and the abdominal cavity. Small abdominal organs —notably the small intestine—may enter the pericardium through these openings (Fig. 18–10, *A* and *B*). These hernias, too, may be confirmed by barium studies of the gastrointestinal tract (Fig. 18–10, *C* and *D*). Megaesophagus, which is a dilation of the esophagus, may also cause compression of the pulmonary parenchyma (Fig. 18–11). Although regurgitation is the most common presenting sign of this condition, dyspnea may also occur when the esophagus is full of food. This condition can be confirmed using a barium esophagogram, but care must be taken not to induce aspiration pneumonia. (*Text continues on page 182*)

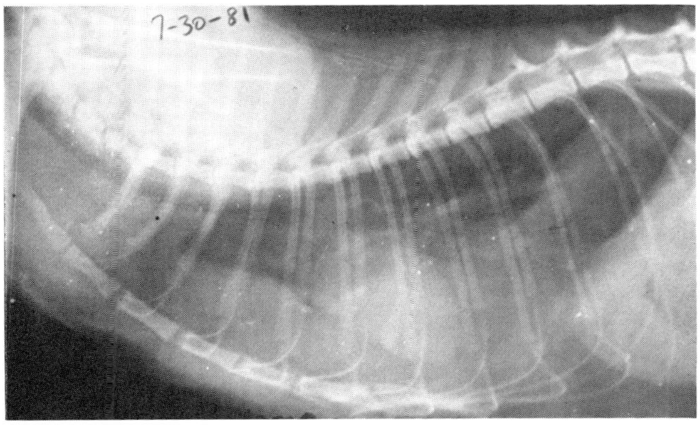

A

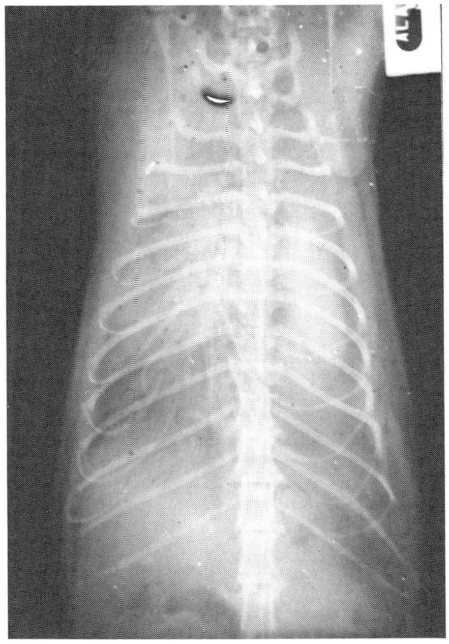

B

Figure 18–6. (*A*) The pulmonary compression seen in this radiograph is the result of a large anterior thoracic mass, a thymoma. This benign tumor is often very chemosensitive and carries a much better prognosis than does lymphosarcoma. (*B*) A ventrodorsal view of the same cat as in Figure 18–6A.

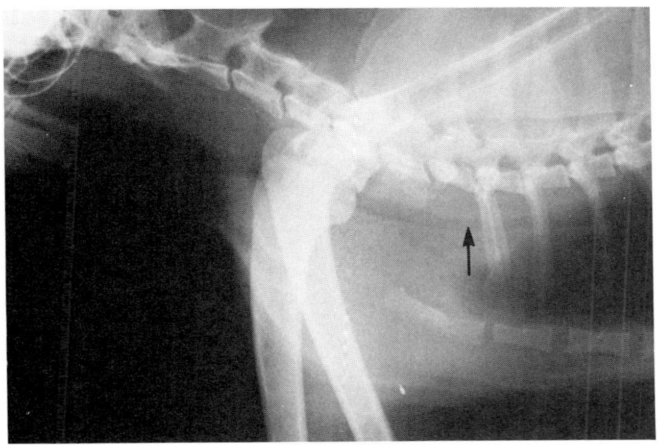

Figure 18–7. The trachea may be collapsed (*arrow*) as a result of congenital anomaly, as is the case in this 1.5-year-old cat. However, this does not occur as frequently in the cat as in the dog.

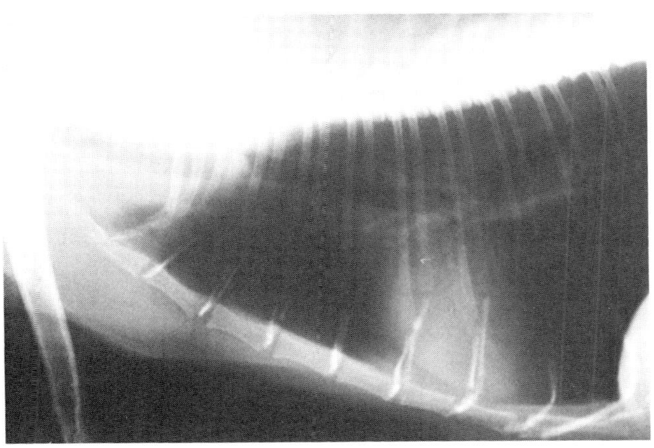

A

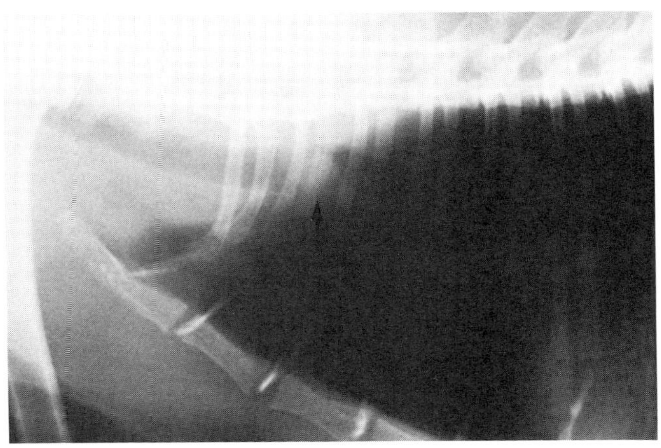

B

Figure 18–8. (*A*) This cat presented with dyspnea, but its lungs were found to be normal. (*B*) An intraluminal mass (*arrow*) was present in the trachea just caudal to the thoracic inlet. Histopathologic study revealed a chrondroma.

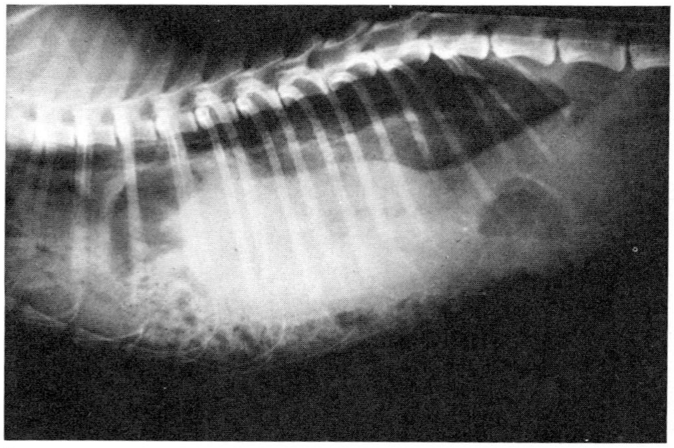

A

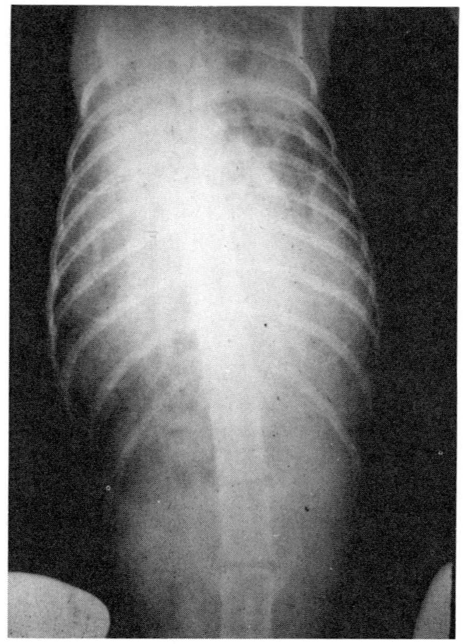

B

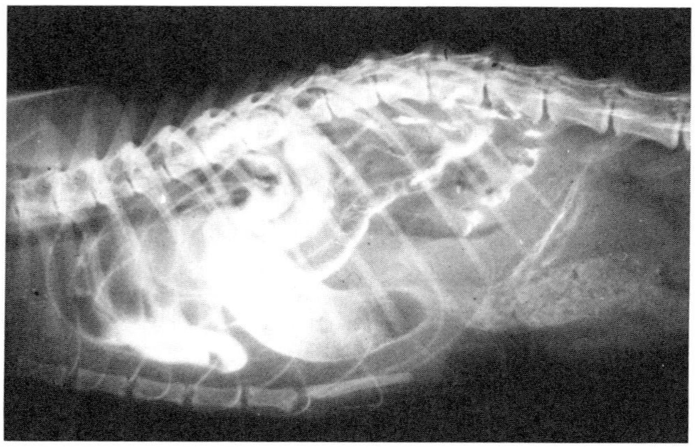

C

Figure 18–9. (*A*) Diaphragmatic hernias are characterized by a loss of the diaphragmatic line, reduced pulmonary expansion, and the presence of soft tissue masses (e.g., the liver) and/or intraluminal gastrointestinal gas in the thorax. The abdomen is often smaller than normal owing to the displacement of abdominal organs into the thorax. (*B*) A ventrodorsal view of the same cat as in Figure 18–9*A*. (*C*) The diagnosis of a diaphragmatic hernia can often be confirmed by a barium study of the gastrointestinal tract. This cat's small intestine and proximal colon are in the thoracic cavity. (*D*) A ventrodorsal view of the same cat as in Figure 18–9*C*. This view demonstrates that this diaphragmatic hernia involves only the right side.

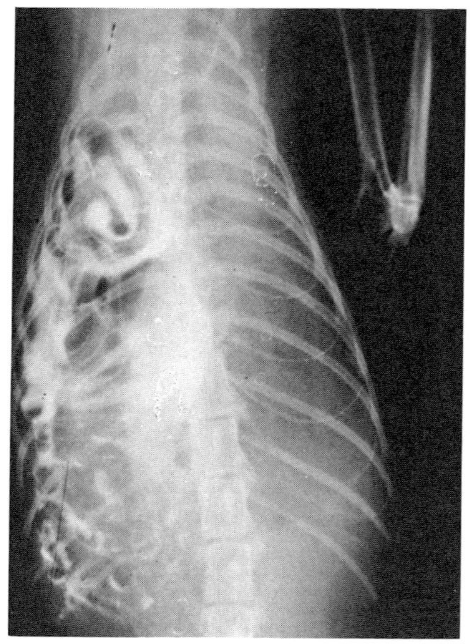

D

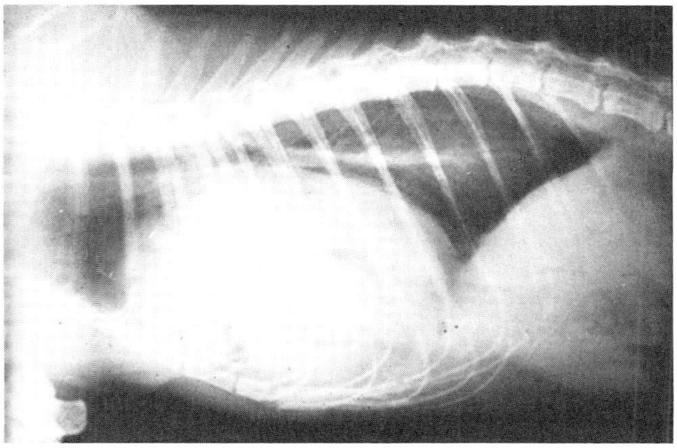

A

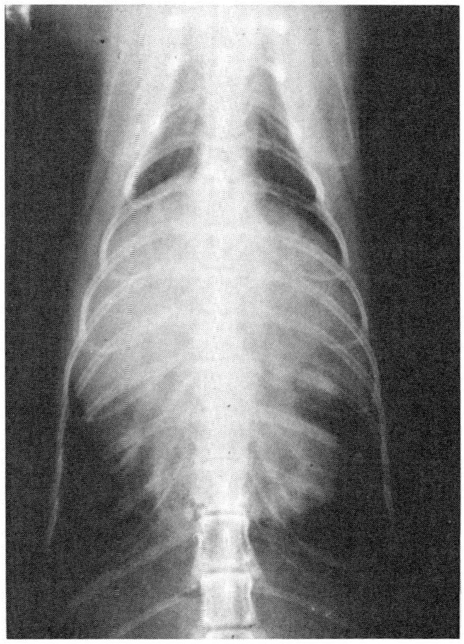

B

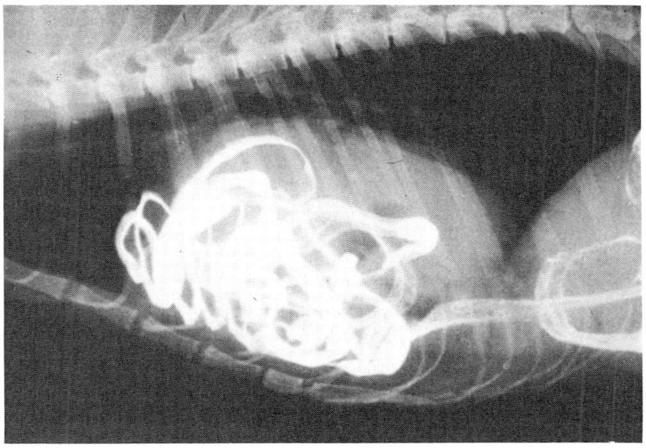

C

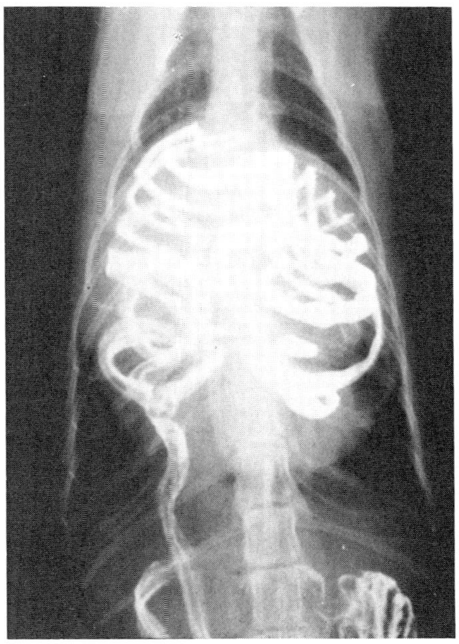

D

Figure 18–10. (*A*) A pericardial diaphragmatic hernia allows abdominal viscera to enter the pericardial sac, causing it to enlarge greatly. Generally, the small intestine is involved, as evidenced by the presence of intraluminal gas. (*B*) A ventrodorsal view of the same cat as in Figure 18–10*A*. (*C*) A suspected pericardial diaphragmatic hernia can be confirmed by a barium study of the intestinal tract. In this case, the small intestines are visible within the pericardium. (*D*) A ventrodorsal view of the same cat as in Figure 18–10*C*.

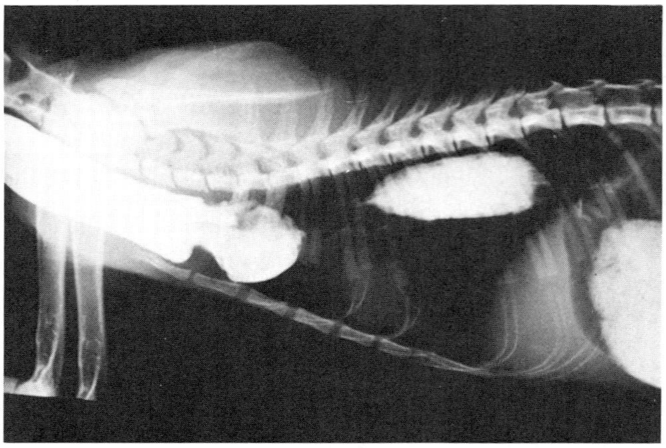

A

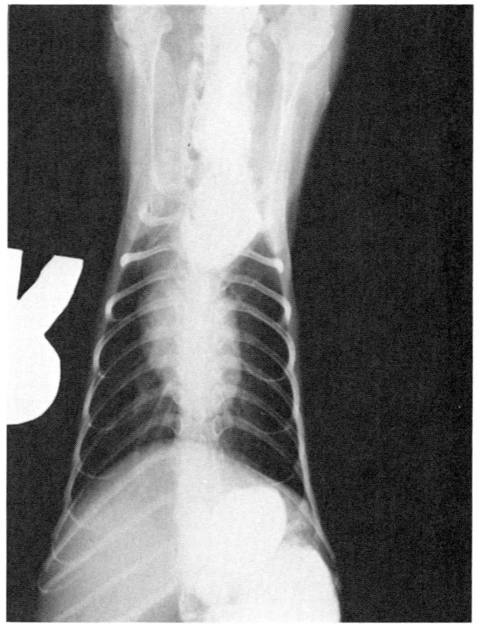

B

Figure 18–11. (*A*) Megaesophagus can be diagnosed with a barium swallow. When filled with food, the esophagus may become large enough to compress the lungs, causing dyspnea. (*B*) A ventrodorsal view of the same cat as in Figure 18–11*A*.

Pulmonary Diseases and Disorders

Pathologic conditions involving the lung parenchyma will cause dyspnea if sufficient lung tissue is affected to reduce pulmonary capacity significantly. *Tearing* of the lung parenchyma may occur as a result of a ruptured intrapulmonary cyst. Such cysts may be traumatically induced (Fig. 18–12), or they may be associated with parasites, such as *Paragonimus kellicotti* (Fig. 18–13). *Lung lacerations* may be caused by trauma or penetrating foreign bodies, or they may be iatrogenically induced during lung aspiration, thoracocentesis, or intrathoracic surgery.

Loss of pleural expansion in cats most often occurs as a result of *pneumothorax* (see Fig. 18–4, *A* and *B*). *Tension pneumothorax* is a variant of this condition, occurring in conjunction with trauma involving the lung parenchyma. In such cases, air flows into the pleural space during inspiration, but is not expelled during expiration. (Fig. 18–12, *A* and *B*), resulting in a rapid increase in intrapleural pressure. Air will often enter the pericardium and dissect its way through the mediastinum into the retroperitoneal space of the abdomen (Fig. 18–12, *C* and *D*). If the tear is not repaired quickly, either spontaneously or surgically, the cat will die.

Lung sclerosis/consolidation may be the result of many chronic diseases, including the dry, pulmonary form of FIP (Fig. 18–14). A similar radiographic pattern can be seen in cases of pulmonary hemorrhage (Fig. 18–15).

The *bronchial pulmonary pattern* is characterized by airstripes and round, end-on bronchi, commonly known as "donuts," caused by the thickened bronchial walls. *Feline asthma* (allergic bronchitis, allergic pneumonitis) is the only common bronchial disease affecting cats (Fig. 18–16). Lung aspiration of a cat with feline asthma may reveal an increased number of eosinophils. More commonly, a peripheral eosinophilia will be noted (see Chapter 25). Other causes of a bronchial radiographic pattern include smoke inhalation and electrical shock.

The *alveolar pulmonary pattern* is characterized by air bronchograms without obvious walls. It is the result of filling the alveoli with fluids or infiltrates. *Pulmonary edema* is the most common alveolar pattern in the cat. It may be caused by drug or transfusion reactions (Fig. 18–17), or by several cardiac diseases, including cardiomyopathy (Fig. 18–18), congenital anomalies, and heartworm disease. *Pneumonia* can also cause an alveolar pattern. Bacterial pneumonia (Fig. 18–19) is uncommon in the cat, so the most common cause of pneumonia is aspiration of fluids or food (Fig. 18–20). *Severe feline asthma* can progress from a bronchial pattern to an alveolar pattern as life-threatening fluid accumulates in the lungs (Fig. 18–21).

The *interstitial pattern* is characterized by generalized or focal areas of consolidation. It has no air bronchograms. The *reticular pattern* is marked by vessels and airways with indistinct margins. The nodular pattern is characterized by the presence of distinct nodules. Typical feline interstitial lung diseases include *primary* or *metastatic neoplasia* (Fig. 18–22), *systemic fungal diseases* (Figs. 18–23 and 18–24), *pulmonary toxoplasmosis* (Fig. 18–25), *parasitic diseases* (see Fig. 18–13), and *pulmonary lymphosarcoma* (Fig. 18–26).

(*Text continues on page 190*)

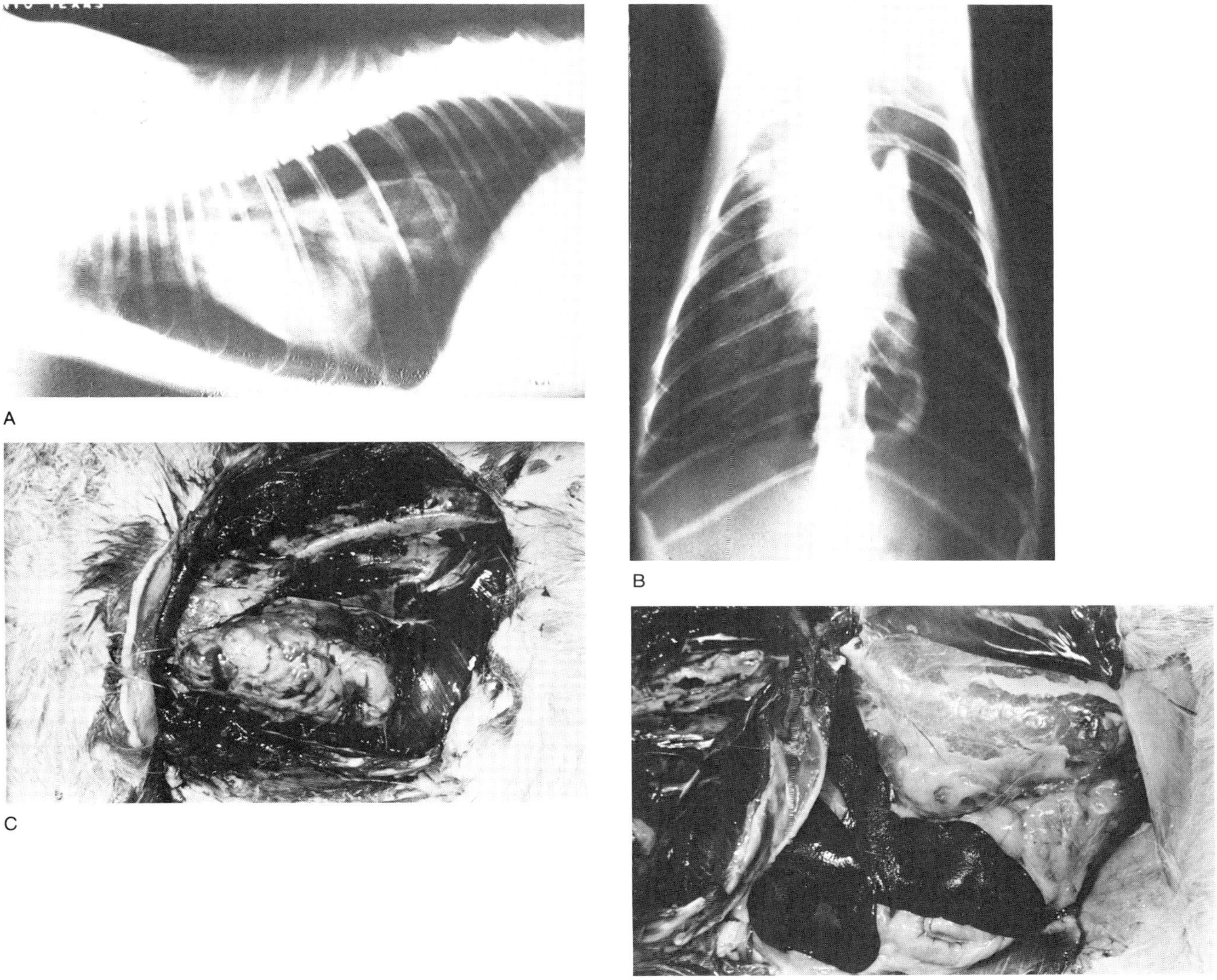

A B C D

Figure 18–12. (*A*) A pulmonary tear resulted in tension pneumothorax. A traumatically induced pulmonary cyst can be seen caudal to the heart. The other signs of pneumothorax are also present (see Figure 18–4, *A* and *B*). (*B*) A ventrodorsal view of the same cat as in Figure 18–12*A*. The traumatic cyst can be seen caudal to the heart and to the right of the midline. (*C*) When the lateral thoracic wall is removed, one can see that air has infiltrated the pericardium and the mediastinum. The cat's head is to the left. (*D*) When the abdomen is opened, one can see that air has infiltrated the retroperitoneal space dorsal to the kidney.

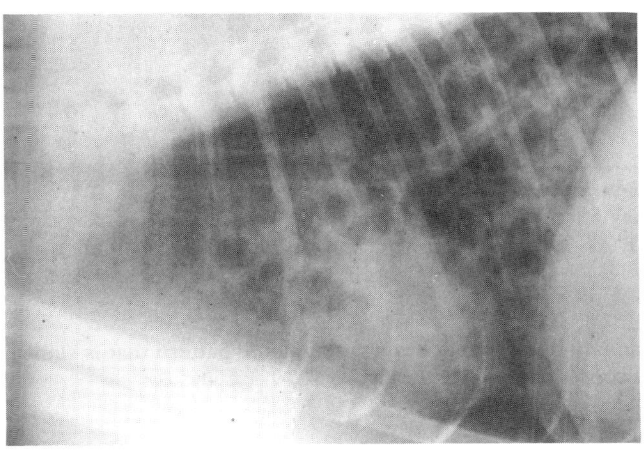

Figure 18–13. Multiple cysts and nodules are visible throughout the pulmonary parenchyma. These were caused by *Paragonimus kellicotti.*

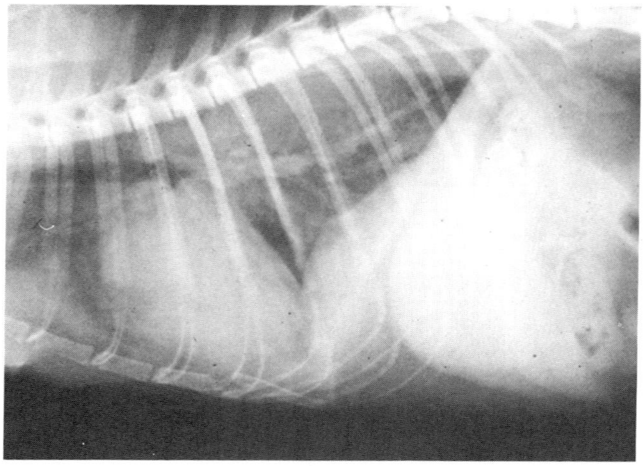

A

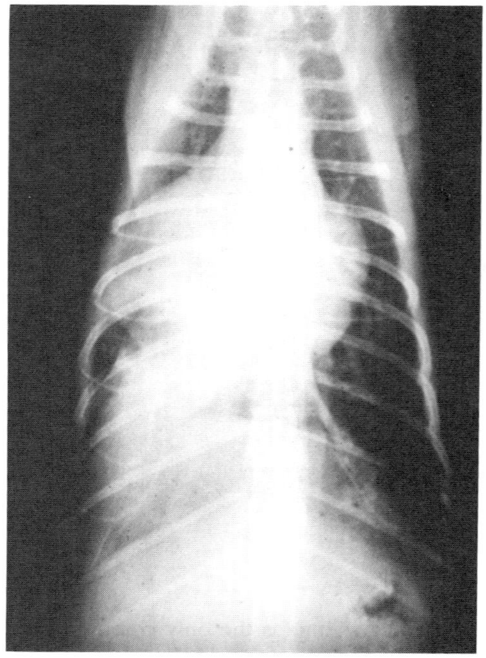

B

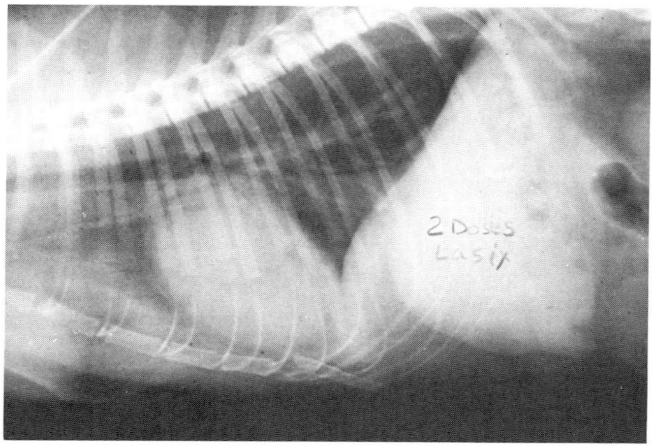

C

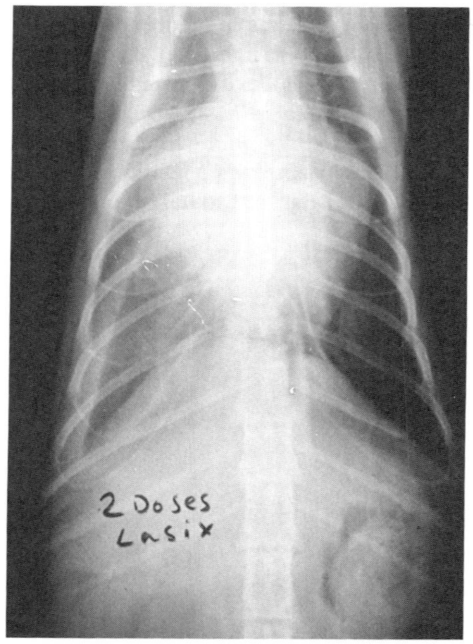

D

Figure 18–18. (*A*) The pulmonary edema in this cat is the result of hypertrophic cardiomyopathy. (*B*) A ventrodorsal view of the same cat as in Figure 18–18*A*. (*C*) Two doses of furosemide were given (2 hours apart), after which repeat radiographs of the chest were obtained in the same cat as in Figure 18–18*A*. Most of the pulmonary edema has been cleared from the lungs, allowing a more exacting evaluation of the cardiac silhouette. The degree of response to furosemide may also help to establish a diagnosis of pulmonary edema. (*D*) A ventrodorsal view of the same cat as in Figure 18–18*C*. The classic valentine-shaped heart of hypertrophic cardiomyopathy is now visible.

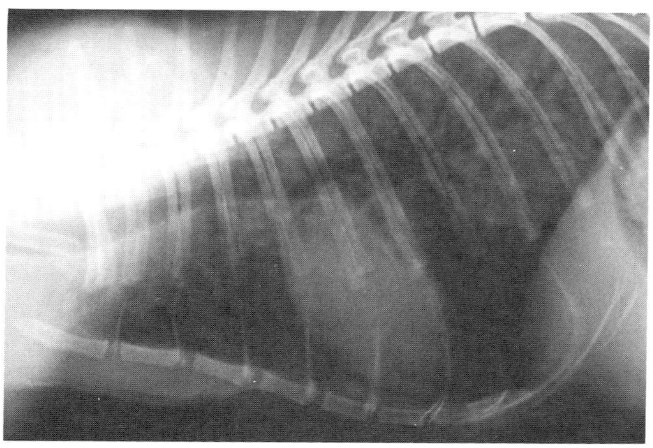

Figure 18–19. Bacterial pneumonia, an uncommon finding in the cat, causes an alveolar radiographic pattern.

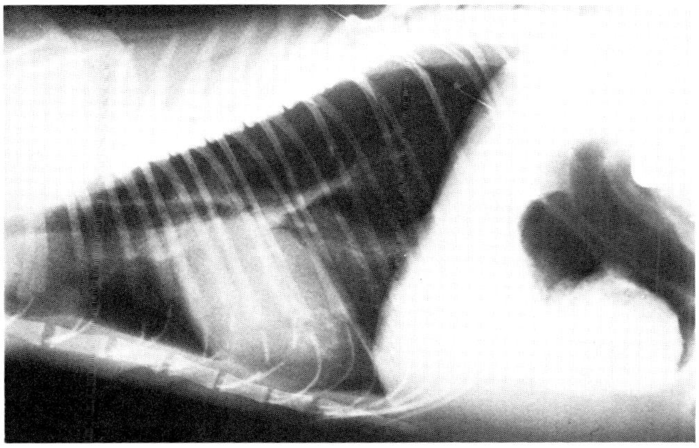

A

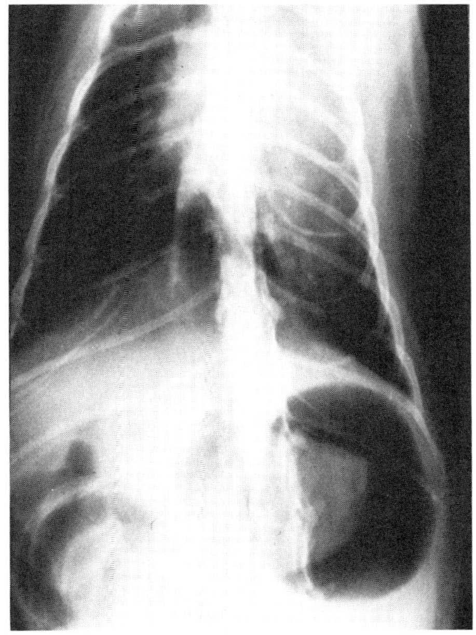

B

Figure 18–20. (*A*) Aspiration pneumonia is characterized by an alveolar pattern. It generally involves the area adjacent to the bifurcation of the trachea. Its occurrence in this case was the result of the cat's attempts to vomit the large hairball that is seen in the stomach. (*B*) A ventrodorsal view of the same cat as in Figure 18–20*A*.

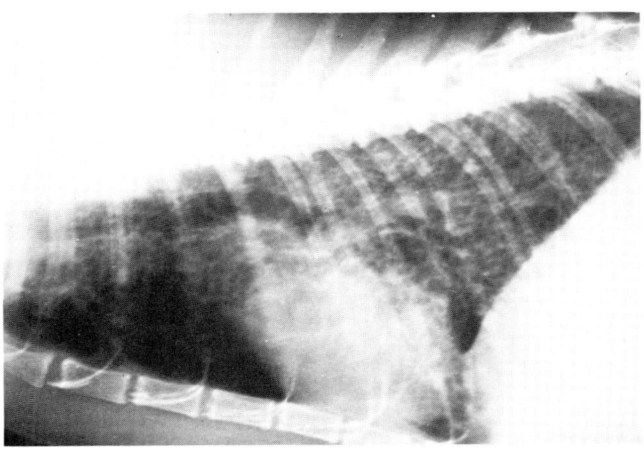

A

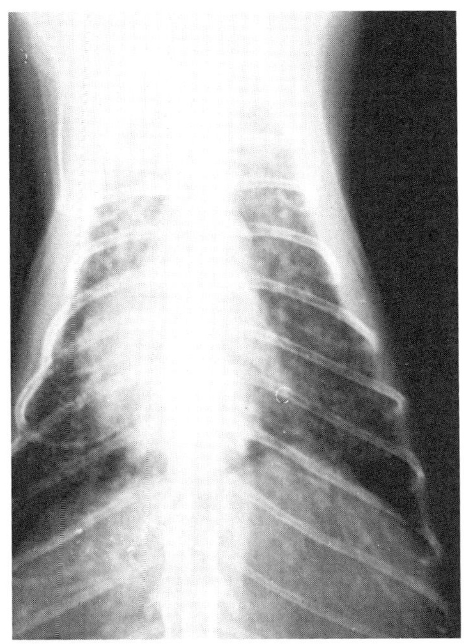

B

Figure 18–21. (*A*) In this case of feline asthma, a bronchial radiographic pattern has progressed to an alveolar pattern as a result of the fluid that has accumulated in the alveoli. (*B*) A ventrodorsal view of the same cat as in Figure 18–21*A*.

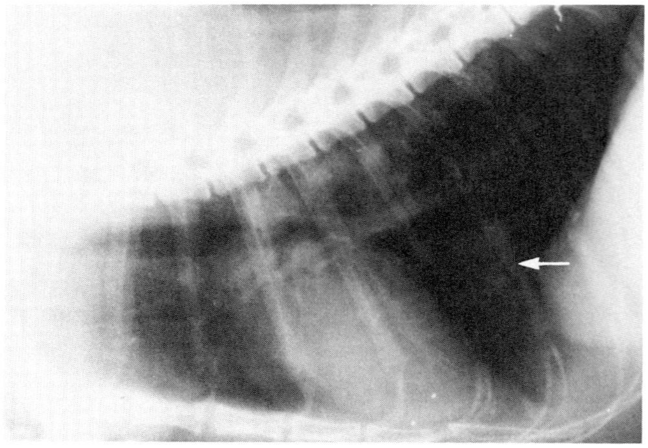

A

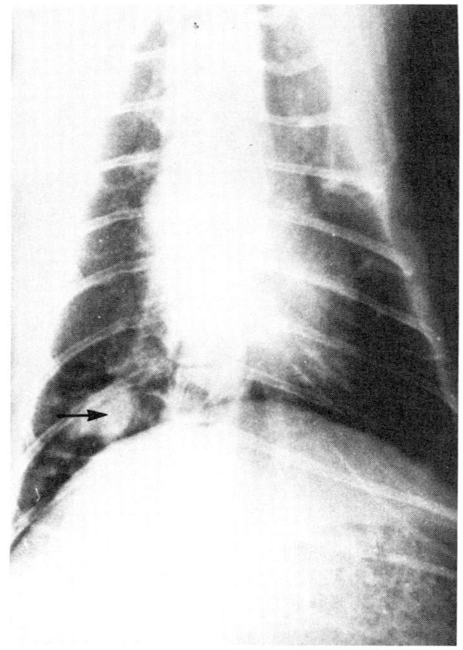

B

Figure 18–22. (*A*) Pulmonary metastasis is characterized by a nodular interstitial radiographic pattern. A single metastatic tumor is evident in the caudal lung lobe (*arrow*). (*B*) A ventrodorsal view of the same cat as in Figure 18–22*A*, showing the single metastatic tumor (*arrow*) in the right caudal lung lobe.

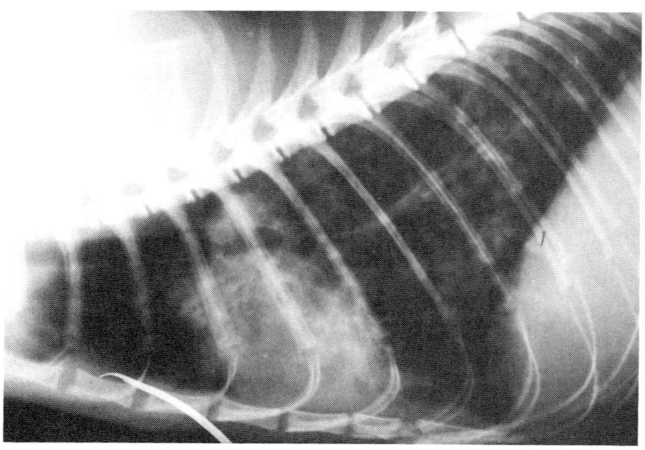

A

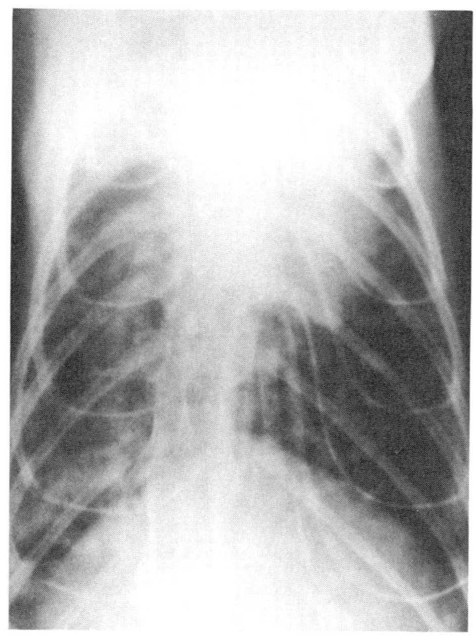

B

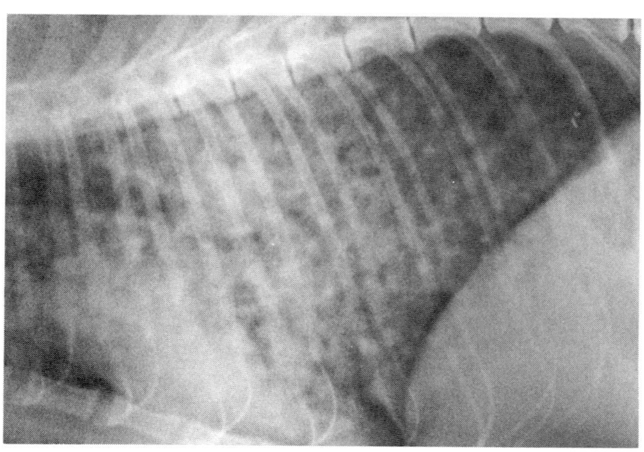

C

Figure 18–23. (*A*) Pulmonary histoplasmosis has a diffuse, nodular, interstitial radiographic pattern. (*B*) A ventrodorsal view of the same cat as in Figure 18–23*A*. (*C*) When pulmonary histoplasmosis is advanced, the nodules appear to coalesce.

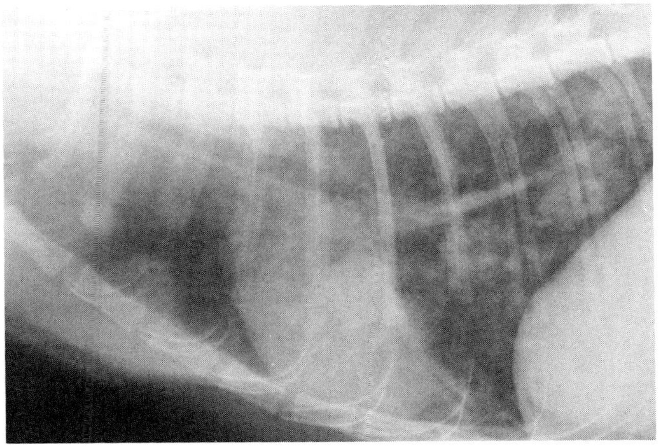

A

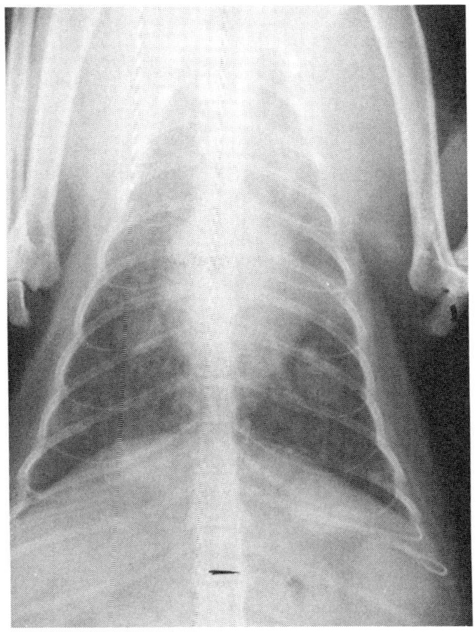

B

Figure 18–24. (*A*) Blastomycosis can produce a diffuse, nodular, interstitial pattern. (*B*) A ventrodorsal view of the same cat as in Figure 18–24*A*.

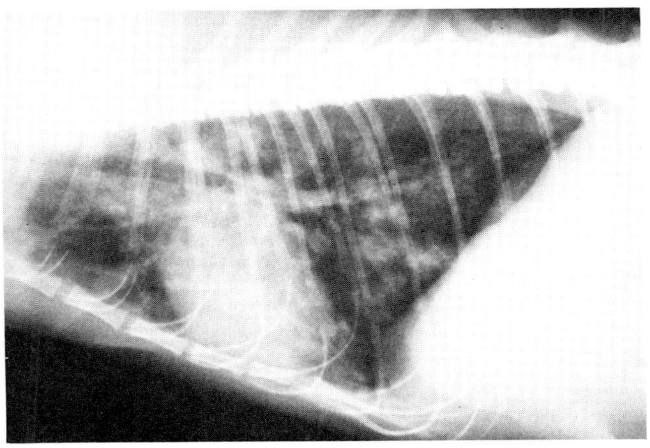

A

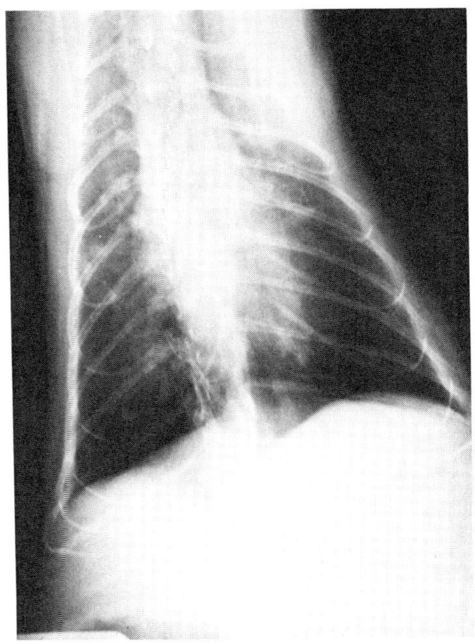

B

Figure 18–25. (*A*) This nodular interstitial pattern is attribut able to pulmonary toxoplasmosis. (*B*) A ventrodorsal view of the same cat as in Figure 18–25*A*.

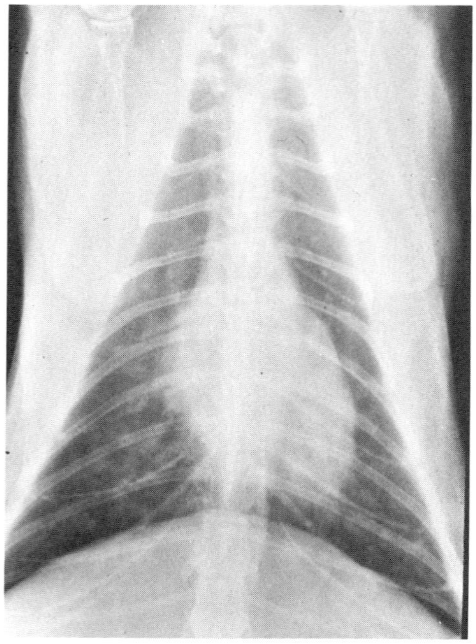

Figure 18–26. This unusual form of lymphosarcoma has a diffuse interstitial radiographic pattern.

Diseases and Disorders Involving Multiple Mechanisms

Several diseases cause dyspnea by multiple mechanisms. For instance, lymphosarcoma may cause lung compression either as a result of an anterior mediastinal mass (see Fig. 18–5) or pleural effusion (see Fig. 18–3). This disease may even occur diffusely within the lungs (Fig. 18–26). Likewise, a diaphragmatic hernia may cause dyspnea by compression of the lungs (see Fig. 18–9) or by the production of pleural fluid. The traumatic pain associated with its cause can also be dyspneogenic. Extreme obesity in cats may cause dyspnea secondary to intrapulmonary fat deposits and the increased effort required to induce inspiration and expiration (Fig. 18–27).

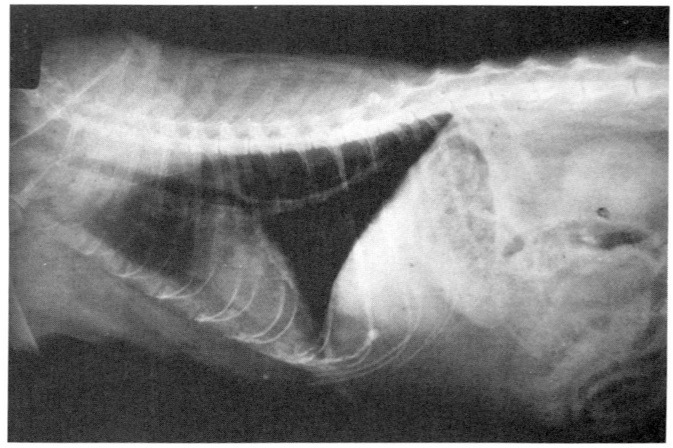

A

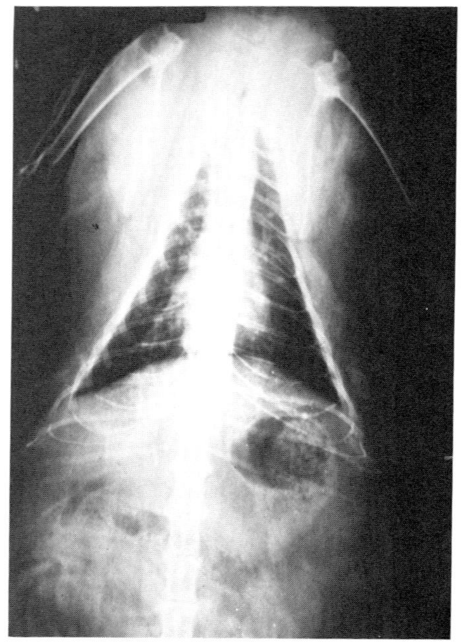

B

Figure 18–27. (*A*) This 23-pound cat was presented for dyspnea secondary to intrapulmonary fat deposits and the increased effort required for inspiration and expiration. This case is similar to the Pickwickian syndrome that is recognized in obese humans. (*B*) A ventrodorsal view of the same cat as in Figure 18–27*A*.

REFERENCES

1. Ware W. Dyspnea: Diagnosis and Management. In: August JR, ed. Consultations in Feline Internal Medicine. Philadelphia: WB Saunders, 1991:147.
2. Center SA, Randolph JF. Eosinophilia. In: August JR, ed. Consultations in Feline Internal Medicine. Philadelphia: WB Saunders, 1991:349.
3. Losonsky JM, Prasse KW, Thrall DE. Dyspnea in the cat. Part I. Radiographic aspects in intrathoracic causes involving the pleural space. Feline Pract 1978;8:35.
4. Thrall DE, Losonsky JM. Dyspnea in the cat. Part II. Radiographic aspects of intrathoracic causes involving the mediastinum. Feline Pract 1978;8:47.
5. Padrid PA, Koblik PD. The techniques used to diagnose feline respiratory disorders. Vet Med 1990;85:956.
6. Hawkins EC, DeNicola DB, Kuehn NF. Evaluation of pulmonary diseases in the dog and cat: The state of the art. J Vet Intern Med 1990;4:267.
7. Kuehn NF, Roudebush P. Dyspnea. In: Allen DG, ed. Small Animal Medicine. Philadelphia: JB Lippincott, 1991:131.

CHAPTER 19

◇ ◇ ◇

Fever of Unknown Origin

James C. Prueter

Definition

Fever of unknown origin (FUO) is a continuous or intermittent febrile disorder that remains undiagnosed following routine historical, physical, and laboratory evaluation for two weeks. The normal temperature for the feline is 100.5° to 102.5°F (38° to 39.2°C). Normal changes in body temperature may be owing to ambient temperatures (up by 5°F or down by 3°F), circadian fluctuations (3°F from morning to evening), exercise (up 5°F), and meals. *Hyperthermia* is a general term for the abnormal elevation of body temperature that is produced without a change in the body's thermoregulatory system. Etiologies for hyperthermia include heat stroke, malignant hyperthermia, exercise, seizures, thyrotoxicosis, drug reactions, and heating pads. These will not be discussed in this chapter. *Fever* is an abnormally high body temperature associated with any disease. A true fever (103° to 106°F) still maintains a balance between heat production and loss, except the thermostat is set at a higher level.

Physiology/Pathophysiology

Body temperature is regulated by a complex sequence of events through a thermostatic system, the hypothalamic thermoregulatory center. The system involves sensors, integrators, and effectors. The sensors include peripheral thermoreceptors in the skin and the central thermoreceptors in the abdomen, spinal cord, and hypothalamus. Their input is relayed by neuronal and humoral means to a central integrating mechanism. Integration is performed by the hypothalamus, the body's thermostat. The hypothalamus receives input from receptors, integrates the information through neuronal networks, and establishes a final set point. This is done rostrally by loss of parasympathetic activity and caudally through production of sympathetic activity. The effectors are multiple physiologic and behavioral mechanisms through which the organism responds because of hypothalamic influence. Effectors function through three mechanisms; heat loss, heat production, and heat conservation. Heat loss occurs through evaporation, sweating and panting, certain postural changes (stretching), seeking a cool environment, and dissipation of heat (spreading saliva over the fur and cutaneous vasodilation). Heat production occurs through the function of certain organs, by muscular activity, through thyroxins, and by sympathetic stimulation. Heat conservation is the result of cutaneous vasoconstriction, piloerection, and postural changes such as curling up and seeking warmth.

This sequence of events is initiated by exogenous pyrogens derived from infectious agents and their products, antigen/antibody complexes, and lymphokines from sensitized lymphocytes, pharmacologic agents, synthetic adjuvants, and cancer cells. Exogenous pyrogens stimulate the release of endogeneous pyrogen (EP) from phagocytic cells (neutrophils, eosinophils, and monocytes) and tissue (Kupffer's cells, splenic sinusoidal cells, alveolar macrophages, peritoneal lining cells, and fixed macrophages). EP is a small polypeptide protein that induces the production or release of various mediators (prostaglandins, monoamine, cholinergics, sodium, and calcium) within the hypothalamus to "reset the thermostat."

Function of True Fever

A true fever is a symptom only, but it should be closely monitored to discover its etiology. It should not be masked during that process. A fever's negative effects (anorexia, metabolic drain, malaise) must be supported, but a fever's positive aspects should be appreciated. Fever causes a decrease in multiplication of some organisms and decreases viral reproduction. It is also important in the activation of the host defense mechanism: it increases immune cell production, the phagocytic ability of white blood cells, and the effects of interferon and interleukin. It has also been shown to increase the antibacterial effects of antibiotics. Fever can be an important clue in disease evaluation and allows an additional parameter when monitoring the effects of therapy. Temperature should be evaluated two to four times daily to differentiate between daily elevations, sustained fevers, and periodic elevations. Response, or lack of response, to therapy is another important reason for frequent temperature monitoring.

Etiology

Human surveys have found an etiologic distribution found in Table 19–1. This is closely paralleled by FUOs in veteri-

Table 19–1. Etiologic Distribution of FUOs in Human Patients

Classification	Incidence (%)
Infectious	40
Immune-mediated disorders	20
Neoplasia	20
Miscellaneous	10
Undiagnosed	10

nary patients. The known feline diseases that may cause fever are listed in Table 19–2.

Diagnosis

A thorough history and physical examination should be performed prior to laboratory testing. The examination should include an ophthalmic and neurologic evaluation. These serve as the basis for determining which tests are appropriate. Because the performance of all of these tests is rarely feasible or necessary, one's clinical judgment and experience become important determinants in the direction that the laboratory evaluation should proceed. Most fever-causing diseases are common diseases that present in an atypical fashion. Testing for the more unusual diseases should be delayed until the common ones have been eliminated.

Table 19–2. Diseases or Organisms Known to Cause Fever in Cats

Infectious Diseases

Viral

Feline leukemia virus (FeLV)
Feline infectious peritonitis
Feline immunodeficiency virus
Upper respiratory viruses—herpesvirus, calicivirus
Feline polyarthritis, usually secondary to FeLV

Bacterial

- Systemic
  - Septicemia
  - Bacterial endocarditis
- Localized
  - External
    - Abscess
    - Cellulitis
  - Intrathoracic
    - Pleuritis
    - Lung abscess
    - Pericarditis
    - Mediastinitis
  - Intraabdominal
    - Pyelonephritis
    - Renal abscess
    - Retroperitoneal abscess
    - Cystitis (rarely)
    - Focal or generalized peritonitis
    - Hepatic abscess
    - Pancreatic abscess or pancreatitis
    - Splenic abscess
    - Endometritis/pyometra
    - Mycobacteria tuberculosis
    - Brucella (rare in cat)
    - Borrelia (Lyme) (rare in cat)
  - Other
    - Septic arthritis
    - Osteomyelitis
    - Diskospondylitis
    - Dental abscess
    - Encephalitis/meningitis
    - Feline plague

Mycotic Diseases

Histoplasmosis
Blastomycosis
Cryptococcosis
Coccidioidomycosis

Parasitic Diseases

Toxoplasmosis
Hemobartonellosis
Heartworm disease
Aberrant larval migrans

Immune-Mediated Diseases

Pemphigus dermatosis
Autoimmune hemolytic anemia
Systemic lupus erythematosus
Polyneuropathy
Polymyopathy
Polyarthritis
Immune-mediated thrombocytopenia

Neoplasia

Primary

Myeloproliferative diseases
Lymphosarcoma
Solid tissue tumors

Secondary

Infection due to destruction of serosal/epithelial barriers to bacterial invasion
Immune suppression predisposing to infection
Anticancer therapy predisposing to infection

Miscellaneous

Cardiomyopathy
Inflammatory bowel disease
Hyperthyroidism
Pansteatitis
Panniculitis
Pancreatitis

History

The history should gather information about the cat's diet, especially the percentage that has been commercial cat food, generic cat food, table food, procured food (e.g., garbage, rodents, and birds) or dog food. Steatitis and congestive cardiomyopathy are among the diet-induced diseases that can cause fever.

Information should be obtained concerning where the cat has lived. This information can be important relative to systemic fungal diseases and certain parasites, including heartworms.

Previous medical diseases and treatments should be considered, especially those that involved vomiting, diarrhea, or weight loss. Some diseases may only appear to be resolved, and others tend to recur. One should inquire about drugs that have been administered, either by a veterinarian or the owner. Their dosage, administration interval, duration, and date most recently given are all important. If this cat has been under the care of another veterinarian, it is important to know about response or lack of response to various forms of therapy. Response to steroids should make one consider immune-mediated diseases. Response to antibiotics should raise one's suspicion for bacterial infections for which therapy was discontinued prematurely. An intermittent fever should not be confused with response to therapy.

One should ask about surgical treatments that have occurred within the last year. Recent surgery could indicate foreign bodies that were incompletely removed, intraoperative contamination, sponges or instruments that may have been left in the patient, or complications related to urinary or intravenous catheters. Catheter-related complications include cystitis, pyelonephritis, and phlebitis.

Physical Examination

The physical examination should begin with an assessment of the severity of fever present. True fevers produce body temperatures of 103° to 106°F. If the temperature is more than 106°F, the causes of hyperthermia should be considered. Next, the cat's age should be considered. Young cats tend to have more infectious diseases; old cats should be suspected of having neoplastic or immune-mediated diseases. The cat's sex is also important, especially as related to being intact or neutered. Intact males tend to roam and fight and contract the previously mentioned diseases. Intact females are prone to infections of the reproductive tract.

A thorough, systematic examination of each organ system is important, especially when an intermittent fever is present. Serial examinations (morning and evening) may be important in some cases.

The ophthalmic examination may reveal indications of systemic mycoses, FeLV, FIP, toxoplasmosis, and neoplasia (see Chapters 38, 39, 51, 61). An examination of the respiratory system begins with an observation of respiratory movements. Dyspnea, hyperpnea, or coughing are notable because they should alert the clinician to consider pneumonia, FeLV, FIP, heartworms, pleural effusions, and intrathoracic masses (see Chapter 41). Cardiac auscultation may reveal a murmur, gallop rhythm, or muffled heart sounds. Each of these is meaningful (see Chapter 18).

The internal and peripheral lymph nodes should be palpated. When they are enlarged, the following should be considered: systemic fungal diseases, lymphosarcoma (LSA), metastatic neoplasia, immune-mediated diseases, and certain infectious diseases such as plague and toxoplasmosis. Palpation should also evaluate other internal organs for enlargement as indicators of immune-mediated diseases, neoplasia, systemic fungal infections, and local infections.

Pain is difficult to elicit in many cats unless it is severe. Its presence may indicate myopathies, myositis, arthritis, diskospondylitis, pyelonephritis, pending abscesses, or other organ dysfunction

It is important that the clinician understand that the physical examination is an ongoing process. It should be performed once or twice daily in order to observe new signs or intermittent symptoms.

Laboratory Evaluation

The laboratory evaluation should begin with a minimum data base consisting of a complete blood count (CBC), serum chemistry profile, urinalysis, and fecal exam; however, the necessary laboratory investigation is usually far more extensive. The CBC may be performed every 2 to 4 days, looking for lymphopenia (LSA), lymphocytosis (LSA, viral disease), eosinophilia (parasitic diseases), monocytosis (fungal, chronic disease, endocarditis, and septicemia), and granulocytopenia (drugs, viral, lupus, leukemia, or myeloproliferative disease). A urinalysis should be followed daily, especially before and after fluid therapy. It may reveal bilirubinuria (significant hepatic disease), pyuria (cystitis, pyelonephritis), hematuria (neoplasia), or casts (pyelonephritis).

Specific serologic tests are available for many feline diseases. Because of expense, many clients cannot afford all of these. Therefore, the history and physical examination should be used to prioritize the tests selected (Table 19–3).

Ancillary Tests

Radiology offers a noninvasive method of evaluating many internal organs. Its use may be indicated by findings in the physical examination or from laboratory results. It may also be used to survey the chest, abdomen, and limbs. Special procedures permit the evaluation of the intestinal tract, urinary tract, and other organs (see Chapter 14).

Ultrasound may also be used to further pursue a specific physical or laboratory finding or for scanning the internal organs. This may be more diagnostic than radiographs because of its ability to evaluate parenchymal disease as well as size or configuration changes (see Chapter 15).

Cytology is an extremely important tool of investigation (see Chapter 13). Fine-needle aspiration of masses and organs may permit a specific diagnosis or may allow differentiation between inflammatory and neoplastic lesions. A buffy coat preparation is useful in identifying abnormal cells, inclusion bodies, and organisms that occur in small numbers (see Chapter 12). Lymph node cytology is indicated in lymphadenopathy and is discussed in Chapter 21. Synovial

Table 19–3. Serologic Tests Available*

Heartworm antigen test
FeLV
FIV (confirm by western blot)
FIP (coronavirus) (questionable significance unless very elevated)
Toxoplasmosis titer (must better define positive titer through enzyme-linked immuno-sorbent assays†)
Protein electrophoresis as an indicator of any chronic inflammatory disease such as FIP, immune-mediated diseases, neoplasia, and stomatitis
Thyroid function testing (T4, T3 suppression test)
Tests for myopathies‡
Immune-mediated tests (antinuclear antibody test and lupus erythematous prep)

*These should be performed following the minimum data base and prioritized based on the history and physical examination.
†Available from MR Lappin, Diagnostic Laboratory, College of Veterinary Medicine and Biomedical Science, Colorado State University, Fort Collins, CO.
‡Available from Diane G. Shelton, Comparative Neuromuscular Laboratory, School of Medicine, University of California, San Diego, La Jolla, CA.

fluid should be examined when joint pain or crepitus is present. In addition to cytology, fluid analysis should include the mucin pH test, total white blood cell count, and total protein count. A bone marrow biopsy is indicated when any blood dyscrasia is present (see Chapter 12). Cerebral spinal fluid analysis is indicated when neurologic signs are present. It may reveal inflammatory or neoplastic disease, although false negatives are common. Any body fluid should be analyzed. Special attention should be given to dyspnea or hyperpnea because of the number of diseases that produce pleural effusion (see Chapter 18). A tracheal wash for cytology and culture is indicated when respiratory signs are present (see Chapter 12).

Cultures are indicated when other tests reveal abnormalities in any organ; however, negative cultures may mean that anaerobic organisms are present. If urinary tract disease occurs, the urine, bladder wall, and urolith should be cultured because different bacteria may be present in each. Quantitative cultures are also important in the urinary tract. Blood cultures are meaningful when positive but may require multiple samples before organisms are found. The cat should be off antibiotics for 3 to 7 days, and the body temperature should be taken every 2 hours to determine when a peak occurs, which is the preferred time for culturing. Sterile collection technique is essential. Culturing of synovium is usually more meaningful than joint fluid.

Many diseases may only be confirmed with histopathology. It is indicated for any organ demonstrating abnormalities by physical examination, laboratory evaluation, radiography, or ultrasound. When skin is biopsied, the specimen should be submitted in Michel's fixative for immunofluorescent testing. Specific examinations are available for muscle and nerve diseases. The synovium is the tissue most likely to contain diagnostic lesions for a joint biopsy sample.

Examinations with fiberoptic endoscopes are indicated when respiratory or digestive signs are present. Fiberscopes permit observation and biopsy of the trachea, tracheal bifurcation, esophagus, stomach, proximal duodenum, colon, and rectum in a noninvasive manner.

Although electromyography and nerve conduction testing are generally only available in referral practices, these tests can reveal neurologic and muscle diseases that are difficult to diagnose in other noninvasive ways. They should be considered when muscle pain or neurologic deficits are present.

Because exploratory surgery is an invasive procedure, it should be reserved as one of the last tests to use, preferably for diagnostic purposes when the possibility that therapeutic measures may also be taken exists. However, exploratory surgery is necessary for strictly diagnostic purposes in some patients and is also indicated to define a neoplasia's type.

REFERENCES

1. August JR. Consultation in Feline Internal Medicine. Philadelphia: WB Saunders, 1991.
2. Ettinger SJ. Textbook of Veterinary Internal Medicine, 3rd ed. Philadelphia: WB Saunders, 1989:23.
3. Greene CE. Infectious Diseases of the Dog and Cat. Philadelphia: WB Saunders, 1989.
4. Pedersen NC. Feline Infectious Diseases. Galeta, CA: American Veterinary Publication, 1988.
5. Sherding RG. The Cat—Diseases and Clinical Management, vol. I, II. New York: Churchill Livingstone, 1989.
6. Wolf AW. Fever of Undetermined Origin in the Cat. Proceedings of the Ninth Annual Veterinary Medical Forum 1991, 1991:125.

CHAPTER 20

◇ ◇ ◇

Icterus

Gary D. Norsworthy

Icterus, or jaundice, is a condition in which there is an increase in serum bilirubin (hyperbilirubinemia) and a deposition of bile pigments in body tissues. Bile pigment deposition is observed most readily in the skin and mucous membranes as yellow coloring in the tissues. In the cat, this is generally visible first in the hard or soft palate as two parallel streaks of yellow. A comprehensive list of the possible causes of icterus in the cat can be found in Appendix F.

Historical Perspective

At one time, it was a common belief among veterinarians that "a yellow cat was a dead cat." Although this generality was expressed somewhat facetiously, 30 years ago, 10% of the cats undergoing necropsy at Angell Memorial Animal Hospital died of a malignant disease of the blood-forming tissues,[1] which included unpreventable hepatic lymphosarcoma; 10 years ago, the predominant feline liver disease was untreatable idiopathic hepatic lipidosis (IHL).[2] As a result of the advent of feline leukemia virus (FeLV) vaccine and our present understanding of the proper treatment for IHL, the number of icteric cats presented for evaluation has decreased, and the number of affected cats that have been treated successfully has increased.

Diagnosis

Cats with a severe degree of icterus (clinical icterus) may readily be identified by the distinct yellow color that is apparent in the thinly-haired areas of the skin, such as the preauricular area above the eyes. Cats with a mild degree of icterus (biochemical icterus) may only be able to be diagnosed by an examination of the serum or plasma. Those whose conditions lie between these two extremes may be diagnosed on the basis of a yellowed hard or soft palate, gingiva, labia of the vulva, or sclera.

Variability

There is probably no other condition that is more difficult to describe and diagnose in concrete terms than icterus. A great deal of variability exists with regard to the clinical signs and laboratory values that accompany this condition. Because of this extreme variability, the statements made in this chapter should be construed as general rules that are subject to a number of exceptions.

Underlying Mechanisms

Three mechanisms can produce hyperbilirubinemia and clinical icterus: hemolysis, hepatocellular disease, and obstruction of bile flow. Differentiation of the cause of the condition is based on a biochemical profile and a complete blood count (CBC) (see Table 20–1). Other appropriate tests include a reticulocyte count and a urinalysis. Additionally, there may be clues in the history and physical examination that may also be very helpful. These include systemic signs of liver disease, such as lethargy, anorexia, and vomiting.[3] Appropriate diagnostic tests for determining the cause of icterus in the cat are listed in Tables 20–2 and 20–3. (See Appendix F for a comprehensive list of causes.)

Hemolysis

Most cats with icterus secondary to hemolysis will present with a history of a sudden onset of lethargy, weakness, and exercise intolerance. Because of the anemia, a holosystolic mitral murmur may be present. The mucous membranes will be pale and often are slightly yellow.

Specific diseases to consider in such cases include:

- Hemobartonellosis (see Chapter 43)
- Heinz-body anemias (secondary to administration/exposure to acetaminophen, methylene blue, phenazopyridine, benzocaine, or propylene glycol) (see Chapter 42)
- Bacteremia/septicemia
- Autoimmune hemolytic anemia

Laboratory findings may include:

- A packed cell volume (PCV) of less than 15%
- Blood smear findings indicating a bone marrow response (see Chapter 16)
  - Macrocytes (reticulocytes)
  - Howell-Jolly bodies
  - Nucleated red blood cells (RBCs)

Table 20–1. Differentiation of the Mechanisms Underlying Icterus on the Basis of Laboratory Values*

Laboratory Test	Hemolysis	Hepatocellular Disease	Biliary Obstruction
Packed cell volume	Decreased	Normal (decreased)	Normal
Alanine aminotransferase	Normal (increased)	Increased	Normal (increased)
Serum alkaline phosphatase	Normal	Normal (increased)	Increased
Total bilirubin	Increased	Increased	Increased
Direct bilirubin	<50% early >50% late	50%–75%	>75%

*These parameters for differentiation should be interpreted as generalities, as there are exceptions.

An increased reticulocyte and nucleated RBC count after 3 to 4 days

An increase in total bilirubin, with more than 50% indirect (unconjugated). (After 3 to 4 days, the direct or conjugated bilirubin may increase to greater than 50%.)

A mild to moderate increase in alanine aminotransferase (ALT) levels, although in many cats this does not occur

A slight increase in urine bilirubin and hemoglobin levels

Additional laboratory tests that should be performed include:

An RBC examination for *Hemobartonella felis*

An RBC examination for Heinz bodies

A blood culture for bacteremia*

A Coombs' test†

Hepatocellular Disease

Cats with icterus secondary to hepatocellular disease are often very ill. Characteristic findings include lethargy, dehydration, anorexia, and vomiting. The degree of icterus will range from mild to severe.

Specific diseases to consider include the following:

FeLV-related diseases (lymphosarcoma, myeloproliferative disorders, reticuloendotheliosis) (see Chapter 39)

Cholangitis/cholangiohepatitis (see Chapter 29)

Idiopathic hepatic lipidosis (see Chapter 47)

Hepatic lipidosis secondary to diabetes mellitus (see Chapter 34)

Feline infectious peritonitis (FIP) (see Chapter 38)

Bacteremia/endotoxemia

Drugs or toxins (including acetaminophen)

Primary or metastatic neoplasia (see Chapter 51)

Systemic fungal diseases (see Chapter 61)

Hepatic shunts (Fig. 20–1)

The laboratory findings in cats with icterus secondary to hepatocellular disease include the following:

PCV

Normal—when the disease is fairly acute and does not directly affect the bone marrow

Decreased—when the disease becomes chronic and produces indirect bone marrow suppression (anemia of chronic disease)

Increased—when dehydration is present in a cat with an otherwise normal PCV

*This test generally has a low diagnostic yield.

†This test is not specific for autoimmune hemolytic anemia because it is often positive in cases of hemobartonellosis. If *H. felis* is not found, the two diseases may be indistinguishable.

Table 20–2. Basic Biochemical Tests for Diagnosing Icterus in the Cat

Packed cell volume
Blood smear examination for:
Hemobartonella felis
Heinz bodies
Howell-Jolly bodies
Macrocytes (reticulocytes)
Nucleated red blood cells
Total and direct bilirubin
Alanine aminotransferase
Alkaline phosphatase
Total protein, albumin, globulin
Glucose

Table 20–3. Other Diagnostic Tests Appropriate for the Icteric Cat

Bile acids, pre- and post-prandial
Liver aspiration biopsy
Abdominal radiography
Reticulocyte count
Feline leukemia virus antigen test
Feline coronavirus antibody test
Abdominal lavage for bile
Urinalysis for bilirubin
Abdominal ultrasonography
Exploratory laparotomy
Blood culture

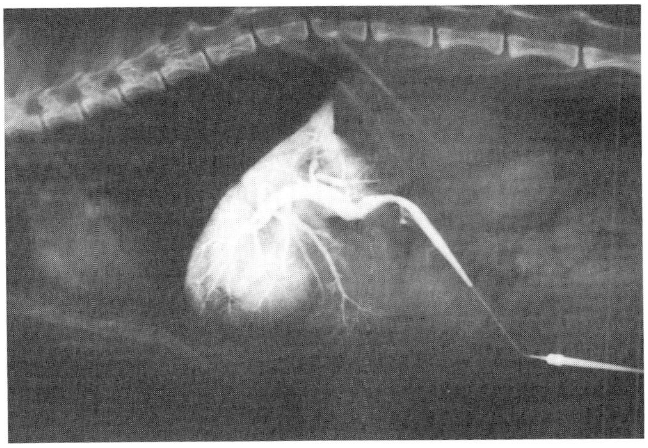

Figure 20–1. If a hepatic shunt is suspected, a splenoportogram may be performed by injecting radiopaque contrast material into the spleen and observing the portal circulation. The results of this study were normal.

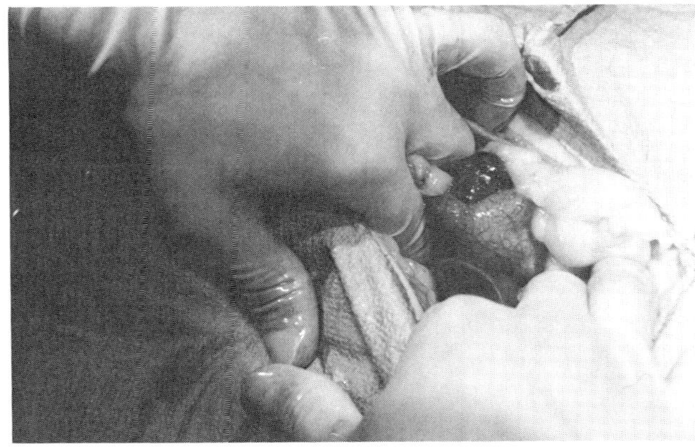

Figure 20–2. The gallbladder may be obstructed by inspissated bile secondary to chronic cholangiohepatitis. In this cat, a greatly distended gallbladder was detected by abdominal ultrasonography and confirmed by exploratory laparotomy.

- Moderate to marked increase in urine bilirubin level
- Increase in total bilirubin level, with more than 50% but less than 75% direct*
- Moderate to marked increase in ALT
- Mild to moderate increase in serum alkaline phosphatase (SAP)
- Variable total protein level
- Normal or decreased albumin level
- Normal or increased globulin level
- Normal or decreased blood urea nitrogen (BUN) level
- Markedly elevated glucose level in cats with hepatic lipidosis secondary to diabetes mellitus

Additional laboratory tests that may be appropriate in affected cats include the following:

- FeLV test
- Liver aspiration or biopsy
- Coronavirus titer
- Blood culture for bacteremia†
- Systemic fungal titers
- Abdominal ultrasonography (see Chapter 15)
- Splenoportogram

Biliary Obstruction

Cats with icterus caused by biliary obstruction are moderately sick. They may exhibit lethargy, decreased appetite, and occasionally, vomiting and weight loss. They are usually profoundly icteric, and the characteristic yellow color will be readily visible in the skin. Biliary obstruction may occur within the parenchyma of the liver, which is termed intrahepatic obstruction, or it may be limited to the gallbladder and bile duct, designated as extrahepatic obstruction.

Specific diseases to consider in the differential diagnosis include the following:

- Cholangitis/cholangiohepatitis (Fig. 20–2) (see Chapter 29)
- Primary or metastatic neoplasia (see Chapter 51)
- Ruptured bile duct or gallbladder (generally secondary to trauma)
- Cholelithiasis (Fig. 20–3) (see Chapter 29)
- FIP (see Chapter 38)

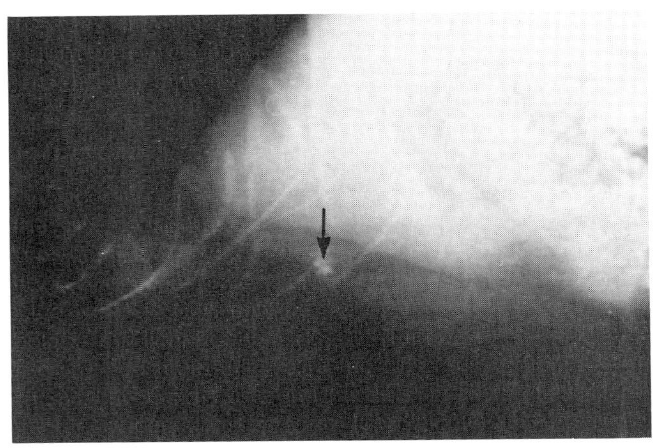

Figure 20–3. The radiodense mass in the area of the liver (*arrow*) is a cholelith. Generally, this condition is caused by chronic cholangiohepatitis.

*This test may be very helpful, but there are exceptions to it.
†This test has a low diagnostic yield.

Laboratory tests in cats with icterus secondary to biliary obstruction may reveal the following:

- Normal PCV
- Moderate to marked increase in urine bilirubin
- Moderate to marked increase in total bilirubin, with greater than 75% direct*
- Mild to moderate increase in ALT
- Moderate to marked increase in SAP

Additional laboratory tests that may be appropriate include the following:†

- FeLV test
- Liver aspiration or biopsy
- Abdominal lavage to detect the presence of bile
- Abdominal radiography to confirm or rule out choleliths
- Coronavirus titer
- Abdominal ultrasonography (see Chapter 15)
- Exploratory laparotomy

*This test may be very helpful, but there are exceptions to it.

†Intrahepatic diseases may obstruct the bile duct, so the same tests that are appropriate for icterus secondary to hepatocellular causes are also appropriate in these cases.

Combined Mechanisms

Cats can have more than one icterus-producing disease concurrently. The most notable combination is hemolysis-producing hemobartonellosis, which frequently is a stress-related disease that occurs secondary to another disease. If a large number of *H. felis* are found in the red blood cells, but a bone marrow response is not occurring, another disease may be affecting the bone marrow. Diseases with the potential to suppress the bone marrow include the chronic form of cholangiohepatitis, lymphosarcoma, systemic fungal diseases, IHL, lipidosis, FIP, and neoplasia.

REFERENCES

1. Holzworth J. Leukemia and related neoplasms in the cat. J Am Vet Med Assoc 1960;136:47.
2. Zawie DA, Garvey MS. Feline hepatic diseases. Vet Clin North Am (Small Anim Pract) 1984;14:1201.
3. Cornelius LM. Icterus. In: Lorenz MD, Cornelius LM, eds. Small Animal Medical Diagnosis. Philadelphia: JB Lippincott, 1987:299.

CHAPTER 21

◇ ◇ ◇

Lymphadenopathy

Rick L. Cowell
and Ronald D. Tyler

Lymphadenopathy may be caused by lymphoid hyperplasia, lymphadenitis, or neoplasia (lymphoid or metastatic). It may be localized or generalized, usually reflecting the extent of the pathologic process. Evaluation of cats with lymphadenopathy should begin with a thorough history and physical examination, which should allow the evaluator to classify the lymphadenopathy as local, regional, or generalized. Generalized lymphadenopathy occurs most commonly due to lymphosarcoma or systemic lymphadenitis/immune stimulation. Rarely, metastatic neoplasia may cause a generalized lymphadenopathy. Local and regional lymphadenopathies occur most commonly secondary to inflammation in the area drained by the enlarged node or nodes. Lymphosarcoma and tumor metastasis are other causes of local and regional lymphadenopathy that must be considered. An algorithmic approach to lymph node aspirate evaluation and interpretation is presented in Figure 21–1. A comprehensive list of causes of lymphadenopathy in the cat can be found in Appendix F.

Sample Collection and Preparation

Before aspirating a peripheral lymph node, the site over the lymph node to be aspirated is prepared as for an injection. However, when aspirating internal lymph nodes, the site of aspiration should be clipped and a surgical preparation applied.

Because lymph nodes readily exfoliate cells, small syringes (5-cc) supply sufficient negative pressure to collect adequate samples. Good lymph node aspirates can be collected using a 21- to 25-gauge needle. Larger gauge needles are less desirable because they tend to collect excessive amounts of blood and may collect cores of tissue that are difficult to smear into a monolayer without causing excessive cell rupturing.

Aspiration Techniques

Peripheral lymph nodes are stabilized for aspiration by holding them between the thumb and forefinger. Once stabilized, the needle with syringe attached is inserted into the enlarged lymph node. Lymphoid cells are aspirated into the bore of the needle by rapidly withdrawing the syringe plunger two-thirds to three-fourths of the syringe barrel-length, to create negative pressure. Several areas of the lymph node should be sampled. If the lymph node is large enough and the animal calm enough to allow the needle to be redirected without fear of the needle exiting the lymph node, negative pressure can be maintained while the needle is redirected. However, if the lymph node is small or the cat is not well controlled, negative pressure should be released before the needle is redirected and then reapplied after repositioning the needle. If the needle exits the lymph node while negative pressure is being applied, perinodal tissue, subcutaneous fat, and various skin layers may be aspirated, inducing artifacts. This may also cause very small samples to be aspirated into the syringe barrel, causing them to be lost for cytologic evaluation. Any time blood becomes visible in the needle or syringe, negative pressure should be discontinued and the needle redirected. Continued aspiration in the previous site may result in excessive blood contamination and dilution of the sample, which could impair cytologic evaluation.

Smear Techniques

After the lymph node has been aspirated in three or four areas, the negative pressure is released and the needle withdrawn. The needle is removed from the syringe and a few milliliters of air are drawn into the syringe barrel. The needle is replaced onto the syringe and the plunger is rapidly depressed, forcing some of the aspirated contents onto a clean, dry glass slide.

The specimen must now be smeared into a monolayer to allow cytologic evaluation; however, lymphocytes, especially lymphoblasts, are fragile cells that rupture easily. Therefore, special care must be taken while spreading the cells to ensure sufficient numbers of cells remain intact to allow accurate evaluation. There are many techniques for smearing specimens into monolayers; whichever technique works best for the person making the smear is the technique of choice. Often, there is sufficient tissue fluid present so that lymph node aspirates can be adequately spread similar to making a blood smear. A combination of procedures may be desirable until the operator learns which technique works best. Combination procedures can be performed on

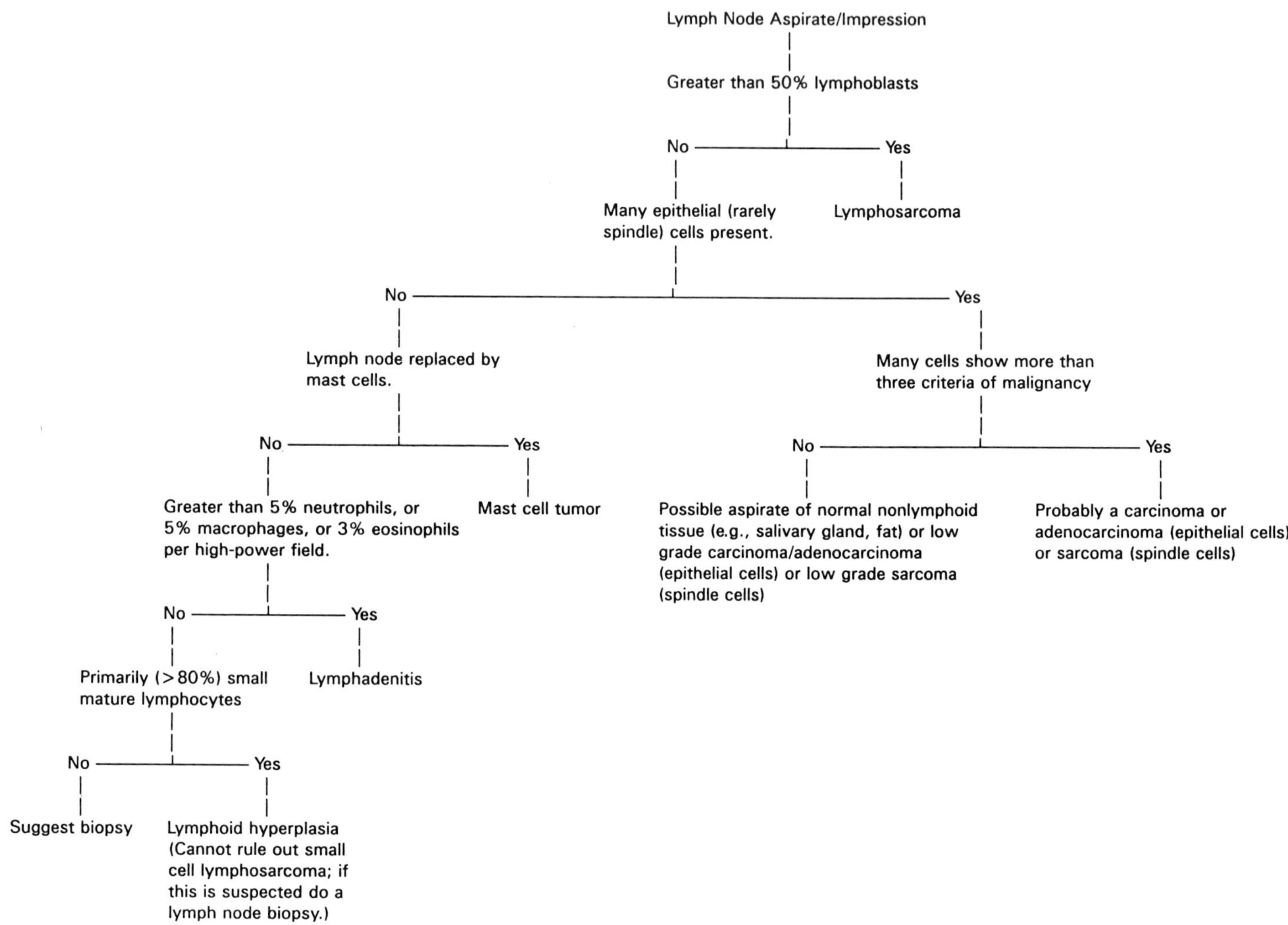

Figure 21–1. A flow chart depicting a logical approach to the cytologic evaluation of lymph node aspirates and impression smears. (Courtesy of Oklahoma State University Clinical Pathology Teaching File.)

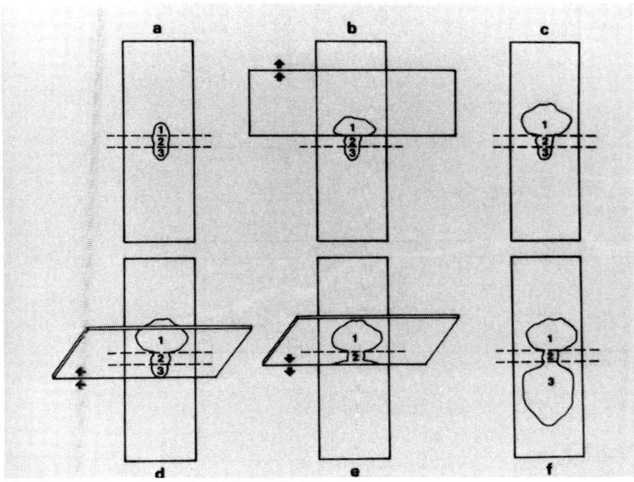

Figure 21–2. Combination cytology preparation. (*A*) A portion of the aspirate is expelled onto a glass microscope slide (prep slide). (*B*) Another glass microscope slide is placed over about one third of the preparation. If additional spreading of the aspirate is needed, gentle digital pressure can be used. Excessive pressure should be avoided. The spreader slide is smoothly slid forward. (*C*) This makes a squash prep of about one third of the aspirate (*area 1*). The spreader slide also contains a squash prep (not depicted). Next, the edge of a tilted glass microscope slide (second spreader slide) is slid backward from the end opposite the squash prep until it contacts about one third the expelled aspirate. (*D, E*) Then, the second spreader slide is slid rapidly and smoothly forward. (*F*) This produces an area (*3*) that is spread with mechanical forces like those of a blood smear preparation. The middle area (*2*) is left untouched and contains a high concentration of cells. (Courtesy of Diagnostic Cytology of the Dog and Cat, American Veterinary Publications.)

the same slide or different slides. A combination procedure performed on the same slide is depicted in Figure 21–2. All cytology smear techniques require some technical skill; however, they can be mastered easily with minimal practice.

Staining

The Romanowsky-type stains (Wright's stain, Giemsa stains, Diff-Quik [AHS del Caribe, Inc., Aguada, Puerto Rico]) are the stains most commonly used on cytologic samples. These stains are readily available, inexpensive, and easy to prepare and maintain by the practicing veterinarian. The Romanowsky-type stains are primarily cytoplasmic stains and, hence, they stain the cytoplasm of cells and most organisms excellently. While nuclear and nucleolar detail is not as clear as with the nuclear stains (e.g., trichrome), cellular morphology is sufficient to differentiate neoplasia from inflammation and evaluate neoplastic cells for cytologic evidence of malignancy.

Each of the different Romanowsky-type stains has a recommended staining procedure. While these procedures should be followed in general, for optimum results they may need to be modified (e.g., altering the time) to adjust for variations in the type and thickness of the smear being stained and to the evaluator's preference. Generally, thinner smears require less staining time and thicker smears require more staining time. By trying variations in the recommended time intervals for the stain, the evaluator can establish which times produce the preferred staining characteristics for various cytologic preparations.

Cell Types

A variety of cell types can be observed in cytologic preparations from lymph node aspirates or impression smears, and include: mature (small) lymphocytes, medium-sized lymphocytes, large lymphocytes (lymphoblasts), plasma cells, macrophages, mast cells, neutrophils, eosinophils, giant inflammatory cells, and metastatic cancer cells. The morphologic characteristics of these cells are described below.

1. ***Small Lymphocyte.*** Small lymphocytes have a round to oval, but indented, nucleus with dense clumps of nuclear chromatin in a coarse to smudged pattern. Nucleoli are not visible in small lymphocytes. The cytoplasm is scanty, clear to light blue, and may contain a few red to purple granules. Small lymphocytes are recognizably smaller than neutrophils but larger than erythrocytes.
2. ***Medium Lymphocyte.*** Medium-sized lymphocytes are approximately the same size as neutrophils. They have a single nucleus that is oval to irregularly shaped, with a stippled to granular chromatin pattern and a moderate amount of bluish cytoplasm that occasionally contains a few red/purple granules. Medium-sized lymphocytes may have nucleoli that are not visible, indistinct, or prominent. However, with lymphosarcoma associated primarily with medium-sized lymphocytes, the nucleoli are usually single, large, and prominent.
3. ***Large Lymphocyte (Lymphoblast).*** Lymphoblasts are larger than neutrophils. They contain a single nucleus that is oval, cleaved, notched, or irregularly shaped with a finely stippled to granular chromatin pattern. Multiple, small to large nucleoli are generally evident. Lymphoblasts have a moderate amount of bluish cytoplasm that may appear somewhat granular but is typically not visible the entire circumference of the nucleus, i.e., it appears to touch the nucleus and run confluent with it at some point. A clear area in the cytoplasm representing the golgi may be evident.
4. ***Plasma Cell.*** Plasma cells are immune-stimulated B-lymphocytes. They have an eccentrically placed, round nucleus with coarse, cord-like nuclear chromatin. Their cytoplasm stains deep blue and a clear area, representing the golgi, is often recognizable between the nucleus and the greatest volume of cytoplasm. Occasionally, clear- or pale-staining vacuoles (Russell's bodies) may fill the cytoplasm of a plasma cell. These cells are sometimes referred to as Mott cells.
5. ***Macrophage.*** Macrophages are larger than lymphoblasts. They have a blue-gray cytoplasm that frequently contains vacuoles and phagocytic debris and a single variably shaped nucleus with a lacy chromatin pattern.
6. ***Mast Cell.*** Mast cells are medium-sized round cells.

They have a moderate amount of cytoplasm that contains metachromatic (red-purple) granules. The nucleus is round to oval and may be partially obscured by the intracytoplasmic granules.

7. ***Neutrophil.*** Neutrophils have a segmented nucleus with coarsely clumped nuclear chromatin and a colorless cytoplasm.
8. ***Eosinophil.*** Cat eosinophils are readily recognized by their numerous, small, rod-shaped, eosinophilic (red), intracytoplasmic granules. Eosinophils are larger than neutrophils and have a segmented nucleus with coarsely clumped nuclear chromatin.
9. ***Giant Inflammatory Cells.*** These cells are very large and multinucleated. They have a moderate to abundant amount of bluish cytoplasm and may contain phagocytized organisms, cells, or debris.
10. ***Metastatic Cancer Cells.*** Nonlymphoid neoplasms are confirmed in lymph node aspirates by recognizing cell types that are not normally present and that have three or more criteria of malignancy. Nonlymphoid neoplasms may also present as a sufficient increase in a cell type that is normally present only in small numbers (e.g., mast cells). Carcinomas and adenocarcinomas (epithelial cell tumors) are the most common metastatic neoplasias found in lymph node aspirates. In general, metastatic carcinoma cells are large, have a high nuclear-to-cytoplasm ratio, coarse nuclear chromatin, large angular nucleoli, and bluish cytoplasm, and may contain cytoplasmic vacuoles. (See Chapter 13.)

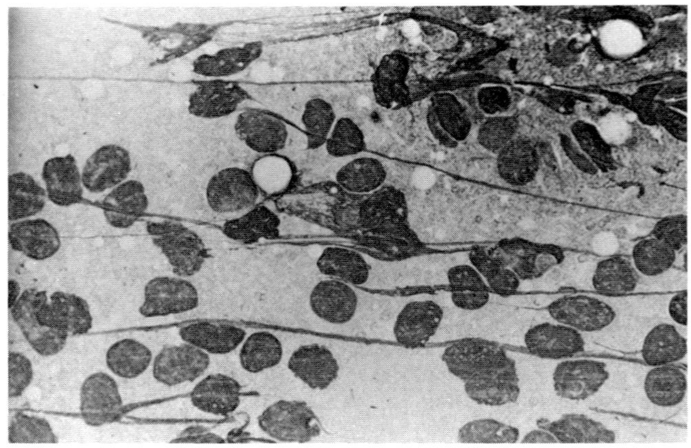

Figure 21–3. **Lymph node aspirate in which excessive cell rupturing has occurred. The cells have been stripped of their cytoplasm and the nuclear chromatin of many cells is forming strands across the slide. Care must be taken to prevent excessive cell rupturing. (Original magnification 250×, Wright's stain.) (Courtesy of Oklahoma State University Clinical Pathology Teaching File.)**

Cytologic Evaluation

Basis for Interpretations

Knowing the normal enables the evaluator to recognize the abnormal and subsequently make interpretations. In normal lymph nodes, small mature lymphocytes are the predominant cell type, being approximately 75% to 95% of the cells present. The remaining cell types, 5% to 25% of the cells present, are an admixture consisting primarily of medium to large lymphocytes with fewer macrophages, plasma cells, and neutrophils. Small, roundish, basophilic structures called lymphoglandular bodies, i.e., cytoplasmic fragments of lymphoid cells, are common findings in all lymph-node aspirates. Lymphoglandular bodies must not be confused with organisms, cells, or parasites (see Figs. 21–4 and 21–13).

Since fine-needle aspiration biopsy samples only a few, small, discrete areas of the lymph node, recognition of one or more processes does not totally rule out the possibility of other processes being present at an unsampled site. However, when a lymph node is enlarged due to lymphosarcoma or lymphadenitis, generally, the node is diffusely infiltrated. Metastatic neoplasia is more likely to have only focal areas of involvement. Depending on the shifts in cell proportions and the presence of abnormal cells, several different interpretations can reliably be made by lymph-node cytology. The bases for those interpretations are the presence of any of the following:

1. ***Excessive Cell Rupturing.*** Lymphoid cells are very fragile and easily ruptured (Fig. 21–3). Determining if excessive cell numbers are ruptured is difficult and varies depending on the population of unruptured cells and the evaluator's experience. If all of the unruptured cells are lymphoblasts, up to 50% of the cells can be ruptured and the slide will still be diagnostic. However, when the intact cell population is pleomorphic and contains a distribution of small lymphocytes as well as lymphoblasts, having 50% of the cells ruptured can make interpretation unreliable. Therefore, the node must be reaspirated.
2. ***Lymphosarcoma.*** If ≥50% of the nucleated cells in the smear are lymphoblasts (large lymphocytes) or prolymphocytes with distinct nucleoli, a diagnosis of lymphosarcoma can be reliably made.
3. ***Lymphadenitis.*** Lymphadenitis may occur as neutrophilic, purulent, eosinophilic, chronic, or granulomatous. While lymphadenitis may be present and recognizable by experienced cytologists at lower concentrations of inflammatory cells than listed below, the concentrations given here are suggested for inexperienced cytologists in an effort to prevent misdiagnosis by overdiagnosing conditions.

    Neutrophilic lymphadenitis is present if a concentration of 5 or more neutrophils appear per 100× objective field (oil power).

    Purulent lymphadenitis is present if a concentration of 20 or more neutrophils appear per 100× objective field (oil power).

    Eosinophilic lymphadenitis is present if a concentration of 3 or more eosinophils appear per 100× objective field (oil power).

    Chronic lymphadenitis is present if a concentration of 5 or more macrophages appear per 100× objective field (oil power).

    Granulomatous lymphadenitis is present if inflammatory giant cells are recognized in the smear.

4. ***Immune Stimulation.*** A concentration of three or more plasma cells appear per 100× objective field (oil power).
5. ***Metastatic Neoplasia.*** Metastatic neoplasia may be recognized by the presence of cell types that have 3 or more criteria of malignancy and that are not normally found within lymph-node aspirates. It may also be recognized if there is a sufficient abnormal increase in the number of a cell type (e.g., mast cells) that is normally present in lymph node aspirates only in very low percentages.

Interpretations

1. ***Lymphoid Hyperplasia.*** Lymphoid hyperplasia occurs when antigens reach the lymph node and stimulate an immune response. This is generally a local reaction stimulating a localized response; however, lymphoid hyperplasia associated with a generalized lymphadenopathy may also occur. Cytologically, hyperplastic lymph nodes generally appear very similar to normal lymph nodes. Hyperplastic lymph nodes consist primarily of small mature lymphocytes (Fig. 21–4), and often increased numbers of plasma cells, indicating immune stimulation, are present. Even in the absence of increased numbers of plasma cells, the term "lymphoid hyperplasia," as opposed to "compatible with normal lymphoid tissue," is used if the lymph node is enlarged clinically.
2. ***Lymphadenitis.*** Lymphadenitis results when inflammatory products are released into a lymph node or gain access to the node by drainage of inflamed tissue. It sometimes, but not always, indicates infection of the lymph node or tissues being drained by the lymph node. Lymphadenitis may be either neutrophilic, purulent, eosinophilic, chronic, granulomatous, or any combination of these reactions. Lymphadenitis may also be classified as primary or secondary. With primary lymphadenitis, the node itself is infected. In secondary lymphadenitis, the node itself is not infected but instead is draining a site of inflammation (not necessarily infection) distant from the node. Secondary lymphadenitis is generally neutrophilic and/or eosinophilic. Plasma cell numbers are generally increased with any cause of lymphadenitis. Typically, lymph nodes infected with bacterial organisms develop a purulent lymphadenitis (Fig. 21–5), while nodes infected with systemic fungal (Figs. 21–6 to 21–8), protozoal (Fig. 21–9), or algal infections develop a granulomatous or pyogranulomatous lymphadenitis. Neutrophilic lymphadenitis is the typical response of lymph nodes draining distant areas

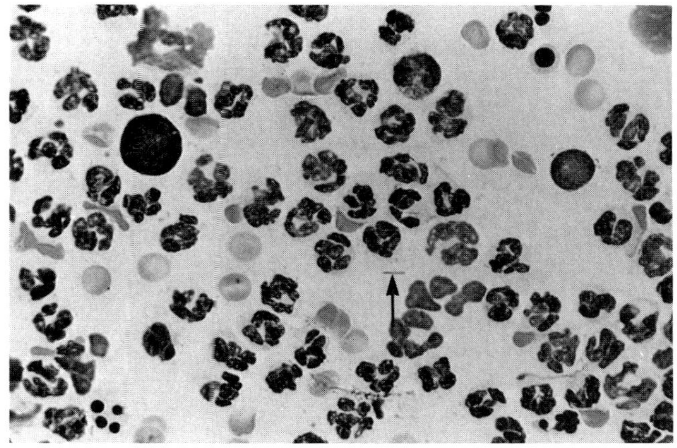

Figure 21–5. Aspirate from an infected lymph node. The slide consists primarily of neutrophils. Scattered bacterial rods (*arrow*) are also present. (Original magnification 250×, Wright's stain.) (Courtesy of Oklahoma State University Clinical Pathology Teaching File.)

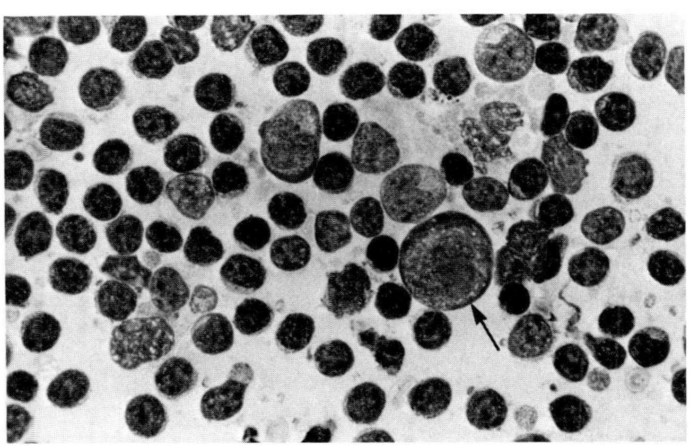

Figure 21–4. Aspirate from a hyperplastic lymph node. Small lymphocytes are the predominant cell type in hyperplastic nodes. Lymphoblasts (*arrow*) are present but comprise less than 50% of the nucleated cell population. (Original magnification 250×, Wright's stain.) (Courtesy of Oklahoma State University Clinical Pathology Teaching File.)

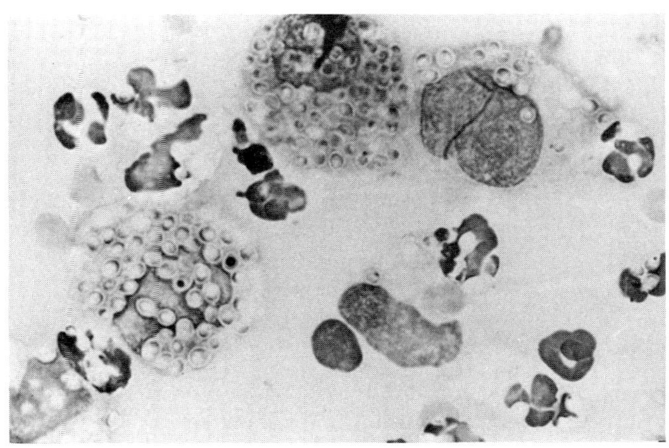

Figure 21–6. Aspirate from a cat with histoplasmosis. Macrophages and neutrophils containing many small (2 to 4 μm), round organisms with thin, clear halos are shown. (Original magnification 330×, Wright's stain.) (Courtesy of Oklahoma State University Clinical Pathology Teaching File.)

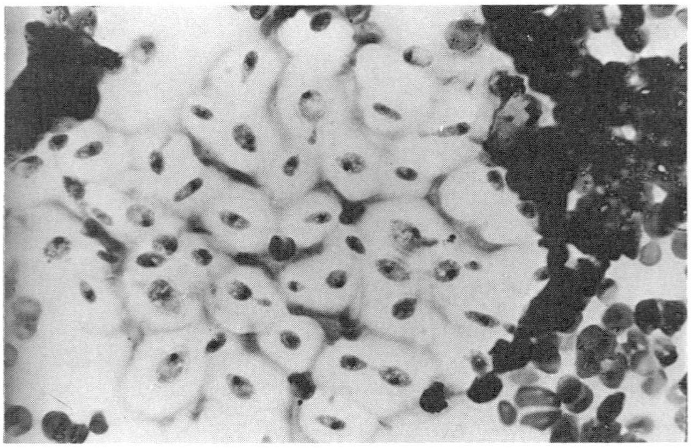

Figure 21–7. Aspirate from a cat with cryptococcosis. Many medium-sized organisms with thick, clear-staining mucoid capsules are shown. Many of the organisms are exhibiting narrow-based budding. (Original magnification 250×, Wright's stain.) (Courtesy of Oklahoma State University Clinical Pathology Teaching File.)

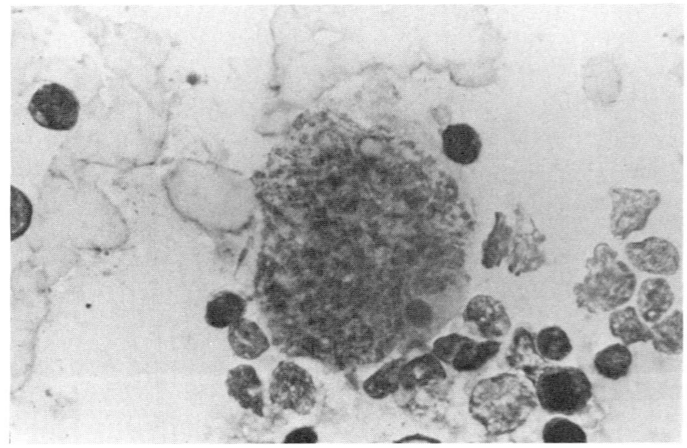

Figure 21–9. Impression smear from a cat with cytauxzoonosis. Scattered lymphocytes and a large mononuclear cell containing developing *Cytauxzoon* organisms are shown. (Original magnification 250×, Wright's stain.) (Courtesy of Oklahoma State University Clinical Pathology Teaching File.)

of inflammation (Fig. 21–10). Eosinophilic lymphadenitis is common in lymph nodes draining the skin, respiratory tract, or digestive tract (Fig. 21–11).

3. ***Lymphosarcoma.*** Lymphosarcoma is the most commonly found neoplasm in feline lymph nodes. Cytologically, lymphosarcoma is identified by recognizing an abnormally increased proportion (50% of the nucleated cell population) of large lymphocytes (lymphoblasts and prolymphocytes) (Fig. 21–12). Cell proportions are evaluated because normal lymph node architecture is lost with cytology smears. Because lymphocytes are fragile, one must be careful not to induce excessive cell rupturing during smear preparation. Traumatized or ruptured cells should not be evaluated. Traumatized lymphocytes of any size may be mistaken for lymphoblasts because they tend to spread out, making their nucleoli visible. Therefore, when evaluating aspirates for lymphosarcoma, only intact, nontraumatized lymphocytes should be evaluated. Usually, traumatized or ruptured cells can easily be differentiated by their loose

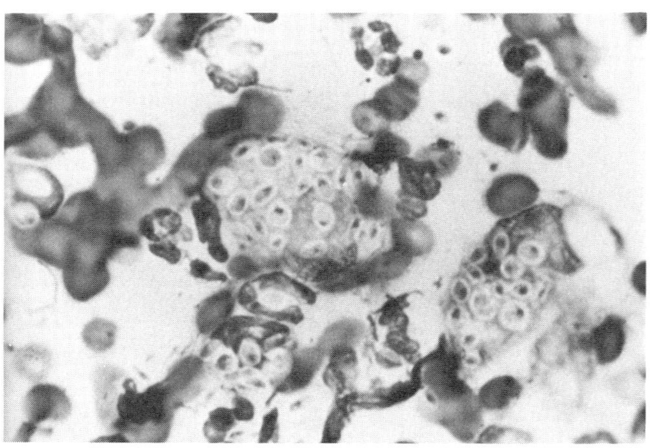

Figure 21–8. Aspirate from a cat with sporotrichosis. Many macrophages and neutrophils containing small (2 to 4 μm) organisms with thin, clear halos are present. The organisms may be round, oval, or fusiform. The fusiform shape of some *Sporotrichum* organisms readily distinguishes them from *Histoplasma* organisms. (Original magnification 250×, Wright's stain.) (Courtesy of Oklahoma State University Clinical Pathology Teaching File.)

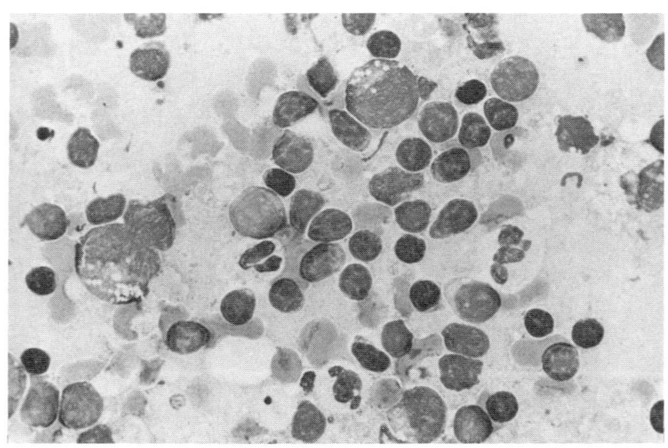

Figure 21–10. Aspirate from a lymph node with neutrophilic lymphadenitis. Small lymphocytes are the predominant cell type; however, neutrophils are present in mildly to moderately increased numbers. (Original magnification 250×, Wright's stain.) (Courtesy of Oklahoma State University Clinical Pathology Teaching File.)

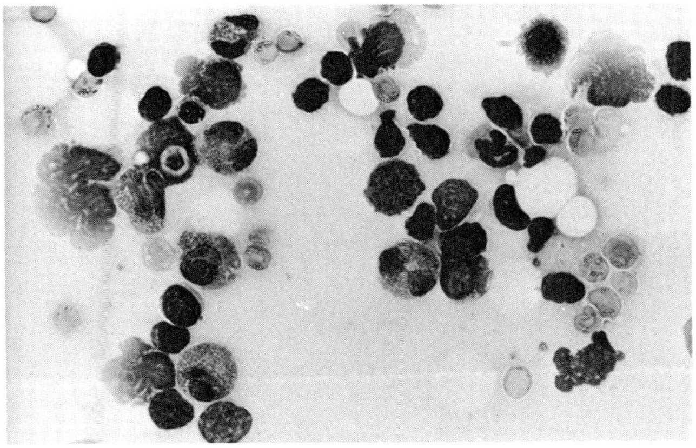

Figure 21–11. Aspirate from a cat with eosinophilic lymphadenitis. Small lymphocytes are the predominant cell type present; however, eosinophils are present in markedly increased numbers. (Original magnification 250×, Wright's stain.) (Courtesy of Oklahoma State University Clinical Pathology Teaching File.)

nuclear chromatin, which stains much more eosinophilic than the nuclear chromatin of intact lymphocytes. Lymphoblasts tend to be more fragile than small lymphocytes and rupture more easily. Therefore, lymphosarcoma may be present, but masked due to a high number of ruptured cells in the smear. Cytologic smears with a high percentage of ruptured lymphocytes limit the cytologic interpretation and, if sufficient number of lymphocytes are ruptured, the lymph node should be reaspirated. If lymphosarcoma cannot be recognized on cytologic smears but is still suspected clinically, an excisional biopsy should be performed. The entire lymph node, incised at one-fourth inch intervals, should be submitted in 10% buffered formalin for histopathologic evaluation. This allows the pathologist to evaluate the nodal architecture that is lost on cytologic smears.

4. ***Nonlymphoid Neoplasia.*** Metastatic neoplasia may be recognized by finding moderate to high numbers of cells that are not normally found in lymph node aspirates and that have 3 or more nuclear criteria of malignancy. They may also be recognized by finding cells that are typically present only in very low numbers but are now present in high numbers. Malignant epithelial cell tumors (carcinomas and adenocarcinomas) and mast cell tumors are the most common type of nonlymphoid neoplasia seen in lymph node aspirates. Finding large epithelial cells with coarse nuclear chromatin and large, prominent, frequently angular nucleoli on cytologic preparations from lymph nodes indicates a malignant epithelial tumor (Fig. 21–13). Epithelial cells may occur singly or in clusters and frequently show marked variation in cell and nuclear size. Evidence of secretory products (vacuolation) may be identified in adenocarcinomas. Mast cell neoplasms are recognized by finding large numbers of round cells with round to oval nuclei that contain high numbers of small, red-purple (metachromatic), intracytoplasmic granules (Fig. 21–14). These granules are characteristic of mast cells.

    Malignant spindle cell tumors (sarcomas) are only rarely identified in lymph-node aspirates. High numbers of cells with cytoplasm that trails away from the nucleus in one or more directions and have many criteria of malignancy indicate a malignant spindle cell tumor.

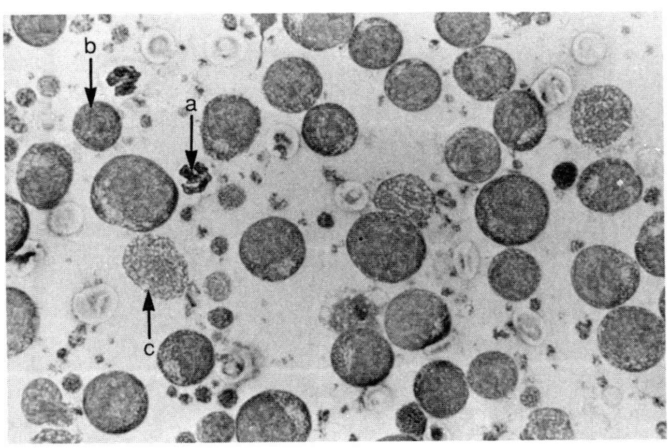

Figure 21–12. Aspirate from a lymph node with lymphosarcoma. Lymphoblasts are the predominant cell type present. Lymphoblasts are larger than neutrophils (*A*). Many lymphoglandular bodies (*B*) and a small lymphocyte (*C*) are also present. (Original magnification 250×, Wright's stain.) (Courtesy of Oklahoma State University Clinical Pathology Teaching File.)

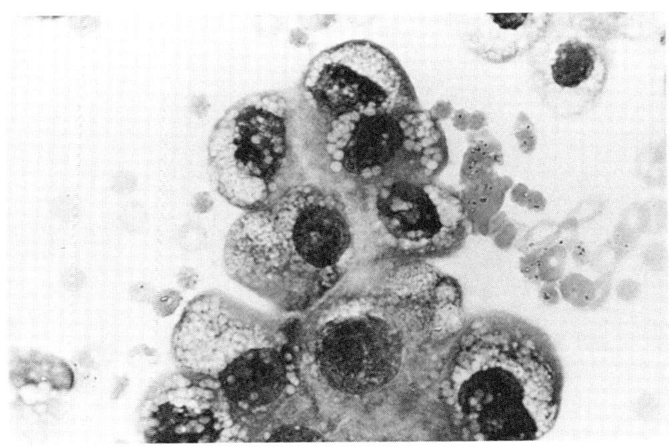

Figure 21–13. Carcinoma cells are large (epithelial) cells. They show marked variation in cell size, nuclear size, have large prominent nucleoli, and basophilic cytoplasm. Evidence of secretory production allows the cells to be classified as adenocarcinoma. (Original magnification 250×, Wright's stain.) (Courtesy of Oklahoma State University Clinical Pathology Teaching File.)

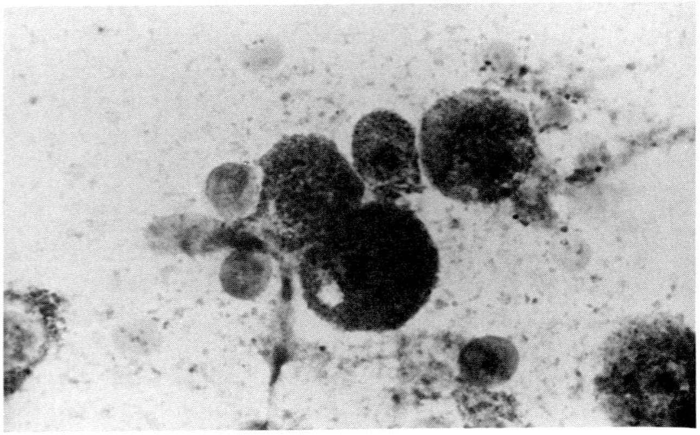

Figure 21–14. Mast cell neoplasms are recognized by finding high numbers of round cells with round to oval nuclei that contain high numbers of small, red-purple (metachromatic), intracytoplasmic granules. (Original magnification 250×, Wright's stain.) (Courtesy of Oklahoma State University Clinical Pathology Teaching File.)

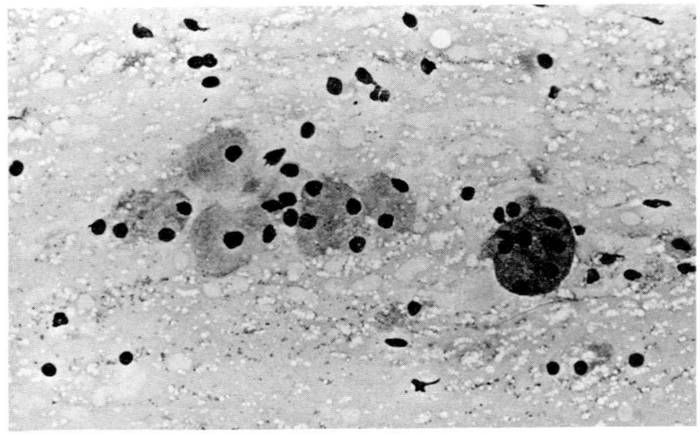

Figure 21–16. Salivary gland aspirates consist of large, uniform cells with abundant, slightly blue, foamy cytoplasm. These cells may be present individually or in clusters. The background consists of heavy eosinophilic, mucoid material. (Original magnification 100×, Wright's stain.) (Courtesy of Oklahoma State University Clinical Pathology Teaching File.)

Aspiration of Nonlymphoid Tissue

Perinodal fat is the most common tissue accidentally aspirated during lymph-node aspiration. Grossly, fat can be recognized on the slide by its wet (oily) appearance and its failure to dry. If all the lipocytes are ruptured or only fat droplets are aspirated (instead of intact fat cells), no material may be identified cytologically because most hematologic stains contain alcohol, which dissolves fat droplets. However, if intact fat cells are aspirated, they are easily recognizable microscopically (Fig. 21–15).

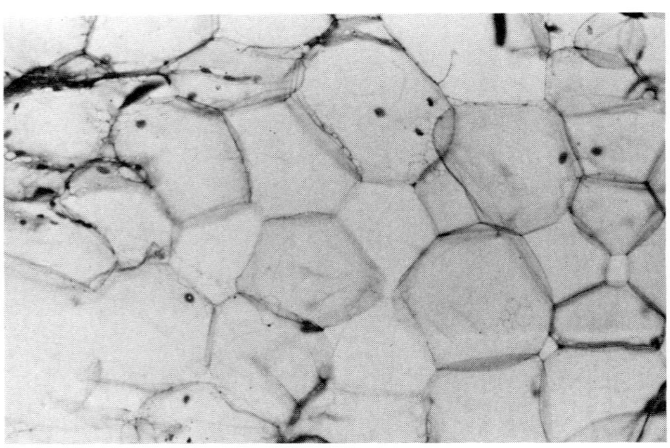

Figure 21–15. Lipocytes are readily recognized as large cells with abundant, clear-staining cytoplasm, and a small, round to oval nucleus. (Original magnification 50×, Wright's stain.) (Courtesy of Oklahoma State University Clinical Pathology Teaching File.)

Salivary gland tissue may be accidentally aspirated when submandibular lymph-node aspirations are attempted. Smears made from salivary gland aspirates usually consist of salivary cells, singly and in clusters, in a background of heavy eosinophilic material (Fig. 21–16). Salivary gland cells are recognized as uniform, medium to large cells that have abundant, slightly blue, foamy cytoplasm. Their nuclei are usually of uniform size and round with dense chromatin. Care should be taken not to confuse these cells with neoplastic cells.

Clinical Application

When a cat is presented with localized, regionalized, or generalized lymphadenopathy, the diagnostic approach should be developed by considering the likely possibilities just discussed. A minimum data base should be performed consisting of a CBC, chemistry profile, FeLV antigen test, and a lymph-node aspiration. If these tests do not render a definitive diagnosis, a lymph node excisional biopsy is indicated.

REFERENCES

1. Duncan JR. The Lymph Nodes. In: Cowell RL, Tyler RD, eds. Diagnostic Cytology of the Dog and Cat. American Veterinary Publications, 1989;93.
2. Perman V, Alsaker RD, Riis RO. Cytology of the Dog and Cat. Denver, CO: American Animal Hospital Association, 1979:11.
3. Rebar AH. Handbook of Veterinary Cytology. St. Louis, MO: Ralston Purina Co., 1980.
4. Tyler RD, Cowell RL, Baldwin CF, Morton RJ. Introduction. In: Cowell RL, Tyler RD, eds. Diagnostic Cytology of the Dog and Cat. American Veterinary Publications, 1989:1.
5. Tyler RD, Cowell RL. Diagnostic Approach to Lymph Node Disorders. In: August JR, ed. Consultations in Feline Internal Medicine. Philadelphia: WB Saunders, 1991:367.

CHAPTER 22

◇ ◇ ◇

Polyuria and Polydipsia

R. Steve Taylor

Water consumption and urine production usually have a direct correlation. Under normal conditions as water consumption increases, urine production increases; as water consumption decreases, urine production decreases. Physiologic variations in the amount of water consumed or the amount of urine produced occur daily as the body makes adjustments to maintain plasma volume and osmolality within normal ranges. Water consumption in excess of 100 mL/kg/day is considered abnormal and is referred to as polydipsia (PD). Urine production above 50 mL/kg/day is considered abnormal and is referred to as polyuria (PU).[1,2] If plasma volume and osmolality are to remain normal, PD must result in compensatory PU, and PU must result in compensatory PD. A condition of either excessive water consumption with resulting excessive urination or vice versa is referred to as the PU/PD syndrome.

The PU/PD syndrome is a pair of related clinical signs that is a manifestation of disease and not a definitive diagnosis.[3] Recognition and documentation of the PU/PD syndrome enables the veterinarian to formulate a list of possible causes that can be differentiated through appropriate testing.

Normal Body Water Regulation

Regulation of the cat's plasma volume and concentration depends on recognition of abnormalities by volume and osmolality sensors, appropriate hormonal release, and response by the thirst center and kidneys. Volume sensors, called baroreceptors, are located in the left atrium, aorta, and the carotid sinus. Hypovolemia and hypotension stimulate the baroreceptors, resulting in the release of antidiuretic hormone (ADH) through stimulation of the supraoptic and paraventricular nuclei of the hypothalamus. The consequence of these actions in the normal cat is the retention of more water by the kidneys, thus expanding the extracellular fluid volume. Plasma concentration receptors, called osmoreceptors, are located in the area of the anterioventral aspect of the third ventricle of the brain. Hemoconcentration, primarily hypernatremia, results in the release of ADH from the hypothalamus. The consequence is the retention of more water by the kidneys, thus reducing plasma osmolality through dilution.

The relationship between increasing plasma osmolality and ADH secretion is linear, while the relationship between decreasing blood volume and ADH secretion is exponential.[4] Under normal physiologic conditions, increases in ADH secretion are not seen until blood volume decreases by 5% to 10%. Because the stimulation for release of ADH is stronger with volume depletion than with increased plasma osmolality, the resulting ADH release is greater, resulting in greater water retention by the kidneys.[4]

Stimulation of the thirst center is also regulated by plasma volume depletion and increases in plasma osmolality. While the release of ADH and the renal response to ADH is rapid, the intake of water and its reabsorption allow a more gradual adjustment of the extracellular fluid volume and osmolality. Although less immediate in its effect, stimulation of the thirst response is often sufficient to prevent severe plasma hypertonicity. Even in the absence of ADH, if the cat has access to sufficient water, drinks, and does not vomit, hypertonicity will not develop.

Causes of Polydipsia and Polyuria

There are many different causes of PU/PD in the cat. These can be classified in a number of different ways. If the causes are classified on the basis of pathophysiology (Table 22–1), the general categories are diabetes insipidus (those disorders associated with decreased production or inappropriate responses to ADH, either primary or secondary), osmotic diuresis, and primary polydipsia (a disorder associated with normal ADH levels and inappropriate water consumption).[4]

Other considerations include recent dietary changes or current drug therapy. Some diets (i.e., Feline Prescription Diet s/d®, Hill's Pet Products, Topeka, KS) and some commercially available cat treats are high in salt and may cause changes in water consumption and urine production. Certain drugs, such as phenobarbital, megestrol acetate, and diuretics, can influence water consumption and urinary output. It would be unusual for dietary or pharmacologic causes to produce true PU/PD; however, they could cause abrupt increases that would be noticed by the owner.

The relative frequency of the different causes of PU/PD is listed in Table 22–2. It is notable that three causes (renal disease, diabetes mellitus, and hyperthyroidism) account for

Table 22–1. Frequency of Diagnoses in 32 Cats with PU/PD[3]

Renal	50%
Diabetes mellitus	33%
Hyperthyroidism	10%
Hyperadrenocorticism	3%
Hepatic	3%

93% of the diagnoses.[3] While these statistics were derived from referral cases and from a small number of cases (32), the data reflect a relatively true frequency of the causes of PU/PD based on the author's experience.

Primary Diabetes Insipidus

Primary diabetes insipidus, central or nephrogenic, is one of the least common causes of PU/PD in the cat.[4] Central diabetes insipidus (CDI) may be partial or complete based on the amount of ADH produced. When the amount of ADH produced is inadequate relative to the stimulus, the condition is termed "partial CDI." Partial production of ADH results in a limited but not maximal urine-concentration response by the kidneys. Complete CDI results in a dilute urine (urine specific gravity: 1.000 to 1.007) irrespective of the state of hydration of the cat.[2,5]

Deficiency in ADH secretion can occur because of congenital/hereditary causes, secondary damage to the neurohypophyseal system (trauma, neoplasia), or idiopathic causes.[6] CDI resulting from congenital/hereditary causes is rare and would be expected in young kittens. Damage to the neurohypophyseal system is usually secondary to trauma.[6,7] Head trauma can cause transient or permanent CDI. Idiopathy is the most common cause.[8]

Primary nephrogenic diabetes insipidus (NDI) is a disorder of the kidneys characterized by renal tubular insensitivity to ADH. The disorder may be partial or complete, but it has never been reported in the cat.

Table 22–2. Pathologic Causes of PU/PD

Primary Diabetes Insipidus

Central
- Partial
- Complete

Nephrogenic*
- Partial
- Complete

Secondary Nephrogenic Diabetes Insipidus

Renal disease
Hyperthyroidism
Pyometra
Hypercalcemia
Hepatic disease
Hypokalemia
Hyperadrenocorticism
Hypoadrenocorticism
Hypercalcemia
Acromegaly

Osmotic Diuresis

Diabetes mellitus
Primary glucosuria
Postobstructive diuresis

Primary Polydipsia

Psychogenic polydipsia

*Not reported in the cat.

Secondary Nephrogenic Diabetes Insipidus

Disorders that affect the kidneys, either resulting in insensitivity to ADH, inability to respond to ADH, or decrease in the hypertonicity of the medullary interstitium (medullary washout), constitute the category of secondary nephrogenic diabetes insipidus.[8] These disorders include renal insufficiency, hyperthyroidism, pyometra, hypercalcemia, hepatic insufficiency, pyelonephritis, hypokalemia, hyperadrenocorticism, hypoadrenocorticism, and acromegaly.

Medullary hypertonicity is necessary for water movement through tubular cells following ADH enhancement of cell membrane permeability.[9] Decreasing medullary hypertonicity causes urine concentrations to fall, even in the presence of excessive ADH.[1] Medullary washout results only in a limitation of the kidney's ability to concentrate nondilute urine and must be considered in the pathogenesis of any chronic polyuric disorder. Unfortunately, medullary washout is a poorly defined entity in the clinical assessment of cat with PU/PD. There is no direct means of determining the amplitude or the degree of loss of the medullary concentration gradient.[9] Decreased medullary hypertonicity is often secondary to other causes of PU/PD; but, even when these other causes are corrected, renal urine concentrating ability will not return to normal until medullary washout is corrected.

Renal Disease

Renal insufficiency is the most common cause of the PU/PD syndrome (Table 22–1). As nephrons are damaged or destroyed and renal reserve is lost, each remaining nephron must adapt in order to accommodate the excretion of increased amounts of solute and water (see Chapter 31). With the increased tubular flow rate reducing the amounts of urea, sodium, and other substances that are reabsorbed, a decrease in the hypertonicity of the medullary interstitium occurs.[8] The production of increased amounts of urine due to decreased urine concentrating ability occurs prior to azotemia in the progression of renal dysfunction. The PU/PD cat in renal failure is often diagnosed because of azotemia, hyperphosphatemia, nonregenerative anemia, and palpably abnormal kidneys. The nonazotemic, polyuric cat with renal insufficiency may require a modified water deprivation test (WDT), endogenous creatinine clearance, and renal biopsy to make a definitive diagnosis.

Pyelonephritis is infrequently documented in the ill or necropsied cat and is an infrequent cause of PU/PD.[19] Infection within the renal pelvis can destroy the countercurrent mechanism in the medulla by decreasing hypertonicity, resulting in polyuria.[8] The cat with pyelonephritis may have fever, pyuria, hematuria, renal pain, and pollakiuria.

Table 22–3. Frequency of Clinical Signs, Abnormal Laboratory Findings, and Abnormal Radiographs in 183 Cats with Pyometra

		Number	Percent
Clinical Signs			
Detected by Owner			
Vaginal discharge		109/183	59
Anorexia		73/183	40
Lethargy		59/183	32
Vomiting		29/183	16
Abdominal distension		32/183	17
Polyuria/polydipsia		17/183	9
Weight loss		6/183	3
Detected by Physical Examination			
Vaginal discharge		126/183	68
Abdominal distention		75/183	40
Palpable uterus		72/183	39
Dehydration		61/183	33
Pyrexia		37/183	20
Laboratory Findings			
Leukocytosis	>15,000 cells/mm^3	109/163	66
Hyperproteinemia	>7.8 g/dL	46/150	30
Normal WBC count		46/163	28
Azotemia	Creat >1.0 mg/dL	19/150	12
Hypokalemia	<3.3 mEq/dL	16/150	10
Increased SGPT	>80 IU/L	11/150	7
Leukopenia	<7,000 cells/mm^3	8/163	5
Anemia	PCV <25%	7/163	4
Hyperbilirubinemia	>1.0 mg/d	13/150	8
Abdominal Radiographs			
Enlarged uterus		138/169	81
Normal		18/169	10
Ascites		9/169	5
Solitary abdominal mass		4/169	2

Used by permission: Kenny KJ, Matthiesen DT, Brown NO, Bradley RL. Pyometra in cats: 183 cases (1979–1984). J Amer Vet Med Assoc 1987;191:1130.

Hyperthyroidism

Hyperthyroidism is the most common endocrinopathy in the cat and the third most common cause of PU/PD.[3] In approximately 50% of the cats with hyperthyroidism, PU/PD is present at the time of the initial examination.[10] Polyuria due to hyperthyroidism is probably the result of an increase in renal medullary blood flow resulting in a decreased medullary hypertonicity. Diagnosis is usually based on an elevation in the serum thyroxine level, a T3 suppression test, or a positive thyroid scan[14] (see Chapter 46).

Pyometra

Pyometra is another infrequent cause of PU/PD. PU/PD was one of the presenting complaints in only about 10% of the 183 cases of pyometra reported in one series.[11] PU is the result of the effect of endotoxins produced by *Escherichia coli* on the distal renal tubules, causing an insensitivity to ADH.[8] In the dog, the endotoxins decrease medullary hypertonicity by interfering with the reabsorption of sodium and chloride.[4] Diagnosis can be made using history, palpation, radiographs, and ultrasound (see Table 22–3 and Chapter 54).

Hypercalcemia

Hypercalcemia is an infrequent cause of PU/PD in the cat because it may occur without PU/PD. In seven cats presented with hypercalcemia (mean value: 15.8 mg/dL), only two had PU/PD.[12] Hypercalcemia has been reported with neoplasia (lymphosarcoma, parathyroid tumors, metastatic bone tumors, myelomas,[13] and squamous cell carcinomas[14]), renal disease, hypoadrenocorticism,[15] and vitamin D toxicosis from ingestion of cholecalciferol-containing rodenticides.[16] Hypercalcemia may induce histologic renal lesions or interfere with the action of ADH on the renal collecting ducts, resulting in PU.[17] Diagnosis is based on demonstration of a persistent hypercalcemia.

Hepatic Disease

Polyuria and polydipsia are reported in the cat secondary to hepatic insufficiency and disease.[4] Because of decreased synthesis of urea in the severely diseased liver, urea concentration in the medullary interstitium is lowered, resulting in a reduction in urine concentrating ability. By the time interstitial hypertonicity is reduced and PU/PD develops, hepatic disease has usually been diagnosed because of the occurrence of other clinical signs such as anorexia, vomiting, or icterus. With hepatic insufficiency, hormones such as renin and cortisol, which normally undergo rapid degradation in the liver, have an increased blood level. While the cat's kidneys do not seem sensitive to cortisol,[18] hyperreninemia may cause hyperaldosteronemia resulting in renal potassium wasting, sodium retention, and thirst stimulation and lead to the development of PU/PD.[4] Diagnosis of hepatic insufficiency is based on decreased BUN and albumin, elevated bile acids and liver enzymes, aspiration cytology, and hepatic biopsy.

Hypokalemia

Hypokalemia can cause polyuria by decreasing renal tubular solute resorption and medullary hypertonicity and by reducing renal tubular response to ADH.[20] Low body potassium is due to lack of potassium intake, loss of potassium, or both. Loss of potassium through urine is particularly important in cats with renal abnormalities.[21] In one study, hypokalemia was the most common electrolyte abnormality in cats with naturally occurring renal disease.[22]

Hyperadrenocorticism

Hyperadrenocorticism in the cat is not characterized clinically by PU/PD.[17] However, hyperadrenocorticism can cause diabetes mellitus through insulin resistance (glucose intolerance). PU/PD develops secondary to the osmotic diuresis associated with the glucosuria. Hyperadrenocorticism is unlikely in a cat presenting with PU/PD without diabetes mellitus. While not common, hyperadrenocorticism should be considered in insulin-resistant diabetes mellitus cases. Diagnosis of hyperadrenocorticism is based on testing of the pituitary–adrenocortical axis using the adrenocorticotrophic hormone (ACTH) stimulation test or the low-dose dexamethasone screening test. Unlike the dog, feline adrenal calcification is generally not indicative of an adrenal tumor[14] (Table 22–4).

Hypoadrenocorticism

Hypoadrenocorticism, a rare disease in the cat, can cause PU/PD. In one study, two of eight cats with hypoadrenocorticism presented with PU/PD.[15] Inappropriate urine specific gravity (less than 1.030) relative to the degree of dehydration and azotemia indicated an impaired urine concentrating ability in four of the five cats tested.[15] Polyuria is the result of sodium wasting due to hypoaldosteronism. Hypoadrenocorticism in the cat should be suspected based on the presence of hyperkalemia, hyponatremia, poor capillary refill time, and weakness. A definitive diagnosis is based on the lack of response to the ACTH stimulation test (Table 22–5).

Acromegaly

Acromegaly, caused by excessive growth hormone (GH), causes PU/PD through either diabetes mellitus secondary to insulin resistance or hypothalamic/pituitary dysfunction secondary to a space-occupying mass. The two cats that the

Table 22–4. Clinical Signs and Abnormal Laboratory Findings in 18 Cats with Hyperadrenocorticism

	Number	Percent
Clinical Signs		
Polyuria/polydipsia	17/18	94
Pot-bellied appearance	17/18	94
Increased appetite	16/18	89
Hair loss	13/18	72
Muscle wasting	12/18	67
Obesity	11/18	61
Hepatomegaly	10/18	56
Infection	7/18	39
Thin skin	6/18	33
Weight loss	2/18	11
Diarrhea	2/18	11
Laboratory Findings*		
Hyperglycemia	14/14	100
Hypercholesterolemia	12/14	86
Glucosuria	14/17	82
Lymphopenia	8/12	67
Eosinopenia	7/12	58
Mature leukocytosis	5/12	42
Increased serum alkaline phosphatase	5/14	36

*Complete laboratory data were not performed in all reported cases.

Used by permission: Petersen ME, Randolph JR. Endocrine Diseases. In: Sherding RG, ed. The Cat: Diseases and Clinical Management. New York: Churchill Livingstone, 1989:1095.

Table 22–5. Clinical Signs and Abnormal Laboratory Findings in Eight Cats with Primary Hypoadrenocorticism

	Number	Percent
Clinical Signs		
Lethargy	8	100
Anorexia	8	100
Weight loss	8	100
Dehydration	7	88
Weakness	6	75
Slow capillary refill-time	5	63
Weak pulse	4	50
Microcardia	4	50
Vomiting	2	25
Polyuria/polydipsia	2	25
Bradycardia	1	13
Laboratory Findings		
Hyperkalemia	8	100
Hyponatremia	8	100
Hypochloremia	8	100
Azotemia	8	100
Hyperphosphatemia	7	88
Lymphocytosis	3	38
Anemia	2	25
Eosinophilia	1	13
Hypercalcemia	1	13

Used by permission: Petersen ME, Randolph JR. Endocrine Diseases. In: Sherding RG, ed. The Cat: Diseases and Clinical Management. New York: Churchill Livingstone, 1989;1095.

Table 22–6. Frequency of Clinical Signs and Abnormal Laboratory Findings in Eight Cats with Acromegaly

	Number	Percent
Clinical Signs		
Polyuria/polydipsia	8	100
Heart murmur	7	88
Cardiomegaly	7	88
Hepatomegaly	7	88
Nephromegaly	5	63
Renal failure	5	63
Large head	5	63
Weight gain	4	50
Arthritis	4	50
Spondylosis	4	50
Large mandible (prognathia inferior)	4	50
Large endocrine organs	3	38
Pot belly	3	38
Large tongue	2	25
Circling	2	25
Laboratory Findings		
Hyperglycemia/glucosuria	8	100
Hyperproteinemia	6	75
Azotemia	5	63
Hyperphosphatemia	4	50
Hypercholesterolemia	3	38
Increased SGPT (alanine aminotransferase)	3	38
Erythrocytosis	3	38
Increased serum alkaline phosphatase	1	13
Ketonuria	1	13

Used by permission: Petersen ME, Randolph JR. Endocrine Diseases. In: Sherding RG, ed The Cat: Diseases and Clinical Management. New York: Churchill Livingstone, 1989:1095.

author has diagnosed and treated had daily insulin requirements in excess of 100 units per day. Acromegaly is uncommon and is caused by a tumor in the hypothalamic-pituitary region. Diagnosis is based on demonstration of an elevated GH level, which does not suppress following glucose administration, or demonstration of a mass in the pituitary region accompanied by insulin-resistant diabetes mellitus and a normal ACTH stimulation test.[23] GH level testing is not commercially available; however, a veterinary endocrinologist should be consulted concerning availability through a veterinary college or research institution (Table 22–6).

Osmotic Diuresis

Polyuria and polydipsia may be caused by a group of disorders characterized by the excretion of osmotically active urine. These disorders are of diabetes mellitus, euglycemic glucosuria, and posturethral obstruction. Renal insufficiency also is characterized by the excretion of osmotically active urine (osmotic diuresis) and a decrease in the hypertonicity of the medulla (secondary nephrogenic diabetes insipidus), thus allowing it also to be classified in either category.

Diabetes Mellitus

Diabetes mellitus (DM) is the second most common cause of PU/PD in the cat (Table 22–1) and the second most common feline endocrinopathy. As the blood glucose concentration exceeds renal tubular capacity for reabsorption (250 to 350 mg/dL), glucosuria results in diuresis because of the osmotic effect of the glucose. Care must be used in interpreting random blood-glucose determinations because of stress hyperglycemia (see Chapter 34).

Euglycemic Glucosuria

Glucosuria without corresponding hyperglycemia is an uncommon cause of osmotic diuresis. This form of glucosuria can be the result of a congenital or transient defect in the proximal renal tubule. Infection and secondary renal damage from certain drugs can cause a transient glucosuria in a euglycemic cat.

Postobstructive Diuresis

Posturethral obstruction diuresis is seen most commonly following urethral blockage in male cats with the feline urologic syndrome. Because of marked elevations in the BUN during the obstructive period, there is a dramatic osmotic diuresis once the obstruction is relieved. When the solute load is excreted, diuresis subsides. Care should be taken to monitor the state of hydration during the diuresis period to prevent dehydration of the patient.

Primary Polydipsia

Primary polydipsia is a rare disorder associated with compulsive water drinking. It is reported in the dog but is not well documented in the cat.[14] The cause is usually psychogenic and seems to follow some change in the cat's environment. This is the only disorder in which polydipsia is the driving force, instead of the compensatory component, in the PU/PD syndrome.

Diagnostic Approach

History

When the presenting complaint is polydipsia, polyuria, or both, a thorough history may provide information as to severity, duration, and even cause. The cat's environment (single- versus multiple-cat household) and life-style (indoors or outdoors) are important factors in evaluating the owner's observations and in determining the best method of verification of the presence of PU/PD. For example, PU/PD may go unnoticed for a prolonged period in an outdoor cat or in a cat in a multiple-cat household. Recent changes in water consumption or urinary habits should be evaluated relative to the patient's physical condition, medication history, and diet. Appropriate physiologic changes in water consumption and urine production may occur in cats with fever, after boarding or hospitalization (water deprivation), with recent dietary changes, or due to certain medications.

Physical Examination

The physical examination in the cat with a historical change in water consumption of urine production is important.

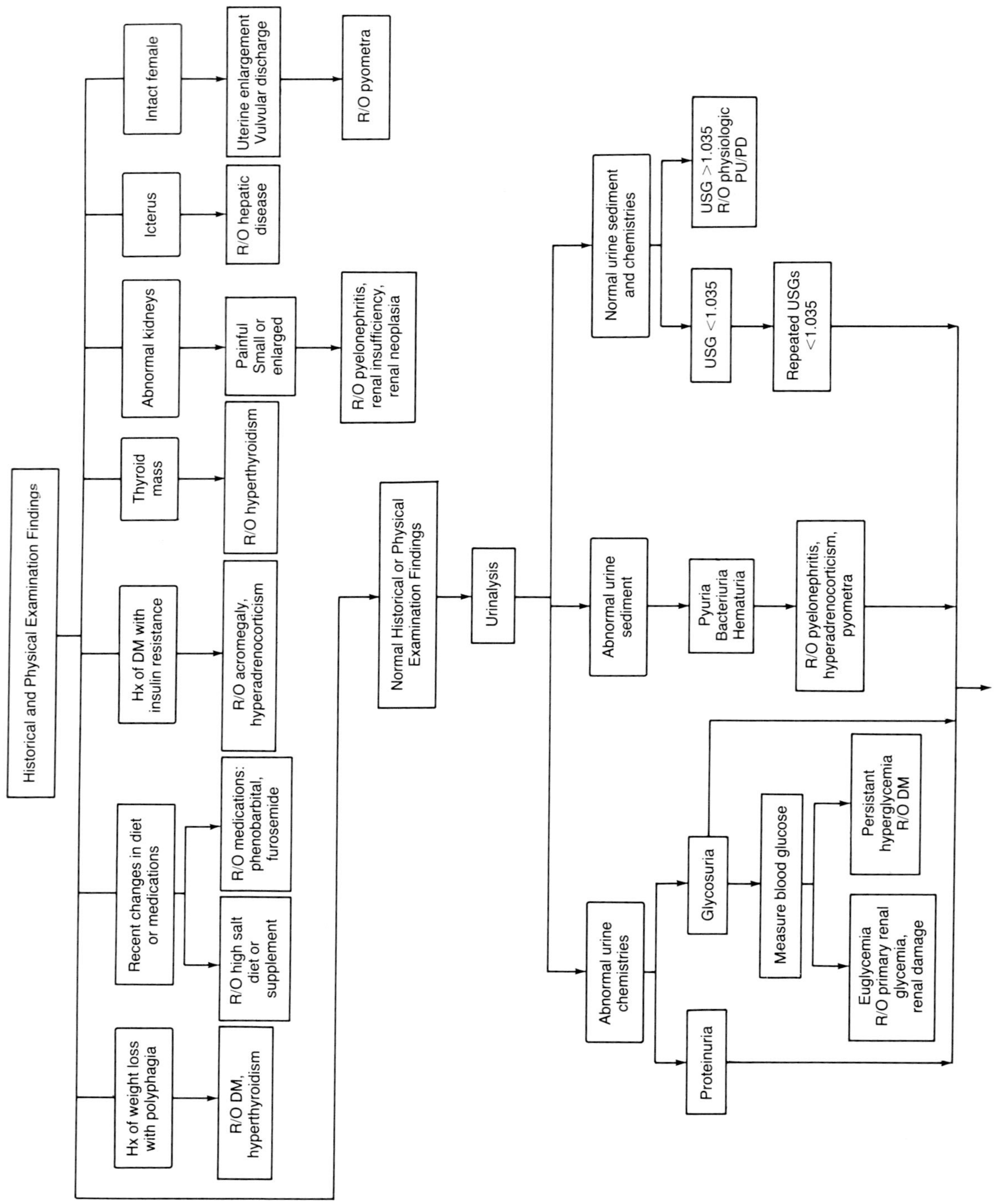
Historical and Physical Examination Findings
Hx of weight loss with polyphagia
R/O DM, hyperthyroidism
Recent changes in diet or medications
R/O high salt diet or supplement
R/O medications: phenobarbital, furosemide
Hx of DM with insulin resistance
R/O acromegaly, hyperadrenocorticism
Thyroid mass
R/O hyperthyroidism
Abnormal kidneys
Painful Small or enlarged
R/O pyelonephritis, renal insufficiency, renal neoplasia
Icterus
R/O hepatic disease
Intact female
Uterine enlargement Vulvular discharge
R/O pyometra
Normal Historical or Physical Examination Findings
Urinalysis
Abnormal urine chemistries
Proteinuria
Glycosuria
Measure blood glucose
Euglycemia R/O primary renal glycemia, renal damage
Persistant hyperglycemia R/O DM
Abnormal urine sediment
Pyuria Bacteriuria Hematuria
R/O pyelonephritis, hyperadrenocorticism, pyometra
Normal urine sediment and chemistries
USG <1.035
Repeated USGs <1.035
USG >1.035 R/O physiologic PU/PD

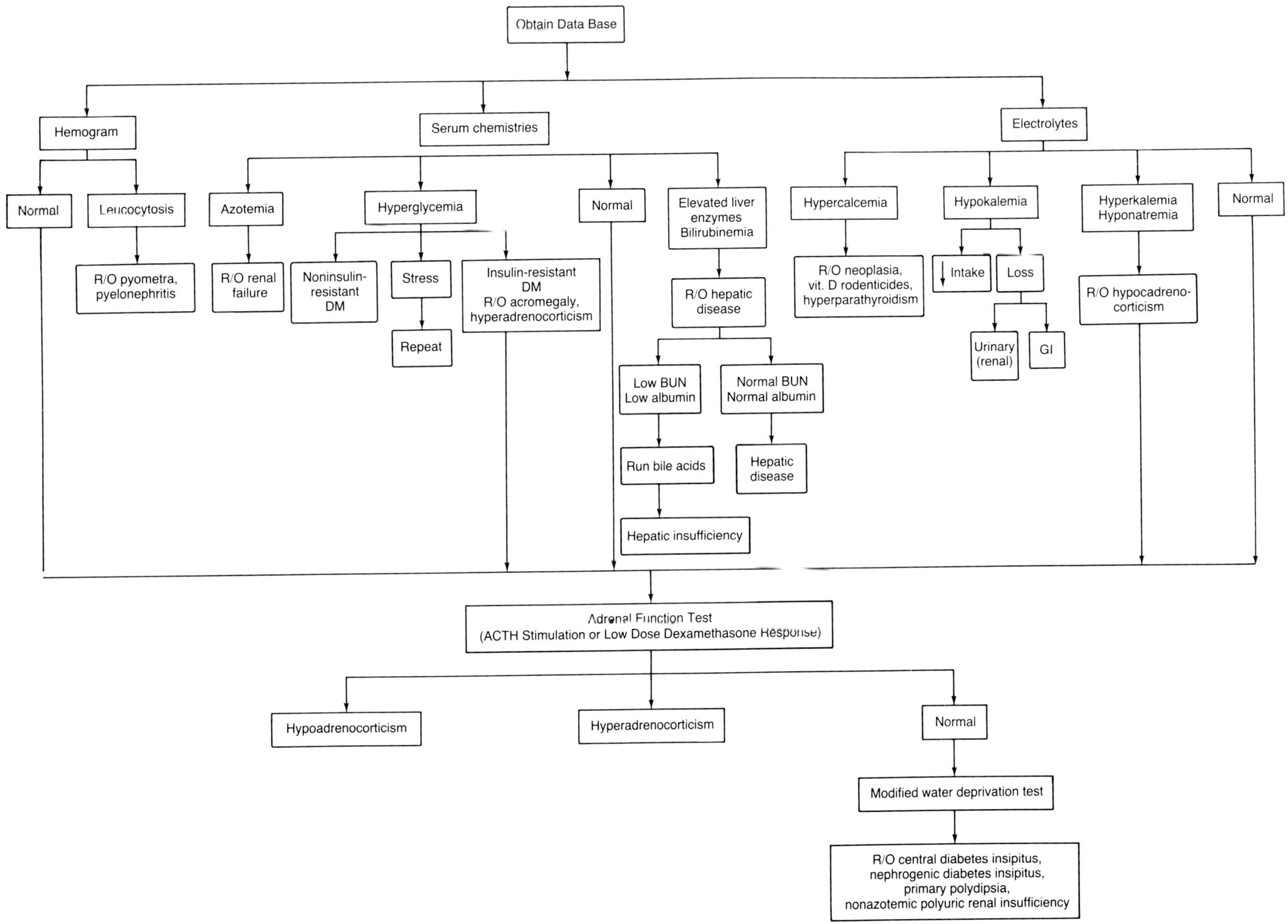

Figure 22–1. Evaluation of a cat with a polyuria/polydipsia complaint.

Some abnormal physical findings may provide enough information to lead to a definitive diagnosis (Fig. 22–1). In addition, the physical examination may identify unrelated but potentially complicating problems such as heart disease or neoplasia.

Verification

If no significant abnormalities are identified by history or physical examination, verification of the PU/PD syndrome should be the next step. Verification can be done through measurement of water consumption or urine production. However, documentation by either method can be difficult in the cat. Fortunately actual measurement of water intake or urine production is not absolutely necessary since PU/PD can be indirectly confirmed in the cat through evaluation of multiple urinalyses. The urinalysis (U/A) can be the major key to establishing the presence of the polyuric state.[5] If the urine is normal (see below) and the urine specific gravity (USG) is greater than 1.035, PU/PD is not present and the increase in water consumption and urinary output is caused by a physiologic rather than pathologic reason. A USG less than 1.035 suggests that a concentration deficit with resulting polyuria is present.[9] If the urinary sediment or chemistries are abnormal (pyuria, glucosuria, hematuria) or if the USG is less than 1.035 on repeated U/As (no less than 3), a minimum data base (MDB) is recommended (Table 22–7).

Table 22–7. Recommended Data Base for Cats with PU/PD

1. Complete blood count (CBC)
2. Serum chemistries and electrolytes

BUN	Alkaline Phosphatase
Creatinine	ALT (SGPT)
Total Protein	AST (SGOT)
Albumin	Total bilirubin
Glucose	Direct bilirubin
Calcium	Triglycerides
Phosphorus	Sodium
Total CO_2	Potassium
CPK	Chloride

3. Complete urinalysis
   - Urine chemistries
     - Glucose
     - Ketones
     - Bilirubin
     - Urobilinogen
     - Protein
     - Blood
   - Urine sediment
     - White blood cells
     - Red blood cells
     - Casts
     - Epithelial cells
     - Crystals
   - Specific gravity
4. T_4

Minimum Data Base

The MDB will identify the majority of the less common causes of PU/PD (Fig. 22–1). A complete urinalysis, including chemistries, USG, and microscopic examination of sediment, provides important information in the PU/PD patient. It may identify potential polyuria before it has been noticed by the owner, especially in a multiple-cat household situation or outdoor cat. Additionally, it may identify renal protein loss leading to detection of early renal disease including glomerulonephritis.

Other Tests

The MDB will generally permit a rapid diagnosis. However, if it does not, PU/PD will likely be caused by diabetes insipidus, nonazotemic polyuric renal insufficiency, primary polydipsia, or hyperadrenocorticism. Hyperadrenocorticism occurring with PU/PD without associated DM is unlikely. If the clinical signs are appropriate for hyperadrenocorticism, an ACTH-stimulation test or low-dose dexamethasone suppression test should be performed before proceeding to a WDT.

Nonazotemic polyuric renal disease or preazotemic chronic renal failure occurs when renal reserve is lost but adequate renal function exists to prevent azotemia. These cats have PU/PD with USGs that are less than 1.035. The urine sediment and urine chemistries may be normal. Physical examination may reveal abnormal renal size or shape; however, without azotemia, a definitive diagnosis is difficult. If nonazotemic polyuric renal disease is suspected, it is safer for the patient if the clinician performs an endogenous creatinine clearance (EnCC) (Table 22–8) than a WDT. The 24-hour urine collection method is more accurate than the 20-minute procedure, but it is also more labor intensive.[24] If the 24-hour protocol is performed, urine may be collected in nonabsorbent kitty litter. The WDT does not differentiate between partial DI and nonazotemic renal disease unless azotemia develops during the test. Fortunately, these diseases are uncommon.

Only eight cases of diabetes insipidus have been reported in the cat.[6,7,25-30] To differentiate between CDI, NDI, nonazotemic polyuric renal disease, and primary polydipsia in the cat requires a water deprivation test and/or administration of ADH or its analogue, desmopressin acetate. The WDT determines whether ADH is produced and released in response to dehydration and whether the kidneys can respond to the ADH. In theory, water deprivation testing should differentiate the above diseases easily. However, the kidneys, in order to respond to ADH maximally, require both adequate levels of ADH and an adequate hypertonicity in the medullary interstitium. Because medullary interstitial tonicity cannot be measured directly and because medullary washout can be caused by prolonged diuresis, the results of the WDT do not always yield clear differentiations of the above conditions. To get the maximum amount of information from the WDT, the effects of potential medullary washout should be minimized. (See Table 22–9 for the protocol for the WDT.)

Table 22–9 includes a recommendation concerning progressive water restriction prior to beginning the WDT to

Table 22–8. Protocol for Determining Endogenous Creatinine Clearance

24-Hour Collection

1. Make sure the urinary bladder is empty, either by voiding or catheterization.
2. Collect all urine produced during a 24-hour period, either by collection in a metabolic cage or periodic voiding or catheterization. Loss of more than a few milliliters of urine will abort the test. The bladder must be emptied at the end of the 24-hour period, preferably by catheterization.
3. Obtain a blood sample for serum creatinine determination approximately 12 hours into the test.

20-Minute Collection

1. Catheterize the urinary bladder and remove all urine (discard); rinse the bladder with saline. The catheter should be secured in the bladder for the duration of the test.
2. Begin the urine collection period immediately after rinsing the bladder. It is best to clamp the catheter for most of the collection period.
3. Obtain a blood sample for serum creatinine determination halfway through the collection period.
4. Begin collecting the urine in the bladder after approximately 18 minutes. Flush the bladder several times with saline; add the saline flushes to the urine collection. *Make sure that all urine and saline have been removed from the bladder.* If in doubt, extend the collection period; the time is not critical as long as the exact duration of the collection period is recorded.

Calculation of Clearance

1. Determine the creatinine concentration of each blood sample and an aliquot of each urine sample.
2. Use the following formula:*

$$C_{creat} = \frac{U_{creat} \times V}{SC \times T \times BW}$$

* C_{creat} = creatinine clearance, mL/min/kg
U_{creat} = urine creatinine concentration, mg/dL
V = urine volume, mL
SC = serum creatinine concentration, mg/dL
T = time of collection period, minutes
BW = body weight, kg

Table 22–9. Procedure for Water Deprivation Test

I. Preparation for the Test
  A. 72 hr prior: limit water intake to 120 mL/kg/day divided over course of the day
  B. 48 hr prior: limit water intake to 90 mL/kg/day divided as above
  C. 24 hr prior: limit water intake to 60 mL/kg/day divided
    1. Hospitalize the cat for 24 hr prior to the onset of water deprivation test (WDT)
    2. Weigh the cat and record weight
    3. Assess hydration throughout the day
    4. If 5% of the body weight is lost (5% dehydration), USG and BUN are checked
      a. if azotemia with a dilute USG (<1.030) develops, cat has renal insufficiency—*Do not do WDT*
      b. if not azotemic, then go directly to Phase II

II. Phase I
  A. Prior to beginning
    1. Withhold all food 12 hr prior to WDT
    2. Withhold all water at least 3 hr prior to WDT
    3. Empty the bladder completely and record USG (save sample)
    4. Obtain and record exact body weight (use same scale throughout the WDT). Calculate weight at which cat has 5% weight loss
    5. Obtain pre-WDT tests
      a. CBC
      b. serum chemistries (save serum)
      c. serum electrolytes
      d. U/A (save)
    6. Assess hydration status prior to beginning the WDT
  B. During the WDT
    1. Completely empty the bladder each time USG is done
    2. Weigh and record weight each time urine is obtained
    3. Time interval between USG/weights is every 2 hr unless weight loss is rapid, then every hour
    4. Check hydration
  C. End of the WDT
    1. When is Phase I of the WDT stopped?
      a. when 5% of body weight is lost
      b. when clinically 5% dehydrated
      c. when have same USG on 3 consecutive samples
      d. when USG is >1.030
    2. At end of phase I obtain the following:
      a. serum chemistries (save serum)
      b. serum electrolytes
      c. U/A (record and save)
      d. accurate weight and record
      e. Do BUN immediately before going to Phase II
    3. If the cat is dehydrated and azotemic, renal insufficiency is present regardless of other causes and the WDT is stopped

III. Phase II
  A. Continue to withhold food and water
  B. Administer aqueous vasopressin IM at rate of 0.5 U/kg
  C. Obtain USG and empty the bladder after each sampling
  D. Sampling should be done every 30 min for 2 hr (0, 30, 60, 90, 120)
  E. Assess hydration and CNS status

IV. After the Test
  A. Introduce small amounts of water (10–20 mL/kg) every 30 min for 2 hr
  B. Monitor patient's hydration and CNS status
  C. If the cat is doing well 2 hr after ending the WDT then return to water free choice

Adapted from: Feldman EC, Nelson RW. Polydipsia and Polyuria. In: Feldman EC, Nelson RW, eds. Canine and Feline Endocrinology and Reproduction. Philadelphia: WB Saunders, 1987:1.

Table 22–10. Disease Differentiation Based on Water Deprivation Test (WDT) and Azotemia

	WDT: Phase I	WDT: Phase II	BUN
CDI	No concentration	Concentration	Normal
NDI	No concentration	No concentration	Normal
Primary Polydipsia	Concentration	No concentration increase	Normal
Nonazotemic Polyuric Renal Insufficiency	Concentration*	No concentration increase	Increases (usually)

Concentration = urine specific gravity > 1.030
No concentration = urine specific gravity < 1.030
BUN = blood urea nitrogen
*Concentration = concentrates to a specific gravity higher than the pretest level but not as high as 1.030.

minimize the effects of medullary washout on the interpretation of results. The latter part of this restriction should be performed in the hospital. The WDT has two phases. During both phases, a urine sample is obtained and the bladder is completely emptied to ensure each sampling is of newly formed urine. Phase I is the creation of a state of dehydration to ensure maximal stimulation for ADH release. Phase II is based on the administration of exogenous vasopressin (ADH) to determine renal response to ADH. Failure of the USG to exceed 1.030 in the nonazotemic cat who has lost 5% of its body weight implies diabetes insipidus.[4]

Cats with complete CDI are unable to concentrate urine during Phase I but respond to exogenous ADH by increasing the USG to greater than 1.030. The cat with complete NDI should have a low USG at the end of Phase I and should not respond to exogenous ADH by increasing USG in Phase II. Partial CDI or NDI show an increase in USGs during Phase I (1.010 to 1.020) and, with the addition of exogenous ADH, can have USGs of 1.020 or greater. Nonazotemic renal insufficiency cannot be differentiated from partial DI unless azotemia develops during the WDT.

Cats with primary polydipsia should be able to concentrate their USGs to greater than 1.030 after water deprivation. Because of the normal level of ADH in a cat with primary polydipsia, an injection of exogenous ADH should not cause an increase in the USG.

The results of water deprivation testing for differentiating CDI, NDI, primary PD, and nonazotemic polyuric renal disease are given in Table 22–10.

Treatment*

Diabetes Insipidus

Cats with DI have significant PU/PD; however, polyuria and polydipsia do not pose a serious hazard to the cat. Treatment may not be necessary unless the polyuria and polydipsia are unacceptable to the owner. If the cat is not treated, access to water must never be restricted. Medical treatments are either hormonal or nonhormonal. Hormone replacement uses vasopressin tannate in oil (Pitressin Tannate in Oil) and synthetic analogues of ADH (desmopressin acetate, DDAVP Nasal Spray). Nonhormonal therapy uses agents such as chlorpropamide (Diabinese) and the thiazide diuretics (HydroDIURIL or Diuril).

*The chapters in this unit are primarily designed to discuss diagnosis, not treatment. However, because this material is not included elsewhere in the book, it is presented here.

Hormone Replacement Therapy

The most effective treatment of ADH deficiency is replacement of ADH. Vasopressin in oil is injected subcutaneously or intramuscularly at the dose of 1 to 2 units per cat q24 to 72h. The drug is difficult to get at this time because it is no longer manufactured.

A synthetic ADH analogue, desmopressin acetate, is considered the treatment of choice in humans for CDI.[30] Experimental studies with normal dogs and spontaneous cases in dogs and cats indicate that the drug is safe for use in small animals.[5] The nasal spray form is administered into the conjunctival sac as an eye drop. The duration of action is reported to be between 8 to 20 hours.[4] Each drop contains approximately 1.5 to 4 μg of desmopressin. A tuberculin syringe can be used for more accurate dosage and ease of administration. One to two drops are administered in alternating eyes once to twice daily. The dosage is adjusted to control polyuria. At one to two drops per day the cost will be $80–$100/cat/month.[15]

Nonhormonal Therapy

Chlorpropamide is an oral sulfonylurea hypoglycemic drug that may help reduce polyuria. The drug is reported to be most effective in partial DI cases because of its actions of potentiating the effect of ADH on the renal tubular cells (enhancing urine concentrating ability) and possible stimulation of the release of ADH.[4] The suggested dose is 10 to 40 mg/kg/day.[5] The response of two cats with partial CDI to chlorpropamide has been reported. In one report, a 3.5-kg cat had remission of PU/PD when treated with 40 mg chlorpropamide once daily for 7.5 months.[6] No response was reported in a 1.6-kg cat treated with 25 mg twice daily. Since chlorpropamide is a potent hypoglycemic agent and toxicity information in the cat is incomplete, caution is warranted in the use of this drug.[15]

The thiazide diuretic, hydrochlorothiazide, and salt restriction have been used to treat CDI and NDI in cats.[4] The benefit of chlorothiazide diuretics is somewhat paradoxical in that they act to cause a natriuretic diuresis.[15] The combination of loss of sodium through decreased intake and the natriuresis leads to a reduction in extracellular fluid (ECF) volume. This results in reduced glomerular filtration rate and increased absorption of sodium and water in the proximal tubules.[5] Because of the reduction in filtrate delivered to the distal tubule and collecting duct (area of ADH sensitivity), there is a reduction in urine production.

Hydrochlorothiazide therapy has been used in three cats with partial CDI. One 6-kg cat did not respond after a short trial of 25 mg once daily.[26] A reduction in water consumption from 700 mL to 450 mL/day was noted in another cat (1.6 kg) treated with hydrochlorothiazide (12.5 mg twice a day).[30] While there was a reduction in PU/PD, nocturia was a persistent problem. A third cat (3.7 kg) was also treated with 12.5 mg twice daily resulting in the elimination of nocturia and a reduction in water consumption from 900 mL to 500 mL/day.[27]

Primary Polydipsia

An increase in water consumption causes an increase in urine production and may result in a decrease in the hypertonicity of the medullary interstitium. Therapy for primary polydipsia consists of restriction of water intake and replacement of medullary solute. The protocol for therapy is patterned after that used in the dog. Water consumption is gradually reduced over several days to prevent dehydration. As water intake is reduced, sodium chloride is added to the food to re-establish the concentration gradient within the medullary interstitium. Though primary PD is not well documented in the cat, other psychologic disorders, such as dermatoses and stress-induced inappetence, would suggest a potential for its occurrence. Behavior modification may be necessary to correct the underlying problem.

REFERENCES

1. Grauer GF. The differential diagnosis of polyuric–polydipsic diseases. Compend Contin Ed Pract Vet 1981;3:1079.
2. Schwartz-Porsche D. Diabetes Insipidus. In: Kirk RW, ed. Current Veterinary Therapy VII. Philadelphia: WB Saunders, 1983:1006.
3. Atkins CE. Polyuria and Polydipsia. In: Ettinger SJ, ed. Textbook of Veterinary Internal Medicine: Diseases of the Dog and Cat, 3rd ed. Philadelphia: WB Saunders, 1987:139.
4. Bruyette DS. Polyuria and Polydipsia. In: August JR, ed. Consultations in Feline Internal Medicine. Philadelphia: WB Saunders, 1991:227.
5. Nichols R. Diabetes Insipidus. In: Kirk RW, ed. Current Veterinary Therapy X. Philadelphia: WB Saunders, 1989:973.
6. Feldman EC, Nelson RW. Polydipsia and Polyuria. In: Feldman EC, Nelson RW, eds. Canine and Feline Endocrinology and Reproduction. Philadelphia: WB Saunders, 1987:1.
7. Rogers WA, Valdez H, Anderson BC et al. Partial deficiency of antidiuretic hormone in a cat. J Am Vet Med Assoc 1977;170:545.
8. Feldman EC, Nelson RW. Diagnostic approach to polydipsia and polyuria. Vet Clin North Amer [Sm Anim Pract] 1989;19(2):327.
9. Breitschwerdt EB. Clinical abnormalities of urine concentration and dilution. Compend Contin Ed Pract Vet 1981;3(5):414.
10. Feldman EC, Nelson RW. Hyperthyroidism and Thyroid Tumors. In: Feldman EC, Nelson RW, eds. Canine and Feline Endocrinology and Reproduction. Philadelphia: WB Saunders, 1987:91.
11. Kenny KJ, Matthiesen DT, Brown NO, Bradley RL. Pyometra in cats: 183 cases (1979–1984). J Amer Vet Med Assoc 1987; 191:1130.
12. Kallet AJ, Richter KP, Feldman EC, Brum DE. Primary hyperthyroidism in cats: Seven cases (1984–1989). J Am Vet Med Assoc 1991;199:1767.
13. MacEwen EG, Mooney S, Brown NO, Hayes AA. Management of Feline Neoplasms. In: Holzworth J, ed. Diseases of the Cat: Medicine and Surgery. Philadelphia: WB Saunders, 1987:597.
14. Klausner JS, Bell FW, Hayden DW et al. Hypercalcemia in two cats with squamous cell carcinomas. J Am Vet Med Assoc 1990;196:103.
15. Petersen ME, Randolph JF. Endocrine Diseases. In: Sherding RG, ed. The Cat: Diseases and Clinical Management. New York: Churchill Livingstone, 1989:1095.
16. Moore FM, Kudish M, Richter K et al. Hypercalcemia associated with rodenticide poisoning in three cats. J Am Vet Med Assoc 1988;193:1099.
17. Feldman EC, Nelson RW. The parathyroid gland–primary hyperthyroidism. In: Feldman EC, Nelson RW, eds. Canine and Feline Endocrinology and Reproduction. Philadelphia: WB Saunders, 1987:328.
18. Nelson RW, Feldman EC, Smith EC. Hyperadrenocorticism in cats: Seven cases (1978–1987). J Am Vet Med Assoc 1988; 193:245.
19. DiBartola SP, Rutgers HC. Diseases of the Kidney. In: Sherding RG, ed. The Cat: Diseases and Clinical Management. New York: Churchill Livingstone, 1989:1353.
20. Fettman MJ. Feline kalopenic polymyopathy/neophropathy syndrome. Vet Clin North Amer [Clin Nutri] 1989;19(3):415.
21. Dow SW, Fettman MJ, LeCouteur RA, Hamar DW. Potassium depletion in cats: Renal and dietary influences. J Am Vet Med Assoc 1987;191:1563.
22. DiBartola SP, Rutgers HC, Zack PM et al. Clinicopathological findings associated with chronic renal disease in cats: 74 cases (1973–1984). J Am Vet Med Assoc 1987;190:1196.
23. Petersen ME, Taylor RS, Greco FD, Nelson RW et al. Acromegaly in fourteen cats. J Vet Int Med 1990;4:192.
24. Ross LA. Assessment of Renal Function in the Dog and the Cat. In: Kirk RW, ed. Current Veterinary Therapy IX. Philadelphia: WB Saunders, 1986:1103.
25. Gregg WA. Diabetes insipidus in the dog and cat. Proc World Vet Cong 1953;2:1117.
26. Green RA, Farrow CS. Diabetes insipidus in a cat. J Amer Vet Med Assoc 1974;164:524.
27. Burnie AG, Dunn JK. A case of central diabetes insipidus in the cat: Diagnosis and treatment. J Small Anim Pract 1982;23:237.
28. Court MH, Watson ADJ. Idiopathic neurogenic diabetes insipidus in a cat. Aust Vet J 1983;24:269.
29. Winterbotham J, Mason KV. Congenital diabetes in a kitten. J Small Anim Pract 1983;24:569.
30. Kraus KH. The use of desmopressin in diagnosis and treatment of diabetes insipidus in cats. Compend Cont Ed Pract Vet 1987;9:752
31. Petersen ME, Randolph JR. Endocrine Diseases. In: Sherding RG, ed. The Cat: Diseases and Clinical Management. New York: Churchill Livingstone, 1989:1095.

CHAPTER 23

◇ ◇ ◇

Seizure Disorders

James R. Cook, Jr.

The epidemiology of feline seizure disorders has undergone a transformation in recent years. In the past, seizures in cats were often an harbinger of progressive and frequently fatal illness. As cats have increased in popularity as pets, however, a perceptible change has occurred in the frequency with which various disease states are diagnosed. In some congested population centers in which cats outnumber dogs as pets, the incidence of idiopathic epilepsy may approach that seen in the canine population (unpublished data). This shift in pet population, as well as recent advances in diagnosis and therapy of neurologic disorders, makes the evaluation and management of feline seizure disorders a more rewarding task.

When classifying seizure disorders, the term "epilepsy" is used frequently and sometimes recklessly. A bewildering number of definitions of epilepsy have evolved. *Primary generalized epilepsy* is the state of having repetitive tonic–clonic seizures without detectable disease conditions that have seizures as part of their symptomatology. This has also been called *idiopathic epilepsy*. *Secondary generalized epilepsy* refers to a situation in which repetitive seizures are occurring due to some pathology in the brain, intoxication, or severe metabolic disease.

In Chapter 17 the reader was introduced to many of the general concepts of problem-solving, diagnosis, and treatment of neurologic diseases. The principles of evaluation and therapy of seizure disorders do not differ significantly from those previously discussed, so in order to avoid redundancy the reader will frequently be referred to Chapter 17 for the review of general information and concepts. This chapter emphasizes more specific information concerning seizure disorders and the common causes of feline seizures. For a comprehensive list, see Table 23–1.

Signalment

The reader should review Chapter 17. Unlike dogs, there are currently no feline breeds strongly suspected of heritable epilepsy; however, certain breed-specific conditions do exist that may have seizures as part of their symptomatology. Table 23–2 contains a partial listing of these; more complete lists may be found in reference textbooks.[1]

History

The reader should review Chapter 17 including the DAMNIT scheme and time–sign progression. Aside from the general concepts introduced in Chapter 17, the clinician should also try to elicit from the owner exactly what type of behavior the patient is showing. Feline seizures may be of several types (Table 23–3) and are frequently bizarre and violent. Two signs that are consistent in seizures are loss of consciousness and abnormal motor function. The clinician needs to differentiate true seizures from those conditions which owners may misinterpret as seizure activity (Table 23–4). Not only is this important in patient safety and management, but it can also prevent embarrassment to the practitioner. The author has on more than one occasion had to explain to an owner that the unusual "seizure" activity for which his young female kitten was referred was actually normal estrus behavior.

Physical Examination

In addition to the general areas of emphasis described in Chapter 17, the practitioner should be alert for significant abnormalities of the head (domed head, open fontanelle, and divergent strabismus of congenital hydrocephalus or evidence of trauma) and for substances or odors that would suggest an acute intoxication. In the case of primary generalized epilepsy, the physical examination in the interictal period should be normal.

Lesion Localization

The principles of neurologic examination (NE) and lesion localization should be reviewed.[2] In primary generalized epilepsy, there should not be detectable neurologic deficits in the interictal period. With secondary generalized epilepsy, neurologic deficits are likely. With primary nervous system disease, forebrain signs (e.g., altered mental state and behavior, contralateral postural deficits, and absence of menace reflex without other cranial nerve abnormalities) will predominate, but the practitioner should remember that many diseases may affect the nervous system in a diffuse

Table 23–1. Comprehensive List of Causes of Feline Seizures

Common	Uncommon	Rare
Feline leukemia virus infection	Rabies	Thallium poisoning
Feline infectious peritonitis, infectious serositis	Aujeszky's disease	Sodium fluoroacetate poisoning
Mycotic infections	Feline immunodeficiency virus infection	
Cryptococcosis	Nocardiosis	
Chemical toxins	Intracranial abscess	
Ethylene glycol toxicity	Aspergillosis	
Organophosphate toxicity	Encephalitozoonosis	
Carbamate toxicity	Toxoplasmosis	
Hypokalemia	Portal systemic shunt (PSS), portal vascular anomalies	
Cranial trauma	Snakebite, snake venom poisoning	
Intracranial neoplasia, brain tumors	Dirofilariasis, heartworm disease	
Idiopathic epilepsy	Chemical toxins	
Hydrocephalus	Chlorinated hydrocarbon toxicity	
Heat stroke	Zinc phosphide poisoning	
Myocarditis	Phosphorus poisoning	
Vegetative valvular endocarditis	Metaldehyde poisoning	
Arterial thromboembolism	Strychnine poisoning	
Ischemic encephalopathy, cerebral vascular accident, stroke	Lead toxicity	
Hepatic cirrhosis, liver cirrhosis	Feline polioencephalomyelitis	
Renal insufficiency, renal failure, uremia, azotemia	Thiamine deficiency	
Kidney anomalies, renal congenital disease	Mucopolysaccharidosis, Hurler's syndrome, Maroteaux-Lamy syndrome	
Hormonal	Glycogenosis, glycogen storage disease	
Hyperinsulinism	Hypoglycemia	
Hypoparathyroidism	Hyperosmolality	
Pituitary neoplasia, tumors	Hypoxia	
Hypersomatotropism,. acromegaly	Cerebral hemorrhage, cerebral vascular accident, stroke	
	Ceroid lipofuscinosis, familial amaurotic idiocy	
	GM2 gangliosidosis, Sandhoff disease	
	GM1 gangliosidosis	
	Puerperal tetany, eclampsia	
	Smoke inhalation	

or multifocal fashion. In these cases, classic forebrain signs may be masked by severe deficits from lower levels of the nervous system. In toxicosis or severe metabolic disease, there may not be specific neurologic deficits, but there will usually be physical evidence of polysystemic disease.

Clinical Presentation

The reader should review Chapter 17, which contains brief discussions of typical patients from each of the categories of the DAMNIT scheme. Those same general descriptions apply to patients with seizure disorders. In addition to those, a brief discussion of the feline patient with primary generalized ("idiopathic") epilepsy follows.

The patient with primary generalized epilepsy is typically young (6 months to 3 years) and has an unremarkable history. Physical examination and NE are usually normal unless performed within a short time following a seizure when postictal depression may be present. The author has also observed transient focal and diffuse NE abnormalities in the immediate postictal period. Routine laboratory data (complete blood count, serum biochemistries, and urinalysis) and all ancillary studies (if performed) are normal or negative (hence the term "idiopathic epilepsy").

Table 23–2. Breed Predilections of Seizuring Disorders

Breed	Seizuring Disorder
Burmese	Encephalocele
Domestic	GM1 and GM2 gangliosidosis, globoid cell leukodystrophy, metachromatic leukodystrophy
Egyptian Mau	Spongiform degeneration
Korat	GM1 gangliosidosis
Siamese	GM1 gangliosidosis, ceroid lipofuscinosis, hydrocephalus

Differential Diagnosis

At this point, the practitioner should be able to develop a reasonable list of differential diagnoses. Table 23–5 provides common differential diagnoses for feline seizure disorders divided by progression of signs with time. References are provided for those readers wishing further information on a particular disease.

Table 23–3. Seizure Types

Tonic-Clonic (Synonyms: grand mal, major motor). This is the most common type of seizure seen in animals. Loss of consciousness and abnormal motor activity (including vocalization, paddling, evacuation of the bladder and colon) are typically seen. Motor activity in feline seizures is frequently very violent.

Absence (Synonym: petit mal). This is rare in cats. A brief lapse in consciousness or awareness occurs, which may or may not have mild associated motor activity.

Partial Motor. Tonic, clonic, or tonic-clonic activity in a specific group of muscles, limb, or set of limbs occurs. There may not be loss of consciousness. It may progress to generalized tonic-clonic seizures. It indicates a focal acquired lesion.

Psychomotor. These are characterized by episodic events of stereotyped behavior (fear, aggression, biting/chewing, compulsive eating behavior, self-trauma, fly-biting, occasional vomiting, diarrhea, or abdominal pain) occurring uncontrollably in inappropriate circumstances. While the behavior may appear deliberate, patients are actually unaware of their actions.

Diagnostic Plan

The reader should review Chapter 17 because the general approach to the seizure-disorder patient is fundamentally the same as that described for ataxia and paresis. An attempt should be made to pinpoint a specific disease or, in the case of primary generalized epilepsy, to eliminate all known diseases that cause seizures. The minimum data base (MDB) collection is followed by specific testing as needed to establish the diagnosis (Table 23–6).

If historical, physical, or NE abnormalities suggest secondary generalized epilepsy or if the patient is from a purebred cattery and has breeding value, a complete laboratory work-up is indicated. If the practitioner is presented with a young cat with a benign history, absolutely no physical or NE abnormalities, and recurrent seizures, it may be difficult to persuade a client to invest in a costly diagnostic evaluation. In these instances, it is not unreasonable to perform a MDB (including feline leukemia virus [FeLV], feline immunodeficiency virus [FIV], feline coronavirus, i.e., feline infectious peritonitis [FIP] testing) for future comparison and to start the patient on anticonvulsant therapy (see the following section). If the seizures are unresponsive, a more convincing argument may be made for a thorough evaluation.

Therapy

The general principles governing therapy of nervous system diseases and specific drug applications are discussed in the therapy section of Chapter 17. This discussion will focus on the emergency treatment of patients having seizures and on maintenance therapy for the patient with primary generalized epilepsy.

Status Epilepticus

This emergency condition exists when there is prolonged and uninterrupted seizure activity (greater than 10 minutes) or when there are multiple short seizures with minimal interictal relief. The pathological changes in brain and systemic physiology resulting from prolonged seizure activity can be extremely detrimental; therefore, it is important that the patient be stabilized as quickly as possible. The author recommends immediately obtaining a blood sample for chemical analysis. (The author has had the unsettling experience of administering heroic amounts of anticonvulsant medications only to find 12 to 24 hours later that the underlying hypoglycemia or other damaging metabolic abnormality had gone undetected.)

Once the blood sample is obtained, 5 mg of diazepam is administered *intravenously*. In order to stop status epilepticus, diazepam must reach a high blood level quickly; this will not happen if it is given intramuscularly. Intravenous (IV) administration will usually provide sufficient time (20 minutes or more) without seizure activity to allow placement of an indwelling IV catheter to facilitate further treatment. Therapy with phenobarbital (2.2 mg/kg oral or parenteral) may be started at this time. If seizures continue, additional diazepam boluses may be given. If after three or more boluses of diazepam seizure breakthrough is still occurring, pentobarbital may be administered. The recommended anesthetic dose of pentobarbital is 25 mg/kg. *If given as a continuous bolus, this dose will almost invariably cause cardiopulmonary arrest.* This is particularly likely when used for seizure control if other drugs have been given that will potentiate its action. Pentobarbital should be given slowly *to effect* and should never exceed the anesthetic dose. Another precaution is appropriate when using this drug. Patients recovering from pentobarbital may display paddling and other motor activity that may be interpreted as seizure activity.

Table 23–4. Behavior or Activity Frequently Mistaken for Seizures

Estrus
Syncope
Acute, severe pain
Hyperesthesia syndrome
Acute vestibular disease
Cervical weakness (seen in polymyopathy and other lower motor neuron syndrome)
Tremors (cerebellar disease, intoxication)

Table 23–5. Differential Diagnoses of Feline Seizure Disorders

Acute, Nonprogressive

Hydrocephalus,[3] encephalocele,[4] feline ischemic encephalopathy,[5] trauma

Acute, Progressive

FIP,[6] toxoplasmosis,[7] FeLV/FIV syndromes,[8] cryptococcosis,[9] bacterial encephalitis/abscess,[10] feline polioencephalomyelitis,[11] parasite migration[12]

Chronic Progressive

Meningiomas,[13] other primary neural tissue tumors (rare), metastatic neoplasia, GM1 gangliosidosis,[14] GM2 gangliosidosis,[15] globoid cell leukodystrophy,[16] ceroid lipofuscinosis,[17] spongioform degeneration,[18] metachromatic leukodystrophy[19]

Variable or Episodic

Hepatic encephalopathy,[20] hyperinsulinism/hypoglycemia,[21] organophosphate toxicosis, lead poisoning, other intoxications, taurine deficiency[22]

If none of the above drugs are available, patients may be anesthetized with halothane or isoflurane. However, phenobarbital should be obtained as quickly as possible because the gaseous anesthetics have no residual anticonvulsant effects. Short-acting barbiturates may actually increase the activity of seizure foci and should not be used to stop status epilepticus unless nothing else is available and impending death from persistent convulsions is likely.

Once the cycle of seizure activity has been broken and the patient has been stabilized, either a diagnostic evaluation or a maintenance anticonvulsant program should be instituted.

Chronic Anticonvulsant Maintenance

Once it has been established that there is not a detectable disease process causing the seizures, maintenance therapy is begun. Client education (Table 23–7) becomes extremely important at this point. Most therapy failures can be traced to a poor understanding of the goals of therapy, inappropriate medication, or both.

Oral phenobarbital is the mainstay of veterinary anticonvulsant therapy and is the only reliable and safe drug for cats. An acceptable starting dose is 2.2 mg/kg b.i.d. While a body-weight dosage is used to initiate therapy, it may be necessary to fine-tune treatment by measurement of serum phenobarbital levels. Individual differences in absorption and rate of metabolism may cause the dose and frequency to vary considerably among patients. Most commercial laboratories can measure blood phenobarbital, and some may provide pharmacokinetic studies as well. The target range is 15 to 40 μg/mL, although the author has found that many patients require stable blood levels above 25 μg/mL. Because there is the potential for hepatotoxicity with chronic administration, a liver function test is recommended every 6 months. Serum phenobarbital should also be measured at this time or whenever there is breakthrough seizure activity.

Oral diazepam has been suggested as a maintenance anticonvulsant in cats at 0.5 to 2 mg/kg divided t.i.d. The increased frequency of administration usually means poorer client compliance.

Other anticonvulsants used in humans and canines include primidone, diphenylhydantoin (Dilantin), and valproic acid. *These are not recommended in cats.*

Taurine may play an important role in feline seizure disorders. Taurine deficiency has not been reported to be causally related to epileptiform seizures in cats but is reported effective in preventing spontaneous seizure activity in epileptic cats.[25] Measurement of serum taurine is not readily available in most commercial laboratories, but if taurine deficiency is suspected or can be documented in a seizuring patient, oral supplementation with 500 mg b.i.d. is recommended.[22]

Table 23–6. Diagnostic Plan: Minimum data base (MDB)

- Blood lead, bile acid assay, cholinesterase levels if indicated by history or MDB abnormalities
- Infectious disease testing (FeLV, FIV, FIP, cryptococcosis, toxoplasmosis) if indicated by history, physical examination, or MDB abnormalities
- Skull radiographs
- Cerebrospinal fluid (CSF) analysis[23]
- Electroencephalogram[24]
- Nuclear imaging (computed tomography, magnetic resonance imaging)
- Cerebral angiography if nuclear imaging is unavailable
- Infectious disease testing, and microbial culture and antibiotic sensitivity if indicated by CSF results
- Biopsy (cerebral cortex, particularly of neoplasms)

Table 23–7. Client Education

- Therapy is lifelong.
- Therapy must be regular and continuous; changes or cessation should occur only under veterinary supervision.
- Treatment is intended to reduce the number and severity of seizures; complete elimination of seizures is an unrealistic expectation. Reduction of frequent seizures to less than two per month should be viewed as reasonably successful.
- Periodic evaluation and dosage adjustment will be needed.

REFERENCES

1. Oliver JE, Hoerlein BF, Mayhew IG. Appendix II. Species and Breed Predisposition for Noninfectious Disease. In: Oliver JE, Hoerlein BF, Mayhew IG, eds. Veterinary Neurology. Philadelphia: WB Saunders, 1987:525.
2. Oliver JE, Lorenz MD. Neurologic Examination. In: Oliver JE, Lorenz MD, eds. Handbook of Veterinary Diagnosis. Philadelphia: JB Lippincott, 1983:19.
3. Silson M, Robinson R. Hereditary hydrocephalus in the cat. Vet Rec 1969;84:477.
4. Zook B, Sostaric BR, Draper DJ, Graf-Webster E. Encephalocele and other congenital craniofacial anomalies in Burmese cats. Vet Clin North Am [Small Anim Med] 1983;78:695.
5. Zaki FA, Nafe LA. Ischemic encephalopathy and focal granulomatous meningoencephalitis in the cat. J Small Anim Pract 1980;21:429.
6. Kornegay JN. Feline infectious peritonitis: The central nervous system form. J Am Anim Hosp Assoc 1978;14:580.
7. Kyle RJ. Toxoplasma encephalitis in a cat. NZ Vet J 1975;23:13.
8. Pedersen NC. Feline Leukemia Virus Infection. In: Pedersen NC, ed. Feline Infectious Diseases. Goleta, CA: American Veterinary Publications, 1988:83.
9. Wilkinson GT. Feline cryptococcosis: A review and seven case reports. J Small Anim Pract 1979;20:749.
10. Fenner WR. Bacterial Infections of the Central Nervous System. In: Greene CE, ed. Infectious Diseases of the Dog and Cat. Philadelphia: WB Saunders, 1990:184.
11. Vandevelde M, Braund KG. Polioencephalomyelitis in cats. Vet Pathol 1979;16:420.
12. Cook JR, Levesque DC, Neuhring LP. Intracranial cuterebral myiasis causing acute lateralizing meningoencephalitis in two cats. J Am Anim Hosp Assoc 1985;21:279.
13. Nafe LA. Meningiomas in cats: A retrospective clinical study of 36 cases. J Am Vet Med Assoc 1979;174:1224.
14. Blakemore WF. GM1 gangliosidosis in a cat. J Comp Pathol 1972;82:179.
15. Cork LC, Munnell JF, Lorenz MD et al. GM2 ganglioside lysosomal storage disease in cats with B-hexosaminidase deficiency. Science 1977;196:1014.
16. Johnson KH. Globoid leukodystrophy in the cat. J Am Vet Med Assoc 1970;157:2057.
17. Greene PD, Little PB. Neuronal ceroid-lipofuschin storage in Siamese cats. Can J Comp Med 1974;38:207.
18. Kelly DF, Gaskell CJ. Spongy degeneration of the central nervous system in kittens. Acta Neuropathol 1976;35:151.
19. Hegreberg GA, Thuline HC, Francis BH. Morphologic changes in feline leukodystrophy. Fed Proc 1971;30:341.
20. Levesque DC, Oliver JE, Cornelius LM et al. Congenital portocaval shunts in two cats: Diagnosis and surgical correction. J Am Vet Med Assoc 1982;181:143.
21. MacMillan F. Insulinoma in a cat (abstract). Proc Am Coll Vet Int Med, 1983:51.
22. da Costa PD, Hoskins JD. The role of taurine in cats: Current concepts. Compend Contin Ed Pract Vet 1990;12:1235.
23. Cook JR, DeNicola DB. Cerebrospinal fluid. Vet Clin North Amer [Small Anim Pract] 1988;18:475.
24. Redding RW. Electroencephalography. In: Oliver JE, Hoerlein BF, Mayhew IG, eds. Veterinary Neurology. Philadelphia: WB Saunders, 1987:111.
25. Tanizawa K, Mizuno T, Ueda K, Koyama I. Taurine treatment for spontaneous epilepsy in the cat. Jpn J Vet Sci 1986;48:1041.

CHAPTER 24

◇ ◇ ◇

Vomiting and Diarrhea

Douglas C. Bronstad and Gary D. Norsworthy

Vomiting and diarrhea may be caused by a multitude of diseases (see Appendix F). Some of these diseases are serious, even life-threatening, in nature. Others are self-limiting, often resolving within 24 hours. Realizing this, the practitioner must make a judgment as to the appropriate diagnostic and therapeutic approach.

Many clinicians look for certain indicators, or groups of indicators, that signal the need for aggressive diagnostic and therapeutic measures. These signs include:

- Repeated vomiting within a 12-hour period
- Marked abdominal pain
- Fever greater than 103.5°F
- Watery, bloody diarrhea
- Dehydration in excess of 5%
- Anorexia for more than 24 hours
- Marked lethargy
- Rapid weight loss

In the absence of these indicators, a conservative approach is generally utilized for the first 24 to 48 hours. The general guidelines for conservative treatment are as follows:

- Subcutaneous (SC) or intravenous (IV) administration of balanced electrolyte fluids to correct/prevent dehydration
- Administration of an injectable drug, such as metoclopramide (Reglan), 0.05–0.15 mg/lb b.i.d. IM, to control vomiting
- Administration of oral medication to control diarrhea, such as diphenoxylate with atropine (Lomotil), ½ tablet (1.25 mg) b.i.d.
- Withholding of food for 12 to 24 hours, followed by a bland diet for 1 to 3 days.

If vomiting or diarrhea continues after 24 to 48 hours of conservative therapy, more aggressive diagnostic measures should be instituted.

If the clinician adopts a conservative approach to treatment, good communication with the client is imperative. The client must understand that other diagnostic or therapeutic measures are available and may be indicated.

Diagnosis

When aggressive diagnostic steps are indicated, the clinician must approach diagnosis in a logical and systematic fashion by ruling out various entities on the basis of the data collected and by developing an appropriate diagnostic plan. The problem-oriented approach to diagnosis offers this format.[1]

Initial data base collection should always begin with an in-depth history and complete physical examination (see Chapter 3). This process allows the clinician to begin establishing a problem list and aids in determining an appropriate diagnostic plan. The diagnostic plan should be individualized according to the presenting clinical status of the patient and whether the condition is acute (duration of less than 3 to 4 days) or chronic (duration of greater than 3 to 4 days).

At a minimum, the data base for severe and chronic conditions should include the results of a fecal examination (flotation and direct saline smear), complete blood count (CBC), biochemical profile (including electrolytes), urinalysis, and survey abdominal radiographs. An attempt should be made to differentiate primary gastrointestinal diseases from nongastrointestinal disorders causing vomiting and diarrhea.

Primary Gastrointestinal Disorders

Dietary Factors

Vomiting and diarrhea in the cat can be a manifestation of dietary indiscretion or allergic gastroenteritis.

Dietary indiscretion is the ingestion of any food, animal products, or foreign material that upsets the normal digestive process. Examples might include table scraps, birds, mice, insects, lizards, garbage, grass, or plant material. Such indiscretions may be the result of an owner's negligence or scavenging behavior in an outdoor cat. The history may lend support to the appropriate etiology. Supportive and symptomatic therapy (e.g., ingesting nothing by mouth, fluid therapy, gastrointestinal protectants, antiemetics, antidiarrheals, prophylactic antibiotics) will usually resolve the problem.

Allergic gastroenteritis in the cat is the result of a hypersensitivity reaction to a specific antigen directly exposed to the gastrointestinal mucosal lining.[2] The offending allergen is usually a food ingredient (e.g., beef, eggs, milk, etc.) or a food preservative. Clinical signs will range from mild to severe depending on the degree and extent of the hypersensitivity reaction. Skin lesions may also be a manifestation of this reaction.[3] The diagnosis is established by ruling out other causes of vomiting and diarrhea, by compiling a minimum data base and by using a hyposensitization diet, if deemed necessary (see Chapter 58). Strict dietary control is essential once the diagnosis is determined.

Intestinal Parasites

Intestinal parasites are more common in kittens and in adult cats kept in a cattery or a multi-cat household setting than in other cat populations. The helminths that most commonly affect cats include hookworms, roundworms, and tapeworms. Less common infestations include stomach worms (e.g., *Physaloptera* species and *Ollulanus tricuspis*). The diagnosis may readily be established on the basis of fecal examinations (i.e., flotation, sedimentation, or direct saline smear) and, in the case of tapeworms, visual observation of segments in the stool or on the hair around the anus. An appropriate anthelmintic should be used to treat the condition.

Protozoal intestinal parasites in the cat usually cause more serious clinical signs. Coccidiosis and giardiasis are the most common conditions caused by these parasites.

Coccidiosis (*Cystoisospora* species), which is the most common of the intestinal protozoal parasitic diseases occurring in the kitten, may be associated with very severe clinical signs. The diagnosis is established by fecal flotation. Coccidia oocysts must be differentiated from toxoplasma oocysts.[4]

Giardiasis (*Giardia lamblia*) is another intestinal disease caused by a protozoal parasite; it occurs most commonly in young cats and those from a multi-cat environment. The Giardia species also has the potential for zoonotic transmission.[5] Clinical signs vary with some cats remaining asymptomatic and others developing severe, chronic diarrhea with weight loss. Diagnosis can be difficult in many cases. Traditionally, the zinc sulfate centrifugation technique and the direct, fresh saline fecal smear have been the diagnostic tests of choice, but the percentage of false-negative results obtained using these techniques has been high. Examination of aspirates of duodenal luminal fluid, obtained by needle aspiration of the duodenum via a celiotomy approach or by endoscopy, is another recommended diagnostic technique. In addition, some laboratories offer an enzyme-linked immunoabsorbent assay (ELISA) that detects Giardia-specific antigen in fresh or preserved (10% formalin) fecal samples. This test will detect Giardia in cats in which cysts cannot be observed.

The diagnostic difficulties associated with giardiasis have prompted many clinicians to treat chronic diarrhea of undetermined cause with a course of oral metronidazole (Flagyl), 5 mg/lb b.i.d. for 5 days. A retrospective diagnosis of giardiasis may then be made based on a response to therapy.

Foreign Bodies

Ingestion of foreign material that becomes lodged in the gastrointestinal tract may produce clinical signs related to bowel obstruction (i.e., vomiting, abdominal pain, abdominal distention, etc.). Commonly ingested foreign matter includes hair (i.e., hairballs), string or yarn (i.e., linear foreign bodies), needles, small toys or parts of toys, cloth, and fish hooks.

Diagnosis of a foreign body is based on the cat's history, clinical signs (i.e., obstructive bowel disease), radiographic studies (survey and/or contrast films), endoscopy, or exploratory celiotomy. If detected early, most cats recover uneventfully from foreign body removal. Delayed diagnosis or undetected foreign bodies, however, may result in bowel necrosis and possibly bowel rupture. For a discussion of the typical radiographic findings in cats with foreign bodies, see Chapter 14.

Infections

Primary infectious bowel disease can be viral, bacterial, or protozoal. Systemic fungi may also involve the bowel, but are usually an extension of the disseminated disease. The most common primary bowel infections occurring in the cat are discussed in this section.

Viral Infections

Viral causes of bowel disease include panleukopenia and feline enteric coronavirus infections. Infections resulting from the feline infectious peritonitis (FIP) virus, feline leukemia virus (FeLV), and feline immunodeficiency virus (FIV) can often cause secondary gastrointestinal symptoms as an extension of the primary disease process (see Chapters 37, 38, and 39).

The panleukopenia virus (feline parvovirus) is a resistant, highly contagious virus that can cause a devastating disease, especially in young cats.[7] Affected cats often present with severe vomiting and diarrhea, weight loss, and varying degrees of dehydration, lethargy, fever, and anorexia. The CBC classically reveals a profound leukopenia, and the animal's prognosis often correlates with the severity of the leukopenia.[7] Diagnosis is usually based on the cat's history and clinical signs, and on the presence of leukopenia; however, electron microscopic examination of the feces, virus isolation, serologic studies, or intestinal biopsies are among the alternative diagnostic modalities.

The two feline coronaviruses—feline enteric coronavirus and FIP—are antigenically related; however, they differ in pathogenicity and prognosis.[8] The feline enteric coronavirus most often causes a mild, rarely fatal, enteritis, predominantly affecting cats younger than 3 months of age.[8] It is usually self-limiting; however, supportive therapy (i.e., fluid administration) is indicated in severe cases. Diagnosis is often speculative owing to the short course of the disease. Coronavirus serum titers are often confusing and nondiagnostic. By contrast, FIP viral infections are usually prolonged, debilitating, and ultimately fatal (see Chapter 38).

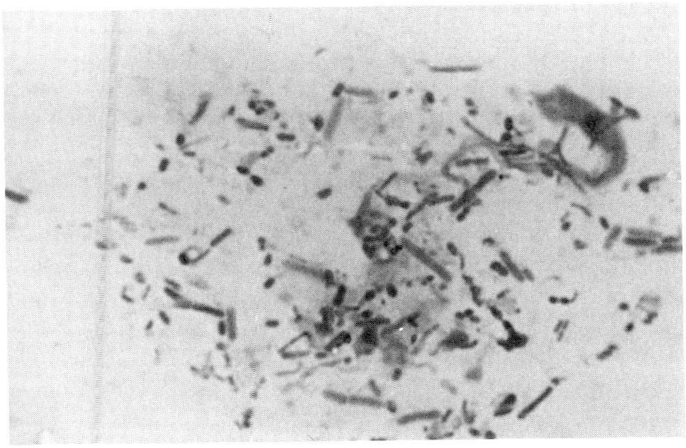

Figure 24–1. The normal bacterial flora of the colon is a heterogeneous population of bacteria of many sizes and shapes.

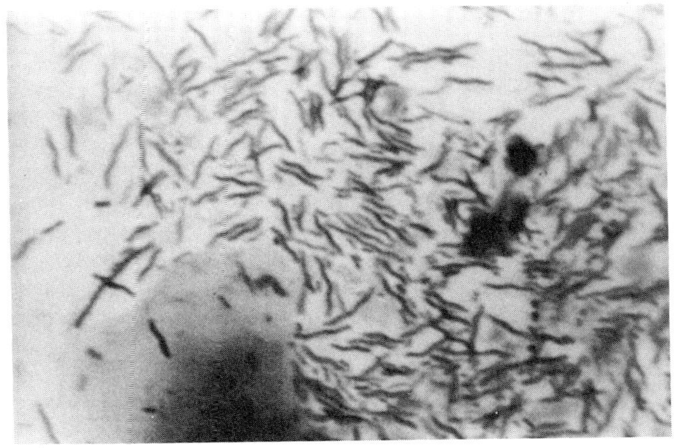

Figure 24–3. The finding of a homogeneous population of spirochetes in a cat with diarrhea is abnormal. This cat's diarrhea responded dramatically to metronidazole.

Bacterial Infections

Bacterial enteritis/colitis is an uncommon disease in the cat. Diagnosis is usually established by a screening cytologic test, as the use of oral antibiotics in the absence of a true bacterial infection will generally increase the severity of diarrhea. A moistened, cotton-tipped applicator is inserted into the rectum and rolled onto the rectal wall. The sample is then smeared on a microscopic slide and stained with Diff-Quik stain (AHS del Caribe, Inc., Aguada, Puerto Rico). The normal bacterial flora is very heterogeneous, consisting of bacteria of varying sizes and shapes (Fig. 24–1). If there is a marked predominance of one bacterium (Figs. 24–2 and 24–3), a rectal culture should be performed to confirm the diagnosis of bacterial enteritis/colitis.

Owing to their potential public health significance, the two bacterial enteritides of greatest concern in the cat are salmonellosis (*Salmonella* species) and campylobacteriosis (*Campylobacter jejuni*). Diagnosis is based primarily on the cat's clinical presentation and on positive fecal cultures. Isolation of *Campylobacter* species requires selective media.

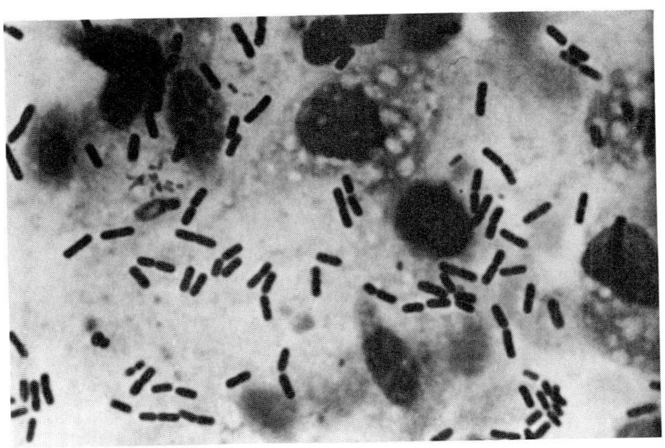

Figure 24–2. If the bacterial flora of the colon contains predominantly one bacterium, bacterial colitis should be suspected and a colon culture should be performed. This cat's colonic culture grew a pure culture of *Salmonella* species.

Protozoal Infections

Protozoal infections in the cat include coccidiosis, giardiasis, toxoplasmosis, cryptosporidiosis, and trichomoniasis. Cryptosporidiosis and trichomoniasis are uncommon infections in the cat. In comparison, toxoplasmosis and giardiasis have much greater public health significance. Toxoplasmosis is discussed in Chapter 64. Coccidiosis and giardiasis are discussed in the section on intestinal parasites that is included in this chapter

Inflammatory Bowel Disease

Inflammatory bowel disease in the cat is a gastrointestinal disorder characterized by the infiltration of inflammatory cells (i.e., lymphocytes, plasma cells, eosinophils, and/or neutrophils) into the mucosal lining of the bowel.[9-11] It is often characterized histopathologically as having a lymphocytic-plasmacytic, eosinophilic, suppurative, or mixed inflammatory response pattern. This disease process is usually chronic, and the cause is often unknown. Diagnosis is made by biopsy of the intestinal mucosa using a fiberoptic endoscopic instrument or by full-thickness intestinal biopsy using a surgical approach. This condition is discussed in Chapter 48.

Idiopathic colitis is an inflammatory process that primarily involves the mucosal lining of the colon and presents with clinical signs of large bowel disease. The clinical signs, which are commonly intermittent, consist of a varying degree of stool consistency and the presence of mucus and/or blood in the stool (often apparent on gross examination). The diagnosis is confirmed by colonoscopic mucosal biopsy. Histopathologic results vary considerably, ranging from minimal to severe inflammatory changes.

Neoplasia

The most common primary neoplasias involving the gastrointestinal tract are lymphosarcoma, carcinoma/adenocarcinoma, and leiomyoma/leiomyosarcoma. In the authors' clinical experience, lymphosarcoma is the most common primary intestinal neoplasia in the cat. Carcinoma/adenocarcinoma is often seen in older cats at the ileocecocolic junction. These disease processes most often involve the submucosa and/or serosa, and a celiotomy is often required in order to obtain a biopsy specimen for definitive diagnosis. If a solitary mass is palpated, percutaneous needle aspiration cytology may aid in the diagnosis. Mast cell tumors can also originate in the gastrointestinal tract, but they more commonly arise in other sites, and the resulting clinical signs, especially vomiting, are attributable to histamine release.

Idiopathic Vomiting Syndrome

The term *idiopathic vomiting syndrome* has been used tc describe an idiopathic syndrome that causes frequent vomiting in an otherwise normal cat. Typically, affected cats have a history of vomiting, first on a monthly, then on a weekly basis. The client may report that, thereafter, the frequency of vomiting increased and the interval between vomiting episodes became shorter, sometimes to the point of daily vomiting.

Such cats are diagnosed as having idiopathic vomiting after all the known causes of vomiting have been ruled out. These cats have a history of eating regularly and consuming normal amounts of food. They do not have fever or weight loss, and are not depressed or lethargic. The vomitus consists primarily of food. The results of multiple gastric and intestinal biopsy studies are normal, thus excluding inflammatory bowel disease. Use of a hypoallergenic diet will produce no results. Cats with this syndrome have normal radiographic studies, even with positive contrast studies. The results of blood profile, serum triiodothyronine (T_3) and thyroxin (T_4), and heartworm antigen tests will be normal.

Because this is a diagnosis of exclusion, a comprehensive diagnostic approach must be utilized. This syndrome appears to occur in a substantial number of cats.

These cats generally do not respond to glucocorticoids or metoclopramide. However, they respond dramatically to megestrol acetate (Ovaban), administered at an initial dose of 5 mg daily for 7 days and then tapered gradually to a maintenance dose of approximately 5 mg every 7 days. Because megestrol acetate is a powerful antiemetic, this drug should not be used indiscriminately, as it has the ability to mask severe underlying disease. It also has a number of significant side effects, discussed in Chapter 7.

Nongastrointestinal Disorders

A variety of clinical disorders affecting the cat can cause vomiting and diarrhea as a secondary complication. These are usually the result of a chemical imbalance that may directly affect the vomiting centers in the brain. An extension of a primary disease process into the bowel may stimulate the afferent receptors that travel via the nerves to the vomiting centers in the brain. Finally, interruption of the normal bowel physiology may create an environment conducive to the development of diarrhea. Conditions creating this type of derangement include metabolic disorders, toxins, systemic fungal infections, and miscellaneous disorders, such as feline heartworm disease and paraneoplastic syndromes.

Metabolic Disorders

The most common metabolic disorders causing vomiting and diarrhea in the cat include liver disease (see Chapters 29 and 47), renal failure (see Chapter 31), ketoacidotic diabetes mellitus (see Chapter 34), and hyperthyroidism (see Chapter 46). Less common causes include hypoadrenocorticism (rare in the cat) and pancreatitis (usually secondary to trauma in the cat and not often a primary disease process). In addition, hypercalcemia occasionally may be seen in association with neoplasia.[12,13]

Diagnosis of a metabolic disorder is made on the basis of the biochemical profile and a urinalysis. These studies should alert the clinician to individual or multiple organ dysfunction and should direct attention toward specific treatment or additional diagnostic modalities deemed necessary to resolve the problem.

Toxic Disorders

Toxin ingestion can result in a variety of clinical signs and organ dysfunction depending on the agent involved, the amount ingested, and the target organ. Toxins may include pharmaceuticals, insecticidal agents, ornamental plants, ethylene glycol, and numerous types of household chemicals. Vomiting and diarrhea are common clinical signs associated with toxin ingestion. It is beyond the scope of this chapter to cover all the potential toxic agents. Rather, the reader is referred to more specific references that focus on this subject[14] and to Chapter 62.

Diagnosis of toxin ingestion is usually based on historical evidence of exposure to the offending agent. In an outdoor cat, diagnosis may also be based on a history of an acute onset of clinical signs that are possibly related to exposure to or ingestion of a toxic substance. Specific organ dysfunction can be determined by a review of the biochemical profile and urinalysis findings. If a specific toxic agent cannot be identified, the clinician must use his or her best clinical judgment in choosing a therapeutic regimen. Most toxic disorders are treated by preventing further exposure to the offending agent and by supportive/symptomatic therapy.

Systemic Fungal Infections

Any mycotic infection that has the potential to disseminate can invade the gastrointestinal tract as an extension of the primary disease process and cause vomiting and diarrhea. Most systemic fungal infections invade other internal organs (i.e., the liver, kidneys, etc.), causing specific organ dysfunction and resulting in a chemical imbalance that produces vomiting and/or diarrhea. There are numerous fungal organisms that can disseminate in this manner.[15] For a more specific review of the most common systemic fungi, see Chapter 61.

Diagnosis of systemic fungal infections is usually based on the cat's history, clinical signs, and radiographic findings, and on organism identification via needle aspiration cytology or histopathologic study. Serologic assays often yield false-negative results and are usually nondiagnostic. Most systemic fungal infections are endemic to certain regions of the country, a factor which may aid the clinician in diagnosing a fungal infection.

Miscellaneous Disorders

Feline Heartworm Disease

Dirofilariasis in cats may be associated with vomiting, the underlying mechanism for which is unknown. Indeed, vomiting and respiratory signs are the most common clinical signs in chronic cases of this disease.[16]

The diagnosis of feline dirofilariasis can often be difficult; in many cases, especially in outdoor cats, it is speculative, based on the cat's history and clinical signs, and the geographic location of heartworms. Specific diagnostic tests should include a CBC (i.e., eosinophilia), microfilaria testing (i.e., modified Knott's and Difil [Evsco Pharmaceuticals, Buena, NJ] tests), thoracic radiography, echocardiography, and serologic testing (e.g., ELISA) (see Chapter 41).

Paraneoplastic Syndromes

Paraneoplastic syndromes are conditions in which chemical substances produced by a tumor cause distant clinical signs.[13] Vomiting and diarrhea are often associated with these syndromes. They occur only rarely in the cat.

The most common of these syndromes causing gastrointestinal clinical signs are hypercalcemia and hyperthyroidism. Hypercalcemia is most commonly associated with lymphosarcoma; however, it can also be associated with parathyroid tumors, multiple myelomas, and metastatic bone tumors. Hypercalcemia is diagnosed on the basis of the biochemical profile. Identification of the offending tumor must be accomplished to confirm a paraneoplastic syndrome.

Hyperthyroidism is the result of excessive production of T_4 by a primary thyroid tumor. Vomiting and diarrhea are common presenting clinical signs and are often accompanied by weight loss, polyphagia, and hyperactive behavior (see Chapter 46).

REFERENCES

1. Lorenz MD. The Problem-Oriented Approach. In: Lorenz MD, Cornelius LM, eds. Small Animal Medical Diagnosis. Philadelphia: JB Lippincott, 1987:1.
2. Strombeck DR. Dietary Allergies, Eosinophilic Gastroenteritis, and Gluten-Induced Enteropathy. In: Strombeck DR, ed. Small Animal Gastroenterology. Davis, CA: Stonegate Publishing Co., 1979:230.
3. Scott DW. The Skin. In: Holzworth J, ed. Diseases of the Cat: Medicine and Surgery, Vol. 1. Philadelphia: WB Saunders, 1987:637.
4. Greene CE, Prestwood AK. Coccidial Infections. In: Greene CE, ed. Clinical Microbiology and Infectious Diseases of the Dog and Cat. Philadelphia: WB Saunders, 1984:824.
5. Kranz JMS. Potential and Newly Recognized Pet-Associated Zoonoses. In: Kirk RW, ed. Current Veterinary Therapy IX. Philadelphia: WB Saunders, 1986:1088.
6. Holzworth J. Other Protozoan Diseases. In: Holzworth J, ed. Diseases of the Cat: Medicine and Surgery, Vol. 1. Philadelphia: WB Saunders, 1987:394.
7. Scott FW. Viral Diseases: Panleukopenia. In: Holzworth J, ed. Diseases of the Cat: Medicine and Surgery, Vol. 1. Philadelphia: WB Saunders, 1987:182.
8. Pedersen NC Coronavirus Diseases. In: Holzworth J, ed. Diseases of the Cat: Medicine and Surgery, Vol. 1. Philadelphia: WB Saunders, 1987:193.
9. Tams TR. Feline Inflammatory Bowel Disease. In: Kirk RW, ed. Current Veterinary Therapy IX. Philadelphia: WB Saunders, 1991:409.
10. Tams TR. Inflammatory Bowel Disease. In: August JR, ed. Consultations in Feline Internal Medicine. Philadelphia: WB Saunders, 1991:409.
11. Sherding RG. Diseases of the Intestines. In: Sherding RG, ed. The Cat—Diseases and Clinical Management. New York: Churchill Livingstone, 1989:976.
12. Carpenter JL, Andrews LK, Holzworth J. Tumors and Tumor-like Lesions. In: Holzworth J, ed. Diseases of the Cat: Medicine and Surgery, Vol. 1. Philadelphia: WB Saunders, 1987:548.
13. MacEwen EG, Mooney S, Brown NO, Hayes AA. Management of Feline Neoplasms. In: Holzworth J, ed. Diseases of the Cat: Medicine and Surgery, Vol. 1. Philadelphia: WB Saunders, 1987:597.
14. Beasley VR. Prevalence of Poisonings in Small Animals. In: Kirk RW, ed. Current Veterinary Therapy IX. Philadelphia: WB Saunders, 1986:120.
15. Holzworth J. Mycotic Diseases. In: Holzworth J, ed. Diseases of the Cat: Medicine and Surgery, Vol. 1. Philadelphia: WB Saunders, 1987:320.
16. Dillon R. Feline Heartworm Disease. In: Kirk RW, ed. Current Veterinary Therapy IX. Philadelphia: WB Saunders, 1986:420.

PART IV

◊ ◊ ◊

Diseases

CHAPTER 25

◇ ◇ ◇

Asthma

Gary D. Norsworthy

Feline asthma is a term used to describe a respiratory disease with an acute onset and a circulating eosinophilia that is responsive to corticosteroids. It has also been called allergic bronchitis, allergic pneumonitis, and eosinophilic pneumonitis. Despite extensive research, its precise cause and pathophysiologic mechanism have not been documented. Some have suggested that these terms be abandoned until a better understanding of this disease is achieved.[1] However, a consistent pattern of clinical signs, diagnostic findings, and therapeutic response occurs in enough cats so that the term seems appropriate at this time.

Pathophysiology

There appear to be many similarities between feline bronchial asthma and that which occurs in humans. Because of these similarities, a number of cross-species assumptions concerning the pathophysiology of the disease have been made.

It is believed that extrinsic or allergic asthma occurs as a result of a Type 1 hypersensitivity reaction that follows exposure to specific, usually undefined, allergens. In cats, the suspected allergens include cat litter dust, perfumes, cigarette smoke, fireplace smoke, and insulation materials. Because of the seasonality of some cases of feline asthma, plant pollens are also considered to be possible allergens.

The hypersensitivity reaction occurs as a result of several important anatomic and physiological factors related to the respiratory tract. Cartilage is a structural component of the airways down to the level of the bronchioles. At that level, bronchial tree support is maintained by elastic tissue and smooth muscle. During an asthmatic event, bronchospasm of the bronchioles, alveolar ducts, and alveoli produces airway obstruction, entrapping air in the alveoli. Because the musculature in the feline bronchial walls is thicker than in most other species, the cat has an increased ability to constrict the bronchial lumen and is thus predisposed to the sequence of events related to bronchial asthma.[3]

The mucociliary apparatus consists of a mucous layer, periciliary fluid, and ciliary movement. This apparatus, in conjunction with tissue macrophages, acts to expel foreign substances from the lower airways. This expulsion process is controlled by the sympathetic nervous system. When allergenic particles cannot be removed, an inflammatory reaction occurs. An exaggerated inflammatory response is thought to be the basis of bronchial asthma. This exaggerated response results in cholinergic (parasympathomimetic) stimulation that produces glandular secretion, contraction of the bronchial musculature, and vasodilation. The airways close as a result of bronchospasm, thickening of the bronchial walls, and tenacious mucous plugs.[3]

Infectious agents are frequently present in the fluids recovered from an affected cat by a diagnostic tracheal wash. When these agents are located on the β_2-adrenergic receptors, they or their metabolities may block the normal response of bronchodilation.[4] Thus, they may precipitate an asthmatic attack. This explains why antibiotics may be indicated as part of the treatment regimen.

In humans, histamine is an important factor in the development of asthma; consequently, antihistamines are useful therapeutic aids in humans. However, owing to antihistamines consistent lack of efficacy in cats, it seems likely that histamine is not a significant component of feline asthma.[3]

Clinical Signs

The major event that contributes to the clinical signs of asthma is expiratory difficulty. Under normal conditions, the airway lumen is smaller during expiration than during inspiration. Thus, partial obstructions secondary to mucus and bronchospasm that occur during inspiration may become complete obstructions during expiration. Thus, the asthmatic cat will often have forced expiration and vesicular emphysema (air trapping). Air can get into the lungs but cannot be removed even with forced expiratory efforts.[3]

The clinical signs of feline asthma are caused by the airway obstruction that results. Coughing is the earliest sign of asthma in the cat and represents mild disease. Affected cats frequently assume a characteristic, crouched position when coughing (Fig. 25–1). Dyspnea with open-mouthed breathing, cyanosis, and a frantic demeanor are the signs of advanced disease and indicate that a major degree of airway obstruction is present. Other clinical signs include increased bronchovesicular sounds, gagging, tachypnea, wheezing, aerophagia, a barrel-shaped chest, abdominal distention, and hysterical clawing movements about the face.

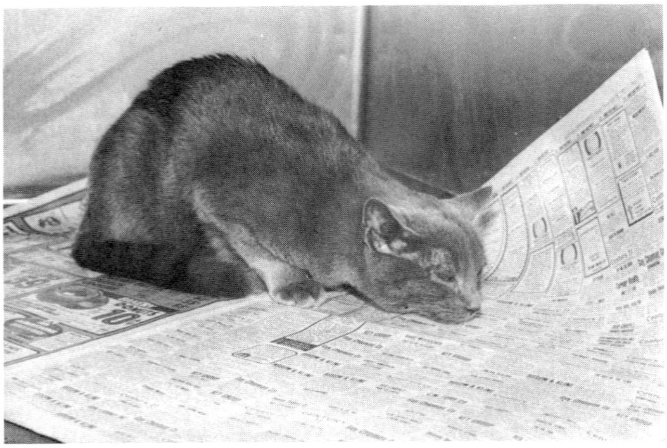

Figure 25–1. Asthmatic cats often assume a characteristic, crouched position when coughing.

A system for staging of feline asthma has been developed (Table 25–1). This classification system is useful in understanding the different levels of disease and how they relate to the differences in clinical signs.

Diagnosis

The diagnosis of feline asthma can often be made on the basis of the cat's history, clinical signs, and response to corticosteroids. If a cat has an intermittent or seasonal, nonproductive cough that responds to corticosteroids, there is a strong likelihood that the cat has asthma. A more complete work-up should include a complete blood count (CBC), heartworm tests (microfilaria and antigen tests), thoracic radiographs, a tracheal wash, and fecal examinations. The CBC will reveal eosinophilia in about 75% of the cases.[5] The heartworm tests should be performed on cats that live outdoors in heartworm endemic areas; asthmatic cats should test negative. Thoracic radiographic findings will vary with the degree of pathology present, but may include trapping of air with increased pulmonary radiolucency, bronchial thickening, increased thoracic volume, flattening of the diaphragm, and aerophagia (Figs. 25–2 and 25–3). Bronchial wall thickenings are typical. A disseminated interstitial pattern will be present if cellular infiltrates or pulmonary edema, or both, are present (Fig. 25–4). Some cats with severe chronic disease even develop pleural effusion (Fig. 25–5). A tracheal wash often reveals an increase in the number of eosinophils and neutrophils. When this proce-

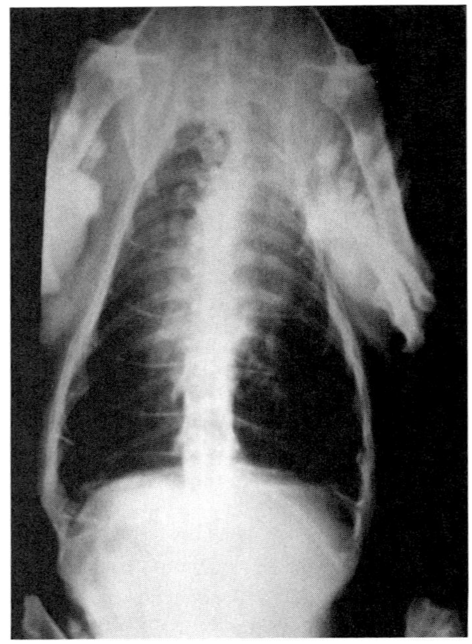

Figure 25–2. Cats with a very early stage of asthma may present without evidence of bronchial thickening, but may exhibit signs of severe dyspnea, including increased pulmonary radiolucency and flattening of the diaphragm.

Table 25–1. Stages of Feline Asthma Based on Clinical Signs

Stage	Clinical Signs
I. Asymptomatic	Asymptomatic; history of previous attack
II. Moderate airway obstruction	Coughing; gagging; increased lung sounds; mild tachypnea; some wheezing
III. Severe airway obstruction	Coughing; gagging; increased lung sounds; marked tachypnea; stress-induced, open-mouthed breathing; wheezing; no cyanosis
IV. Hypoxemia	Increased lung sounds; open-mouthed breathing; forced expiration; aerophagia; barrel-shaped thorax; cyanosis; anxiety
V. Status asthmaticus	Increased lung sounds; open-mouthed breathing; cyanosis; gasping; marked aerophagia; abdominal distention; frantic clawing at face; death

Adapted from Moise NS, Spaulding GL. Feline bronchial asthma: Pathogenesis, pathophysiology, diagnostics, and therapeutic considerations. Compend Contin Educ Pract Vet 1981;3:109.

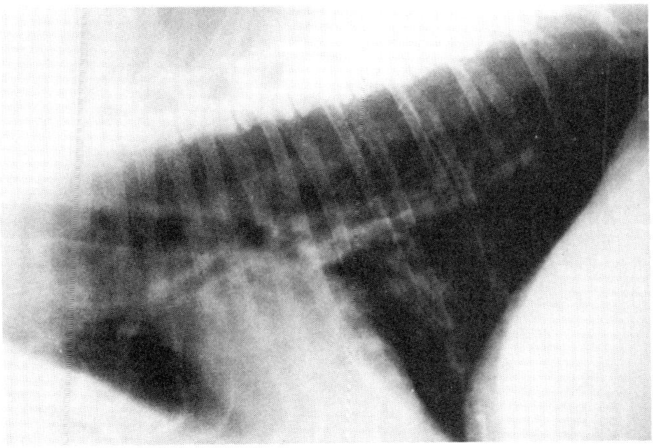

A

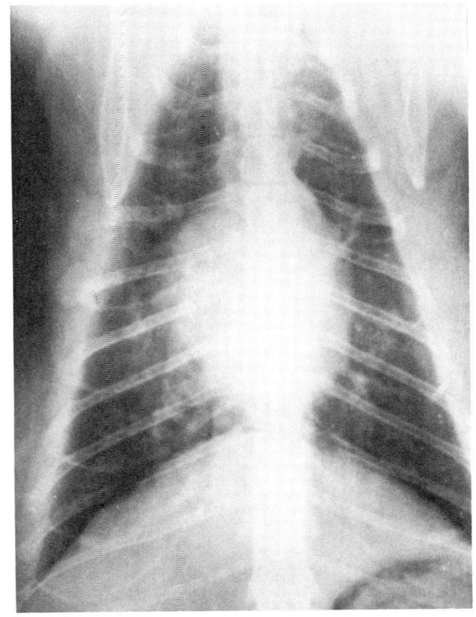

B

Figure 25–3. (*A*) A lateral thoracic radiograph of a cat with the early chronic stage of asthma reveals increased pulmonary radiolucency and bronchial wall thickening. This is the only common feline disease that produces a bronchial pattern. Other diseases producing the same radiographic pattern are electric shock and smoke inhalation. (*B*) A ventrodorsal view of the same cat as in Figure 25–3*A*.

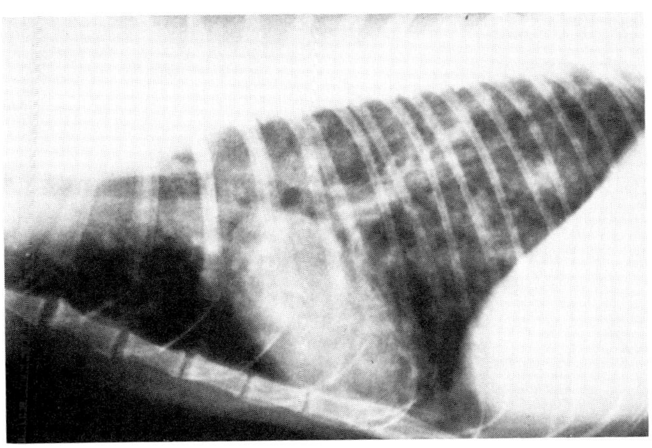

A

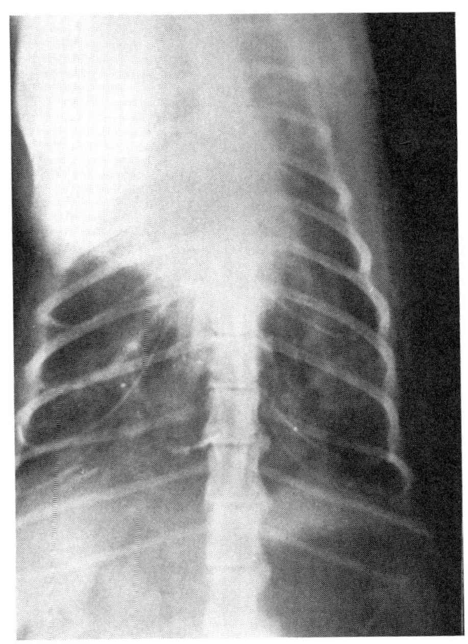

B

Figure 25–4. (*A*) A lateral thoracic radiograph of a cat with the advanced chronic stage of asthma reveals a disseminated interstitial pattern that is secondary to cellular infiltrates. (*B*) A ventrodorsal view of the same cat as in Figure 25–4*A*.

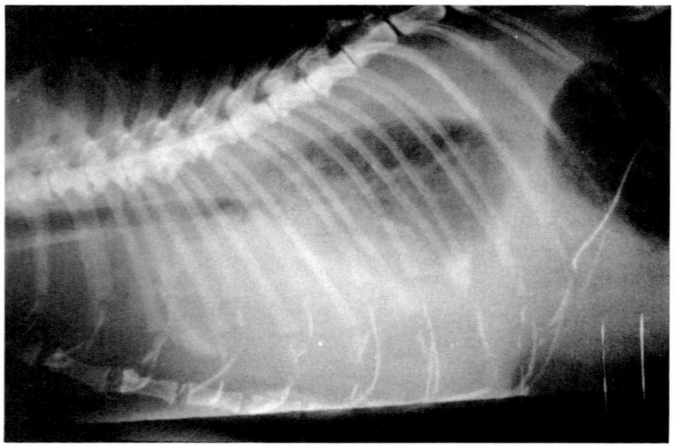

Figure 25–5. **Advanced asthma may result in pleural effusion, as evidenced by this radiograph.**

dure is performed, a bacterial culture should also be performed on the recovered fluid in order to confirm or rule out the possibility of a bacterial infection acting as a primary contributing factor or as a secondary factor. Flotation and Baermann fecal examinations are also appropriate in order to rule out migrating intestinal parasites and lungworms.[2,3]

Treatment

For most cats with asthma, periodic treatment is all that is needed. Because asthma is often a seasonal condition, many cats have only one to three bouts of asthma per year. However, cats with nonseasonal asthma that have frequent episodes may require continuous therapy.

If the cat is extremely dyspneic, oxygen administration may be required before any other drugs are given or any diagnostic tests are performed. The use of a face mask is discouraged because severely dyspneic cats may die struggling to resist the mask. Placing the cat in an oxygen cage for a few minutes to a few hours may be adequate for stabilization.

There are three goals of treatment in severe cases of feline asthma:[6]

- To block and/or present the hypersensitivity reaction
- To relieve bronchospasm
- To treat a bacterial infection, if present

In Stage II disease, only the first goal may need to be met, whereas in Stage V disease, all three goals must be attained. Blocking the hypersensitivity reaction involves the use of corticosteroids. Stage II asthma may be treated with an injection of a long-acting drug, such as methylprednisolone acetate (Depo-Medrol) or triamcinolone (Vetalog), or with a 1- to 4-week regimen of prednisolone. Cats with Stage III, IV, or V disease will require rapid-acting drugs, such as dexamethasone (Dexamethasone Sodium Phosphate Injection) or prednisolone sodium succinate (Solu-Delta-Cortef) (see Table 25–2).

Preventing the hypersensitivity reaction involves removing the offending allergen. Dusty cat litter should be replaced with newspaper or aquarium gravel on a trial basis.

Table 25–2. Drugs for Treating Feline Asthma

Drug	Dosage
Initial Corticosteroids	
Dexamethasone (Dexamethasone Sodium Phosphate Injection)	0.1–1.0 mg/lb/day IV or IM
Prednisolone sodium succinate (Solu-Delta-Cortef)	0.45–1.4 mg/lb IV or IM
Maintenance Corticosteroids	
Prednisolone	0.45–0.9 mg/lb orally b.i.d. or t.i.d., then 2.5–5.0 mg/cat every other evening
Methylprednisolone acetate (Depo-Medrol)	0.23 mg/lb IM q6–8 wk
Triamcinolone (Vetalog)	0.23 mg/lb IM or SC q3–4 wk
Initial Bronchodilators	
Epinephrine (Adrenalin)	0.5–0.75 mL of 1:10,000 solution IM or SC
Aminophylline (Aminophyllin)	50 mg/cat orally t.i.d. or 0.5–1.5 mg/lb/day IM, or by slow IV infusion
Terbutaline (Brethine)	2.5 mg orally t.i.d.
Atropine	0.02 mg/lb IM or SC
Maintenance Bronchodilators	
Terbutaline (Brethine)	1.25 mg/cat orally b.i.d.
Aminophylline (Aminophyllin)	50 mg/cat orally t.i.d.
Theophylline elixir (Elixophyllin)	0.05 mL/lb orally q6–12h
Theophylline (sustained) (Theo-Dur)	50–100 mg/cat orally s.i.d.

Adapted from Moise NS, Spaulding GL. Feline bronchial asthma: Pathogenesis, pathophysiology, diagnostics, and therapeutic considerations. Compend Contin Educ Pract Vet 1981;3:109, and Kuehn NF, Roudebush P. Allergic Lung Disease. In: Allen DG, ed. Small Animal Medicine. Philadelphia: JB Lippincott, 1991:423.
Abbreviations: IV, intravenous; IM, intramuscular; SC, subcutaneous.

The cat's environmental exposure to cigarette smoke, fireplace smoke, strong perfumes, insulating materials, and plant allergens should be curtailed or eliminated. Furnace and air conditioner filters should be replaced. Air purifying filters may be helpful. Unfortunately, these measures are rarely successful.

The alleviation of bronchospasm, which is usually necessary in Stage III, IV, and V disease, may be accomplished with one or more of several drugs. Epinephrine (Adrenalin, 1:1000) should be considered in the most severe cases; however, this agent should be used with caution because it may produce tachycardia and arrhythmias. Terbutaline (Brethine) is a pure β_2 stimulator but has a slower onset of action than epinephrine because it must be given orally. Atropine has proved useful in treating resistant bronchospasm, but it should not be used for long-term therapy because it thickens airway secretions. When dyspnea is relieved, bronchodilation may be sustained by administering aminophylline (Aminophyllin or Aminophyllin Injection), theophylline (Elixophyllin or Theo-Dur), or terbutaline. These drugs may be continued on a long-term basis if needed (see Table 25–2).

If pyrexia suggests a bacterial infection, or if the results of a bacterial culture are positive, antibiotic therapy is indicated. Until the results of culture and sensitivity are available, treatment with antibiotics having a high affinity for the respiratory tract, a wide spectrum of activity, and minimal side effects in cats should be considered. These include gentamicin (Gentocin), amikacin (Amiglyde-V), enrofloxacin (Baytril), and amoxicillin (Amoxi-Tabs and Clavamox).

Fractious or panicked cats may benefit from mild sedation. Ketamine (Ketaset) has been found to block bronchospasm and would thus be a good choice at a dose of 10 to 20 mg intramuscularly (IM) or subcutaneously (SC). The phenothiazine tranquilizers, such as acepromazine (Acepromazine Maleate Injection), have α-adrenergic blocking properties and would also be acceptable.[3]

Prognosis

Intermittent feline asthma carries a good prognosis. Even if the allergen is never identified, many cats can be treated successfully with periodic steroid therapy for many years. However, the prognosis is not so favorable for cats that require continuous therapy. Progressive bronchial thickening will eventually lead to emphysema and pulmonary fibrosis. Cats exhibiting this progression should be treated aggressively and continuously with corticosteroids and bronchodilators to minimize the inflammatory response and to prolong adequate airway function.

REFERENCES

1. Perhman RD, Jr. Newer knowledge of feline bronchopulmonary disease. Vet Clin of North Am (Small Anim Pract) 1984;14(5): 1007.
2. Hawkins EC, Ettinger SJ, Suter PF. Diseases of the Lower Respiratory Tract (Lung) and Pulmonary Edema. In: Ettinger SJ, ed. Textbook of Feline Internal Medicine, 3rd ed. Philadelphia: WB Saunders Co., 1989:816.
3. Moise NS, Spaulding GL. Feline bronchial asthma: Pathogenesis, pathophysiology, diagnostics, and therapeutic considerations. Compend Contin Educ Pract Vet 1981;3:109.
4. Weiss EB. Bronchial asthma. Clin Symp 1975;27(1/2):3.
5. Carpenter JL. Bronchial Asthma in Cats. In: Kirk RW, ed. Current Veterinary V. Philadelphia: WB Saunders Co., 1974:208.
6. Kuehn NF, Roudebush P. Allergic Lung Disease. In: Allen DG, ed. Small Animal Medicine. Philadelphia: JB Lippincott, 1991:423.

CHAPTER 26

◇ ◇ ◇

Behavior Problems

Amy R. Marder

One of the most important reasons that people enjoy keeping cats is that they like the way they behave. However, when a cat's behavior begins to interfere with a person's comfortable life-style, the cat is no longer enjoyable and problems develop. Unfortunately, all too often pets with behavior problems are abandoned, given up to shelters, or euthanized. In fact, behavior problems and the resulting disruption of the human–companion animal bond are one of the leading causes of death (through enthanasia) of our pets. In many cases, these behavior problems could have been prevented or successfully treated.

Veterinarians are in a perfect position to diagnose, treat, and help prevent behavior problems. The private practitioner is usually the first person asked for advice about the proper rearing of pets and about unusual and problem behaviors that develop during an animal's life. Since the majority of behavior problems are not due to abnormal behavior, but rather due to normal species-typical behaviors that are incompatible with human behavior, it is essential that a veterinarian understand the normal behavior of companion animals. Knowing about companion animal behavior is just as important as knowing about the gastrointestinal tract when caring for the welfare of the entire animal. Any information the veterinarian is able to give a client is invaluable to both owner and pet. The clinician may be able to offer advice before a problem develops that will help prevent it, or he or she may give advice early in the course of the problem that will eliminate it or stop its progression. In addition, once a problem is established the veterinarian should be able to make an educated differential diagnosis in order to treat the problem or refer the client to an appropriate behavioral specialist.

The feline species has become increasingly popular in recent years and has surpassed the canine species as America's favorite pet. But cats, being members of the feline species, come with their own set of species-typical behaviors that are just waiting to inconvenience owners. Some of the most common complaints that owners have about their cats concern elimination, clawing, and aggression.

Elimination Behavior Problems

Housesoiling is the most common feline behavior problem seen by veterinary animal behaviorists.[1] Although more cat owners in general may be bothered by scratching and walking on countertops, these types of problems are usually tolerable and do not often cause owners to give up a pet. A daily greeting of fresh feces or urine in the corner of the living room, however, often ruins a previously good human–feline relationship and ends in pet relinquishment.

Causes

A cat who is urinating or defecating outside of the litterbox may be doing so for either medical or behavioral reasons. Cystitis and diseases that cause polyuria (e.g., diabetes mellitus) often lead to inappropriate urination. Diarrhea often leads to litterbox problems as well. Although most cats with medical problems have other signs in addition to housesoiling (i.e., polydipsia or stranguria), some either do not or have not been observed by their owners. Therefore, in order to rule out disease, a complete urinalysis and/or fecal exam is necessary. If a cat is both urinating and defecating in inappropriate areas, the cause is most likely behavioral, although neurogenic incontinence should be considered.

After the possibility of disease has been ruled out, a behavioral diagnosis must be pursued (Fig. 26–1). A cat who is urinating and/or defecating in objectionable locations may be marking or merely eliminating. Urine marking is an innate, genetically based behavior that occurs in territorial, agonistic, sexual, or other highly arousing situations. It is most often performed in a spraying posture (standing, with tail upright and quivering while urine is sprayed onto vertical surfaces) but may also be done while squatting. The expression of marking behavior is influenced by many factors, hormonal and environmental stimuli being the most important. Androgens and estrogens facilitate urine marking, while progestins are inhibitory. Intact male cats mark more frequently than castrated males and intact female cats more than spayed females (primarily during estrus). The sights, odors, and sounds of outdoor cats may cause a cat to mark as does competition among indoor cats. Often, a male (intact or castrated) cat may start to mark if a queen in the house or neighborhood goes into estrus. The marking function of feces has not been clearly demonstrated in domestic cats. However, the fact that it serves a communication function in many other species makes a marking function in some situations likely (such as when feces are deposited on countertops and beds).

Cats who are urinating and/or defecating outside of

SCIENCE SUMMARY

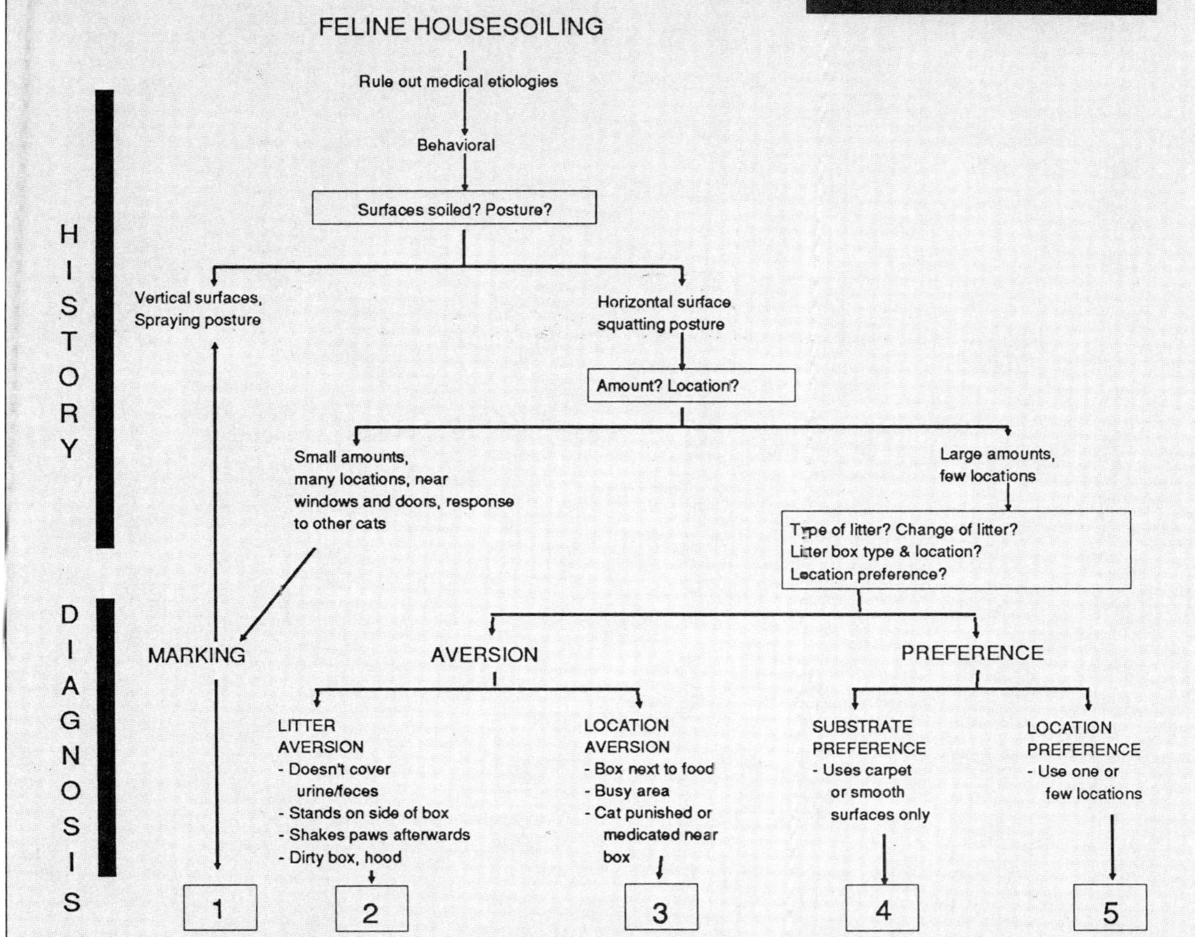

1. Dx: Marking

Management:

- Neuter intact cat.
- Environmental manipulation:

❒ Limit exposure to outdoor cats (pull blinds).

❒ Increase or decrease time spent outdoors.

❒ Change significance of marking areas (food, toys).

❒ Make marking areas aversive (foil, lemon scent).

- Drug therapy:

❒ Progestins.

❒ Diazepam.

❒ Other anxiolytics.

2-5. Note: Aversions and preferences often occur simultaneously. Thus, the basic management approach is to make the litterbox inviting *and* the inappropriate locations unpleasant.

2. Dx: Litter aversion

Management:

❒ Use plain clay or sand-like clay (2-3 in.).

❒ Scoop urine and feces daily; change at least weekly, using only plain soap and water.

❒ Remove hood.

❒ Provide one box per cat in multi-cat households.

❒ Give choice of substrate.

3. Dx: Location aversion

❒ Move box to quieter area.

❒ Separate box from feeding area.

❒ Don't punish then put in box.

4. Dx: Substrate preference

❒ Alter substrate/surface—cover carpet with thick plastic, leave water in bathtub; remove alteration gradually.

❒ Place preferred substrate next to non-aversive litter.

❒ Make preferred location aversive (with foil, lemon scent); remove aversive substance gradually.

5. Dx: Location preference

❒ Change significance of preferred location (with food, toys).

❒ Make preferred location aversive (with foil, lemon scent); remove aversive substance gradually.

❒ Place the litter box at preferred location; gradually return to original location.

Figure 26–1. Flowchart for diagnosis of feline housesoiling. (Used with permission from Marder A. Feline housesoiling. Pet Veterinarian 1989;1;11.)

the litterbox merely for the purpose of elimination use a squatting posture. They use locations other than their litterbox because of the instinctive urge of cats to eliminate in many substrates and locations (loose dirt, leaves, sand, etc.) combined with learned aversions and preferences. Cats often will faithfully use the box for one form of excrement but avoid the box for the other. A cat may avoid using the litterbox if the litter or the box area is or has been associated with something aversive, e.g., new litter, hood on box, dirty box, deodorizer, punishment, loud noise, feeding near box, or a bout of painful cystitis. Whether or not a cat clearly demonstrates a litter aversion, most cats with elimination problems also show either a location or surface preference. Cats with location preferences generally choose areas that are quiet and somewhat secluded (e.g., the corner of the dining room). The most common surface preference is for carpeting, although some cats choose smooth surfaces such as bathtubs, sinks, and linoleum. It is controversial whether cats are drawn back to an area because of the odor there. In fact, a dirty litterbox or very soiled area may be more likely to deter cats than attract them. In the author's experience, emotional causes of housesoiling problems are not as common as popularly believed. Separation anxiety and the introduction of new household members (such as a new baby) do however occasionally cause cats to mark or eliminate outside of the litterbox.

Diagnosis

A thorough history, physical examination and appropriate laboratory tests (urinalysis and fecal exam) are necessary in order to make a diagnosis (Table 26–1).

Table 26–1. Diagnosis of Feline Elimination Problems

Diagnosis	**Urination**
Posture	Squat
Location	Horizontal surfaces
Amount	Usually large volume
History	Occurs when cat needs to empty bladder. Cat usually scratches before and after. Cat often shows signs of litter or box aversion: does not dig or cover, stands on the sides of the box, runs from the box. Obvious causes for aversion: dirty box, hood, food close to box, inaccessibility, noisy area, perfumed litter. Cat shown location or substrate preference (carpet, sinks). Usually urinates in only a few locations. Cat often uses box for feces.
Diagnosis	**Defecation**
Posture	Squat
Location	Horizontal surfaces
Amount	Normal bowel movement
History	Occurs when cat has urge to defecate. Same as urination. Cat will often use box for urine.
Diagnosis	**Marking**
Posture	Spray
Location	Vertical surfaces
Amount	Usually small volume
History	Often occurs in many locations. Occurs in contact of territorial, sexual, or competitive interactions or other highly arousing circumstances. Often seasonal. Often occurs at exit points, e.g., doors and windows. May be initiated by introduction of new family member (baby, spouse) or animal.
Diagnosis	**Marking**
Posture	Squat or semi-squat
Location	Horizontal surfaces
Amount	Usually small volume
History	Occurs in same circumstances as spray. Often occurs on objects, beds, and clothing.
Diagnosis	**Fecal marking**
Posture	Squat
Location	Horizontal surfaces
Amount	Normal bowel movement
History	Very little is known, but may occur in same circumstances as urine marking.

Treatment

Before any behavioral therapy is initiated, physical disorders (i.e., cystitis, diarrhea) must first be corrected.

Marking

Because marking behavior is influenced by a number of hormonal, environmental, and behavioral variables, there are a variety of treatment techniques that may be effective. Manipulation of the environment is the least invasive of all techniques and is sometimes helpful. If a cat is marking in only a few locations, changing the significance of the areas by feeding or playing with the cat there may at least stop the problem in those locations. Making the locations unpleasant by placing citrus-scented air fresheners or aluminum foil at the spots may also help. Preventing access to outdoor cats (closing a shade or door) or changing (increasing or decreasing) the amount of time a cat spends outdoors may reduce or eliminate marking in the home. For some unknown reason, providing cats who are marking with one form of the sandlike (clumping) litters reduces the incidence of marking.[2] Behavior modification in the form of reward and punishment are rarely if ever effective.

Although some cats may no longer mark in the owner's presence, they continue to do so at other times. Surgical therapies include neutering, ischiocavernosus myectomy, and olfactory tractotomy. Castration has a 90% probability of reducing spraying in male cats, regardless of age performed or the duration of spraying.[3] Spaying is likely to reduce marking by a female cat if the incidence of marking is related to the estrus cycle. Removal of the cat's sense of smell through an olfactory tractotomy is reported to reduce or stop spraying in about 50% of cats refractory to castration and progestin drug therapy.[4] Recently, researchers have described the surgical procedure of severing the ischiocavernosus muscle as a treatment for spraying.[5]

The most effective treatment for marking in already neutered cats is drug therapy. The progestins, diazepam, amitriptyline, and other antianxiety drugs have been shown to be effective in reducing or eliminating marking behavior.[6] When using drug therapy, owners should be advised that no drugs are approved or marketed for treatment of behavioral problems in cats. Drug therapy of any kind should be gradually stopped every 1 to 2 months to determine if the cat is still motivated to mark, as many cats are seasonal sprayers. As there seems to be a wide range of minimum therapeutic doses, the lowest effective dose should be used.

Diazepam (Valium) at a dose of 1 to 2 mg PO b.i.d. significantly reduces spraying in more than 70% of cats.[7] Side effects include increased appetite and affection, sedation, and ataxia. In addition, cats develop a tolerance to the drug and thus should be gradually withdrawn when discontinuing therapy. Two progestins have been used. Megestrol acetate (Ovaban) is generally used at a dose of 5 mg PO s.i.d. for 7 to 10 days, then 5 mg PO once weekly for 1 month, then 2.5 mg PO once weekly for another month.

Medroxyprogesterone acetate (Depo-Provera) has been used at a dose of 10 to 20 mg/kg SC repeated as needed for a maximum of three injections per year. These drugs reduce or eliminate marking in about 30% of cats.[8] Potential side effects include increased appetite, lethargy, transient hyperglycemia, diabetes mellitus, aspermatogenesis, mammary gland hyperplasia, mammary adenocarcinoma, and pyometritis. If used, blood glucose, mammary gland development, and body weight should be carefully monitored during the course of therapy (see Chapter 7). Oral therapy is preferred because it is slightly more effective and can be rapidly withdrawn if side effects occur.[9]

Urination or Defecation Problems

When a cat chooses a new area in which to eliminate, the new behavior becomes ingrained, somewhat like a bad habit.[10] At this point, just changing the initiating cause (such as cleaning a once dirty litterbox) is unlikely to correct the problem. The factors that are operating to maintain the problem at the present time as well as the initiating factors must be considered when designing a program for inappropriate elimination problems. (In many cases, the original cause is no longer present.[1])

Two treatment techniques, which are commonly prescribed but are rarely effective, are punishment and confinement. Punishment many hours after the fact, followed by putting the cat in the box, is more likely to cause a litterbox aversion than cure an elimination problem. Confinement forces the cat to use the box, but at the same time does not allow access to the inappropriate area. Once the cat is again permitted into the area, however, it usually resumes eliminating there.

A simple way to approach elimination problems is to make the litterbox desirable from the cat's point of view and make the inappropriate areas unpleasant. If done simultaneously, in most cases both the initiating and maintaining factors are addressed.

Ways to make litter boxes more desirable generally correct the initiating factors. These may include eliminating the hood if present, using plain clay litter rather than deodorized or perfumed types (the new sandlike clumping litters are best),[12] keeping the box clean by scooping both the feces and urine-soaked litter daily and changing the entire box weekly, keeping 2 to 3 inches of litter in the box at all times, moving the box to a more accessible or quieter location, moving it to the inappropriate area (if the cat has a strong location preference), providing at least two boxes and one box per cat (within limits), feeding the cat a distance from the box, or providing another type of substrate such as newspaper or wood shavings (if the cat does not seem to like clay at all).

At the same time that the changes in the box are made, the inappropriate area must be made relatively intolerable. This usually eliminates the maintaining factors. Ways to do this may include covering a carpeted area with a thick plastic drop cloth in order to change the feeling of the substrate, putting a citrus-scented solid air freshener in the area, feeding the cat or playing with it at the problem location, and leaving a few inches of water in the bathrub or sink. Sometimes rewarding the cat with praise and a special treat every time it uses the box is also helpful.

Once the cat begins to use the box again, things should not be changed too quickly back to the way the owner might prefer them. If the owner progresses too quickly, the cat usually goes back to its old habits. Things should be left in place for one month, then changes can be made. For instance, the owner might start to cut away the plastic, move the box a few inches each day back to a more desirable location, and begin mixing in clay litter with wood shavings over a period of another month. Most households are back to normal within 3 months. Special care should be taken not to initiate the problem again or the process may start all over.

Although relapses are common, in the majority of elimination problem cases cats can be converted back to using the litterbox. Unless environmental factors radically change, marking behavior is rarely completely "cured." It can usually be well controlled, however, and kept to a tolerable minimum.

Clawing

Cats' instinctive urge to scratch and claw has ruined many a couch and stereo speaker. Some simple advice based on feline normal scratching behavior may not only save your clients' furniture but also enable your patients to keep their claws.

Causes

Scratching is a normal species-typical behavior of cats. The act of scratching not only removes the sheaths from the claw but also serves a visual and olfactory territorial marking function. Outdoor cats claw trees and wood and frequently return to the same marking posts. Indoor cats, if not provided with an adequate surface, usually choose furniture and woodwork.

Diagnosis

The diagnosis of destruction by scratching is easily made by taking a history. Owners usually have either observed the behavior directly or have seen the results of the behavior numerous times.

Treatment

Problem scratching can be treated either by behavioral or surgical means. Most owners will want to try behavioral methods before surgery. Owners should first be advised to provide a natural and desirable scratching post, preferably from the time of kittenhood. Simple posts made of securely supported soft logs are often eagerly used and are inexpensive. Of the scratching posts that can be purchased, those made of sisal seem to be preferred by many cats. Since many cats claw soon after awakening, the post or posts should be placed close to the cat's sleeping area. Toys and catnip may be used to initially attract the cat. After the cat begins to use the post, a combination of olfactory and visual cues, texture, and location act to draw the cat back again. Food rewards and verbal praise may be added following usage of the post if necessary. If a cat has already started to claw inappropriate surfaces, some form of punishment must be used. Loud noises (whistles, airhorns, handclaps, screams) and water sprayed at the cat may be used by the owner; however, this does not prevent scratching when the owner is not present. Double-sided cellophane tape placed on the surfaces that the cat is clawing is an easily applied deterrent that is usually effective. Once the post has been used exclusively for a period of a few months, the tape can be gradually removed.

Every effort should be made to make the scratching post more desirable than the furniture. (If the owner is considering reupholstering, a tightly woven or smooth fabric should be chosen. The old clawed fabric can then be used to cover the post.) If behavioral methods are not effective, some owners are interested in trying products, which when applied to the cat's nails, allow the cat to claw without being destructive. Since these products are glued to the cat's claws and need to be replaced as the claws grow, only compliant cats are able to be fitted with them. Clients should be made aware of their availability, however.

Surgical declawing is often thought of as a last resort because of ethical considerations and fears of behavioral and "psychological" consequences. Critics of declawing claim that the surgery may trigger physical ailments, such as cystitis, asthma, and skin disorders, and a weakening of the muscles of the forelimbs and shoulders. They also state that hunting, balance, fighting, climbing, and feline social relationships are adversely affected. It is also widely believed that declawed cats bite more and suffer more litterbox problems. Recent studies have indicated, however, that declawing had no adverse behavioral effects and successfully satisfied owners' expectations. In addition, many cats continued to go outdoors without any problems (41% of 276 in one study). Owners claimed that their cats continued to hunt, climb, and defend themselves without difficulty after being declawed. The studies also indicated that declawed cats were no more likely to bite and did not have any more inappropriate elimination problems than clawed cats.

Other than a short period of postsurgical discomfort, medical complications of declawing were minimal. Many owners reported that they could not have kept their cats had they not been declawed.[10] Considering the results of these studies, declawing should be considered an effective and safe treatment for a clawing problem that has not responded to a behavior modification program.

Aggression

Aggression[11] directed to people or other cats is another common behavioral complaint of cat owners. Cat bites and scratches, although not usually severe, may potentially lead to serious infections in both people and cats. Signs of aggression (stalking, chasing, pouncing, scratching, biting, growling, and hissing) are often quite frightening to owners and are commonly misinterpreted.

Causes and Classification

Aggression is a complex, multidimensional phenomenon that is influenced by numerous factors including genetic predisposition, early experience, maturation, sex, age, size, learning, hormonal status, physiologic state, and external stimuli. It is not surprising, therefore, that the classification of aggression has often been the subject of controversy among behaviorists. A functional classification scheme, based on an analysis of sequences and patterns of behaviors and the circumstances in which they occur, seems to be most useful when making a diagnosis and setting up a treatment plan.

When presented with an aggressive cat, it is most important to understand that the majority of aggressive cats are exhibiting normal and appropriate species-typical behavior that is unacceptable or dangerous in a human household. Some diseases, however, do cause some cats to exhibit truly abnormal behavior patterns that are not consistent with species-typical behavior. Although most organically caused behavior changes are accompanied by other signs of disease that are evident on a thorough physical examination, a good knowledge of normal feline behavior is essential in order to make an accurate diagnosis (Tables 26–2 and 26–3).

Interfeline Aggression

Intermale Aggression

As males reach adulthood, they often start to threaten each other over territory and mates.[12] Sometimes these encounters lead to fighting. Aggressive interaction usually begins with a threat ritual and is accompanied by growls and loud howls. If an attack occurs, it often results in only one bite, but if infection ensues it may be serious.

Treatment

Castration has a 90% probability of stopping or reducing intermale aggression regardless of age or duration of the problem. It may also be reduced by progestins (megestrol acetate or medroxyprogesterone acetate). If the problem persists after castration, separating the male cats is the best prevention.

Territorial Aggression

Aggression occurring between two cats in defense of territory generally involves an aggressive pursuit accompanied by growling and hissing. One cat is usually the aggressor

Table 26–2. Intercat Aggression Problems

Diagnosis	**Intermale aggression**
Age	Onset 2 to 3 years
Sex	Male
History	May be sudden or gradual onset.
Behavioral Description	Yelling, yowling, scratching, hissing, attacking other male cats. Usually accompanied by ritualized threat displays.
Diagnosis	**Territorial aggression**
Age	Onset 2 to 3 years
Sex	Either
History	May be sudden or gradual onset.
Behavioral Description	Characterized by one cat pursuing the other, growling, chasing, attacking, scratching, and biting.
Diagnosis	**Fear-induced aggression**
Age	Any age
Sex	Either
History	Sudden onset. May begin after frightening event or redirected aggression.
Behavioral Description	Both cats assume defensive attitudes (ears back, body hunched, dilated pupils, paw blows, piloerection). Cats usually do not seek each other. Cats seem to misinterpret each other's signals.
Diagnosis	**Redirected aggression**
Age	Any age
Sex	Either
History	Sudden onset. Usually occurs after some type of aggressive event.
Behavioral Description	Same as fear-induced.

and relentlessly pursues the other cat, attempting to chase it away. In a house, the aggressor often lies in wait behind a closed door growling at his victim.

This is one of the most difficult feline problems to treat, and the prognosis is poor. Recommending relocation to a new home for one of the cats, preferably the aggressor if in a multi-cat household, is often the best plan for both cats and owner. Drug therapy either with progestins or tranquilizers is rarely if ever curative. A program consisting of counterconditioning and habituation techniques may be attempted if the owner is motivated. There have been a few reports of successful treatment with these techniques. The cats are initially separated and then gradually introduced using a cage at first and then leashes. They are first exposed to each other at a long distance (20 feet, for instance) and only during feeding time. The intercat distance is gradually shortened and the time of exposure is then gradually lengthened. If at any time during the process there are signs of aggression, they are separated again or they are kept together with one in a cage until the aggression ceases. Owners should be advised to use a pillow or blanket when handling an aggressive cat, as many will redirect their aggression to owners.

Table 26–3 Feline Aggression Toward People

Diagnosis	**Play aggression**
Age	Usually <3 years (but may be <1 year)
Sex	Either
History	Usually occurs in single-cat households or with young cat and older unplayful cat. Directed toward one or several family members.
Behavioral Description	Predatory-like behavior (stalking, chasing, pouncing, biting, and scratching). Bites are usually not severe. Cat goes for moving body parts such as hands and legs. Pupils often dilate. Does not growl.
Diagnosis	**Redirected aggression**
Age	Any
Sex	Either
History	Occurs suddenly. Happens when person approaches or touches cat in aggressive mood. May be elicited by smell.
Behavioral Description	Usually involves hissing, growling, biting, and scratching. Cat may even pursue person.
Diagnosis	**Fear-induced aggression**
Age	Any
Sex	Either
History	Usually directed toward new person. Problem is frequently made worse with punishment.
Behavioral Description	Cat assumes fearful/defensive posture (crouch, flattened ears, piloerection), hiss, and growl. May bite and scratch if approached or touched.
Diagnosis	**Territorial**
Age	Any
Sex	Either
History	Directed toward visitors. Usually very friendly to family.
Behavioral Description	Cat assumes offensive attack posture. Ears forward, sometimes swiveled outward, body erect. Often accompanied by a growl. Cat follows person.
Diagnosis	**Aggression while being petted or hugged.**
Age	Any
Sex	Either
History	Directed toward anyone who pets or hugs the cat.
Behavioral Description	Cat enjoys or tolerates petting up to a point, may even purr, but then bites and runs away. May also resist being held and petted. Bites are inhibited.
Diagnosis	**Idiopathic aggression**
Age	Any
Sex	Either
History	Sudden attack with no apparent eliciting stimulus.
Behavioral Description	Severe and repeated attacks and biting, scratching, and sometimes chasing.

Fear-Induced or Defensive Aggression

A cat that is frightened often defends itself by being aggressive. A defensive cat will crouch, flatten its ears, hiss, spit, and exhibit piloerection. If approached, the cat is likely to attack. Sometimes two cats within the same household will suddenly begin fighting after a frightening incident occurs. For instance, two cats that were previously friendly become aggressive to each other after a lamp falls off a table.

Treatment

Unlike territorial aggression, fear-induced aggression has a good prognosis. The two cats must first be separated so that they are unable to see each other. When the two cats are no longer in an obviously aggressive state (as when they start to play with each other under a closed door) a gradual introduction program should be initiated as described under territorial aggression. The program must proceed slowly to avoid provoking aggression and may last anywhere between one week and several months. Occasionally, a tranquilizer such as diazepam (1 to 2 mg/cat s.i.d. or b.i.d.) is helpful and may shorten the length of treatment.

Redirected Aggression

Redirected aggression[13] is a common cause of intercat aggression. Cats often redirect aggression onto another cat if interfered with while in an aggressive state. A typical example is the cat who becomes aggressively aroused on seeing an outdoor cat and attacks its housemate who is walking by.

Treatment

Redirected aggression between cats is treated in the same manner as territorial aggression or fear-induced aggression. The prognosis is good. Owners must be aware that the treatment may last as long as six to eight weeks and that the problem could recur. All attempts should be made to eliminate the original stimulus of the aggression. Reducing or eliminating access to outdoor cats is often helpful, as they are common initiators (e.g., keeping shades closed, trapping strays, keeping cat indoors, spraying outdoor cats with water, or putting mothballs outside in cloth sacs).

Introducing a New Cat to a Household

Another common concern of cat owners is how to go about introducing a new cat into a household that already has a resident cat.[11] When giving advice on this matter, the word to stress is *gradual.* If they are introduced too rapidly, they may attack each other, disturbing the owner and risking injury to both cats and owners. The cats should be kept separately at first for a few days. They may be alternated among different rooms in the home so that they become familiar with each other's odor. After the hissing and growling subsides, they may be allowed to see each other during feeding time while they are fed at a distance. They are gradually fed closer and closer together until they can eat next to each other without becoming aggressive. At this point, all is well and they can be allowed to be with each other. If signs of aggression occur, however, they should be separated again and the process repeated. Although the introduction procedure usually takes only two to three days, it may occasionally take weeks.

Aggression Toward People

Play Aggression

Although often misinterpreted, aggression as a part of play is probably the most common type of aggressive behavior that cats exhibit toward their owners.[11] Young mammals in general spend a considerable portion of their day engaging in play. Normal play consists of behaviors that closely resemble components of predation and fighting (stalking, pouncing, scratching, and biting). During play they "practice" to help them prepare for hunting and intercat disputes later in life.

Treatment

As play aggression usually occurs in single-cat households and in cats under one year of age, the easiest method of treatment for some owners is just to get another cat of approximately the same age. If a feline playmate is present, the young playful patient usually prefers the cat over the human. If getting another cat is not convenient or possible, a program consisting of daily vigorous and appropriate play combined with mild punishment should be initiated. String toys that can be pulled across the floor, Ping-Pong balls, and balls of crumpled paper or foil are effective ways to get a cat to play vigorously. Paper bags and boxes often stimulate exploration and play. Bird feeders placed on windows also keep bored cats occupied. If the cat's playful attacks can be predicted, as they often can, the attack can be redirected to a moving toy first. For example, the owner can dangle a string while stepping out of the shower, or throw a Ping-Pong ball before coming down the stairs. Punishment, when used, must be combined with active play, as the cat needs to play. Sometimes, a water sprayer or loud air horn is an effective method of punishment. Whatever is used, it must be used every time the cat begins the play attack. Owners should be warned not to hit or otherwise physically punish playfully aggressive cats, as they are likely to become defensive and injure their owners. The prognosis for play aggression is good.

Redirected Aggression

Aggression is also sometimes directed toward people if a cat is interfered with while aggressively motivated. Redirected aggression often occurs unexpectedly in otherwise friendly and affectionate cats. Owners are commonly attacked while trying to soothe an aggressive cat.

Treatment

The best method of treating redirected aggression is prevention. Owners often try to calm an aggressive cat by petting. They should be advised that it is dangerous to approach or handle an aggressive cat. Owners should always wait until the cat is out of its aggressive state before interacting with it. Physical punishment is contraindicated, as it often makes the cat more aggressive. Occasionally, the cat's aggressive state lasts for days. In these cases, tranquilizers (diazepam 1 to 2 mg/cat b.i.d.) are helpful. Separation from the cat, except during feeding time, usually solves the problem. Petting the cat should be avoided until the cat has clearly demonstrated that it is no longer aggressive. The prognosis is good, but the problem may recur.

Fear or Defensive Aggression

Cats who are frightened may also aggressively defend themselves from a person. A typical example is a cat who is disciplined for hissing at a house guest out of fear and responds aggressively.

Treatment

A problem that occurs often is when a cat living with a single person must accept a new person (such as a roommate, boyfriend, or girlfriend). The best method of treatment is to avoid all behaviors that frighten the cat (loud voices, forced petting, punishment) and encourage those that the cat enjoys. The easiest way to desensitize the cat's fear of a person is to associate that person with delicious food and play. The cat should at first eat its favorite food at a distance from the person. Gradually, the cat should eat closer and closer to the person until it will eat directly from the person's hand. Pulling string toys along the floor is a good method of initiating play in fearful cats. The prognosis is good.

Aggression Related to Being Petted

Some cats do not like to be held or petted excessively and may respond to these activities by biting or scratching. In most cases these are just signals to tell their owners to stop. Often owners, because of previous experience and expectations, have difficulty accepting the fact that they just do not own a huggable cat.

Treatment

Probably the most important part of the treatment for this type of aggression is to get the owner to accept that their cat does not like excessive petting. They must understand that it is not that their cat does not like them, it is just that some cats like physical contact and others do not. Physical punishment should be avoided as it is likely to provoke a defensive response. Rather than punishing after the bite, owners should carefully observe the cat for signs of discomfort before the actual bite and stop petting first. Owners should also interact with their cats in ways that the cats clearly enjoy, such as play. Most owners find that when they stop trying to force physical affection on their cats, their cats start to become more affectionate in other ways. For example, many begin to sit next to their owners more often and sleep with them. In general, the prognosis is good.

Idiopathic Aggressive Behavior

There have been occasional reports of cats becoming suddenly aggressive with no warning and without any identifiable eliciting stimulus. Many of these cats are probably cases of redirected or defensive aggression, but they have been euthanized before a good behavioral history could be taken. Psychomotor epilepsy should be considered an etiology (see Chapter 23).

Treatment

In many cases of seemingly unprovoked aggressive attacks, a thorough behavioral history reveals a cause, such as redirected or defensive aggression. But if no medical or environmental reason for the attacks can be determined, they cannot be treated. Sudden, unprovoked feline attacks are extremely dangerous and euthanasia must be considered.

Territorial Aggression

Although rare, some cats defend their homes from people. This sometimes occurs when owners are away and catsitters enter the house to care for the cat.

Patient Monitoring

All cases of feline aggression must be treated as serious problems. Follow-up evaluations are generally done by telephone on a weekly basis to monitor both the progress of the cat and owner. The treatment program is altered if necessary. The length of treatment varies according to the type and severity of the aggression and the motivation of the owner. When and if the problem is controlled, owners are told to call if it recurs.

Prevention of Behavior Problems

Although not always possible, the best way to treat a behavior problem is by preventing it from occurring. Owner education in the early kitten visits may not only prevent problems but also makes owners more aware (even if unconsciously) of their pet's behavior so that they can detect problems sooner. By discussing behavior at the beginning and also at regular yearly check-ups, owners know that their veterinarian is interested and knowledgeable about behavior and are more likely to seek help early.

REFERENCES

1. Borchelt PL, Voith VL. Elimination behavior problems in cats. Compend Contin Ed Pract Vet 1986;8:197.
2. Borchelt PL. Cat elimination behavior problems. Vet Clin North Am (Small Anim Pract) 1991;21(2):257.
3. Hart BL, Barrett RE. Effects of castration on fighting, roaming, and urine spraying in adult male cats. J Am Vet Med Assoc 1973;163:290.
4. Hart BL. Olfactory tractotomy for control of objectionable urine spraying and urine marking in cats. J Am Vet Med Assoc 1981;179:231.
5. Komtebedde J, Hauptman J. Bilateral ischiocavernosis myectomy for urine spraying in cats. Vet Surg 1990;19:293.
6. Marder AR. Psychotropic drugs and behavioral therapy. Vet Clin North Am (Small Anim Pract) 1991;21(2):337.
7. Marder AR, Voith VL. Effectiveness of diazepam for the treatment of spraying in cats. Paper presented at the Animal Behavior Society Meeting, Raleigh, 1985.
8. Hart BL. Objectionable urine spraying. Urine marking in cats: Evaluation of progestin treatment in gonadectomized males and females. J Am Vet Med Assoc 1980;177:529.
9. Henik RA, Olson PN, Rosychuk RA. Progestagen therapy in cats. Compend Cont Ed Pract Vet 1985;7:132.
10. Landsberg GM. Feline scratching and destruction and the effects of declawing. Vet Clin North Amer (Adv Companion Anim Behav) 1991;21(2):265.
11. Borchelt PL, Voith VL. Aggressive behavior in cats. Compend Cont Ed Pract Vet 1987;9:49.
12. Voith VL, Borchelt PL. Diagnosis and treatment of elimination behavior problems in cats. Vet Clin North Am (Small Anim Pract) 1982;12(4):673.
13. Chapman BL, Voith VL. Cat aggression redirected to people: Cases (1981–1987). J Am Vet Med Assoc 1990;196:947.

CHAPTER 27

◊ ◊ ◊

Cardiomyopathy and Thromboembolic Disease

Gary D. Norsworthy

Overview

Cardiac diseases may be the result of valvular, ischemic, congenital, or other cardiovascular structural abnormalities. Feline cardiomyopathy is the result of myocardial dysfunction or failure.[1] Many forms of feline cardiomyopathy have been described, but four dominate the literature. Each form has unique characteristics, as well as characteristics that overlap with the other types. Differentiation is essential, as the ideal therapy is based on the specific disease form. Table 27–1 offers a brief comparison of the three most common forms.

Most cardiomyopathy is primary and idiopathic. However, two secondary forms have been identified. Hyperthyroidism has been identified as a cause of hypertrophic cardiomyopathy as well as occasional cases of dilated cardiomyopathy.[2] Taurine deficiency has also been documented to cause dilated cardiomyopathy.[3]

Each of the forms of cardiomyopathy has the potential to progress to thromboembolism, which often causes the presenting clinical sign of paresis or paralysis. Such a cat's thromboembolic disease must be treated, but one must not overlook the underlying cardiomyopathy that invariably accompanies it.

The incidence of cardiac disease in the cat is considerably greater than was recognized prior to 1970 when the first report of feline cardiomyopathy was published.[4] That report sparked a search for a better understanding of feline heart disease. Based on nearly 5,000 consecutive necropsies of feline patients at The Animal Medical Center, an 8.5% incidence of cardiomyopathy was reported.[5] Increased diagnostic capabilities later increased this estimated incidence to 12% to 15%.[1] Since the discovery of taurine-related cardiomyopathy and the subsequent fortification of commercial cat foods with that element, the incidence is now somewhat lower.

Hypertrophic Cardiomyopathy

The most common type of feline cardiomyopathy is the hypertrophic form. In this form of the disease, the left ventricular free wall and often the ventricular septum thicken and encroach upon the left ventricular chamber (Fig. 27–1). This results in decreased left ventricular filling capacity, hyperdynamic function, and left-sided diastolic dysfunction or failure. Primary hypertrophic cardiomyopathy is idiopathic, but a reversible form of the disease occurs secondary to hyperthyroidism.

Signalment

Hypertrophic cardiomyopathy is not necessarily a disease of older cats, as it has been reported in cats as young as 5 months of age. However, it may also affect geriatric cats; the mean age of onset is 5 to 7 years.[5-7] Domestic shorthair cats, domestic longhair cats, and Persians seem to be predisposed to this form of the disease.[8] It occurs only rarely in Siamese, Burmese, and Abyssinians.[9]

Clinical Signs and Findings

There are three typical presentations for cats with hypertrophic cardiomyopathy: dyspnea, paresis or paralysis of one or more legs (generally both of the rear legs), and sudden death. The former is attributable to pulmonary edema or occasionally, to pleural effusion. The latter two are the result of thromboembolic disease. In addition to these dramatic clinical signs, anorexia and vomiting may also occur, preceding the other signs.

Auscultation may reveal tachycardia, a diastolic gallop rhythm, rales, mild murmurs, and arrhythmias. If pleural or pericardial effusion is present, the heart and lung sounds may be muffled.

Because hypertrophic cardiomyopathy causes a state of cardiac hyperdynamic function, hypertension may result. Clinical signs of hypertension include hyperemia of the pinna of cats with white hair coats, a short capillary refill time (<2 sec), a heartbeat that is palpably prominent on the chest wall, and salient femoral pulses. In addition, venous blood may often be drawn into a syringe more easily in these cats than in those that are unaffected. This is especially noticeable when blood is drawn from the cephalic veins.

Table 27–1. A Comparison of the Three Major Forms of Feline Cardiomyopathy

	Hypertrophic	Dilated	Restrictive
Incidence	Common	Uncommon	Rare
LVC	Decreased	Increased	Normal/decreased
LVW	Thickened	Normal	Normal/increased
Apex location*	On midline	Left of midline	Left of midline
Heart shape	Valentine	Globoid	Valentine
Failure type	Diastolic	Systolic	Diastolic
Left-sided failure	Yes	Yes	Yes
Right-sided failure	Uncommon	Possible	Uncommon
Pulmonary edema	Yes	Yes	Yes
Pleural effusion	Uncommon	Common	Uncommon
Emboli	Yes	Yes	Yes

Abbreviations: LVC, left ventricular chamber size as determined by angiography and/or echocardiography; LVW, left ventricular wall thickness as determined by angiography and/or echocardiography.
*Apex of the heart as viewed on a true ventrodorsal radiograph.

Diagnosis

Diagnosis is based on electronic and radiographic methods of cardiac evaluation. Diagnostic methods that allow quantification of the left ventricular myocardium and chamber are necessary.

Plain film radiography often demonstrates mild to moderate left ventricular enlargement accompanied by moderate to severe left atrial enlargement. When atrial enlargement is severe, a valentine-shaped image occurs on the ventrodorsal view, with the cardiac apex aligning on the midline (Fig. 27–2). Interstitial densities of pulmonary edema and slight pleural effusion may be seen. In advanced hypertrophic cardiomyopathy, generalized cardiomegaly with severe pulmonary edema, pleural effusion, and hepatomegaly may occur[1,10-12] (Fig. 27–3).

The most sensitive method for identifying hypertrophic cardiomyopathy is echocardiography. This technique provides a noninvasive means of assessing the morphologic characteristics of the left ventricular wall and chamber, as well as evaluating cardiac function[9] (Fig. 27–4). If available, this is the diagnostic test of choice.

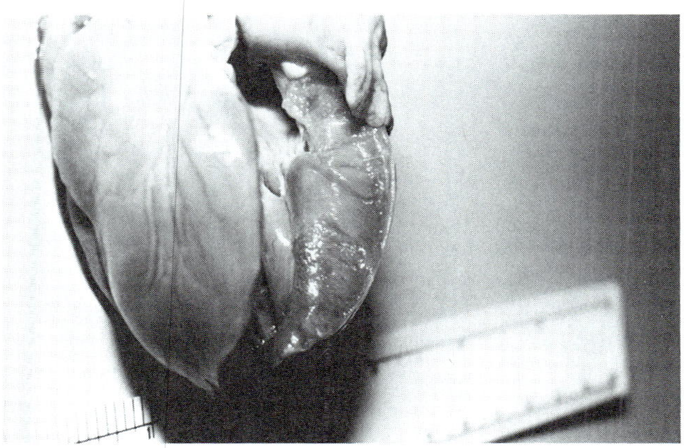

Figure 27–1. **The left ventricle has been opened to expose the greatly thickened left ventricular free wall in this cat with hypertrophic cardiomyopathy.**

Nonselective angiocardiography allows one to visualize the left atrium and ventricle. The left ventricular free wall will appear greatly thickened, and the left ventricular chamber often is reduced in size to a mere slit (Fig. 27–5). Left atrial enlargement may also be demonstrated. The pulmonary veins may be tortuous owing to increased left atrial and ventricular end-diastolic pressures.[1,9-11] This procedure is safe except in the presence of severe cardiac failure, as evidenced by the presence of pleural effusion or severe dyspnea. For a more detailed explanation of this procedure, see Chapter 14.

An electrocardiogram (ECG) will reveal abnormalities in cats with hypertrophic cardiomyopathy 35% to 70% of the time.[8,10] The most common findings are conduction disturbances, left ventricular enlargement patterns (QRS > 0.04 ms; lead II R waves > 0.9 mV), and arrhythmias.[9] This is the least sensitive and least cost-effective diagnostic method that specifically evaluates the heart.

Treatment

The goals of treatment in cats with hypertrophic cardiomyopathy are as follows:[12]

- Reduction of anxiety and activity
- Restoration of arterial oxygenation
- Removal of alveolar fluid
- Improvement of cardiac output
- Correction or management of the underlying causes
- Prevention of thromboembolism

These goals are accomplished with a variety of drugs and procedures that are chosen based on the pathologic abnormalities present and the individual response of the cat.

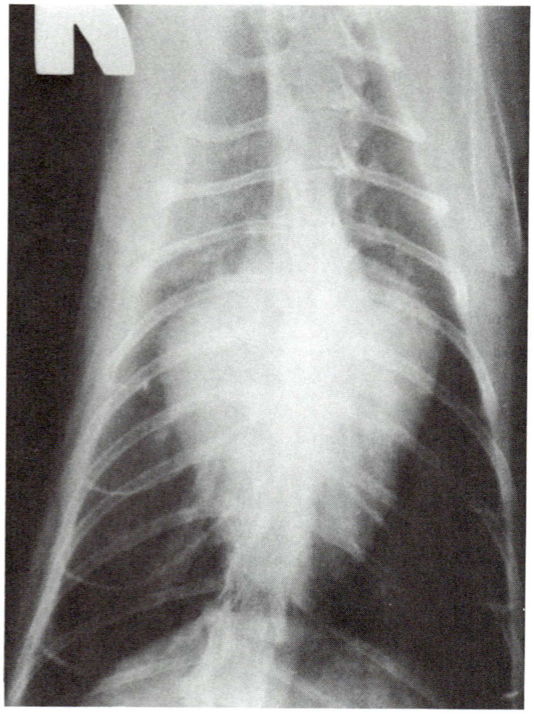

A

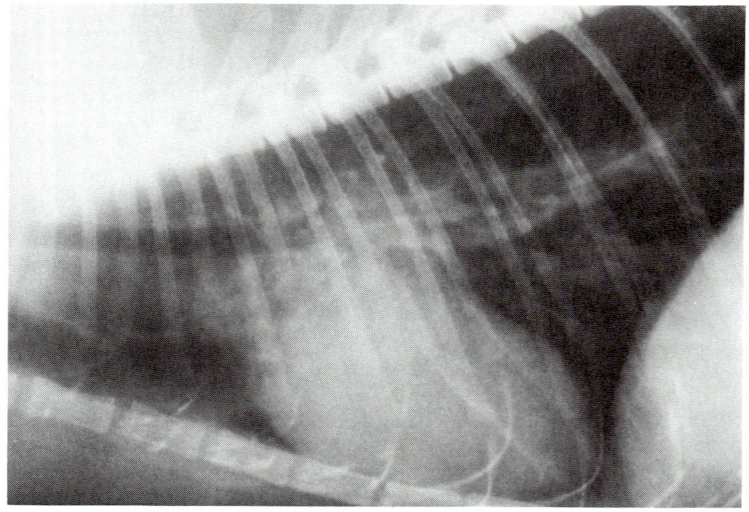

B

Figure 27–2. (*A*) A valentine-shaped heart is typical in cats with hypertrophic cardiomyopathy. (*B*) A lateral view of the same cat as in Figure 27–2*A*.

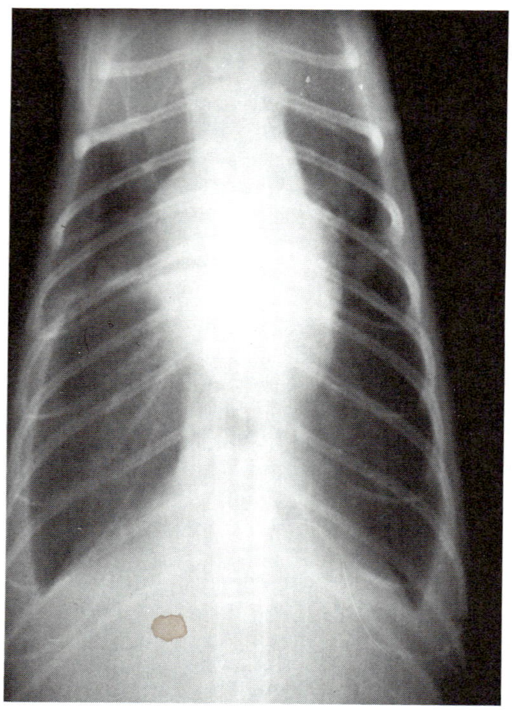

A

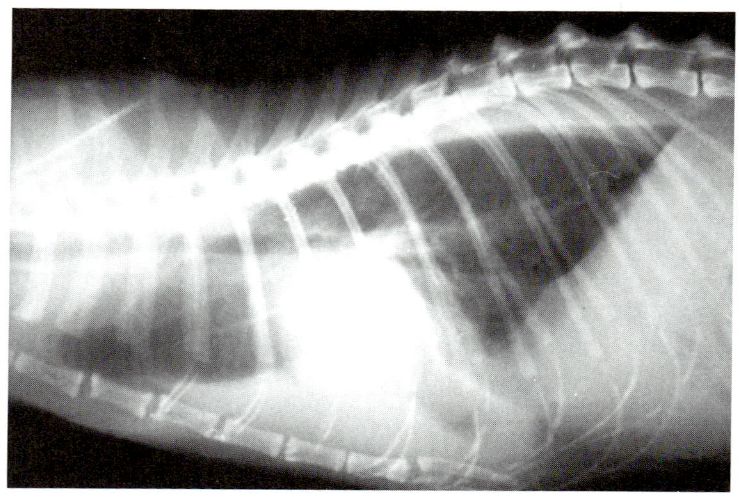

B

Figure 27–3. (*A*) Pleural effusion is evident in this cat with advanced hypertrophic cardiomyopathy. (*B*) A lateral view of the same cat as in Figure 27–3*A*.

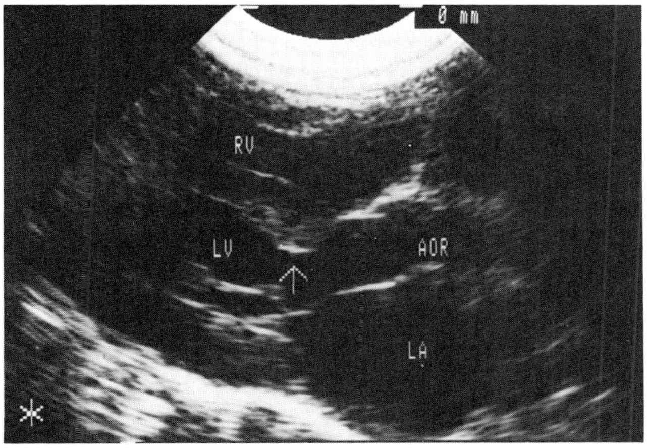

Figure 27–4. **Echocardiogram in a cat with hypertrophic cardiomyopathy. Note the decreased volume of the left ventricle (LV) as compared to that shown in Figure 27–8. (Courtesy of Dr. R. W. Green, Texas A & M University, College Station, TX.)**

Those treatment modalities that are most often chosen are as follows:[9,12]

- Administration of oxygen and cage confinement—Increasing the oxygen supply to the tissues can be accomplished by increasing the atmospheric oxygen content. Confinement of the cat to a cage will reduce the oxygen demand.
- Airway suctioning—This procedure is employed if froth is present in the trachea. Affected cats are nearly terminal, so sedation is generally not required.
- Acetylpromazine (Acepromazine)—Very mild sedation may reduce anxiety and promote peripheral redistribution of blood. If overdosed, hypotension and hypothermia may occur. The appropriate dose is 0.02 to 0.1 mg/lb subcutaneously (SC).

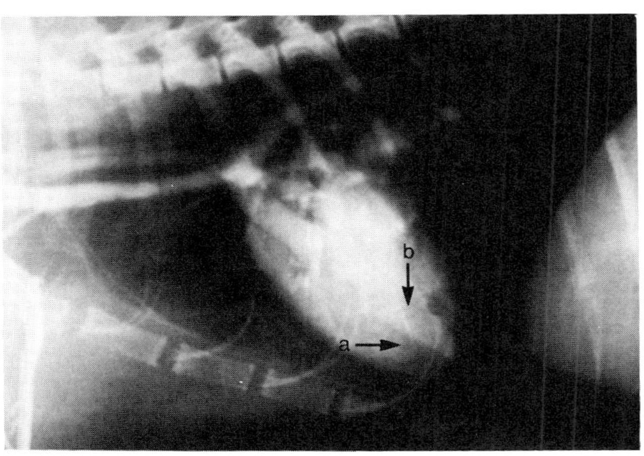

Figure 27–5. **The left ventricular chamber is a narrow slit (*a*) and the left ventricular free wall is thickened (*b*) in this nonselective angiogram of a cat with hypertrophic cardiomyopathy.**

- Furosemide (Lasix)—This diuretic is used to eliminate edema and effusion. The initial dose is dependent on the degree of edema or effusion that is present. Most cats will respond to 0.5 mg/lb intravenously (IV) or intramuscularly (IM) every 8 to 12 hours. Cats with hypertrophic cardiomyopathy may require up to 2.0 mg/lb every 8 hours. If the cat is refractory to the high dose, a second diuretic should be added.
- Hydrochlorothiazide (Hydrozide Injection)—This diuretic may be added to a regimen of furosemide at a dose of 0.5 to 1.0 mg/lb orally every 12 hours. When combination therapy is used, the cat must be monitored closely for azotemia, hyponatremia, and hypokalemia.
- Aminophylline (Aminophyllin)—This drug has bronchodilating effects in addition to mild diuretic and positive inotropic actions that are beneficial to critical cases. The correct dose is 2 to 4 mg/lb orally b.i.d. or 1 to 3 mg/lb IV b.i.d.
- Nitroglycerin, 2% (Nitrostat Ointment 2%)—This drug is effective in reducing preload and is indicated for fulminant pulmonary edema. A strip of ointment that is ⅛ to ¼ inch in length is applied cutaneously to any hairless area (generally, inside the pinna) every 4 to 6 hours for the first 24 to 36 hours. Gloves should be worn when applying this ointment to avoid absorption by one's own skin.
- Phlebotomy—When fulminant pulmonary edema does not respond to furosemide and nitroglycerin therapy, phlebotomy may be beneficial. Blood should be removed at a rate of 3 to 5 mL/lb.
- Diltiazem (Cardizem Tablets)—This drug has replaced propranolol as the drug judged to be most effective in supporting the myocardium in the short- and long-term. Like propranolol, diltiazem reduces cardiac contractility, heart rate, systolic pressure gradient, and myocardial oxygen demand. In addition, it directly improves myocardial relaxation, relieves coronary vasospasm, and dilates the coronary vessels. It is used at whatever dosage is sufficient to correct tachycardia, which may range from 3.75 to 15 mg every 8 to 24 hours. The dosage should be adjusted at least weekly by the veterinarian or the owner so that the resting heart rate remains below 180 bpm. The owner can be shown how to palpate the heart beat on the thoracic wall in order to ensure maintenance of a normal heart rate. Once stabilized, many cats can be maintained on this drug alone.
- Aspirin (Bayer Children's Aspirin)—As cats with hypertrophic cardiomyopathy are predisposed to thromboembolism, long-term aspirin therapy should be instituted to minimize the possibility of this complication. The appropriate dose is 5 to 12 mg/lb (or about 1.25 gr for a 10-lb cat) twice weekly.

Do not use the following for treatment of hypertrophic cardiomyopathy:

- Hydralazine (Apresoline)
- Captopril (Capoten) (both may worsen outflow obstruction)
- Digoxin (Lanoxin) (except for cats with biventricular failure without dynamic outflow obstruction)

Prognosis

Hypertrophic cardiomyopathy secondary to hyperthyroidism is generally reversible when the primary disease is corrected or controlled. Therefore, this form of the disease has a good prognosis. However, primary hypertrophic cardiomyopathy is a nonreversible form of myocardial failure. With aggressive medical therapy and restricted exercise (living indoors), though, cats have survived for 6 years or more.[9] However, with this form of cardiomyopathy, the possibility of sudden death secondary to thromboembolism remains constant.

Dilated Cardiomyopathy

Dilated cardiomyopathy was a common form of cardiomyopathy until the discovery that most cases were the result of taurine deficiency.[3] Commercial cat foods have since been fortified with taurine with the result that this disease has a greatly reduced incidence.[13] Dilated cardiomyopathy is a form of systolic (pump) failure. The ventricular wall is generally normal in thickness; however, in some cats it may become abnormally thin. The left ventricular chamber is greatly dilated (Fig. 27–6), and the papillary muscles and trabeculae are atrophied. The left auricle is also dilated.[9]

Signalment

The taurine-deficiency form of dilated cardiomyopathy occurs in young to middle-aged cats, with the average age being 7.5 years.[14] All breeds are affected, and sex distribution is about equal.[11]

Clinical Signs and Findings

The presenting clinical signs may be dyspnea, or paresis or paralysis of one or more legs (generally both rear legs). The former is the result of pulmonary edema or pleural effusion, whereas the latter is attributable to thromboembolic disease. These signs may be preceded by subtler signs, such as lethargy, inappetence, anorexia, or vomiting.

On physical examination, most of these cats are lethargic, depressed, and mildly dehydrated. Hypothermia is common. A gallop rhythm and a left and/or right systolic heart murmur are frequently found on auscultation. If pulmonary edema is present, crackles may be heard. If pleural effusion occurs, the heart and lung sounds may be muffled. If biventricular failure occurs, ascites and hepatomegaly may result.[9]

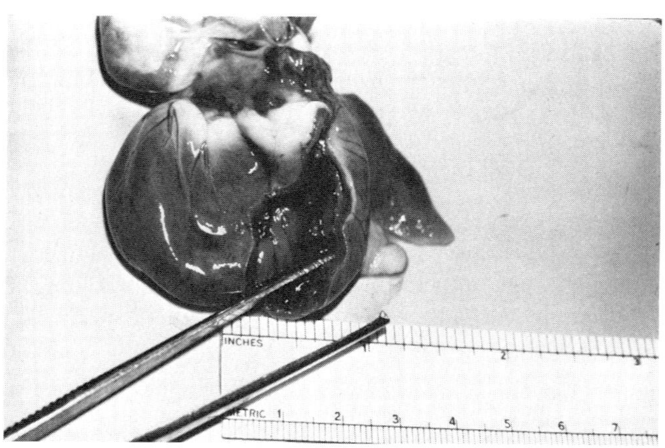

Figure 27–6. **The left ventricle has been opened to expose the thin left ventricular free wall and the dilated chamber of this cat with dilated cardiomyopathy.**

Diagnosis

As with hypertrophic cardiomyopathy, the diagnosis of dilated cardiomyopathy is based on electronic and radiographic methods of cardiac evaluation. Methods that allow quantification of the left atrium and ventricle are necessary. In addition, cats with dilated cardiomyopathy are more likely to have abnormalities that are revealed by a blood profile than are cats with HCM. These abnormalities may include prerenal azotemia, indicated by a blood urea nitrogen (BUN) level of 35 to 60 mg/dL, and mild hyperglycemia. If thromboembolism is present, serum lactic acid dehydrogenase (LDH), creatinine phosphokinase (CPK), alanine aminotransferase (ALT), and aspartate aminotransferase (AST) levels may be elevated, and coagulopathies may be evident.

Plain film radiography will demonstrate mild to severe left atrial and ventricular enlargement or severe, generalized cardiomegaly. A characteristic round, globoid-shaped ventricular apex may be seen on ventrodorsal radiographs. The apex is generally to the left of midline (Fig. 27–7). Mild pulmonary edema and mild to moderate pleural effusion are often present.[11,15]

The most sensitive method for diagnosing dilated cardiomyopathy is echocardiography. This technique allows an assessment of the morphologic characteristics of the left atrial and ventricular chambers, as well as of ventricular wall thickness (Fig. 27–8). It also provides a noninvasive means of evaluating cardiac function.[9] If available, this is the diagnostic test of choice.

Nonselective angiocardiography allows visualization of the left atrium and ventricle in cats with dilated cardiomyopathy. The left ventricular free wall will generally be of normal thickness. The left and right ventricular chambers will be greatly dilated, and the left atrium will be enlarged (Fig. 27–9). Because dilated cardiomyopathy is a form of systolic failure, the aorta may appear to be smaller in diameter than usual.[1,10,16] This procedure is safe except in cats with severe cardiac failure, as evidenced by severe dyspnea or pleural effusion. This procedure is described in greater detail in Chapter 14.

An ECG will reveal a normal rhythm in about 50% of cats with dilated cardiomyopathy. The reported incidence of left ventricular enlargement patterns (QRS $>$ 0.04 ms; lead II R waves $>$ 0.9 mV) is 25% to 39%.[10,11] Ventricular premature complexes have been reported in nearly 50% of affected cats.[14] As with hypertrophic cardiomyopathy, this is the least sensitive and least cost-effective diagnostic method that specifically evaluates the heart.

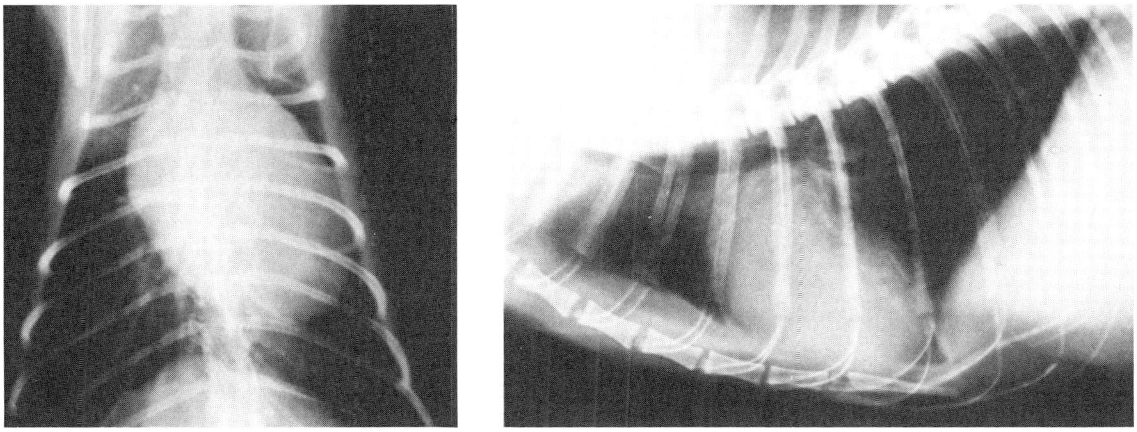

A B

Figure 27–7. **(*A*) A rounded cardiac apex located to the left of the midline is typical for cats with dilated cardiomyopathy. (*B*) A lateral view of the same cat as in Figure 27–7A.**

Treatment

The goals of treatment in dilated cardiomyopathy are to:[12]

- Improve pulmonary function by eliminating pulmonary edema and pleural fluid
- Increase cardiac contractile strength
- Optimize cardiac output

These goals are accomplished with drugs and procedures that are chosen on the basis of the pathologic abnormalities present and the individual response of the cat. Those treatment modalities that are generally employed include the following:[9,12]

- Administration of oxygen and cage confinement—Increasing tissue oxygenation may be accomplished by increasing the atmospheric oxygen content. Cage confinement will reduce the oxygen demand.
- Thoracocentesis—In cats with pleural effusion, thoracocentesis can improve pulmonary function very quickly. As much as 300 mL of fluid may be removed from some cats.
- Furosemide (Lasix)—This diuretic is used to eliminate edema and effusion. The initial dose depends on the degree of edema and/or effusion present. Most cats will respond to a dosage of 0.5 to 1.0 mg/lb every 8 hours. As cats with dilated cardiomyopathy are likely to have difficulties with hydration, renal function, electrolyte imbalances, and peripheral perfusion, the dose should be tapered quickly to the lowest effective dose and frequency.
- Digoxin (Lanoxin Elixir)—This drug is used for its positive inotropic effects. Because of the cat's sensitivity to

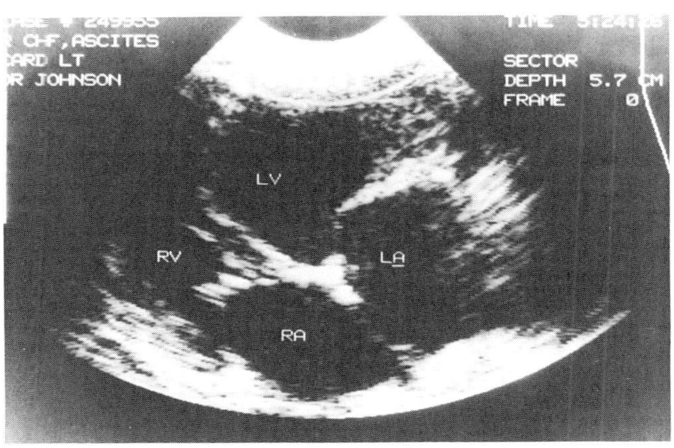

Figure 27–8. **Echocardiographic results in a cat with dilated cardiomyopathy. Note the increased volume of the left ventricle (LV) as compared to that shown in Figure 27–4. (Courtesy of Dr. R. W. Green, Texas A & M University, College Station, TX.)**

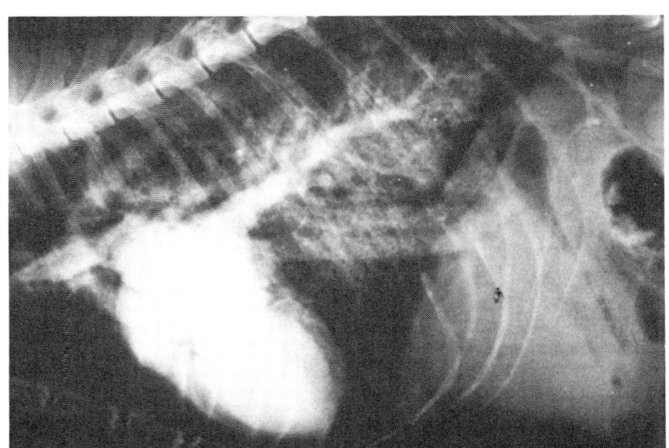

Figure 27–9. **A nonselective angiogram of a cat with dilated cardiomyopathy reveals a dilated left ventricular chamber and a normal or thin left ventricular free wall.**

this drug, extreme caution should be exercised when administering digoxin IV for rapid digitalization, and only those cats with severe cardiac dysfunction should be so treated. An IV dose of 0.001 mg/lb (lean body weight) may be administered, followed in 1 hour by a dose of half that amount. The latter dose can be repeated in another hour if there are no clinical or electrocardiographic signs of digitalis toxicity. Once the cat is stabilized, the following maintenance dosages are recommended:[15]

Weight	Dosage
<3 kg	1/4 of a 0.125-mg tablet q2–3 days
3–6 kg	1/4 of a 0.125-mg tablet q1–2 days
>6 kg	1/4 of a 0.125-mg tablet q12–24h

- Digoxin elixir should not be used in cats because most cats object to its taste and because serum concentrations may be as much as 50% greater than that achieved with a comparable tablet dose.[12]
- For cats that develop digitalis toxicity even with low maintenance doses, captopril (Capoten) may be used for maintenance therapy at a dosage of 2.0 to 3.0 mg/cat t.i.d. or 3.0–6.25 mg/cat b.i.d. If anorexia occurs, the dose should be reduced by 50%. This agent should not be combined with furosemide.
- Fluid therapy—Fluid therapy may be necessary because the prescribed diuretics may reduce cardiac filling and predispose the cat to circulatory shock. Administration of SC or small IV doses of half-strength saline, 2.5% dextrose, or any low-sodium fluid may be initiated at a rate of 10 to 16 mL/lb/day. One should be alert to the development of hypokalemia.
- Vasodilation—Cardiac output can be improved with peripheral vasodilation; however, overtreatment can result in hypotension. Vasodilation can be achieved by administering 2% nitroglycerin (a 1/8- to 1/4-inch strip cutaneously q6–8h), hydralazine (0.2–0.4 mg/lb q12h), or captopril (3.0–6.25 mg/cat q8–12h).
- Taurine supplementation—Even if a cat is receiving a taurine-sufficient diet, taurine supplementation is still recommended at the rate of 500 mg every 12 hours for 1 to 2 months.[15] If there is radiographic evidence of a significant improvement in heart shape, taurine should probably be continued indefinitely.
- Taurine-fortified diet—The owner should be questioned about the cat's diet. If a commercial cat food is not being consumed, every effort should be made to change the cat to such a diet, even though this is often impossible owing to lack of compliance by the owner or intolerance of a dietary change by the cat. The ideal diet is one that is taurine-fortified and low in sodium, such as Prescription Diet Feline h/d (Hill's Pet Products, Topeka, KS).
- Aspirin (Bayer Children's Aspirin)—Because cats with dilated cardiomyopathy are predisposed to thromboembolism, aspirin should be administered as long-term therapy to minimize the risk of this complication. A dosage of 5–12 mg/lb (or about 1.25 gr for a 10-lb cat) twice weekly is appropriate.

Prognosis

If dilated cardiomyopathy is induced by taurine deficiency and if taurine supplementation can be achieved on a long-term basis, the prognosis is good. Otherwise, the prognosis is guarded, although some cats have survived for more than 4 years with this condition. Thromboembolism is a constant threat.

Restrictive Cardiomyopathy

Restrictive cardiomyopathy is another form of cardiomyopathy that results in diastolic failure. Sometimes termed intermediate cardiomyopathy, it has a lower incidence than either hypertrophic cardiomyopathy or dilated cardiomyopathy. It is characterized by endocardial, subendocardial, or myocardial fibrosis, which prevents both stretch (compliance) of the left ventricular wall and ventricular filling. This leads to reduced preload and cardiac output. Extensive endomyocardial fibrosis may reduce the left ventricular chamber to a size comparable to that seen in hypertrophic cardiomyopathy.[9]

Signalment

Restrictive cardiomyopathy can occur at any age, having been reported in cats ranging in age from 8 months to 19 years.[5,17-19] Its sex distribution is approximately equal.[10]

Clinical Signs and Findings

The clinical signs of restrictive cardiomyopathy are similar to those associated with both hypertrophic cardiomyopathy and dilated cardiomyopathy. Affected cats are typically either dyspneic as a result of pulmonary edema or pleural effusion, or have paresis or paralysis secondary to thromboembolism. Anorexia or vomiting may precede these signs by a few days. Upon presentation, these cats are often hypothermic. Auscultation may reveal either muffled heart sounds secondary to pleural effusion or crackles resulting from pulmonary edema. Gallop rhythms, arrhythmias, and/or mild to moderate systolic murmurs occur frequently.[10,11,14]

Diagnosis

As with the other forms of cardiomyopathy, diagnosis is based on electronic and radiographic methods of cardiac evaluation. Methods that allow quantification of the left atrium and left ventricle are necessary.

Plain film radiography often demonstrates mild to moderate left atrial enlargement accompanied by left ventricular enlargement. Pulmonary edema is a common finding. When biventricular failure exists, pleural effusion or pericardial effusion, or both, may occur. If the latter is present, the heart will have a globoid appearance. The pulmonary veins are frequently prominent and tortuous. Hepatomegaly and ascites may also be present.[10,11,14]

Echocardiography usually demonstrates hypertrophy of the left ventricular septum and free wall, and left atrial enlargement. The irregularities of the left ventricular chamber are often able to be visualized.[9]

Nonselective angiocardiography is the most sensitive test for restrictive cardiomyopathy Left ventricular hypertrophy with an irregular ventricular chamber, often having the appearance of filling defects, will be evident. In severe cases, the ventricular chamber will be nearly obliterated. The left atrium will be seen to be enlarged.[10,11,14] This procedure is described in greater detail in Chapter 14.

Abnormal ECG findings have been reported in 31% to 70% of affected cats. Often, there is evidence of left atrial and left ventricular enlargement. In addition, ventricular and supraventricular arrhythmias are common.[9,10] However, none of these findings is specific for restrictive cardiomyopathy. As with the other forms of cardiomyopathy, an ECG is the least sensitive and least cost-effective diagnostic approach.

Even when a nonselective angiocardiogram is performed, subtle irregularities of the left ventricular chamber may elude detection. Because of their similarities, restrictive cardiomyopathy can be mistaken for hypertrophic cardiomyopathy. This may account for some of the treatment failures reported in cats diagnosed as having hypertrophic cardiomyopathy. Indeed, accurate diagnosis may only be possible at necropsy.

Treatment and Prognosis

The therapeutic goals and treatment regimens appropriate for restrictive cardiomyopathy are the same as those applicable to hypertrophic cardiomyopathy, as both result in diastolic failure. The prognosis is generally poor; uncomplicated left-sided failure carries the best prognosis. Thromboembolism is always a threat.

Excessive Moderator Bands

Moderator bands are normal structures within the right ventricle of the cat and several other species, including the dog.[20] They transport Purkinje fibers from the atrioventricular bundle.[21] When an excessive number of these bands is present, a form of cardiomyopathy occurs that may result in left-sided or right-sided cardiac failure.

Clinical Signs and Diagnosis

The anatomic aspects of this condition vary greatly, resulting in a number of different clinical signs that overlap with the signs of other forms of cardiomyopathy. The typical clinical features may include one or more of the following: dyspnea, paresis or paralysis secondary to thromboembolic disease, pulmonary edema (left-sided failure), pleural effusion (right-sided failure), gallop rhythms, and systolic murmurs. These are often preceded by a few days of anorexia. Left ventricular hypertrophy is the predominent finding in younger cats, whereas left ventricular dilatation is more typical for older cats.[9]

The diagnostic approaches are the same as for the other forms of cardiomyopathy. An ECG may reveal any of a number of abnormalities, none of which are pathognomonic for this disease A nonselective angiocardiogram generally does not identify the abnormal moderator bands, although it may indicate left ventricular hypertrophy or dilatation. The most sensitive test is an echocardiogram, which often will allow visualization of the abnormal structures. Some cases are only diagnosable by necropsy.

Treatment and Prognosis

The treatment regimens that are appropriate for either hypertrophic cardiomyopathy or dilated cardiomyopathy are also applicable to excessive moderator bands, depending on whether the condition is associated with left ventricular hypertrophy or dilatation. The prognosis is generally very guarded.

Establishing a Presumptive Diagnosis

Factors Used to Establish a Presumptive Diagnosis

Cats presenting with dyspnea or a sudden onset of paresis or paralysis should be suspected of having cardiomyopathy. Plain film thoracic radiographs may be adequate to diagnose cardiomyopathy and to differentiate between hypertrophic cardiomyopathy and dilated cardiomyopathy. If not, a nonselective angiocardiogram or echocardiogram should be performed before initiating therapy. If these are not available or are prohibitively expensive, two factors—incidence and diet—can be useful in establishing a presumptive diagnosis. First, hypertrophic cardiomyopathy is significantly more common than either dilated cardiomyopathy or restrictive cardiomyopathy. If the cat has a history suggestive of hyperthyroidism (polyuria/polydipsia/polyphagia/weight loss), hypertrophic cardiomyopathy is the most likely diagnosis. Second, the cat's diet should be considered. If it is a taurine-adequate diet (i.e., if the cat is fed a commercial cat food), hypertrophic cardiomyopathy is the most likely diagnosis. However, if the diet is taurine-deficient (consisting primarily of table food, dog food, or a home-made preparation), dilated cardiomyopathy is likely.

Treatment Based on a Presumptive Diagnosis

If therapy must begin based on a presumptive diagnosis, the owner should be advised of the grave consequences of treating the wrong form of cardiomyopathy. However, because some of the drugs and procedures that are used are common to all forms of cardiac failure, these can be employed without hesitation. These treatment modalities include the following:

- Furosemide for pulmonary edema
- Thoracocentesis for pleural effusion
- Cage rest and oxygen administration
- Nitroglycerin for preload reduction

If the cat can be stabilized using just these measures, the clinician may elect to continue this therapeutic approach on a long-term basis. This strategy is also appropriate to use while arrangements for further diagnostic tests are being made. However, if the cat's condition does not stabilize and other tests are impractical to perform, the selection of other drugs should be based on the presumptive diagnosis, as mentioned previously.

Thromboembolic Disease

Thrombosis is the formation of a blood clot within the heart or a vessel, generally an artery. As a rule, thrombi form in the heart, dislodge, and are then carried by normal blood flow to a randomly selected artery. They may become lodged when the arterial luminal diameter becomes smaller than the clot's diameter.

Thromboembolism has been recorded frequently in cats.[17,22,23] In one study, thromboemboli were found in 10 of 21 (48%) cats with cardiomyopathy that underwent necropsy,[24] although the incidence of clinical thromboembolism is considerably less.[9] There is such a strong correlation between thrombi and cardiomyopathy that any cat with cardiomyopathy is at great and constant risk of a thromboembolic event, and nearly all cats with thromboembolism have some form of cardiomyopathy.

Pathophysiology

Although an embolus may cause total obstruction of the affected artery, vasoconstrictive substances released from the clot have a major effect on the formation of collateral circulation. If the iliac arteries are surgically ligated, function of the rear legs will return within 72 hours. If an embolus is present, functional return as a result of collateral circulation will take 7 to 10 days. This difference is attributable to serotonin and other vasoactive substances. Antiprostaglandin drugs, such as aspirin, are important in counteracting the effects of these substances.[25-28]

Loss of circulation also results in damage to the peripheral nerves distal to the lesion. When iliac embolization occurs, the nerve lesions typically begin in the mid-thigh region. The nerves below the stifle are especially affected. The cranial tibial muscles are affected more severely than the gastrocnemius muscles, primarily resulting in flexion deficits. The distal limb loses sensory perception.[29,30]

Clinical Signs

When an embolus escapes the left side of the heart, it enters the ascending or descending aorta. When it escapes the right side of the heart, it enters the pulmonary artery and causes dyspnea or death (Fig. 27–10). The most common form of feline thromboembolism is the saddle thrombus. This is an embolus that occludes the trifurcation of the descending aorta (Fig. 27–11). Cats with a saddle thrombus have an acute onset of paresis or paralysis of both rear legs. The degree to which the legs are affected is determined by the degree of occlusion of the iliac arteries. These cats typically present with extreme pain, cyanosis of the rear foot pads (within a few hours), absence of the femoral pulses, and cold extremities. They can flex or extend the hips, but are paralyzed from the hocks distally. The anterior tibial and gastrocnemius muscles become firm or very hard within 12 to 18 hours.[9] A thrombus may also enter the descending aorta and lodge in one or both of the renal arteries, or in a mesenteric artery.

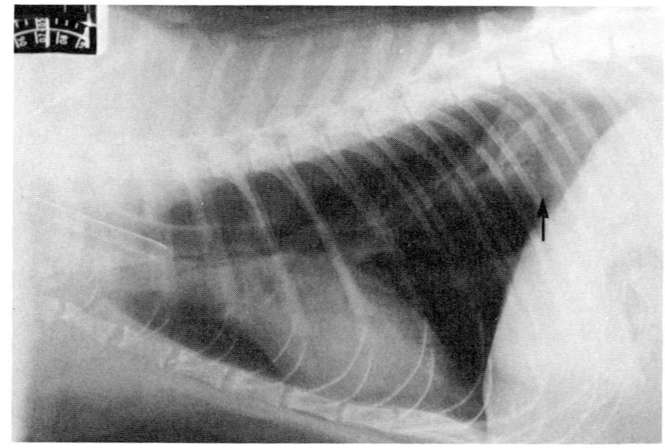

Figure 27–10. **The congestion that is seen in the caudal pulmonary lobe (*arrow*) is the result of an embolus escaping the right side of the heart and entering the pulmonary artery.**

If an embolus is carried cranially, the cat may experience unilateral paresis or paralysis of a front leg, or a stroke-like event. If a thrombus develops in the right side of the heart, it will enter a pulmonary artery. Some cats will have multiple thrombi and will develop lesions in several locations. Thrombi that enter the renal arteries, the mesenteric arteries, or the pulmonary arteries can result in sudden death or death within a few hours.

Diagnosis

Several changes in the biochemical profile are consistent with thromboembolism and the resulting skeletal muscle inflammation and necrosis. Levels of aspartate aminotransferase (formerly, SGOT) will be elevated within 12 hours, and will peak by 36 hours postembolization. LDH and CPK

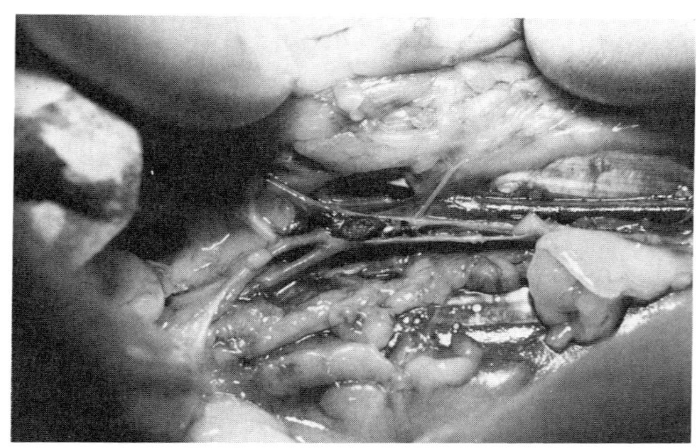

Figure 27–11. **A saddle thrombus is extruding from the opened aortic trifurcation.**

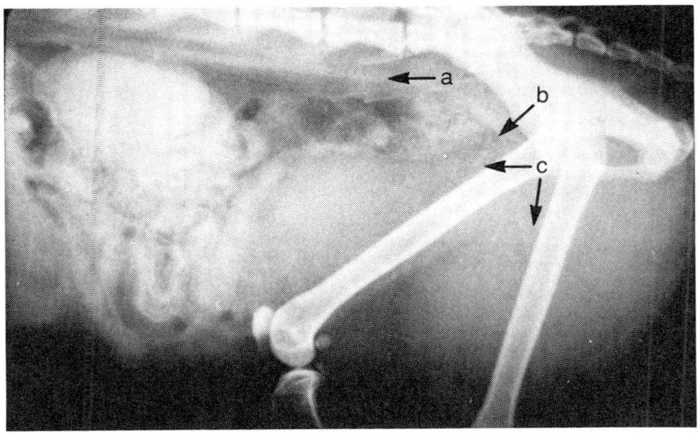

A

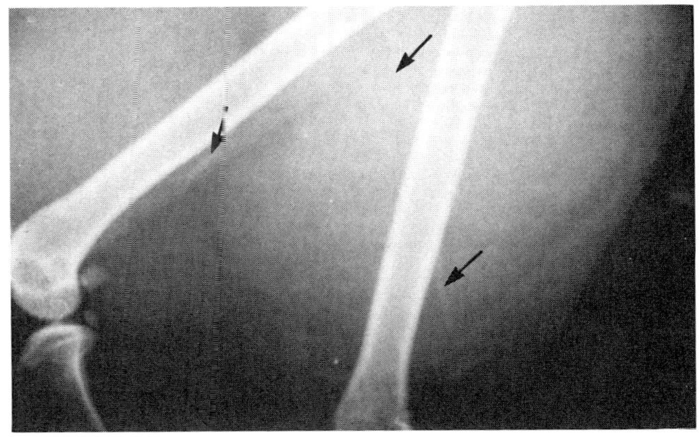

B

Figure 27–12. (*A*) This nonselective angiogram, performed in a normal cat, reveals contrast material in the aorta (*a*), the aortic trifurcation (*b*), and the iliac arteries (*c*). (*B*) A close-up of the nonselective angiogram pictured in Figure 27–11*A* shows normal circulation at the different levels of the iliac arteries (*arrows*).

levels will be greatly elevated within a few hours, and will remain elevated for weeks.[9]

The clinical signs of a saddle thrombus are often diagnostic. However, many cats will exhibit only one or more of the typical clinical signs. In such cases, a nonselective angiogram will allow visualization of the blood flow to the rear legs (see Chapter 14) (Figs. 27–12 and 27–13). Unexplained front or rear leg lameness or signs of a stroke should raise one's index of suspicion for a thrombus. Because affected cats invariably have concomitant cardiomyopathy, dyspnea, tachycardia, murmurs, and/or a gallop rhythm may also be present. A thoracic radiograph should be included in the work-up.

Treatment

Cats experiencing paresis of one or two legs or those having stroke-like manifestations generally recover to a normal or near-normal state within a few days. Treatment may require only cage confinement and aspirin therapy for prophylaxis.

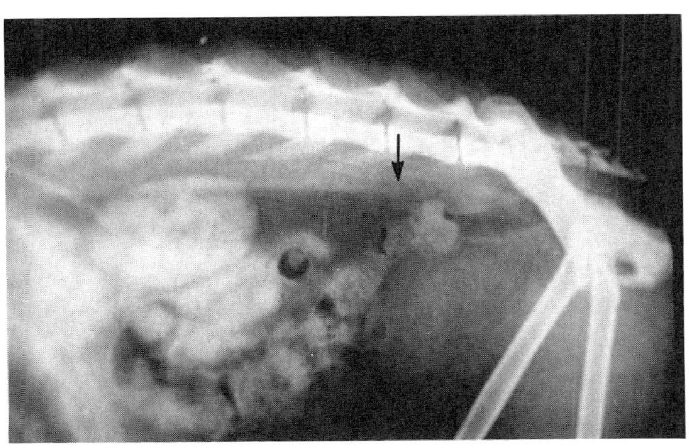

Figure 27–13. Contrast material is seen to stop abruptly (*arrow*) cranial to the aortic trifurcation in this cat with a saddle thrombus.

Cats that develop posterior paralysis secondary to a saddle thrombus require aggressive medical therapy. Treatment must be directed at relieving the extreme pain experienced by some cats, reversing the effects of the thrombus, preventing future thrombi, and controlling the underlying cardiomyopathy. Although propranolol has been used for hypertrophic cardiomyopathy or restrictive cardiomyopathy, it should not be used in cats with a thrombus because of its peripheral vasoconstrictive properties.

In the past, the surgical removal of thrombi, especially saddle thrombi, was a common approach to treatment. Although this procedure was effective in rapidly restoring circulation, it was associated with a very high mortality rate. Those cats that underwent such surgery often died of cardiac failure during or shortly after the procedure.[11,15,31] For this reason, this treatment approach has largely been abandoned. Cats for whom such an operation is still indicated are those with a thrombus in one or both renal arteries (Fig. 27–14). As the kidneys have no potential for collateral circulation, their function must be restored within a few hours or terminal renal failure will occur.

Cats presenting with extreme pain may receive morphine at a dose of 0.05 mg/lb IM or SC as needed (caution, very low dose), or butorphanol (Torbugesic) at a dose of 0.1 to 0.2 mg/lb IM or SC t.i.d. Reversal of the effects of the thrombus may be facilitated in two ways. First, administration of acetylpromazine (Acepromazine) (0.5 to 1.0 mg/cat every 8 hours) is recommended because its peripheral vasodilator effects may hasten collateral circulation. Diltiazem (3.75–15 mg every 8 to 24 hours to maintain heart rate below 180 bpm) may be used for the same purpose in cats with hypertrophic cardiomyopathy or restrictive cardiomyopathy. However, these drugs should not be used concurrently. Frequent application of hot packs to the legs, followed by muscle massage, may also help to stimulate collateral circulation. Second, although heparin has not been shown to

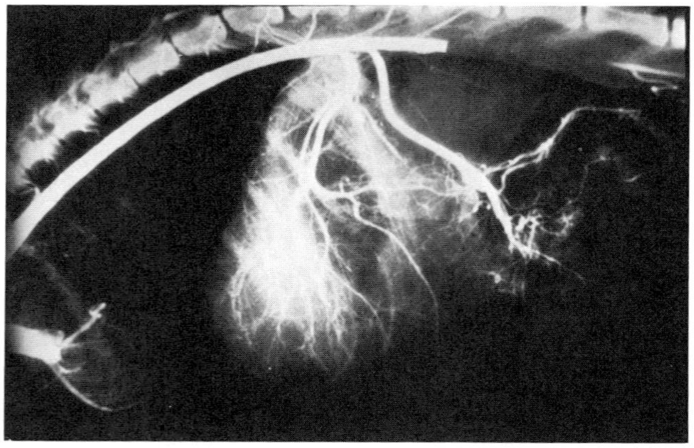

Figure 27–14. **Contrast material is seen to stop abruptly cranial to the renal arteries in this cat with an aortic thrombus. (Courtesy of Dr. Kenneth W. Knauer, Texas A & M University, College Station, TX.)**

have any effect on an established thrombus, it is indicated as a means of preventing thrombus formation. Initially, the appropriate dose is 1,000 U.S.P. units IV. Three hours later a dose of 25 U.S.P. units/lb may be administered SC; this dose is then repeated every 6 to 8 hours thereafter.[14] Because bleeding can be a complication, heparin use is not recommended for more than 24 hours. Aspirin has been shown to be effective in inhibiting platelet function and in aiding collateralization.[28] When heparin is discontinued, aspirin therapy should be initiated at a dose of 1.25 gr/cat every 3 days.[9]

At the same time that these treatment measures are instituted, the cardiac manifestations of this disease must be aggressively addressed. Appropriate tests (as previously outlined) must be performed to establish an accurate diagnosis that specifies the form of cardiomyopathy that is present.

Prognosis

The short-term prognosis in thromboembolic disease depends on whether the cardiac failure associated with the underlying cardiomyopathy can be alleviated or controlled. If that effort is unsuccessful, the cat may die within a few hours or days.

Cats exhibiting paresis or stroke-like symptoms generally recover within 7 to 10 days, and typically regain full function. Cats experiencing paralysis secondary to a saddle thrombus have a guarded to good prognosis, but take considerably longer to recover. Motor ability in these cats should begin to return within 10 to 14 days. By 21 days postembolus, motor function should approach normal, although many cats will exhibit a greater degree of lameness in one leg than in the other. By 4 to 6 weeks, recovery is generally complete, even though the cat may not have returned to a normal state. However, most cats do achieve an acceptable functional level of locomotion by that time.[9,11,15]

Likewise, the long-term prognosis is also governed by the manageability of the cardiomyopathy and by any recurrence of thromboembolic events. Most cats will experience more of these events within a few months to a few years of the first episode.

A retrospective study of 74 cats with a clinical diagnosis of hypertrophic cardiomyopathy found a median survival of all cats of 732 days and that one-third were alive after 5 years. Of those cats that were not exhibiting clinical signs at the time of diagnosis, over two-thirds were alive after 5 years. Cats presenting with heart failure had a median survival time of 92 days; forty percent were alive more than 6 months, and twenty percent survived more than 3 years. The duration of survival was increased if the cat was not tachycardic on initial presentation. Cats presenting with signs of thromboembolism had a median survival of 61 days, and all were dead by 6 months.

REFERENCES

1. Bond BR, Fox PR. Advances in feline cardiomyopathy. Vet Clin North Am (Small Anim Pract) 1984;14(5):1021.
2. Feldman EC, Nelson RW. Hyperthyroidism and Thyroid Tumors. In: Feldman EC, Nelson RW, eds. Canine and Feline Endocrinology and Reproduction, 1st ed. Philadelphia: WB Saunders Co., 1987:91.
3. Pion PD. Myocardial failure associated with low plasma taurine levels in cats and its reversal with oral taurine. Science 1987; 237:764.
4. Liu S-K. Acquired cardiac lesions leading up to congestive heart failure in the cat. Am J Vet Res 1970;31:2071.
5. Liu S-K. Pathology of feline heart diseases. Vet Clin North Am (Small Anim Pract) 1977;7(2):323.
6. Maron BJ. Spontaneously Occurring Hypertrophic Cardiomyopathy in Dogs and Cats: A Potential Animal Model of a Human Disease. In: Kaltenbach M, Epstein SE, eds. Hypertrophic Cardiomyopathy. Berlin: Springer-Verlag, 1982:73.
7. Liu S-K. Feline hypertrophic cardiomyopathy: Gross anatomic and quantitative histologic features. Am J Pathol 1981;102:388.
8. Tilley LP. Primary myocardial disease in the cat: A model for human cardiomyopathy. Am J Pathol 1977;87:493.
9. Fox PR. Myocardial Diseases. In: Ettinger SJ, ed. Textbook of Veterinary Internal Medicine, 3rd ed. Philadelphia: WB Saunders Co., 1989:1097.
10. Harpster NK. Feline Myocardial Diseases. In: Kirk RW, ed. Current Veterinary Therapy IX. Philadelphia: WB Saunders Co., 1986:380.
11. Fox PR. Feline Cardiomyopathy. In: Bonagura JD, ed. Contemporary Issues in Small Animal Practice: Cardiology, Vol. 7. New York: Churchill Livingstone, 1987:157.
12. Ware WA. Dyspnea: Diagnosis and Management. In: August JR, ed. Consultations in Feline Internal Medicine, 1st ed. Philadelphia: WB Saunders Co., 1991:147.
13. Harpster NK. Cats Don't Have Heart Disease. Proceedings, 1990 Academy of Veterinary Cardiologists. San Francisco: American Animal Hospital Association, 1990:22.
14. Harpster NK. The Cardiovascular System. In: Holzworth J, ed. Diseases of the Cat. Philadelphia: WB Saunders Co., 1986: 820.
15. Fox PR. Feline Myocardial Diseases. In: Fox PR, ed. Textbook of Canine and Feline Cardiology. New York: Churchill Livingstone, 1988:435.

16. Owens JM, Twedt DC. Nonselective angiocardiography in the cat. Vet Clin North Am (Small Anim Pract) 1977:7(2);309.
17. Fox PR. Feline Myocardial Diseases. In: Kirk RW, ed. Current Veterinary Therapy VIII. Philadelphia: WB Saunders Co., 1983: 337.
18. Fox PR. The Cardiovascular System. In: Pratt PW, ed. Feline Medicine. Santa Barbara: American Veterinary Publications, 1983: 249.
19. Tilley LP. Myocardial Disease. In: Ettinger SJ, ed. Textbook of Veterinary Internal Medicine, 2nd ed. Philadelphia: WB Saunders Co., 1983:1029.
20. Truex RC, Warshow LJ. The incidence and size of the moderator band in man and animals. Anat Rec 1942;82:361.
21. Sandusky GE, White SL. Scanning electron microscopy of the canine atrioventricular bundle and moderator band. Am J Vet Res 1985;46:249.
22. Tilley LP, Liu SK. Cardiomyopathy and thromboembolism in the cat. Feline Pract 1975;5:32.
23. Harpster N. Feline Cardiomyopathy. Vet Clin North Am (Small Anim Pract) 1977;7:355.
24. Liu SK. Excessive moderator bands in the left ventricle of 21 cats. J Am Vet Med Assoc 1982;180:1215.
25. Imhoff RK. Production of aortic occlusion resembling acute aortic embolism syndrome in cats. Nature 1978;192:979.
26. Schaub RG. Inhibition of feline collateral vessel development following experimental thrombolic occlusion. Circ Res 1976; 39:736.
27. Schaub RG. Serotonin as a factor in depression of collateral blood flow following experimental arterial thrombosis. J Lab Clin Med 1977;90:645.
28. Schuab RG. Effect of aspirin on collateral blood flow after experimental thrombosis of the feline aorta. Am J Vet Res 1982; 43:1647.
29. Griffiths IR, Duncan ID. Ischaemic neuromyopathy in cats. Vet Rec 1979;104:518.
30. Fox PR Feline thromboembolism associated with cardiomyopathy. Proceedings, 5th Annual Veterinary Medicine Forum, Boston, 1987:92.
31. Flanders JA. Feline aortic thromboembolism. Compend Contin Educ Pract Vet 1986;8:473.
32. Atkins CE, Gallo AM, Kurtzman ID, Cowen P. Risk factors, clinical signs, and survival in cats with a clinical diagnosis of idiopathic hypertrophic cardiomyopathy: 74 cases, 1985–1989. J Am Vet Med Assoc 1992;201:613.

CHAPTER 28

◇ ◇ ◇

Cervical Ventroflexion

R. Steve Taylor

Cervical ventroflexion is a pronounced bending of the neck (Fig. 28–1). This clinical sign has been associated with many disease entities including thiamine deficiency, polymyopathies, and myelopathies.[1] Although cervical ventroflexion is not pathognomonic for any disease, when accompanied by other signs, such as muscle pain, abnormal gait, and generalized muscle weakness, it becomes highly suggestive of a polymyopathy often associated with hypokalemia.[2] While other primary myopathies and neuromuscular junction diseases may cause similar signs, hypokalemic polymyopathy is the most common cause of the cervical ventroflexion/muscle weakness (CVF/MW) complex.[2]

Clinical Signs

Cats presenting with CVF/MW will often have the chin close to the sternum, frequently with the head slightly cocked to one side. The cat usually cannot lift its head; it may only move the neck stiffly from side to side. The gait is characteristically stiff and stilted, with a pronounced rolling of the shoulders (excessive scapular motion).[1] The generalized muscle weakness is exacerbated with exercise. Some cats will walk a short distance and then assume a praying position with the chin on the floor, the front legs crouched, and the rear legs elevated (Fig. 28–2). The weakness and decreased tone of the cervical muscles is obvious when the chin is lifted and released; it falls to the sternum without resistance. In many instances, pain is noted on palpation of any of the muscles, particularly those of the appendicular skeleton. Many of the author's hypokalemic polymyopathy patients have had pyrexia at the time of presentation.

Reported Cases

CVF/MW was first reported in a series of 24 cats in Massachusetts diagnosed with a primary muscle disorder. The diagnosis of polymyopathy was based on clinical signs (muscle weakness, muscle pain), elevations in muscle enzyme levels, electromyographic abnormalities, and histopathologic lesions in skeletal muscle biopsies. In this series, muscle pathology was found in 13 of 16 biopsies; however, only four of the 16 muscle biopsies revealed inflammation. In addition, approximately two-thirds of the cats were hypokalemic with no history of gastrointestinal signs. Mild elevation of serum urea nitrogen and creatinine was noted in approximately one-third of the cats, and an unexpected increase in the incidence of interstitial nephritis was noted in those cats necropsied. Autoimmunity was postulated to be a potential etiologic factor because of the lymphocytic myositis in some cats and the resolution of clinical signs after glucocorticoids.[3] In a report from Colorado, six cats presented with CVF/MW signs.[1] These cats had muscle pain, elevations is muscle enzymes, hypokalemia, mild to moderate metabolic acidosis, and persistent azotemia. Diffuse muscle membrane electromyographic (EMG) abnormalities were present, although muscle biopsies were normal or revealed only mild myonecrosis.[5] A relative absence of inflammation was noted. Hypokalemia was apparently caused by the combined effects of urinary potassium loss and dietary potassium deficiency.[5] The nephropathy resulted in increased urinary fractional clearance of potassium even though the serum potassium was low.[6] It was concluded that hypokalemia was the cause of the polymyopathy (hypokalemic polymyopathy).[4]

Another report of the CVF/MW complex, hypokalemia, and polymyopathy noted periodic muscle weakness in Burmese kittens in the United Kingdom.[7] Polymyopathy with associated hypokalemia was also reported in cats with renal distal tubular acidosis and primary hyperaldosteronism.[7] Episodic weakness and cervical ventroflexion were prominent signs in another series of young Burmese cats in Australia; however, serum potassium levels were not measured.[7] In another report of one cat, extreme hypernatremia subsequent to hypodipsia caused muscle dysfunction that clinically was indistinguishable from hypokalemic polymyopathy.[7]

Etiology

The etiologies of CVF/MW currently include, in order of incidence: hypokalemic polymyopathy (apparently immune mediated), steroid-responsive myositis, and hypernatremic myopathy. In most of the reported cases of cats with CVF/MW, hypokalemia is present. Normal feline muscle function is sensitive to changes in extracellular electrolyte concentrations, especially sodium and potassium.[2] The incidence of hypokalemia in hospitalized sick cats at one institution over a 3-year period was 37%.[2] Generally, hypokalemia resulting

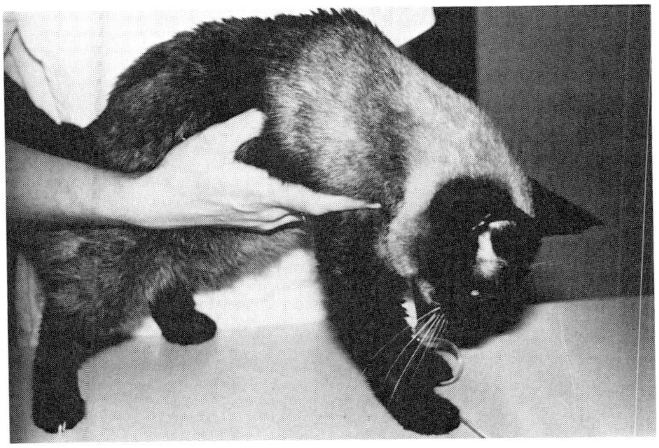

Figure 20–1. The typical cat with signs of the CVF/MW complex presents with excessive, passive flexion of the neck.

from a decrease in total body potassium occurs over a period of weeks to months, with the sustained hypokalemia leading to eventual neuromuscular dysfunction.[13] Because of the high incidence of chronic potassium depletion in cats, any disease entity that further reduces body potassium can result in the CVF/MW complex.

Pathogenesis of Hypokalemia

Potassium depletion may be relative or absolute. In the former situation, there is a normal total body potassium level present, but an abnormal amount is redistributed intracellularly, resulting in low serum levels. In the latter situation, total body potassium stores are depleted so the serum level is abnormally low. Studies have found the most likely causes of relative hypokalemia to be rare in the cat, although metabolic alkalosis should be considered with each patient.

Absolute hypokalemia results from decreased intake, increased loss, or both of potassium.[2] One study found that some commonly fed commercial diets were marginally low in potassium.[6] Correction of the potassium levels in these diets resulted in a decrease in the numbers of cats with normal renal function presenting with hypokalemia.[5] Urinary acidifiers may decrease gastrointestinal potassium absorption and thus contribute to hypokalemia.[13] Cats with renal dysfunction were found to be 14 times more likely to have significant hypokalemia than cats without renal disease.[6] In addition, hypokalemia was found to be the most common electrolyte abnormality in a study of naturally occurring renal disease.[14] Based on the response to potassium supplementation (reduction of azotemia and hyperkaluria), it was considered likely that cats with pre-existing renal disease were initially predisposed to potassium depletion and that renal disease was further complicated by the resultant hypokalemia.[5]

Pathogenesis of Myopathy

The exact mechanism by which feline hypokalemia causes muscle dysfunction is not proven. It has been postulated that severe potassium depletion causes a decrease in muscle-cell

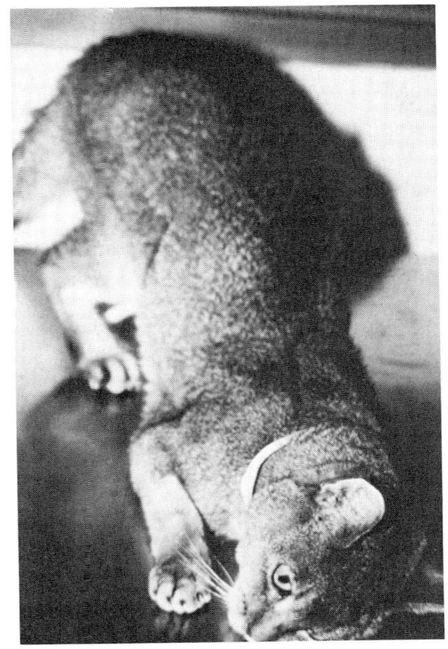

Figure 20–2. The generalized muscle weakness is exacerbated with exercise. Some cats will walk a short distance then assume a praying position with the chin on the floor, the front legs crouched, and the rear legs elevated.

transmembrane potential and results in clinical muscle weakness, as occurs in humans and dogs. Hypokalemia also results in a decrease in muscle glycogen synthesis, intracellular glycogen content, and muscle blood-flow during exercise. These effects of hypokalemia on muscle, especially during exercise, may explain the muscle damage. Muscle damage is evidenced by elevations in serum creatine kinase (CK) levels and biopsy findings.[13]

Decreased taurine levels, and the associated congestive cardiomyopathy, have been noted in several experimentally potassium-depleted cats. Plasma taurine levels were also low in the cats with naturally occurring hypokalemic polymyopathy reported in the original Colorado study.[4] Intracellular concentrations of potassium and taurine are interrelated; it has been postulated that decreased intracellular taurine levels may be linked to the pathogenesis of feline hypokalemic polymyopathy.[13]

Some naturally occurring cases of hypokalemic polymyopathy seen by the author have presented with pyrexia. This sign was also noted in 25% of the polymyopathy cats in a clinical report.[3] The cause of the pyrexia is unknown. The fever is not usually associated with significant leukocytosis or with biopsy-confirmed polymyositis. It may be associated with protein release from damaged muscles.

Diagnosis

The diagnosis of hypokalemic polymyopathy is dependent on the presence of the following:

1. Clinical signs of CVF/MW
2. Hypokalemia

3. Evidence of muscle dysfunction (muscle pain, EMG abnormalities, serum creatine kinase elevation, noninflammatory myopathy on biopsy)
4. A favorable response to potassium supplementation.[2]

Cats may exhibit some of these signs, and they may be subtle. The severity of clinical signs varies among patients, but generally signs are more severe with lower serum potassium levels. Potassium levels in severely affected cats are usually below 3 mEq/L; however, cats with levels between 3 and 3.5 mEq/L have been reported to have severe signs.[13] It is important to obtain pretreatment laboratory values (complete blood count, serum chemistries including CO_2 and CK levels, and urinalysis) at the time of presentation. It is also important to identify the presence of metabolic alkalosis, which can induce significant intracellular redistribution of potassium and hypokalemia.[14] Hemoconcentration may cause serum potassium to appear higher than actual—an important consideration in treatment.

Evidence of muscle dysfunction and a favorable response to potassium supplementation are also diagnostic criteria that must be evaluated. Muscle dysfunction may be measured by creatine kinase levels, which may be in the range of 5,000 to 10,000 units/L, and Burmese cats have been reported to develop much higher CK levels than do other breeds.[13] However, the CK levels should always be evaluated in relation to muscle pain because the level of CK does not always reflect the severity of the condition. Muscle pain may even be present without diagnostic CK levels in some cats. Response to adequate potassium supplementation should occur within 24 hours[2]; however, improvement of muscle strength is gradual and may not return to normal for several days.[13]

Differential Diagnosis

The signs of the CVF/MW complex appear to be primarily the result of severe, generalized muscle weakness. In some cats, the dorsal cervical muscles seem to be disproportionately involved, resulting in cervical ventroflexion. Cats presenting with pronounced CVF/MW signs typically have hypokalemic polymyopathy; however, CVF/MW signs may be subtle or overlap with signs caused by other conditions. The cause and degree of generalized weakness and muscle pain may be difficult to assess in some cats, especially if aggressive or timid. Therefore, a diagnosis of hypokalemic myopathy based on clinical signs alone may be erroneous.

The differential diagnoses of cats with cervical ventroflexion or generalized muscle weakness include thiamine deficiency, myopathies (primary and electrolyte induced), myelopathies, polyneuropathies, neuromuscular junction diseases (myasthenia gravis, organophosphate toxicosis, spider bite), ethylene glycol, generalized sepsis, and severe anemia. Thiamine deficiency produces a cervical ventroflexion that is active (i.e., the ventral cervical muscles are contracted) as opposed to the passive cervical ventroflexion of hypokalemic polymyopathy. In addition, thiamine deficiency results in excessive muscle tone, dilated, nonresponsive pupils, torticollis, and seizures.[2] Primary inflammatory myopathies (immune-mediated,[3] myositis ossificans,[14] and toxoplasmosis myositis[2]) may require a muscle biopsy, serum potassium levels, and toxoplasmosis titer for differentiation. Myopathies secondary to extreme hypernatremia or hypophosphatemia can usually be distinguished with serum electrolyte levels and response to correctional therapy. Myelopathies (fibrocartilaginous embolization, intervertebral disc herniation, and spinal lymphosarcoma) may be ruled out by the use of the neurologic examination (i.e., reflex changes, localized or lack of hyperpathia versus generalized muscle pain), and lack of hypokalemia. Polyneuropathies (long-standing diabetes mellitus, vincristine therapy, and idiopathic polyradiculopathy)[2] can be differentiated by history, motor nerve-conduction testing, and neurologic examination (i.e., lower motor neuron signs). Neuromuscular junction diseases can sometimes be difficult to distinguish clinically from hypokalemic polymyopathy; however, a history of exposure to organophosphates or pyrethins, the presence of low acetylcholinesterase levels (organophosphate toxicosis), appropriate response to edrophonium chloride (myasthenia gravis), serologic evidence of autoantibodies against acetylcholine receptors (myasthenia gravis), and evidence of local soft-tissue swelling or necrosis (spider bite) aid in the evaluation. Ethylene glycol can be differentiated with a history of exposure, presence of oxalate crystals in the urine, severe renal failure, and poor response to potassium supplementation. Generalized sepsis can be differentiated by elimination of a potential source of infection (pyometra) using physical examination, radiographs, and urinalysis, evaluation of white blood cells for toxicity, blood culture, and the elimination of immunosuppressive diseases (notably the feline leukemia virus and feline immunodeficiency virus). The degree to which anemia contributes to generalized muscle weakness is dependent on the severity and rate of onset.

Treatment

The hypokalemic polymyopathic cat has sustained negative potassium balance over weeks to months, resulting in a total body potassium depletion.[13] The patient's ability to conserve potassium or to compensate for hypokalemia is exhausted, and reserve potassium stores have been depleted. Therefore, the margin of error in treatment is narrow. The replacement of potassium must be appropriate relative to the severity of the signs; its rate and route of administration are critical. Extreme hypokalemia (<2 mEq/L) not only results in severe generalized muscle weakness but also can lead to respiratory insufficiency or failure because of respiratory muscle weakness. If parenteral fluids are inappropriately low in potassium, the patient's condition may decline.[2] If parenteral fluids containing high levels of potassium are given too rapidly, fatal cardiac arrhythmias may occur.[13]

Serum measurements of potassium usually do not reflect the true severity of hypokalemia in the dehydrated cat. When the extracellular compartment is expanded with parenteral fluids, the extracellular potassium level is diluted. Because hypokalemic compensatory mechanisms have already been exhausted, the effects of sudden dilution can be dramatic and severe. In addition to dilutional effects, expansion of the extracellular volume may accelerate renal tubular potassium excretion.[13] Initial fluid administration to most dehydrated animals is empirical regarding electrolyte concentrations; adjustments are made when pretreatment laboratory results are obtained. However, in hypokalemic polymyopathic cats, the administration of fluids that are inappropriately low in potassium may actually exacerbate clinical signs.[2] Therefore, a patient with CVF/MW signs should have serum electrolytes determined prior to beginning subcutaneous or intravenous fluid therapy, if possible.

The route, concentration, and rate of potassium supplementation are dependent on the severity of the CVF/MW signs (initially and during potassium therapy), competency of the respiratory efforts, initial serum potassium level (relative to the state of hydration), and serial potassium determinations during potassium therapy. The severity of generalized muscle weakness is an approximate, but clinically useful, estimate of functional potassium concentrations at the cellular level. Generally, the more severe the CVF/MW signs, the lower the functional potassium level and the more aggressive that therapy needs to be.

With severe weakness of the intercostal muscles and diaphragm, the cat is unable to move adequate air volumes. Clinically, respiratory competency is difficult to assess. However, it can be estimated based on lateral thoracic radiography during inspiration and expiration, mucous membrane color, and respiratory effort. If available, blood gases are a more reliable indicator.

Routine Potassium Supplementation

Hypokalemic cats are treated with 7 to 20 mEq of potassium chloride (KCl) in 250 mL of an isotonic intravenous fluid (Table 28–1). (Allowance should be made for potassium in the fluid. Lactated Ringer's solution [LRS] contains 1 mEq/250 mL; 0.9% sodium chloride contains none.) However, the initial serum potassium value should be interpreted relative to the cat's state of hydration, as judged by skin turgor, total serum protein, hematocrit, and serum sodium. Fluid diuresis for rehydration will cause a further decline in serum potassium; therefore, the next higher level of potassium in Table 28–1 should be used for dehydrated cats. Following initial therapy, potassium supplementation is also based on Table 28–1.

Table 28–1. Guidelines for Intravenous Potassium Supplementation*

Serum Potassium (mEq/L)	mEq KCl to Add per 250 mL of Fluid†	Maximal Infusion Rate (mL/kg/hr)‡
<2.0	20	6
2.1–2.5	15	8
2.6–3.0	10	12
3.1–3.5	7	16

*From Dr. R.C. Scott, Animal Medical Center, New York, NY.
†Assume a potassium-free fluid (e.g., 0.9% NaCl). Adjust amount of potassium added according to potassium contents of fluid used.
‡Do not exceed 0.5 mEq/kg/hr.
Used by permission: Bell FW, Osborne CA. Treatment of hypokalemia. In: Kirk RW, ed. Current Veterinary Therapy IX, Philadelphia: WB Saunders, 1989:25.

Table 28–2. Components of Fluid Therapy

1. Hydration Deficit (Replacement Requirement)
   Body weight (lb) × % dehydration as a decimal × 500*
   = deficit in milliliters
   Body weight (kg) × % dehydration as a decimal
   = deficit in liters
2. Maintenance Requirement (20–40 mL/lb/day)
   Sensible losses (urine output): 12–20 mL/lb/day
   Insensible losses (fecal, cutaneous, respiratory): 6–10 mL/lb/day
3. Contemporary (Ongoing) Losses
   Vomition, diarrhea, polyuria

*500 mL = 1 lb of fluid.
Used by permission: Muir WW, Dibartola SP. Fluid Therapy. In: Kirk RW, ed. Current Veterinary Therapy VIII. Philadelphia: WB Saunders, 1987:25.

Intense Potassium Supplementation

Intense potassium supplementation is indicated if an acute, life-threatening muscle weakness or paralysis develops,[13] if the serum potassium level drops 1 mEq/L (or greater) compared with the pretreatment value, or if the serum potassium value drops below 2 mEq/L.[2] Intense potassium supplementation consists of the administration of high concentrations of KCl in minimal amounts of parenteral fluids at a rapid rate. The typical KCl concentration is 182 mEq of KCl/L of LRS or 45 mEq of KCl/250 mL of LRS; the rate should approach but not exceed 0.5 mEq/kg of body weight/hour. At this concentration and the maximal rate, KCl in LRS would be administered at a maintenance rate of 66 mL/kg/day or 2.75 mL/kg/hour).[13] By giving KCl in a minimal amount of fluid, potassium loss via renal tubular excretion is minimized. An infusion pump and constant electrocardiographic (ECG) monitoring are recommended when administering solutions with high potassium levels (>20 mEq/250 mL of fluid).[13] Serum potassium levels should return to normal after 2 to 4 hours of constant intravenous infusion of the above solution. Once the serum potassium reaches normal, the concentration of the potassium-containing fluid is reduced to 80 mEq/L (20 mEq/250 mL of LRS).[13] The amount of fluids required to correct the hydration deficit and to meet the maintenance fluid requirement is calculated and given over the next 24 hours at a rate not to exceed 0.5 mEq/kg/hr (Table 28–2). Serum potassium levels should be monitored every 2 to 3 hours after intense potassium supplementation for the first 24 hours, if possible. After the first 24 hours, adjustments in potassium supplementation are based on the recommendations in Table 28–1.

Long-Term Potassium Supplementation

Cats with hypokalemic polymyopathy or subclinical hypokalemia that are eating or that can be fed via an orogastric tube should be supplemented with oral potassium gluconate (Kaon Elixir or Tumil-K). It should be dosed at 5 to 10 mEq/cat/day until the serum potassium is normal. The latter product in powder form is designed to be administered in food.[13] The oral route is the safest form of potassium supplementation and should be used as early in the treatment of hypokalemia as possible. Long-term oral potassium supplementation is usually required in hypokalemic polymyopathy cats with renal dysfunction because continued accelerated renal potassium excretion will likely cause a recurrence of the disease. However, it is generally not required if renal function is normal.[13] The amount of potassium required for maintenance averages 2 to 6 mEq/cat/day but must be individualized by periodic measurements of serum potassium levels until an appropriate dose is found. Hypokalemic cats with normal renal function should receive potassium gluconate for at least 2 months after release from the hospital. If normokalemia is maintained over several weeks without oral supplementation, it may be discontinued.

REFERENCES

1. Fenner WR. Neurologic Disorders. In: Sherding RG, ed. The Cat: Diseases and Clinical Management, vol. 2. New York: Churchill Livingstone, 1989:1163.
2. Dow SW, LeCouteur RA. Hypokalemic Polymyopathy of Cats. In: Kirk RW, ed. Current Veterinary Therapy X, Philadelphia: WB Saunders, 1989:812.
3. Schunk KL. Feline Polymyopathy. In: Proceedings of the Second Annual ACVIM Forum and Twelfth Annual Scientific Program, 1984:197.
4. Dow SW, LeCouteur RA, Fettman MJ, Spurgeon TL. Potassium depletion in cats: Hypokalemic polymyopathy. J Amer Vet Med Assoc 1987;191:1563.
5. Fettman MJ. Feline kaliopenic polymyopathy/nephropathy syndrome. Vet Clin North Am [Small Anim Pract], 1989;19(3):415.
6. Dow SW, Fettman MJ, LeCouteur RA, Hamar DW. Potassium depletion in cats: Renal and dietary influences. J Am Vet Med Assoc 1987;191:1563.
7. Blaxter A, Lievesley P, Gruffydd-Jones T, Wotton P. Periodic muscle weakness in Burmese kittens. Vet Rec 1986;118:619.
8. Drazner FH. Distal renal tubular acidosis associated with chronic pyelonephritis in a cat. Calif Vet 1980;34:15.
9. Eger CE, Robinson WF, Huxtable CRR. Primary aldosteronism (Conn's syndrome) in a cat: A case report and review of comparative aspects. J Small Anim Pract 1983;24:293.
10. Mason K. A hereditary disease in Burmese cats manifested as an episodic weakness with head nodding and neck ventroflexion. J Am Anim Hosp Assoc 1988;24:147.
11. Dow SW, Fettman MJ, LeCouteur RA et al. Hypodipsic hypernatremia and associated myopathy in a hydrocephalic cat with transient hypopituitarism. J Am Vet Med Assoc 1987;191:217.
12. Dow SW, Fettman MJ, Curtis CR et al. Hypokalemia in cats: 136 cases (1984–1987). J Am Vet Med Assoc 1989;194:1604.
13. Dow SW, LeCouteur RA. Potassium-Depletion Myopathy. In: August JR, ed. Consultations in Feline Internal Medicine. Philadelphia: WB Saunders, 1991:519.
14. DiBartola SP, Rutgers HC, Zuck PM et al. Clinicopathologic findings associated with chronic renal disease in cats: 74 cases (1973–1984). J Am Vet Med Assoc 1987;190:1196.
15. Dow SW. Studies of potassium depletion in cats. In: Proceedings of the 12th Annual Kal-Kan Symposium for the Treatment of Small Animal Diseases, Feline Medicine. 1988:61.
16. Kornegay JN. Feline Neurology. In: Kay WJ, Brown NO, eds. Problems in Veterinary Medicine. Philadelphia: JB Lippincott, 1991;3(3):378.
17. Bell FW, Osborne CA. Treatment of Hypokalemia. In: Kirk RW, ed. Current Veterinary Therapy IX. Philadelphia: WB Saunders, 1989:25.
18. Muir WW, DiBartola SP. Fluid Therapy. In: Kirk RW, ed. Current Veterinary Therapy VIII. Philadelphia: WB Saunders, 1987:25.

CHAPTER 29

◇ ◇ ◇

Cholangitis/Cholangiohepatitis Syndrome

Gary D. Norsworthy

The cholangitis/cholangiohepatitis syndrome (CCHS) is among the two or three most common liver diseases affecting the cat.[1-4] Because of the frequency with which it occurs, it should be considered in any icteric cat. Although relatively common, the causes and pathogenesis of CCHS are poorly understood. Currently, it is divided into three disease types: suppurative cholangitis/cholangiohepatitis; chronic, nonsuppurative (lymphocytic) cholangitis/cholangiohepatitis; and biliary cirrhosis.[2,3,5,6] Some authors have speculated that this syndrome represents three stages of one progressive disease; however, the available evidence indicates that CCHS is more likely to be two separate diseases that may or may not terminate in biliary cirrhosis.

The term *cholangitis* is used to describe inflammation which is confined to the biliary tree, without hepatic lobular invasion,[7] and which is limited to the bile ducts within the parenchyma of the liver. *Cholangiohepatitis* is an inflammatory process that involves the intrahepatic bile ducts and that has also spread to adjacent hepatocytes. *Biliary cirrhosis* is characterized by hepatocyte replacement by fibrous connective tissue.[8]

Suppurative Cholangitis/ Cholangiohepatitis

Etiology

The first type of CCHS is an acute disease that may be a cholangitis or a cholangiohepatitis. Many authorities believe that this disease process has a bacterial etiology in most cats. It is presumed that bacteria from the duodenum ascend the common bile duct, enter the gallbladder, and eventually progress into the intrahepatic bile ducts and the adjacent hepatocytes. Indeed, most of the bacteria cultured from the hepatic parenchyma are coliforms, supporting the assumption that they are duodenal in origin. Rarely, other infectious agents have been recovered, including *Toxoplasma* species and *Bacillus piriformis*.[3] In some cats, bacterial cultures have been negative. In those cats, other pathologic processes are usually present and thought to be etiologically significant. Those processes may include chronic pancreatitis, cholecystitis, thickened inspissated bile, cholelithiasis, and regional enteritis.[1,2] There is also speculation that the predisposing diseases just listed may actually be secondary to the cholangiohepatitis.[8]

Clinical and Examination Findings

Many cats with suppurative cholangitis are symptomatic. In the presence of suppurative cholangiohepatitis, some cats will be clinically asymptomatic or will have nonspecific signs of illness such as lethargy or decreased appetite. In these cats, leukocytosis may be the only hematologic abnormality. These cats typically recover spontaneously or with antibiotic therapy. However, most cats with liver involvement manifest clinical signs that are typical of hepatic disease, including anorexia, vomiting, fever, weight loss, depression, drooling, and icterus. Prior to presentation, some cats may have been ill for 1 to 2 weeks with a progression of clinical signs; others may become acutely ill. Some cats also present with a history of several prior episodes of illness that subsequently resolved. The physical examination is generally unremarkable except for icterus and occasionally, dehydration.

Radiographic and Laboratory Findings

There are no consistent diagnostic radiographic findings in this disease, but one should observe the gallbladder for evidence of cholelithiasis. Because this is a relatively acute disease, the liver is normal in size and shape. The biochemical profile will generally reveal findings typical of many acute liver diseases, including an increase in the serum levels of bilirubin, alkaline phosphatase (SAP), and alanine aminotransferase (ALT). However, in some cats, SAP and ALT levels may be normal. Bilirubin and urobilinogen may be found in the urine.[8]

Diagnosis

A presumptive diagnosis can be established on the basis of a fine needle aspiration biopsy of the liver which may reveal either a bacterial or a sterile suppurative pattern. However, a number of other diseases and conditions, such as feline infectious peritonitis (FIP), blunt liver trauma, and hepatotoxicosis, can produce the same findings. A definitive diagnosis requires a liver biopsy. The biopsy sample may be taken via a laparotomy, percutaneous needle technique, or laparoscopy. The laparotomy has the advantages of permitting an examination of the gallbladder, common bile duct, and pancreas and of allowing culturing of the liver and bile. If other biliary disease is detected, corrective measures may be taken at that time. However, the laparotomy is more stressful to the patient and more expensive to the client than the other methods. The characteristic histologic findings include a periportal hepatitis and the presence of purulent material within dilated intrahepatic biliary ducts. The purulent material will contain a predominance of neutrophils, distinguishing this disease from the chronic lymphocytic form.

Treatment

Supportive and symptomatic care is important in very ill cats. Correction of dehydration with an isotonic intravenous (IV) fluid is essential. Control of vomiting is also important. This may be accomplished with the use of antiemetics, such as metoclopramide (Reglan), administered at a dose of 0.05–0.15 mg/lb every 12 hours IM or SC. Because of the strong likelihood of a bacterial etiology, antibiotics are definitely indicated. If a liver biopsy is obtained, aerobic and anaerobic bacterial cultures should be performed on the biopsy specimen to aid in the selection of a specific antibiotic. If cultures are not available, antibiotics that reach high concentrations in bile and that are likely to affect hepatic anaerobes and enteric coliforms should be chosen.[8] Ampicillin (Polyflex), amoxicillin (Amoxi-tabs), β lactamase-resistant antibiotics (e.g., Clavamox), enrofloxacin (Baytril), and chloramphenicol (Medicol) are excellent choices. Another excellent choice is metronidazole (Flagyl), which may be used concurrently with ampicillin, amoxicillin, Clavamox, or chloramphenicol. Treatment should continue until the cat's fever and neutrophilia are resolved, but for no less than 2 weeks. Most cats require antibiotic therapy for 3 to 6 weeks.

There are several additional antibiotics that would appear to be good choices for this disease owing to their ability to produce high biliary concentrations, or to their spectrum of activity. However, each has certain disadvantages in cats with CCHS. Erythromycin (Erythromycin Stearate Tabs) is often ineffective in combatting gram-negative bacteria and often causes anorexia and vomiting. Tetracycline hydrochloride often causes fever and anorexia and has been shown to induce hepatic lipidosis. Aminoglycosides, such as gentamicin (Gentocin), and first- and second-generation cephalosporins, such as cefadroxil (Cefa-tabs), are not excreted in bile in an active form.[7,8]

Corticosteroids are not indicated for this form of CCHS. Dehydrocholic acid (Decholin) has been touted as an agent that improves bile flow. However, this claim has not been documented in humans or in cats. Additionally, there are some drugs that stimulate bile flow by bile salt-independent mechanisms.[9] These include furosemide (Lasix), theophylline (Elixophyllin), phenobarbital, and hydrocortisone. Their efficacy in this disease in the cat has not been documented.

Prognosis

In the short term, many cats recover completely, even if antibiotic therapy is not instituted. However, the short-term prognosis for many others is guarded to fair. The long-term prognosis is highly variable and often poor. Many cats have long periods of remission that are followed by severe exacerbations. Other have chronic disease that progresses into biliary cirrhosis.[1,10]

Lymphocytic Cholangitis/ Cholangiohepatitis

The second disease classification within the CCHS is lymphocytic cholangitis/cholangiohepatitis. It is the most commonly reported form of the disease. Most cats diagnosed with this form of the disease are younger than 4 years of age, but cats ranging in age up to 10 years have been reported to be affected.[5]

Clinical and Laboratory Findings

These cats are generally less ill than those with the suppurative form of CCHS. Typically upon presentation, they are not vomiting or febrile, and they do not appear to be lethargic. Icterus is a quite variable sign; in one series of cats, it was present in only 50% of affected animals.[5] An uncommon but striking clinical feature in some of these cats is the presence of ascites, a finding not common in other feline liver diseases. Hepatomegaly may also be evident on radiographic studies or on palpation.

The biochemical profile will reveal an elevation in the serum levels of bilirubin (primarily direct), SAP, and ALT, similar to that which occurs with the suppurative form. However, these cats often will exhibit hyperglobulinemia and hypoalbuminemia, as do many cats with chronic inflammatory diseases, such as FIP.[5]

Diagnosis

As with the suppurative form of the disease, a presumptive diagnosis can be made on the basis of a fine needle aspirate that reveals an acute or subacute inflammatory pattern predominated by lymphocytes and plasmacytes (Fig. 29–1). In contrast to the suppurative form, the inflammatory pattern will be consistently sterile. A definitive diagnosis depends upon a liver biopsy. Nodules of liver tissue separated by fibrous connective tissue septa are typical. The periportal area will contain a large number of lymphocytes, and hyperplasia of the bile ductules is common.[7] Some biopsy studies also reveal significant numbers of plasmacytes. If a laparotomy or percutaneous liver biopsy is performed, the liver tissue should be cultured for aerobes and anaerobes, if possible. This should be a standard procedure for liver disease, as the exact diagnosis is generally not known at the time of biopsy.

Treatment

Unless bacteria are identified, antibiotics are unlikely to be helpful. However, a broad-spectrum antibiotic, such as

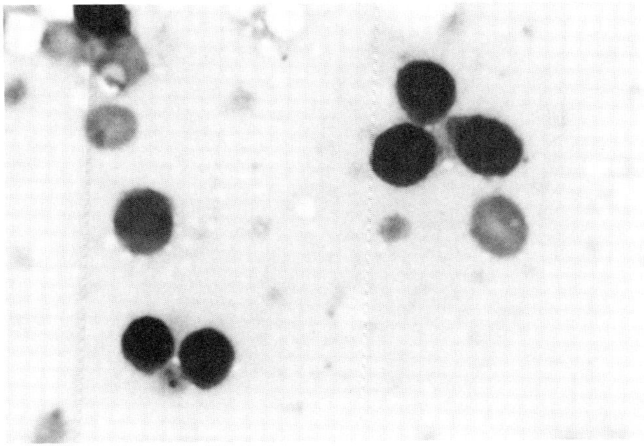

Figure 29–1. **Lymphocytic cholangitis/cholangiohepatitis is characterized by a liver aspirate in which lymphocytes and plasmacytes predominate. There are six mature lymphocytes in this field.**

amoxicillin, is generally recommended. The cornerstone of therapy is the use of corticosteroids. Prednisolone tablets should be used at immunosuppressive doses (1 to 2 mg/lb/day) until remission occurs; the dosage should then be tapered over a period of 30 to 60 days.[8] When prednisolone is discontinued, the cat should be monitored closely because relapses may occur.[6,10]

Prognosis

Although some cats will recover, most have clinical or biochemical relapses of disease. It has been demonstrated experimentally that the immune system can perpetuate some forms of chronic inflammation in the liver. The release of antigens from damaged hepatocytes may activate immunocompetent cells that cause damage to additional hepatocytes. This cycle then repeats itself, causing extensive liver damage.[1] This is probably how this type of disease progresses to biliary cirrhosis. Therefore, these cats should be monitored with periodic biochemical profiles. At the first indication of a recurrence, corticosteroid therapy should be reinstituted. Despite careful monitoring, many affected cats will progress to biliary cirrhosis.

Biliary Cirrhosis

Biliary cirrhosis is the least common form of CCHS because many cats die before reaching this stage of end-stage liver disease. Because the cirrhosis is generalized within the liver, these cats are typically terminally ill. They often present with icterus, lethargy, vomiting, and a history of weight loss. The liver is often contracted (Fig. 29–2), and ascites is common. In many ways, the laboratory findings in biliary cirrhosis are similar to those reported with the two other forms of the disease. However, cats with biliary cirrhosis may have marked elevations in the hepatic enzymes, and enough liver damage may have occurred to result in coagulopathies. A liver biopsy will reveal extensive fibrosis and bile duct hyperplasia.[8]

Because these cats have functional, irreversible hepatic failure, their prognosis is grave. Despite supportive care, most die within a few days or weeks.[7]

Sequelae and Complications

There are several sequelae and complications that may occur as a result of either the suppurative or the lymphocytic form of CCHS. Sludging of bile is the most common. This may occur in the gallbladder, common bile duct, or the intrahepatic channels. Cholestasis and bacterial infections alter the consistency of the bile so that it becomes viscid and cannot flow through the biliary system. When this occurs, the gallbladder becomes distended (Fig. 29–3) and the prognosis worsens.

Surgical removal of the inspissated bile from the gallbladder or common bile duct is recommended. However,

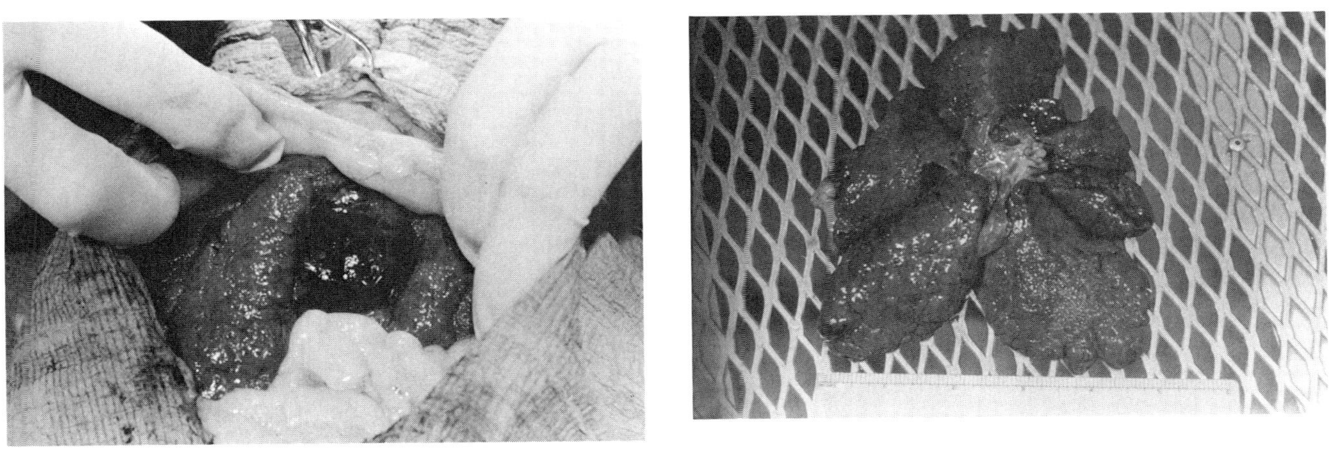

A B

Figure 29–2. **(*A*) Biliary cirrhosis causes contraction of the liver, as seen in this intraoperative photograph. (*B*) At necropsy, the generalized cirrhosis of the liver seen in Figure 29–2A is apparent.**

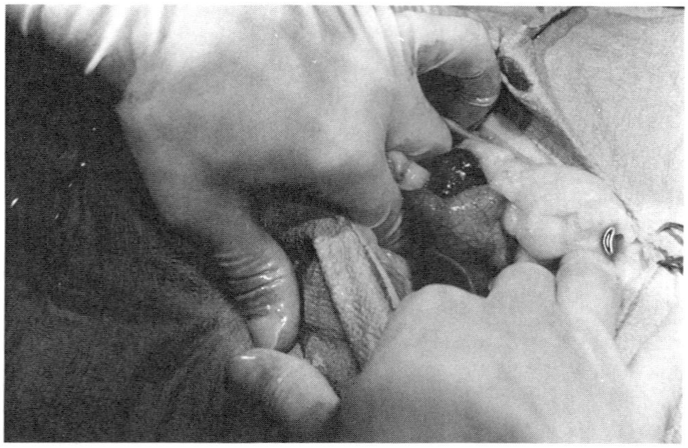

Figure 29–3. Bile sludging causes the gallbladder to become greatly distended.

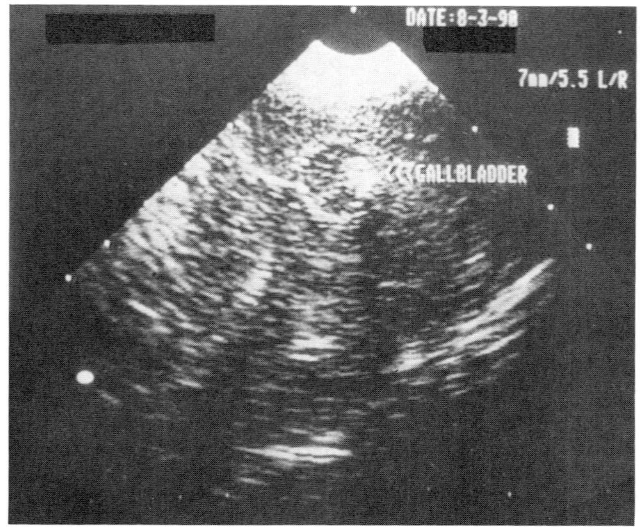

Figure 29–5. A sonogram of the same cat as in Figure 29–4 clearly reveals the cholelith within the gallbladder.

if the intrahepatic channels are blocked, little will be accomplished. Because there is no drug currently available that has been clinically proven to decrease the bile's specific gravity or to move it through the biliary system, this is a serious complication that often signals impending terminal disease.[7] As mentioned, dehydrocholic acid has not been proven to be efficacious in humans or cats and is contraindicated in complete biliary obstruction.[11]

Cholelithiasis occurs when choleliths form either in the gallbaldder or the common bile ducts. They are typically radiolucent (Figs. 29–4 and 29–5) and are composed primarily of bile pigments. Most authorities believe that they are the final stage of the bile sludging process. If diagnosed, they should be removed surgically, but this is not considered an indication for cholecystectomy.[1]

The so-called *white bile syndrome* has been reported by a few authors. When the gallbladder is opened, it may be found to contain a clear, thick fluid that is devoid of bile pigments, hence the "white bile." This material is actually the fluid and mucus that has been secreted by the gallblad-

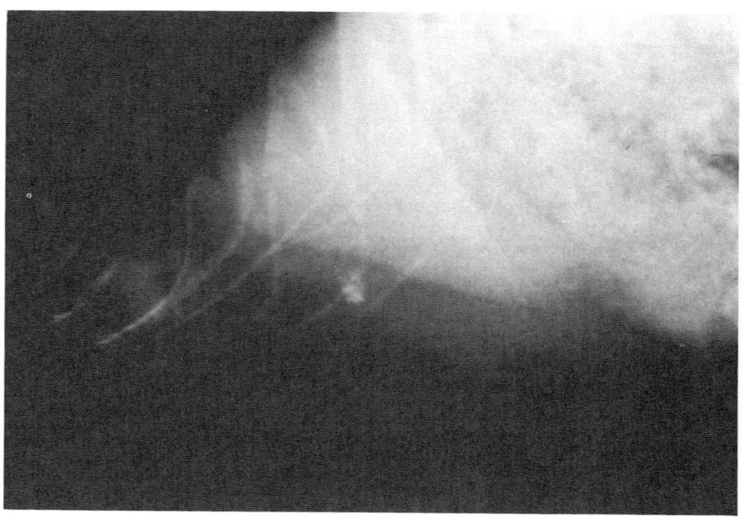

A

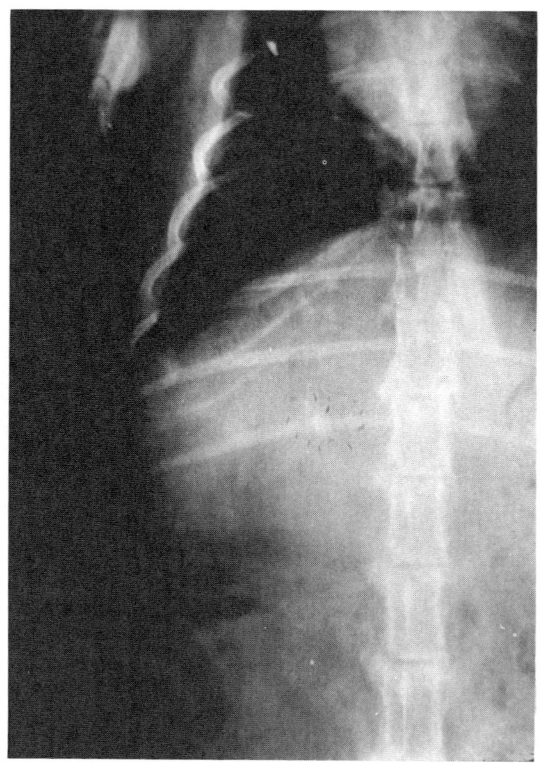

B

Figure 29–4. (*A*) A cholelith can be seen at the level of the 12th rib in this lateral radiograph. (*B*) A ventrodorsal view of the same cat as in Figure 29–4A demonstrates the cholelith at the level of the 13th rib, just to the right of the midline.

der itself. This phenomenon occurs as a result of bile flow obstruction; no bile is able to enter the gallbladder. Consequently, this is a poor prognostic sign.[2,12]

Hepatic encephalopathy is a rare occurrence in cats with CCHS. It is unlikely to occur because most cats die of end-stage liver failure prior to its occurrence. However, if it is diagnosed, IV fluid therapy should be instituted to maintain a normal glucose, fluid, acid–base, and electrolyte status. Azotemia, hypoglycemia, hypokalemia, and alkalosis are likely sequelae. Dietary protein should be restricted by the use of a low-quantity, high-quality protein diet, such as Feline Prescription Diet k/d (Hill's Pet Products, Topeka, KS). Lactulose (Cephulac) should be used to acidify the colon and to create a gentle osmotic diarrhea. The appropriate oral dose is 1.5 mL (1 g)/10 lb t.i.d. Treatment with metronidazole is indicated to decrease the colonic bacterial population and thus reduce the production of circulating ammonia. The oral dose is 3.4 mg/lb t.i.d.[13]

REFERENCES

1. Zawie DA, Garvey MS. Feline hepatic disease. Vet Clin North Am (Small Anim Pract) 1984;14(6):1201.
2. Hirsh VM, Doige CE. Suppurative cholangitis in cats. J Am Vet Med Assoc 1983;182:1223.
3. Rogers KS, Cornelius LM. Feline icterus. Compend Contin Educ Small Anim Pract 1985;7:391.
4. Hitt ME. The feline liver: Identifying and treating its diseases. Vet Med Small Anim Clin 1987;82:139.
5. Lucke VM, Davies JD. Progressive lymphocytic cholangitis in the cat. J Small Anim Pract 1984;25:249.
6. Prasse KW. Chronic lymphocytic cholangitis in three cats. Vet Pathol 1982;19:99.
7. Zawie DA, Shaker E. Diseases of the Liver. In: Sherding RG, ed. Diseases of the Cat. New York: Churchill Livingstone, 1989: 1015.
8. Hardy RM. Diseases of the Liver and Their Treatment. In: Ettinger SJ, ed. Textbook of Veterinary Internal Medicine, 3rd ed. Philadelphia, WB Saunders Co., 1989:1479.
9. Papich MG, Davis LE. Drugs and the liver. Vet Clin North Am (Small Anim Pract) 1985;15(1):17.
10. Center SA. Feline liver disorders and their management. Compend Contin Educ Small Anim Pract 1986;8:889.
11. American Medical Association: AMA Drug Evaluations, 4th ed. Chicago: American Medical Association, 1980:809, 1002, 1452.
12. O'Brien JR, Mitchum GD. Cholelithiasis in a cat. J Am Vet Med Assoc 1970;155:1015.
13. Tams TR. Hepatic encephalopathy. Vet Clin North Am (Small Anim Pract) 1985;15:177.

CHAPTER 30

◇ ◇ ◇

Chronic Nasal Discharge

Gary D. Norsworthy

Chronic purulent nasal discharge (Fig. 30–1), usually accompanied by sneezing, is a relatively common occurrence in cats. It may be caused by a number of disease processes, as listed in Table 30–1. The disease process causing the disorder may originate in the nose, in the frontal sinuses, or both. Regardless of the focus of infection, the cat will sneeze violently, propelling purulent material into the cat's immediate environment.[1] This is often poorly tolerated by the owner, resulting in many of these cats being banned to the outdoors or euthanized.

Etiology

Chronic rhinitis may be caused by a number of disease processes. Nasal foreign bodies (Fig. 30–2), benign nasal (inflammatory) polyps (Fig. 30–3), malignant nasal tumors (Fig. 30–4), disease involving the roots of the maxillary teeth, chronic fungal infections (most commonly secondary to *Cryptococcus neoformans*), and chronic viral infections are the most common primary causes.[2] Each of these may be complicated by a secondary bacterial infection caused by a variety of pathogens.[2,3]

Chronic viral rhinitis is a common sequela of infections with the feline herpesvirus (rhinotracheitis virus) and the feline calicivirus. Cats infected with either virus often become chronic carriers. This form of rhinitis often is associated with a secondary infection caused by a number of pathogenic bacteria.[1-4] If these bacteria ascend into the frontal sinuses, a chronic, purulent sinusitis may occur.[5] This will result in a persistent purulent nasal discharge that often becomes intolerable to the owner. Systemic antibiotic, antihistamine, and steroid therapy will usually provide relief of the clinical signs of chronic sinusitis, but only temporarily. Except for the chronic sneezing and nasal discharge, these cats are generally healthy. There are no systemic effects, even when the disease is present for several years, except for infrequent episodes of fever and depressed appetite.

History

Acute viral and bacterial nasal infections may cause a heavy, purulent discharge. If treated aggressively with antibiotics, these infections will resolve in a few days. When taking the history of a cat with a purulent nasal discharge, the clinician should determine the duration of the problem. If the duration is less than 4 weeks, it should be considered an acute disease, and a diagnostic work-up such as the one described below is not justified. However, if the nasal discharge has been present for more than 2 months, a more thorough diagnostic evaluation is warranted.

It is also important to establish whether the discharge is unilateral or bilateral, and whether blood is a component of the discharge.

Anatomy

The nasal cavity is composed of a maxillary and an ethmoid region. The former is located immediately dorsal to the nasal cavity. These two regions are not separated, but communicate freely (Fig. 30–5*A*).

The frontal sinuses are hollow cavities located below the dorsal surface of the skull 1 to 2 cm caudal to the eyes (Fig. 30–5*B*). They are lined with a mucous membrane and communicate with the ethmoid region of the nasal cavity through an ostium (Fig. 30–5*C*).

Diagnosis

Because of the variety of possible etiologies the clinician should evaluate a cat that presents with a chronic nasal discharge with several diagnostic modalities, including radiographs, cytologic studies, culture, and serologic tests.

Radiographic Studies

Radiographs of the skull must be of high quality to allow visualization of the fine structure of the turbinates. In order to obtain the needed information, specific views, using proper positioning, are essential. The following views are necessary:

- Lateral view of the skull (Fig. 30–6)
- Rostral-caudal (skyline) view of the skull with the frontal sinuses exposed (Fig. 30–7)
- Ventrodorsal view of the nasal cavity without superimposition of the mandible (Fig. 30–8)

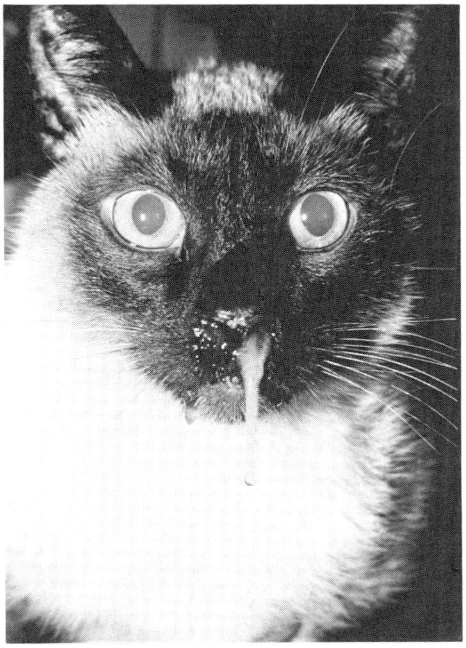

Figure 30–1. A chronic nasal discharge can be of a long duration and be extremely copious, and yet not produce systemic signs of illness. This cat was otherwise healthy despite a nasal discharge of 6 years' duration.

Table 30–1. Likely Causes of Chronic Nasal Discharge in the Cat

Purulent Discharge
Chronic viral infection with secondary bacteria
Bacterial infection, especially *Pseudomonas aeruginosa*
Fungal infection, especially *Cryptococcus neoformans* and *Histoplasma capsulatum*
Foreign body
Traumatic injury with secondary bacteria
Oronasal fistula
Abscess of roots of maxillary teeth, especially the canines
Neoplasia, especially adenocarcinoma and squamous cell carcinoma
Nasopharyngeal (inflammatory) polyps
Mucoid to Mucopurulent Discharge
Fungal, especially *C. neoformans* and *H. capsulatum*
Neoplasia, especially adenocarcinoma and squamous cell carinoma
Sanguinopurulent Discharge
Neoplasia, especially adenocarcinoma and squamous cell carcinoma
Bacterial infection as above
Foreign body
Abscess of roots of maxillary teeth, especially the canines

Adapted from Kuehn NF, Roudebush P. Nasal Discharge. In: Allen DG, ed. Small Animal Medicine. Philadelphia: JB Lippincott, 1991:383.

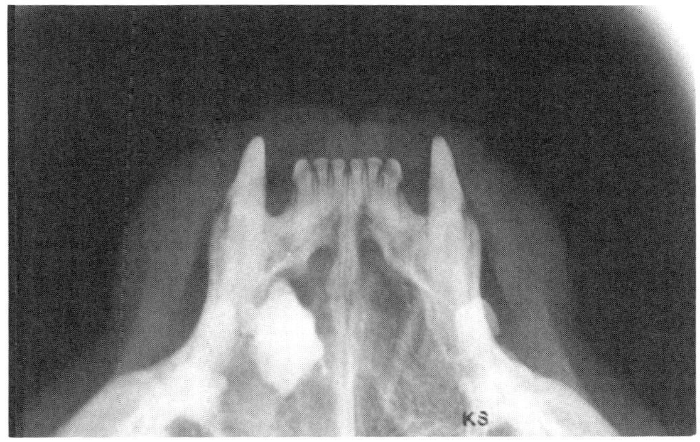

Figure 30–2. A rock-like material was present in this cat's right nasal cavity, producing a unilateral, chronic nasal discharge. (Courtesy of Dr. Henry Weir, San Antonio, TX.)

The lateral view of the skull may be obtained without sedation. However, anesthesia is essential for the skyline view of the frontal sinuses and the ventrodorsal view of the nasal cavity.

It is important to understand the location(s) of any pathology. Increased density in the frontal sinuses is easily visible on the lateral view; however, only by taking the skyline view can one determine whether the disease process is unilateral or bilateral. Proper positioning (see Fig. 30–8) will allow one to obtain radiographs of the nasal cavity without superimposing the mandible. If rare earth or very fine-screened film is used, the fine bone structure in the nasal cavity may be visualized.

Analysis of the Nasal Discharge

The discharge that exits the nasal opening(s) is not ideal for cytologic study or culture. However, if the nasal flushing procedure described in this section cannot be performed, cytologic and culture studies should be performed on the discharge material obtained from the nose. A pure culture of a pathogenic bacterium should be interpreted as being significant. It is preferable to remove any collected discharge, allow the cat to sneeze, then collect fresh discharge just as it exits the nasal opening.

The preferred sample for cytologic study and culture is collected by a flushing technique. This method allows collection of material that has not yet drained from the nose and thus has not been contaminated with incidental organisms. Two flushing methods are acceptable:

- *Method A.* The cat is anesthetized and a 3.5-French open-ended catheter is inserted approximately ½ inch into the nasal cavity. Then, 2 to 5 mL of saline solution are flushed through the catheter into the nasal cavity. As much fluid as possible is immediately aspirated back through the catheter or is collected on a gauze square as described below.
- *Method B.* The cat is anesthetized, and a cuffed endotracheal tube is passed into the trachea. A sterile gauze

(*Text continues on page 272*)

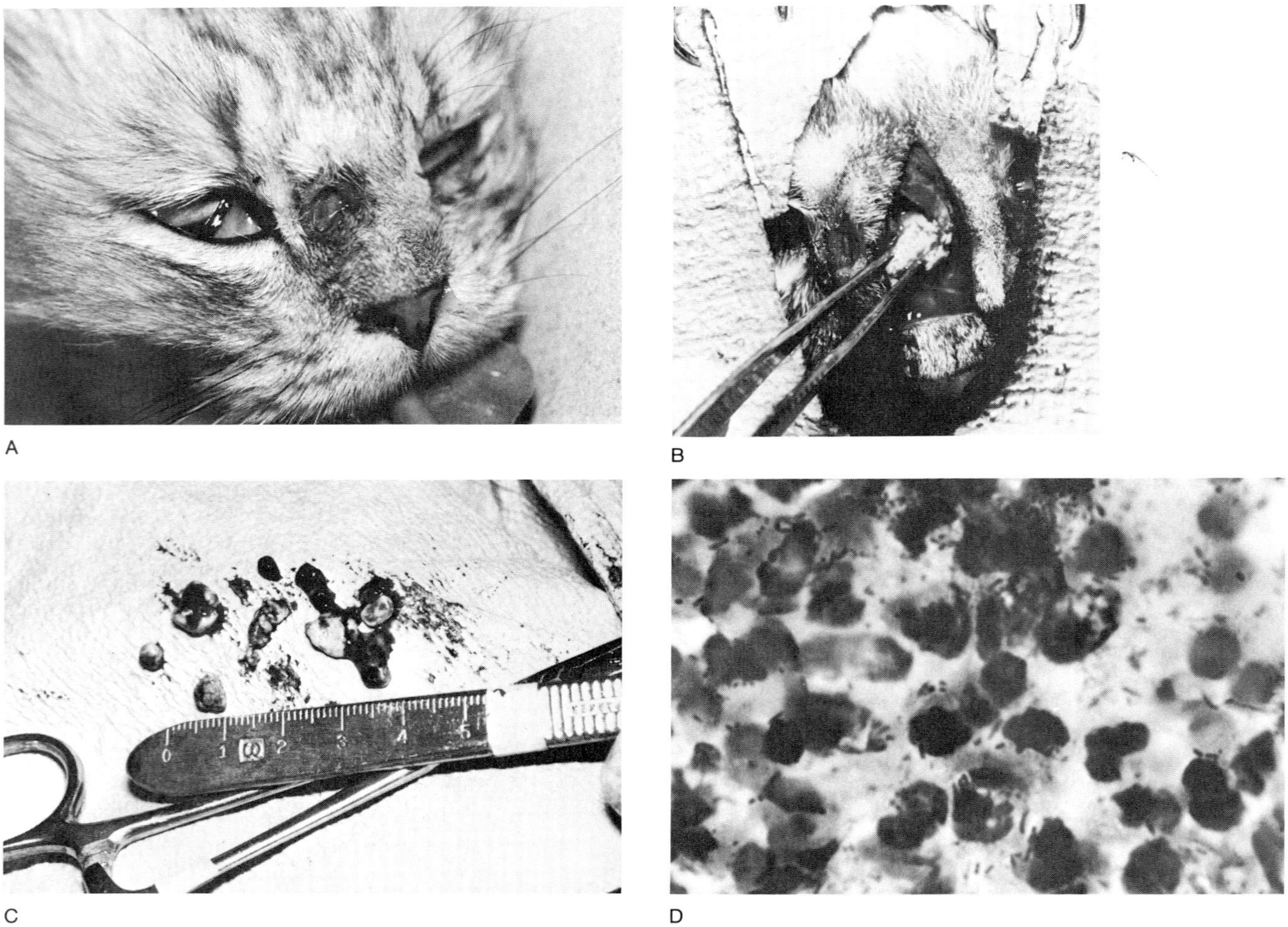

Figure 30–3. (*A*) This cat had a unilateral (left) chronic nasal discharge and a draining fistula through the nasal bones. (*B*) An inflammatory polyp was removed through the fistula in the nasal bones of the same cat as in Figure 30–3*A*. (*C*) Multiple inflammatory polyps were removed (same cat as in Figure 30–3*A*). (*D*) An impression smear made from one of the inflammatory polyps see in Figure 30–3*C* revealed a septic inflammatory pattern. Copious amounts of bacteria were found. The results of a culture were reported as normal nasal flora.

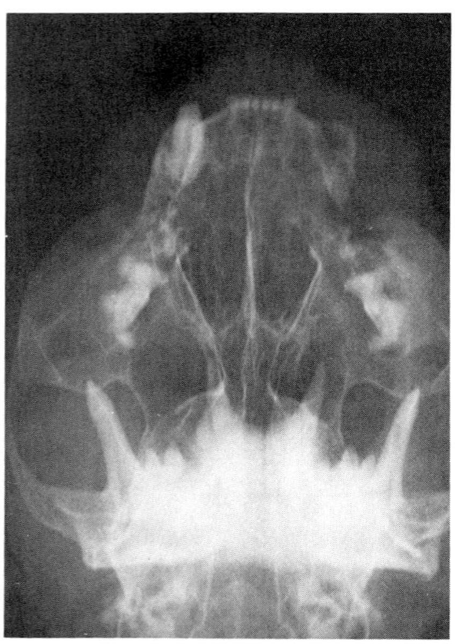

Figure 30–4. Lysis of bone and loss of the left upper canine tooth are typical findings in nasal malignant disease.

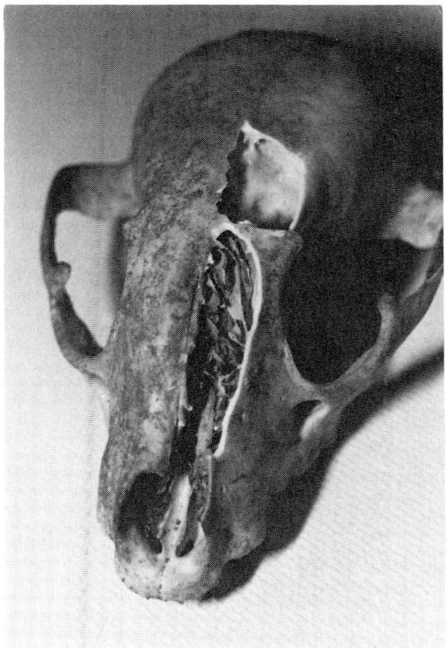

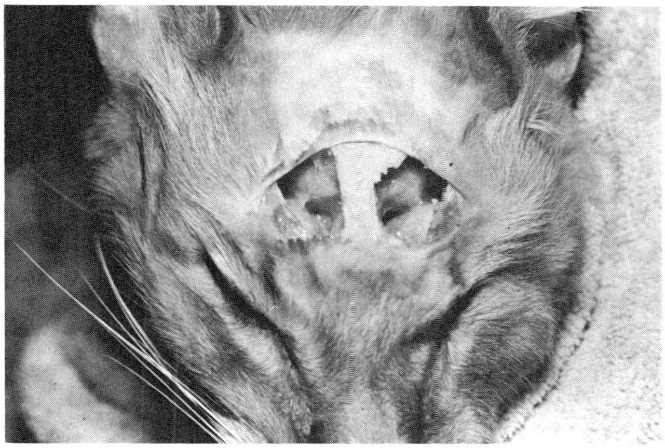

B

A

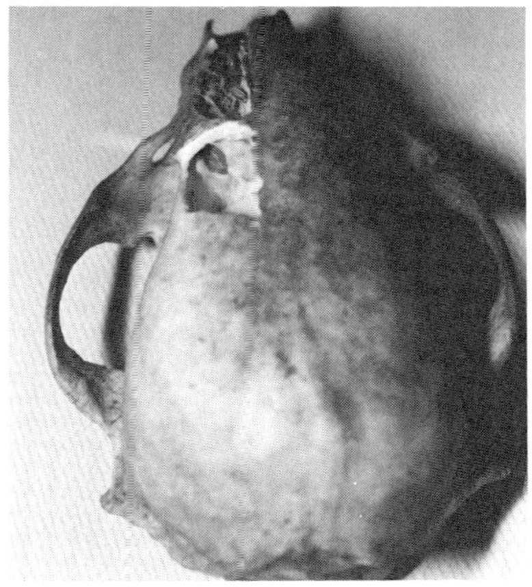

Figure 30–5. (*A*) The left turbinate bones are exposed in this cut-away view of a cat's skull. Note their lacy, intricate anatomic pattern. The left frontal sinus is also opened. (*B*) Both frontal sinuses are opened, allowing their size to be estimated and their anatomic relationship to other cranial structures to be demonstrated. (*C*) When the left frontal sinus is opened, the ostium connecting it to the left nasal cavity can be seen.

C

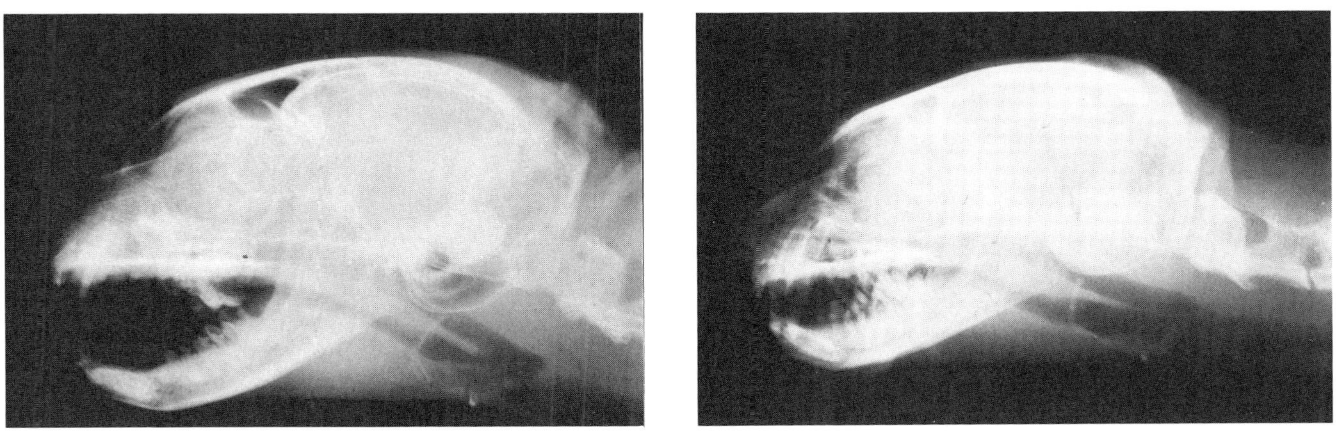

A B

Figure 30–6. (*A*) Normally, the frontal sinuses are air-filled. They may easily be seen on a lateral radiograph. (*B*) When the frontal sinuses are filled with purulent material, they are no longer visible on a lateral radiograph.

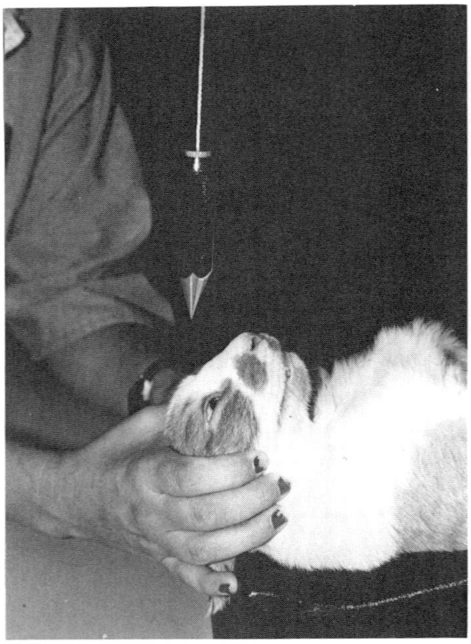

A

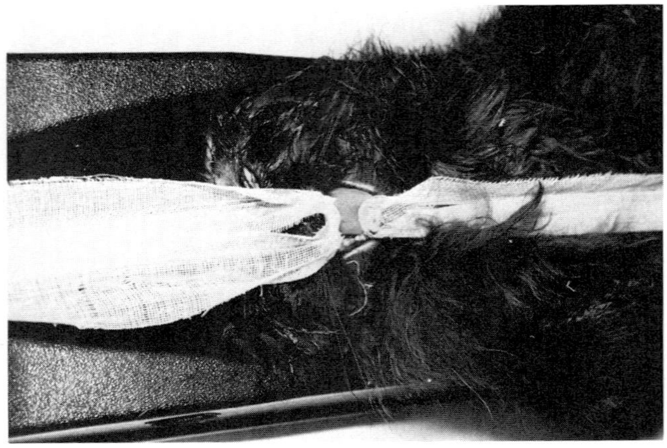

B

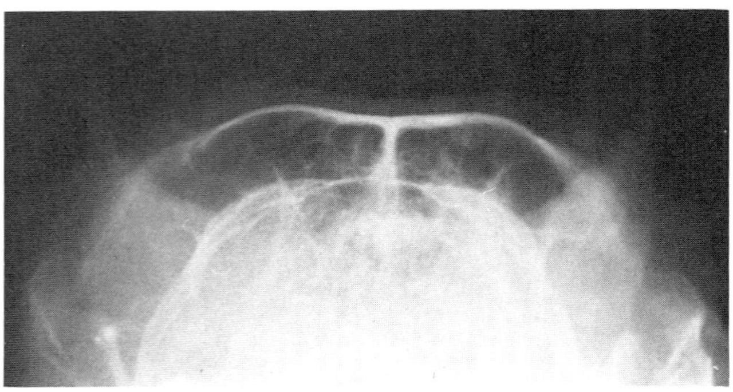

C

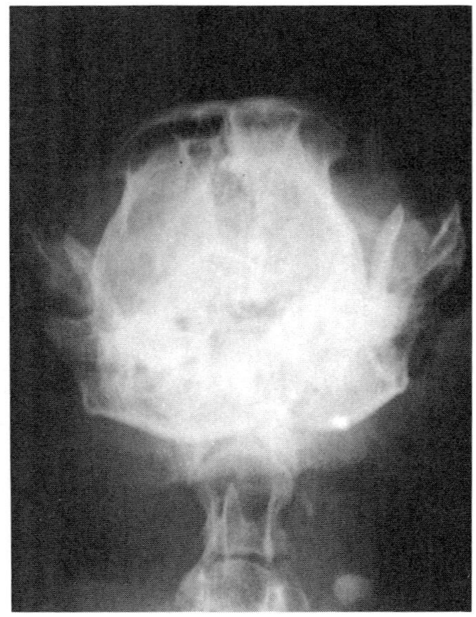

D

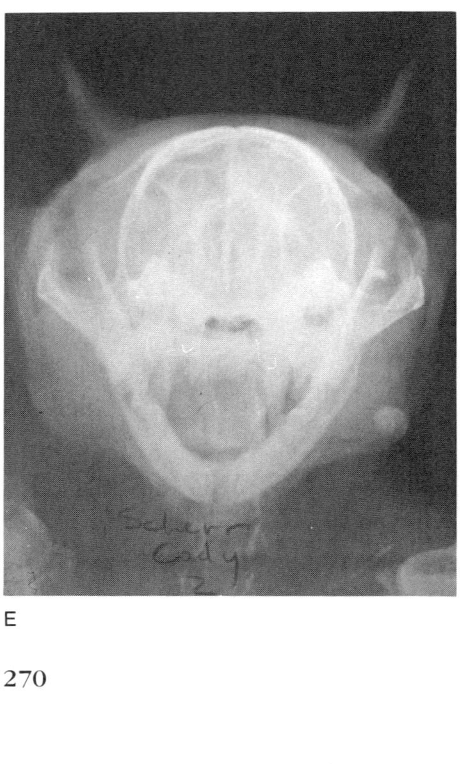

E

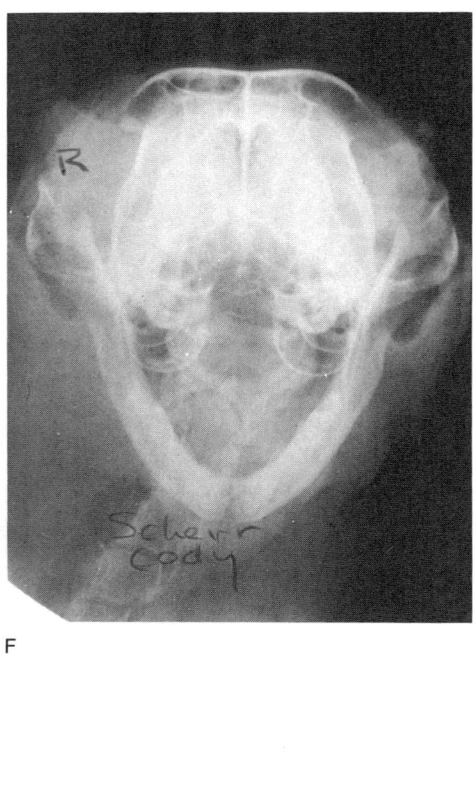

F

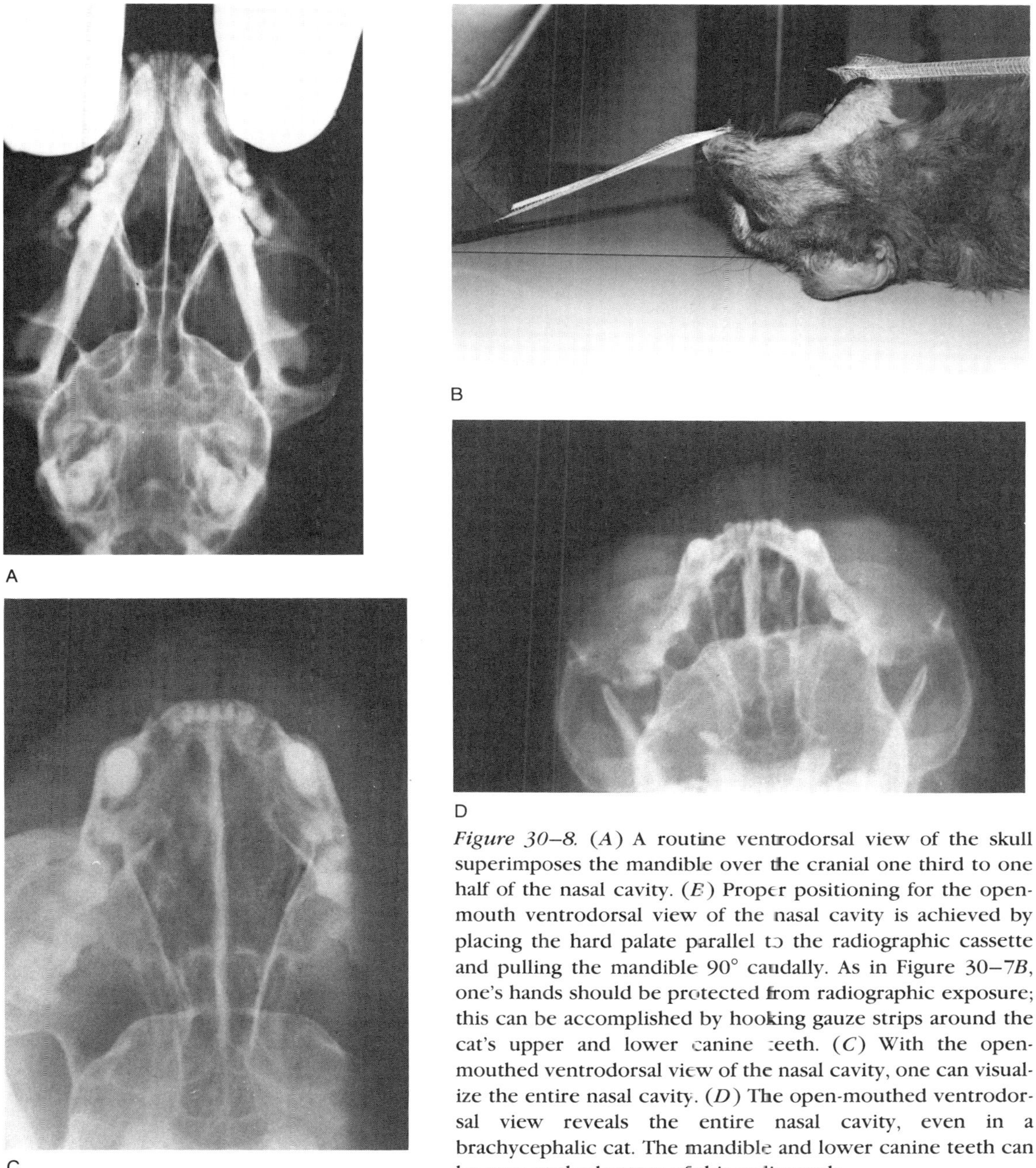

Figure 30–8. (*A*) A routine ventrodorsal view of the skull superimposes the mandible over the cranial one third to one half of the nasal cavity. (*E*) Proper positioning for the open-mouth ventrodorsal view of the nasal cavity is achieved by placing the hard palate parallel to the radiographic cassette and pulling the mandible 90° caudally. As in Figure 30–7*B*, one's hands should be protected from radiographic exposure; this can be accomplished by hooking gauze strips around the cat's upper and lower canine teeth. (*C*) With the open-mouthed ventrodorsal view of the nasal cavity, one can visualize the entire nasal cavity. (*D*) The open-mouthed ventrodorsal view reveals the entire nasal cavity, even in a brachycephalic cat. The mandible and lower canine teeth can be seen at the bottom of this radiograph.

◄ *Figure 30–7.* (*A*) The frontal sinuses should be radiographed using the skyline (rostral-caudal) view. The plumbline simulates the radiographic beam as it passes through the properly positioned frontal sinuses. (*B*) Proper positioning for the skyline view can be achieved without exposing one's hands to radiation by using gauze strips hooked over the canine teeth. This is an anteroposterior view. (*C*) The skyline view reveals that normal frontal sinuses are air-filled structures. (*D*) This cat's left frontal sinus is filled with purulent material (water density). It should be compared with the normal right frontal sinus, which has a gas density. (*E*) If the positioning is slightly incorrect on the skyline view, the frontal sinuses will not be visualized. (*F*) This is the same cat as in Figure 30–7*E*. The frontal sinuses are seen because the positioning is correct.

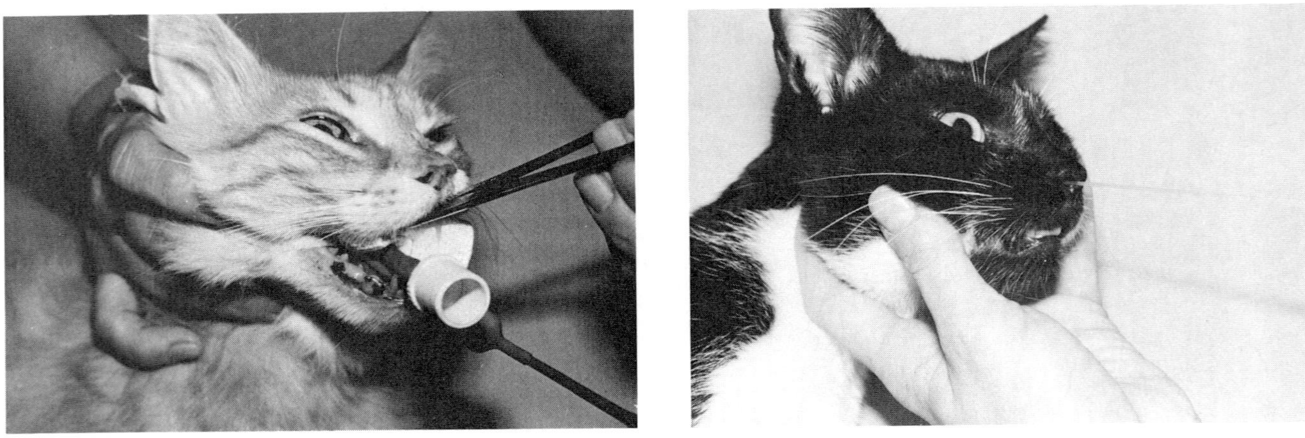

A B

Figure 30–9. (*A*) To perform a nontraumatic, diagnostic nasal flush, one should first administer anesthesia to the cat, after which a cuffed endotracheal tube may be placed. A sterile gauze square is then positioned in the pharynx. (*B*) A 3.5-French catheter is inserted 0.75 to 1 inch into the nasal cavity, and 5 to 10 mL of sterile saline are flushed through the catheter. Nasal material is filtered by the gauze in the pharynx.

square (2″ × 2″) is packed into the pharynx using a pair of small hemostats. Purulent material is removed from the nasal opening. Once this has been done, 5 to 10 mL of sterile saline solution are flushed rapidly through a 3.5-French-open-ended catheter that has been inserted 0.75 to 1.0 inch into the nasal cavity. The gauze square is then removed. The material from the nasal cavity that is present on the gauze square is then used for cytologic and culture studies (Fig. 30–9).

For cytologic examination, the material should be stained with a modified Wright's stain (Diff-Quik, AHS del Caribe, Inc., Aguada, Puerto Rico). The examination will probably reveal a septic inflammatory pattern with numerous bacteria engulfed in neutrophils or macrophages (Fig. 30–10). This is typical for bacterial rhinitis/sinusitis. One should examine the cytolic specimen carefully for tumor cells, *Cryptococcus neoformans* (Fig. 30–11), and *Histoplasma capsulatum.* Because fungi cannot be detected by routine culture techniques, it is especially important that the cytologist check carefully for their presence. Sometimes, *C. neoformans* can be best demonstrated with a Gram's stain.[6]

Serologic Studies

Because of the difficulty in identifying *C. neoformans* in a cytologic preparation, it is advisable to submit a serum sample for the purpose of testing for this organism. However, it must be noted that serologic tests may be positive only in the earlier stages of infection. When the infection is well-established, the patient often becomes seronegative.[7] *H. capsulatum* is much easier to detect by cytologic means, is less often a cause of nasal discharge, and is regionalized; therefore, serum testing for this organism is optional.

Treatment

Proper diagnosis is essential for effective treatment. Most cases of chronic nasal discharge are attributable to bacterial infection. However, if bacteria are not present or are secondary to chronic viral or fungal infections, antibiotic therapy alone will fail.

Proper localization is also essential. Even if aggressive surgical modalities are employed, they must be directed at the correct location. Surgical treatment involving the nasal cavity will not be successful if disease is also present in the frontal sinuses.

Medical Intervention

Medical treatment of nasal discharges of several months' duration is palliative, and produces only temporary relief. Suggested treatment protocols include the long-term use of antibiotics selected on the basis of culture and sensitivity studies, antihistamines (administered orally and intranasally), humidification of the cat's atmospheric environment,

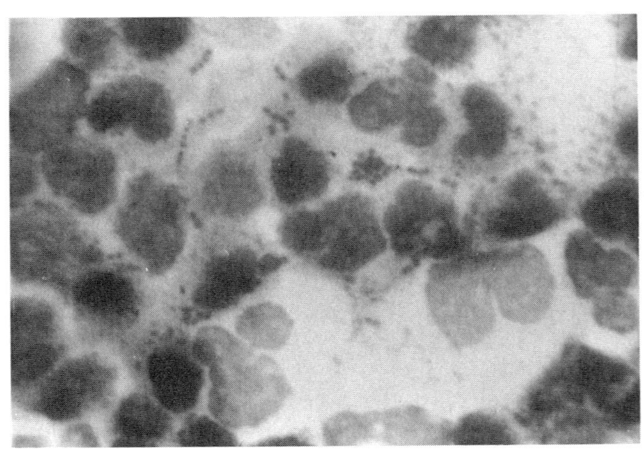

Figure 30–10. Typical chronic bacterial rhinitis/sinusitis has a septic inflammatory pattern. Copious bacteria and neutrophils will be evident.

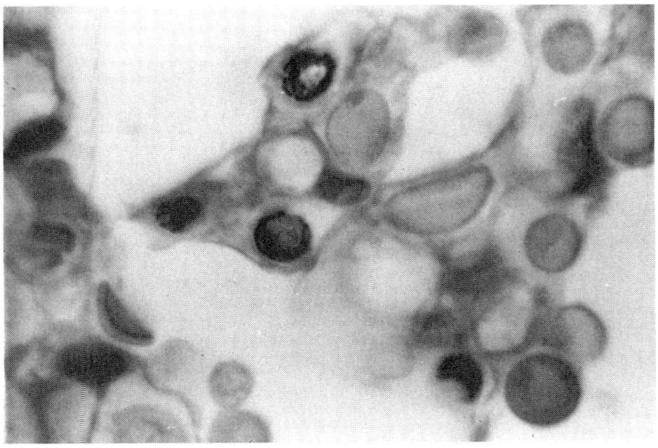

Figure 30–11. **Cryptococcus neoformans may infect the nasal cavity. The prominent, dark-staining organisms are readily visible.**

and nasal flushes using a variety of drugs, including antibiotics, steroids, and DMSO (Domoso Solution).[6,8]

The author has found the use of an injectable penicillin G procaine/penicillin G benzathine combination (Ambi-Pen) to be as effective as oral antibiotics in many cats. The appropriate dose for a 10-lb cat is 2 mL, administered subcutaneously (SC). Most cats will have a good response for 30 to 45 days, at which time the treatment can be repeated. A large percentage of cats will respond better to this than to oral antibiotics, and may be able to be maintained reasonably well for several months or even years.

Surgical Treatment[9]

Medical treatment for chronic bacterial rhinitis is generally unsuccessful because of the anatomic structure of the nasal cavity. The turbinate bones in the maxillary and ethmoid regions of the nasal cavity entrap bacteria and purulent material. If a frontal sinusitis exists, constant drainage of purulent material through the nasal cavity perpetuates the infection.

The frontal sinuses are hollow cavities that become a focus for purulent material. Frontal sinusitis is also resistant to medical therapy because of inadequate antibiotic perfusion and drainage of the infected site. Therefore, surgical drainage and sinus obliteration is often necessary to produce long-term results. The author's preferred procedure is described in Chapter 55.

Because the turbinates become chronically infected with bacteria, the removal of these bones may be necessary. Bilateral turbinectomy does not cause chronic anorexia, as some have feared. The procedure is described in detail in Chapter 55.

Nasal surgical exploration may be indicated for diagnostic and therapeutic purposes, as nasal polyps, foreign bodies, neoplasia, and *C. neoformans* may elude diagnosis or treatment by other methods. The procedure described in Chapter 55 permits access to and removal of most abnormal tissue within the nasal cavity. Material removed from the nasal cavity should then undergo histopathologic examination.

The nasal cavity and frontal sinuses may be surgically treated sequentially. However, the author prefers to perform both procedures simultaneously.

Prognosis

The prognosis for cats with a chronic nasal discharge that is medically treated is poor. Usually, only a temporary response will be elicited upon institution of antibiotic, antihistamine, and/or steroid therapy.

The prognosis for cats whose chronic nasal discharge is treated surgically varies depending on the etiology of the condition. Generally, primary bacterial infections and nasal foreign bodies are associated with a good prognosis. The results of treatment of viral rhinitis and inflammatory polyps are often mixed; some cats improve greatly, whereas others improve only slightly. The prognosis for cats with malignant tumors of the nasal cavity depends upon the tumor type and the use of other treatment modalities, such as radiation therapy and chemotherapy (see Chapter 51).

Conclusions

A proper diagnostic evaluation should be performed in cats with a chronic nasal discharge. This work-up should include radiographs and culture, cytologic, and serologic studies. Because cats with a chronic nasal discharge rarely respond to medical treatment alone for more than a few days or a few weeks, the frontal sinus and/or nasal cavity surgical procedures described in Chapter 55 should be performed for diagnostic and therapeutic purposes.

REFERENCES

1. Ford RB. The Respiratory System. In: Pratt PW, ed. Feline Medicine. Santa Barbara: American Veterinary Publications, 1983:306.
2. Bright RM, Nasal Foreign Bodies, Tumors, and Rhinitis/Sinusitis. In: Bojrab MJ, ed. Pathophysiology in Small Animal Surgery. Philadelphia: Lea & Febiger, 1981:335.
3. Lane JG. Rhinitis and Sinusitis in the Cat. In: Kirk RW, ed. Current Veterinary Therapy VI. Philadelphia: WB Saunders Co., 1977:228.
4. Anderson GI. The treatment of chronic sinusitis in six cats by ethmoid conical curettage and autogenous fat graft sinus ablation. Vet Surg 1987;16:131.
5. Ford RB. Viral upper respiratory infection in cats. Compend Contin Educ Pract Vet 1991;13:593.
6. Vaden S, Ford RB. Medical Management of Upper Respiratory Tract Disease. In: Kirk RW, ed. Current Veterinary Therapy X. Philadelphia: WB Saunders Co., 1989:337.
7. Jacobs RM. Interpretation of Serum Titers. In: Allen DG, ed. Small Animal Medicine. Philadelphia: JB Lippincott, 1991:1019.
8. Kuehn NF, Roudebush P. Nasal Discharge. In: Allen DG, ed. Small Animal Medicine. Philadelphia: JB Lippincott, 1991:383.
9. Norsworthy GD. Surgical treatment of chronic nasal discharge in the cat. Vet Med (in press).

CHAPTER 31

◇ ◇ ◇

Chronic Renal Disease

R. Steve Taylor

Chronic renal failure (CRF) is the insidious, irreversible deterioration of the kidneys resulting in their progressive failure. Diseases involving the kidneys that can lead to progressive renal dysfunction include toxicities, neoplasia, infections, immune-mediated disorders, hereditary disorders, thromboembolic/vascular disorders, anomalies, and traumatic damage. These collectively constitute chronic renal disease (CRD).[1,2] At the time of recognition, CRF has usually resulted in the loss of 75% of the functional capacity of both kidneys.[3] In many instances the original insult is not identifiable. Instead, one only identifies the result, chronic interstitial nephritis (CIN), the progression of which leads to renal failure. In other instances, the disease process or abnormality is identifiable (i.e., glomerulonephritis, amyloidosis, neoplasia, polycystic disease,[4] and renal pseudocysts.[5] Nevertheless, renal failure is often the end result.

The nephrons are responsible for numerous functions that help maintain body homeostasis (Table 31–1).[6] Normally the kidneys have adequate nephrons to exceed the body's requirements; this excess is called renal reserve.[7] When the renal reserve is lost, the remaining nephrons adjust their function to compensate. This adaptive alteration in function requires each remaining nephron to increase its excretory function relative to fluids and electrolytes (*fractional excretion*). This results in the modification and ultimate loss of the ability to conserve body fluids even when conservation is required for maintenance of homeostasis.[8] *Renal insufficiency* begins with loss of renal reserves which occurs when 66% of the functional capacity of both kidneys is gone. *Renal failure* exists when 75% of functional renal capacity is lost (Table 31–2).[9] Decreased renal function occurs when elevated levels of blood urea nitrogen (*BUN*) and creatinine are present (*azotemia*) with inappropriately dilute urine. When the levels of retained metabolic wastes are high, a group of clinical signs (Table 31–3) develop that are collectively known as the *uremic syndrome.*[10,11] The severity of the clinical signs are related to the rate of build up, as well as the actual level of the toxins. *End stage renal failure* occurs when the remaining nephrons, through their maximum adaptive alteration in function, cannot prevent the build up of nitrogenous by-products, such as urea, in the blood (*uremia*)[7] and the uremic syndrome cannot be relieved.

Diagnosis

The diagnosis of CRD is made with the aid of clinical history, physical examination, and appropriate laboratory tests. Many of the clinical signs associated with CRD are nonspecific. The most common presenting signs, inappetence, weight loss, and lethargy, are typical "sick cat signs."[2]

History

The usefulness of the clinical history in the diagnosis of CRD is complicated by many factors. By nature, the cat is secretive, often hiding clinical signs until late in the course of disease. Because the cat is often part of a multi-cat household, signs such as polydipsia, polyuria, and decreased appetite easily go unnoticed. Because many cats with CRD are older, the owners may dismiss or fail to mention early clinical signs because they are thought to be the result of aging. A further complication is the insidious progression of CRD, often leaving the clinician with a poor correlation between the state of the presenting patient and the history of the onset of signs.

The history should identify the reason the cat was presented for examination. This may provide a clue to the cause of the acute decompensation of this chronic state and aid in treatment. The history should also identify any recent changes in the cat's environment or routine that may have exacerbated CRD, the cat's state of health prior to the development of the presenting signs, and the relative adaptation of the cat to the chronic uremic state.

Physical Examination

Through a complete physical examination, the veterinarian is able to assess the patient's overall physical state and to evaluate the status of the individual organ systems. Objective evaluation of weight loss, hydration, and nutritional status is important in the determination of the seriousness of the presenting problems. Individual organ system evaluation may provide the information needed to understand the disease process. For example, the cat with an abnormal gait, a normal neurologic examination, and small kidneys may be hypokalemic.[12] The sudden onset of retinal hemorrhage and

Table 31–1. Renal Contributions to Homeostasis

1. Regulation of volume and concentration of body fluids
2. Maintenance of acid-to-base balance
3. Preservation of the concentration in the body fluids of critical solutes like potassium and phosphorus
4. Excretion of the waste products of metabolism
5. Major source of erythropoietin
6. Regulation of blood pressure

detachment in a cat with small kidneys may be due to high blood pressure secondary to renal disease.[13] Information may be obtained that will identify contributing factors to the apparent sudden onset of clinical signs of chronic renal failure. These factors include cardiovascular dysfunction, anemia, intestinal bleeding, dental problems, and fever. The physical signs of uremia (Table 31–3) may be recognized by the owner as the first signs of disease. For example, halitosis, oral bleeding or ulcers, or muscle tremors may be evident with no history of polyuria or polydipsia (PU/PD).

The cat's kidneys are readily palpable. Generally, one expects to find small, firm, irregular kidneys in CRD. However, in one university study of 74 cats with CRD, small kidneys were found only slightly more often than enlarged kidneys. Kidney size was abnormal on physical examination about 75% of the time.[4] Abnormal renal size, even in asymptomatic cats, should prompt further testing of renal function.

Laboratory Testing

The purposes of laboratory tests are to confirm the suspected diagnosis, determine the extent of the disease, identify causative or contributory factors, and aid in the formulation of a treatment plan. Minimally, these tests should include a complete blood count (CBC), serum chemistries, and a urinalysis. The serum chemistries should include the basic tests in Table 31–4. If anemia is present, a determination of whether it is regenerative or nonregenerative should be made (see Chapter 16). Ideally, laboratory results should be obtained prior to starting treatment. Enough urine should be obtained to permit culture and sensitivity, urine protein-to-creatinine ratio determination and, if needed, electrolyte determinations.

The blood profile in the CRD cat is ever changing as the body attempts to maintain homeostasis. As renal compensatory mechanisms reach their limits or as other disease processes limit these mechanisms, blood values often change rapidly and dramatically. One common example is a cat with isosthenuric urine with otherwise normal preanesthetic blood tests that becomes severely azotemic after a procedure involving anesthesia. Another example is the older cat that becomes uremic after the stress of an office visit

In a suspected CRD cat, the amount of blood that is drawn should only be that required for the needed tests. Most of these animals present with a nonregenerative anemia. Because of this preexisting erythrocyte deficit, serial tests should be used judiciously.

Table 31–2. Progression of Renal Disease

1. Progressive nephron loss up to 65%	Increased fractional clearance of electrolytes
2. Loss of >66% of nephrons in both kidneys	Loss of urine concentrating ability Onset of PU/PD
3. Loss of >75% of nephrons in both kidneys	Elevation of BUN/creatinine with dilute urine

Table 31–3. Clinical Manifestations of Uremia

Gastrointestinal System
- Uremic gastroenteritis
  - Anorexia, diarrhea, vomiting, weight loss*
- Uremic stomatitis
  - Uremic ulcers, fetid breath

Hemolymphatic System
- Anemia*
  - Pallor of mucous membrane, fatigue, listlessness, lethargy, weakness, anorexia
- Hemorrhagic diathesis
  - Hemorrhage from gums, bleeding after venipuncture, blood in stool/vomitus

Cardiovascular/Pulmonary Systems
- Systemic hypertension
- Hyperpnea due to metabolic acidosis
- Pulmonary edema
  - Uremic pneumonitis, overhydration
- Pneumonia due to immunosuppression

Musculoskeletal System
- Renal osteodystrophy*
  - Rubber jaw/loose teeth, skeletal resorption, pathologic fractures
- Soft tissue calcification
- Hypokalemic myopathy

Urinary System
- Altered urinary volume
  - Polyuria, oliguria, anuria (urinary obstr)
- Altered kidney size
  - Small kidneys,* renomegaly
- Distended urinary bladder, (urinary obstruction)

Nervous System and Eyes
- Uremic encephalopathy and neuropathy
  - Dullness, drowsiness, lethargy, tremors, tetany, gait imbalance, myoclonus, seizures, stupor/coma
- Scleral and conjunctival injection
- Hypertensive retinopathy
  - Retinal hemorrhages, dilated/tortuous retinal vessels, hyphema, retinal detachment

Integumentary System
- Impaired wound healing
- Poor haircoat*
  - Reduced skin pliability due to dehydration

*Primarily occurs with chronic renal failure.

Adapted from: Polzin DJ. Spectrum of Clinical and Laboratory Abnormalities in Uremia. In: Kirk RW, ed. Current Veterinary Therapy X. Philadelphia: WB Saunders, 1989:1133.

Table 31–4. Serum Chemistries with Uremic Patients

Alkaline phosphates	Blood urea nitrogen	Potassium
AST or SGOT	Creatinine	Sodium
ALT or SGPT	Total CO_2	Phosphorous
Total bilirubin	Glucose	Calcium
Total Protein	Cholesterol	Chloride
Albumin		Triglycerides

Urinalysis

Interpretation of the urinalysis depends on the state of hydration. A urine sample should be collected at the time of initial blood sampling. Because total protein has been shown to correlate more accurately with the state of hydration than with skin turgor, especially in older cats, a urine specific gravity (USG) with a serum protein level offers a more accurate assessment of renal function than either alone.[14] If urine is obtained after treatment has begun, the influence of fluids on the urinary values must be evaluated. This can be difficult.

Urine gives valuable information concerning the health of the kidneys, as well as provides clues about the underlying pathologic processes. Significant proteinuria (a urine protein-to-urine creatinine ratio above 1) is present with glomerulonephritis, is sometimes present with amyloidosis, and is usually present with pyelonephritis.[15,16,17] If the serum glucose is below the renal threshold (300 mg/dL) and no evidence of a urinary tract infection exists, glucosuria may indicate severe renal dysfunction. This should be confirmed on more than one sample. If a urine sample is obtained by cystocentesis, the presence of white blood cell casts or pyuria (>10 leukocytes/450 × field)[18] indicates urinary tract infection and warrants a urine culture. In suspected polyuric cats that are nonazotemic, multiple urine samples, preferably with documented amounts of water consumption, allow a more accurate evaluation of urine concentration than a single sample.

Many laboratory abnormalities in renal disease may be predicted based on failure of normal renal functions (Table 31–1).[6] The failing kidney loses its ability to conserve body water in times of need.[3] As a result, the kidneys respond inappropriately to the need for water conservation when the patient is dehydrated by producing a less than maximally concentrated urine (USG <1.035).[3,19] Although experimentally cats can concentrate urine even with large functional loss, in naturally developing CRD, the USG tends to be inappropriately low for the cat's state of hydration.[2,20] In those instances in which the appropriateness of the USG is in question, the kidney size of the patient will help in evaluation of CRD.[21] Because the loss of urine concentrating ability precedes the loss of the ability to excrete metabolic waste, an inappropriately low USG will precede azotemia in most cats. This is important in preanesthetic or geriatric evaluations.

Electrolytes

Increased fractional clearance (FC) of electrolytes also precedes azotemia in the progression of renal dysfunction (Table 31–2).[7,22] Creatinine clearance (CrCl) is a crude estimate of glomerular filtration rate (GFR). Because an overall decrease in GFR is present in CRD, a decrease in creatinine clearance is also present in CRD. Endogenous creatinine clearance is used to identify nonazotemic polyuria or early renal insufficiency (see Chapter 22). Because the residual nephrons adapt their function to allow for increased fractional excretion of individual electrolytes to maintain homeostatis, demonstration of increased FC above that expected at a given GFR (or creatinine clearance) may indicate renal adaptation secondary to increased electrolyte levels from one of the following: renal damage, food intake, or parenteral therapy.[23,24]

Many factors influence the serum levels of electrolytes in chronic renal disease. These factors include GFR, dietary intake of the electrolyte, acid base status, other disease processes, and other compensatory or trade off mechanisms used by the body to control electrolyte levels. Thus, it is very difficult to make comments concerning what levels of electrolytes to expect in CRD.

Urea Nitrogen and Creatinine

An elevation in the metabolic waste products, BUN and creatinine, is expected in chronic renal failure. One must decide whether the cause of azotemia is prerenal, renal, postrenal, or a combination (Table 31–5). Prerenal azotemia is caused by decreased vascular perfusion of the kidneys. This decrease in delivery can be the result of a decrease in extracellular fluid volume (vomiting, diarrhea, hypoalbuminemia), shock (cardiogenic, hypovolemic, or circulatory), or cardiovascular dysfunction (congestive heart failure and arrhythmias). Prerenal azotemia should be accompanied by a USG greater than 1.035. In addition, the prerenal azotemic patient responds dramatically to the correction of the underlying cause, resulting in a resolution of azotemia. Postrenal azotemia is associated with urethral obstruction or rupture

Table 31–5. Types of Azotemia

Type	Physiology	Laboratory Findings
Prerenal	Decreased renal blood flow, dehydration, shock, increased blood pressure	Concentrated USG (>1.035) T. Protein and PCV increased
Renal	Decreased functional capacity: permanent or temporary	Dilute USG (<1.035) Increased fractional clearance Exogenous creatinine clearance
Postrenal	Decreased ability to excrete urine from the body Trauma Neoplasia Calculi	Variable USG (1.015–1.060) Peritoneal effusion Elevated creatinine in fluid

Table 31–6. Differentiating Features Among Causes of Uremic Crises

Cause	Renal Osteo-dystrophy	Kidney Size	Potassium (mEq/L)	Urine Specific Gravity	PCV	BUN (mg/dL)	Creatinine	PO_4	History of PU/PD*	History of Anuria/ Oliguria	Urine Sediment
Prerenal azotemia with normal kidneys	NO	Normal	3.5–5.5	>1.030	35–60	60–100	1.8–4.5	4.5–7	NO	YES	Normal casts
Prerenal azotemia complicating chronic renal failure	YES No	SMALL Normal	3.5–6.5	1.007–1.015	25–45	100–250	4.5–15.0	7.5–12	YES	Yes NO	Usually little sediment
Acute renal failure	NO	Large NORMAL	6–9	1.007–1.015	25–45	75–250	5–15	7–20	NO	YES No	May be casts, >RBC, >WBC
Acute renal failure complicating chronic renal failure	YES No	SMALL Normal	6–9	1.007–1.015	25–45	75–250	5–15	7–20	YES	Yes NO	May be casts, >RBC, >WBC
Postrenal azotemia	No	NORMAL Large	4–10	1.015–1.060	35–60	50–300	2–25	6–20	NO	YES	Variable; often >WBC and >RBC
Terminal chronic renal failure	YES	SMALL	4–7.5	1.007–1.015	10–20	150–250	12–20	12–25	YES	NO Yes	Usually little sediment

*PU/PD = polyuria/polydipsia

Notes: Usual or commonly encountered laboratory values are listed. Results outside of these ranges may be found. Answers in capital letters indicates most common situation.

Used with permission from: Low DG, Cowgill LD. Emergency Management of the Acute Uremic Crisis. In: Kirk RW, ed. Current Veterinary Therapy VIII. Philadelphia: WB Saunders, 1983:981.

of ureters, bladder, or urethra. Physical examination and history are usually helpful. If an abdominal effusion due to a disruption of the lower urinary tract is present, the creatinine in the effusion should be higher than the creatinine in the blood.[25]

Azotemia occurs when 75% or greater of the functional capacity of both kidneys is lost. The BUN is affected by diet and any process that induces protein catabolism, including hemorrhage into the gastrointestinal tract, fever, corticosteroid administration, infection, and tetracycline administration.[3,27,28] In states of dehydration and decreased renal blood flow, urea diffuses back across the renal tubules and increases the BUN. Because it is affected by so many nonrenal factors, the BUN may not reflect renal function as efficiently as creatinine. Although there is a correlation between the level of the BUN and creatinine and the degree of renal damage, there is no absolute value above which the patient must be euthanized. The degree of elevation of the BUN and creatinine is not as important as the degree of change after the patient is challenged with fluids (Tables 31–6 and 31–7).

Red Blood Cell Count

Another common laboratory abnormality is the nonregenerative anemia that occurs when erythropoietin production is impaired. The presence of this type of anemia usually indicates the loss of 75% of the functional capacity of both kidneys. The severity of the anemia may be increased by a compromised nutritional state, a decreased number of red blood cell (RBC) precursors in the bone marrow as a result of uremic toxins, and decreased RBC survival time.[29] Correction of the anemic state by transfusion is generally not recommended because the results are temporary and the transfused protein increases renal excretion demands.

Radiology and Ultrasonography

The contribution of survey radiographs in the evaluation of individual CRD patients varies widely. In the emaciated cat, the lack of radiographic contrast rarely reveals any additional information over that obtained by palpation concerning size, shape, or contour. When the renal silhouettes are easily seen, radiographs allow objective information about kidney size. Normal renal size is 2.5 to 3 times the length of the second lumbar vertebra (L_2).[21] Kidneys affected by chronic interstitial nephritis are small. Enlarged kidneys indicate neoplasia, polycystic disease, pseudocysts, and hydronephrosis. Survey radiographs can also contribute by identifying radiopaque renal or cystic calculi.[30] Dystrophic calcification of renal tissue or the lining of the stomach sometimes appears on survey radiographs, suggesting chronicity (see Chapter 14).

Survey thoracic radiographs in CRD patients may also permit early identification of other disease processes. Car-

Table 31–7. Changes in Some Differentiating Features Among Causes of Uremic Crises Following Treatment for Hypotension and Hypovolemia*

	Potassium (mEq/L)	Urine Specific Gravity	PCV	BUN (mg/dL)	Creatinine (mg/dL)	PO_4 (mg/dL)	Increased Urine Volume	Biopsy
Prerenal azotemia with normal kidneys†	3.5–5	1.010–1.035	30–45	10–20	1–1.5	3.5–5	YES	Unnecessary
Prerenal azotemia complicating chronic renal failure	3.5–5	1.007–1.015	20–40	50–120	1.8–6	4.5–10	YES	Unnecessary
Acute renal failure	6–9	1.007–1.015	20–40	75–250	5–15	7–20	NO Yes	Useful
Acute renal failure complicating chronic renal failure	6–9	1.007–1.015	20–40	75–250	5–15	7–20	NO Yes	Useful
Postrenal azotemia†	3.5–5	1.007–1.035	30–45	10–20	1–1.5	3.5–5	YES	Unnecessary
Terminal chronic renal failure	4.5–7.5	1.007–1.015	9–18	100–200	10–20	10–25	Slight increase	Unnecessary

*Compare with pretreatment values in Table 31–6.
†After relief of primary problem plus restoration of fluid balance.
Notes: Usual or commonly encountered laboratory values are listed. Results outside of these ranges may be found. Answers in capital letters indicate most common situation.
Used with permission from: Low DG, Cowgill LD. Emergency Management of the Acute Uremic Crisis. In: Kirk RW, ed. Current Veterinary Therapy VIII. Philadelphia: WB Saunders, 1983:981.

diomyopathy without an auscultable murmur is common. Cats with normal cardiac size but with severely compromised extracellular fluid volume may reveal their cardiomegaly only after rehydration. Early identification of heart disease is important in fluid management and in prognosing suspected CRD patients. Early pleural or peritoneal effusions, not found on physical examination, may be identified or suspected after radiographs and lead to other appropriate diagnostic tests.

Generally in chronic renal failure, excretory urography is not needed or recommended. In the severely azotemic cat or in the cat with a low USG, the quality of the study is often poor and noncontributory. Although a good excretory urogram provides anatomic and pathologic information about the kidneys, ureters, and bladder, it provides only limited information about renal function. Excretory urography is most useful when one or both kidneys are enlarged or when the clinician needs to verify bilateral versus unilateral function. Excretory urography permits the clinician to visualize the structure of the enlarged kidney, which aids in the diagnosis of polycystic kidneys, pseudocystic kidneys, neoplasia, hydronephrosis, and obstructive uropathies secondary to radiolucent renal calculi or blood clots. If contrast urography is warranted, the patient should be well hydrated prior to the procedures (see Chapter 14).[30]

Ultrasonography is a relatively new diagnostic tool in veterinary medicine.[31] Like many diagnostic tools its contribution is directly related to its availability and the skill of the operator. Renal enlargement or large irregularities of the kidneys are readily detected by ultrasonography. Fluid accumulations perirenally, as in renal pseudocysts, or intrarenally, as in polycystic disease or hydronephrosis, are most easily identified with ultrasound. Renal calculi can also be readily identified. Changes in renal parenchymal density may be discrete, as in renal carcinoma, or diffuse, as in some renal lymphosarcomas or feline infectious peritonitis (see Chapter 15).

In many instances, excretory urography and ultrasonography both contribute to the diagnosis of renal disease. These diagnostic aids are especially indicated when the kidneys have an increased size or an abnormal shape. Excretory urography and ultrasonography may allow the clinician to identify the cause before having to proceed to invasive procedures such as renal biopsy. These diagnostic aids may also help in determining not only if, but where, a renal biopsy should be taken. The availability of a qualified ultrasonographer, the degree of renal dysfunction of the cat, the history, and the thoroughness with which the kidneys can be palpated determine which modality is used or needed.[30]

Renal Biopsy

In most cases of chronic renal disease, renal biopsy is not helpful in identifying underlying causes, in establishing a treatment plan, or in determining prognosis. In fact, in many instances the information obtained does not justify the potential risk to the patient. End stage renal failure, regardless of the underlying cause, often appears the same histopathologically. Prior to end stage and in special instances, renal biopsy may help guide the clinician in making recommendations to the owner. Renal biopsy can be justified in mildly azotemic, renomegaly cats with significant proteinuria, in suspected renal neoplasia, and in suspected renal feline infectious peritonitis (FIP). Renal biopsy of patients with significant proteinuria allows differentiation of amyloidosis and glomerulonephritis.[2] Although both disease processes have a guarded prognosis, renal biopsy should help in patient assessment and prognosis. Identification of the type of renal neoplasia provides rational treatment alternatives and prognosis. The identification of granulomatous inflammation in a febrile cat is suggestive of the dry form of FIP in the kidney and the prognosis is poor. However, in some instances, both renal neoplasia and FIP can be identified by aspiration cytology alone.

Treatment

Initial Care

Fluid Therapy for Dehydration

Initial fluid therapy should be administered intravenously (IV) to correct dehydration. Subcutaneous fluids will not be adsorbed in sufficient amounts to meet these requirements.[32] The degree of dehydration should be determined clinically by evaluating skin turgor, moistness of the mucous membranes, capillary refill time (Table 31–8), the hematocrit, total plasma protein level, and plasma electrolyte levels (Table 31–9). The hydration deficit (Table 31–10) is calculated based on an estimate of the percent of dehydration of the cat multiplied by its weight in pounds at the time of the initial examination (dehydration weight).[33]

If the cat does not appear clinically dehydrated but is azotemic, a loading fluid amount equal to 3% to 5% of body weight should be given. This hydration deficit is replaced more rapidly in an azotemic cat than in a cat with normal renal function. It should be replaced in 4 to 6 hours in severe dehydration with normal cardiac function[34] or in 6 to 8 hours in moderate dehydration or with compromised cardiac function.[32] This is done to prevent further renal damage from ischemia and to get a general idea of urinary output.[32]

If after rehydration the cat has not urinated, does not have a full bladder, or is not producing at least 1 to 2 mL/kg/hr of urine, either the fluid deficit replacement was un-

Table 31–8. Clinical Signs of Dehydration

Dehydration (%)	Clinical Signs
<5	Not detectable
5–6	Subtle loss of elasticity of skin
6–8	Definite delay in return of skin to normal position Slight prolongation of capillary refill time Eyes possibly sunken in orbits Possibly dry mucous membranes
10–12	Tented skin stands in place Definitive prolongation of capillary refill time Eyes sunken in orbits Dry mucous membranes Possibly signs of shock (tachycardia, cool extremities, rapid and weak pulses)
12–15	Definite signs of shock Death imminent

Adapted from: Cornelius LM. Fluid Therapy in Small Animal Practice. J Am Vet Med Assoc 1980;176:110.

Table 31–9. Interpretation of Hematocrit and Plasma Protein Values

PCV (%)	Total Plasma Protein (gm/dL)	Interpretation
Increased	Increased	Dehydration
Increased	Normal or decreased	Splenic contraction Polycythemia Dehydration with pre-existing hypoproteinemia
Normal	Increased	Normal hydration with hyperproteinemia Anemia with dehydration
Decreased	Increased	Anemia with dehydration Anemia with preexisting hyperproteinemia
Decreased	Normal	Non-blood loss anemia with normal hydration
Normal	Normal	Normal hydration Dehydration with pre-existing anemia and hypoproteinemia Acute hemorrhage Dehydration with secondary compartment shift
Decreased	Decreased	Blood loss Anemia with hypoproteinemia Overhydration

Used with permission from: Muir WW, DiBartola SP. Fluid therapy. In: Kirk RW, ed. Current Veterinary Therapy VIII. Philadelphia: WB Saunders, 1983:28.

Table 31–10. Components of Fluid Therapy

1. Hydration deficit (replacement requirement)
   Body weight (lb) × % dehydration as a decimal × 500* = deficit in milliliters
2. Maintenance requirement (18–30 mL/lb/day)
   Sensible losses (urine output): 12–20 mL/lb/day
   Insensible losses (fecal, cutaneous, respiratory): 6–10 mL/lb/day
3. Contemporary (ongoing) losses (e.g., vomition, diarrhea polyuria)

*500 mL fluid = 1 lb body weight.

Used with permission from: Muir WW, DiBartola SP. Fluid Therapy. In: Kirk RW, ed. Current Veterinary Therapy VIII. Philadelphia: WB Saunders, 1983:28.

Table 31–11. Biochemical Similarities and Differences in Patients with Polyuric and Oliguric Primary Renal Failure

Factor	Polyuria	Oliguria
Urine SG	1.007 to 1.034	1.007 to 1.034
Urea nitrogen (serum)	Increased	Increased
Creatinine (serum)	Increased	Increased
Sodium (serum)	Usually normal	Variable
Sodium (total body)	Variable	Variable
Potassium (serum)	Usually normal	Increased
pH (blood)	Normal to decreased	Marked decrease
Phosphorus (serum)	Usually increased	Usually increased
Calcium (serum)	Usually normal to decreased*†	Usually normal to decreased*†

*Unless renal failure is caued by hypercalcemia.

†Occasionally hypercalcemia occurs in patients as a sequela to primary renal failure.

From: Osborne CA, Finco DR, Low DG. Pathophysiology of Renal Diseases, Renal Failure, and Uremia. In: Ettinger SJ, ed. Textbook of Veterinary Internal Medicine, 2nd ed. Philadelphia: WB Saunders, 1983:1760.

derestimated (physiologic oliguria) or the renal damage is severe (pathologic oliguria). With physiologic oliguria, adequate fluid replacement results in good urinary output. If the urinary output is adequate after rehydration, the cat is in polyuric renal failure and diuresis is begun. If urinary output is inadequate, the cat is in oliguric renal failure and diuresis is not begun until urinary output is adequate (Table 31–11), although this may not occur in some cats.[35]

The cat's weight after rehydration (base weight) should be recorded and used for comparison when re-evaluating fluid therapy, regardless of which type of renal failure is present. If the potassium levels are high, the fluid of choice for replacement therapy is normal saline. Otherwise the fluid of choice is lactated Ringer's solution (LRS).

Oliguric Renal Failure

Oliguric renal failure or pathologic oliguria of primary renal origin occurs during the early stages of ARF and in the terminal stages of CRF. It is characterized by a small urine volume of low specific gravity following rehydration. Postrenal causes can result in apparent oliguria in which urine is lost outside the urinary system.[25] Diagnosis is made with the aid of history and repeated physical examinations as discussed earlier.

Treatment of oliguric CRF consists of stimulating urinary output through the use of diuretics, administering fluids to replace continued fluid losses and urinary output, and correcting hyperkalemia and acidemia.

Diuretics are given to stimulate urinary output, which facilitates the excretion of excessive electrolytes, acids, and renal toxins. Osmotic (hypertonic dextrose and mannitol) and loop (furosemide) diuretics are both advocated for pathologic oliguria after patient rehydration.[32] Hypertonic dextrose (10% or 20%) is often preferred to mannitol and furosemide because it also provides calories to the catabolic patient, is inexpensive, and is readily detectable in the urine when its effects begin.[35] Guidelines for the use of dextrose are included in the section on intense diuresis. Mannitol (0.25 to 0.5 g/lb of body weight) given intravenously over 15 to 20 minutes will, if effective, increase urine flow within 1 hour. Mannitol is contraindicated in oliguric cats that are overhydrated. Furosemide (1 to 2 mg/lb of body weight given as an intravenous bolus) is considered by some as the initial diuretic of choice in oliguric renal failure. Furosemide should increase urine output within 30 minutes. If it does not, the dose should be doubled, and then tripled at hourly intervals. One author suggests that doses above 2 mg/lb may not be any more effective.[32] If diuretics fail to correct pathologic oliguria, continued administration is usually to no avail and signals a terminal state.

Fluid administration after rehydration must be undertaken knowing that iatrogenic volume overload can occur if excessive fluid is given or if it is given too rapidly. After rehydration, fluid therapy in the oliguric patient should consist of the replacement of fluids from insensible losses (10 mL/lb divided over 24 hours, given in 6 hour increments), plus estimated ongoing gastrointestinal losses (adjusted and given every 6 hours) and urinary output (adjusted and given every 6 hours).[34] Once urinary output is above 1 mL/lb/hr, the cat is treated as a polyuric CRF patient. If diuresis is not established within 24 hours, the condition is usually terminal.

Potassium levels and acidosis must be monitored in oliguria. Treatment of severe hyperkalemia (serum potassium >8 mEq/L with electrocardiographic changes) should consist of either intravenous calcium gluconate (0.25 mg/lb), bicarbonate (0.25 to 0.5 mEq/lb) or insulin/dextrose (1 unit of regular insulin/4 mL of 50% glucose with a total dose of 4 units in an acute crisis). Treatment of moderate hyperkalemia and acidosis should be undertaken cautiously with fluids and bicarbonate.

Diuresis

Types and Indications

When hydration is complete and adequate urinary output is established, treatment must concentrate on increased excretion of uremic toxins by maintaining adequate renal blood flow and by enhancing urine flow. This is done through diuresis with either parenteral fluids alone (fluid diuresis) or with diuretics being added to the amounts of fluids needed for maintenance and ongoing losses (intense diuresis). Intense diuresis (ID) permits uremic toxins to be removed more rapidly.[36]

The method of diuresis used will depend on a number of factors including:

1. The severity and stability of the patient's condition
2. Urinary output
3. Adequacy of the patient's response to fluid therapy alone
4. Presence and type of complicating conditions
5. Available time commitment of the veterinarian
6. Level of training of the staff.

Fluid therapy exceeding rehydration and replacement of ongoing losses and maintenance will induce a fluid diuresis in the polyuric CRD cat, but the diuresis may take hours to begin.[36] If time is not critical, fluid diuresis (FD) should be adequate to manage a uremic crisis. In CRD cats that have severe uremic signs (altered mentation, hypothermia below 99°F, severe emaciation), that are marginally stable, and in which survival is in question, ID should be used. If an oliguric cat resumes normal urine production following rehydration, it should be treated with ID. ID should also be considered if correction of dehydration does not reduce the BUN significantly within 24 hours and moderate the signs of uremia within 2 days.[34]

Patients with heart disease or hypertension may have difficulty handling the large volume expansion of the extra cellular fluid compartment associated with ID. In these patients, FD administered over a longer period may be safer as long as patient monitoring occurs frequently. Properly performed ID requires greater time commitment by the veterinarian and a staff whose level of training is more advanced than that required for FD.

Monitoring

Diuresis monitoring requires either direct measurement of urinary output through an indwelling urinary catheter and closed collecting system (Fig. 31–1) or indirect measurement through reassessment of the state of hydration. The latter is achieved by comparison of current weight versus base weight, clinical assessment, and laboratory assessment. The level of monitoring depends on the patient's condition and availability of intensive care monitoring. If ID is needed or if oliguria is present or suspected after rehydration, an indwelling urinary catheter and collecting system is used; otherwise, an indirect measurement is used. Problems with urinary catheterization include initial placement, infection, maintenance of patency and flow, and patient tolerance. Although the catheter is placed as aseptically as possible, this author administers antibiotics as well. (Other authorities avoid this practice due to possibility of the emergence of resistant bacteria.) The tip of the catheter is also cultured after removal from the patient. The catheter is usually left in place only during ID. If a catheter cannot be placed or maintained, indirect measurements should be used along with monitoring of central venous pressure, especially in critical patients (cardiac patients, oliguric patients).[34]

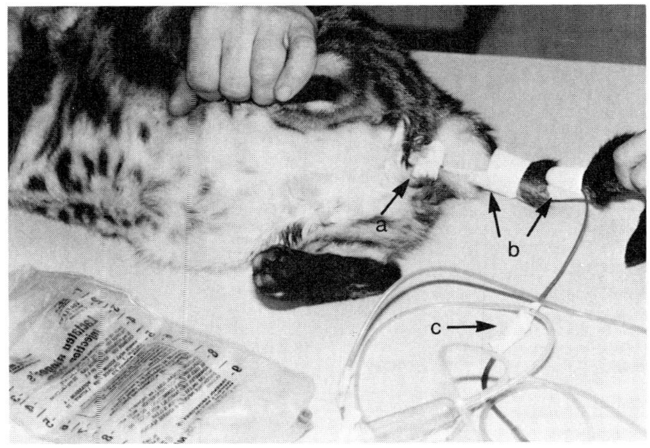

Figure 31–1. **A closed urinary collecting system consists of a 3.5- or 5-French, soft urinary catheter (Feeding Tube and Urethral Catheter [Monoject, Division of Sherwood Medical, St. Louis, MO]), an IV set (with the roller value removed), and an empty IV fluid bag. The catheter is passed into the bladder, sutured to the skin with a tape butterfly to the dorsal prepuce (*a*), taped to the tail in two places (*b*), and attached to the IV set (*c*). When the cat is placed in a cage, the bag should be placed beneath the cat's level so that gravity will assist fluid flow. Some cats tolerate this system well; others need an Elizabethan collar.**

Fluid Diuresis

After correction of dehydration, fluid diuresis (without diuretics) must provide enough fluid to include maintenance requirements (approximately 30 mL/lb/day) and an estimate of continued fluid losses. The fluid losses must include those associated with vomiting, diarrhea, and urinary loss.[33] An additional fluid volume of 45 to 90 mL/lb/day should be added to the fluid calculation used to meet maintenance requirements and ongoing loss. This additional volume promotes diuresis. The total volume is given over the next 24 hours.[32] Prior to further fluid therapy, the patient's hydration is reassessed by physical examination criteria (Table 31–8), comparison with the base weight, and evaluation of the packed cell volume (PCV) and total protein.

Intense Diuresis

Intense diuresis is begun only after the cat has been rehydrated and urinary output is deemed adequate. A urinary catheter is placed; the amount of fluid needed for rehydration is administered; then the bladder is emptied. A 20% dextrose solution is administered intravenously to a total dose of 10 to 30 mL/lb. Give at a rate of 2 mL/min for 10 to 15 minutes then decrease the rate 1 mL/min. Newly formed urine is tested for glucose with a urinary dipstick. Glucosuria develops within minutes in polyuric cats; in severely oliguric cats it does not. By the time one-half of the glucose has been administered, glucosuria should occur. If it does not or if urine production does not reach the rate of 1 to 4 mL/min by the time one-half of the glucose is given, the administration should be stopped to prevent overhydration.

If urine production is not adequate, the cat should be re-evaluated for oliguria. If urine production is adequate, the entire calculated amount of the dextrose solution should be given.

After initial rehydration and an adequate response to osmotic (dextrose) diuresis, the cat is loaded with LRS equal to 3% to 5% of the body weight over a 1-hour period followed by the administration of dextrose again. (One pound of body weight equals 500 mL of fluid.) This cycle of fluid loading followed by osmotic (dextrose) diuresis is usually repeated 2 to 3 times every 24 hours.[36]

Nutritional Support

Because the cat experiences less nausea and vomiting than the dog, forced alimentation is feasible in many CRF patients as early as Day 2 of treatment. The strength gained from a balanced diet can be a tremendous asset to recovery. Furthermore, the likelihood of hypokalemia is minimized. The use of an orogastric tube and a blenderized, low protein feline diet should be considered (see Chapter 5).

Patient Monitoring

Regardless of the diuresis method used, after the initial 24 hours, the cat should be reweighed, the clinical status reassessed, and the blood checked for azotemia. Weight loss from the weight after hydration (base weight) is because the urine production is greater than fluid administration and requires further rehydration of the patient. Weight gain from the base weight indicates that fluid administration has exceeded urinary output and requires decreasing the amount of fluid. In addition, furosemide should be administered or the dose increased.[35]

If the patient's clinical status declines in any way, serum electrolytes, PCV, and serum protein levels should be rechecked. Diuresis without intake of potassium can lead to hypokalemia and severe weakness. A decrease in the hematocrit because of blood loss or secondary to dilution may alter the cat's clinical state. Marginal serum protein values may become very low with rehydration and affect tissue perfusion dynamics. Re-evaluating cardiac function may also be warranted. If BUN and creatinine values do not decline after 1 to 2 days of ID, the cat is probably in terminal renal failure.[35]

The kidneys' ability to respond to diuresis is finite because of the overall decrease in GFR and the diminished number of functional nephrons. The kidneys have an end point for the amount of dilute urine that they are able to produce late in the course of CRD. At this point, further diuresis will not continue to reduce the azotemia.[8] This level of maximal reduction in azotemia reflects the amount of renal function remaining and is usually reached within 2 to 4 days from the beginning of diuresis. If more fluid is given parenterally than can be excreted, overhydration results.[37] This constitutes a serious therapeutic error that is extremely difficult to correct because the body's main eliminators of fluid, the kidneys, are severely compromised. Therefore, until the cat is drinking water, fluid administration should not exceed urinary output, whether it is measured directly or indirectly.

Hypokalemia is one of the most common problems encountered in diuresis of anorectic cats. The greater the amount of replacement fluids given, the greater the risk of inducing hypokalemia. The amount of potassium in LRS approximates normal serum levels but is low relative to the amount of potassium lost in the urine during diuresis. Hypokalemia may result in generalized muscle weakness, cervical ventroflexion, and muscle tenderness. Potassium should be supplemented to parenteral fluids based on the patient's needs (see Chapter 28).

In severely ill patients, the acid-to-base status should always be checked. While renal failure often results in metabolic acidosis, excessive loss of hydrogen, potassium, and chloride ions through vomiting or adequate extrarenal buffering of hydrogen may result in a normal to nearly normal acid-to-base status.[35] The bicarbonate deficit associated with metabolic acidosis should only be assessed after the cat is rehydrated, except in cases of severe acidosis. As a general rule, unless the serum bicarbonate level is 18 mEq or lower, no therapy is recommended. Some cats will have enough renal function left to regulate acid-to-base balance if they are provided adequate hydration and appropriate electrolytes. Overly aggressive bicarbonate administration can lead to metabolic alkalosis.

If bicarbonate replacement is warranted, the deficit is calculated as follows:

$$HCO_3 \text{ deficit (mEq)} = \text{body wt (kg)} \times 0.5 \times (25 - \text{serum } HCO_3)$$

Half of the calculated amount is infused over the first 4 hours, and the patient is re-evaluated with blood values. If blood values are not available, the rest of the calculated dose should be given over the next 24 hours.[38] Other formulas found in the literature use other coefficients (0.4 or 0.3); these allow the bicarbonate to be given more rapidly (one-half over 1 hour, then the remainder over the next 6 hours).[37] Except in extreme circumstances, a bolus of bicarbonate is not necessary or recommended. How accurately and frequently the clinician can monitor the acid-to-base status will determine (or limit) the aggressiveness of bicarbonate therapy.

Long-Term Medical Management

Because chronic renal disease is irreversible and progressive, the goals of therapy must include the following: slowing disease progression, decreasing or minimizing signs of uremia, maintaining a positive nutritional state, and minimizing stress. Each of these goals is important because the patient's own compensatory mechanisms are already operating at maximum limits.

Slowing Disease Progression

Slowing the progression of the disease must include the following: maintaining adequate renal perfusion, decreasing dietary protein, decreasing dietary phosphorus, preventing infections, and preventing nephrotoxin exposure.[29]

Because of its high-energy production and consumption requirements, the renal tubular cells are especially susceptible to the effects of ischemia or decreased renal perfusion. Causes of renal hypoperfusion must be corrected or managed quickly to ensure that renal damage is minimized. Anticipation of circumstances that could result in renal hypoperfusion is the first step in prevention of ischemia.[37] Obligatory loss of water in the urine of CRD cats predisposes them to the rapid development of dehydration if water intake does not replace this urinary loss. Any condition that limits or prevents adequate water intake requires parenteral fluid support.

At the other extreme, hyperperfusion and high-protein diets can cause hyperfiltration resulting in glomerular damage and progression of renal failure. The frequency of hypertension in CRD cats is unknown. One retrospective study found that 3% of CRD cats had hypertension.[1] Two other studies found the incidence to be 65% to 69% in CRD cats.[39,40] Blood pressure measurement depends on the type of equipment used and the experience of the operator. The cost of the equipment and the difficulty in quality control of the measurements prevent most primary care veterinarians from using blood pressure in their management of the CRD cat. In the future, blood pressure determinations may influence the management of renal disease and may help in the early detection of renal failure.

The level of protein in the diet and its relationship to the progressive deterioration of renal function is controversial,[46,47] and research concerning feline renal function and protein levels is incomplete. Recommendations concerning appropriate dietary protein levels for cats are based on data obtained using experimental models of renal failure, not naturally occurring disease models.

Cats are unique in that they have higher protein requirements than many other species. This higher protein need is because of a unique requirement for one or more essential amino acids and because a significant amount of dietary protein is used as a caloric source. Formulating a diet for the uremic cat requires limiting potentially toxic waste products of protein metabolism. Ideally, the amount of protein offered to the CRD patient should be as high as possible, while maintaining the BUN below 60 mg/dL. Currently recommendations are that diets for the CRD cat contain a minimum of 3.3 to 3.8 g/kg (1.5 to 1.7 g/lb) of body weight per day of high quality natural protein. This is about 20% of the total dietary calories needed and is equivalent to approximately 8% protein for canned food and 20% to 22% protein for dry food.

Reducing dietary phosphorus is important in treating the CRD cat and in slowing the progression of the renal failure.[29,41,42] Most of the phosphorus in the diet is found in the protein component, and as a result, protein restriction also restricts phosphorus intake. Phosphorus should be restricted if the fractional clearance exceeds 30%. Phosphate binders, agents that bind phosphorus in the food to prevent absorption from the intestinal tract, have not been shown to consistently reduce serum phosphorus levels in the cat.[42] These binders add to the palatability problem of the protein restricted diet; they cause constipation in some cats. If phosphate binders are used, best results have been achieved mixing the aluminum carbonate gel in powder form with the food.[29] The contents of Basaljel capsules may be mixed with food at an initial dose of 15 to 45 mg/lb/day. The dosage should be regulated based on serum phosphorus levels.

Other considerations in slowing the progression of renal failure include early identification of urinary tract infections and prevention of exposure to nephrotoxins, including therapeutic drugs. CRD cats that have a history of recurring urinary tract infections should have a urinalysis performed at intervals appropriate to the incidence of the problem or at least every 3 months. Conditions that increase the likelihood of a urinary tract infection, such as urethral catheterization or a perineal urethrostomy, should prompt a urinalysis and, if appropriate, antibiotics.

Controlling the Signs of Uremia

The next goal in long-term management of the chronic renal failure patient is to decrease or minimize the signs of uremia. This requires reducing protein and phosphorus in the diet, maintaining adequate hydration, limiting the severity of the associated anemia, reducing nausea and vomiting, and limiting the severity of the acidemia.

The nonregenerative anemia associated with chronic renal failure can contribute subtly or dramatically to the overall manifestations of the uremic syndrome. The causes of the anemia are multiple, but lack of erythropoietin production is generally agreed to be the most significant contributor. In the cat, erythropoietin is produced mainly in the kidneys and to a lesser degree from the carotid bodies. With diminished renal tissue in chronic renal disease, there is a decreased production of erythropoietin. Ideally, replacing the erythropoietin would substantially improve the anemia.[29]

A formulated recombinant erythropoietin product has been developed for humans by using specific segments of human DNA that are responsible for coding of endogenous erythropoietin to cause cultured mammalian cells to manufacture a replica hormone, recombinant human erythropoietin (r-HuEPO) Clinical trials in humans have demonstrated that r-HuEPO reverses the anemia and normalizes the hematocrit, hemoglobin concentration, and red blood cell count. Concomitant with the hematologic benefits, patients report improvements in their sense of well-being, appetite, strength, and exercise capacity.

This r-HuEPO is also used in uremic cats.[43] Hematologic benefits have included dramatic increases in red blood cell count, hemoglobin concentration, and hematocrit. The hematocrit often normalized in most patients within 3 to 4 weeks. Clinical improvement in well-being, appetite, and water consumption were noted. The correction or dramatic improvement of many of the nonspecific manifestations of uremia, such as inappetence, weakness, fatigue, lethargy, and social apathy, document the significance of anemia in the uremic cat. The negative side of r-HuEPO includes local and systemic allergic reactions (2 of 17 dogs and cats),[43] improvement followed by a progressive anemia associated with anti-r-HuEPO antibodies (7 of 17% to 41% uremic dogs and cats),[43] and expense. The benefits of treatment must always be weighed against the potential risk. When the cat's anemia is profound and associated with overt clinical signs, the risks of r-HuEPO treatment are acceptable and the results beneficial. In patients with mild anemia, a more cautious approach is in order. The veterinarian must also re-

Table 31–12. Preliminary Recommendations for the Use of r-HUEPO (Epogen) in the Cat[43]

Initial Dosage (100 U/kg)

Subcutaneous injection
Administer 3 times/week
Maintain the starting dosage until a target hematocrit of 30–40% is achieved (goal)

Adequate Response (goal achieved)

Maintenance dosage: 100 U/kg 2 times/week
If cat develops polycythemia on the maintenance dosage, reduce to once weekly.
If anemia redevelops with either once or twice weekly injections:
- Reinstitute initial dosage and interval.
- If inadequate control cannot be maintained, increase the dosage progressively by increments of 25–50 U/kg with a dosage interval of 1–3 times weekly.
  - The dosage that achieves the target hematocrit is maintained.
  - Generally, doses of 75–100 U/kg 2–3 times weekly are sufficient.

Inadequate Response (goal not achieved in 8–12 weeks)

Evaluate the cat for:
- Iron deficiency (most cats need iron supplementation)
- External blood loss
- Hemolytic disease
- Neoplasia
- Inflammatory disease

If the evaluation for the above diseases is negative:
- Increase the dosage in 50 U/kg increments, but do not change any more often than every 2–3 weeks because of lag time from dosage change to hematocrit change.
- If polycythemia develops, treatment is temporarily stopped until the goal is attained again.

Monitoring the Cat

Hematocrit is monitored weekly until goal is reached and an appropriate dosage regimen has been determined to maintain a stable hematocrit for at least 4 weeks.
Once the goal is reached, a CBC, serum iron, and total iron binding capacity are performed monthly.

Treatment is Stopped if:

An increase in blood pressure occurs
Pain, inflammation, or discoloration develops at the injection sites
A refractory anemia develops despite an adequate dosage of r-HUEPO and normal iron metabolism
- May indicate the development of anti-r-HUEPO antibodies
- An increase in the bone marrow myeloid-to-erythroid ratio is a sensitive monitor of antibody development and may precede decreases in the hematocrit.

member that r-HuEPO is neither licensed for use in the cat nor does the manufacturer endorse its administration to cats. The protocol and dosages are listed in Table 31–12.[43]

Anabolic steroids are advocated in uremic animals to correct anemia. Subjective clinical evaluation of the therapeutic efficacy of anabolic steroids in dogs and cats with renal failure is favorable; however, documentation of efficacy is limited.[44] Some anabolic steroids appear to be more efficacious than others; however, clinical trials in the cat are lacking.[29] If anabolic steroids are used, the choices include nandrolone decanoate (Deca-Durabolin) (0.45 mg/lb every 7 days IM), stanozolol (Winstrol-V) (1 mg/cat b.i.d. PO), oxymethalone (Anadrol-50), testosterone proprionate, and testosterone enanthate.

Vomiting in the uremic CRD cat is not as common a clinical problem as in other species. Studies have shown an incidence of 27.4% and 9.9%.[1,2] Uremia can cause vomiting either through toxic stimulation of the chemoreceptor trigger zone or through local gastric irritation associated with increased gastrin and hydrochloric acid levels. To counteract the effect of uremic toxins on the central nervous system, drugs such as phenothiazine tranquilizers like acetylpromazine (PromAce), 0.1 mg/kg, intramuscularly or orally every 12 hours, or metoclopramide (Reglan), 0.1 to 0.3 mg/kg, intramuscularly or orally every 12 hours may be needed.[42] Metoclopramide is considered the drug of choice for vomiting associated with renal failure. Uremic gastritis can be treated with H_2 antagonists such as cimetidine (Tagamet) (doses reported as 2 mg/lb every 6 hr, 2.3 mg/lb every 8 hr, and 2.3 mg/lb every 12 hr)[45,46] or famotidine (Peptid) (doses reported as 1–2 mg s.i.d. PO; it is best administered by using the oral suspension).[49]

Nausea probably contributes to anorexia as much as vomiting. Because of the inability of the kidneys to conserve water and the resulting obligatory polydipsia in the CRD cat, lack of water intake causes dehydration and increased uremia. Fluid diuresis is the most efficacious and safest treatment of nausea: it promotes excretion of uremic toxins and gastrin.

In chronic renal failure, the degree of acidemia is variable. Generally, treatment is not required unless the serum bicarbonate levels are below 18 mEq/L or the urine pH is below 6.[29] If supplementation is required, sodium bicarbonate should be cautiously administered at a dosage of 4 to 8 mEq/lb orally two times a day. Baking soda is usually used for bicarbonate therapy; 1 g (⅓ teaspoon) of baking soda contains 12 mEq of sodium bicarbonate.[27] The goal of treatment is to maintain the serum bicarbonate level between 18 to 24 mEq/L. If the urine pH increases above 7 or the serum bicarbonate increases above 20 mEq/L, supplementation should be discontinued or decreased. If the cat is hypertensive, blood pressure should be monitored during supplementation because of the sodium content of sodium bicarbonate.[29]

Positive Nutritional State

The maintenance of a positive nutritional state is vital in the long-term management of a CRF cat. A proper diet is only effective if the cat will eat it; feline diets that are most palatable are those high in animal fat and protein. In trying to maintain a positive nutritional state the veterinarian should strive to remove or moderate all causes of inappetence including medical causes (nausea, dehydration, uremia, fever, nasal congestion), psychological causes (environmental stresses, fear), and dietary causes (protein and fat levels, texture, odor). The removal or moderation of medical causes of inappetence may include both symptomatic and specific therapy.

Increasing dietary palatability is aided by adding poultry fat or clam juice. Warming the food, especially food that has

Table 31–13. Feline Restricted-Protein Diet

¼ lb (115 g) liver
2 large eggs (100 g, hard cooked)
2 cups (350 g) cooked white rice without added salt
1 tablespoon (15 g) vegetable oil
1 table: (5 g) calcium carbonate

Also, add a balanced supplement that fulfills the feline MDR for all vitamins and trace minerals, and 250 mg taurine/day.
Dice and braise the meat, retaining fat.
Combine all ingredients and mix well.
This mixture is somewhat dry and the palatability may be improved by adding some water (not milk). Yield: 1¼ lb.

Calcium Carbonate Sources: Ground Egg Shells, Drug and Health Food Stores

Analysis	As Fed
Protein	7.3%
Fat	5.3%
Carbohydrate	15.8%
Moisture	70.0%
*Metabolizable energy	635 Kcal/lb

*This diet supplies 21% protein calories, 35% fat calories, and 44% carbohydrate calories.

Used with permission from: Lewis LD, Morris ML, Jr, Hand MS. Small Animal Clinical Nutrition III. Topeka, KS: Mark Morris Assoc. 1987:A3–3.

been refrigerated, can be effective. Because cats seem to prefer foods that have a low pH, the benefits of adding bicarbonate (baking soda) must be weighed against a potential decrease in palatability.[47]

A commercially formulated diet designed for the CRF feline patient is the diet of choice, if the cat will eat it.

Because of the fixed preferences of many cats, commercial diets will not be accepted by all. Changing the dietary form (dry versus canned) will be successful for some cats; using the previously mentioned palatability techniques may be helpful. The greatest advantage of commercial diets is the balance provided for vitamins, essential amino acids, and minerals.

CRF cats must eat well in order to remain compensated. If commercial diets are not accepted by the cat, homemade diets should be tried. Table 31–13 contains a recipe for a homemade low protein, low phosphorus diet.[48] The owner should be instructed to follow the recipe closely so that imbalances do not occur. The inclusion of a balanced vitamin, mineral, and taurine supplement is essential for long-term use. In addition, special attention should be paid to calcium, potassium, and phosphorus levels.

When the CRF cat is reluctant to eat any of the prescribed foods, the use of benzodiazepine derivatives should be tried to stimulate the appetite. Diazepam (Valium) and oxazepam (Serax) have proven useful (Table 31–14). For further suggestions, see Chapter 5.

Minimizing Stress

Another important goal in the management of the CRD cat is to minimize stress. Changes in the cat's environment can cause a renal failure patient to decompensate. These include hospitalization, moving, boarding, and obtaining a new dog or cat. A reduction in the cat's intake of water or calories can lead to decompensation. Even medical care may be stress-inducing. The owner, veterinary staff, and veterinarian must appreciate the effects of stress on the cat's ability to maintain homeostasis. Stressful situations should be avoided when possible. When medical treatments are necessary, the cat should be treated as an outpatient, if at all possible. Aggressive supportive care, fluid therapy, and forced nutritional support should be provided when stress induces decompensation.[29]

Table 31–14. Benzodiazepines Used to Stimulate Appetite in Anorectic Cats

Agent	Dose (mg/kg)	Route	Frequency	Dose Form
Diazepam (Valium)	0.2–0.3	Oral IV	Every 12–24 hr	2 mg tablet 5 mg/mL
Oxazepam (Serax)	0.2–0.4	Oral	Every 12–24 hr	10 mg/caplet* 15 mg/caplet†

*Dissolve the contents of one capsule in ½ oz 5% dextrose, then give 1 dropperful b.i.d.
†Dissolve the contents of one capsule in 1 oz 5% dextrose, then give 1 dropperful b.i.d.

REFERENCES

1. Krawiec DR, Gelberg HB. Chronic Renal Disease in Cats. In: Kirk RW, ed. Current Veterinary Therapy X. Philadelphia: WB Saunders, 1989:1170.
2. DiBartola SP, Rutgers HC, Zack PM, Tarr MJ. Clinicopathological findings associated with chronic renal disease in cats. J Am Vet Med Assoc 1987;190:1196.
3. Osborne CA, Polzin DJ. Azotemia: A review of what's old and what's new part I. Definition of terms and concepts. Compend Contin Ed Pract Vet (Small Anim Pract) 1983;5:497.
4. Crowell WA, Hubbell JJ, Riley JC. Polycystic renal disease in related cats. J Am Vet Med Assoc 1979;175:286.
5. Brace J. Perirenal Cyst (Pseudocysts) in the Cat. In: Kirk RW, ed. Current Veterinary Therapy VIII. Philadelphia: WB Saunders, 1983:980.
6. Leaf A, Cotran RS. Chronic Renal Disease. In: Renal Pathophysiology. New York: Oxford University Press, 1976:183.
7. Grauer GF. Management of Chronic Renal Failure. In: Proc Am Anim Hosp Assoc, 58th Annual Meeting. 1991:383.
8. Morrison G, Murray TG. Electrolyte, acid-base, and fluid homeostasis in chronic renal failure. Med Clin North Am 1981;65:429.

9. Grauer GF, Allen TA. Chronic renal failure in the dog. Compend Contin Ed Pract Vet (Small Anim Pract) 1981;3:1009.
10. Polzin DJ. Spectrum of Clinical and Laboratory Abnormalities in Uremia. In: Kirk RW, ed. Current Veterinary Therapy X. Philadelphia: WB Saunders, 1989:1133.
11. Bovee KC. The uremic syndrome. J Am Anim Hosp Assoc 1976;12:189.
12. Dow SW, LeCouteur RA. Hypokalemic Polymyopathy of Cats. In: Kirk RW, ed. Current Veterinary Therapy X. Philadelphia: WB Saunders, 1989:812.
13. Morgan RV. Systemic hypertension in four cats: Ocular and medical findings. J Am Anim Hosp Assoc 1986;22:615.
14. Breitschwerdt EB. Clinical abnormalities of urine concentration and dilution. Compend Contin Ed Pract Vet (Small Anim Pract) 1981;3:414.
15. Hoerauf A, Reusch C, Minkus G, Hermanns W. On the significance of the urine/protein ratio for distinguishing between feline nephropathies—A laboratory diagnostic–bioptic comparative study. In: Proceedings of the Eighth Annual Veterinary Medical Forum. 1990:1134.
16. Adams LG, Polzin DJ, Osborne CA. Urine protein/creatinine ratio and twenty-four hour urinary protein loss in normal and chronic renal failure cats (abstract). In: Proceedings of the Seventh Annual Veterinary Medical Forum. 1989:1043.
17. Russo EA. Assessment of Proteinuria in the Dog and Cat. In: Kirk RW, ed. Current Veterinary Therapy IX. Philadelphia: WB Saunders, 1986:1111.
18. Lees GE, Osborne CA. Feline Urinary Tract Infections. In: Kirk RW, ed. Current Veterinary Therapy VIII. Philadelphia: WB Saunders, 1983:1058.
19. Barsanti JA. Azotemia. In: Proc Am Anim Hosp Assoc, 49th Annual Meeting. 1982:135.
20. Ross LA, Finco DR. Relationship of selected clinical renal function tests to glomerular filtration rate and renal blood flow in cats. Am J Vet Res 1981;42:1704.
21. Barsanti JA. Renal failure in the dog and cat. In: Proc Am Anim Hosp Assoc, 49th Annual Meeting 1982:197.
22. DiBartola SP, Chew DJ, Jacobs G. Quantitative urinalysis including 24-hour protein excretion in the dog. J Am Anim Hosp Assoc 1980;16:537.
23. Finco DR, Barsanti JA. Clinical Evaluation of Renal Function. In: Kirk RW, ed. Current Veterinary Therapy X. Philadelphia: WB Saunders, 1989:1123.
24. DiBartola SP, Rutgers HC. Diseases of the Kidney. In: Sherding RG, ed. The CAT: Diseases and Clinical Management. New York: Churchill Livingstone, 1989:1353.
25. Osborne CA, Finco DR, Low DG. Pathophysiology of Renal Disease, Renal Failure, and Uremia. In: Ettinger SJ, ed. Textbook of Veterinary Internal Medicine, 2nd ed. Philadelphia: WB Saunders, 1983;1733.
26. DiBartola SP, Buffington CA, Chew DJ, Sparks RA. Chronic metabolic acidosis, potassium depletion, and renal function in adult cats. In: Proceedings of the Ninth Annual Medical Forum, 1991:765.
27. Allen TA. Management of Advanced Chronic Renal Failure. In: Kirk RW, ed. Current Veterinary Therapy X. Philadelphia: WB Saunders, 1989:1195.
28. Barsanti JA. Azotemia. In: Proc Am Anim Hosp Assoc, 49th Annual Meeting. 1982:197.
29. Osborne CA, Polzin DJ. Conservative Management of Feline Chronic Polyuric Renal Failure. In: Kirk RW, ed. Current Veterinary Therapy VIII. Philadelphia: WB Saunders, 1983:1008.
30. Ackerman N. Radiology and Ultrasound of Urogenital Diseases in Dogs and Cats. Ames: Iowa State University Press, 1991:7.
31. Walter PA, Feeney DA, Johnston GR, O'Leary TP. Ultrasonographic evaluation of renal parenchymal diseases in dogs: 32 cases (1981–1986). J Am Vet Med Assoc 1987;191:999.
32. Ross LA. Fluid therapy for acute and chronic renal failure. Vet Clin North Amer (Small Anim Pract). 1989;3:343.
33. Muir WW, DiBartola SP. Fluid Therapy. In: Kirk RW, ed. Current Veterinary Therapy VIII. Philadelphia: WB Saunders, 1983:28.
34. Cowgill LD. Management of Oliguric and Anuric Renal Failure. In: Kirk RW, ed. Current Veterinary Therapy VII. Philadelphia: WB Saunders, 1980:1087.
35. Cornelius LM. Fluid Therapy in the Uremic Patient. In: Kirk RW, ed. Current Veterinary Therapy VIII. Philadelphia: WB Saunders, 1983:989.
36. Finco DR, Low DG. Intensive Diuresis in Polyuric Renal Failure. In: Kirk RW, ed. Current Veterinary Therapy VII. Philadelphia: WB Saunders, 1980:1091.
37. Low DG, Cowgill LD. Emergency Management of the Acute Uremic Crisis. In: Kirk RW, ed. Current Veterinary Therapy VIII. Philadelphia: WB Saunders, 1983:981.
38. Schaer. The Diagnosis and Treatment of Metabolic and Respiratory Acidosis. In: Kirk RW, ed. Current Veterinary Therapy IX. Philadelphia: WB Saunders, 1986:60.
39. Ross LA, Labato MA. Use of Drugs to Control Hypertension in Renal Disease. In: Kirk RW, ed. Current Veterinary Therapy X. Philadelphia: WB Saunders, 1989:1201.
40. Kobayashi DL, Graves TK, Nichols CE. Blood pressure is elevated in hyperthyroid cats and cats with renal disease (abstract). In: Proceedings of the Sixth Annual Veterinary Medical Forum, 1988;723.
41. Osborne CA, Polzin DJ, Abdullahi S, Klausner JS, Rogers QR. Role of diet in management of feline chronic polyuric renal failure: Current status. J Am Anim Hosp Assoc 1982;18:11.
42. Finco DR, Brown SA. Newer Concepts and Controversies on Dietary Management of Renal Failure. In: Kirk RW, ed. Current Veterinary Therapy X. Philadelphia: WB Saunders, 1989: 1198.
43. Cowgill LA. Clinical Experience and Use of Recombinant Human Erythropoietin in Uremic Dogs and Cats. In: Proceedings of the Ninth Annual Veterinary Medical Forum. Blacksburg, VA: Amer Col Vet Inter Med, 1991:147.
44. Papich MG. Drugs Used in the Treatment of Gastrointestinal Disease. In: August JR, ed. Consultation in Feline Internal Medicine. Philadelphia: WB Saunders, 1991:463.
45. Ross LA. Feline Renal Failure. In: Breitschwerdt EB, ed. Contemporary Issues in Small Animal Practice: Nephrology and Urology. New York: Churchill Livingstone, 1986:109.
46. Chew DJ. Acute Renal Failure. In: Van Marthens E, ed. Seventh Annual Kal Kan Symposium for the Treatment of Small Animal Diseases. Vernon, CA: Kal Kan Foods, 1983:9.
47. Lewis LD, Hand MS. Gastrointestinal, pancreatic, and hepatic diseases. In: Proc, Am Anim Hosp Assoc, 55th Annual Meeting, 1988:336.
48. Hodgkins EM, Franks PT. Nutritional Requirements of the Sick Cat. In: August JR, ed. Consultations in Feline Internal Medicine. Philadelphia: WB Saunders, 1991:37.
49. Center S. Feline Hepatobiliary Diseases. Proceedings of the American Association of Feline Practitioners, Fall Meeting, Scottsdale, AZ, 1992.

CHAPTER 32

◇ ◇ ◇

Chylothorax

Gary D. Norsworthy

Chylothorax, the presence of chyle in the pleural space, is one of the common types of pleural effusions in the cat. It was once assumed that chylous fluid escaped from a traumatically ruptured thoracic duct into the pleural space; however, lymphangiography has shown that the thoracic duct is generally not ruptured in chylothorax. Instead, chyle typically leaks from dilated but intact cranial mediastinal lymphatics, a condition called lymphangiectasia.[1]

Etiology

Several primary intrathoracic diseases have been found in cats with chylothorax (Table 32–1). These diseases are presumed responsible for thoracic duct rupture or lymphangiectasia. However, most cases are not associated with primary disease and are thus considered idiopathic.[2]

Clinical Signs

In a study of 37 cases of feline chylothorax, the following clinical signs were noted[2]:

- Dyspnea (78%)
- Coughing (30%)
- Lethargy/depression (16%)
- Anorexia (14%)
- Weight loss (11%)
- Gagging (5%)
- Regurgitation/vomiting (5%)
- Exercise intolerance (5%)
- Cyanosis (3%)
- Salivation (3%)
- Posterior paresis (3%)

It is notable that coughing was present in 30% of the cases and was the only clinical sign in 11%. Although coughing in cats is generally not associated with pleural effusions—it is most commonly due to feline asthma, heartworms, or lungworms—one should consider chylothorax in cats with a history of coughing. Thoracic radiography should be part of the diagnostic evaluation.

Physical Examination

In the same study of 37 cases of chylothorax, the most consistent findings on physical examination were increased bronchovesicular sounds (46%) and muffled heart sounds (41%). Tachycardia was found in 16%; 86% had normal body temperatures. These findings are typical of many cats with pleural effusion, regardless of the cause.

Diagnosis

Laboratory Tests

Hematologic analyses are variable and not diagnostic. The white blood cell (WBC) count may range from about 6,000 cells/μL to as high as 33,000 cells/μL. Many cats have a WBC count in the normal range; lymphopenia is the most consistently found abnormality in WBC differentiation.[2] Affected cats are typically not anemic, and the values on a biochemical profile are usually normal. Because of the underlying diseases associated with chylothorax, other appropriate tests include a feline leukemia virus antigen test and an occult heartworm test.

Radiography

Thoracic radiography is an important part of the diagnostic process. It allows the detection of pleural fluid and the differentiation of unilateral from bilateral disease (Fig. 32–1*A*,*B*). Because cardiac disease is a predisposing factor in some cats, the pleural fluid should be removed and the chest radiographed again so that the size and shape of the heart can be evaluated. Radiography following fluid removal also permits detection of anterior mediastinal masses, another predisposing factor in chylothorax.

Chylous Fluid

A diagnosis of chylous fluid is based on gross, biochemical, and cytologic findings (Tables 32–2 and 32–3). The most reliable test is the cholesterol-to-triglyceride (C:T) ratio. The C:T ratio is generally less than 1.0 in a chylous fluid and greater than 1.8 in a pseudochylous fluid. The specific gravity and total protein level of pleural effusions are commonly

Table 32–1. Intrathoracic Diseases Thought to Cause Chylothorax[2,6]

Neoplasia, especially lymphosarcoma
Cardiac disease, especially cardiomyopathy and heartworm disease
Trauma, as evidenced by rib fractures and/or diaphragmatic hernia
Inflammation around the thoracic duct
Venous thrombi
Congenital malformation of the lymphatic-venous junction
Fungal granulomas
Lung lobe torsion
Lobectomy

obtained as part of the analysis. However, refractometry is not a reliable means of performing these tests because it falsely elevates the specific gravity of fluids containing lipids.[3]

Fluid Cytology

Cytologic examination of the pleural effusion can be very helpful in making a diagnosis of chylothorax. The typical finding is a large number of mature lymphocytes with the approximate diameter of red blood cells (Fig. 32–2). Once these are identified, one should continue to examine the sediment for evidence of an underlying disease.

Treatment

Before treatment begins, one must attempt to define any primary intrathoracic disease that may underlie the chylothorax. If found, its treatment must be considered along with that for chylothorax. The primary disease must also be considered when a prognosis is formulated.

Initial treatment should be thoracocentesis to remove the life-threatening effusion. Generally an in-dwelling thoracostomy tube is indicated, because fluid production will likely continue for several days to weeks (see Chapter 55). Strict attention should be paid to preventing sepsis, since cats with chylothorax seem prone to developing pyothorax. A low-fat diet such as Prescription Diet Feline r/d or Prescription Diet Feline w/d (Hill's Pet Products, Topeka, KS) may be helpful in resolving chylothorax.[2] Fat supplementation with medium-chain triglycerides is beneficial, because they are absorbed directly into the portal system, bypassing the thoracic duct. An example of a commercial preparation of medium-chain triglycerides is MCT oil, which is given at 1 to 2 mL/kg/day. Its main disadvantage is its unpalatability.

Chylothorax secondary to diaphragmatic hernia is reported to spontaneously resolve when the diaphragmatic hernia is surgically corrected.[4] The author treated a cat for heartworm disease and observed spontaneous resolution of chylothorax. These findings suggest that cats should be treated with chest drainage and a low-fat diet for 2 to 4 weeks before the surgical options listed below are considered.[2]

Ligation of the thoracic duct has been attempted by a number of surgeons. Death during either anesthetic admin-

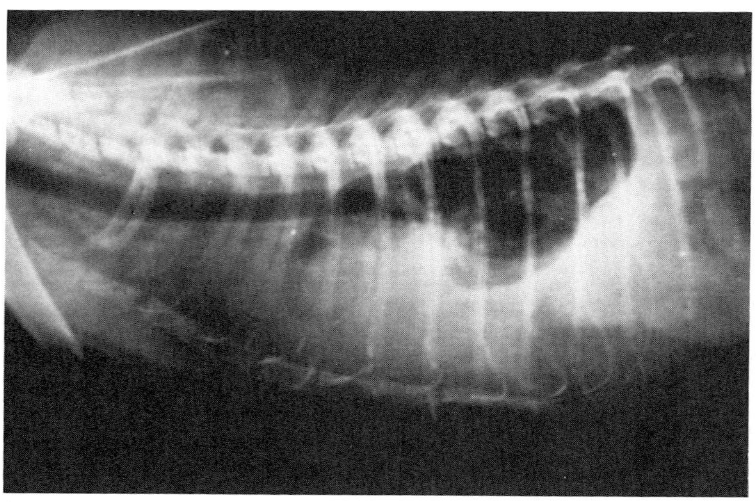

A

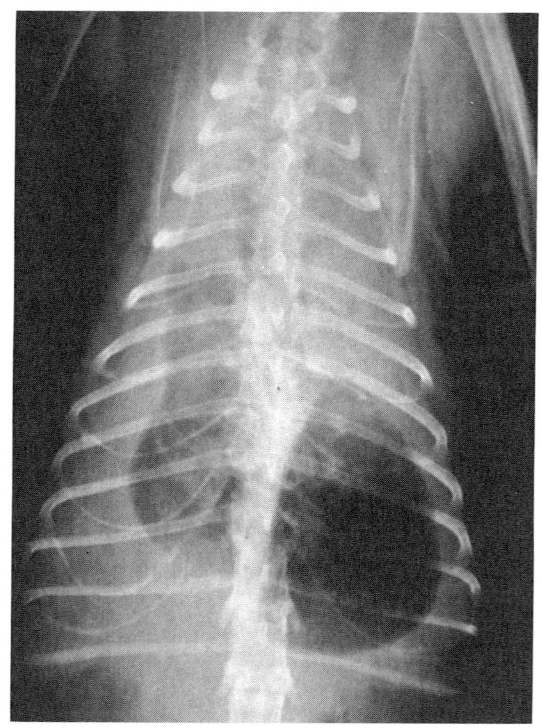

B

Figure 32–1. (*A*) Chylothorax produces pleural effusion. On the lateral radiograph, this is seen as ventral scalloping of lung borders and obscuring of the cardiac and diaphragmatic silhouettes due to the extrapulmonary fluid present. (*B*) The signs of pleural effusion on the ventrodorsal radiographic view include the appearance of fissure lines between the lung lobes, rounding of the lung borders at the costophrenic angles, mediastinal widening, obscuring of the cardiac and diaphragmatic silhouettes, and separation of the lung margins from the thoracic wall.

Table 32–2. Characteristics of Chylous Fluid[2,7]

Most Reliable
Has a cholesterol-to-triglyceride ratio of less than 1.0
Generally Reliable
Has the gross appearance of skimmed milk
Does not clear when centrifuged
Contains fat that will stain with Sudan III stain
Lipoprotein electrophoresis demonstrates chylomicrons
Milky color will not clear when mixed with diethylether and alkali (ether clearance test) (see Table 32–3).
Usually contains lymphocytes as the predominant cell, although neutrophils may predominate in some cats. The lymphocytes are mature and approximately the size of red blood cells (see Fig. 32–2)

istration or surgery has been a significant problem. One report of five cats treated conservatively and five cats treated surgically had equal success rates (40%).[5] Another study reported complete resolution in only two of 14 (14%) cats that underwent thoracic duct ligation.[2]

Other attempted surgical treatments include the implantation of a pleuroperitoneal shunt to actively pump thoracic fluid into the abdomen, the implantation of mesh in the diaphragm to allow passive drainage of thoracic fluid into the abdomen, and the decortication of pleural tissue. None has produced consistently satisfactory results.[2] A new procedure of fenestrating the diaphragm has shown promising results: twenty 4-mm holes are surgically introduced into the diaphragm to allow the chylous fluid to flow into the peritoneal cavity.

Pleurodesis has had limited trial as a treatment for chylothorax. In the procedure, tetracycline hydrochloride or oxytetracycline hydrochloride is injected into the pleural space in an attempt to obliterate it by causing adhesions to form between the visceral pleura and the parietal pleura. In a study involving three cats, two died as a result of the oxytetracycline, and pleural effusion continued in the third, given tetracycline. Pleurodesis is also very painful.[2]

Table 32–3. Ether Clearance Test

Place one part of the suspect fluid in each of two test tubes.
Add 2 drops of 10% potassium hydroxide to each tube.
Add one part water to one tube and one part diethylether to the other.
Mix both tubes by inverting.
If the fluid is chyle, the fluid in the diethylether tube will remain milky. (The tube with water is a control. It will remain milky.)
If the field is pseudochyle, the fluid in the diethylether tube will become transparent. (The tube with water is a control. It will remain milky.)

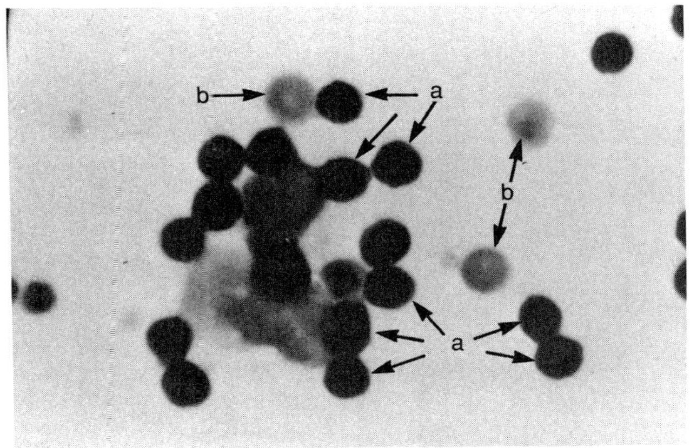

Figure 32–2. **The typical cytologic finding of chylothorax-induced pleural effusion is the presence of large numbers of mature lymphocytes (*a*) that have the approximate diameter of red blood cells (*b*).**

Prognosis

Although some cats have a spontaneous recovery once the primary disease is treated, the overall success rate is less than 50%, regardless of the form of therapy utilized. Therefore, cats with chylothorax should be given a poor to guarded prognosis.

REFERENCES

1. Fossum TW, Birchard SJ. Chylothorax. In: Kirk RW, ed. Current Veterinary Therapy X. Philadelphia: WB Saunders, 1989:393.
2. Fossum TW, Forrester SD, Swenson CL, et al. Chylothorax in cats: 37 cases (1969–1989). J Am Vet Med Assoc 1991;198:672.
3. Fossum TW, Jacobs RM, Birchard SJ. Evaluation of chylous and nonchylous pleural effusions using serum and pleural fluid cholesterol and triglyceride concentrations. J Am Vet Med Assoc 1986;188:49.
4. Meincke JE, Hobbie WV, Barto LR. Traumatic chylothorax with associated diaphragmatic hernias in the cat. J Am Vet Med Assoc 1969;155:15.
5. Harpster NK. Chylothorax. In: Kirk RW, ed. Current Veterinary Therapy IX. Philadelphia: WB Saunders, 1986:295.
6. Forrester SD, Troy GC, Fossum TW. Pleural effusions: Pathophysiology and diagnostic considerations. Compend Contin Ed Pract Vet 1988 121.
7. Bauer T. Mediastinal, Pleural, and Extrapleural Diseases. In: Ettinger SJ, ed. Textbook of Veterinary Internal Medicine, 3rd ed. Philadelphia: WB Saunders, 1989:883.

CHAPTER 33

◇ ◇ ◇

Dental Diseases

Robert B. Wiggs and Heidi B. Lobprise

This chapter explores the range of diseases and pathology associated with tooth structure.* An understanding of the basics of examination and anatomy enhance the study of clinically significant abnormalities.

Physical Examination

A thorough examination and a working knowledge of anatomy and function are the basis of diagnostics in most oral and dental problems. The examination is a multistaged activity, beginning with a thorough history and followed by an external and oral examination. In all cases, recognition of normal anatomy is essential.

History

The patient history is the foundation of the examination. It relies on the owner's direct personal involvement and provides information that is a valuable aid in directing the physical, oral, and laboratory examination. A complete history provides more than the vaccination status; details of diet, levels of professional and home dental care, past disease problems and treatments, current problems and treatments in progress, exposure to infectious diseases, traumatic incidents, and behavioral changes help the clinician fully evaluate the patient. Even closer attention should be paid to the actual oral symptoms, including onset, duration, degree of severity, and recurrence profile.[1]

External Examination

The external physical examination is essential to the evaluation of obvious oral problems. Observe the face, mandible, and head for swellings that can indicate neoplastic enlargements, cellulitis, and abscesses. Cellulitis and abscessation can be caused by foreign bodies, fight wounds, periodontal disease, or periapical disorders; fistulous tracts, with or without purulent drainage, may be present. Neoplasia and manifestations of the eosinophilic granuloma complex may result in raised ulcerative lesions of the lip or gingiva or enlargement of the mandibular lymph nodes.

Asymmetry of the face or head can be present in hereditary or congenital mutations, inflammatory disease, neoplasia, dislocations, fractures, and nerve damage. The most common of these causes are dislocation of the temporomandibular joint (TMJ) and maxillary or mandibular fractures. Open mouth disorders are usually a result of trauma to the TMJ, fracture of the maxillary or mandibular bones, or nerve damage (see Chapter 52).

Oral Examination

The oral examination is a two-part procedure, a portion accomplished with the cat awake and a portion requiring sedation or anesthesia. The degree of oral examination that can be accomplished in the conscious, alert animal varies significantly with the individual. Before proceeding, the practitioner must evaluate the personality of the patient as well as the degree of discomfort an oral exam may cause. A complete oral examination can only be performed on an anesthetized animal.

A detailed systematic approach is necessary for a complete oral examination. It begins with appraisal of the lips and proceeds to the vestibules, tongue, hard palate, pharynx, tonsils, gingivae, and teeth.[2,3] Soft tissues should be examined for trauma, ulcerations, inflammation, swelling, masses, discoloration, and foreign materials. Inspection of the ventral tongue is facilitated by pushing a finger into the temporomandibular space.[1] The gingival sulcus should be examined with a periodontal probe for abnormal pocket depths and with an explorer for indication of cervical line lesions, subgingival plaque, and calculus. Finally, the teeth should be inspected for plaque, calculus, fractures, discoloration, cervical line lesions, appropriate number, and occlusion. Correct assessment of a cat's oral and dental health relies on familiarity with normal anatomy.

Oral Anatomy

The major facial bones associated with dental structures are the incisive bone (rostral part of the upper jaw), maxilla,

*The procedures described in this chapter should not be undertaken until one understands them and has proper instrumentation. Veterinarians who have attended seminars and wet labs in dental procedures will find this material practical and helpful.

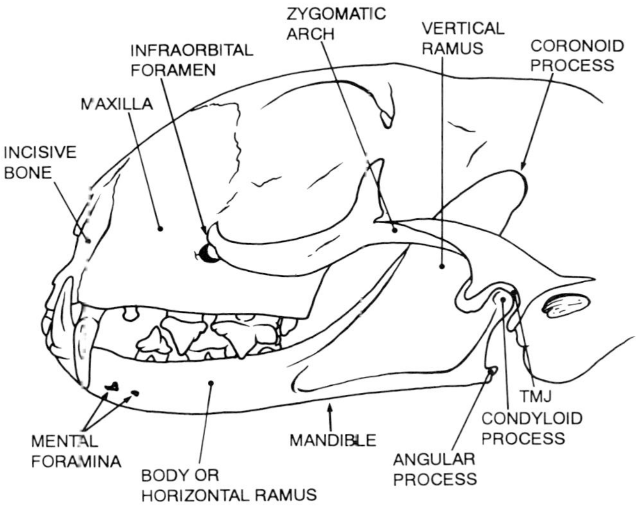

Figure 33–1. **Normal skull and mandibular anatomy.**

and mandible (Fig. 33–1). The tooth consists of a crown (above the gumline) covered with enamel, the hardest substance in the body, and a root (below the gumline) covered by cementum, a modified bone structure (Fig. 33–2). The crown and root join at the cementoenamel junction or neck. The bulk of the tooth is comprised of dentin (under the enamel and cementum), which is a dynamic, living tissue that continues to grow and is permeated with dentinal tubules containing odontoblastic extensions from the central pulp cavity. The pulp cavity is the entire inner cavity, consisting of the pulp chamber in the coronal portion and the root canal within the root. This area is filled with nerves, blood vessels, and connective tissue[4] and is lined with odontoblasts that can secrete secondary dentin. The supportive structure of the tooth is the periodontium, made up of the gingiva (gums), periodontal ligament (a bacterial barricade and "shock absorber" between cementum and alveolar bone), and the alveolar bone (socket). The gingival margin is the edge of tissue that usually lies closely against the tooth near the neck. The gingival sulcus is a groove or theoretical space between this margin and the tooth; it can be up to 0.5 mm in depth normally, although quite often is negligible in cats. Sulcus or pocket depth is measured with a calibrated periodontal probe. It should be held securely against the

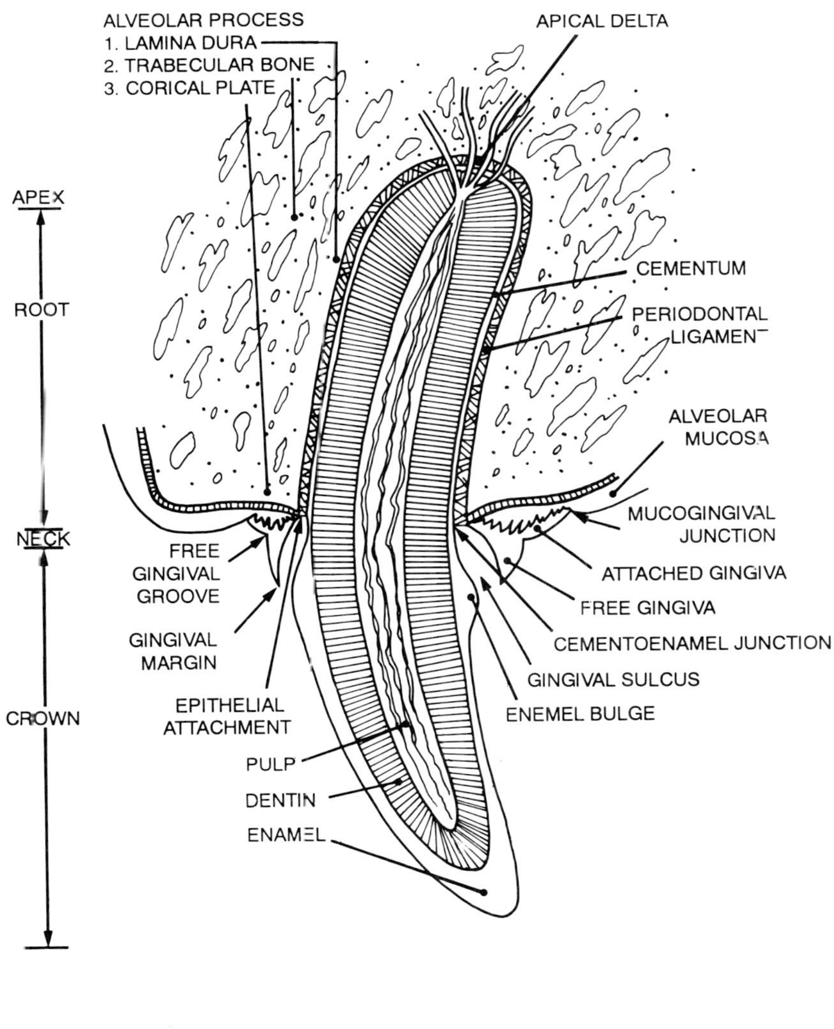

Figure 33–2. **Normal dental and paradental anatomy. (Used with permission: Manfra Marretta S: The common and uncommon clinical presentations and treatment of peridontal disease in the dog and cat. Sem Vet Med Drug (Small Anim) 1987;2:2300.)**

Table 33–1. Dental Terms

Palatal: surface of the tooth toward the palate (upper)
Lingual: Surface of the tooth toward the tongue (lower or upper)
Labial: Surface of the tooth toward the lips
Buccal: Surface of the tooth toward the cheek
Facial: Labial or buccal surface
Occlusal: Surface of the tooth facing a tooth in the opposite jaw
Interproximal: Surface between two teeth
Mesial: Surface of the tooth toward the front midline
Distal: Surface of the tooth away from the front midline
Apical: Toward the apex (root)
Coronal: Toward the crown

tooth and inserted gently into the sulcus until resistance is met. At that point the depth should be read. Three facial and three lingual measurements of each tooth should be made by walking the probe circumferentially around the tooth. These are taken at the mesial, midfacial/midlingual, and distal line angles, both facially and lingually. Any sulcus deeper than 0.5 mm should be recorded on the chart.

Descriptive terms are necessary to ensure accurate information regarding dental conditions (Table 33–1).

Knowing the correct dental formulas of both deciduous and permanent teeth, as well as eruption times, will help one to recognize abnormalities such as missing teeth, supernumerary (extra) teeth, and retained deciduous teeth, which generally should be extracted.[5,6] Identifying the tooth type is essential for good charting. These are listed with feline dental formulae in Table 33–2 and illustrated in Figure 33–3. Eruption times are listed in Table 33–3.

Many methods of dental charting are possible, but one should be selected and used consistently. The authors denote the tooth type by the described abbreviations, then indicate the position and number by superscripts and subscripts:

^{1}C: Upper left canine

P_3: Lower right third premolar

S^1P^1: Supernumerary right and left upper first premolar

Table 33–2. Dental Nomenclature and Formulae

I: Incisor	Id or i: Deciduous incisor
C: Canine or cuspid	Cd or c: Deciduous canine/cuspid
P: Premolar	Pd or p: Deciduous premolar
M: Molar	Md or m: Deciduous molar
S: Supernumerary	

Deciduous: (Id 3/3, Cd 1/1, Pd 3/2) × 2 = 26
Permanent: (I 3/3, C 1/1, P 3/2, M 1/1) × 2 = 30

In a cat, it is currently accepted that the premolars "missing" are actually the ones in front; that is, the upper premolars should be numbered from 2 to 4, and the lower premolars should be numbered 3 and 4.[7] Nomenclature rulings may name the first visible upper premolar as either 1 or 2, and the upper molar as either 1 or 3.

Table 33–3. Eruption Times

	Deciduous (weeks)	Permanent (months)
Incisors	2–3	3–4
Cuspids	3–4	4–5
Premolars	3–6	4–6
Molars		4–6

The American Veterinary Dental College Nomenclature and Classification Committee has suggested the use of the Triadan tooth-numbering system, which uses three-digit numbers without commas. The first number designates the quadrant location and whether a tooth is primary or secondary. The number sequence is upper right, upper left, lower left, and lower right. The adult dentition uses numbers 1 to 4 and primary dentition uses numbers 5 to 8. In each quadrant the first incisor is always 1, with incisors numbered 1 to 3, cuspids numbered 4, premolars numbered 5 to 8 (except when not present), and molars numbered 9 to 11 (except when not present). This numbering is based on a fully phenotypic dentition of (I 3/3, C 1/1, P 4/4, M 3/3) × 2 =

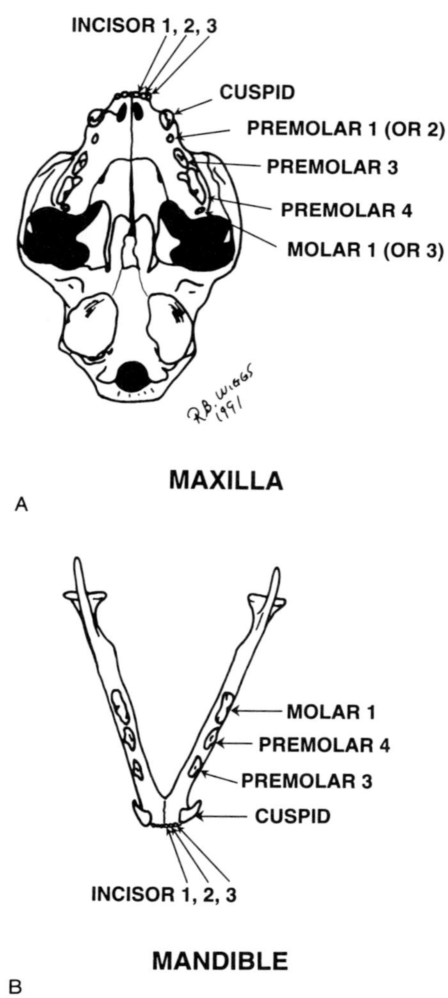

Figure 33–3. Tooth identification.

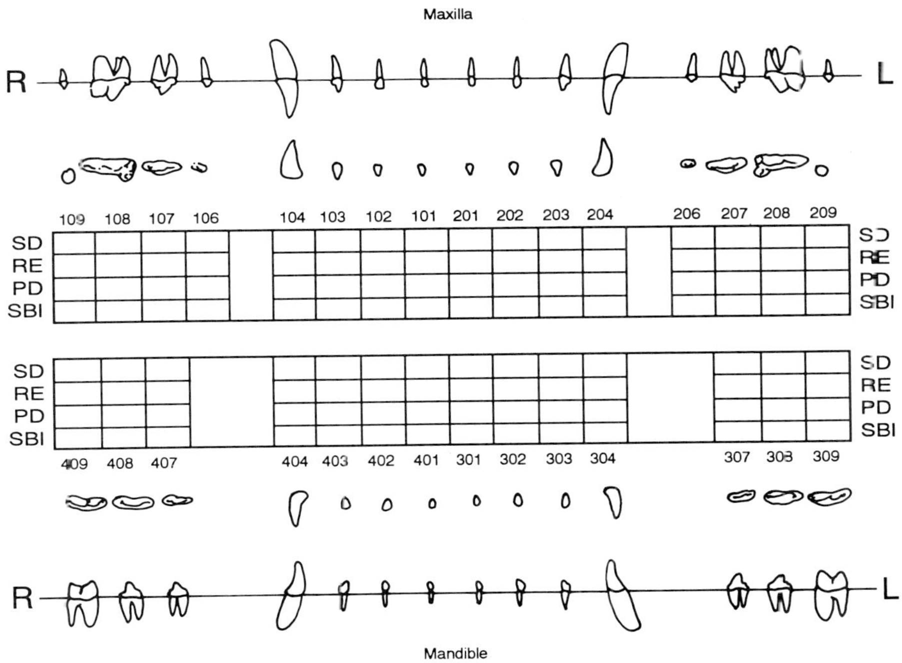

Figure 33–4. **Feline dental chart.**

44, as in swine. The cat's numbering is suitably altered (Fig. 33–4).

upper right 1/5	upper left 2/6
lower right 4/8	lower left 3/7

It is also useful to have a dental chart on the permanent record, either a stamped impression, sticker, or separate sheet. One chart can be used for recording the examination, assessment, and pathology with a second to denote the specific treatment, or a single diagram may be used as a combined report form. Some common notations used in dental charts are listed in Table 33–4.

The number of root tips is also important, particularly in exodontia (extractions) and endodontics (root canal procedures):

One root: All incisors, canines, and lower second premolars

Three roots: Upper fourth premolars

Two roots: All others

Cervical Line Lesions

Cervical line lesions (CLL) of feline teeth have also been referred to as cervical neck lesions (CNL), cervical line erosions, cervical line resorptions, subgingival resorptive lesions, initiocircocervical desmodentiopathy, and buccal cervical root resorptions.[4,5,8] CLL is currently the most common disease of the domestic feline tooth structure.[5] The disease was virtually unrecognized until the mid-1970s; the first published description was in 1976.[8,9] Retrospective examination of feline skulls into the late 1800s revealed a low incidence of the disease,[10] and one text by Colyer in 1936 failed to describe any lesions of this nature.[4] This information differs significantly from the relatively high rate recorded during the last decade.

In early published reports, the lesions were thought to be of a carious, decay-type nature.[4,11,12] Later, they were described as being progressive, subgingival, resorptive lesions with osteoclastic involvement.[4,9] Histologically, lesions at the cementoenamel junction (CEJ) are concave defects lined by odontoclasts,[13] with normal surrounding dentin and no inflammation of the pulp tissue in early stage lesions.[4,14] Root resorption can occur with more advanced lesions and is most commonly found in the cat with periodontal disease complications.[9,14] Although one study indicated that Siamese and Persians were more susceptible to these lesions,[15] the authors' clinical experience has not reflected this.

Periodontal disease and plasmacytic–lymphocytic stomatitis are commonly associated with CLL.[16] Many feline leukemia virus (FeLV) infected cats have periodontal disease and CLLs, but the majority of CLL patients are negative for the FeLV.[17,13] Some patients have increased immunoglobulins, while others have immune deficiencies.[17] One study has demonstrated that a high percentage of CLL patients are positive for the feline calicivirus,[18] but the significance of this has not been determined. Human bulimia patients demonstrate a similar form of CLL that results from the chronic exposure of the CEJ to stomach acids. Because many cats have periodic episodes of vomiting, some associated with hair, stomach acids may play a part in certain individuals in further exacerbation of lesions, as osteoclasts work best at a low pH.[19]

These studies may reflect the role that inflammation of the periodontal ligament (with fibroelastic activity and cellular differentiation into cementoclasts and odontoclasts)

Table 33–4. Abbreviations Used in Dental Charts

AM or AF	Amalgam filling	N/CNL/CLL	Cervical line lesion[f]
AT	Attrition	O	Missing tooth
C	Calculus	OA	Orthodontic appliance
CA	Cavity	OB/B	Orthodontic button
CI	Calculus index[a]	P/PP	Periodontal pocket
CF	Composite filling	PD	Periodontal disease[g]
CR	Crown restoration[b]	PE	Pulp exposure
E	Enamel lesion	PI	Plaque index[h]
EP	Epulis	RT	Rotated tooth
F	Furcation exposure[c]	RC	Root canal
Fx	Fracture	RD	Retained deciduous tooth
G	Gingivitis	RE	Root exposure
GG	Gingivectomy	RR	Root resorption
GI	Gingivitis index[d]	SBI	Sulcus bleeding index[i]
GF/GIF	Glass ionomer filling	SD	Sulcus depth
GH/H	Gingival hyperplasia	V/VP	Vital pulpotomy
GR	Gingival recession	X	Extraction
M	Mobile tooth[e]		

[a]Calculus index: rate 0–3; none, slight, moderate, abundant.
[b]Crown restoration: CRC—composite, CRM—metal, CRP—porcelain.
[c]Furcation exposure: rate 1–3; exposed, undermined, through and through communication. Additionally, F, L. M, D (facial, lingual, mesial, distal) can be used to denote furcation. For example, F2–F = furcation exposure and undermined on facial surface of the tooth.
[d]Gingivitis index: rate 0–3; none, mild, moderate, severe.
[e]Mobile tooth: rate 0–3; none, slight, moderate, severe.
[f]Cervical neck lesion/cervical line lesion: rate as stages 1–5.
[g]Periodontal disease: rate 1–4; gingivitis, early, moderate, severe.
[h]Plaque index: rate 0–3; none, slight, moderate, severe.
[i]Sulcus bleeding index: rate 0–5; 0 = none on probing, 5 = spontaneous.

plays in the external resorptive process. If such is the case, CLLs may be an extension of a form of periodontal disease more specific to the feline,[14,20-23] but some think the inflammation is secondary to the resorptive lesion.[9] Feeding raw liver was found by some researchers to increase the rate of incidence of these lesions.[4,11,24] This has led some to suspect a calcium–phosphorous imbalance as a possible causative agent, but diet is not generally considered to be a primary factor because of the occurrence of lesions even in captured cats found living in the wild.[4,11] The use of calcium-regulating hormones has been considered in an attempt to control the process of reparative bone-cementum tissue that leads to root ankylosis.[13]

Clinical Signs

Cervical line lesions are common in the domestic feline; recent studies have shown that 52% to 65% of cats display at least one lesion and, periodontal disease is commonly associated.[15,16,25] They are often covered with hyperplastic or hyperemic gingiva, plaque, or calculus.[26] Normally the lesions begin at the cementoenamel junction below the gum line; therefore, most lesions identified in the early stages are located with a dental explorer during routine prophylaxis. The advanced lesions may be more obvious on simple oral examination. The authors have found a reduced incidence of the lesions on the lingual or palatal aspect of the teeth, with the vast majority located on the facial and proximal surfaces. The lesions are most frequently encountered on the premolars, molars, cuspids, and incisors, respectively.

Various presenting signs have been observed from slight to severe gingival inflammation with gingival hypertrophy and hyperemia to gingival recession with bone loss and loose teeth. As the lesions advance, root resorption and loss of the crown may occur as the tooth structure is weakened. A simple gingival swelling where a tooth once existed may indicate possible root retention below the gum line following crown loss.

Halitosis is a common component of the patient's history. Teeth may be sensitive in early lesions but sensitivity is more pronounced when pulpal irritation causes overt pain. Similar lesions in the CEJ area of humans are known to be very sensitive.[27] In the cat, this sensitivity may lead to anorexia, ptyalism, lethargy, dysphagia, and weight loss.[19] Head shaking, sneezing, and excessive lingual movement has been seen in maxillary cuspid tooth involvement.

Diagnosis and Treatment

Most lesions are diagnosed during routine prophylaxis. Even under general anesthesia, a sensitivity response (involuntary twitch) may occur when a dental explorer or probe is drawn across or near a lesion. The probe should be gently inserted into the gingival sulcus and the tooth probed for any surface irregularities. If the explorer end is used, care should be taken with the pointed tip to not lacerate the epithelial attachment at the bottom of the sulcus.

Generally, teeth should be saved when possible, but exodontia (extraction) is the most common treatment method employed by the primary care veterinarian. If restoration is considered as an alternative, radiographs should always be taken.[28] What appears to be an early stage of the disease by visual and tactile probe examination may prove to be a more advanced lesion radiographically. In addition, the authors have found that teeth more prone to restorative failures typically have indications of apical external resorption or internal pulp cavity resorption even if the CLL does not appear to communicate with these lesions.

Using G.V. Black's modified cavity classification,[29] the lesions' incidence of occurrence would be class V (gingival third of labial or lingual surface), class II (proximal surface premolars or molars), or class III (proximal surface cuspids or incisors without involving incisal angle). They may also be classified into five stages for diagnostic and therapeutic purposes:

Stage I: Into cementum or enamel only

Stage II: Through the cementum/enamel into the dentin

Stage III: Through the dentin into the pulp cavity

Stage IV: Extensive structural damage, fragile tooth

Stage V: Crown lost, roots still present

Stage I

These lesions are shallow with extension only into the cementum or enamel (Fig. 33–5). They appear early in the progression of the disease and should be treated, not extracted, unless radiographs indicate complicating factors. Treatment is simple; after routine prophylaxis, the sulcus is gently burnished with a gingival packer or other blunt instrument dipped into a hemostatic solution to control gingival hemorrhage. If additional sulcus exposure is needed, gingival retraction cord should be packed into the sulcus. *Do not use epinephrine-type cord on patients with cardiac or endocrine disease, especially hyperthyroidism.* The lesion should be root planed thoroughly with a dental curette, polished with a nonfluoride prophylaxis paste, rinsed, and dried. A fluoride varnish is applied to the dry tooth surface using a cotton swab or small brush.[15,28,30]

Stage II

Lesions of this nature have penetrated into the dentin and require treatment evaluation and selection of either restoration or exodontia (extraction). If extraction is chosen, care must be exercised during the process, as these teeth may be fragile from the structural loss. Some roots may be ankylosed to the surrounding alveolar bone, making simple extraction impossible. These conditions should be apparent on radiographs taken during initial assessment (see Exodontia).

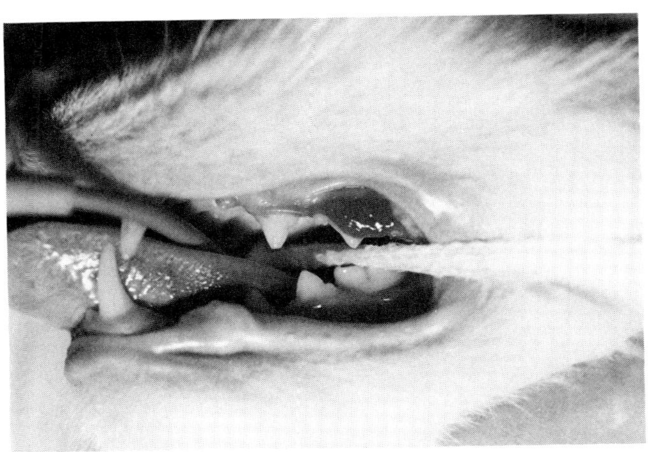

Figure 33–5. **Stage I cervical line lesion. The hyperplastic gingiva was the only obvious clinical sign.**

Restoration of these teeth in cats is performed differently than in most other species due to the limited dental structures present. The extensive cavity preparations required for amalgam and composites are not practical in most of the feline's diminutive teeth. For these reasons, glass ionomer restoratives that can chemically attach to the hard dental tissues (enamel, cementum, and dentin) are typically the restorative of choice. Glass ionomers come in ADA type I luting cements and type II base restoratives. The ADA type II glass ionomers are used for restoration of CLLs. Additionally, these are available in auto-cure (self-curing) and visible light cure. The auto-cure glass ionomers are chemically activated during the mixing of the base and catalyst and self-cure or harden. Light-cure restorative glass ionomers require a visible light (450 to 500 nm) source. This is a blue light similar to ultraviolet (320 to 365 nm) but in a different wavelength range. Certain safety precautions must be observed because visible light can result in damage to the lens and retina of the patient or operators if viewed unprotected. Therefore, patients' eyes should be closed or covered, and operators should make use of visible-light safety shields or glasses. Use of light-cured restorative materials can noticeably reduce procedural time; however, it can greatly increase initial set-up costs because of the expense of the special instruments, light-cure source, and safety equipment.

For restoration, the lesion is initially prepared as in the stage I treatment, except the fluoride varnish is omitted. The following describes treatment using a self-curing glass ionomer. An auto-curing type II glass ionomer is prepared according to the individual manufacturer's specifications and placed in the lesion. It should be covered with Mylar or cocoa butter to prevent moisture contamination while setting up. Moisture exposure during the setting stage of the glass may result in untimely deterioration of the glass or failure to adhere. Once set up, most material irregularities can be corrected by gently using a sharp curette. When the finish is acceptable, a coat of waterproof varnish is applied for a few hours to prevent dehydration of the restorative. All restorations should be rechecked for weakening or loss approximately two weeks after treatment.

A kit containing all materials and instructions needed for restoration is marketed as Restore FL-1 (VRx Products, Harbor City, CA).

Stage III

Lesions of this type have pulpal exposure and are generally candidates for exodontia (extraction) by most practitioners (Fig. 33–6). If restoration is attempted, a root canal is required; this is practical only in the cuspids (canine teeth), although other of the larger teeth can be treated. Root canal procedures are performed with a zinc oxide/eugenol sealer and gutta-percha as core material or with a calcium hydroxide sealer and then filled with a calcium hydroxide paste (see Root Canals). These lesions should be evaluated carefully by visual examination, palpation, and radiography prior

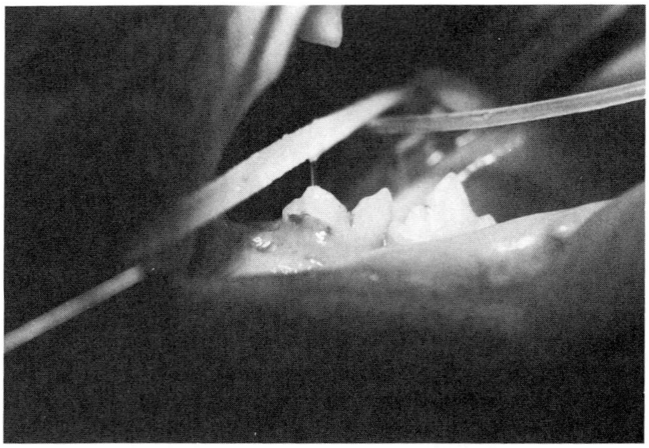

Figure 33–6. **Stage III cervical line lesions with extensive structural damage and hyperplastic gingiva occluding the defect.**

to consideration for restorative procedures. After endodontic therapy, the restoration should be performed as described previously.

Stage IV

Due to the structural instability of stage IV lesions, these lesions are candidates for exodontia only (Fig. 33–7). In most cases when elevators are applied, the tooth crown fractures or disintegrates rapidly. Radiographically, most show ankylosed roots that defy normal extraction attempts. In many cases, pulverization with a high-speed dental handpiece and a round number 2 burr will be the only practical removal method, with radiographic confirmation of complete removal.

Stage V

These are lesions that have progressed until only roots of teeth are left behind. In most cases the gingiva cover the roots, leaving an appearance of a small bulge. Diagnosis can only be confirmed by radiographs. The majority of these roots will be ankylosed and require pulverization for removal.

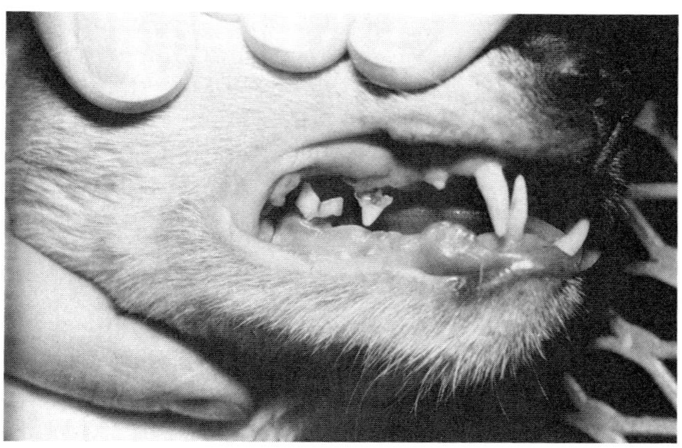

Figure 33–7. **Stage IV cervical line lesions with extensive structural damage. The crown is nearly fractured from the root at the neck. (Photo courtesy of Dr. Gary D. Norsworthy, San Antonio, TX.)**

After Care

The cat is placed on appropriate antibiotics for 2 weeks and then rechecked for gingival inflammation and loss of restoration. Even if the lesions are controlled with no further indications of problems, they should still be checked at 3- to 12-month intervals according to the stage and treatment. Restorations should be reradiographed at 9 to 12 months following treatment to determine if lesions are active or dormant. Professional prophylaxis to aid in the control of any periodontal disease is recommended at least yearly. Scaling around the restoration should be done carefully with hand instruments because ultrasonic, Roto-Pro, and sonic scalers can disrupt glass ionomer restorations. The teeth should be cleaned, root planed, and fluoride treated. Fluoride aids by reducing tooth sensitivity and preventing deterioration of enamel by certain agents, such as some acids from bacterial by-products. Topical fluoride gels are applied to the teeth and left in place for 5 minutes then wiped off (do not rinse the gel from the mouth or allow the cat to drink water for 30 minutes following treatment, as this will reduce the effectiveness of sodium-type fluoride products).

Home Care

Home care must be tailored to the individual client and patient in accordance with the degree of problem and other complicating factors. Based on results of current studies, diet and home dental care are the two primary areas in which the client can help with control of progression of CLLs.[4] Ingesting large amounts of raw liver and possibly other meats may aggravate the condition; therefore, these should be avoided when possible. Chronic vomiting may also play some part in the progression of lesions. For this reason, medical investigation and management of such conditions with appropriate medication and dietary changes are warranted (see Chapter 24). Although dry food has been shown to reduce the rate of accumulation of plaque on the teeth, felines are discriminating eaters, and owners sometimes have difficulty changing the textures of their pets' diets.

Direct dental care by the owner should be approached in a gentle and caring way to create a stress-free activity for both parties. Some anxious and distraught animals cannot have home care performed without risk of injury to client or patient. The owner should be consulted concerning this matter in order to assess their ability and willingness to perform such tasks in a safe and productive manner. Initially, using only a finger dipped in water saved from a can of tuna, gently rubbing the facial surfaces of the anterior teeth should be attempted. Once this can be performed in an amiable fashion, a piece of cloth wrapped around the finger is incorporated. From this point, appropriate oral hygiene products can gradually be substituted for the tuna water and a small feline tooth brush for the cloth.

There are many therapeutic oral hygiene products on

the market, from solutions to pastes. For routine daily to twice weekly use, any of the nonfluoride products may be selected. Frequency of use must be adapted to the degree of oral disease and the ability and commitment of the owner. The use of fluoride gels in the treatment of CLLs is common. Stannous fluoride (0.4%) gels such as Gel Kam (Gel Kam Corp., Dallas, TX) and QyGel (Veterinary Products Laboratories, Phoenix, AZ) are some of the more effective and popular. The use of fluoride in the mouth should be regulated closely by the practitioner, to minimize effects on body systems from long-term ingestion. Generally only a small amount of gel should be applied to the teeth once weekly.

Tooth Fractures (Traumatic Dental Injuries)

Traumatic injuries to the teeth are common in the cat,[4] usually due to external trauma if the teeth are otherwise healthy. These occur primarily in male cats living outside.[4] The canine teeth (cuspids) have the highest incidence of this type of trauma, and the fractures are usually horizontal. Pulpal exposure is common but does not occur in every case. If the pulp canal is exposed by the break, signs of pain and discomfort may be demonstrated but seldom persist longer than a few days. Cats do not generally have the same chewing habits as dogs, so fractures due to occlusal trauma are less likely.[31] Additionally, metal crowns may be appropriate to avert further deterioration of remaining dental structure, restore function, or improve the oral appearance.[32]

When teeth are diseased, occlusal activity can commonly cause dental fractures. The majority of problems of this nature are associated with teeth affected by cervical line lesions. Most of these animals demonstrate signs of discomfort in advanced CLL disease, often for some time before the tooth fractures (see Cervical Line Lesions).

Clinical Signs

If the fracture does not expose the pulp chamber or injure the pulp directly, few or no signs of discomfort normally occur. Should the pulp be exposed, bacterial contamination occurs, resulting in pulpitis and the eventual death and necrosis of the pulp. Degradation of the pulp spreads to the apical structures through the delta or foramen opening. Eventually, periapical abscessation or cyst formation occurs, leading to resorption of supporting bone and possibly the root apex.[5] Abscess formation at the apex may or may not fistulate into the oral cavity or facial surface with purulent drainage. Exophthalmos may be observed in some cases of abscessation involving the maxillary premolars. With time, the loss of supporting structures typically results in the loss of the tooth.

With an acute episode of pulp exposure, discomfort is common and lasts from 1 to 7 days. Pawing at the mouth, drooling, and reluctance to eat are clinically observed in many cases.[5] Visually, the fracture appears pink or a red dot indicating the acutely exposed pulp may be apparent, in contrast to the dark spot in the center of the fracture in a chronic exposure. A periodontal explorer, endodontic explorer, or an endodontic pathfinder should be used to palpate for the open canal if canal exposure is suspected because visual inspection may be inconclusive. Some canal exposures and periapical pathology can only be diagnosed radiographically. A fracture or traumatized tooth without canal exposure can still result in pulpitis from the trauma to vascular structures, thermal irritation, or bacteria migrating through open dentinal tubules.

Diagnosis

Visual examination, palpation, and radiography are the primary diagnostic tools used to detect dental fractures. Most cases are discovered during oral examination by visual assessment. It must be determined whether or not the pulp cavity is open and if irreversible pulpitis has occurred. If a pink or bleeding pulp is seen, acute exposure has occurred; recent injuries (only several hours old) may indicate the possibility of the tooth still being vital. If an open central area is seen and dark material is exposed, chronic exposure has occurred and the tooth is nonvital.

When the fracture appears deep but the pulp cavity cannot be seen because of a small opening, a pathfinder or periodontal explorer can be used to physically palpate and probe for the opening. This may require sedation or anesthesia in some animals if the lesion is still painful or if the animal is fractious. The tooth should also be digitally palpated to check for looseness, which may indicate considerable loss of bony support, fractures involving the roots or supporting bone, or inflammation within the alveolus.

Radiology is the third part of the examination triad. Standard radiographs of the entire oral cavity can be diagnostic, but intraoral films can greatly enhance diagnostic capabilities by better isolation of the suspected tooth or teeth. Radiographs allow examination of the tooth for root fractures, apical root resorption, widening of the periodontal ligament, periapical bone loss, densities at the apex, and radiolucencies at the apex, indicating possible abscess or cyst formation. Should complete endodontic therapy (root canal) be initiated, radiographs are a necessity to determine correct file working-length and master file depth and to verify correct fill. Without radiographs, the fill may be short or the apex perforated by the file.

Intraoral films can be used with standard radiographic units, but positioning is greatly simplified with a dental radiographic unit. Intraoral films are available in many sizes. The DF 54, DF 56, and DF 58 are the films most useful in feline intraoral radiography. Most exposures are taken using the bisecting angle technique.[33] This is done to obtain as correct an image as possible within the cat's mouth. Once the film is in place, the angle between the tooth and the film is bisected. The radiographic beam is oriented to intersect this bisecting line at a 90° angle. Using a standard radiographic unit, the technique uses 7.5 to 10 mAs at 50 to 60 kvp, with a focal distance of 40 cm (10 to 12 inches) from machine to film.[1,29] Dental films can be processed in standard developing and fixing solutions, in automatic processors attached (taped) to a larger film, or by using rapid dental developer and fixer solutions in a chair-side developer or in small containers in the darkroom.

Treatment: Chipped Tooth with No Canal Exposure (Vital)

Most of these go untreated in general practice and may never have serious complications, however, fractures should be smoothed when possible to reduce plaque and calculus accumulation and to prevent self-trauma by the ragged edges. This is done with a bullet or egg-shaped 12-fluted burr, a heatless, white stone burr, a diamond burr, or even a simple crosscut-type burr on a high or low speed dental handpiece. The dentinal tubules are sealed to prevent bacterial migration. The use of a true dentinal sealer and conditioner such as Tenure (Den Mat Corp., Santa Maria, CA) or an application of a thin-layer cavity varnish such as a copal varnish with fluoride is recommended. The area must first be cleaned and dried before varnish is applied. With a small brush or cotton swab, briskly coat the area lightly with the varnish and allow it to dry. Application of several coats is preferable.

Treatment: Fractured Tooth with Acute Pulpal Exposure

Once this condition is diagnosed, there are four appropriate treatment modalities: extraction, pulpotomy, complete endodontic therapy (root canal), or a crown following a root canal. Selection of treatment plan must be based on the clinician's experience and equipment available.[5]

Extraction. Extraction (exodontia) is the treatment of choice in fractures of most incisors, premolars, and molars. The canine tooth should be extracted if the fracture line extends subgingivally or if excessive structural damage has occurred.[4] Before extraction teeth should be radiographed to determine any complicating factors such as ankylosed roots. In most cases, these teeth will require root pulverization with a high-speed dental handpiece. Numbers 1/2, 1, 2, and 4 round-ball burrs, especially the number 2, are useful in pulverization. Teeth with healthy root structures are much easier to remove. The epithelial attachment is first severed with an elevator or number 11 blade. Multirooted teeth are sectioned with a dental handpiece into their corresponding rooted section; it is best to extract single-rooted sections. The 699L tapered crosscut burr is most often used for sectioning feline teeth. The elevator is placed into the gingival sulcus and lightly twisted back and forth as it is pressed forward. The process is continued around the tooth's circumference until the tooth section becomes loose and can be easily removed with an extracting forceps. Extracting forceps should not be used forcibly, as this usually results in a fractured tooth structure. Once the tooth has been removed, the socket is curetted and bony prominences or spicules reduced, in order to simplify closure. A simple gingival flap is used to cover the extraction site. Absorbable suture material in simple, interrupted sutures with large bites is recommended to diminish chances of dehiscence.

Occasionally cuspids and other teeth that are not ankylosed may need additional root exposure to ease extraction. This is accomplished by creating releasing incisions just beyond the proximal gingiva and down the facial gingival surface and alveolar mucosa to the approximate extent of the root structure. The gingiva is reflected with a number 2 Molt periosteal elevator to uncover the buccal cortical bone plate lateral to the root(s). A 699L burr is used to cut through the bone plate on both sides of the root structure. The plate is elevated away from the surface of the tooth with the Molt. If the plate is not elevated excessively, it may remain attached at the uncut apical border, which facilitates replacement. The tooth is rolled out laterally with a dental elevator, such as a 301 apical or a number 2 Molt. Removal of the lower cuspids may cause the tongue to protrude from the mouth in some cats. Additionally, if the empty socket of the upper cuspid is not filled with an osteogenic or osteoconductive material (tricalcium phosphate, ADD [Osmed Inc., Costa Mesa, CA], and hydroxyapatite) and the flap is not properly closed, the socket may collapse. This occasionally results in an alteration in facial features, objectionable to some owners.

Pulpotomy. A pulpotomy is performed in an attempt to maintain the vitality of a tooth fractured less than 4 to 6 hours previously (Fig. 33–8). This is done by stimulating odontoblasts to bridge secondary dentin over the exposure, thereby sealing the pulp. The pulpotomy must be examined later because a high percentage of these eventually fail and require complete endodontic treatment or extraction.[34] For this reason, many practitioners prefer to do a complete root canal initially.

Feline teeth are small and, in many cases, do not easily lend themselves to pulpotomy. First, some pulp material is removed to provide access for the cavity preparation materials. A number 1/2- to number 2-round burr on a low- or high-speed handpiece is used to excavate canal pulp contents to the level of the cementoenamel junction of the pulp chamber. Bleeding is not unusual and normally can be controlled using a dry paper point inserted with gentle pressure. If the pulp continues to bleed over 5 minutes, it has

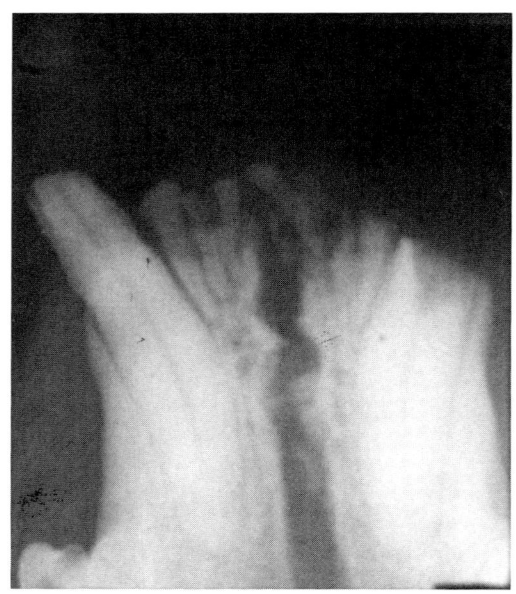

Figure 33–8. **Radiograph of fractured lower cuspids with pulp exposure.**

probably proceeded to irreversible pulpitis, and extraction or complete endodontics is warranted.[29]

Once the access is made, calcium hydroxide powder (USP) is placed to stimulate the dentinal bridging.[29] Its high pH is antibacterial, and it lightly irritates the pulp, stimulating the odontoblasts to cover the area with secondary reparative dentin. The powder can be placed into the canal with the aid of a small spatula or an amalgam carrier. It is gently packed against the pulp with a sterile plugger or similar blunt-ended probe. It should not be packed tightly, as excessive pressure on the pulp can result in necrosis.

Dycal (Caulk Densply, Milford, DE), a calcium hydroxide based paste catalyst, is placed over the calcium hydroxide powder. A small amount of each of the two pastes is mixed together on a pad and placed into the canal with a pitch placer or other blunt instrument. The mixture hardens within a few minutes so it must be placed quickly. Exposure to moisture results in a faster setting time. Some of the Dycal can be removed if necessary to make room for closure of the access opening with a type II or III glass ionomer or a composite restorative; however, the latter will adhere to enamel but not to dentin or cementum.

Root Canal. A complete endodontic or root canal procedure is performed to maintain or retain an endodontically compromised tooth.[4] In domestic cats, this is usually the canine or cuspid teeth.

Access to the canal can normally be made through the open canal at the fracture site, due to minimal curvature of the root system as compared with the dog. Radiographs are taken at four intervals during the procedure: the survey film, working length film, master file film, and master cone film.

The scout or survey film is taken to check for radicular and periradicular pathology prior to the procedure.[8] The smallest file available (size 8, 10, 15, or pathfinder) is inserted into the access opening of the canal. Coating the file with Premier RC Prep (Medical Products Laboratories, Philadelphia, PA) will facilitate file movement. The file is moved in a simple up and down shallow motion to clean and enlarge the canal opening. The file is removed, and a barbed broach gently placed into the canal and rotated 180° to entangle the pulp material. The file is slowly removed with the pulp. On occasion, this step must be repeated to remove necrotic or friable pulp, and in some cases, the pulp will have to be removed with the files during instrumentation. Once the pulp has been removed, the file is reinserted (with an endostop marker on the file) and pressed into the canal until a stricture is felt with the tactile sense of the file. The second radiograph is taken with the file in place in the canal to confirm proper working length. The endostop (a small piece of rubber) is adjusted down the file to the level of the access opening before removing the file from the canal. The distance from the endostop to the file tip can be measured and recorded. Endostops should be placed on all the other files to be used at this predetermined working length. This ensures that all files reach full working length in debriding the canal and do not perforate through the apex. The canal is systematically enlarged with the files. The file, coated in RC Prep, is placed at or near the working length and moved in a push–pull action until it reaches full working length and moves freely within the canal. K-type files and reamers can also be used in a rotary fashion to facilitate the process. Between each change of file size, the canal should be flushed or irrigated to remove debris. These files should be inserted, rotated only a quarter turn, and removed. Too much rotation can result in a broken file tip. The two irrigants commonly used are full- or half-strength bleach (5.5% or 2.6% sodium hypochlorite) and normal sterile saline. The authors routinely use the half-strength sodium hypochlorite to reduce chances of periapical inflammatory response should small amounts pass through the apical foramen. The irrigants are introduced into the canal with a 3-cc syringe and 25- or 27-gauge needle. The needle should not occlude the entire orifice; solution must be able to flow back around the needle to flush debris from the canal. The bleach is used first, as it aids in dissolving organic material and helps sterilize the canal, and this is immediately followed by the saline solution. If there is any indication of a root fracture, open apex, or other pathology that would allow an irrigant to flow out of the tooth into the periradicular tissue, *bleach should not be used.* In these cases, use only saline as the irrigant and rely on the RC Prep to aid in sterilization of the canal. Once clean, white filings are returned when the file has a firm fit, master file size has been reached. A third radiograph should be taken with the master file at full depth to confirm proper instrumentation (Fig. 33–9). The master canal size and depth should be noted on the patient record.

The canal should receive its final saline irrigation and

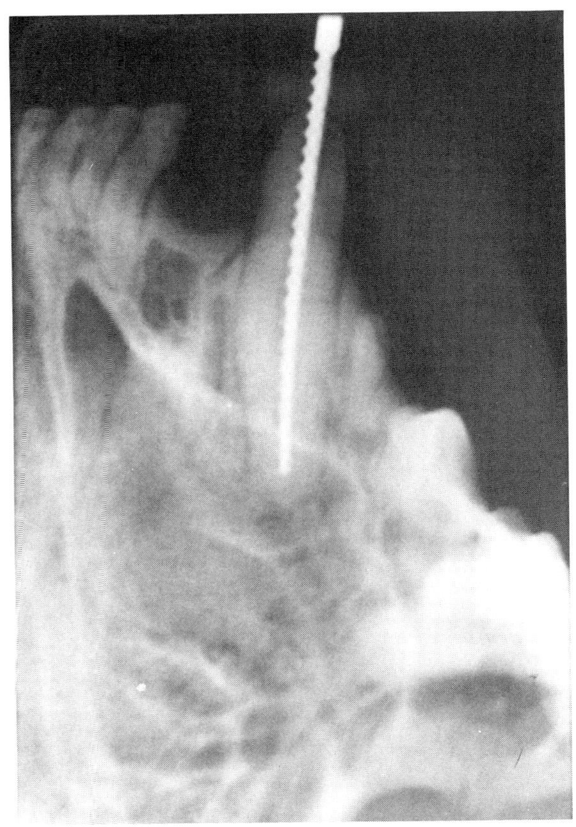

Figure 33–9. **Radiograph of master file to full working length.**

then be dried, by first aspirating excess fluid with the syringe as the needle is withdrawn. *Do not attempt to blow dry the canal by forcing air in with the syringe; this can result in air being forced out the apex and into the adjacent vessels, leading to air emboli.* Once excess moisture is removed, absorbent paper points can be introduced into the canal to complete the drying process.

Obturation of the canal with a positive seal concludes the root canal procedure. The most common dental sealer cements currently used in feline dentistry are the ZOE (zinc oxide and eugenol) types. The zinc oxide powder is mixed with the eugenol liquid with a small spatula on a glass slab or mixing pad. The consistency preferred is one that allows a string of the cement to stretch approximately 1 inch before breaking. The sealer cement is placed in the canal with a spiral filler or simply with the master file. The tip of the master file is dipped into the cement and is inserted full depth into the canal. It is rapidly rotated counterclockwise as it is removed to coat the apical third of the canal. Gutta-percha points can be used as the core material. A gutta-percha point the same size as the master file is placed to the full depth of the canal. Endodontic spreaders may be inserted into the canal beside the gutta-percha point and gently pressed toward the apex while slightly rotating the spreader back and forth. Once space is made with the spreader, an auxiliary gutta-percha point is inserted into this space and the procedure repeated until no new points can be placed. The tooth is radiographed once again to verify a good fill (Fig. 33–10). The excess gutta-percha is removed using a flat instrument heated to melt the material even with the tooth. A small round or pear-shaped burr can be used to make an undercut in the access site for placement of the final restorative material, such as a composite.

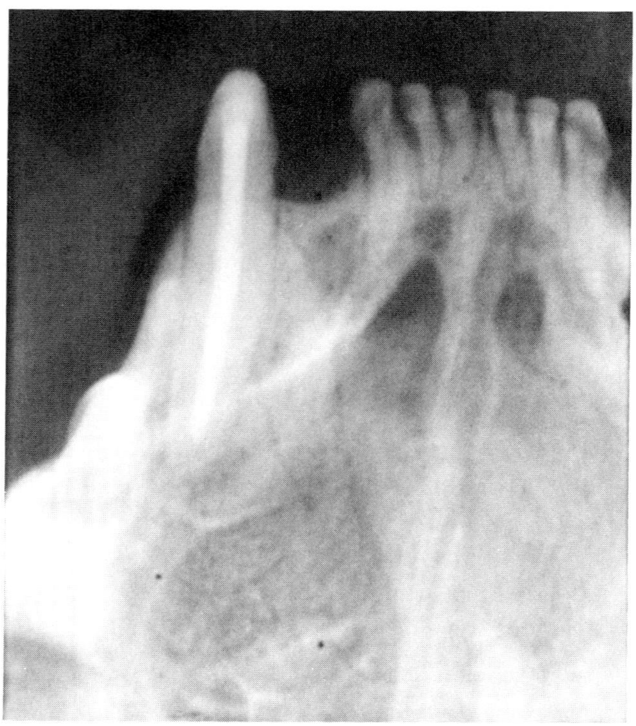

Figure 33–10. **Radiograph of completed ZOE–gutta-percha obturation.**

Crown. Endodontically treated teeth gradually become brittle with time and, therefore, may be at higher risk for further damage.[32] Even teeth not endodontically compromised that have fractures may benefit from restoration of function. Furthermore, some clients may request such purely for aesthetic reasons. Currently, only the cuspid (canine) teeth have had crown work performed.

Gold and high noble metals have demonstrated superb biocompatability in the feline.[32] These metals have good working characteristics and excellent strength. Little work has been done with porcelain jackets or ceramometal crowns in the cat because of the bulky size. Cemented crowns can be lost for various reasons.

A minimum of 6 mm of good tooth structure above the gumline is required to retain a crown properly. Little crown preparation is required or prudent for the cuspid in the cat—only undercuts and unsupported structure should be removed. Standard crown preparation with margins can lead to excessive structural reduction and compromised strength. A high-speed dental handpiece and a crown preparation diamond burr are routinely used, although a crosscut-type burr can be used. Teeth with vertical fractures greater than one-third the width of the tooth or extending more than 3 to 4 mm below the gumline are structurally compromised, and extraction is usually the treatment of choice. Crown lengthening procedures can be performed on some teeth to enhance the tooth's acceptability for crowning. This is done by making four releasing incisions around the tooth and connecting them circumferentially within the sulcus. Full thickness mucoperiosteal flaps are reflected using a number 2 Molt periosteal elevator to expose the tooth root. A slow-speed burr, preferably, or rongeurs can be used to remove the bone 2 to 4 mm below the apical extent of the fracture. The flaps can be closed with absorbable suture material at this apically repositioned location. Undercuts should be smoothed. The canine tooth has a natural taper or bevel that allows a crown to be drawn easily onto the tooth in most cases. Ideally, all sides of the tooth should taper toward the axial plane by approximately 6°.

Impressions of the tooth structure for the dental laboratory to make models and construct the crown should be made with a polysiloxane impression material, which provides excellent detail, remains stable for long periods of time, resists distortion, and demonstrates little or no shrinkage. If the practitioner plans to pour his or her own models, an improved type III dental stone, such as Die Keen (Columbus Dental Co., St. Louis, MO) should be used. Additional full upper and lower impressions (standard alginate is often adequate) and models with articulation marked or with a bite registration of wax or polysiloxane must accompany the individual crown work. Initially, attempt to work with dental laboratories currently providing veterinary dental services, and consult with them prior to undertaking such an enterprise to reduce confusion and complications.

Malocclusions

Malocclusions are not common in most breeds of domestic cats.[4] This is probably due in part to the limited variation in skull and jaw types in comparison to dogs. The classical scissor bite is the correct occlusion of the domestic cat, with the lower incisors fitting slightly behind the uppers and the lower canine teeth fitting between the upper corner incisor and the upper canine teeth. Even the brachycephalic feline breeds maintain this proper occlusal pattern. Persians, with their brachycephalic head types, are the breed that most frequently develop malocclusions,[4] due in part to the lack of proper dental interlock between the canine and incisor teeth, allowing variables to occur during development. A portion of these malocclusions has been attributed to hereditary involvement.[4] Malocclusion can also develop due to various oral traumas or retained deciduous teeth.[35] Ethics should always be considered if orthodontic treatment is to be used.

Clinical Signs

Often malocclusions are observed as early as 5 to 7 weeks (Fig. 33–11), even prior to full eruption of the deciduous dentition. In brachygnathic or overjut individuals (mandible shorter than maxilla), it is common for the lower canine teeth to contact other teeth, the hard palate, or the gingiva. This trauma may result in excessive dental wear or periodontal disease.[4] In prognathia, with an underjutting jaw (mandible longer than maxilla), the anteriorly displaced lower canine teeth may injure the lips, hold the lips open, or disrupt normal lip function and occlusion.[5] In the brachycephalic breeds with prognathia, the most probable cause is a retrusive maxilla.

Another form of malocclusion is wry mouth, the misalignment of the central midline of the upper and lower incisors.[8] Usually noticeable in the young patient, it results from the disproportionate growth of one or the four quadrants of the oral cavity, leading to asymmetrical growth patterns in the skull and jaws. In some cases, an open bite may result from occlusal interference; in others, protrusion of one of the lower canines from under the lip may cause ulceration of the lip (see Wry Mouth).[8]

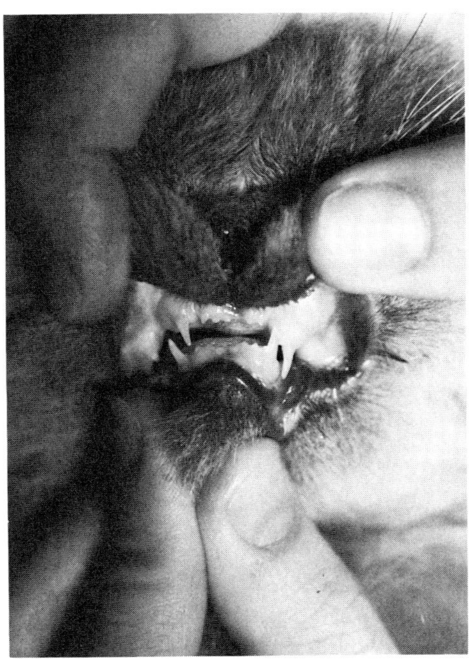

Figure 33–11. Malocclusion evident in young cat.

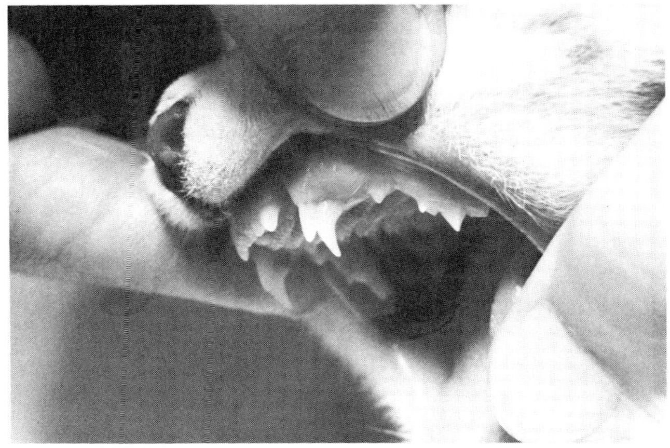

Figure 33–12. Retained upper deciduous cuspid with permanent tooth erupting rostrally to correct position.

Supernumerary and missing teeth sometimes affect occlusion. Supernumerary teeth often result in crowding and misalignment of the teeth,[35] often accompanied by resulting periodontal disease. Missing teeth may result in changes in the occlusion during the growth stages. Lack of appropriate interlock can lead to misalignment and drifting of teeth into abnormal positions.

When the deciduous teeth are retained, the permanent teeth are deflected lingually with the exception of the maxillary canine teeth, which are deflected rostrally (Fig. 33–12). Rostrally displaced canine teeth in the cat frequently result in traumatic occlusion with the lower canine teeth, shown by excessive wear or displacement of the lower canines.

The clinical manifestations of acquired malocclusions are as varied as the trauma that induces them. Jaw fracture repairs that do not address proper occlusion during reduction can result in successful stabilization but abnormal tooth position with serious complications (see Chapter 52). Electrical burns, tooth avulsions, temporomandibular dislocations, symphyseal fractures, as well as other physical trauma, appear to be the most common causes.[29]

Prognathic Malocclusions

Persians and other felines with brachycephalic head types are more prone to this type of malocclusion. There are two basic treatment stages in accordance with the developmental stages of the malocclusion. In the young kitten with deciduous teeth and a malocclusion, interceptive orthodontics is the only course of action that may aid in the correction of the problem. Interceptive orthodontics is the selective extraction of teeth in hopes of relieving a developing orthodontic problem. The permanent teeth tend to follow the path of the deciduous teeth, if still present. Therefore, the removal of deciduous teeth involved in a malocclusion allows the permanent teeth to follow an alternative path, hopefully of a normal occlusal pattern. Furthermore, if an early deciduous malocclusion causes the upper incisors to be located behind the lower incisors (anterior crossbite), the resulting interlock may prevent the maxilla from growing to its full potential length. Extraction of the upper incisors will not necessarily change the genetic capacity of the jaw length, but it will remove any impedance the interlock may have caused in disrupting its growth pattern.

In Persians with malocclusions, it is common to use interceptive orthodontics as early as six weeks of age. The earlier treatment is begun, the better chances of improvement. Selective extractions only a few days or weeks prior to the eruption of the permanent teeth results in a reduced likelihood of movement toward normal patterns. Extractions of deciduous teeth should be done carefully and gently. Pressure or trauma by instruments or inflammation due to swelling or blood by-products can result in injury or alteration to the permanent tooth buds. These usually demonstrate themselves when permanent teeth erupt by displaying discoloration and enamel hypoplasia-type lesions in the teeth in the immediate area of extraction. In some cases, when trauma is severe, the tooth bud will not erupt due to resorption or will erupt in grossly abnormal locations.

In older prognathic animals with the permanent dentition fully erupted, the treatment option is different. In a majority of cases, the protruding lower canine teeth hold open the lips or cause trauma to them. Occasionally tooth-to-tooth trauma is involved causing attrition, periodontal disease, or dental movements. Treatment usually proceeds in one of three directions: exodontia (extraction), orthodontia (tooth movement), or endodontia (crown amputation and pulp capping).[5,8] Exodontia is the removal of the offending tooth and the common treatment choice (see Extraction).

Orthodontically, many cases are treated with a combination of direct bond buttons and power chains.[6] Small, base-direct bond buttons are often attached with the aid of orthodontic bonding adhesives to the teeth. Buttons are placed on the lower canine teeth to be moved, approximately half way up the labial aspect (toward the lip), and on the lingual (toward the tongue) aspect of the ipsilateral lower first molars near the neck of the tooth. The power chain is attached to the two buttons and tightened only one notch initially. Orthodontic movement of teeth should be slow and gradual to prevent damage to the periodontal structures and dental circulation. The chain can be tightened one notch at a time as appropriate progress occurs. Once the desired movement has been attained, the power chain should be left in place in a dead pull position (without tension) to act as a retainer until the tooth becomes stable in its new occlusal pattern. Orthodontia is the movement of teeth and not the lengthening or shortening of a jaw. Actual jaw lengths are not changed in treatment, and teeth cannot be moved to unsupported sites. Abnormal jaw lengths sometimes necessitate genetic counseling.

In other cases, endodontia in the form of crown amputation, pulpotomy, and pulp capping may be the treatment of choice.[6] In this surgical endodontic procedure the crowns of teeth that were initiating an orally disruptive condition are removed. This is generally accomplished with a low-speed dental handpiece and a diamond disc or a high-speed dental handpiece and a carbide burr. In performing this process, the pulp cavity is normally exposed. A pulpotomy, removal of a small amount of the pulp, and a pulp capping procedure are required. Failure to address the exposed pulp results in endodontic infection and associated complications (see Pulpotomy). The pulp is capped with a combination of calcium hydroxide, sealers, and restoratives. These should be monitored because some endodontic failures are to be expected in any species.[34]

Brachygnathic Malocclusions

In brachygnathia the maxillary dental arcade overshoots the mandibular arcade. This can result in the canine teeth of the shorter mandible producing damage to the soft tissues of the hard palate or associated periodontal structures (Fig. 33–13).[5] Genetics may be involved in these conditions, and reproductive counseling is encouraged. In early stages in which the deciduous teeth have just erupted, interceptive orthodontics may help the condition. This generally entails the selective extraction of the lower deciduous canine and

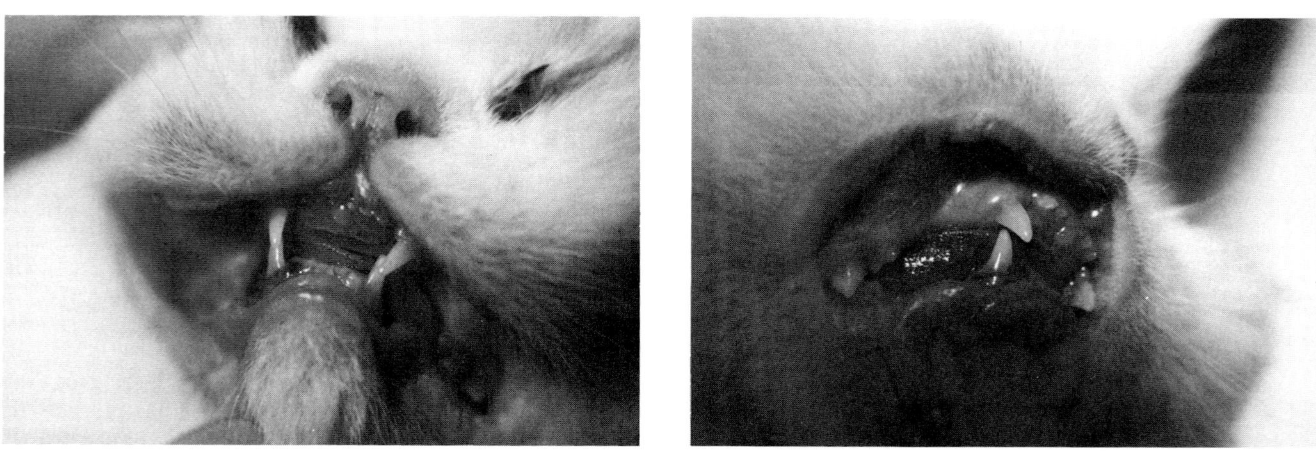

A B

Figure 33–13. (*A*) Brachygnathic malocclusion in a Persian. (*B*) Side view showing lower cuspid traumatizing upper cuspid.

incisor teeth that are interlocking in an improper manner. As always, care should be exercised in extractions to reduce the chances of damage to the permanent tooth buds. Interceptive orthodontics will not resolve all cases, and a substantial number of these will not improve, requiring additional treatment once the permanent teeth have erupted.

In therapy of adult cats with brachygnathic malocclusions, the three basic treatment regimens are exodontia, endodontia, and orthodontia, with exodontia being the extraction of offending teeth. Endodontia entails crown amputation and pulp capping of the same teeth. Orthodontia is a more time-consuming process and customarily only used to initiate movement if only one of the upper canine teeth is involved in traumatic malocclusion. Arch bars attached to the upper third and fourth premolars and unaffected canine tooth are used as a base for the use of elastics to attach to the canine tooth desired for movement. Generally a dental laboratory produces the appliance for most practitioners. Only a posterior or distal orthodontic movement of the lower canine teeth is possible in most cases, using direct bond brackets and power chains. This can provide some benefit on occasion, but more often is of little advantage.

Wry Mouth

Wry mouth is a skeletal malocclusion in which one or more of the four quadrants of the jaws is growing or in which one has grown disproportionately to the others. The result is that the midlines of the arcades do not align properly. Facial disfigurement is common, with a twisted or crooked appearance of the lower jaw or maxilla and nose. Genetics are a consideration in these animals.[4] Treatment is purely symptomatic to provide as functional a bite as possible. Selective extractions or crown amputations and pulp capping is frequently the treatment of choice, although many cases require no intervention.

Deciduous Teeth

In cases of retained deciduous teeth, two rules apply. First, if there is no permanent counterpart as confirmed radiographically and if the tooth is causing no pathology, leave it in place. Second, if there is a permanent counterpart, extract the deciduous tooth as soon as the permanent has begun eruption into the oral cavity.[6] No two teeth should be allowed to contend for the same space, as only crowding and malocclusion will occur.

Congenital Disorders

Congenital abnormalities occur in the cat but are uncommon.[31] Malocclusions are discussed in detail previously in this chapter. Variations in the number of teeth occur frequently, as shown by a recent survey.[4] In conditions of supernumerary teeth, there are two treatment choices. If the additional tooth is causing no pathology, it can be left in place. Should the tooth be evoking a disease process, such as crowding, periodontal disease, or malocclusion, extraction should be considered at the earliest possible opportunity.[5] Missing teeth seldom cause problems with the cat, although occlusion is affected in some cases. The domestic feline copes well without teeth; therefore, missing teeth are of no major consequence, except for aesthetics, showing, and breeding purposes. Anodontia, the total lack of any teeth, has been reported in a young adult cat.[36] Fusion teeth arise from two tooth buds merging together during development. Teeth of this nature are rarely a problem. Alternatively, gemination teeth are the consequence of a single tooth bud attempting to divide into two teeth (twinning effect) (Fig. 33–14). These teeth occasionally precipitate crowding in the arch and periodically require extraction. Fusion and gemination teeth are observed infrequently. Supernumerary roots are sporadically encountered and sometimes in association with gemination teeth (Fig. 33–15).

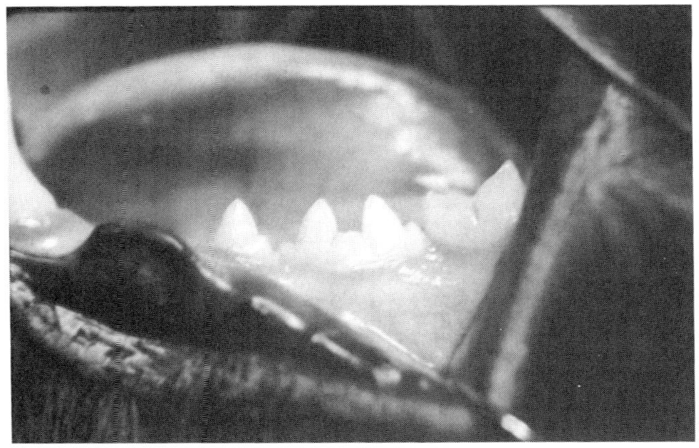

Figure 33–14. Gemination tooth.

Acquired Disorders

Acquired disorders of the teeth are common. Fractures, cervical line lesions, and malocclusions are discussed in detail earlier in this chapter. Enamel hypoplasia, with weak and thin enamel lesions varying from chalky white to tan or brown in color, is uncommon in the domestic cat. The lesions result from systemic or localized insult to the tooth bud during the enamel formation stage of tooth development. If treatment is undertaken, crowns and veneers are

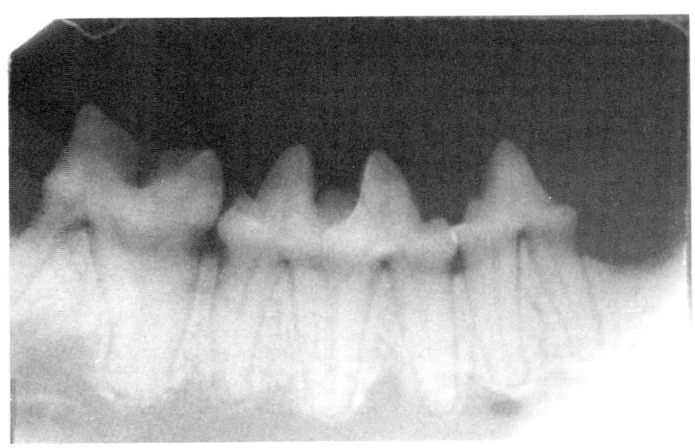

***Figure 33–15.* Radiograph of gemination tooth showing supernumerary roots.**

seldom appropriate for most of the teeth, and little can be done for incisors. The diseased enamel is scrubbed off the teeth with light pressure using a high-speed dental handpiece and a flame-shaped Roto Pro burr (Ellman International Mfg Co., Detroit, MI). Care should be taken not to remove excessive structure. The tooth surface is treated with an enamel and dentinal bonding agent, and an opaque pit and fissure sealant is applied. These teeth will require periodic treatment because the composite wears, chips, or deteriorates with time. Teeth of this nature typically show attrition and degeneration at an accelerated rate as compared with healthy dentition.

Tetracycline staining of the teeth is the result of ingestion or treatment with a tetracycline during the formative stage of the tooth buds, under 4 weeks of age for deciduous teeth and 4 weeks to 4 months for permanents. Discoloration of the teeth varies from light yellow, to dark orange, to gray-blue according to the type of tetracycline, amount, duration of administration, and exposure to light, which may gradually darken the color. In addition to the discoloration, dental structure may be compromised due to hypoplastic enamel formation caused by the original disease process treated by the antibiotic. No treatment is necessary or generally recommended for affected deciduous teeth, and permanent teeth are seldom treated. But, if the teeth are otherwise healthy, vital bleaching with 37% hydrogen peroxide and a dental bleaching unit can be undertaken with striking improvements in some cases.[37] Extreme care should be exercised in this process because of the risks to patient, practitioner, and assistants when using heating elements, high-intensity lights, acids, and caustic agents.[37]

REFERENCES

1. Burrows CF, Harvey CE. Oral Examination and Diagnostic Techniques. In: Harvey CE, ed. Veterinary Dentistry. Philadelphia: WB Saunders, 1985:23.
2. Gruffydd-Jones TJ, Evans RJ, Gaskell CJ. The Alimentary System. In: Pratt PW, ed. Feline Medicine. Santa Barbara, CA: American Veterinary Publishers, 1983:202.
3. Holzworth J, Stein BS. The Sick Cat. In: Holzworth J, ed. Diseases of the Cat. Philadelphia: WB Saunders, 1987:4.
4. Frost P, Williams CA. Feline dental disease. Vet Clin North Amer (Small Anim Pract) 1985;16:851.
5. Frost P. Feline Dentistry. In: Canine Dentistry, 3rd ed. Nabisco Compendium, 1990:60.
6. Lyons KF. An Approach to Feline Dentistry. Compend Cont Ed Pract Vet 1990;12:493.
7. West L. The enigma of feline dentition. J Vet Dent 1990;7(3):167.
8. Holmstrom SE. Feline Dentistry. In: Small Animal Dental Symposium. Am Anim Hosp Assoc Proc 1989;4:12.
9. Schenck GW, Osborn JW. Neck lesions in the teeth of cats. Vet Rec 1976;99:100.
10. Harvey CE. Dental disease in cat skulls acquired before 1960. Am Vet Dent College/Acad Vet Dent Forum 1990;11:41.
11. Joshua JO. The Clinical Aspects of Some Diseases of Cats. London: W. Heinemann, 1965:51.
12. Wilkinson GT. Diseases of the Cat. Oxford: Pergammon Press, 1966:47.
13. Okuda A, Harvey CE. Histopathological Findings of Features of Odontoclastic Resorptive Lesions in Cats Teeth with Periodontitis. Am Vet Dent College/Acad Vet Dent Forum 1991;9:141.
14. Reichert PA, Durr UM, Triadan H, Vickendey G. Periodontal disease in the domestic cat. J Periodont Res 1984;19:67.
15. Beard GB, Beard DM. Geriatric dentistry. Vet Clin North Amer (Small Anim Pract) 1989;19:67.
16. Eisner E. Chronic subgingival tooth erosion in cats. Vet Med 1989;84:378.
17. Johnesse JS, Hurvitz A. Feline plasmacell gingivitis/pharyngitis. J Am Anim Hosp Assoc 1983;19:179.
18. Thompson RR, Wilcox GE, Clark WT, Jansen KL. Association of calicivirus with chronic gingivitis and pharyngitis. J Small Anim Pract 1984;25:207.
19. Lyons KF. Feline dental disease—Classification and treatment. Vet Focus 1990;2(1):27.
20. Rossman LE, Garber DA, Harvey CE. Disorders of Teeth. In: Harvey CE, ed. Veterinary Dentistry. Philadelphia: WB Saunders, 1985:84.
21. Seltzer S, Sinai I, August D. Periodontal effects of root perforations before and during endodontic procedures. J Dent Res 1970;49:332.
22. Birkendahl-Hansen H. External root resorption caused by luxation of rat molars. Scand J Dent Res 1973;81:47.
23. Reichart PA, Althoff J, Eckhardt W, Rippel W. ^{224}Ra and ^{226}Ra experimentally induced dental changes in rats. J Oral Path 1979;8:157.
24. Von Schlup D. Epidemiologische und morphologische Untersuchungen am Kazengebib. I. Mitteilung: Epidemiologische Untersuchungen. Kleinterpraxis 1982;27:87.
25. Coles S. Prevalence of buccal cervical root resorptions in Australian cats. J Vet Dent 1990;7(4):14.
26. Hawkins BJ. Cervical line lesions (neck lesions) in the cat. Acad Vet Dent 1987:11.
27. Addy M, Dowell P. Dentine hypersensitivity—A review: Clinical and in-vitro evaluation of treatment agents. J Clin Periodontol 1983;10:351.
28. Emily P. Restoring cervical erosion lesions. Vet Forum 1988, Oct:22.
29. Emily P, Penman S. Handbook of Small Animal Dentistry. Oxford: Pergammon Press, 1990:55.
30. Hawkins BJ. Desensitization and treatment of feline cervical line lesions in the cat. World Vet Dent Congress 1990:28.
31. Sams DL, Harvey CE. Oral and Dental Diseases. In: Sherding RG, ed. The Cat—Diseases and Clinical Management. New York: Churchill Livingstone, 1989:875.
32. Grove TK. Functional and aesthetic crowns for dogs and cats. Vet Med Report 1990;85:409.
33. Emily P. Intraoral radiology. Vet Clin North Amer [Small Anim Pract] 1986;165:801.
34. Wiggs RB. Pulpotomy failure in a Rhesus monkey. J Vet Dent 1990;7(1):15.
35. Eisner E. Malocclusions in cats and dogs: Recognizing dental alignments. Vet Med 1988:83;1006.
36. Elzay RP, Hughes RD. Anodontia in a cat. J Am Vet Med Assoc 1969;154:667.
37. Wiggs RB. Bleaching vital teeth in canines. J Vet Dent 1988; 5(4):15.

CHAPTER 34

◇ ◇ ◇

Diabetes Mellitus

Gary D. Norsworthy

Diabetes mellitus (DM) is the second most common endocrine disease in the cat. It is a metabolic illness resulting from an absolute or relative insulin deficiency that is usually due to an age-related amyloid deposition in the pancreatic islet cells.[1] The most notable laboratory finding in DM is hyperglycemia, although it is not a life-threatening component of this disease. The seriously ill diabetic cat suffers from a group of potentially fatal complications that includes fluid, electrolyte, and acid-base balance disturbances.

DM occurs in two syndromes. *Uncomplicated DM* is relatively easily controlled with insulin or oral hypoglycemic drugs and dietary restrictions. *Complicated DM* requires extensive hospitalization and intensive care because it is accompanied by severe metabolic derangements that result in ketoacidosis, electrolyte abnormalities, depression, or death. Although these syndromes are distinct, the former may turn into the latter as the blood glucose level rises and as time passes.

Some cases of uncomplicated DM are a challenge to regulate because of the unique characteristics of the feline form of this disease, which are discussed later. The long-term complications that frequently occur in humans (e.g., retinopathy, glomerulopathy, neuropathy, and vascular disease) rarely occur in cats.[2]

History and Clinical Findings

The classic clinical signs of DM are polydipsia, polyuria, polyphagia, and weight loss. These may develop rather slowly, so that the owner is not aware of their severity until they are quite advanced. For example, upon presentation to the veterinarian, the cat may show a profound weight loss. Many such cats remain relatively stable until a concomitant disease process occurs. The stress of the second disease may cause the cat to exhibit a variety of clinical signs not typically associated with DM, such as anorexia, dyspnea, coughing, lethargy, vomiting, diarrhea, dysuria, or weakness.[3] Diseases such as cardiomyopathy, cystitis, pancreatitis, and hepatic lipidosis are often the stressors that complicate DM.

The findings on physical examination are nonspecific. In early DM, obesity is often present; in advanced DM, often the cat is very thin. Icterus and dehydration may be seen. An uncommon finding is diabetic neuropathy, which can cause a diabetic cat to walk with a plantigrade posture (Fig. 34–1).

A recent epizootiologic study of diabetic cats revealed that the risk factors for this disease are a higher body weight (greater than 6.8 kg), advanced age (greater than 10 years), the male gender, and neutering; Thus, the "typical" diabetic is an old, fat, neutered male cat.[5]

Differential Diagnosis

A diagnosis of DM should be considered in any cat exhibiting all or most of the four classic clinical signs. However, other feline diseases may cause these same abnormalities. For example, weight loss accompanied by a normal or increased appetite may also be associated with hyperthyroidism or primary gastrointestinal disease, especially lymphosarcoma and inflammatory bowel disease.[2,6] Similarly, hyperadrenocorticism and acromegaly may cause insulin antagonism, resulting in the clinical signs of DM. Although these conditions are rare in the cat, they should be considered, especially if the signs are very difficult to regulate with insulin. Renal disease can lead to polydipsia, polyuria, and weight loss, and liver disease can produce weight loss. Because DM and several other diseases share these clinical signs, it is essential to include a biochemical profile in the diagnostic evaluation.

Transient Hyperglycemia

The cat's fight-or-flight mechanism is highly refined. When a cat senses danger, a chain of physiologic events occurs to

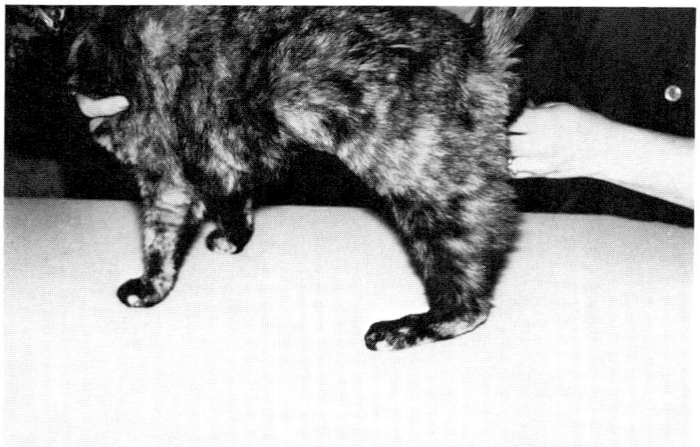

Figure 34–1. **Diabetic neuropathy is an uncommon finding in DM that causes a cat to walk with a plantigrade posture.**

prepare for self-preservation. Stress and excitement cause the release of epinephrine, resulting in a sudden release of glucose from the liver and a simultaneous inhibition of insulin utilization at the cellular level.[7]

A routine trip to the veterinary hospital is often enough to cause a physiologic hyperglycemia. Consider the following scenario: The cat is awakened and placed in a pet carrier, which signals a trip to either the veterinary hospital or the boarding kennel. Then the cat is placed in the car—cats generally do not like the unsettling movement. On arrival at the veterinary hospital the cat's carrier is placed on the floor of a reception room near other dogs and cats.

The cat is then placed on a cold examination table, where the cat is palpated from head to tail; a thermometer is thrust into the cat's rectum. Finally, the cat is restrained for blood collection, and a needle pierces the skin of the foreleg or the neck.

From the time the cat is placed in the pet carrier until blood is drawn, as much as 1 hour may elapse. This allows adequate time for the cat's defensive mechanisms to activate and for physiologic hyperglycemia to develop.

There are other nondiabetic causes of hyperglycemia in the cat. These include:

- The administration of glucose-containing fluids, either intravenously or subcutaneously
- The administration of progestogens, notably megestrol acetate
- The administration of anticonvulsants, notably phenobarbital
- The administration of corticosteroids
- Estrus

Clinical Pathology

Persistent hyperglycemia, with the fasting blood glucose greater than 200 mg/dL, accompanied by glucosuria is the classic clinical pathologic finding in DM. Fat mobilization in the diabetic cat often results in lipemia. Fat deposition in the liver leads to hepatomegaly and mild or moderate elevations of alanine aminotransferase (ALT, formerly SGPT), alkaline phosphatase, and serum cholesterol. A small percentage of diabetic cats are icteric and thus have elevations in total bilirubin. Alterations in serum sodium and potassium may occur. The dehydration that occurs in some diabetic cats results in prerenal azotemia, hyperproteinemia, hyperalbuminemia, and an increase in the packed cell volume. Diabetic cats are predisposed to bacterial cystitis due to the presence of glucose in the urine. An examination of urine sediment or a urine culture may reveal bacteria.

Diagnosis

To be diagnosed with DM, the diabetic cat should be persistently hyperglycemic, with a fasting blood glucose greater than 200 mg/dL, and have glucosuria. Mild to moderate hyperglycemia is not pathognomonic of DM, because of the cat's susceptibility to stress- and drug-related hyperglycemia. The absence of glucosuria in an acutely stressed cat often signals transient hyperglycemia instead of DM.

In addition to hyperglycemia and glucosuria, the cat's history must reveal at least three of the four typical signs of polydipsia, polyuria, polyphagia, and weight loss.[2] This is another means of differentiating DM from transient hyperglycemia; its importance cannot be minimized.

Treatment

DM has three main forms: insulin-dependent diabetes mellitus (IDDM), also called Type I diabetes; non–insulin-dependent diabetes mellitus (NIDDM), also called Type II diabetes; and transient diabetes mellitus, a variant of Type I or Type II diabetes. IDDM is the classic form associated with a severe or absolute insulin deficiency. It is treated with exogenous insulin. NIDDM is treatable with dietary restrictions and oral hypoglycemic agents. Recent studies indicate that as many as 50% of diabetic cats may need exogenous insulin to survive, and as many as 35% may be responsive to oral hypoglycemic therapy.[8] Transient diabetes is treated with exogenous insulin on an as-needed basis accompanied by careful monitoring.

Successful treatment of diabetic cats requires the recognition of the IDDM versus the NIDDM form and recognition of the uncomplicated state versus the complicated, ketoacidotic state. Cats with the NIDDM form generally do not develop the complicated, ketoacidotic state.

Exogenous Injected Insulin

The cornerstone of treatment for most diabetic cats is exogenous insulin by injection. The veterinarian must understand the types of insulin available and their differences. Furthermore, the metabolism of each form of insulin varies greatly from one cat to the next. Published dosages are based on averages, and so the effects of insulin in any given cat should be documented with frequent blood glucose determinations.

Insulin is no longer available in the concentration of 40 U/mL. Since most cats require less than 10 units per dose, the clinician is strongly urged to dilute U-100 insulin 1:9 with an insulin diluent. However, diluted insulin has a refrigerated shelf life of 4 to 8 weeks. The insulin manufacturers (Eli Lilly and Novo Nordisk) will supply the appropriate diluents to the clinician, generally at no charge. These should be used instead of normal saline, because they have the correct pH, preservative, isotonic agent, and buffer. In addition, insulin diluted with normal saline has a shelf life of only 7 days. The owner should be closely instructed on the modified use of insulin syringes, since the insulin will now have a concentration of 10 U/mL. An alternative is the use of microdose insulin syringes. They are available in ⅓ and ½ cc sizes and calibrated in units according to the U-100 concentration. These syringes can be used to accurately measure in 1-unit increments.

Insulin Types by Length of Action

The action of *regular insulin* has an immediate onset when given subcutaneously or intramuscularly. It peaks in about 30 minutes and has a maximum duration of 6 hours. Regular insulin is indicated in the ketoacidotic cat with an extremely high blood glucose or with life-threatening hyperkalemia. Its use should be under conditions in which frequent blood glucose determinations can be made.[9] Commonly used products include Regular Insulin, Semilente, Novolin R, and Humulin R.

Intermediate-acting insulins have an onset of action in 30 to 60 minutes and reach a peak effect in 1 to 2 hours. They last 6 to 10 hours in most cats.[9] However, their effects are so brief that they are not suitable for most diabetic cats.[2] Commonly used products include NPH, Lente, Novolin L, Novolin N, Humulin L, and Humulin N.

Long-acting insulins have an onset in 1 to 3 hours. They peak in 1 to 8 hours and have a duration of 8 to 20 hours. These insulins are suitable for most diabetic cats.[9] Ultralente and Humulin U Ultralente are commonly used products.

Insulin Types by Source

Insulin can be extracted from the bovine and porcine pancreases. Some brands are from only one of these; other brands are from a combination of the two. Insulin may also be synthesized in a nonpathogenic laboratory strain of *Escherichia coli* that has been genetically altered by the addition of the human gene for insulin. This is known as human-derived insulin (Table 34–1).

Insulin Use by Owners

The practitioner must spend adequate time educating the owner so that therapeutic success is not jeopardized by an improper injection technique. Obtaining proper doses for the cat can be difficult because all forms of insulin are prepared in concentrations suitable for use in humans. Diluting insulin to 1:10 can make dosing much easier. Saline can be used for dilution purposes, but special diluting solutions are preferred. It is not recommended that diluted insulin be stored for longer than 8 weeks.[2] Vigorous shaking of insulin is prohibited on most insulin bottles. Although shaking has no effect on the efficacy of the drug,[10] the bubbles that result make accurate measurements difficult. The owner must be instructed to properly fill the syringes so air bubbles are not present. In addition, the owner must understand the meaning of the calibration marks on the side of the syringe.

Table 34–1. Comparison of Insulins

Trade Names	Origin	Manufacturer
Short Acting		
Regular Insulin	Pork	Novo Nordisk
Semilente	Beef	Novo Nordisk
Regular Purified Pork	Pork	Novo Nordisk
Semilente Purified Pork	Pork	Novo Nordisk
Novolin R	Human	Novo Nordisk
Humulin BR	Human	Lilly
Humulin R	Human	Lilly
Intermediate Acting		
NPH	Beef	Novo Nordisk
Lente	Beef	Novo Nordisk
Lente Purified Pork	Pork	Novo Nordisk
Novolin L	Human	Novo Nordisk
Novolin N	Human	Novo Nordisk
NPH Purified Pork	Pork	Novo Nordisk
Humulin L	Human	Lilly
Humulin N	Human	Lilly
Long Acting		
Ultralente	Beef	Novo Nordisk
Ultralente Iletin I	Beef/ Pork	Lilly
Humulin U Ultralente	Human	Lilly

Finally, the owner should be instructed in the proper subcutaneous injection technique at the preferred sites (neck or lumbar areas). If owner compliance or understanding seems to be a problem, it is helpful to have the individual come to the hospital with insulin, syringes, and needles for a demonstration of their injection technique.

Treatment of the Uncomplicated Form

Because we are currently unable to differentiate between Type I and Type II diabetics by laboratory tests, a trial of an oral hypoglycemic agent is currently recommended by this author. Glipizide (Glucotrol) is dosed initially at 5 mg orally b.i.d. accompanied by a high fiber diet (see below). After 2–4 days a fasting blood glucose is determined. If improvement from pretherapeutic levels is achieved, the drug is continued and the dose modified according to blood glucose levels. If no improvement occurs, insulin therapy is initiated.

Some authors recommend that the goal of insulin administration should be to keep the blood glucose between 100 mg/dL and 200 (maximum 250) mg/dL throughout each 24-hour period.[2] However, this is not easily achieved. Fortunately, most cats will be clinically normal even if the blood glucose peaks around 300 mg/dL. Attaining adequate regulation requires choosing the appropriate type of insulin, determining the correct dosage, and achieving the appropriate interval of administration.

The initial dose of insulin is generally 0.25 to 0.50 U/lb of body weight of Ultralente given once daily in the morning. The choice between 0.25 U/lb and 0.50 U/lb depends on the cat's blood glucose level. It should be administered for 2 to 3 days before the glucose curve is performed, if the cat's physical condition will permit a delay. Concurrently the cat is placed on a high-fiber diet.

A high-fiber diet can be a valuable part of treatment for the diabetic cat. Consumption of fiber delays carbohydrate (sugar) absorption from the digestive tract. This dampens the postprandial glycemia, which may be extreme. High-fiber diets also promote weight reduction in obese cats. The ideal diet contains greater than 15% fiber and slightly less than 50% complex carbohydrates. The following diets (available from Hill's Pet Products, Topeka, KS) are the most desirable; they are listed in order of preference[11]:

Dry Prescription Diet Feline r/d
Dry Prescription Diet Feline w/d
Dry Science Diet Feline Maintenance Light
Canned Prescription Diet Feline r/d
Canned Prescription Diet Feline w/d

Changing to one of the high-fiber diets is often met with resistance from the cat, because cats tend to become fixed on their diets. Since most diabetic cats are older, they are often particularly reluctant to change. A gradual diet change, by mixing the high-fiber diet with the cat's preferred diet, may be necessary. Some cats do not accept a high-fiber diet, so their management must be based on insulin administration. A diabetic must not eat any of the semi-moist foods, since they contain large amounts of sugar.

Treatment of the Complicated, Ketoacidotic Form

Treatment of the ketoacidotic cat can be very challenging. A number of the attendant disorders of body fluid, serum electrolyte, and major organ functions may be life-threatening. If misused, the drugs used in treatment can also be life-threatening. Therefore the following general rules should be observed[12]:

1. *Do not overtreat the patient.* Diabetics usually present with hyperglycemia, metabolic acidosis, dehydration, hyperosmolarity, and hypokalemia. If the cat is overtreated, hypoglycemia, iatrogenic metabolic alkalosis, overhydration, hypo-osmolarity, and/or hyperkalemia (or aggravated hypokalemia) can result.
2. *Do not regulate the patient too quickly.* Many of the drugs used are potentially detrimental. If the proper treatments are administered too quickly, they may kill the patient.
3. *Do not try to overregulate the patient.* It is not necessary to achieve constant euglycemia in animals with diabetes mellitus. It is better to allow the patient to be mildly hyperglycemic than to take a chance on life-threatening hypoglycemia.

Table 34–2. Estimation of Degree of Dehydration

7–8%	Skin becomes noticeably inelastic. Globe is slightly depressed into the orbit.
10–12%	Skin in markedly inelastic. Globe is noticeably depressed into the orbit.
12–15%	Shock begins. Death is imminent.

Treatment of the complicated, ketoacidotic patient must be tailored according to the results of complete biochemical profiling. There are so many possible complications associated with DM that treatment without a biochemical assessment of the patient is medically unacceptable. The following issues must be assessed and addressed.

Fluid Balance

Fluid therapy is an important aspect of treatment for seriously ill diabetics, especially those that are vomiting, anorectic, or dehydrated. Choosing a fluid that is isotonic and has approximately the same constituents as normal plasma water is best. A balanced electrolyte solution such as Ringer's solution or lactated Ringer's solution (LRS) is appropriate for nearly all situations involving complicated DM.

Proper fluid therapy should be appropriate for the patient's degree of dehydration, the daily maintenance requirement, and the contemporary loss related to DM. The calculated 24-hour amount should be provided steadily throughout the entire 24-hour period. Only if dehydration is severe should rapid infusion be considered. In this situation, the fluids should be provided rapidly at the beginning of therapy then slowed to last 24 hours.

Assessing the degree of dehydration should be made on the basis of skin turgor and mucous membrane moistness (Table 34–2). The packed cell volume and plasma protein level are not reliable indicators in diabetics because of the glucose-mediated hemodilution that occurs. The following formulas are used to determine the fluid volume appropriate for the first 24 hours:

Amount for rehydration

$$= \text{body weight (lb)} \times \%\ \text{dehydration} \times 500\ \text{mL}$$

plus

$$\text{Daily maintenance requirement} = 30\ \text{mL/lb}$$

plus

$$\text{Contemporary loss}^{*} = 20\text{–}25\ \text{mL/lb}$$

Sodium

Sodium controls the movement of intracellular and extracellular water; therefore, it can control its own concentration by determining surrounding water levels. However, in DM the regulatory mechanisms controlling the amount and concentration of plasma sodium and vascular volume may be overwhelmed by the osmotic effect of increased blood and urine glucose.

*Contemporary loss is the fluid loss due to the direct effects of DM.

If *hyponatremia* occurs it is generally dilutional hyponatremia directly related to the osmotic pull of glucose in the vascular space. Generally it is not severe enough to be life-threatening and corrects itself as the blood glucose returns to normal.

Hypernatremia is more serious than hyponatremia. Treatment consists of slow correction with an intravenous, isotonic-balanced electrolyte solution, such as LRS. Rapid correction with a hypotonic fluid should be avoided because of the danger of inducing fatal cerebral edema.

Potassium

Altered serum potassium concentrations affect the function of the muscles, including the myocardium. Hypokalemia may cause dramatic skeletal muscle weakness, complicating an already-weak patient. Hyperkalemia may also cause muscle weakness, notably affecting the myocardium. Cardiac arrhythmias may progress to atrial standstill, idioventricular rhythms, and complete asystole.

A diabetic in oliguric renal failure may experience *hyperkalemia*. This may be confirmed by electrocardiography (Table 34–3 and Fig. 34–2 *A* to *C*). Treatment consists of the administration of intravenous fluids and insulin. Normal saline is the fluid of choice, since it contains no potassium; however, the small amount of potassium in LRS also makes the latter very acceptable. The intravenous fluids serve to correct hyperkalemia by their dilutional effects and by promoting renal excretion. Insulin drives potassium intracellularly, especially in the liver and skeletal muscles. The treatment plan is as follows:

1. Administer Regular insulin at a dosage of 0.1 U/lb IM.
2. Check blood glucose in 1 hour; if it is above 250 mg/dL, repeat at 0.1 U/kg IM. Continue hourly monitoring and administration until the level falls below 250 mg/dL.[6]
3. At that time, administer NPH or Ultralente at 0.12 to 0.25 U/lb SC.

Table 34–3. ECG Findings in Hyperkalemia[19]

Serum K level (mEq/L)	ECG Findings
5.5	Tall peaked T waves
6.5	Decreased height of R wave, ST depression; prolonged QRS complexes and P waves; mild bradycardia
7.0	Decreased height and increased duration of P wave; QRS complex and QT interval lengthen; moderate bradycardia
8.5	No P waves (atrial standstill)
10.0	Wide and biphasic QRS complex; ventricular flutter, fibrillation, or asystole

Hypokalemia is quite common in complicated diabetics. It results from a decreased potassium intake caused by anorexia and vomiting, and an increased potassium loss as a result of vomiting and polyuria. One should closely observe the diabetic cat for the development of hypokalemia, because the administration of intravenous fluids and insulin contributes to a decrease in serum potassium. Since treatment of DM generally begins before a serum potassium level is determined, the following treatment plan serves to minimize the production of hypokalemia:

1. Rapidly administer LRS intravenously in an amount needed to correct dehydration. Do not add potassium to intravenous fluids given rapidly.
2. Once the cat is rehydrated, reduce the fluids to a maintenance administration rate. Add potassium chloride at the concentration of 5 to 7 mEq per 250 mL of fluids.
3. Insulin can then be administered, either as Ultralente subcutaneously or as regular insulin intramuscularly.

The maximal rate of potassium administration should be 0.5 mEq/kg/hr. If that rate is exceeded, fatal hyperkalemia may likely result.

Hyperosmolarity

Hyperosmolarity is a potential problem in diabetics for two reasons: first, hyperglycemia causes a direct increase in serum osmolarity; second, polyuria may lead to hypernatremia by causing a net free-water loss. Hypernatremia has a profound effect in increasing osmolarity.

Treatment of hyperosmolarity consists of administration of an isotonic, balanced electrolyte solution. The administration of a hypotonic fluid, such as 0.45% saline or 5% dextrose in water, is dangerous. The appropriate fluids should not be administered rapidly to avoid producing fatal cerebral edema.

As the blood glucose is lowered, the serum osmolarity is reduced. One should not lower the blood glucose more than 50% in the first 12 to 24 hours. This can be difficult, since rehydrating the diabetic may lower the blood glucose by as much as 30% even without the administration of any insulin

Acidosis

Acidosis can be established by demonstrating the presence of ketones with urine dipsticks. If ketonuria exists, the patient's serum bicarbonate (total CO_2) level and degree of compensation (as evidenced by the degree of hyperventilation) can be used to estimate the arterial pH (Table 34–4). This is essential for understanding proper therapy.

Treatment consists of the administration of sodium bicarbonate; however, it should not be administered indiscriminately or rapidly, because it is a hypertonic solution. The osmolarity of a 7.5% solution is six times greater than that of normal serum. Sodium bicarbonate may also induce paradoxic central nervous system acidosis if administered improperly.

As a rule, a diabetic whose blood pH is below 7.1 is facing death due to acidosis. This cat should be treated with

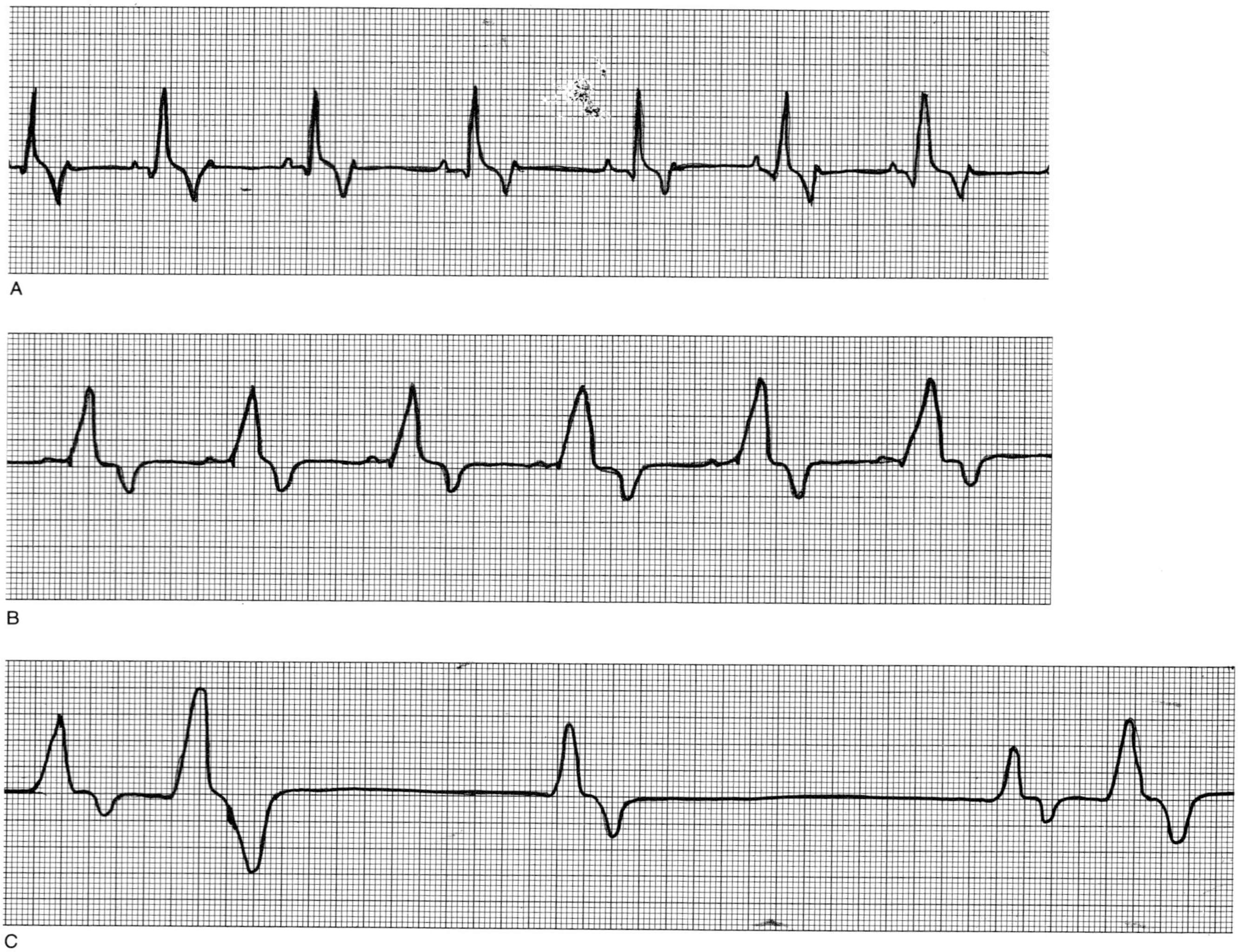

Figure 34–2. (*A*) Tall peaked T waves are the first ECG indication of hyperkalemia. This occurs when the serum potassium is in the range of 5.5 to 6.0 mEq/L. (*B*) When the serum potassium is in the range of 6.5 to 7.5 mEq/L, the P waves are shortened and their duration is increased. The QRS complexes and the QT intervals are lengthened. (*C*) At 8.5 to 10.0 mEq/L, there are no P waves and the QRS complexes are wide and biphasic.

Table 34–4. Estimation of Arterial pH Based on Serum Total CO_2 and Degree of Hyperventilation

	Level of Compensation* (Degree of Hyperventilation)			
Serum Total CO_2 (mEq/L)	**None ($pCO_2 \pm 40$)**	**Mild (pCO_2 30–35)**	**Moderate ($pCO_2 \pm 25$)**	**Maximal ($pCO_2 \pm 20$)**
20	7.32†	—	—	—
15	7.20	7.28†	—	—
10	7.02‡	7.12	7.22†	—
5	6.72‡	6.82‡	6.93‡	7.02‡

*No values are listed from some combinations because the stimulation for hyperventilation increases with the degree of acidosis.

†Do not treat with sodium bicarbonate.

‡Treat with $NaHCO_3$.

Adapted from Garvey MS. Complications of diabetes mellitus. In: Proceedings: Eastern State Veterinary Conference, Orlando, FL, January 1986:87.

sodium bicarbonate. A patient whose blood pH is above 7.2 should not be treated with sodium bicarbonate. Based on Table 34–4, the following generalities can be made:

1. If the total CO_2 is greater than 15 mEq/L, sodium bicarbonate should not be given.
2. If the total CO_2 is less than 10 mEq/L, bicarbonate treatment is usually needed.

If one deems sodium bicarbonate therapy appropriate, the following dosage schedule is recommended:

Amount of sodium bicarbonated (mEq)
$= 0.3 \times$ body weight in kilograms $\times$ [24 − total CO_2]

Half of the calculated amount should be given over the first 6 hours and the remainder, if needed, over the next 6 to 24 hours.

The Glucose Curve

The cornerstone of proper insulin administration is based on the glucose curve, also called the insulin tolerance test. The glucose curve allows one to understand how the various types of insulin are metabolized in an individual diabetic patient.

The cat should receive insulin for 2 to 3 days. The initial choice should be 0.25 to 0.5 U/lb s.i.d. of Ultralente SC. The test should begin early in the morning. The first blood glucose reading is made, and the insulin is administered. The cat is fed the food he or she will be eating when regulated and in the amount the cat would be expected to eat. Feeding is essential, even if it must be via an orogastric tube.

Blood glucose readings are made every 2 hours until three things can be determined:

- The level of the peak insulin effect.
- The time lapse from insulin administration to the peak insulin effect.
- Whether the maximum blood glucose level is likely to rise above 250 mg/dL.

The insulin dosage should be adjusted until the peak level is between 80 and 120 mg/dL.[9] The time elapsed until the peak insulin effect is reached allows one to determine the appropriate type of insulin as well as the dosing frequency —either once or twice daily. Ideally, the insulin type and administration frequency should be chosen so that the highest blood glucose reading for the 24-hour period is about 200 (maximum 250) mg/dL. However, acceptable regulation is achieved if the blood glucose peaks at 300 mg/dL.

Repeated venipunctures can be a problem in a cat because of the small size of the accessible veins. These suggestions should prove helpful:

- Use a 25-gauge needle.
- Make the first venipuncture as distally as possible in a cephalic vein.
- Make subsequent venipunctures progressively proximal to the previous sites.
- Alternate cephalic veins between venipunctures.
- Place tape over the venipuncture site each time to prevent hematoma formation and to preserve the veins.

Glucometers

A glucometer is a device used to determine glucose readings. There are several types of glucometers. The Beckman Glucose Analyzer is one of the standard machines used in commercial laboratories. A number of serum chemistry units that include a test for glucose are available for use in veterinary hospitals. A third type is the hand-held reflectance meter.

Hand-held reflectance meters are marketed for use by humans with DM. If a serum chemistry unit is not available, this is a practical, inexpensive alternative. One or two drops of blood are placed on a glucose reagent stick, the glucose strip is inserted in the reflectance for 30 seconds, and the meter produces a digital read-out. The operating time is less than 1 minute, the cost is minimal (about $100.00), and the results are reliable.[13] In one study, three reflectance meters were compared with the Beckman Glucose Analyzer. They were all found to be acceptable, but the Accu-Chek II meter (Boehringer Mannheim, Indianapolis, IN) utilizing Chemstrip bG reagent strips (Boehringer Mannheim, Indianapolis, IN) gave the most reliable results.[13]

Rebound Hyperglycemia

One aspect of the cat's survival ability is its compensation for severe hypoglycemia. This is termed *rebound hyperglycemia* or the Somogyi Overswing.

The following events occur when the blood glucose falls below 65 mg/dL[14]:

1. Diabetogenic hormones, epinephrine and glucagon, are released. These hormones promote gluconeogenesis and glycogenolysis in the liver and decrease the utilization of glucose by peripheral tissue.
2. The blood glucose level rises rapidly.
3. Cortisol and growth hormone are released, which further increase the production of and release of glucose.
4. The blood glucose level increases even more rapidly.
5. Because the cat is diabetic, levels of insulin adequate to respond to the glucose rise are unavailable.
6. Therefore, the blood glucose rises to uncontrollable levels, as high as 600 mg/dL.

A typical example of rebound hyperglycemia is illustrated in Figure 34–3*A*.

Mental dullness followed by seizures (typical clinical signs of hypoglycemia in the dog) occur in the cat only if glucose stores are depleted. Therefore, in most cats the hypoglycemic phase cannot be recognized on the basis of the typical canine criteria. When the hyperglycemic phase develops, the cat begins to exhibit the typical clinical signs, especially polydipsia and polyuria, accompanied by glucosuria. The insulin dosage should *not* be increased, as such a response would only aggravate the problem.

In order to diagnose rebound hyperglycemia, it is necessary to perform a glucose curve. If the blood glucose level falls below 30 mg/dL, rebound hyperglycemia should be anticipated. Following the blood glucose levels for a few more hours will allow one to determine if the rise is extreme.

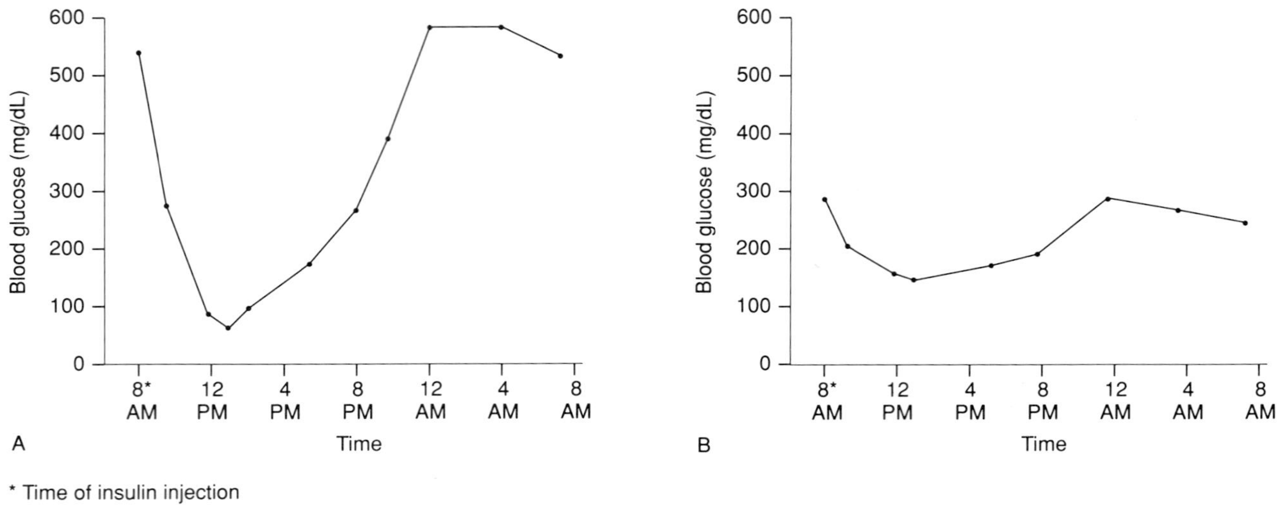

Figure 34–3. (*A*) **Blood glucose concentrations in a 9-pound Siamese cat receiving subcutaneous injections of 19 units of ultralente zinc insulin (2.1 U/lb).** (*B*) **Blood glucose concentrations in the same 9-pound Siamese cat receiving subcutaneous injections of 5 units of ultralente insulin (0.55 U/lb). Note that the serum glucose determinations performed at 5:00 PM were the same in both cases, although only the one in Figure 34–3*B* was properly regulated.**

Treatment for rebound hyperglycemia is the reduction of the dosage of insulin. Most cats require a reduction by 50% to 75% of the previous dosage. The desired response is illustrated by Figure 34–3*B*.

Veterinary Monitoring

Once adequate glucose curves have been performed to achieve regulation, the cat should be monitored every 1 to 3 months. At that time a blood glucose level should be determined about 8 to 10 hours following insulin administration and feeding. If the cat is receiving insulin twice daily, the test must be performed prior to an insulin injection. The desired blood glucose level is approximately 100 to 150 mg/dL. If there is any question as to the regulation status, a glucose curve should be obtained. Any dosage adjustment should be followed in 2 to 3 days by another glucose curve.[2]

Home Monitoring

Due to the unstable nature of the "regulated" diabetic, periodic changes in insulin dosage are to be expected. Ideally, changes should be based on a glucose curve. However, the economics of this procedure can make this unfeasible to some owners. The more the owner can contribute to glucose monitoring, the more likely changes in insulin utilization can be detected before the cat's condition deteriorates.

The ideal form of glucose monitoring is having a blood sample read by a *glucometer*. Pricking the marginal ear vein for a blood sample has proven workable for some owners. However, the logistics of this procedure makes it prohibitive for all but exceptional owners.

Urine glucose monitoring should be attempted by the owner. This may be performed with urine glucose dipsticks after urine has been collected from the litter box. This may be accomplished by replacing the normal litter with Non-Absorbable Cat Litter (Veterinary Concepts, Inc., Spring Valley, WI), aquarium gravel, the paper tracts from computer paper, or Uro-Collect (Jorgensen Laboratories, Loveland, CO). These will not absorb urine so the test strip can be dipped into the urine while it is still in the litter pan. Another alternative is to use material that is added to normal litter and reacts to glucose, CatScan G (Health-Check, Buford, GA).

However, urine glucose monitoring has some definite limitations for the feline patient. The renal threshold in the cat is much more variable than in the dog. It may vary from 200 mg/dL to 290 mg/dL.[2] Therefore, a urine sample that is negative for glucose may mean the cat is reasonably regulated, or it may mean that the cat is not well-regulated. Another limitation of urine sampling is the inability to have a cat "urinate on command," which can be achieved in many dogs. Since the regulated cat may urinate only two or three times per day, the urine in the bladder at any given time may represent many hours of urine collection.

In spite of its limitations, urine monitoring can alert the owner to seek veterinary care if the urine is consistently positive for glucose or if ketones are detected. However, it should not be used as a basis for changing the insulin dosage.

A third method of home monitoring is to observe for the clinical signs of DM. This is certainly not as accurate as blood glucose readings, but it may be useful in some situations. A normal cat or a well-regulated diabetic cat will generally drink water no more than 3 times per day. If the cat's water consumption exceeds that, the owner should have the cat's fasting blood glucose level determined. When a cat is unregulated, the other classic signs of DM may also be present. If the cat exhibits polyuria, polyphagia, or weight loss, a fasting blood glucose determination should be made.

Some owners may not be able to afford more scientifically preferred, but also more expensive, methods of home monitoring than urine glucose and clinical signs. Even with their limitations, they are preferred to euthanasia.

Hypoglycemia

Although hypoglycemia is less likely to happen in the cat than in the dog, it can be induced. Two scenarios are possible. In the most likely one the diabetic cat stops eating while the owner continues to administer insulin. The owner should be instructed to discontinue insulin or reduce the insulin dosage if a meal is missed or if the cat's appetite is reduced. In the second scenario, the cat's insulin requirements change. Unfortunately, this may occur at any time and is the basis for much frustration in dealing with feline DM.

The hypoglycemic cat typically exhibits an attitude change. If hypoglycemia is mild, the cat becomes very quiet. This generally corresponds with the peak of insulin activity. As the insulin activity wanes the cat may return to normal activity, especially if food is consumed. Severe hypoglycemia may stimulate the rebound hyperglycemia phenomenon to occur, or it may cause profound depression or even death. Seizures are unlikely.

The cat owner should be forewarned of the possibility of hypoglycemia. If the cat becomes unusually quiet several hours after insulin administration, veterinary care should be sought to make an insulin dosage adjustment. If severe depression occurs, the owner should administer about 1 teaspoon of a saturated sugar solution or a sugar-based syrup orally. If there is no response in 10 minutes, it should be repeated. If there is no response in another 10 minutes, the owner should quickly seek veterinary assistance. When the cat recovers, the reason for hypoglycemia should be determined.

Feline Peculiarities

The feline form of DM has two peculiarities not found in other species. The first one is *transient diabetes*. Affected cats are regulated for a few weeks to a few years, then gradually or suddenly lose the need for insulin. They will experience rebound hyperglycemia if insulin administration contiues. They often regain their need for insulin, so they must be monitored every 3 or 4 months.[6]

It has been speculated that these cats may experience NIDDM in a pattern similar to that of humans with NIDDM. Humans can exist in a compensated state without signs of DM, and do not require insulin until a stressful event occurs. If this is what happens in the cat, episodes of stress may cause decompensation and result in clinical DM with the need for insulin. With resolution of the stress factor (e.g., a concomitant disease), the cat becomes asymptomatic and no longer needs insulin.[2,15] Diabetic cats with a history of spontaneous remission should be suspected of having NIDDM, especially if weight reduction brings on remission.[9]

The other feline peculiarity is *DM related to megestrol acetate* (Ovaban), which causes insulin antagonism. This drug is commonly used to treat a variety of feline diseases, often being the only or most effective drug to control certain ailments (see Chapter 7). Cats taking this drug, especially if they have NIDDM, may develop clinical DM. This may occur at any dosage for any duration, but most commonly occurs at doses over 5 mg/wk for several months. When megestrol is discontinued, most of these cats become asymptomatic within a few days. However, others may take several weeks to become asymptomatic, or they may become long-term diabetics if pancreatic exhaustion occurs. They should be monitored closely to determine if insulin therapy is needed. Owners whose cats are receiving this drug should be instructed to watch for the classic clinical signs of DM and report such promptly.

Causes of Regulation Difficulties

The diabetic cat is significantly more difficult to regulate than the diabetic dog. If regulation proves difficult to achieve and/or maintain, several factors should be considered (Fig. 34–4).

Failure to Perform a Glucose Curve. If the cat is started on insulin without first performing a glucose curve, one will be guessing about what type of insulin to use, how to dose the insulin, and at what interval to administer it. The insulin dose that can produce rebound hyperglycemia is highly variable and unpredictable. It can be verified only with a glucose curve, because the cat does not exhibit the typical clinical signs of hypoglycemia. Some cats also have an unusually early insulin peak. This phenomenon and rebound hyperglycemia can be differentiated only with a glucose curve.

Failure to Administer Insulin at Prescribed or Consistent Doses. The owner's understanding of measuring and injecting insulin should be verified.

Vigorously Shaking Insulin. Insulin manufacturers instruct patients (owners) to mix insulin by rolling the bottle between the hands. Vigorously shaking the insulin can result in inaccurate measurements due to foam production.

Estrus and Pregnancy. Progestogens cause major fluctuations in insulin utilization. Female cats must be spayed.

Failure to Feed the Cat Consistently. The quantity of the cat's daily food (calorie) intake has a direct bearing on the amount of insulin needed. If the quantity varies from day to day, the insulin requirement also varies.

Failure of the Cat to Eat Two to Four Meals per Day. If given the opportunity, the typical cat eats 12 to 20 times per day, one mouthful at a time. Dry foods offer several advantages over canned foods, including the availability on a free-choice basis. Many diabetic cats have been on this feeding schedule and do not wish to change to interval feeding. However, interval feeding is the preferred method for controlling DM. Two, or up to four, feedings are the most desirable.

Improper Diet. There are many advantages of high-fiber diets for the diabetic cat. However, not all cats will eat high-

Inadequate diabetic control
and
Insulin dose >2.5 U/kg/day

↓

Review insulin mixing and administration

↓

Review diet, feeding habits, activity swings

↓

Review multi-cat household & boarding problems

↓

Rebound Hyperglycemia—Glucose curve—Rapid insulin metabolism

↓

Steroids, ovaban, glucose—Drug history

↓

Intact female—Estrus, pregnancy

↓

Correct diet—Yes—Obese (>15% ideal body wt)

↓

Minimum data base—R/O Infection, liver, kidney

↓

Other tests—R/O Acromegaly, Cushings, hyperthyroidism

↓

Change insulin (from pork to beef to human)

Figure 34–4. **Flow chart for causes of regulation difficulties in diabetic cats.[20] (Adapted with permission from Wolfsheimer KJ. Insulin-Resistant Diabetes Mellitus. In: Kirk RW, ed. Current Veterinary Therapy X, Philadelphia: WB Saunders, 1989:1011.)**

fiber diets. Cats tend to become fixed on their diet and frequently will not change. Semi-moist foods contain large amounts of sugar and should be avoided for diabetic cats.

Irregular Activity Levels. The amount of the cat's exercise and activity will influence caloric utilization and thus the need for insulin. This is generally not a significant problem in older cats. It is desirable for diabetic cats to live indoors all the time.

Concomitant Disease. Liver diseases, especially hepatic lipidosis, can alter the liver's utilization of glucose. Abnormal elevations of thyroid hormone (hyperthyroidism) increase glycogenolysis and gluconeogenesis. Polyuria associated with early renal failure causes rapid elimination of insulin. In advanced renal failure, metabolic clearance of insulin may decrease. These, and other metabolic diseases, contribute to or complicate the management of DM.[16]

Need for Steroids or Megestrol. Corticosteroids and megestrol acetate can induce insulin antagonism or pancreatic exhaustion.[16] These should not be administered to diabetic cats. However, some diseases can be controlled only by the use of these drugs, making DM in these cats very difficult to control.

Multi-Cat Households. Consistently feeding the cat the same food and the same amount of food each day is more difficult than in a single-cat household; the diabetic cat must generally be fed individually. Multi-cat households also make monitoring of urine glucose, water consumption, and the other clinical signs more difficult.

Prolonged or Frequent Boarding. The changes in eating habits and activity levels associated with boarding make it difficult for the diabetic cat. If the owner must be gone frequently, it is preferable to arrange for some type of in-home care.

Obesity. Insulin resistance is caused by obesity due to several mechanisms. It has been demonstrated that some diabetic patients lose their need for exogenous insulin if obesity is corrected.[6]

Hyperadrenocorticism. Hyperadrenocorticism results in insulin antagonism. Fortunately this disease is rare in cats.[17]

Acromegaly. Acromegaly results in insulin antagonism. Fortunately this disease is also rare in cats.[18]

Insulin Incompatibility. Some cats develop antibodies to beef or pork insulins. Many of these can be regulated with one of the human insulins, such as Novulin or Humulin, although their lack of antigenicity has not been proven.

Insulin Resistance. True insulin resistance is rare in the cat. It is defined as the cat having a persistent blood glucose of over 300 mg/dL in spite of the administration of greater than 1.2 U/lb/day.[6] It may be due to abnormal insulin receptors, a low number of receptors, altered receptor affinity, a postreceptor defect, or antibodies produced against the insulin.[2]

Boarding a Diabetic Cat

Boarding a diabetic cat requires some careful planning and attention to maintain proper regulation of DM. However, even with the finest care, dysregulation is a constant threat.

Prior to admission of any diabetic cat, the staff must understand some of the basic principles concerning management of DM: the importance of (1) a consistent, proper diet and the possible influence of a reduced activity level, (2) observing for polydipsia, polyphagia, and anorexia, and (3) regular insulin administration at the proper dosage and time.

Upon admission of the diabetic cat, the staff needs to gather the following information:

- The brand and quantity of the cat's food.
- How often and when (in relation to insulin administration) the cat eats.
- How much exercise the cat normally gets (indoor versus outdoor).
- The type, dose, and interval of insulin administered.
- An emergency phone number where the owner can be reached.
- If the owner cannot be reached by phone, their desires in the event that a diabetic crisis occurs.

The staff should understand that anorexia can have serious consequences. If the cat is not eating properly, hand or force feeding may be necessary. A blood glucose determination should be made at about the time of peak insulin activity for the first 2 days and on any day that the cat's food consumption is not proper.

It is always better for the blood glucose to be too high than too low. If adjustments in insulin dosage are made, that principle should be kept in mind.

Because of the possibility of dysregulation, one should be prepared to obtain at least a partial glucose curve at any time. The owner should understand that the charges for boarding may vary considerably, depending upon the special care and laboratory tests needed.

Conclusion

The diabetic cat can be a challenge to regulate. Understanding the differences between DM in cats and that of other species is essential Properly educating the client and soliciting his or her full cooperation is also essential.

Successful regulation should begin with a glucose curve. This serves as the basis for determining the proper type, dosage, and interval of administration for insulin.

Although the successful management of a diabetic cat is demanding, it can also be very rewarding to the veterinarian and the owner. Properly managed cats can remain cherished pets for many years.

REFERENCES

1. Chastain CB, Ganjam VK. Diabetes Mellitus. In: Clinical Endocrinology of Companion Animals. Philadelphia: Lea & Febiger, 1986:257.
2. Feldman EC, Nelson RW. Feline Diabetes. In: Feldman EC, Nelson RW, eds. Canine and Feline Endocrinology and Reproduction. Philadelphia: WB Saunders, 1987:264.
3. Schaer M. A clinical survey of thirty cats with diabetes mellitus. J Am Vet Med Assoc 1977;170:23.
4. Kramek BA, Moise NS, Cooper B, Raffe MR. Neuropathy associated with diabetes mellitus in the cat. J Am Vet Med Assoc 1984;184:42.
5. Panciera DL, Thomas CB, Eicker SW, Atkins CE. Epizootiologic patterns of dibetes mellitus in cats: 333 cases (1980–1986). J Am Vet Med Assoc 1990;197:1504.
6. Wolf AM. Management of geriatric diabetic cats. Compend Contin Ed Pract Vet 1989;11:1088.
7. Hamburg S, Hendler R, Sherwin RS. Influence of small increments of epinephrine on glucose tolerance in normal humans. Ann Intern Med 1980;93:566.
8. Ford S, Feldman E, Nelson R. Intensive evaluation of glipizide therapy in the management of feline diabetes mellitus (DM). In: Proceedings of the Ninth Annual Veterinary Medical Forum. Am Coll Vet Intern Med, May 28–31, 1991:234.
9. Wallace MS, Kirk CA. The Diagnosis and Treatment of Insulin-Dependent and Non-Insulin-Dependent Diabetes Mellitus in the Dog and Cat. In: Nichols R, ed. Problems in Veterinary Medicine, Endocrinology. Philadelphia: JB Lippincott 1990; 2(4):573.
10. Brange J. Insulin Preparation. In: Brange J, ed. Galenics of Insulin. Berlin Springer-Verlag, 1987:17.
11. Nelson RW. The role of fiber in managing diabetes mellitus. Vet Med 1989;84:1156.
12. Garvey MS. Complications of diabetes mellitus. In: Proceedings: Eastern State Veterinary Conference, Orlando, FL, January 1986:87.
13. Joseph RJ, Allyson K, Graves TK, Rondeau MJ, Peterson ME. Evaluation of two reagent strips and three reflectance meters for rapid determination of blood glucose concentrations. J Vet Intern Med 1987;1:170.
14. McMillan FD, Feldman EC. Rebound hyperglycemia following overdosing of insulin in cats with diabetes mellitus. J Am Vet Med Assoc 1986;188:1426.
15. Peterson ME, Randolf JF. Endocrine Diseases. In: Sherding RG, ed. The Cat: Diagnosis and Clinical Management. New York: Churchill Livingstone, 1989:1095.
16. Wolfsheimer KJ. Problems in Diabetes Mellitus Management: Insulin Resistance. In: Nichols R, ed. Problems in Veterinary Medicine: Endocrinology. Philadelphia: JB Lippincott, 1990; 193:591

17. Nelson RW, Feldman EC, Smith MC. Hyperadrenocorticism in cats, seven cases (1978–1987). J Am Vet Med Assoc 1988; 193:245.
18. Peterson ME, Taylor RS, Greco DS, et al. Acromegaly in 14 cats. J Vet Intern Med 1990;4:192.
19. Frenier SL, Dhein CR. Diagnosis and Management of Acute Renal Failure. In: August JR, ed. Consultations in Feline Internal Medicine. Philadelphia: WB Saunders, 1991:281.
20. Wolfsheimer KJ. Insulin-Resistant Diabetes Mellitus. In: Kirk RW, ed. Current Veterinary Therapy X. Philadelphia: WB Saunders, 1989:1011.

CHAPTER 35

◇ ◇ ◇

The Eye: Extraocular Diseases

Art J. Quinn and Virginia A. Schultz

Diseases of the Orbit

The bony orbit of the cat is formed by seven bones: frontal, lacrimal, zygomatic, maxilla, presphenoid, basisphenoid, and palatine.[1] The bony orbit is incomplete because the lateral aspect is composed of a dense orbital ligament that extends from the zygomatic process of the frontal bone to the frontal process of the zygomatic bone. There is no bony orbital floor in the cat except for a small shelf of tuberous maxillary bone above the molar teeth. The floor of the orbit is composed primarily of supportive soft tissue. The open orbit of carnivores may allow greater jaw movement and power in seizing prey.[1]

The orbital contents are enclosed in a conical, fibrous, periorbital membrane (orbital cone) with its apex attached firmly to the orbital wall around the optic foramen and with its base attached to the orbital margin and orbital ligament. This anatomic relationship is important to understanding the effects of disease processes of the orbit because the orbital cone effectively separates the orbital contents from the surrounding tissues. The long axis of the orbital cone passes ventroposteriorly and medially. The orbital cone comprises the retrobulbar tissues (including the extraocular muscles, cranial nerves II, III, IV, VI, and the ophthalmic branch of V), autonomic nerves, arteries, veins, smooth muscles, and fat. The orbital cone should be regarded as a potential space rather than a hollow cone since the space between structures within the cone is composed of fat and loose connective tissue. The lacrimal gland is contained in the periorbital membrane in close proximity to the supertemporal aspect of the globe.

Orbital disease may result from congenital disorders, traumatic injury, inflammatory disease, or space occupying lesions. Clinical signs vary depending on which of the anatomic compartments is involved in the pathologic process. The compartments are defined as follows: within the extraocular muscle cone, outside the muscle cone but within the periorbita, and within the orbit but outside the periorbita.[2]

The clinical signs of orbital disease include exophthalmos, enophthalmos, strabismus, impaired globe movements, protrusion of the membrana nictitans, chemosis, swelling of the eyelids, periorbital swelling pain on opening the mouth, exposure keratitis, optic nerve impairment with vision loss, and decreased pupillary light reflexes.

Congenital Disorders

Anophthalmia and microphthalmia with an absent or smaller than normal globe and a narrow palpebral fissure with incomplete development of the orbit are reported in the cat. Anophthalmia is reported in cats after griseofulvin was administered to queens during the first half of gestation.[3] A shallow bony orbit with resulting physiologic exophthalmos is observed in brachycephalic breeds such as the Persian.

Traumatic Injuries

Orbital trauma frequently accompanies contusive accidents (automobiles), projectiles (bullets), and wounds (animal fights). The usual findings are retrobulbar and subconjunctival hemorrhages. Passive congestion may cause eyelid swelling, chemosis membrana nictitans protrusion, and exophthalmos, with accompanying lagophthalmus and exposure keratopathy. Because of the anatomic globe–orbit configuration in the cat, proptosis occurs with difficulty; therefore, when present, it usually represents more serious trauma to the globe and related structures. Tearing or avulsion of the medial rectus and inferior oblique muscles occurs frequently. Optic nerve damage and avulsion, accompanied by other severe posterior segment trauma including retinal hemorrhage, tearing, and detachment, may be present. Globe rupture occurs with more severe contusional trauma.

Traumatic proptosis is truly an ophthalmic emergency, and management depends on etiology, extent of damage, and duration (Figs. 35–1 and 35–2). The eye should be kept moist and may be gently bathed with warm saline solution or cleansed with moist gauze to remove debris and dirt. Evaluation of the proptosed eye should include determination of the condition of the extrinsic muscles, the integrity of the globe and internal structures, and evaluation of pupillary size. Eyes with extensive internal injuries are more susceptible to becoming either glaucomatous or phthisical. If extensive damage to the extrinsic muscles causes the eye to hang loosely from the orbit, enucleation is necessary. A pinpoint pupil may have a more favorable prognosis than a dilated pupil, which usually signals a guarded to unfavorable prognosis. In general, when the outcome is uncertain, enucleation can always be performed if other treatments fail.

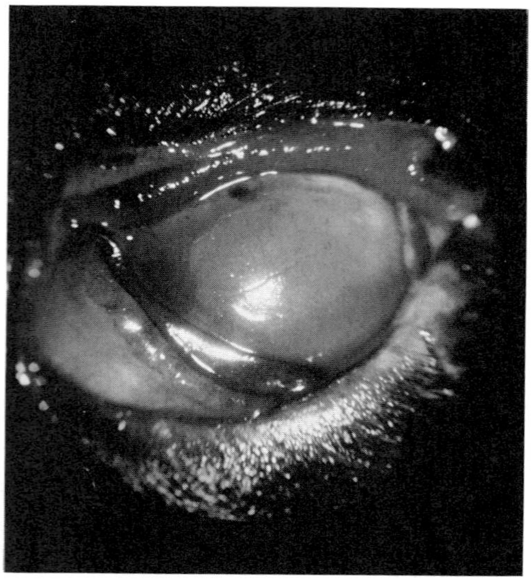

Figure 35–1. **Traumatic proptosis, immediately after replacement, with eyelid swelling, subconjunctival hemorrhage, and edema of the membrane nictitans. Corneal ulceration and hyphema are also present. A temporary tarsorrhaphy was performed.**

As a result of the proptosis, the globe becomes entrapped in front of the eyelids. Under anesthesia, muscle hooks or scalpel handles are inserted under the eyelids at the nasal or temporal canthus. With gentle pressure on the globe and "rimming" of the eyelids, the globe will return to normal position if there has not been excessive orbital hemorrhage or edema and muscle avulsion. Alternatively, Allis tissue forceps may be used to pull the lids cranially as pressure is applied to the globe. If the proptosis is uncomplicated, the globe will return to its normal position with minimal circulatory compromise, eyelid swelling, chemosis,

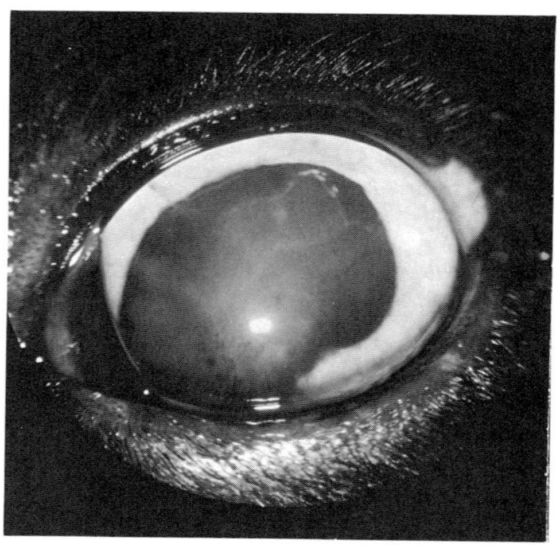

Figure 35–2. **Three weeks after trauma, the adnexal trauma has resolved. Posterior synechia is present in the inferior medial portion of the pupil, and vitreal–retinal hemorrhage persists. Although the eye was blind, cosmesis was maintained.**

and corneal irritation or damage. In this situation, a temporary tarsorrhaphy is usually not necessary. In contrast, a temporary tarsorrhaphy is always indicated if the proptosis is complicated by lagophthalmos.

The postprocedural medical regimen includes a broad-spectrum systemic antibiotic. Topical application of an antibiotic ointment is indicated for corneal injury. The antibiotic may be applied between the eyelids at the nasal canthus if a temporary tarsorrhaphy was necessary. Atropine ointment should also be applied in the same manner if anterior uveitis is present.

Premature removal of the temporary tarsorrhaphy is frequently a complication. Removal should not occur prior to resolution of hemorrhage, edema, and swelling of the orbital tissue and return of complete eyelid function. Unresolved keratopathy secondary to exposure from the lagophthalmos, corneal damage incurred at the time of proptosis, or neurotropic keratitis secondary to ophthalmic nerve damage may require extended use of the tarsorrhaphy. Secondary glaucoma or phthisis bulbi from extensive intraocular trauma may result. Deviation of a normal gaze or lateral strabismus from tearing, damage, or avulsion of the medial muscles may be sequelae. Medial tarsorrhaphy to prevent exposure keratopathy may be required while waiting for correction of the strabismus. If the strabismus is severe and persists 6 to 8 weeks after the insult, muscle surgery is indicated. Optic nerve and vascular damage leading to blindness are common.

The prognosis is guarded for the return of complete ocular functions in all but the acute, minimally traumatized patient. In general, when in doubt about the outcome, replace the globe for the cosmetic effects: results are often better than expected.

Inflammatory Diseases

Periorbital cellulitis, retrobulbar abscess, and orbital cellulitis are terms that describe inflammation in the orbit. Inflammations in the retrobulbar space are rare. Most of the retrobulbar abscesses encountered in cats are actually located in the periorbital tissues outside the orbital cone, perhaps because the periorbital cone acts as a formidable barrier to extension into the retrobulbar space.

The etiology often remains speculative or obscure and is frequently unconfirmed. Probable causes include foreign bodies that penetrate the skin or conjunctiva or that lodge and penetrate through the mouth behind the last upper molar tooth. Bite and claw wounds that gain access into the periorbital region and the spread of infections from hematogenous or regional disorders (sinus or teeth) are other possibilities. Another regional source is the zygomatic (orbital) salivary gland located outside the periorbital region on the ventral aspect of the orbit; it can be the site of the inflammation and abscessation.

Clinical Signs

Clinical signs vary in intensity and onset. In general, an abscess has an acute onset, while cellulitis is more gradual. Abscessation may result from cellulitis. The accompanying clinical signs of eyelid swelling, chemosis, exophthalmos, membrana nictitans protrusion, orbital edema, limited ocu-

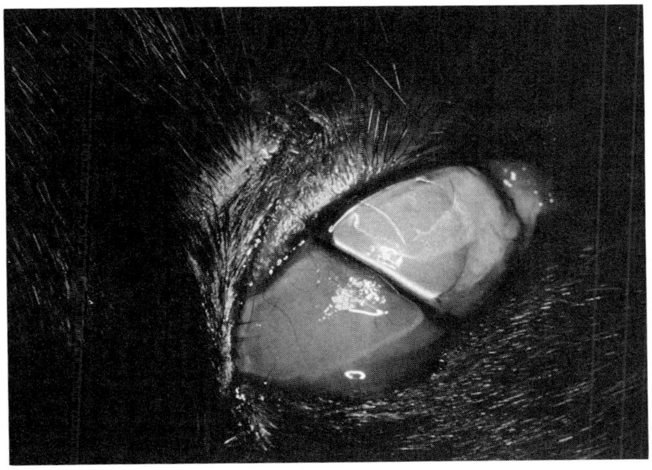

Figure 35–3. Cellulitis producing eyelid swelling, chemosis, and membrana nictitans protrusion.

lar movement, exposure keratopathy, and pain are observed in both conditions (Fig. 35–3). Fever and pain on opening the mouth are usually more evident with abscessation. Papilledema and retinal hemorrhage are observed with orbital cellulitis.

Diagnosis

An orderly examination of the orbit, globe, and adjacent structures is essential. Visual inspection and digital palpation are performed. The mouth is examined for swelling or a draining tract caudal to the last molar tooth. Opening the mouth may create pain of such magnitude that sedation or general anesthesia may be required to perform the examination.

Biopsy samples of the tissues and exudates for histologic and cytologic evaluation and culture may be collected. Aspiration may be attempted using a 20-gauge, 1-inch needle with syringe vacuum. The needle should be directed posterior and dorsal to the angle formed by the orbital ligament and the zygomatic arch.[4] Draining tracts may be explored with a blunt instrument.

Routine radiography may reveal abnormalities. Several other assessment techniques have been developed such as orbital venography[5] and arteriography,[6] pneumorbitography,[4] positive contrast orbitography,[7] optic thecography,[8,9] and magnetic resonance imaging.[10] Ultrasonography is also used to diagnose inflammatory and neoplastic diseases.[11] The use of these specialty techniques is limited to larger referral centers or teaching institutions.

A definite etiologic diagnosis is the exception rather than the rule. The usual approach is to establish drainage behind the last upper molar. This is accomplished, under general anesthetic, by making a small incision in the mucus membrane posterior to the last molar tooth; a blunt instrument, such as a hemostat, is directed dorsally to the posterior aspect of the globe in an attempt to reach a pocket of exudate. It may be redirected, but excessive trauma should be avoided. If an abscess is present, purulent exudate may erupt; however, more commonly, only serosanguinous material appears at the incision site. In either circumstance, this material should be collected for cytology and culture. Tissue can also be collected for histopathology. Rarely is a foreign body identified. The wound should be gently irrigated with an aqueous antibiotic solution but not with iodine or other cauterizing agents. A broad spectrum systemic antibiotic should be administered for 7 to 10 days. Hot packs on the orbital area are beneficial. If excessive swelling of the eyelids, chemosis, or exophthalmos prevent proper closing of the eyelids with resulting exposure keratopathy, a temporary tarsorrhaphy should be performed and remain in place until normal function is restored.

Sequelae may include enophthalmos from muscle and periorbital tissue atrophy, keratoconjunctivitis sicca from inflammatory atrophy of the lacrimal gland, neurotropic keratopathy from damage of the ophthalmic branch of the trigeminal nerve, and blindness from retinal and optic atrophy.

Orbital Neoplasia

Orbital signs associated with neoplasia are usually unilateral and slowly progressive but not painful. Exophthalmos and protrusion of the membrana nictitans usually result. Diagnostic techniques previously mentioned will aid in the differential diagnosis of orbital neoplasia.

Diseases of the Eyelids

The eyelids are delicate, pliable folds of integument designed to protect the eye, to secrete and distribute precorneal tear film, and to provide access to the drainage apparatus. There are four layers comprising the eyelids: (1) the external cutaneous layer, (2) the muscular layer containing the orbicularis oculi, levator palpebrae superioris, and some smooth muscle fibers,[12] (3) the tarsus with its tarsal glands, and (4) the palpebral conjunctiva.

According to some authors, cilia are lacking in the cat.[13] Less distinct cilia can be demonstrated on gross and histologic examination[14] from the medial third of the upper eyelid laterally.[15] Stimulation of the cilia results in a blink reflex controlled by a branch of the fifth cranial nerve. The orbicularis oculi is innervated by the seventh cranial nerve to control eyelid closure. Closure proceeds from lateral to medial.[14]

The levator palpebrae superioris muscle opens the eyelid and is innervated by the third cranial nerve. The smooth muscle fibers, which also aid in opening the eyelids, are under sympathetic innervation. The third eyelid of the cat has muscle fibers innervated by the sixth cranial nerve and can be voluntarily elevated.[16]

Diseases affecting the feline adnexa are not as common as in the dog. The conditions encountered are categorized as either congenital or acquired. Many of the conditions are identical in appearance and treatment may be similar; they differ only in their origin.

Many of the acquired conditions affecting the feline adnexa are the result of trauma, infectious agents (either viral or bacterial), or parasites. Initial treatment is to remove the inciting agent if known. Treatment, if varied from that of the congenital condition, is described with each entity (Table 35–1).

Table 35–1. Conditions Affecting the Eyelid and the Third Eyelid, and the Most Prevalent Breeds Affected

Condition	Breed (Reference)
Agenesis/atresia/coloboma of eyelid	Burmese (13,17); domestic cats and captive tigers (14)
Ankyloblepharon	Blue Persians (12,15,16,19)
Autonomic polyganglionopathy or Key–Gaskell syndrome	Blue Persians (12,20,21)
Bilateral Protrusion of the third eyelid	Blue Persians (12,15,22)
and Haw's syndrome	Blue Persians (12,13,15,21)
Blepharitis	Blue Persians (14,15)
Chalazion	Blue Persians (14)
Dermoids	British Birmans (15)
Distichiasis	Abyssinians (12,14,23)
Ectropion	Abyssinians (15,16)
Entropion	Persians (14,15)
Eversion of cartilage of third eyelid	Persians (12,22,24)
Facial paralysis	Persians (22)
Horner's syndrome	Persians (13–16,21,25)
Hyperplasia/inflammation of follicles of third eyelid	Persians (14,15,22)
Lacerations	Persians (12,22)
Lagophthalmos	Persians (19,21,25)
Microblepharon/microphthalmia	Persians (25)
Neoplasms	Persians (12,15,22,25)
Premature opening of eyelid	Persians (13)
Prolapse of gland of third eyelid	Persians (13,22)
Trichiasis	Persians (rare, 25)

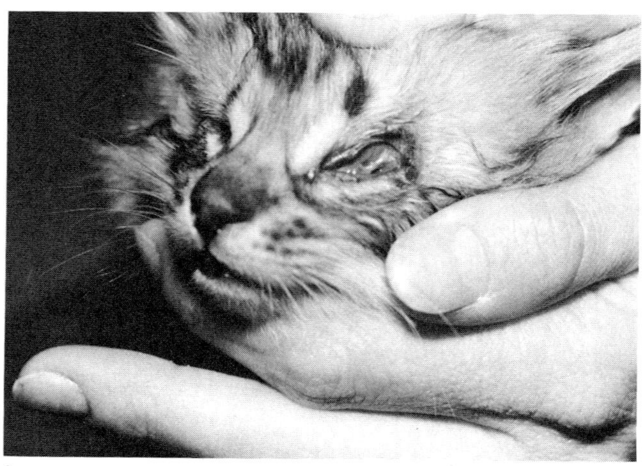
A

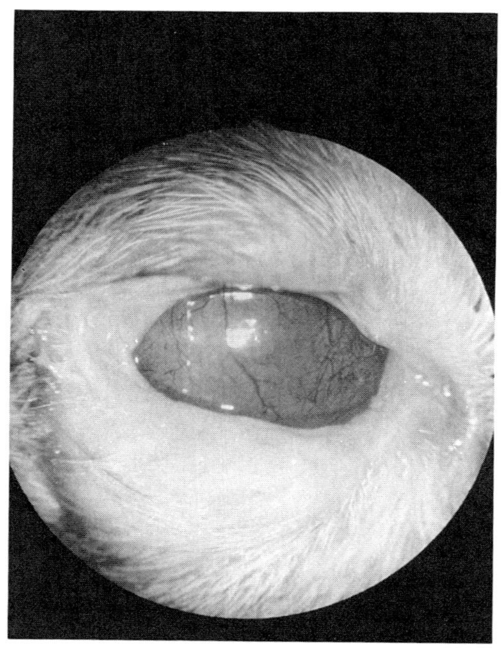
B

Figure 35–4. (*A*) Agenesis of the upper temporal eyelid. (*B*) Agenesis of the upper temporal eyelid. Distichiasis with irritation and vascularization is also present.

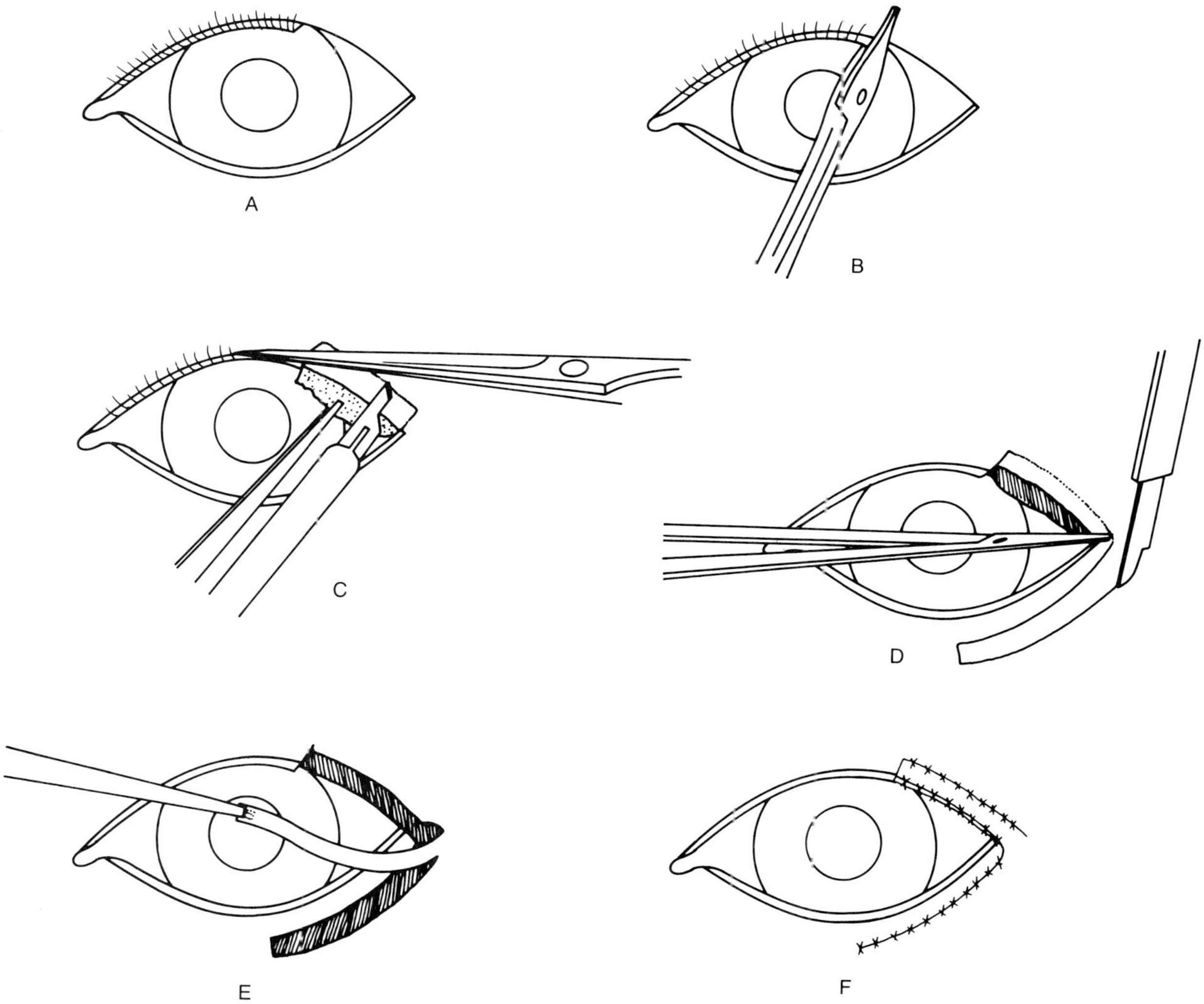

Figure 35–5. (*A*) Repair of eyelid agenesis (coloboma). (*B*) The margin of the upper lid is prepared by splitting it into a skin portion and a conjunctival portion to receive the pedicle. (*C*) The pedicle is obtained by incising the skin and orbicularis oculi parallel to the lower lid margin, leaving the lateral canthus intact. (*D*) A second incision, which parallels the first, is made slightly wider than the defect to be repaired and joins the first incision nasally. (*E, F*) This flap is rotated into the prepared site and sutured in place.

Agenesis

Eyelid agenesis, or coloboma, is often bilateral and occurs most commonly on the upper temporal lid (Fig. 35–4). Exposure keratitis and trichiasis may be secondary conditions. The cat should be carefully examined for other anomalies of the iris and lens.[17] Treatment involves surgical reconstruction (Fig. 35–5). A modified pedicle flap can be used for correction. Some authors also advise preparing a pedicle strip of conjunctival defect.[18] The pedicle flap hair tends to grow downward and may need to be retained by applying a thin layer of petrolatum to redirect the hairs.[12]

Ankyloblepharon

Ankyloblepharon, a condition in which a membrane joins the upper and lower lids, was reported by Smythe in 1958 in Blue Persians.[19] Ankyloblepharon is a normal condition for the first 10 to 12 days of the kitten's life. If the lids do not separate after this period of time or if a mucopurulent discharge is noted from the medial canthus (Fig. 35–6), the lids should be gently separated with a *blunt* instrument. The cornea should be examined for ulceration, and a broad spectrum antibiotic should be applied for several days. The most frequent cause of ankyloblepharon is neonatal keratoconjunctivitis associated with an upper respiratory infection.[16]

Autonomic Polyganglionopathy

Autonomic polyganglionopathy, Key–Gaskell syndrome, has been described in American and British cats. These are usually young, adult male domestic short-hairs.[12,20] Ocular

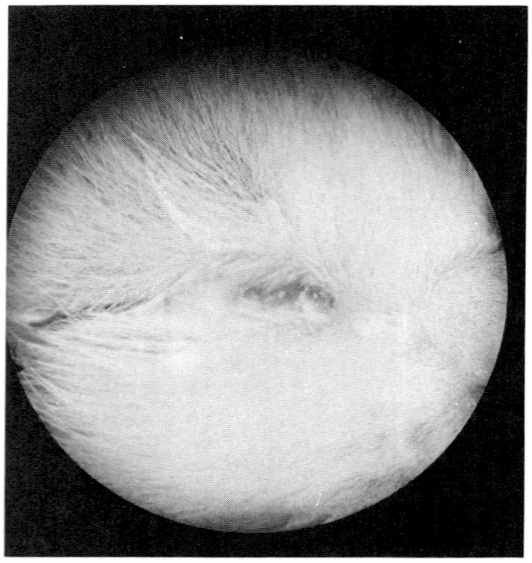

Figure 35–6. Neonatal conjunctivitis prior to lid separation.

symptoms include persistent pupillary dilation, decreased tear formation, and bilateral protrusion of the third eyelid. Another frequent feature is megaesophagus. A specific etiology is yet to be determined, but denervation hypersensitivity of both parasympathetic and sympathetic systems has been demonstrated.[13,20] Treatment is symptomatic with oral pilocarpine drops daily and stool softeners.[21] The disease is usually fatal.

Bilateral Protrusion of the Third Eyelid

Bilateral protrusion of the third eyelid, or haws, occurs most commonly in cats under 3 years of age. Cats usually have a history of viral infections, transient gastroenteritis,[15] or heavy intestinal parasitism, especially tapeworms.[12] If the owner is unaware of the presence of diarrhea, the anal–perianal area should be observed for inflammation or adherent fecal material. Another proposed cause is anterior cervical sympathetic ganglionitis.[22] Besides protrusion of the third eyelid, increased peristalsis is often noted and results in softer than normal stools lasting 2 to 12 weeks.[22] An application of 1% to 2% topical epinephrine or 2.5% ophthalmic phenylephrine (Neo-Synephrine) administered three to four times daily may produce temporary response. However, this is usually not necessary because the condition is self-limiting in weeks to months.

Blepharitis

Blepharitis has many initiating agents. These and their symptoms and treatments are summarized in Table 35–2.

Chalazion

When a meibomian gland becomes obstructed, adjacent tissue becomes inflamed and is termed a "chalazion." The condition is usually nonpainful, although the overlying conjunctiva is reddened. The recommended treatment is surgical drainage.

Dermoids

Dermoids are usually limbally oriented on the conjunctiva, cornea, eyelid, or third eyelid. Signs are related to the resulting irritation. Surgical excision is the treatment of choice.

Distichiasis

Distichia are additional cilia or rows of cilia emerging from the tarsal glands (see Fig. 35–4*B*) and are rare in the feline. If the distichia are coarse, irritation, keratitis, and possible ulceration result. Cryoepilation has proven to be the best method for permanent removal.

Acquired distichiasis is rare but may be a sequelae of blepharitis. Cryoepilation, described by Wheeler and Severin, appears to be the best treatment.[23]

Ectropion

Ectropion is usually related to facial wounds, chronic inflammation, or surgery near the eyelid (Fig. 35–7). Surgical correction usually involves the V-to-Y technique (Fig. 35–8). Other techniques, such as removal of a triangle of skin from the eyelid margin have also been advocated.[22]

Entropion

Entropion in Persians is reportedly due to a lid deformity.[14] It is usually located on the lateral lower lid (Fig. 35–9). Clinical signs include blepharospasm, epiphora, and ulceration. Treatment involves surgical removal of a wedge of eyelid adjacent to the involved area to evert the offending lid. Microphthalmia is reported as a cause of entropion.[16]

Following a fight, any breed of cat may acquire entropion. Treatment is identical to that for congenital entropion.

Epiphora

Persians are the breed most affected with epiphora. Epiphora is often related to the configuration of the Persian, i.e., a prominent globe with a shallow orbit and constriction of the lacrimal duct.[12] Severe epiphora has been treated with a conjunctivorhinostomy to provide an alternate route for excretion.[12] Instead, many clinicians prefer to treat the discoloration with daily administration of 5 to 10 mg of oral tetracycline.[16]

Eversion of the Cartilage of the Third Eyelid

Two cases of everted cartilage of the third eyelid in Burmese cats are described.[24] Clinically, the cats appeared to resemble dogs with a prolapsed gland of the third eyelid. The cause was determined to be a deterioration between the cartilage and deep orbital fascia. Correction in one cat was accomplished by suturing with 5-0 silk through the gland, cartilage, and the ventral oblique muscle. The second cat had the cartilage incised to allow straightening.[24]

Table 35–2. Blepharitis

Agent	Symptoms	Treatment
Bacterial[15]		
Staphylococcus	Moist exudate, red lid margins, chronic alopecia	Warm packs, topical antibiotics Severe: parenteral antibiotics
Chalazion[14]	Chronic tarsal distension and inflammation	Incise swelling, curretage, antibiotics systemically for 2–10 days
Allergic[12]	Pruritus, erythema, lid margin mutilated Biopsy: mast cells and eosinophils	Alternate day steroids
Autoimmune[14]		
Pemphigus vulgaris	Severe mucocutaneous involvement, febrile, systemic illness, acute intraepidermal bulla	Immunosuppressive doses of steroids, antibiotics
Parasitic[14,15]		
Notoedres cati	Hyperemia, scaliness, alopecia, pruritis	Rotenone or 2% sulfur ointment or eserine ointment
Demodex folliculorum	Nonpruritic blepharitis, circular alopecia	Rotenone
Dermatologic[12]		
Microsporum canis	Patchy (circular) alopecia	Griseofulvin
Mechanical[12]		
Burns	Necrotic tissue	Topical antibiotics

Facial Paralysis

Traumatic facial paralysis may result in several abnormalities including facial distortion, flaccid lips, and lagophthalmos. Treatment involves keeping the cornea moist with artificial tears.

Horner's Syndrome

Horner's syndrome occurs in cats as a result of sympathetic denervation (Fig. 35–10).[25] The most common sites are the T_1-T_3 ventral roots of the cranial thoracic and cervical sympathetic trunks.[12] Lesions may occur anywhere from the hypothalamus to the effector muscle.[13]

The common causes for Horner's syndrome are cervical or brachial plexus injury, surgery, otitis media, middle ear polyps, and mediastinal or retrobulbar neoplasia.[12,13] Unilateral disease may be the result of neoplasms, cellulitis, keratitis, or conjunctivitis.[21] Uncommon causes of bilateral disease include certain tranquilizing agents and loss of orbital fat from trauma, infection, or previous myositis.[21] Radiographs of the cervical and thoracic areas should be performed due to the incidence of lymphosarcoma associated with a cranial mediastinal mass.[13]

Treatment is symptomatic and elective; topical 1% to 2% epinephrine or 2.5% ophthalmic phenylephrine may be administered three to four times daily. Many cases induced by surgery or trauma resolve in 6 to 12 weeks.[25]

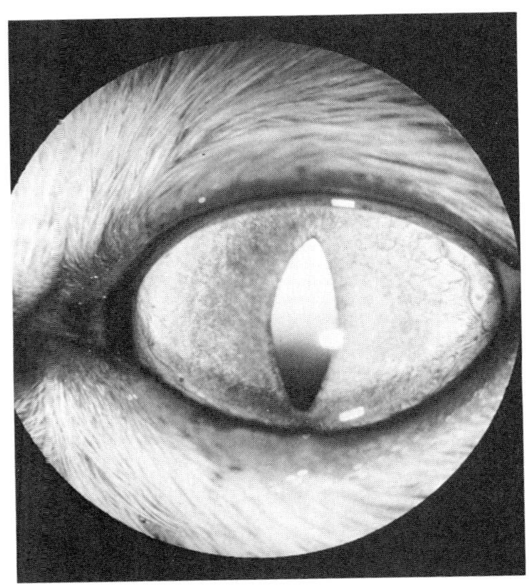

Figure 35–7. Ectropion of the lower lid.

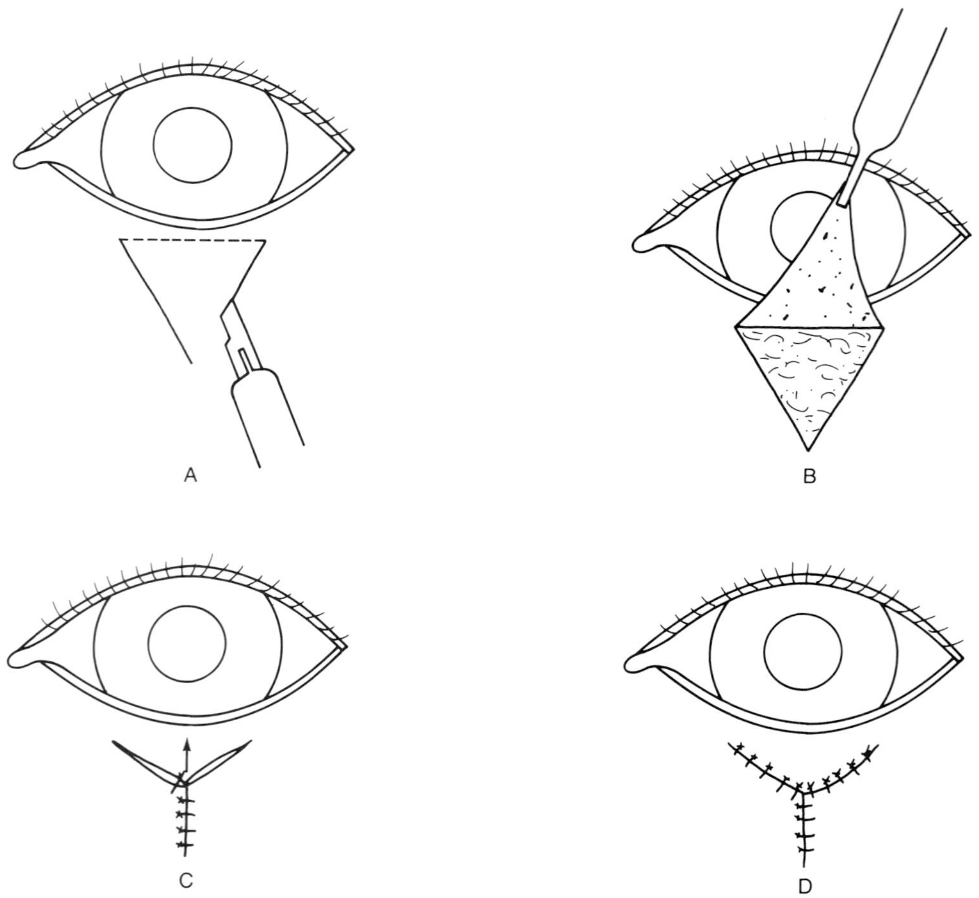

Figure 35–8. Surgical correction of ectropion may use the V-to-Y technique. (*A*) A V-shaped wedge of skin and orbicularis oculi muscle is incised in the area of ectropion. (*B*) The flap is undermined and the wound is sutured from the V's point until the lid has a normal position (*C*). (*D*) The sides of the incision are sutured to create a "Y."

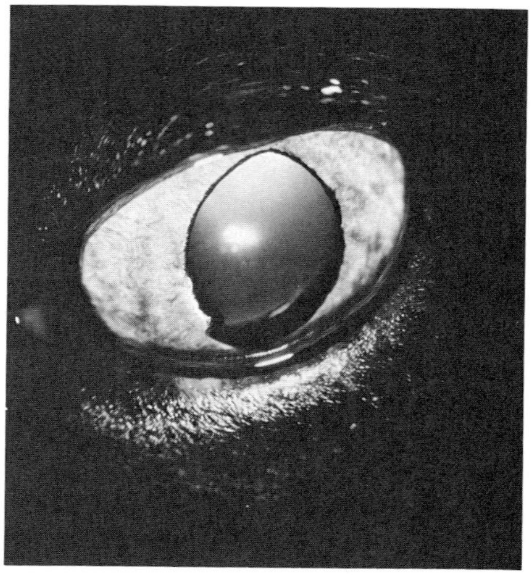

Figure 35–9. Entropion of the lower lid.

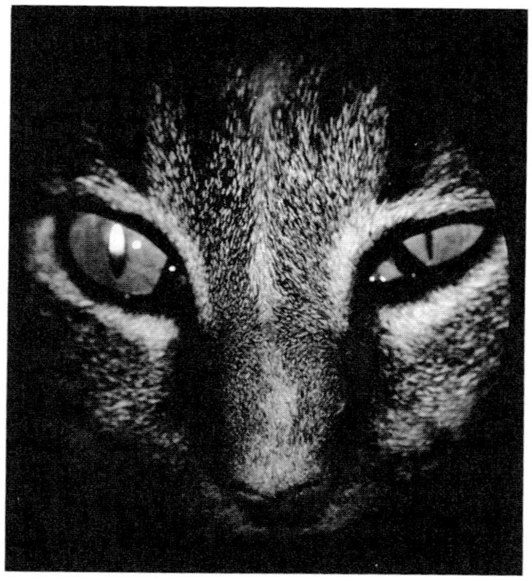

Figure 35–10. Horner's syndrome involving the left eye.

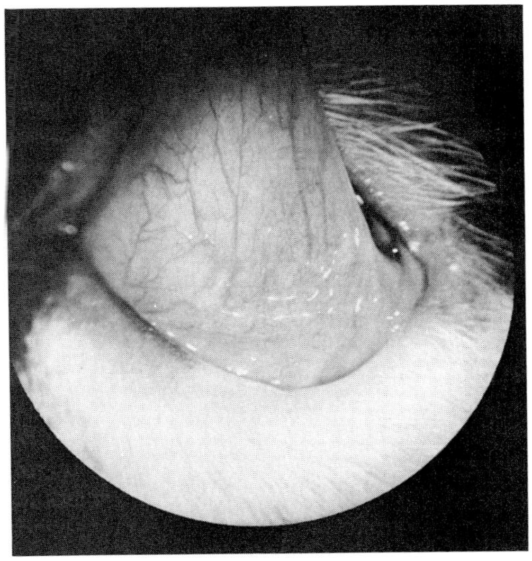

Figure 35–11. Follicular conjunctivitis due to chlamydia.

Hyperplasia of Follicles

Hyperplasia or inflammation of the third eyelid follicles is uncommon in cats; the most common etiology is chlamydial conjunctivitis (Figs. 35–11, 35–12).[22] Chronic irritation or immunologic stimulation results in the lymphoid follicles on the posterior third eyelid becoming hyperplastic. They will perpetuate themselves if the initiating cause is not quickly removed.[22]

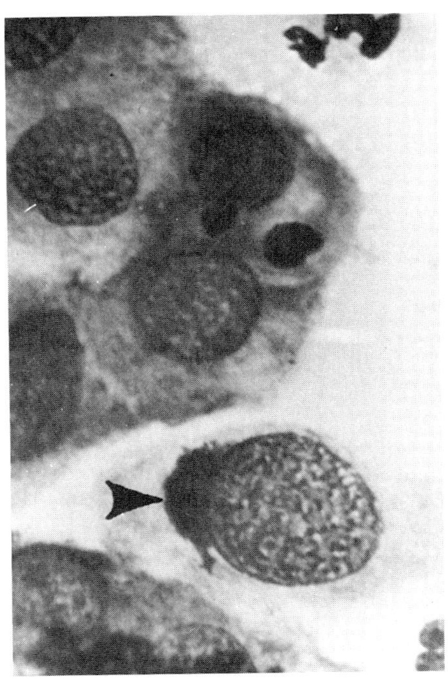

Figure 35–12. Conjunctival scrapings demonstrating the cytoplasmic inclusion of chlamydia (*arrow*).

A mucoid discharge may be the only clinical sign. Examination of the posterior side of the third eyelid reveals red, roughened follicles.

Three methods of follicle removal are proposed: (1) rubbing the follicles with a gauze sponge soaked in a mild cauterizing agent such as iodine, ether, or dilute silver nitrate; (2) scraping the follicles with a dull blade or sterile gauze; (3) rubbing the follicles with copper sulfate crystals to cauterize them, followed by liberal irrigation and the application of an antibiotic-steroid ointment q4 to 6h for 2 days then q8h until symptoms resolve. Copper sulfate crystals will cause severe corneal damage if they contact the cornea.[14,22,25] Many consider follicle scraping the treatment of choice.

Lacerations

Lacerations in the lids should be repaired early to prevent scarring with contracture.[12] If the conjunctiva is lacerated, it should also be cleaned and minimally debrided before it is sutured. Suturing should begin at the lid margin and proceed outward. The sutures should be buried to prevent irritation to the cornea.[22] Systemic antibiotics should be considered.

Lagophthalmos

Lagophthalmos is the inability to close the eyelids associated with an eyelid coloboma or hydrophthalmia. Lagophthalmos may be acquired as a result of facial wounds, scars, tumors, or diseases causing paralysis of the orbicularis oculi muscle secondary to facial nerve damage.[25] It may also be secondary to keratoconjunctivitis sicca[22] and is a temporary state during unconsciousness and anesthesia.[25]

Treatment varies according to the etiology. A partial tarsorrhaphy or surgical reconstruction may suffice, but the cornea must be protected from drying with administration of artificial tears. Some traumatically induced paralysis recovers in 4 to 6 weeks without treatment. A permanent partial tarsorrhaphy may be performed at the lateral canthus to preserve tears. Scar tissue may be relieved with a canthoplasty technique to lengthen the eyelid (Fig. 35–13 A-D).[22]

Neoplasm

Eyelid neoplasia is less common in cats than dogs. The common tumors include lymphosarcomas, dermoids, carcinomas, adenomas, lipomas, and melanomas. Although these tumors are often malignant, they have minimal tendency to metastasize with the exception of lymphosarcoma.[25] Many orbital tumors are the result of extension from adjacent areas. All growths should be examined histologically for malignancy.[22]

Cats with orbital tumors may show symptoms of proptosis. The cat remains afebrile until the tumor outgrows its blood supply and necrosis begins.[25] Malignant tumors appear to enlarge more rapidly than benign ones.

Lymphosarcomas are reported on the third eyelid, and surgical removal with chemotherapy is a necessity. Squamous cell carcinoma is most frequently seen in cats with

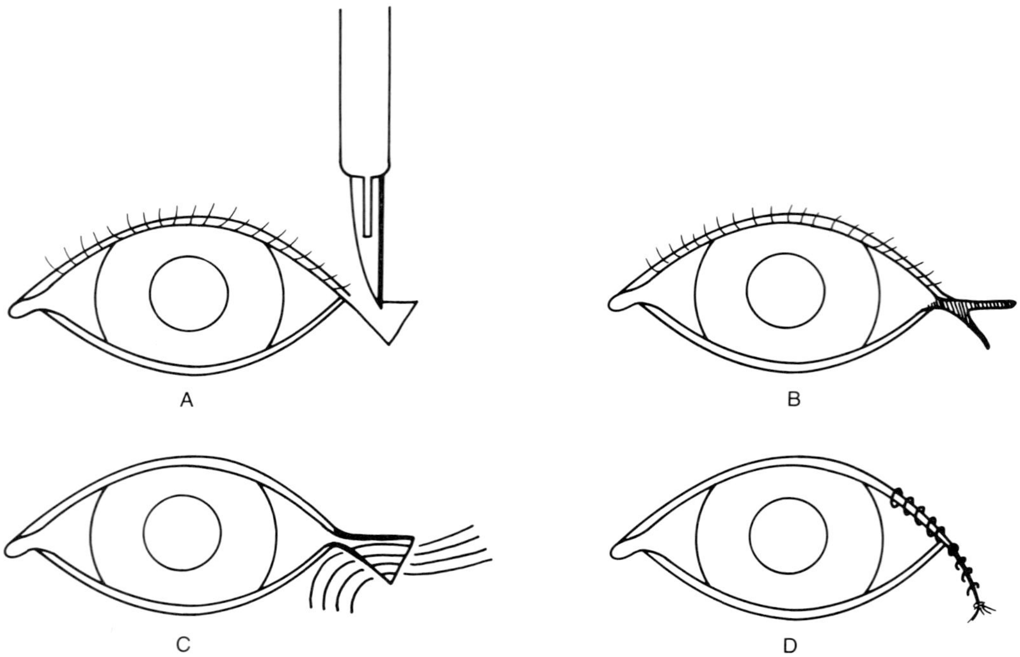

Figure 35–13. (*A*) In order to lengthen the upper lid and thus correct lagophthalmos, a V-shaped wedge of tissue is excised at the lateral canthus. (*B*) The adjacent tissue is undermined. (*C*) The conjunctiva is incised along the V's side. The superior edge of the triangle's length will increase the upper eyelid length. (*D*) The sides of the triangle are sutured together.

eyelids and nictitating membranes lacking pigment (see Chapter 59 and Fig. 35–14). Most tumors require surgical excision or cryosurgery. Chemotherapy and radiation therapy may be combined with surgery depending on the tumor type (see Chapter 51).

Geriatric-associated lid ulcers are resistent to most treatment; supportive care to relieve itching is indicated.

Premature Opening of the Eyelids

In contrast to ankyloblepharon, premature opening of the eyelids may result in corneal desiccation, ulceration, and possible perforation. Treatment consists of a temporary tarsorrhaphy for 7 to 10 days and administration of an antibiotic ointment and artificial tears through a gap at the medial canthus.[13]

Prolapse of the Gland of the Third Eyelid

Protrusion of the third eyelid gland is often termed "cherry eye." This condition is not due to primary inflammation, neoplasia, or hyperplasia[13] but rather to a lack of connective tissue holding the gland to the periorbita. Following trauma to the third eyelid or orbit or superficial irritation, the eye retracts into the orbit and the gland everts; it becomes irritated, inflamed, and enlarged. Cats undergoing surgical excision of the gland have a high incidence of keratoconjunctivitis sicca in later years. Current recommended treatment is surgical replacement by suturing the gland to the periosteum of the inferior orbital margin.[13] An alternative procedure is to place a vertical mattress suture starting at the palpebral surface of the base of the third eyelid, going through the third eyelid to the bulbar side, proceeding up the gland, and then reversing the steps. Nylon suture material (5-0 or 6-0) is recommended. The suture is tied and the knot buried on the palpebral surface so its removal is not necessary.

Trichiasis

Trichiasis is the presence of cilia that contact the cornea or conjunctiva to cause irritation, blepharospasm, and possible ulceration. Generally, the offending cilia originate from normal cilia locations. Although the condition is rare in the cat,[25] correction is surgical removal of the offending cilia, whether on the lid margin or from a prominent nasal fold.

Diseases of the Lacrimal Apparatus

Abscess of the Lacrimal Gland

Abscess of the lacrimal sac is uncommon and usually unilateral. Clinically, the abscess is located below the medial canthus. The inciting agent is usually dacryocystitis leading to necrosis of the lacrimal sac.[15] Treatment involves drainage and irrigation of the abscess and antibiotic therapy. Recurrence may require removal of the sac, but this often results in epiphora.[15]

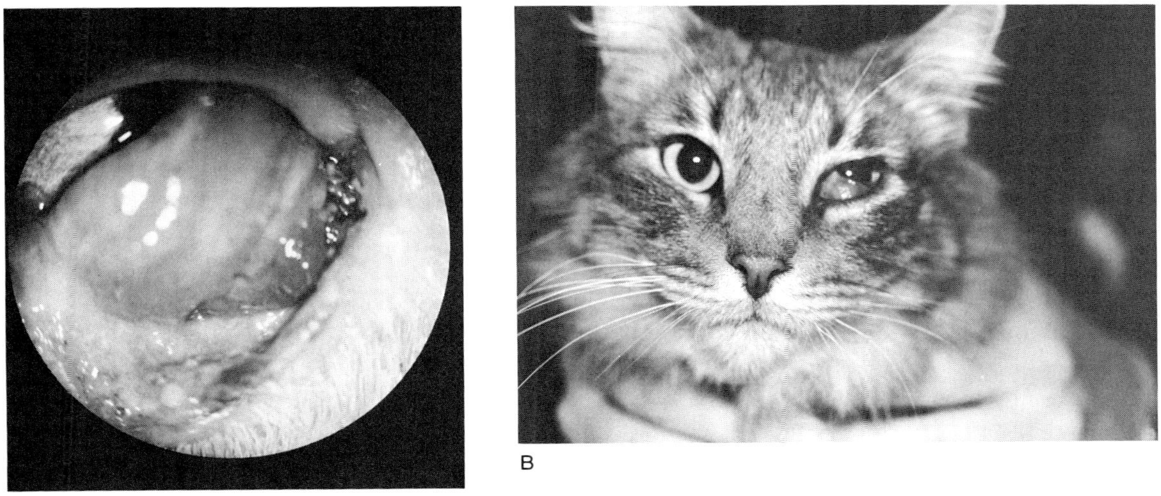

Figure 35–14. (*A*) Squamous cell carcinoma of the lower eyelid and third eyelid. (*B*) Lymphosarcoma of the third eyelid. This cat was FeLV positive and had ipsilateral enlargement of the submandibular and prescapular lymph nodes.

Adenitis

Inflammation of the lacrimal gland, adenitis, is rare. Symptoms include decreased tear production and cellulitis. Management of the keratoconjunctivitis sicca and adenitis are necessary.

Atresia

Lacrimal punctum atresia is rare; the most common clinical sign is epiphora. Treatment consists of cannulating the present punctum, usually the superior punctum, and irrigating with saline to expose the conjunctiva overlying the punctum. The conjunctiva is incised to establish drainage. Nasolacrimal irrigation may also reveal absence of the canaliculus. Treatment of atresia of the canaliculus is more complex, usually requiring a conjunctivoralostomy. A 3- to 4-mm polyethylene tubing is threaded through an opening created through the lower conjunctival fornix and upper fornix of the lips. The ends of the tubing are sutured to the conjunctiva and mucosa with 4-0 silk. The tubing remains in place at least 2 months so a permanent fistula may develop.

Dacryocystitis

Chronic epiphora and a mucoid conjunctivitis are symptoms of dacryocystitis or inflammation of the lacrimal sac and nasolacrimal duct.[15] The sac may have been penetrated by a foreign object or infected by bacteria. Irrigation of the lacrimal puncta with normal saline and administration of systemic antibiotics are effective treatments.

Keratoconjunctivitis Sicca

Keratoconjunctivitis sicca (KCS) is decreased tear formation. In the cat, this is usually characterized by a chronic keratoconjunctivitis with ulceration.[15] KCS may be secondary to upper respiratory viral infections (especially herpesvirus) or a chronic ocular infection. A neurogenic form may result from facial or orbital trauma. Transient KCS may result from the administration of greater than therapeutic levels of sulfonamides[12]; a geriatric form may be due to spontaneous atrophy of the third eyelid gland.[22] KCS may be surgically induced by removal of the prolapsed gland.[13] Autoimmune KCS results from destruction of the lacrimal gland; however, the majority of cases are idiopathic.

Symptoms include unilateral or bilateral chronic KCS with corneal vascularity superficially and recurrent ulceration [12] a thick, tenacious, mucopurulent exudate, a "lusterless" cornea, and pain and blepharospasm prior to keratinization. Diagnosis is based on appropriate clinical signs and a Schirmer tear test result of less than 10 mm/min; however, some normal cats may have Schirmer test values less than 10 mm. Therefore, if there are no clinical signs of KCS, treatment is not indicated.

Treatment consists of lubricating the eye. Medical treatments include the use of artificial tears 4 to 6 times/day, antiviral ophthalmic agents (for the herpetic form), and 1% to 2% cyclosporine applied topically. Surgical treatments provides long-term management. The preferred procedure is a parotid duct transposition as described by Severin[22] or Bistner.[26]

Diseases of the Conjunctiva

Conjunctival Emphysema

Conjunctival emphysema causes crepitus and subconjunctival swelling. Air enters the periorbita from the paranasal sinuses following trauma. Radiographs of the sinuses should be taken. Air is resorbed in 1 to 2 weeks in the absence of other lesions.[13]

Conjunctivitis

Inflammation of the conjunctiva is one of the most common ocular conditions in the cat. Conjunctivitis can be unilateral or bilateral and acute or chronic. Unilateral conjunctivitis is usually related to dacryocystitis or foreign body irritation, and the bilateral form is related to systemic or infectious disease.[15] Common signs are hyperemia, chemosis, and ocular discharge. Unless the cornea is involved, pain is absent. Table 35–3 shows the varieties of conjunctivitis with their common symptoms and treatment.

Subconjunctival Hemorrhage

Subconjunctival hemorrhage is usually a sequela to trauma. Some bleeding disorders may underlie spontaneous subconjunctival hemorrhage when trauma is not present. Pain is usually absent. Blood is usually resorbed in 2 weeks or less, so treatment is not necessary in uncomplicated cases. However, if the conjunctiva protrudes at the point of the hemorrhage, a temporary tarsorrhaphy may prevent desiccation.

Symblepharon

Symblepharon, adhesion between the bulbar and palpebral conjunctiva with the third eyelid involved, is most often seen in the Siamese.[15] Clinical signs are usually limited to cosmetic asymmetry. Treatment is surgical incision of the adhesions; however, success may be elusive because the conjunctiva tend to regrow over the excised tissue creating new areas of adhesion.

Diseases of the Cornea and Sclera

The cornea and sclera form the tough protective envelope that encloses the ocular tissues. This fibrous tunic consists of the opaque posterior sclera, the corneal–scleral junction (limbus), and the transparent anterior cornea. The transparent cornea of the cat occupies 30% of the anterior portion of the globe.[1] The feline cornea is oval with a horizontal diameter of 16 mm and a vertical diameter of 15.5 mm.[27] This elliptical appearance is owing to the wide superficial scleral shelf at the limbus of the vertical meridian.[28] Corneal diameter serves as a guide to globe size, which enlarges in chronic glaucoma or decreases in microphthalmia. The cornea has four histologic layers: epithelium, stroma, posterior limiting membrane (Descemet's membrane), and endothelium. The anterior limiting membrane (Bowman's) is histologically indistinct in the cat.[28]

The sclera covers the posterior aspect of the globe. It is continuous anteriorly with the cornea and posteriorly with the external optic nerve sheath.

Scleral Disease

Diseases of the sclera are rare.[27] Scleral stretching with thinning is observed in buphthalmia resulting from chronic glaucoma. Perforating wounds and neoplasia may also affect the sclera.

Corneal Disease

Corneal diseases in the cat share many of the same characteristics as other species; however, several are unique. Clinical signs of corneal disease include lacrimation, blepharospasm, conjunctival hyperemia, transparency loss, cellular infiltration, ulceration, neovascularization, aqueous flare, anterior uveal spasms, and pigmentation.

Bacterial Keratitis

Bacterial keratitis caused by traumatic disruption of the corneal epithelium is uncommon in the cat.[29] The same therapeutic measures as those for other species are entirely satisfactory. There is no restriction for the use of atropine to combat pain secondary to the ciliary spasms, but many cats exhibit excessive salivation if they taste atropine. This is less likely to happen if the ointment form is used.

Feline Herpesvirus Keratitis

The feline herpesvirus is the only known virus to cause keratitis in cats.[29,30] This viral disease is reported in neonatal, juvenile, and adult cats. The keratitis may be unilateral or bilateral and appears most frequently in the adult.[30] The first sign of initial involvement is the development of fine granular lesions in the corneal epithelium followed by aggregation with vesicle formation. Fissures develop in the epithelium and, when they appear in the linear pattern, are called dendritic ulcers. These fissures will stain with fluorescein, but the stain may undermine the adjacent epithelium since it has become loosely attached to the underlying stroma. If the disease becomes progressive and chronic, the fissures broaden and coalesce to form larger irregular ulceration. Interstitial keratitis and uveitis, as well as vascularization and granulation, occur with chronicity and recurrence (Fig. 35–15).

Diagnosis. Presumptive diagnosis is made from the clinical ocular signs. Rose bengal and fluorescein stain are helpful in identifying the epithelial lesions. Confirmation is by identification of the viral antigen by the fluorescent antibody technique. Virus isolation and serum neutralizing titer testing are also available.

Treatment. Treatment response has been unpredictable at best.[29] Response depends on the duration, extent, and complications. Topical antiviral drugs, including idoxuridine, adenine arabinoside, and trifluridine are most frequently used. The latter seems to produce the most consistent results. The recommended frequency of administration is hourly during the day and every 2 hours at night for the drops, and at least 5 times daily for ointments. The usual duration of treatment is a minimum of 2 to 3 weeks and at least 1 week after the signs have abated. Corticosteroids are known for their ability to aggravate viral infections and stimulate epithelial to stromal keratitis.[31] Dilute aqueous organic iodine (1:20) with saline applied as a topical medication 4 to 6 times daily is reported to produce good results in refractory cases.[32]

Table 35–3. Conjunctivitis

Etiology	Symptoms	Dx and Rx
Infectious		
Herpesvirus	Uni- or bilateral, serous and mucopurulent, epiphora, blepharospasm, pseudodiphtheritic membrane—only respiratory virus involving cornea	Cytology, virus isolation, response to Rx, self-limiting, antivirals, topical antibiotics
Calicivirus	Serous exudate, mild to moderate conjunctivitis, ulceration of tongue and pharynx, 7–10 day course	Signs, tissue, culture, FA test, prophylactic immunization artificial tears, topical antibiotics
Reovirus	Bilateral, serous discharge photophobia, mild conjunctivitis, respiratory signs unusual, mucopurulent exudate	Tissue culture, HA test, symptomatic Rx
Chlamydial	All ages, uni- or bilateral, severe chemosis at onset, serous epiphora, purulent conjunctivitis	Conjunctival scrapings intracytoplasmic inclusion bodies, follicles on bulbar or palpebral conjunctiva, tetracyclines
Mycoplasmal	Ulilateral serous and mucoid becoming bilateral, pale conjunctiva, pseudomembrane	Culture of conjunctival scrapings, chloramphenicol, erythromycin
Bacterial	Purulent ocular discharge, blepharospasm	Culture and sensitivity, topical and systemic antibiotics
Mycotic	Rare, chronic catarrhal conjunctiva. Conjunctiva: hyperemic, dry, thick. Cornea: focal, white-yellow plaques	Scraping, biopsy, histopathology, antifungals
Parasitic		
Thelazia	Catarrhal conjunctivitis with hyperemia	Observation, remove mechanically under topical anesthesia
Allergic	Serous discharge, moderate to intense hyperemia, mild chemosis, general dermatologic manifestations, may be seasonal	Presumptive Dx after steroid therapy, removal of irritating agent, topical steroids
Follicular	Lymphoid follicles on conjunctiva	Signs, follicle removal, topical antibiotics
Mechanical		
Endogenous/exogenous	Mild hyperemia, serous to mucoid discharge	Removal of irritation, topical antibiotics

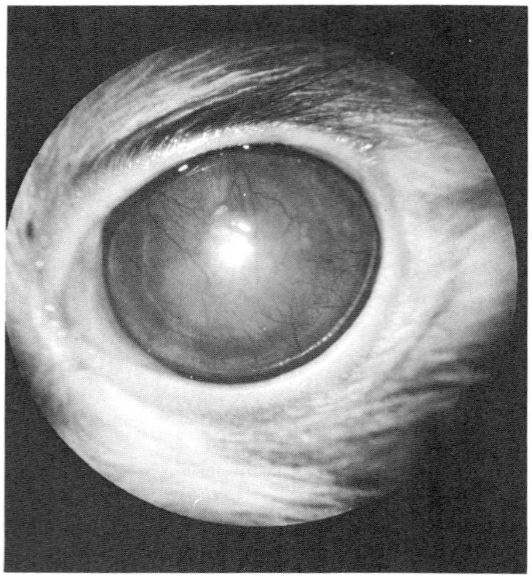

Figure 35–15. Herpes keratitis and uveitis with interstitial corneal neovascularization.

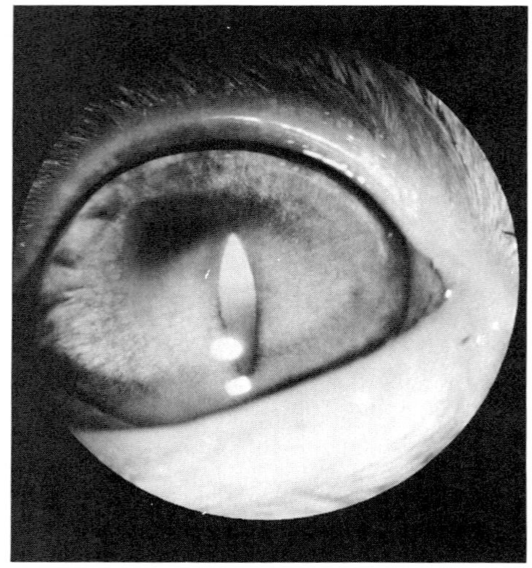

Figure 35–17. Type II corneal sequestration.

Corneal Sequestrum

Corneal sequestrum is unique to cats and is characterized by the degeneration of collagen and an accumulation of brown pigment.[15,33] A variety of terms are used to describe this distinct degeneration in the cornea of the cat including mummification, corneal nigrum, focal degeneration, isolated black lesions, and sequestration. The clinical appearance is a chronic pathologic process characterized by a unilateral, sometimes bilateral, brown to black subepithelial plaque. The etiology is unknown, but history of previous corneal insult may be reported. Corneal sequestrum is reported in all breeds, but the Persian, Siamese, Himalayan, and Burmese breeds have higher incidences. The lesions are circular to oval and central or paracentral.

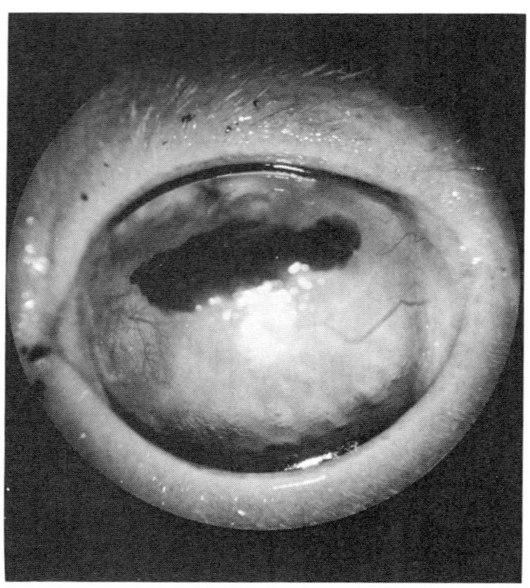

Figure 35–16. Type I paracentral corneal sequestration. This is somewhat atypical because the usual lesion is more ovoid in shape.

Diagnosis. Two types have been described. Type I is a well-defined, dark brown to black plaque with elevation above the corneal surface (Fig. 35–16). Type II is less distinct with less blackness and less surface elevation (Fig. 35–17).[15]

Treatment. Surgical removal by superficial keratectomy usually resolves Type I plaque. However, if the plaque is showing evidence of separating from the underlying corneal stroma, it may be treated with topical antibiotics to promote sloughing. The Type II lesion usually resolves over a period of time so no treatment is necessary.

Eosinophilic Keratitis

Eosinophilic keratitis in the cat is a proliferative granulomatous corneal infiltration.[34] Clinically it presents as unilateral or bilateral lesions that are proliferative with an irregular, white to pink, vascularized surface (Fig. 35–18). It most commonly arises from the temporal limbus and invades that corneal quadrant; however, with chronicity it may affect the entire cornea.

Diagnosis. Eosinophilic keratitis must be differentiated from corneal neoplasia and other granulomatous lesions. The diagnosis is confirmed by corneal scraping or biopsy with the identification of large numbers of eosinophils and mast cells.

Treatment. Eosinophilic keratitis may respond to topical ophthalmic corticosteroid therapy with 1% prednisolone acetate suspension or 0.1% dexamethasone ointment. In refractory cases, the condition is controlled with megestrol acetate. The usual dose regimen is 5 mg daily for 1 week followed by 5 mg on alternate days until regression, and then 5 mg weekly to prevent recurrence.[35] Side effects of megestrol acetate are discussed in Chapter 7.

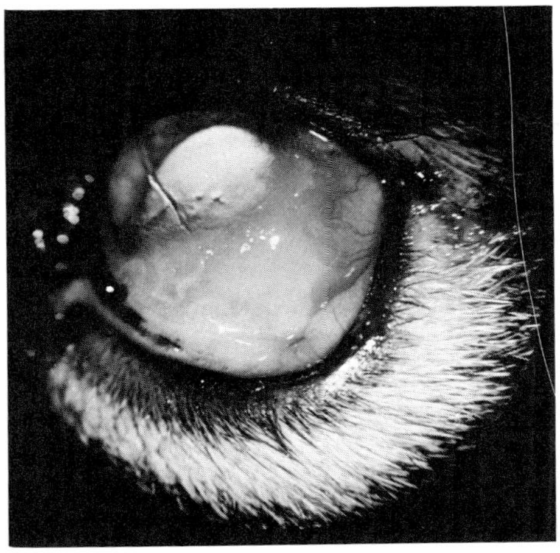

Figure 35–18. **Eosinophilic keratitis appears as an irregular proliferative lesion of the ventral portion of the cornea.**

Miscellaneous Corneal Diseases

To complete the differential diagnosis of corneal disease the following conditions should be considered. Keratomycosis is rare in the cat.[36] Various corneal dystrophies and degenerations are infrequently described.[15,37] The lysosomal storage diseases (gangliosidosis, mannasidosis, and mucopolysaccharidosis) have produced corneal haze, cloudiness, and opacities associated with the inborn metabolic errors.[29] Squamous cell carcinoma and melanoma can invade the cornea; however, they are rare.

REFERENCES

1. Prince JH. Anatomy and Histology of the Eye and Orbit in Domestic Animals. Springfield: Charles C Thomas, 1960.
2. Slatter DH, Chambers ED. The Orbit. In: Slatter DH, ed. Textbook of Veterinary Surgery, vol. II. Philadelphia: WB Saunders, 1985:1549.
3. Scott FW. Teratogenesis in cats associated with griseofulvin therapy. Teratology 1975;11:79.
4. Betts DM. Diseases of the Orbit. In: Kirk RW, ed. Current Veterinary Therapy VIII, Small Animal Practice. Philadelphia: WB Saunders, 1983:577.
5. Oliver JE. Cranial sinus venography in the dog. J Am Vet Rad Soc 1969;10:70.
6. Ticer JW. Radiographic Techniques in Small Animal Practice. Philadelphia: WB Saunders, 1975:278.
7. Munger RJ, Ackerman N. Retrobulbar injections in the dog. A comparison of three techniques. J Am Anim Hosp Assoc 1978;14:490.
8. Davis JP. Cat optic nerve imaging with metrizamide. Invest Ophthalmol Vis Sci 1979;18:273.
9. LeCouteur RA. Indirect imaging of the canine optic nerve using metrizamide (optic thecography). Am J Vet Res 1982;43:1424.
10. Quinn AJ, Frantz K. Magnetic resonance imaging (MRI) in tumor diagnosis. Proc Annu Meet Am Int Soc Vet Ophthalmol San Francisco: 1990;60.
11. Morgan RV. Ultrasonography of retrobulbar diseases in the dog and cat. J Am Anim Hosp Assoc 1989;25:393.
12. Szymanski C. The Eye. In: Diseases of the Cat. Holzworth J, ed. Philadelphia: WB Saunders, 1987:681.
13. Slatter D. Fundamentals of Veterinary Ophthalmology. Philadelphia: WB Saunders, 1990:147.
14. Wyman M. Manual of Small Animal Ophthalmology. New York: Churchill Livingstone, 1986:67.
15. Peiffer RL. Feline Ophthalmology. In: Gelatt KN, ed. Veterinary Ophthalmology Philadelphia: Lea & Febiger, 1981:521.
16. Brightman AH. The Eye. In: Pratt PW, ed. Feline Medicine. Santa Barbara: American Veterinary Publications, 1983:609.
17. Koch SA. Congenital ophthalmic abnormalities in the Burmese cat. J Am Vet Med Assoc 1979;175:90.
18. Dziezyc J, Millichamp N. Surgical correction of eyelid agenesis in a cat. J Am Anim Hosp Assoc 1989;25:513.
19. Symthe RH. Veterinary Ophthalmology, 2nd ed. Baltimore: Williams & Wilkins, 1958.
20. Griffith IR, Nash AS, Sharp NJH. The Key-Gaskell syndrome: The current situation. Vet Rec 1982;118:532.
21. Peiffer RL. Small Animal Ophthalmology: A Problem-Oriented Approach. Philadelphia: WB Saunders, 1989:145.
22. Severin GA. Veterinary Ophthalmology Notes, 2nd ed. Fort Collins: Colo State Univ, 1986.
23. Wheeler CA, Severin GA. Cryosurgical epilation for the treatment of distichiasis in the dog and cat. J Am Anim Hosp Assoc 1984;20:877.
24. Albert RA, Garrett PD, Whitley RD. Surgical correction of everted third eyelid in two cats. J Am Vet Med Assoc 1982; 180:763.
25. Roberts SR, Lipton DE. The Eye. In: Catcott EJ, ed. Feline Medicine and Surgery. Santa Barbara: American Veterinary Publications, 1975:491.
26. Bistner SI. Aguirre G, Batik G. Atlas of Veterinary Ophthalmic Surgery. Philadelphia: WB Saunders, 1977.
27. Blogg JR. The Eye in Veterinary Practice—Extraocular Disease. Philadelphia: WB Saunders, 1980:376.
28. Martin CL, Anderson BG. Ocular Anatomy. In: Gelatt KN, ed. Veterinary Ophthalmology. Philadelphia: Lea & Febiger, 1981:23.
29. Nasisse MP. Bacterial Keratitis. In: Gelatt KN, ed. Veterinary Ophthalmology, 2nd ed. Philadelphia: Lea & Febiger, 1991:567.
30. Bistner SJ. Ocular manifestations of feline herpesvirus infection. J Am Vet Med Assoc 1971;159:1223.
31. Nasisse MP. Experimental ocular herpesvirus infection in the cat: Sites of virus replication, clinical features, and effects of corticosteroid administration. Invest Ophthalmol Vis Sci 1989; 30:1758.
32. Severin GL. Personal communication, 1991.
33. Pentlarge VW. Corneal sequestration in cats. Compend Contin Ed Pract Vet 1989;11:24.
34. Brightman AH. Chronic eosinophilic keratitis in the cat. Feline Pract 1979;9:21.
35. Ketring KL. Eosinophilic Keratitis in Cats. Proc Am Spc Vet Ophthalmol Am Acad Vet Dermat 1991.
36. Schmidt GM. Mycotic keratoconjunctivitis. Vet Med Small Anim Clin 1974;69:1177.
37. Bistner SI. Hereditary corneal dystrophy in the Manx cat: A preliminary report. Invest Ophthalmol Vis Sci 1976;15:15.

CHAPTER 36

◇ ◇ ◇

The Eye: Intraocular Diseases

Art J. Quinn and Virginia A. Schultz

The Anterior Uvea

The uvea is composed of the iris, ciliary body, and choroid. It comprises the middle of the three tunics of the eye and is of prime functional importance. It has a rich complement of blood vessels and is often the locus of inflammatory changes. It reacts to microorganisms, toxins, and systemic infections. The uvea is frequently the site of allergic reactions and functions as a lymph node, producing T-lymphocytes, plasma cells, and antibodies. The uvea in the cat is a sensitive indicator of many systemic abnormalities in the body.

Diseases of the uveal tract are some of the most interesting and perplexing problems. In some instances the cause is clear and concise, such as an acute episode of trauma; in others, such as systemic diseases or hypersensitivity or autoimmune reactions, it is obscure.

Uveitis

Uveitis appears to be the result of an antibody-dependent disease. Uveitis is more complicated than simple mechanical injury to cells. It occurs when an immune complex response becomes the primary initiator of an inflammatory reaction. Mediators in the inflammatory response include prostaglandins, lymphokines, and immunoglobulins. When the uveal tract becomes immunocompetent intraocular antigen passes into the systemic circulation. The antigen stimulates distant lymphoid tissue; subsequently, sensitized lymphocytes migrate toward the antigen-producing tissue (uvea) and cause cell-mediated antibody production, resulting in the inflammatory reaction. Further exposure to the same antigen causes a more rapid and severe response; the uvea behaves as an accessory lymph node.

Another inflammatory reaction is thought to be neuronal in origin, such as that associated with minor corneal damage. Corneal nerve trauma initiates the inflammatory reaction. Small numbers of inflammatory cells enter the aqueous in response to anterior uveal vessel dilatation secondary to the axon-mediated response. This response is transient and produces no structural change.

Clinical Signs

Pain results from irritation of the ciliary nerves and is aggravated by exposure to light and by pressure.

Photophobia is most common in acute uveitis and more severe when keratitis is present.

Lacrimation is associated with photophobia and pain.

Congestion is circumcorneal and within the conjunctiva, owing to the extension of the uveal inflammation of the anterior ciliary vessels at the limbus.

Keratopathy arises by extension into the peripheral cornea from the limbal circulation or through damaged corneal endothelium and Descemet's membrane. Prolonged inflammation leads to persistent edema, folds in Descemet's membrane, and vesicle formation in the corneal epithelium.

Keratic precipitates, deposits of inflammatory cells on the corneal endothelium, occur in acute and chronic uveitis and vary in size, number, character, and position.

Damage to the corneal endothelium favors deposition. They are usually located in the lower cornea because of the aqueous convection currents.

Aqueous flare is produced by light passing through the protein-rich aqueous.

Aqueous cells are due to inflammation of the iris and ciliary body; they pass either by diffusion or by active migration into the aqueous.

Precipitates may be observed on the trabecular meshwork in the anterior chamber angle and on the anterior surface of the iris and lens.

Fibrin clots are due to an excessive amount of fibrin and coagulation of the exudate in the anterior chamber.

Hemorrhage is more often associated with trauma; however, some primary types of iritis produce hemorrhage. The exact reason is unknown. Absorption is rapid if the outflow channels are not impaired.

Iris atrophy results from prolonged inflammation of the iris stroma and epithelium. Fibrosis, scarring, and pigmentary changes are common.

Synechiae result when heavy exudation of protein-rich aqueous causes adhesions of the iris to adjacent structures (lens or cornea).

Cataract formation results from the toxic effects of uveal inflammation.

Low intraocular pressure (hypotony) is characteristic of acute uveitis. The exact method by which decreased aqueous production by the ciliary body results in lowered tension is unknown.

Increased intraocular pressure (glaucoma) may develop as an early or late manifestation caused by obstruction of the outflow channels by the inflammatory process in the trabeculae. The spaces are occluded by cellular debris and exudate or sequelae of the prolonged inflammation, producing degeneration and fibrosis of the outflow channels and synechiae.

Miosis is moderate to marked.

The clinical signs often lead to a diagnosis of anterior uveitis. However, since posterior uveitis frequently accompanies anterior uveal inflammation, the examination should include the choroid for the following findings:

Vitreous opacities are produced by inflammatory cells, erythrocytes, tissue cells, and protein-rich fluid penetrating the vitreous.

Chorioretinitis is observed as grayish white areas containing fluid and cells during active disease. Pigmentation may occur within the lesion as healing occurs.

Optic nerve changes appear as a swelling of the optic disk due to the effects of irritation on it.

Retinal degeneration occurs secondary to retinotoxic effects of the inflammation.

Retinal detachment is usually secondary to retroretinal choroidal exudate and cellular infiltration or from contraction of vitreous traction bands.

Causes

Historically, anterior uveitis in cats has been viewed as a manifestation of multisystemic disseminating disease. Those of most frequent occurrence include the systemic mycoses, feline leukemia virus (FeLV) or feline immunodeficiency virus (FIV) infection, feline infectious peritonitis (FIP), and toxoplasmosis.

Systemic Mycoses. Disseminating mycotic agents are saprophytes that become opportunistic pathogens after gaining entrance to the body. The fungal agents more commonly reported to cause intraocular manifestations are *Blastomyces dermatitidis,*[1,2] *Cryptococcus neoformans,*[3-5] *Coccidioides immitis,*[6] and *Histoplasma capsulatum.*[7-10] The responses in organs, including the eye, are extensive proliferation and infiltration of reticuloendothelial cells, macrophages, and epithelial cells (Fig. 36–1; see Chapter 61).

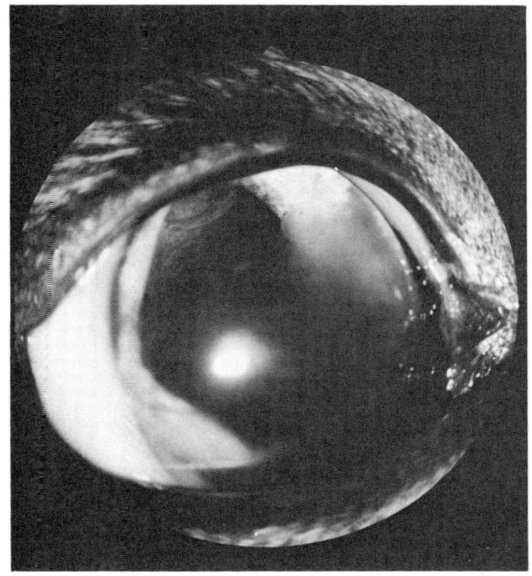

Figure 36–1. **Anterior uveitis, hyphema, and anterior chamber fibrin caused by histoplasmosis.**

Feline Leukemia Virus. Lymphoid neoplasia is the most common malignancy of cats and is considered the most prevalent intraocular neoplasm.[11] Anterior segment change is a frequent clinical sign; however, it is not unusual to find disease only in the posterior segment. Anterior segment findings include keratopathy, hypopyon, keratic precipitates, aqueous cells and flare, hemorrhage, lymphoid proliferative iritis, and synechiation (Fig. 36–2; see Chapters 39 and 51).

Feline Immunodeficiency Virus. An association between FIV infection and intraocular inflammation was recently demonstrated.[12-14] Chronic anterior uveitis with aque-

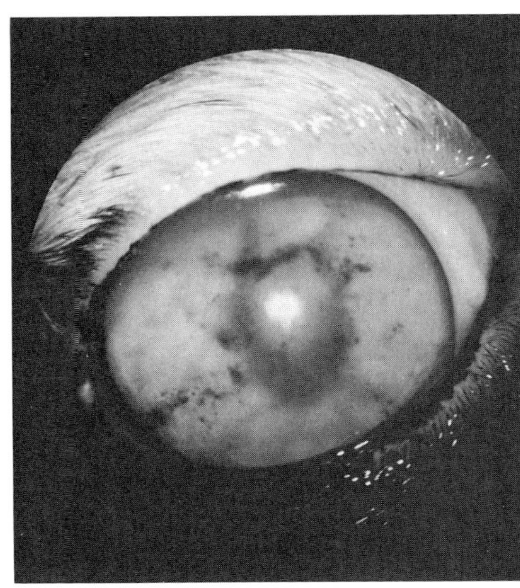

Figure 36–2. **Aqueous flare and cells, keratic precipitates, iris hyperemia and hemorrhage, and posterior synechia associated with the FeLV.**

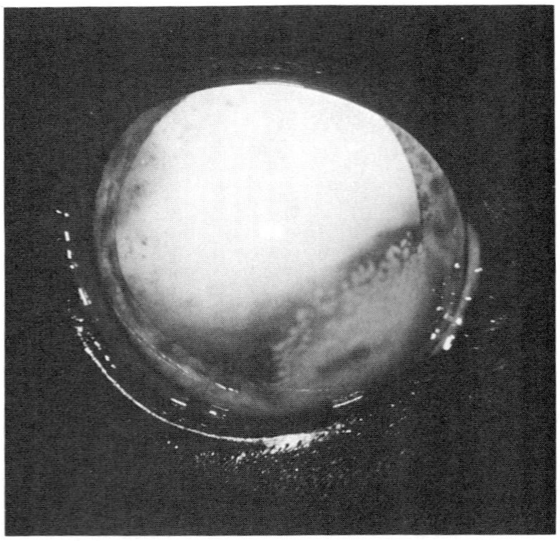

Figure 36–3. **Keratic precipitates, aqueous flare, iritis, mydriasis, and glaucoma (IOP 60 mm Hg). The cat had FIV antibodies.**

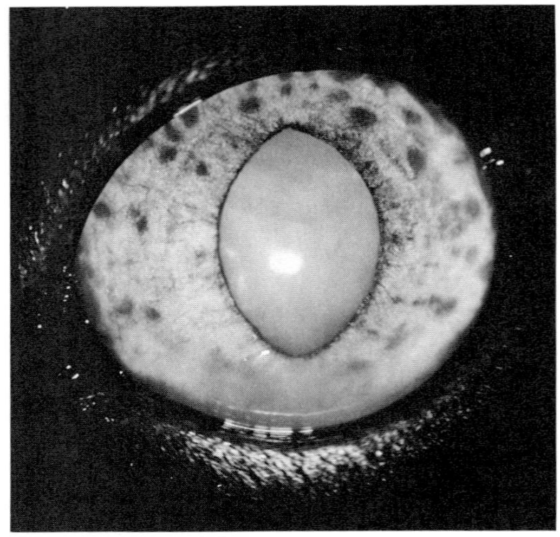

Figure 36–5. **Anterior uveitis caused by toxoplasmosis. Keratic precipitates are present on the inferior aspect of the cornea. Note the multifocal hyperpigmented areas of the iris and secondary inflammatory cataract.**

ous flare, keratic precipitates, iris hyperemia and congestion, posterior synechia, and glaucoma have been observed associated with this disease (Fig. 36–3; see Chapter 37).

Feline Infectious Peritonitis. The systemic signs of FIP are those of chronic, multisystemic, progressive, debilitating disease. The vasculitis caused by the coronavirus leads to increased diffusion and effusion through the vessel walls, resulting in accumulation of fibrin and fluid. Damage to the uveal blood vessels allows exudation of cells and proteinaceous material to accumulate in the intraocular tissues. With additional disruption of the ocular hemodynamics uveal degeneration occurs as the disease progresses.

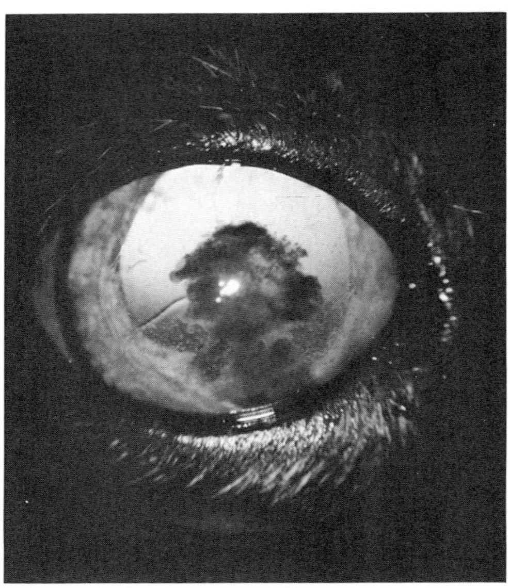

Figure 36–4. **Fibrinohemorrhagic clot and fibrin strands in the anterior chamber. Histopathologic examination confirmed FIP.**

The clinical signs most commonly associated with FIP-induced anterior uveitis are corneal edema, keratic precipitates, aqueous flare, fibrinohemorrhagic clot formation, miosis, and posterior synechia.[15,16] The ocular media opacities often preclude posterior segment examination (Fig. 36–4; see Chapter 38).

Toxoplasmosis. Toxoplasmosis is caused by *Toxoplasma gondii,* an obligate intracellular protozoan parasite. Ocular lesions are found in both asymptomatic and clinically affected cats. Anterior segment involvement may produce a nongranulomatous hypersensitivity reaction or a granulomatous response to actual infection (Fig. 36–5).[11]

Diagnosis

Careful history, meticulous systemic and ophthalmic examination, and laboratory procedures should be exhausted in the attempt to identify the cause of uveitis. In some cases it will remain a mystery, regardless of extensive diagnostic evaluations. Overt clinical signs of uveitis may not be present; the following findings may be of value:

- Red eye is characterized by congestion of the ciliary vessels at the limbus with the corneal-scleral flush.
- The iris may exhibit edema, hyperemia, and discoloration or dullness with loss of fine architecture.
- Pupillary light reflexes are abnormal. The direct pupillary light reflex is sluggish or absent, even when the pupil is not miotic.
- The tropicamide response is diminished: instillation of 1% tropicamide produces little or no pupillary dilatation.
- Hypotony is characteristic of uveitis. Tonometry should be performed initially and to monitor progress.

- Changes in the liquid media occur. Transillumination with magnification often reveals evidence of flare, cells, and precipitates.

Treatment

The extent of ocular inflammation, the duration of disease, and the cause dictate the medical regimen. Early and vigorous treatment is required to prevent permanent ocular damage. The basis of treatment is an etiologic diagnosis, elimination of the causative agent, iridocycloplegia, and suppression of inflammation.

Cycloplegics (parasympatholytics) are indicated when pain or miosis is present. The goals of therapy are to obtain a slightly larger pupil, thereby reducing posterior synechia formation, and to relieve pain from ciliary and pupillary spasms. The cycloplegic of choice is topical atropine (1 to 3%) in ointment form. The dosing schedule should be based on clinical response. Careful monitoring of intraocular pressure during the first 48 to 72 hours is necessary to minimize the possibility of angle closure. When the initial pain and outpouring of inflammatory cells are arrested dosing with the cycloplegic should be reduced or discontinued, allowing normal pupillary action. A dark environment is beneficial because it reduces reflex parasympathetic stimulation of the iris and ciliary body.

Corticosteroids are the drug of choice to reduce inflammation and its serious sequelae, to preserve ocular tissue, and to maintain normal physiologic function. They decrease cellular and fibrinous exudation, decrease tissue infiltration, inhibit fibroblastic and collagen-forming activity, retard epithelial and endothelial regeneration, diminish postinflammatory neovascularization, and restore normal permeability of inflamed capillaries. Thus, corticosteroids prevent further extensive damage to the ocular tissues.

The exact mechanisms by which corticosteroids act in suppressing ocular inflammation are incompletely understood. Their effects also include lysosomal stabilization, reduction of lymphoid elements, and reduction or inhibition of antibody production, thereby limiting immune reactions. Corticosteroids of choice include these:

Topical: Prednisolone acetate, 1% (Pred Forte); apply up to six times daily.

Subconjunctival: Betamethasone (Betasone), 7 mg/mL; one 3.5-mg (0.5-mL) injection, *or* methylprednisolone acetate (Depo-Medrol), 40 mg/mL, one 10-mg (0.25-mL) injection.

Systemic: Prednisolone, 0.5 mg/lb b.i.d., *or* dexamethasone, 0.1 to 0.2 mg/lb s.i.d.

Precautions must be taken when corticosteroids are administered because they can cause serious complications and side effects. They do not eliminate infectious agents, can mask signs, and can further reduce host resistance to bacteria, viruses, and fungi. They should not be used in the presence of such infections except in conjunction with an effective antibiotic or other appropriate antimicrobial agent.

Prostaglandins play a significant role in ocular inflammations by causing protein leakage from inflamed uveal vessels. Prostaglandin inhibition reduces the release of protein and decreases immune reactions by reducing antibody production, and thus fibrin production. Prostaglandin inhibitors such as aspirin, 8 mg/lb every 3 days, and topical use of flurbiprofen (Ocufen) is beneficial when corticosteroids are contraindicated.

Complications in the treatment of uveitis occur most frequently when the ocular inflammation is not recognized or not controlled until late in the course of the disease, resulting in irreversible ocular changes. Common sequelae include endothelial damage with permanent corneal edema and deep interstitial keratitis, protein leakage resulting from altered vasculature, synechia formation and iris atrophy, glaucoma associated with anterior synechia and closure of the filtration angle, secondary cataract formation, retinal degeneration and separation with optic neuritis and atrophy, phthisis bulbi, and total loss of vision.

The cause of uveitis is usually obscure, which often makes early diagnosis and treatment very difficult. The most desirable results are achieved when a diagnosis is made and treatment is instituted prior to the appearance of marked clinical signs. Uveitis is often diagnosed as conjunctivitis or keratitis, so treatment measures are inappropriate. The main errors in treatment include delayed initiation of therapy and administering anti-inflammatory agents in subtherapeutic doses or for an inadequate period.

Inflammatory uveal tract disease is a devastating disease, often of obscure or unidentified cause. The prognosis must be guarded, owing to its many sequelae.

Melanoma of the Iris

A common entity of the iris is diffuse melanoma. Usually a slow migration of melanocytes into the iris stroma causes grossly visible darkening of the iris. It may progress to cause thickening of the iris and exfoliation of pigment cells into the anterior chamber. The melanocytic infiltration can go into the angle and cause secondary glaucoma. There is a higher incidence of metastasis when glaucoma occurs.

Affected eyes should be followed with tonometry and gonioscopic examination to monitor the progression of melanocytosis. When the angle becomes pigmented and there is a rise in intraocular pressure, enucleation is advisable. Prior to surgery a thoracic radiograph is recommended to detect possible metastasis.

Diseases of the Lens

The crystalline lens is a biconvex transparent structure whose function is to focus light upon the retina.[17] The lens is suspended by the zonular ligaments, which connect the ciliary body with the lens capsule at the equator of the lens. The lens is suspended behind the iris and separates the aqueous humor from the vitreous humor. A patellar fossa is formed as a depression in the anterior surface of the vitreous humor by the posterior surface of the lens. The circumference of the lens, the equator, is not a smooth surface but has irregularities which represent the attachment of the zonular fibers. The anterior pole is the center of the anterior surface of the lens; the posterior pole is the corresponding farthest posterior surface of the lens. The lens consists of a capsule, anterior cuboidal epithelium, lens fibers, and an amorphous cement material.[18]

The lens capsule is a semipermeable membrane through which all metabolites readily pass. The epithelial layer immediately beneath the anterior lens capsule provides a barrier between the aqueous humor and the lens proper. The oxygen content of the lens is limited primarily to the epithelium and the outer cortex. The metabolic rate of the lens is slow, and the metabolism is limited primarily to glucose utilization. Most of the metabolism is limited to anaerobic glycolysis, which produces lactic acid. The lens is composed primarily of protein, 33% of its total weight, a greater proportion than in any other organ of the body.[19] The other metabolites are present in levels similar to those in the aqueous. The lens proteins are primarily (85%) soluble α-, β-, and γ, crystallin. The remaining 15% is insoluble albuminoid. The α crystallin is in higher concentration in the outer cortical portion, whereas the insoluble albuminoid is in higher concentration in the nuclear portion. In cataracts and with natural changes of aging, the insoluble albuminoid fraction increases. Because of their location in the avascular lens, the lens proteins are recognized as foreign protein by the immune system. The antigenicity of the lens proteins is clinically significant; an inflammatory response can be expected to follow escape of lens proteins.[19] Lens proteins leaking into the aqueous can stimulate antilens antibody production, resulting in severe uveitis.

The diseases commonly encountered are classified as developmental abnormalities, opacities, displacements, or ruptures.[18,20] The lens in the adult cat cannot become inflamed, owing to its isolated position and lack of blood supply; therefore, its reaction to disease is manifested as changes in transparency, in position (ectopia lentis), and in size through intumescence or resorption.[21]

Cataracts

The lens fiber's transparency is affected by swelling and coagulation. As the fiber swells from the imbibition of water the size of the protein mycelle changes, and opacities develop because of the change in continuity. This opacity is reversible. Vacuolization and coagulation cause the protein to become more insoluble. This opacity is irreversible; once the process of coagulation begins, it is generally progressive and leads to clinical cataract formation. Changes in transparency of the lens may be primary, or intrinsic: changes observed when there is no evidence of local or systemic disease. Secondary causes are extrinsic factors causing alterations in the lens proteins through other ocular or systemic diseases.

Lens transparency depends on maintaining normal levels of metabolites. Being avascular, it depends upon metabolite diffusion through the capsule from the aqueous and vitreous. Removal of metabolic waste products utilizes the same structures. Toxic substances entering the aqueous or the vitreous can disturb metabolism in the lens. Theories have been advanced on the mechanism of primary or intrinsic cataract formation, but the exact physiochemical mechanism that produces the denatured lens protein and abnormal arrangement of the lens fibers remains undefined.

The processes by which the lens reacts to certain disease conditions can be classified as biologic, immune-mediated, local, and systemic disturbances. The pathologic

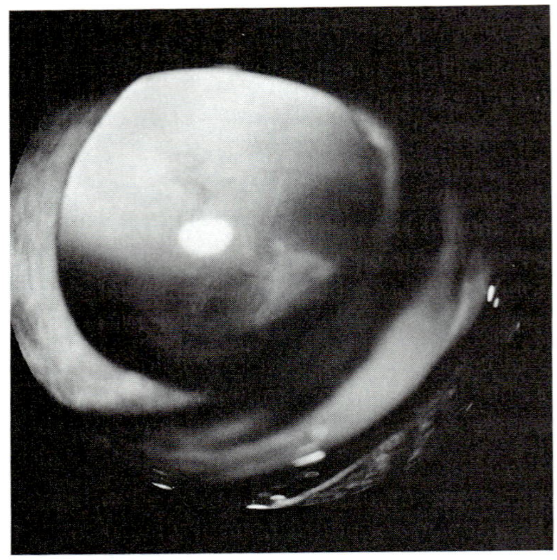

Figure 36–6. **Posterior capsular and Y suture (triangular) cataractous opacities.**

biologic changes include congenital cataracts, posterior lenticonus, and the other developmental disturbances of the eye that affect the lens. The nonpathologic biologic changes include nuclear sclerosis. The sclerotic nucleus, strictly speaking, is a cataract; however, it does not interfere with visualization of the fundus as do the opacities of cataracts, and there is little if any disturbance of vision.

Immune-mediated disturbances include phagolytic uveitis. During cataract development leakage of the lens protein into the aqueous humor causes secondary inflammation of the uveal tract. Another immune-mediated type of cataract results from inflammation of the surrounding uveal tissue induced by local or systemic disease. Other conditions such as glaucoma, ocular trauma, radiation, and chemical toxins have produced cataracts.

Cataracts are the most common of the lenticular diseases of cats (Fig. 36–6).[22] In contrast to dogs, cats rarely have genetically influenced developmental cataracts.[22] Cataracts in cats are usually secondary and are attributable to other underlying ocular disease. Traumatic cataracts are frequently observed in cats secondary to penetrating ocular injuries and are usually located in the area of the lens adjacent to the ocular insult (Fig. 36–7). The traumatic cataract is generally slow to progress (Fig. 36–8). Serious uveitis may occur secondarily if sufficient lens protein escapes from a large capsular tear. Diabetic cataracts are uncommon; they progress more slowly than diabetic cataracts of dogs.[23]

Changes in lens position have been described by the terms dislocation, displacement, ectopia lentis, and luxation. Ectopia lentis is further defined as subluxation or luxation. A lens is subluxated if it is partially dislocated from its normal position but remains in the patellar fossa in a plane behind the iris (Fig. 36–9). Lens luxation is defined as dislocation from the normal position. With the iris in close apposition to the lens, luxation leads to iris tremor, iris wobble, or iridoneisis. The tremor may be noted when the patient moves its head. An aphakic crescent is formed when the lens becomes dislocated, and the lens is visible as a crescent

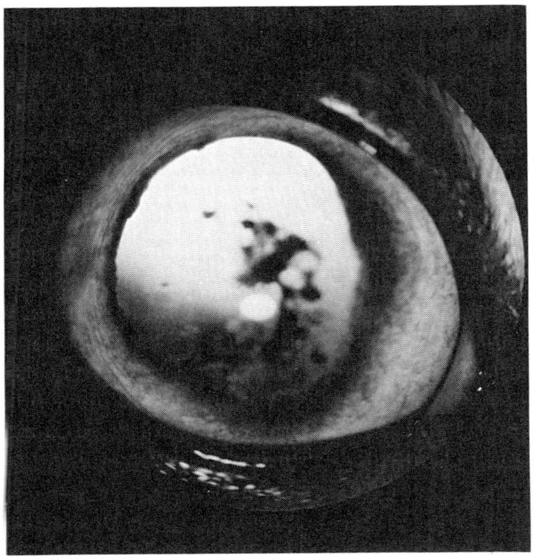

Figure 36–7. Posterior synechia (7 o'clock position) with pigment on the anterior lens capsule. A lenticular opacity is present at the 6 o'clock position. There are changes secondary to previous perforating corneal trauma.

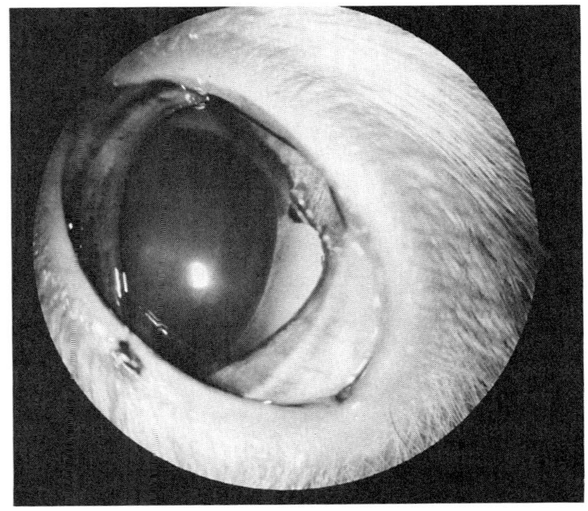

Figure 36–9. Subluxation of the lens. Note the superior aphacic crescent.

in the pupillary margin. Anterior luxation results in the lens being moved forward; posterior luxation describes a lens that has fallen into the vitreous.

Trauma, chronic glaucoma, generalized degenerative disease of the globe, chronic uveitis, intraocular neoplasms, and aging contribute to zonular degeneration, weakness, stretching, and rupture of the zonules. These lead to lens displacement. Following luxation the transparent lens frequently becomes rapidly cataractous because of its inability to sustain normal metabolism (Fig. 36–10).

When the lens is moved forward it can mimic keratitis, anterior uveitis, or produce secondary glaucoma due to pupillary block. An increase in the depth of the anterior chamber occurs with posterior luxation. Iris tremor may be observed, and vitreous protrudes through the pupil. Secondary glaucoma is the most serious complication. Retinal degeneration, detachment, or hemorrhage may also occur. In posterior luxation, the image is not reflected from the anterior lens surface. If the lens is cataractous it may be seen in the vitreous as a dark circular area or as a dark-rimmed globule magnifying the retina if it is transparent.

Treatment is surgical removal of the cataractous lenses. Careful ocular examination is recommended prior to surgery to rule out secondary, inflammatory causes of cataracts; these would significantly reduce the success rate. The prognosis is also worse if cataracts are associated with lens luxation, glaucoma, or lens trauma.

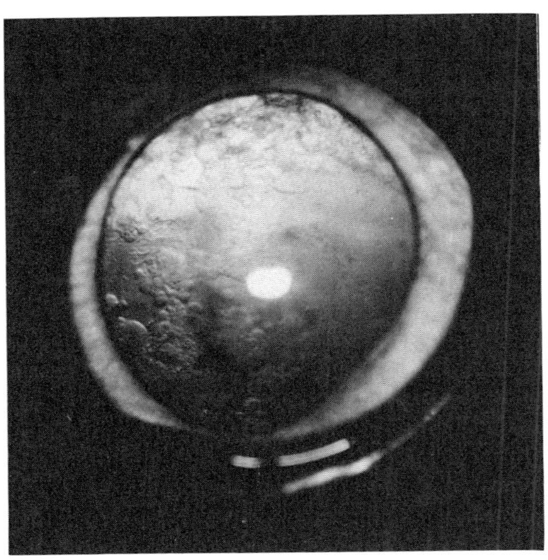

Figure 36–8. Cataract developing (vascularization) resulting from trauma. This was made 6 months later of the cat in Figure 35–1.

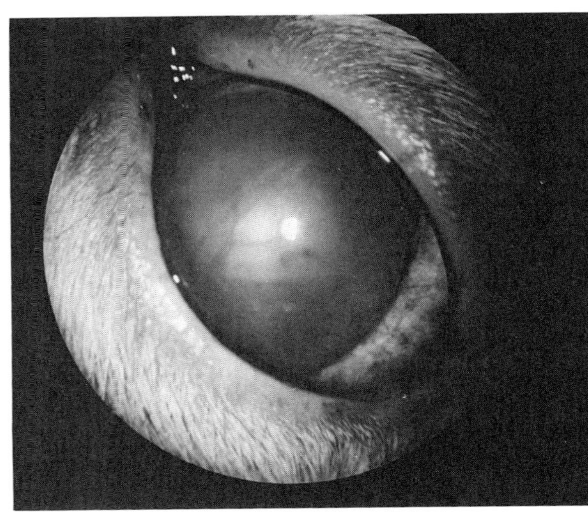

Figure 36–10. Anterior lens luxation. The lens has become opaque (cataract).

The surgical procedure is the same as for dogs. Surgery is recommended when the cataracts are bilateral and cause marked visual deficit. In general, cataract surgery is more successful in cats than in dogs. Postsurgical uveitis occurs less frequently and is more responsive to treatment.

The Vitreous

The vitreous, the largest structure in the eye, occupies about 75% of its volume. If fills the posterior compartment of the globe from the posterior lens surface to the retina. The vitreous is composed of about 98% water, with a skeleton of collagen fibers (hyalocytes) and mucopolysaccharide. Clinical examination of the vitreous is difficult, and routine histologic techniques are inadequate since dehydration during processing leaves an empty space with only a few collagen fibrils.[24]

Examination should be performed after mydriasis in a darkened environment utilizing direct illumination and magnification, direct and indirect ophthalmoscopy, and slit lamp biomicroscopy. The anterior vitreous and zonules may be observed posterior to the lens; the zonules attach to the lens equator. With the biomicroscope the branching fibrils appear white in the anterior cortex. An optically empty, funnel-shaped space, the primary vitreous, is observed immediately posterior to the lens. Cloquet's canal appears as an undulating, posteriorly extending structure. In young animals the hyaloid vessels may be patent, spanning the vitreous from the optic disk to the posterior lens capsule. The posterior vitreous should be examined by ophthalmoscopy. The cornea must be neutralized with another lens system if the vitreous is to be studied with the slit lamp biomicroscope.[25]

Congenital Anomalies

The most common anomaly is retention of the primary vitreous. The hyaloid artery should be atrophied by 9 weeks of age.[26] Varying amounts of the persistent hyaloid artery appear as a red or a white spot extending from the optic disk a variable distance into the vitreous or coursing the entire distance from the optic disk to the lens. Extensive primary vitreous results in the development of a retrolental fibrovascular mass that interferes with vision. The proliferating mass is termed persistent hyperplastic primary vitreous. Cataracts, retinal separation, microphthalmia, and glaucoma may accompany this condition.

Pathologic Conditions

The range of vitreous reactions is limited because of the relatively simple structure and the lack of lymphatic and vascular components. Liquefaction, cicatrization, vascularization, infection, and inflammation are the changes that occur in cats.

Liquefaction may occur to the vitreous (syneresis) in response to a variety of stimuli because of its high water content. Following liquefaction, the vitreous separates from the retina, encouraging retinal separation. Vitreous syneresis alone does not result in visual abnormalities, but it may occur as a sequela to lens subluxation or luxation, glaucoma, or inflammation of surrounding structures.

Cicatrization (scar tissue formation) may occur in the vitreous after inflammation or infection of the surrounding tissues. These bands (vitreous traction bands) have the capacity to contract, causing retinal separation.

Vascularization in the vitreous may occur from an inflamed or malformed retina. (The normal vitreous has no blood supply.) These vessels are frequently incompletely developed and bleed into the vitreous.

Injection and inflammation result. Because of the lack of vitreous vasculature, inflammation cannot occur in the same manner as in other vascularized ocular tissues; however, opacification and cellular exudates have been observed.

Vitreous infection can follow perforating ocular injuries and in systemic bacterial and fungal infections.

Hemorrhage into the vitreous may occur with retinitis, retinochoroiditis, ocular trauma, acute hypotony, chronic glaucoma, or intraocular neoplasms. Systemic diseases such as hypertension, hypercholesterolemia, hyperlipemia, and multisystem disease caused by microorganisms can also cause vitreous hemorrhage.

Asteroid hyalosis is defined as small, fixed, refractile bodies of a calcium-lipid complex in the vitreous frequently observed in older animals. They are not associated with other ocular problems, and vision is not affected.

Synchysis (liquefaction) scintillans of the vitreous occurs with small, yellow opacities of cholesterol settling to the ventral aspect of the vitreous. If the head is moved, the particles are distributed in the vitreous, but they settle again. Their formation and significance is unknown, and vision is rarely affected.

Vitreous opacities (floaters) are a relatively frequent occurrence, especially in aged cats. Increased numbers have been seen after intraocular inflammation, particularly uveitis.

Glaucoma

Glaucoma is defined as elevation of intraocular pressure (IOP) beyond the limits of the health and function of the eye.[27] Glaucoma occurs less frequently in cats than in dogs,[21] presumably because of the relatively large iridocorneal angle and ciliary cleft.[23]

Aqueous is produced by the ciliary body by active and passive processes. Aqueous enters and fills the posterior chamber, flows through the pupil, and enters the anterior chamber. It exits the anterior chamber at the iridocorneal angle between the pectinate ligaments into the ciliary cleft. From that point it returns to the blood circulatory system. This delicate balance between formation, circulation, and return back into the general circulation is measured as IOP. An IOP of 15 to 25 mm Hg is considered normal for cats.

Glaucoma is not one disease entity but the result of any of many entirely different diseases. Many diseases of the eye obstruct the flow of aqueous after it is produced by the ciliary body and before its exit from the eye. Glaucoma is a sign, and every effort should be made to find the cause of the elevated pressure.[28] Differentiation of the various types of glaucoma by thorough ophthalmic examination is necessary to formulate a rational basis for treatment.

Glaucoma has been divided into two broad groups, primary and secondary. By definition, primary glaucoma is unrelated to other ocular disease.[29] Secondary glaucoma occurs as a consequence of another recognizable ocular abnormality or disease such as intraocular tumor, inflammation, vascular disorder, or injury.[29]

Primary glaucoma appears to be infrequent in cats. In a histopathologic study of 131 glaucomatous cat eyes, primary glaucoma was suspected in only three.[30]

Secondary glaucoma is more common in cats.[21,30] The most common causes appear to be inflammation, trauma, and neoplasms.[21,30] In one study glaucoma was caused by iris melanoma in 38 of the 131 eyes.[29] Any infectious disease that causes uveitis has the potential to cause secondary glaucoma. FeLV, FIV, FIP virus have been associated with secondary glaucoma resulting from uveitis. Trauma to the globe with inflammation and scarring that interferes with normal aqueous outflow can result in secondary glaucoma.

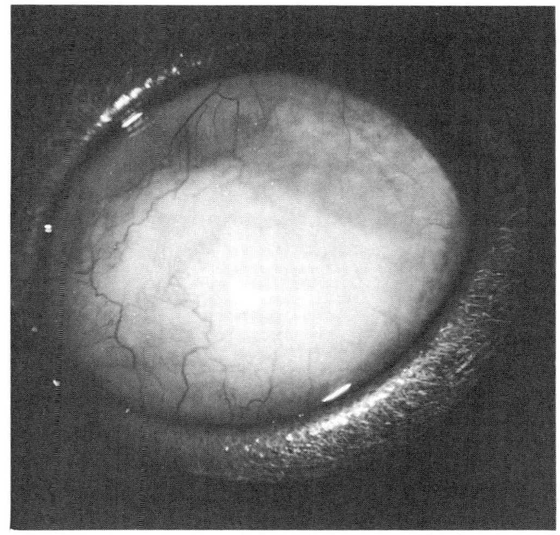

Figure 36–12. **Buphthalmia, megalocornea, neovascularization, and corneal scarring. All are the result of chronic glaucoma.**

Clinical Signs

Glaucoma in cats usually has an insidious onset. Even with acute disease the clinical signs may be subtle, consisting of epiphora, mild episcleral injection, and a somewhat dilated pupil with sluggish pupillary light reflexes (Fig. 36–11).[31] Cats generally do not display the intense corneal edema and episcleral injection observed in dogs.[23,32] Buphthalmia (enlargement of the globe), megalocornea (corneal enlargement), and exposure keratopathy commonly occur as the disease progresses (Fig. 36–12). In chronic glaucoma, lens luxation and retinal degeneration are also frequent findings.

An increase in IOP above the normal range is the cardinal sign of glaucoma. IOP is measured with a tonometer. Digital tonometry is only a crude estimation of IOP; only extremes in tension may be estimated. The Schiotz tonometer is inexpensive and is a reliable instrument for the diagnosis of glaucoma. Readings from the normal and affected eyes should be compared. The variation between two normal eyes in a given animal rarely exceeds 5 mm Hg.

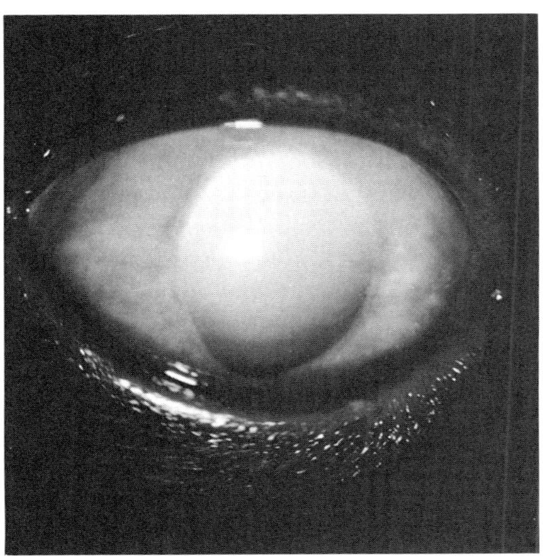

Figure 36–11. **Corneal edema. The pupil is partially dilated with glaucoma.**

Corneal edema related to the elevation of intraocular pressure is less common in cats, but when present it must be differentiated from other causes such as anterior lens luxation, anterior uveitis, corneal cellular infiltration, corneal dystrophy, and scarring.

Venous injection and congestion of the episcleral vessels are not as remarkable as in dogs. The conjunctival and scleral vessels are congested and enlarged from the limbus to the fornix and usually do not shrink after glaucoma is controlled. The index of suspicion should increase when a "red eye" is unresponsive to therapy for conjunctivitis or uveitis or an episode of red eye has persisted several days or weeks. Vascular congestion from anterior uveitis is primarily perilimbal, owing to lower intraocular pressure. When conjunctivitis is present only the superficial conjunctival vessels are congested.

A semidilated to dilated pupil that is unresponsive to light is very suspect for glaucoma. Mydriasis becomes more absolute as the duration of glaucoma increases. Overdiagnosis can occur, owing to interruption of parasympathetic innervation from the oculomotor nerve to the iridal sphincter muscles, synechiae, generalized retinal atrophy, and iatrogenic causes such as parasympatholytic drugs.

Although glaucoma may be painless, it may also be painful. Manifestations including lacrimation, photophobia, and blepharospasm. Pain may be displayed by rubbing of the eye, reluctance to be touched around the eye, or reduction of activity and appetite. Pain is thought to be due to irritation of sensory nerve endings in the fibrous tunic, and it is not relieved by topical anesthetics. Ironically, decreased corneal sensation may also be present.

Prolonged increased intraocular pressure results in the fibrous tunic becoming stretched, resulting in buphthalmos. The cornea becomes enlarged (megalocornea). Striate keratopathy is caused by breaks in Descemet's membrane, commonly called Descemet's striae (streaks). Megalocornea leads to other keratopathies resulting from the inability of the eyelids to properly cover the cornea and distribute tears. Corneal vascularization, pigmentation, and ulceration occur as a result of improper lid closure. Buphthalmia must be differentiated from exophthalmia that is due to retrobulbar abscessation, cellulitis, or neoplasia.

Loss of vision is due to the effects of increased IOP on the retina and optic nerve plus ischemia due to the pressure on the vascular system. Because the feline optic papilla normally lacks myelin, optic nerve cupping is often difficult to visualize.[23]

Diagnosis

Diagnosis of glaucoma is based on clinical signs, examination findings, and increased IOP above 25 mm Hg or a disparity greater than 5 mm Hg between the two eyes as confirmed by tonometry. The underlying cause of glaucoma must be established before a rational regimen of therapy can be instituted. All therapy, whether medical or surgical, is directed toward reducing IOP by decreasing aqueous production or increasing aqueous outflow.

Medical Treatment

Medical treatment is aimed at increasing the outflow or decreasing the production of aqueous.[33] Increasing outflow ability is accomplished with miotic agents; carbonic anhydrase inhibitor diuretics or hyperosmotic agents, or both, are used to accomplish the latter. Because topical administration alone rarely controls glaucoma additional systemic medication must be administered. It is important to hospitalize the patient with glaucoma to monitor the reduction of intraocular pressure and to determine the patient's other responses to therapy.

The primary function of a topical miotic is to contract the ciliary muscles, which open the iridal corneal angle and increase the outflow of aqueous. In general, the miotics are divided into two groups based on mechanisms of action. The first group mimics acetylcholine, the second group inhibits the acetylcholinesterase enzyme, prolonging the action of locally produced acetylcholine.

Pilocarpine is probably the most frequently used miotic. It is available in 0.5% to 10% solutions; the 2% solution is used most frequently. It is administered two to four times daily. Pilocarpine solutions more concentrated than 4% usually produce vomiting. Pilocarpine may be given every 10 to 15 minutes for three to four doses; however, when it is applied this frequently side effects may be noticed. Pilocarpine is effective because it acts directly at the myoneural junction and does not require the neurotransmitter to produce miosis. However, when the IOP approaches 60 mm Hg it usually fails to produce pupillary constriction. In this situation another topical agent or a diuretic is used.

A longer-acting topical agent, echothiophate (Phospholine Iodide), is available in 0.06%, 0.125%, or 0.25% solution. Begin with the weaker solution and increase, if necessary, to produce the required effect. It is a long-acting miotic that can be administered once or twice daily in the 0.125% or 0.25% strength to sustain the desired effect. Demecarium bromide (Humorsol), is another organic phosphate anticholinesterase miotic. It is stable in water and is relatively long acting. It is available in concentrations of 0.125% ad 0.25% and is administered once or twice daily.

In cats, β-blockers and epinephrine compounds have not produced consistent reduction of IOP. Because dilated pupils in acute glaucoma may be completely refractory to all types of miotics additional therapy must be instituted to reduce IOP if the sphincter muscle is to respond.

Carbonic anhydrase inhibitor diuretics and osmotic agents are also useful in treating glaucoma. Chlorothiazide, hydrochlorothiazide, and furosemide are not effective in reducing IOP. The carbonic anhydrase inhibitor diuretics are effective in reducing aqueous formation by as much as 50% after systemic use. Methazolamide (Neptazane) and dichlorphenamide (Daranide) are equally effective and can be safely administered to cats at the rate of 1 to 2 mg/lb two or three times daily. If they are given long-term or in large doses a mild acidosis or hypokalemia may occur.

Mannitol and glycerin are the osmotic agents used for glaucoma control. Their activity is determined by their molecular size and their inability to traverse cell membranes; therefore, these osmotic agents poorly penetrate the blood-aqueous barrier. Mannitol and glycerin shrink the vitreous, increasing anterior chamber outflow. Mannitol is commonly given intravenously (IV) at the rate of 1 to 2 g/kg to reduce the IOP prior to intraocular surgery and as the initial therapy for acute congestive glaucoma. The reduction of IOP occurs within 30 to 60 minutes and has an effect from 6 to 10 hours. Glycerin is administered orally; it begins to reduce the intraocular pressure within 10 minutes and has maximum effect in about 30 minutes. Its duration of action is approximately 5 hours. Glycerin is an inexpensive hyperosmotic agent that can be given orally and can be used on a continued basis for control of chronic glaucoma. The dose of glycerin is 1 to 2 g/kg, and it may be administered in divided doses. Glycerin is rather unpalatable; it can be mixed with flavored agents or milk to enhance its acceptability. Retching, vomiting, and diarrhea sometimes are observed.

Initially acute glaucoma is treated with pilocarpine and mannitol. Mannitol is given once to rapidly reduce the IOP then replaced with a carbonic anhydrase inhibitor. The carbonic anhydrase inhibitor and a topical miotic are used long term and given at whatever intervals are necessary to keep IOP below 25 mm Hg. Chronic glaucoma is treated as is the acute form, but without mannitol. Surgical intervention should be considered when medical therapy fails initially to lower IOP below 25 mm Hg or fails to sustain such a pressure level on a long-term basis.

If glaucoma is secondary to anterior uveitis corticosteroids are recommended for their antiinflammatory effect. Systemic assessment of the patient with glaucoma is mandatory, and the cause of the glaucoma must be diagnosed before corticosteroids are recommended.

Pharmacologic ablation of the ciliary epithelium by intravitreal gentamicin injection is contraindicated for cats because of the potential for sarcoma formation.[23]

Surgical Treatment

Numerous surgical procedures have been advocated for the reduction of increased IOP.[33] No one procedure is entirely satisfactory for the control of glaucoma in all feline patients. Because there are many causes of increased IOP numerous considerations must be addressed prior to surgical intervention. It is even more difficult to properly assess the success of glaucoma surgery, since the criteria for evaluation of success depend on whether the only purpose is to remove the pain, retain a cosmetically acceptable eye, or restore vision. As a result, assessment of each individual surgical procedure is extremely difficult. The surgical procedures commonly used in veterinary ophthalmology can be divided according to whether they attempt to reduce aqueous formation, increase the capacity for outflow, or both.

Since primary glaucoma is rare in cats, the success of the various surgical procedures to reduce aqueous production or increase outflow are rarely critically evaluated in comparison to cyclocryothermy, cyclodiathermy, laser cyclocoagulation, and filtering implants.

Lens extraction for subluxation or luxation must be weighed against the duration and underlying cause. Evisceration of the intraocular contents accompanied by an intraocular implant to retain the globe's shape is a possible consideration for a blind, painful, buphthalmic eye, but only after the cause has been determined and if no ocular neoplasm is present.[34] Enucleation becomes the surgical procedure of choice in the majority of patients because most of them have an underlying neoplasm.

Diseases of the Posterior Segment

The posterior segment refers to the retina, the arteries and veins, the optic nerve, the tapetum, and the nontapetum. Direct ophthalmoscopy is used most frequently in general veterinary practice to examine the posterior segment, although indirect ophthalmoscopy permits better retinal visualization. Because of the cat's extremely light-sensitive pupil, constriction must be ameliorated by the use of a short-acting mydriatic such as tropicamide. Other diagnostic tools such as electroretinography, ultrasonography, and fluorescein angiography can be utilized to aid in diagnosis, though the equipment may not be readily available. Ophthalmoscopy remains the primary technique for most primary care veterinarians.

Afflictions of the retina may be divided into congenital anomalies, trauma, circulatory disturbances, inflammation, detachment, tumor, and degenerations[35] (Table 36–1).[35] Congenital or hereditary anomalies are relatively rare in cats; changes are usually related to the other categories.

Feline Retinal Dysplasia

The feline panleukopenia virus (FPL) and FeLV have been shown to be capable of infecting the developing retina and causing retinal dysplasia.[36,37] Experimentally, the developing retina is susceptible to the FPL virus in utero and during the first few days of life.[37] The ophthalmoscopic appearance of lesions due to either of these viruses is that of nonspecific multifocal areas of tapetal hyperreflectivity or hyporeflectivity (Fig. 36–13). Confirmation of diagnosis is histologic findings of outer nuclear layer folding and rosettes[38] and optic nerve degeneration.

Retinal Degenerations

Retinal degenerations of cats are divided into feline central retinal degeneration (FCRD) and generalized retinal degeneration, based on findings at ophthalmoscopic and histologic examination.

Feline Central Retinal Degeneration

FCRD appears ophthalmoscopically as an oval to elliptical area of hyperreflectivity in the area centralis superior, temporal to the disk (Figs. 36–14, 36–15). The rim of the lesion may appear hyporeflective or darker and grayish green if the angle of incidence of the illuminating light source changes. As the lesion expands, a hyperreflective linear streak may extend from the area centralis superior to the optic disk into the nasal retina (Fig. 36–16), or a second circumscribed isolated focal area may appear in the nasal retina. Continued progression leads to generalized degeneration of the retina, and when viewed with the ophthalmo-

Table 36–1. Retinopathies of Cats

Cause	Active	Quiescent	Ant	Post	Dx	Rx	Prevention
Mycosis	+	+	+	+	±	±	−
FIP	+	+	+	+	+	±	+
FeLV	+	−	+	+	+	±	+
FIV	+	−	+	−	+	±	−
Toxoplasma gondii	+	+	+	+	+	±	−
FPL	−	+	−	+	+	±	+
Anemia	+	+	±	+	+	+	±
Secondary tumor	+	−	+	+	±	−	−
Hereditary	−	+	−	+	+	−	+
Nutritional	−	+	−	+	+	+	+

Ant, anterior segment involvement; Post, posterior segment involvement; Dx, diagnostic tests available; Rx, therapy available.

Modified from Bellhorn RW. Feline retinopathy and systemic disease. Proc Am Soc Vet Ophthalmol, 1977:4.

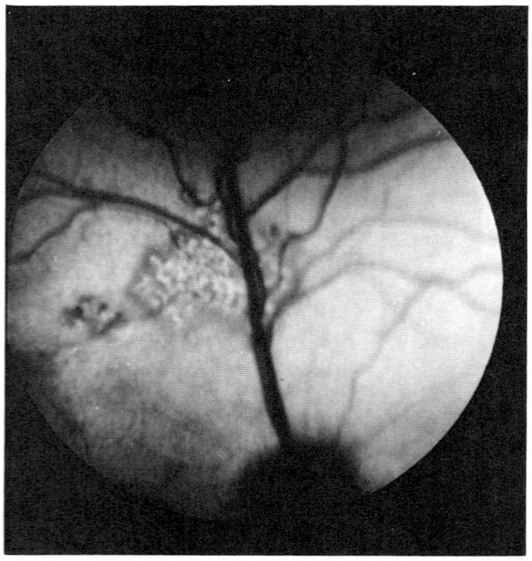

Figure 36–13. Irregularly shaped area of tapetal hypo- and hyperreflectivity located in the midsuperior tapetum as a result of neonatal FPL.

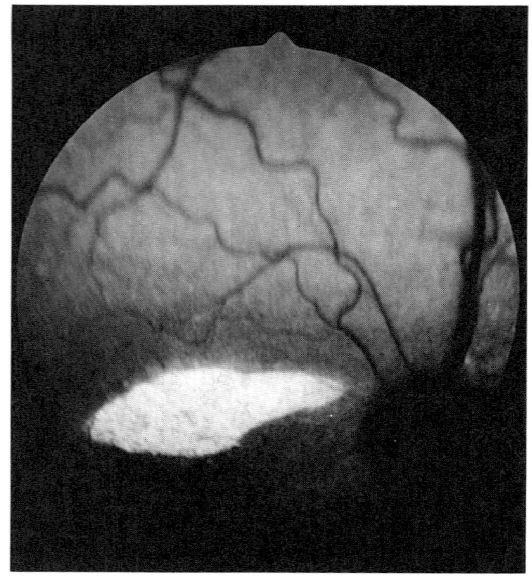

Figure 36–15. Expanded area of FCRD (right eye).

scope, severe diffuse tapetal hyperreflectivity, vascular attenuation, and optic nerve degeneration are seen (Fig. 36–17).

Studies have demonstrated that this lesion can be reproduced by feeding a taurine-deficient diet.[39,40] It is theorized that the cat has very limited capacity to convert cysteine to taurine and, so, must rely on dietary sources—red meat, seafood, and milk. If the dietary deficiency is corrected prior to extensive retinal degeneration the lesions remain static but do not improve.

Generalized Retinal Degeneration

Generalized retinal degeneration in cats has been described as hereditary[41,42] and nutritional.[43] Ophthalmoscopic findings are generalized tapetal hyperreflectivity due to the overall retinal thinning, vascular attenuation, and nontapetal pigment changes.

Hypertensive Retinopathy

Hypertensive retinopathy has not been reported as a frequent condition in cats; it is more common in older cats. The presenting sign is sudden blindness. Examination may reveal hyphema, but more often only posterior segment disease is present. Ophthalmoscopic examination reveals retinal and vitreous hemorrhages of various sizes and shapes, retinal vascular engorgement with tortuosity, and

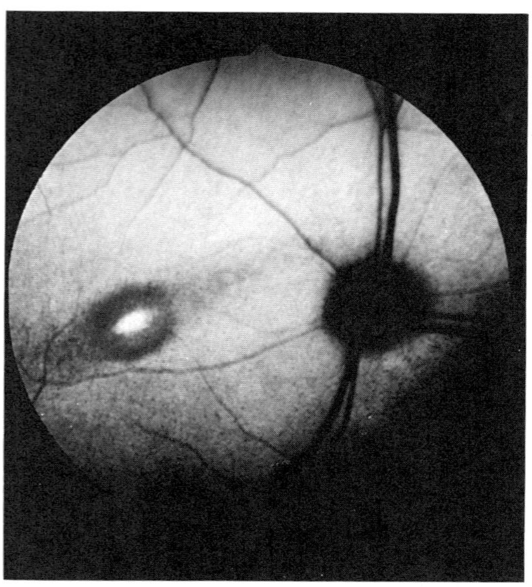

Figure 36–14. FCRD. There is minimal area of reflectivity in the area centralis (right eye).

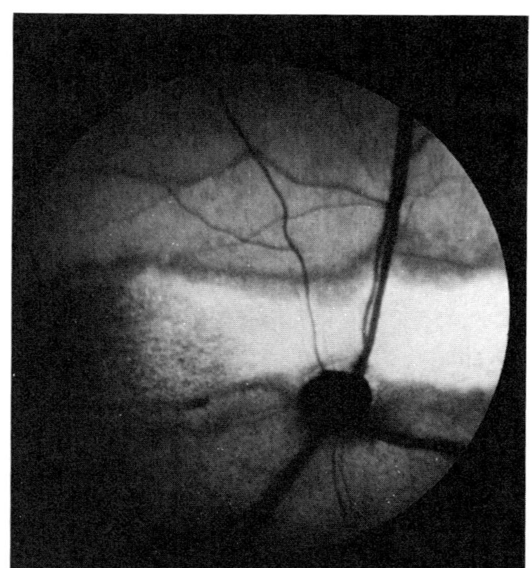

Figure 36–16. Linear streak extends from temporal to nasal retina (right eye).

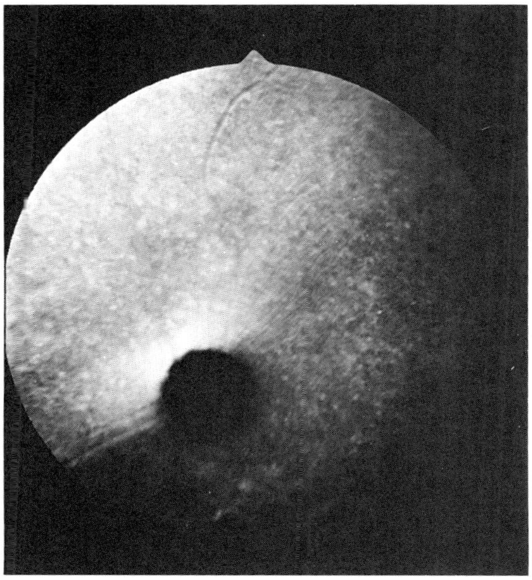

Figure 36–17. **Generalized degeneration with intense tapetal hyperreflectivity, vascular attenuation, and optic nerve degeneration. The cat had been fed dry dog food for 7 years.**

various degrees of retinal detachment from focal to complete (Fig. 36–18).[44] Systolic arterial blood pressure in cats with hypertensive retinal disease is typically greater than 200 mm Hg (normal is less than 150 mm Hg).[23] Cardiac and renal abnormalities are also frequently associated with the hypertensive retinopathy. The relationship of these abnormalities is ill-understood at this time. Therapy is directed toward the renal or cardiac disease through feeding a sodium-restricted diet and giving diuretics and antihypertensive drugs. Usually, the ocular disease is so extensive and so advanced that the likelihood of therapy achieving return of visual function is questionable or poor. However, the use of hydrochlorothiazide (HydroDIURIL), 12.5 mg b.i.d., may in about 50% of cases, allow the detached retina to return to a normal location, with return of vision.

Retinal Hemorrhage

Cats are apparently predisposed to the development of posterior segment hemorrhage. Hemorrhages occur preretinally, intraretinally, and subretinally. Characteristic ophthalmoscopic shapes or appearances help locate sites of hemorrhage. Keelboat-shaped hemorrhages appear in the preretinal area, intraretinal hemorrhages are flame shaped if within the inner layers (Fig. 36–19) or dot shaped in the outer layers of the retina (Fig. 36–20), and a subretinal location is typically irregularly shaped and very dark.

When retinal hemorrhages are noted during ophthalmoscopic examination systemic evaluation, hematologic tests, serum chemistries, bone marrow evaluation, and specific systemic disease titers must become part of the diagnostic work-up.

Anemia and retinal hemorrhages are the characteristic findings in the condition known as anemic retinopathy.[45] Affected cats have nonspecific bone marrow suppression and a nonregenerative anemia with hemoglobin levels of 6 g/dl or less. Hemorrhages occur in all levels of the retina and, as the hemorrhage is absorbed secondary degeneration is seen as tapetal hyperreflectivity or nontapetal hypopigmentation. Retinal hypoxia secondary to anemia stimulates various compensatory mechanisms. These attempt to maintain retinal perfusion, resulting in vascular dilatation, increased capillary fragility, and retinal hemorrhage. The condition may be further aggravated by FeLV and concurrent thrombocytopenia.

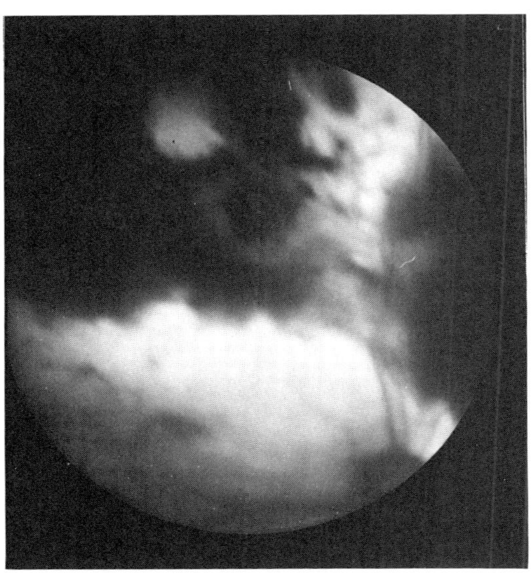

Figure 36–18. **Vitreal and retinal hemorrhages resulting from hypertension.**

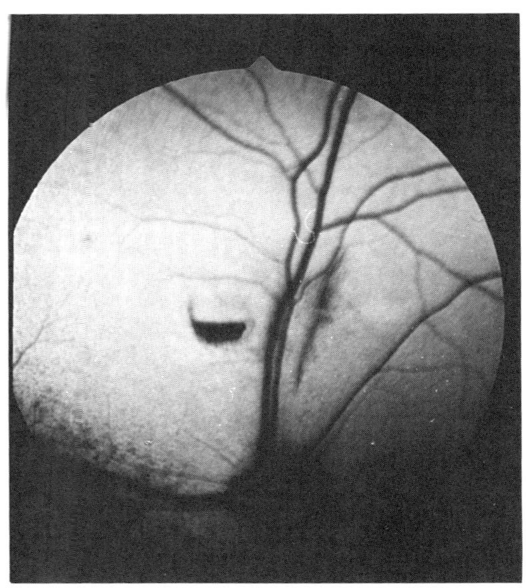

Figure 36–19. **Keelboat- and flame-shaped hemorrhages.**

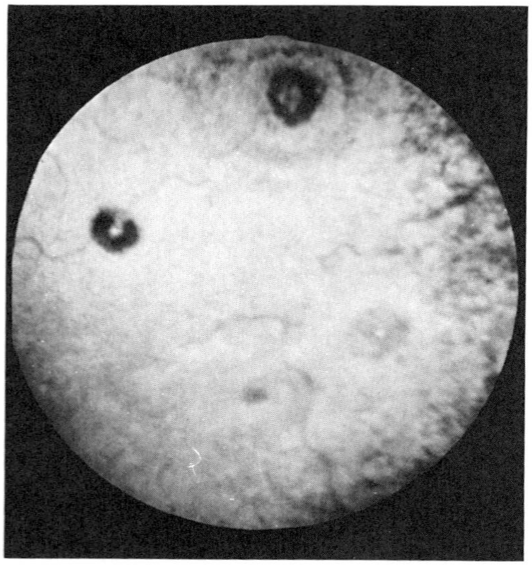

Figure 36–20. Dot-shaped hemorrhages. Note retinal degeneration in the surrounding area as characterized by changes in tapetal reflectivity.

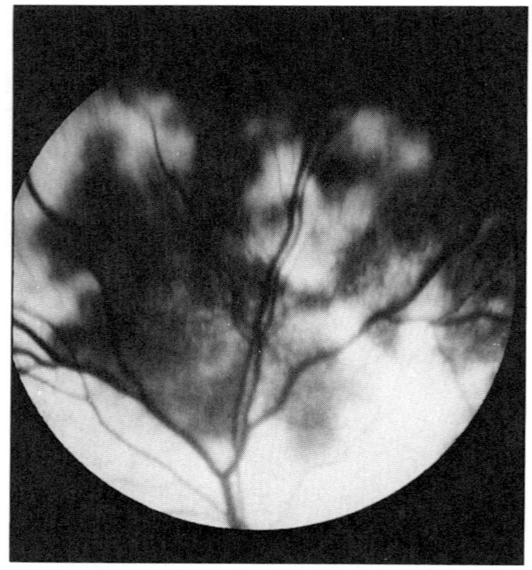

Figure 36–21. Multifocal hyperpigmentation of the tapetum.

Multisystem Disseminating Diseases

Systemic Mycoses

Disseminating mycotic agents are saprophytes that become opportunistic pathogens after gaining entrance to the body. The respiratory tract appears to be the most likely portal by which fungal spores gain entry. Hematogenous dissemination allows the organism to reach the eye.

Histoplasma capsulatum[7,46], *Blastomyces dermatitidis*[2], *Cryptococcus neoformans*[5,47], and *Coccidioides immitis*[6] have caused intraocular disease of cats. Histoplasmosis and cryptococcosis are more frequently seen in the U.S. Midwest and South, blastomycosis in the East, and coccidioidomycosis in the Southwest. With today's transient population, however, the endemic geographic distribution should not rule out these diseases in any cat.

The responses in organs are extensive proliferation and infiltration of reticuloendothelial cells, macrophages, and epithelial cells. Ocular mycotic disease is characterized by granulomatous inflammation, principally in the uvea. Multifocal, circumscribed, and irregular-shaped hyperreflective, or hyperpigmented areas are seen in the tapetal fundus (Fig. 36–21). Irregular multifocal areas of hypopigmentation, interspersed with gray exudates, occur in the nontapetum (Fig. 36–22). Irregular-shaped, elevated, pink to red, granulomatous lesions (Fig. 36–23) and bullous retinal separations have been observed (Fig. 36–24). The loss of posterior segment function is proportional to the space-occupying lesions and their secondary effects on the adjacent tissues.

Histologic examination is characterized by granulomatous inflammation in the anterior and posterior uvea. The cellular infiltrate is usually confined to the choroid in the posterior segment and is composed of macrophages containing the organisms, neutrophils, plasma cells, and lymphocytes.

Diagnosis by serologic mycotic titers has not been consistent nor reliable. Since the mycotic organisms are primarily confined to the uvea, aqueous, and vitreous, aspiration for cytologic identification of the organisms are usually unrewarding. Cytologic examination of bone marrow aspirate has provided the most consistently positive results.

The prognosis for disseminating mycotic disease is usually grave. As in the eye, severe compromise of the lungs, liver, kidneys, lymph nodes, and bone marrow occurs, and the granulomatous inflammation leads to multisystem organ malfunction.

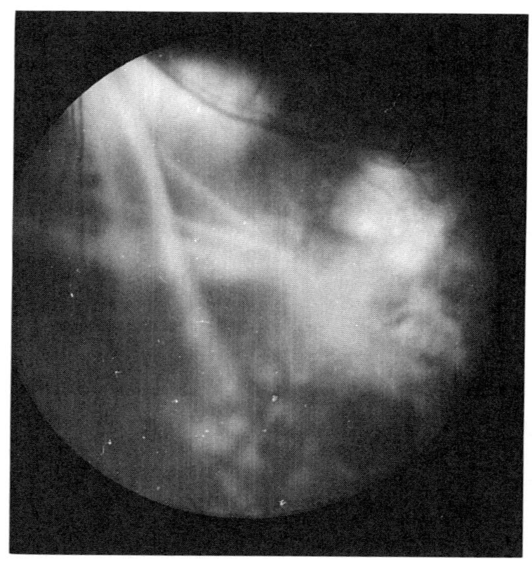

Figure 36–22. Vitreous traction bands, areas of hypopigmentation, and gray exudates in the nontapetum.

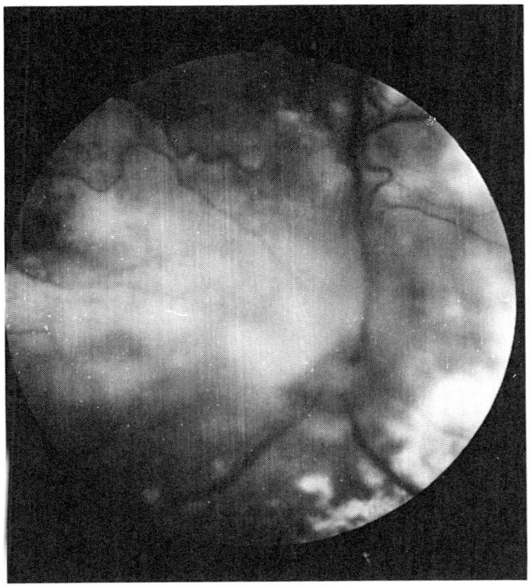

Figure 36–23. **Irregularly shaped, elevated, granulomatous lesion in the tapetum. Retinal separation is present adjacent to the optic disk (10 to 11 o'clock position).**

Various antifungal agents and regimens have been advocated and treatments tried. Amphotericin B has been used, but compromised kidney function and the nephrotoxicity of the drug limit its usefulness. Ketoconazole has also been used, with inconsistent results. Supportive medical regimens of intravenous fluids, blood transfusions, antibiotics, and forced alimentation must be considered for debilitated patients, depending on clinical signs and laboratory findings. If it is determined that the ocular disease is only unilateral, enucleation of the affected eye appears to be of benefit. For a further discussion of systemic fungal diseases and their treatment see Chapter 61.

Toxoplasmosis

Toxoplasma gondii is a protozoal parasite for which cats are the definitive host.[48] The incidence of apparent clinical disease is undetermined. Naturally occurring ocular toxoplasmosis has been described in ten cats, of which the consistent lesion was retinitis, recognized by focal dark spots in the tapetal fundus and white to gray lesions in the nontapetum.[49] *Toxoplasma* organisms were histologically demonstrated in the retina where the inflammation was present.

The diagnosis of toxoplasmosis has relied upon demonstration of oocysts in the feces or infected tissues or immunoglobulin G (IgG) antibodies to the organism. These procedures have not been reliable. Recently enzyme-linked immunosorbent assay (ELISA) technology for the detection of circulating *Toxoplasma* antigen and an IgM assay have been developed.[50,51] The presence of an IgM titer or a positive antigen detection test is considered suggestive of recent clinical infection when combined with accompanying clinical signs.

Toxoplasmosis has been treated in the past with sulfonamides and pyrimethamine. Recently, oral clindamycin hydrochloride (25 mg/kg/day in divided doses) has been shown to effectively control *Toxoplasma* retinitis.[52,53]

Feline Infectious Peritonitis

FIP, caused by a coronavirus, is a multisystemic, progressive, debilitating disease.[54] The ophthalmic clinical sign most commonly associated with FIP is anterior uveitis.[15,16] The ocular media opacities often preclude posterior pigment examination; however, in some cases only changes in the posterior segment have been observed. Vitreous flare and opacities, retinal vascular sheathing, edema, and hemorrhage have been observed (Fig. 36–25). Retinal separation has not been a consistent finding.

Examination of pleural or peritoneal fluids is helpful in diagnosing FIP. A positive coronavirus titer supports the

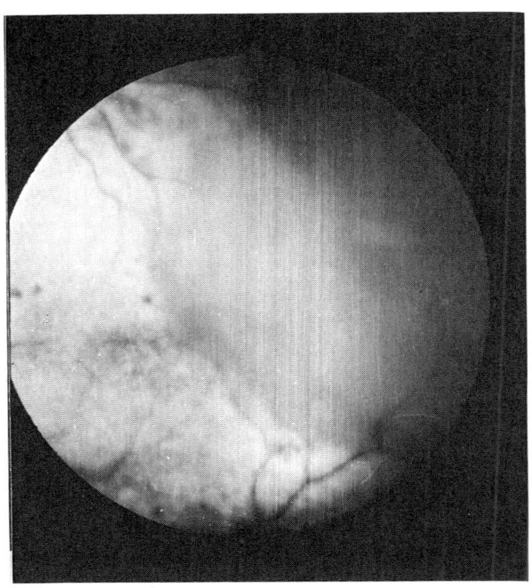

Figure 36–24. **Bullous retinal separation of the superior temporal tapetum.**

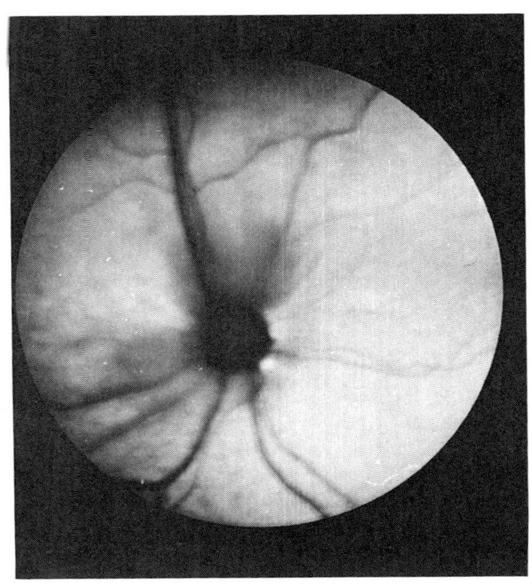

Figure 36–25. **Peripapillary retinal vascular sheathing and edema, also present in the nasal and superior tapetal areas.**

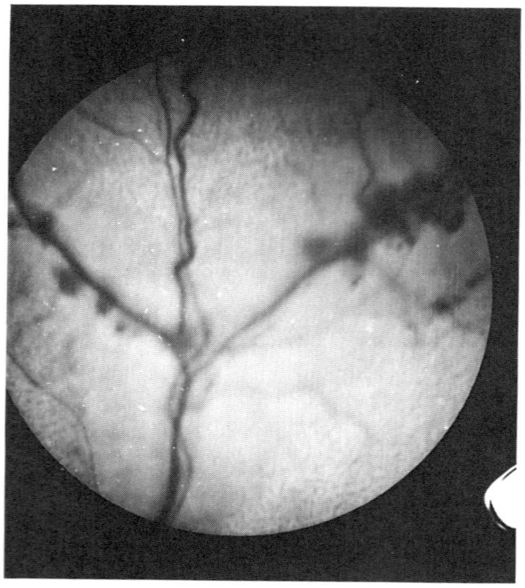

Figure 36–26. **FeLV retinal changes noted are vascular cuffing and sheathing, retinal edema, and hemorrhage.**

diagnosis, but because of the cross-reactivity with the enteric coronavirus, this test lacks specificity. Currently, there is no known effective treatment against the viral infection (see Chapter 38).

Feline Leukemia Virus

Lymphoid neoplasia is the most common intraocular neoplasm.[11] Anterior segment change is a frequent clinical sign; however, posterior segment disease only is not an infrequent finding. Retinal changes include paleness of the retinal vessels (anemia), hemorrhage, vascular cuffing and sheathing, and neovascularization (Fig. 36–26). Retinal separation is not an uncommon finding during the initial examination (Fig. 36–27). Histopathologic examination of a separated retina reveals a severely degenerated retina with subretinal fibrillar material. The choroidal vasculature is usually infiltrated with neoplastic lymphoid cells (see Chapter 39).

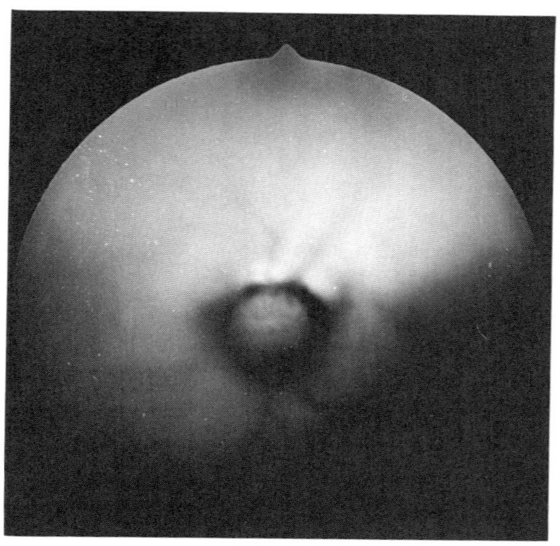

Figure 36–27. **Bullous retinal separation in an FeLV-positive cat.**

Lysosomal Storage Diseases

These are a group of rare, inherited diseases that result from defects in metabolism caused by deficiencies of certain lysosomal enzymes. An abnormal accumulation of the specific deficient enzyme substitute in the lysosomes of the affected cells results in disease.

Mucopolysaccharidosis (MPS_1 and MPS_6) has been described in cats.[55,56] MPS_1 is a defect in α-L-iduronidase. MPS_6 has been more frequently reported as a recessive genetic disease due to a defect in glycosaminoglycan metabolism. Skeletal and facial deformities (broad face, short ears and nose, protruding forehead) mark the disease. The accumulation of polysaccharides results in corneal opacities, aqueous and vitreous cloudiness, and retinal pigment epithelial changes. Blindness occurs in the later stages.

Gangliosidosis 1 (GM_1) is a deficiency of β-galactosidase, and GM_2 a deficiency of β-D-*N*-acetylhexosaminidase. They cause glycolipid buildup, observed as corneal opacities and pale gray areas in the retina.[57,58] Continued accumulation in the retinal ganglion cells results in blindness.

α-Mannosidosis is a defect in α-mannosidase. It is the third category of lysosomal storage diseases reported in cats.[59] Mottling of the tapetum is the typical ophthalmoscopic finding in affected cats.

Confirmation of diagnosis of the lysosomal storage diseases is based on enzyme assays for evidence of a lysosomal enzyme deficiency.

REFERENCES

1. Alden CL, Mohan R. Ocular blastomycosis in a cat. J Am Vet Med Assoc 1974;164:527.
2. Nasisse MP, van Ee RT, Wright B. Ocular changes in a cat with disseminated blastomycosis. J Am Vet Med Assoc 1985;187:629.
3. Fisher CA. Intraocular cryptococcosis in two cats. J Am Vet Med Assoc 1971;158:191.
4. Wilkinson GT. Feline cryptococcosis: A review and seven case reports. J Small Anim Pract 1979;20:749.
5. Blouin P, Cello RM. Experimental ocular cryptococcosis: Preliminary studies in cats and mice. Invest Ophthalmol Vis Sci 1980;19:21.
6. Angell J. Ocular coccidioidomycosis in a cat. J Am Vet Med Assoc 1985;187:167.
7. Mahaffey E. Disseminating histoplasmosis in three cats. J Am Anim Hosp Assoc 1977;13:46.
8. Peiffer RL, Jr, Belkin PV. Ocular manifestations of disseminated histoplasmosis in a cat. Feline Pract 1979;9:24.
9. Percy DH. Feline histoplasmosis with ocular involvement. Vet Pathol 1981;18:163.
10. Clinkenbeard KD, Cowell RL, Tyler RD. Disseminated histoplasmosis in cats: 12 cases (1981–1986). J Am Vet Med Assoc 1987;190:1445.
11. Peiffer RL Jr. Ocular Manifestations of Systemic Disease. Part I: Dog and Cat. In: Gelatt K, ed. Veterinary Ophthalmology. Philadelphia: Lea & Febiger, 1981:719.
12. Friedman DS. Panuveitis and gingivitis in a cat with lentivirus. Trans Am Coll Vet Ophthalmol 1988:105.

13. English RF. Uveitis associated with lentivirus infection in cats. J Am Vet Med Assoc 1990;196:116.
14. Davidson MG. Feline anterior uveitis: A study of 53 cases. J Am Anim Hosp Assoc 1991;27:77.
15. Doherty MJ. Ocular manifestations of feline infectious peritonitis. J Am Vet Med Assoc 1971;159:417.
16. Campbell LH, Reed C. Ocular signs associated with feline infectious peritonitis in two cats. Feline Pract 1975;5:32.
17. Quinn AJ. Embryology, anatomy, and physiology of the lens. J Canine Pract 1981;8:19.
18. Quinn AJ. Examination of the lens. Proc Am Anim Hosp Assoc 1979;46:335.
19. Cotlier E. The Lens. In: Moses RA, ed. Adler's Physiology of the Eye. 7th ed. St. Louis: CV Mosby Co, 1981;277.
20. Gwin RM, Gelatt KN. The Lens. In: Gelatt K, ed. Ophthalmology. Philadelphia: Lea & Febiger, 1981;435.
21. Blogg JR. Diseases of the Lens. In: The Eye in Veterinary Practice. North Melbourne: VS Supplies Ltd, 1975;480.
22. Peiffer RL, Gelatt KN. Cataracts in the cat. Feline Pract 1974;4:34.
23. Nasisse MP. Feline Ophthalmology. In: Gelatt KN. Veterinary Ophthalmology. 2nd ed. Philadelphia: Lea & Febiger, 1991;558.
24. Gloor BP. The Vitreous. In: Moses RA, ed. Adler's Physiology of the Eye. 7th ed. St. Louis: CV Mosby Co, 1981;225.
25. Quinn AJ. The vitreous. Proc Am Anim Hosp Assoc 1986;53:447.
26. Blogg JR. Vitreous. In: The Eye in Veterinary Practice. North Melbourne: VS Supplies Ltd, 1975;508.
27. Spencer WH. Glaucoma. In: Ophthalmic Pathology, An Atlas and Textbook. Vol. I. Philadelphia: WB Saunders, 1985;480.
28. Quinn AJ. Some observations on glaucoma. J Okla Vet Med Assoc 1977;29:94.
29. Scheie HG, Albert DM. Glaucoma. In: Textbook of Ophthalmology. Philadelphia: WB Saunders, 1977;522.
30. Wilcock B. The causes of glaucoma in cats. Vet Pathol 1990;27:35.
31. Peiffer RL Jr. Small Animal Ophthalmology: A Problem-Oriented Approach. Philadelphia: WB Saunders, 1989;67.
32. Peiffer RL Jr, Gelatt KN. Feline Ophthalmology. In: Gelatt KN, ed. Veterinary Ophthalmology. Philadelphia: Lea & Febiger, 1981;547.
33. Quinn AJ. Some Observations on Glaucoma. Part II: Medical and Surgical Treatment. J Okla Vet Med Assoc 30;1:2.
34 Brightman AH II. Intraocular prosthesis in the dog. J Am Anim Hosp Assoc 1977;13,4:481.
35. Helper LC. Diseases of the Vitreous, Retina, and Optic Nerve. In: Magrane's Canine Ophthalmology. 4th ed. Philadelphia: Lea & Febiger, 1989;238.
36. Albert DM, Lahav M, Colby ED, et al. Retinal neoplasia and dysplasia. I. Induction by feline leukemia virus. Invest Ophthalmol 1977;16:325.
37. MacMillan AD. Retinal dysplasia and degeneration in the young cat: Feline panleukopenia virus as an etiological agent. PhD thesis. Davis: University of California at Davis, 1974.
38. Silverstein AM, Osburn BI, Prendergast RA. The pathogenesis of retinal dysplasia. Am J Ophthalmol 1971;72:13.
39. Hayes KC, Carey RE, Schmidt SY. Retinal degeneration associated with taurine deficiency in the cat. Science 1975;188:949.
40. Aguirre GD, Schmidt SY. Retinal degeneration in cats fed dog food. Proc Am Coll Vet Ophthalmol 1976;6:129.
41. Rubin LF, Lipton DE. Retinal degeneration in kittens. J Am Vet Med Assoc 1970;157:1415.
42. Narfstrom K. Hereditary progressive retinal atrophy in the Abyssinian cat. J Hered 1983;74:273.
43. Scott PP, Greaves JP, Scott MG. Nutritional blindness in the cat. Exp Eye Res 1964;3:357.
44. Morgan RV. Systemic hypertension in four cats: Ocular and medical findings. J Am Anim Hosp Assoc 1986;22:615.
45. Fischer CA. Retinopathy in anemic cats. J Am Vet Med Assoc 1970;156:1415
46. Quinn AJ. Granulomatous chorioretinitis of disseminated histoplasmosis in cats. Proc Am Soc Vet Ophthalmol and Int Soc Vet Ophthalmol 1982:159.
47. Gwin RM. Ocular cryptococcosis in a cat. J Am Anim Hosp Assoc 1977,13:680.
48. Piper RC, Cole CR, Shaddack JA. Natural and experimental ocular toxoplasmosis in animals. Am J Ophthalmol 1970;69:662.
49. Vainisi SJ, Campbell LH. Ocular toxoplasmosis in cats. J Am Vet Med Assoc 1969;154:141.
50. Lappin MR. Diagnosis of recent *Toxoplasma gondii* infection in cats by use of an enzyme-linked immunosorbent assay for immunoglobulin M. Am J Vet Res 1989;50:1580.
51. Lappin MR. Enzyme-linked immunosorbent assay for the detection of circulating antigens of *Toxoplasma gondii* in the serum of cats. Am J Vet Res 1989;50:1586.
52. Lappin ML. Clinical feline toxoplasmosis: Serologic diagnosis and therapeutic management of 15 cases. J Vet Intern Med 1989;3:239.
53. Lappin MR. Feline Toxoplasmosis. In: Kirk RW, ed. Current Veterinary Therapy X. Philadelphia: WB Saunders, 1989:1112.
54. Hardy WD, Jr, Hurvitz AI. Feline infectious peritonitis: Experimental studies. J Am Vet Med Assoc 1971;158:994.
55. Haskins ME. Mucopolysaccharidosis in a domestic short-haired cat: A disease distinct from that seen in the Siamese cat. J Am Vet Med Assoc 1979;175:384.
56. Breton L, Guerin P, Morin M. A case of mucopolysaccharidosis VI in a cat. J Am Anim Hosp Assoc 1983;19:891.
57. Blakemore WF. GM_1 gangliosidosis in a cat. J Comp Pathol 1972;82:179.
58. Cork LC, Munnell JR, Lorenz MD. The pathology of feline GM_2 gangliosidosis, Am J Pathol 1978;90:723.
59. Blakemore WF. A case of mannosidosis in the cat: Clinical and histopathological findings. J Small Anim Pract 1986;27:447.
60. Bellhorn RW. Feline Retinopathy and Systemic Disease. Proc Am Soc Vet Ophthalmol 1977.

CHAPTER 37

◇ ◇ ◇

Feline Immunodeficiency Virus Diseases

Gary D. Norsworthy

The feline immunodeficiency virus (FIV) was first identified in 1986 in a California cattery in which chronic and recurring infections were observed. It was originally named the feline T-lymphotropic virus (FTLV) because of its affinity for T-lymphocytes.[1] It has also been referred to as the "feline AIDS virus" because the acquired immunodeficiency syndrome that occurs in cats is in many ways similar to the analogous syndrome in humans caused by the human immunodeficiency virus (HIV).

FIV is a lentivirus and clearly different from the feline leukemia virus (FeLV), which is an oncornavirus. However, FIV shares many similarities with the lentiviruses that affect other veterinary species, including sheep, goats, cattle, and horses, as well as the lentivirus that affects humans, HIV. Lentiviruses are typically characterized as producing a prolonged asymptomatic period of latency followed by a stage of clinical disease that is usually life-threatening.[2,3] Lentiviruses are also species-specific; FIV has not been found to infect primary human, mouse, or dog peripheral blood lymphocytes or T-lymphocytes.[4] Eighteen people exposed to FIV through either bite wounds or laboratory accidents have remained seronegative for FIV.[5]

Incidence

Several recent surveys have been done to determine the incidence of FIV in the cat population of the United States. One survey demonstrated an incidence of 14% in ill cats versus 1.2% of healthy cats.[5] Another survey found that 12% of sick cats at a veterinary teaching hospital were seropositive for FIV antibodies.[5] A recent national survey of nearly 28,000 cats from a population that was primarily symptomatic and at risk established an incidence of 7.4%.[7]

Risk Factors

Outdoor free-roaming cats are at the greatest risk of FIV infection; the incidence is two to three times higher in males than in females. It has been found more often in domestic cats than in purebred cats and in short-haired cats rather than long-haired ones. The average age of an FIV-positive cat is 5 to 6 years.[4] The incidence of FIV infection increases with age; however, this apparently does not reflect an age-related susceptibility but is more likely a consequence of the extended latent period.[8] Although the virus was initially isolated from cats in a cattery, the overall incidence in catteries is thought to be low.[4]

Transmission

Biting is the most commonly documented method of natural transmission. Cat fight wounds seem to be an efficient means of spreading the virus between cats.[9] Two studies have reported transmission via milk to nursing kittens. However, this finding appears to be restricted to situations in which the queen becomes infected *during* pregnancy presumably because the virus level is high in the early stage of infection.[10,11]

Casual contact between cats, including eating and drinking from common bowls and grooming each other, does not appear to be an efficient means of transmission. Thus, cats that do not fight may coexist for months to years with a minimal chance of transmission. The virus is not stable in the external environment, so prolonged contamination of the premises is not a factor in transmission.[9,12] Evidence to date indicates that neither in utero nor genetic, vertical transmission occurs.[13,14]

FIV occurs in high levels in the blood of seropositive cats following the initial infection (acute stage) and with the onset of terminal disease (chronic stage). Its levels in the blood are much lower during the period of time that the cat does not exhibit clinical signs (latent stage).[13] Therefore, it is likely that the contagion is greatest during the acute and chronic stages, and is least during the latent stage.

Clinical Findings

Studies of experimentally inoculated cats and observations of naturally infected cats have revealed three stages of infection: (1) the acute stage (primary illness), (2) the latent stage, and (3) the chronic/terminal stage.

1. *Acute Stage (Primary Illness).* This stage begins 4 to 6 weeks after infection has occurred and generally lasts about 2 to 3 weeks, but may last up to 9 months. Cats in this stage exhibit fever that may have a duration of

TABLE 37–1. **Diseases and Lesions Associated with Terminal-Stage FIV Infection**[4,16]

1. Stomatitis/gingivitis/periodontitis (Fig. 37–1)
2. Chronic weight loss/poor weight gain
3. Lymphadenopathy
4. Chronic diarrhea
5. Chronic upper respiratory infections
6. Chronic dermatitis
7. Fever of unknown origin
8. Purulent otitis externa
9. Bacterial cystitis
10. Unusual neoplasms: Non–FeLV-associated lymphosarcoma and myeloproliferative disease, hepatic myelolipoma, and aggressive nasal adenocarcinoma
11. Non-healing abscesses/wounds (Fig. 37–2)
12. Nonregenerative anemia
13. Chronic rhinitis
14. Neurologic signs: dementia, aggression, convulsions, etc.
15. Increased incidence of squamous cell carcinoma
16. Presence of unusual infections/parasites: *Toxoplasma gondii, Cryptococcus neoformans, Dirofilaria immitis, Candida albicans,* atypical mycobacteriosis, poxvirus infection, *Demodex cati, Notoedres cati,* and *Hemobartonella felis*

up to 14 days, neutropenia for 4 to 9 weeks, and lymphadenopathy characterized by lymphoid hyperplasia for 2 to 9 months.[13] Some cats show no clinical signs during this stage. On the other hand, if the cat has been previously infected with FeLV, this stage may result in fulminant disease.[15]

Cats in this stage are usually seropositive for FIV.

2. ***Latent Stage.*** This stage lasts several months to several years. During this time, cats show no clinical evidence of disease.

   These cats should be seropositive for FIV.

3. ***Chronic/Terminal Stage.*** This stage may last for a few weeks to a few months and is characterized by a variety of diseases and lesions related to immunodeficiency. These may take the form of opportunistic or unusual infections, unusual tumors, or neurologic signs. Virtually any organ system may be involved. Table 37–1 is a list of diseases that have been observed in association with FIV. Two of these diseases—stomatitis/gingivitis and nonhealing abscess—are illustrated in Figures 37–1 and 37–2. One should note that this is a dynamic list to which other diseases will undoubtedly be added as our experience with FIV progresses. Nearly all of these diseases have also been associated with the immunosuppressive effects of FeLV.

   As a rule these cats are seropositive. However, a few have been observed to become seronegative. This occurs if increased antigen production results in antigen to antibody complexing, so that free antibodies fall below detectable levels.

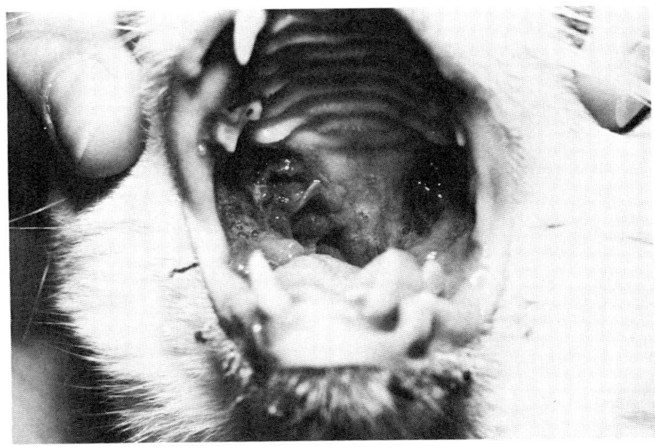

Figure 37–1. **Chronic stomatitis and gingivitis are found in many FIV-infected cats. The ulcerative lesions at the angle of the jaw are typical findings in these cats.**

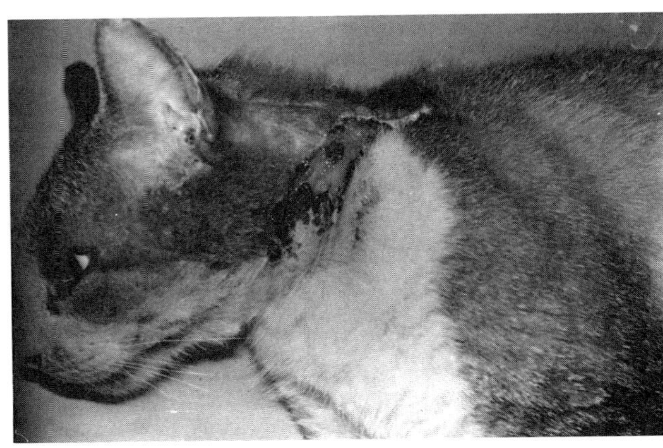

Figure 37–2. **Nonhealing abscesses and bite wounds are characteristic of FIV cats. The wound on this cat's neck had been present for 6 months when the FIV was detected.**

Unusual forms of neoplasia have been observed in FIV-infected cats. These include non–FeLV-associated lymphosarcoma and myeloproliferative disease, hepatic myelolipoma, and aggressive nasal adenocarcinoma.[5,13,16,17] These findings may represent the results of the immunosuppressive effects of FIV or may be due to an undefined oncogenic property of FIV.[5] An increase in the incidence of squamous cell carcinoma has been noted, as has an unusual interaction of FIV and griseofulvin. In one study, six of seven FIV-infected cats given griseofulvin developed a non–dose-related neutropenia in which the neutrophil count was less than $400 \times 10^3/mm^3$.[18]

The additive effects of FeLV are clinically significant. When FIV and FeLV coexist, serious and often fatal disease results. Since both viruses are immunosuppressive, their combined effects on the cat can be more devastating and occur more rapidly than the effect of either alone.[4]

Diagnosis

The presence of the antibody to any lentivirus in any species is equivalent to lentivirus infection.[4] Several methods are currently available to detect FIV antibody in cats. The most commonly used method is the enzyme-linked immunosorbent assay (ELISA) (CITE FIV antibody test kit and CITE COMBO FeLV antigen/FIV antibody test kit [IDDEX Corp, Portland, ME]). Generally, this is considered a reliable test; however, one study showed a 25% to 33% rate of false-negative results due to cross-reactivity.[19] If results of the ELISA are inconsistent with sound clinical observation (e.g., a positive test result in a young, healthy cat), they should be checked against a Western blot (WB) test (Hansen Veterinary Immunology, Dixon, CA; New York State Diagnostic Laboratory, Cornell University, Ithaca, NY; and National Veterinary Lab, Franklin Lakes, NJ).

The time from FIV infection until levels of antibody are detectable is typically 2 to 6 weeks.[5] However, there is evidence that it may be months or even years.[4] Therefore, false-negative results may occur in cats less than 1 to 2 years of age. False-negative results may also occur in cats in the terminal stages of disease if the antibody level falls below that detectable by the currently available tests.[4,13] Positive test results in a young kitten may be due to maternal antibodies;[20] the kitten should be tested again after 12 weeks of age.

Treatment

Currently there is no effective treatment for any lentivirus infection in any species. Therefore, treatment is palliative and supportive. Some cats, especially those with opportunistic infections, may respond initially to appropriate antibiotic, antifungal, or antiparasitic therapy. However, relapses are not unusual. Most cats die within 6 months to 3 years after entering the chronic stage of disease.[21]

FIV-infected cats survive longest if protected from the opportunistic agents listed in Table 37–1 and from FeLV. This is best accomplished by strictly confining them to the indoors. Indoor confinement also minimizes transmission of FIV to free-roaming cats.

Research for specific treatment of lentivirus infections is multifaceted; it currently covers six areas: (1) biologic response modifiers; (2) reverse transcriptase inhibitors, including the drug AZT; (3) target cell toxins; (4) virus receptor blockage; (5) bone marrow transplantation; and (6) gene therapy.

Prevention

Ideally prevention would be accomplished with a vaccine against FIV. However, lentiviruses have several characteristics that make them defiant of effective vaccine production. A great deal of research is under way to develop a vaccine against HIV.[22] If this is accomplished, an FIV vaccine will likely follow. Until then, the only form of prevention that we can offer is to recommend avoidance of cat fights with FIV-infected cats.

1991 Colloquium on FIV

On March 1 to 3, 1991, a colloquium on FeLV and FIV was held in Orlando, Florida. Wide-ranging issues related to these viruses were discussed. The following conclusions and recommendations concerning tests are among those developed by a panel of distinguished veterinary scientists and reported in the Journal of the American Veterinary Medical Association.[23]

1. Available FIV diagnostic tests (ELISA, IFA, and WB) detect antibodies against the virus. Tests are only diagnostic for FIV infections that have stimulated detectable antibody—they are not diagnostic for clinical disease. There is a high correlation between antibodies to FIV and persistent viremia. The FIV antibody–positive cats should be assumed to be persistently viremic and a persistent source of virus.
2. Maternally derived immunity in young kittens can interfere with diagnostic antibody tests for FIV. If positive test results are obtained in kittens <12 weeks old, kittens must be retested after the age of 12 weeks to assure that antibodies detected were not maternally derived.
3. As with FeLV, positive results for FIV should be confirmed by use of another test if euthanasia of a healthy cat is contemplated. Results of ELISA can be confirmed by IFA testing or by WB. The panel encourages more diagnostic laboratories to make available the WB assay for FIV as a confirmatory test.

REFERENCES

1. Pedersen NC, Ho EW, Brown ML, Yamamoto JK. Isolation of a T-lymphotropic virus from domestic cats with an immunodeficiency-like syndrome. Science 1986;235:790.
2. Narayan O, Clements JE. Biology and pathogenesis of lentiviruses. J Gen Virol 1989;70:1617.
3. Haase AT. Pathogenesis of lentivirus infections. Nature 1986; 322:130.
4. Sparger EE. Feline Immunodeficiency Virus. In: August JR, ed. Consultations in Feline Internal Medicine. Philadelphia: WB Saunders, 1991:543.
5. Yamamoto JK, Hansen H, Ho EW. Epidemiologic and clinical aspects of feline immunodeficiency virus (FIV) infections in cats from the continental United States and Canada and possible mode of transmission. J Am Vet Med Assoc 1989;194:213.
6. Zenger E. Clinical findings in cats with feline immunodeficiency virus. Fel Pract 1990;18:25.
7. The National FeLV/FIV Awareness Project, IDDEX Corp, Portland, ME, 1990.
8. Wolf A. Report on the National FeLV/FIV Awareness Project. Diag Cit IDEXX Corp 1991; Summer:1.
9. Connaughton D. What you need to know about the feline immunodeficiency virus (interview with NC Pederson). J Am Vet Med Assoc 1989;194:169.
10. Wasmoen T, Armiger-Luhman S, Egan C, et al. Transmission of feline immunodeficiency virus from infected queens to kittens

(abstract). First International Conference of FIV Researchers. University of California, Davis, CA, Sept 4–7, 1991.
11. Callanan JJ, Hosie MJ, Jarrett O. Natural transmission of feline immunodeficiency virus in kittens. (abstract). First International Conference of FIV Researchers. University of California, Davis, CA, Sept 4–7, 1991.
12. Barr MC, Barlough JE. Feline immunodeficiency virus. Cornell Fel Health Cent Info Bull 1989;10:1.
13. Yamamoto JK, Sparger EE, Ho EW. Pathogenesis of experimentally induced feline immunodeficiency virus infection in cats. Am J Vet Res, 1988;49:1246.
14. Ueland K, Nesse LL. Vertical transmission of naturally acquired feline immunodeficiency virus infection (abstract). First International Conference of FIV Researchers. University of California, Davis, CA, Sept 4–7, 1991.
15. Pedersen NC, Torten M, Rideout B. Feline leukemia virus infection as a potentiating cofactor for the primary and secondary stage of experimentally induced feline immunodeficiency virus infection. J Virol 1990;64:598.
16. Sparger EE, Luciw PA, Elder JH. Feline immunodeficiency virus is a lentivirus associated with an AIDS-like disease in cats. AIDS 3 1989;(suppl 1):43.
17. Hooper CD, Sparkes AH, Gruffy-Jones TJ. Clinical and laboratory findings in cats infected with feline immunodeficiency virus. Vet Rec 1989;125:341.
18. Shelton GH, Grant CK, Linenbarger ML, Abkowitz JL. Severe neutropenia associated with griseofulvin therapy in cats with feline immunodeficiency infection. J Vet Intern Med 1990;4:317.
19. Hardy WD Jr, Zuckerman EE. Comparison of ELISA, IFA, and immunoblot tests for detection of FIV infection (abstract). First International Conference of FIV Researchers. University of California, Davis, CA, Sept 4–7, 1991.
20. Shelton G, Hoskins J, Barlough JE, et al. Stopping the spread of FeLV and FIV. Vet Forum 1991;8:44.
21. Sparger EE. Feline Immunodeficiency Virus. 12th Annual Kal Kan Symposium, 1988:35.
22. Yamamoto JK, Okuda T, Ackley CD, et al. Efficacy of experimental feline immunodeficiency virus vaccines (abstract). First International Conference of FIV Researchers. University of California, Davis, CA, Sept 4–7, 1991.
23. Scott FW, Hancock B, Hardy WD Jr, et al. Panel report on the Colloquium on Feline Leukemia Virus/Feline Immunodeficiency Virus Tests and Vaccinations. J Am Vet Med Assoc 1991;199:1273.

CHAPTER 38

◇ ◇ ◇

Feline Infectious Peritonitis

Gary D. Norsworthy

Feline infectious peritonitis (FIP) can produce a clinical disease so dramatic and unique that it can be diagnosed correctly by the most inexperienced clinician. It can also produce a clinical disease so difficult that to diagnose it causes frustration and embarrassment for the clinician with advanced knowledge and experience.

Feline Coronaviruses

To understand FIP, one must first understand coronaviruses. There are four coronaviruses that can produce seroconversion in cats: the feline infectious peritonitis virus (FIPV), the feline enteric coronavirus (FECV), the porcine transmissible gastroenteritis virus (TGEV), and the canine coronavirus (CCV). Although only the first two cause disease in cats, all four are antigenically related.

FIPV is fairly heat labile, although it may survive at room temperature on dry surfaces for as long as 3 to 7 weeks. The amount of infectious virus decreases rapidly with time, and relatively large quantities of virus are needed for transmission. Therefore, even if no disinfection measures are taken, the level of environmental contamination is not likely to remain significant for more than 2 to 3 weeks.[1] The virus can be destroyed by many household disinfectants and detergents; for example, 1 cup of Clorox Bleach (The Clorox Company, Oakland, CA) in 1 gallon of water is effective against all strains of FIPV.[2]

FECV has the same heat-labile properties as FIPV. It, too, is susceptible to household disinfectants and detergents. It replicates within enterocytes and is limited to the cat's gastrointestinal tract and the mesenteric lymph nodes.

About 25% of free-roaming cats in the United States have been or are infected with FECV.[3] Catteries where FECV is endemic may have infection rates of up to 100%. Cats are believed to become infected by the oral route. Infected adult cats generally show a subclinical infection. Infected kittens may have subclinical infection or a clinical syndrome of low-grade fever, neutropenia, vomiting, and diarrhea. The diarrhea results from lesions in the jejunum and ileum that reduce absorptive capacity; it lasts 2 to 5 days and is rarely fatal even without symptomatic treatment.[4] A definitive diagnosis of this virus can be made only by electronmicroscopy of the feces. The virus may be visible 7 to 13 days after infection occurs.

An FECV infection is clinically significant because (1) it causes a clinical diarrhea in kittens; (2) it produces antibodies that are detectable by the commonly used feline coronavirus test; and (3) most importantly, it may sensitize a cat to subsequent FIPV challenge.[5]

The similarities between FIPV and FECV have led to two theories of origin. One states that both are altered biotypes of the same virus, differing in pathogenicity.[6,7] According to the other theory, FIPVs arise periodically as mutants of FECVs.[8] Regardless of their origin, both viruses show a seropositive response to the commonly used feline coronavirus test, which creates considerable difficulty in distinguishing them.

Viral Strains

The spectrum of pathogenicity for various FIPV strains is more diverse than that for most feline viruses, ranging from the FIPV-79-1146 strain with a mortality rate of 100% to the FIPV-UCD2 strain with a mortality of 0%. Mortality rates for other strains are evenly distributed between those two extremes (Table 38–1).[4] This variation has greatly complicated our ability to predict the outcome for cats exposed to the FIPV or for cats with FIP.

Furthermore, some cats with FIP also have intestinal lesions. At least one FIPV strain can produce both FIP and enteritis after experimental inoculation.[4]

Transmission

It is unlikely that cats with clinical FIP are the only—or even the primary—source of FIPV for other cats.[3] Because of the instability of the virus in vitro and its susceptibility to detergents and disinfectants, it is also unlikely that many cats are infected environmentally or via fomites.[9] Therefore, the source of most FIPV is thought to be asymptomatic carriers, also known as immune carriers. For about 10 days following infection, transmission may occur via feces, urine, or oronasal secretions.[3,10] Thereafter, the potential exists for virus to be shed any time that stress occurs.[10] This means that cats

Table 38–1. Pathogenicity for Various FIPV Strains

Isolate	No. of Cats That Developed FIP	Mortality Rate (%)
FIPV-79-1146	6/6	100
FIPV-NOR 15 (FIPV-DF2)	30/33	91
FIPV-UCD1	18/21	86
FIPV-TN-406/Black	6/8	75
FIPV-HR	2/3	67
FIPV-NW1	19/42	45
FIPV-UCD4	3/12	25
FIPV-UCD3	2/9	22
FIPV-Yayoi	4/36	11
FIPV-UCD2	0/16	0
FIPV-TN-406/Black (attenuated)	0/5	0

Adapted from Stoddart CA, Barlough JE. Feline Coronaviruses: Spectrum of Virus Strains and Clinical Manifestations of Infection. In: August JR, ed. Consultations in Feline Internal Medicine. Philadelphia: WB Saunders, 1991:551.

sharing litter boxes, food bowls, and water bowls with asymptomatic carriers are at risk. Grooming each other, breeding, and fighting, also place cats at risk. Asymptomatic carriers typically do not shed virus continuously; therefore, casual contact is much less likely to produce contagion opportunity than continuous exposure to the immune carrier.

Transmission may also occur between queens and their kittens. Some authorities believe that as many as 90% of FIPV-infected cats are infected in this manner.[2] Some believe that this may occur in utero or during the neonatal period. Some in utero–infected kittens are reported to be born sick, although others are normal.[3] A few coronavirus-negative queens appear to have passed FIPV to their kittens.[2] However, more recently other authors have presented convincing evidence that vertical transmission from queens to kittens does not occur. Rather, they report that transmission to kittens occurs horizontally after FIPV maternal antibodies have waned. This transmission may be from the kittens' mother or from other cats in the household or cattery.[11]

The greatest amount of virus shedding occurs within the first few days or weeks of the initial infection. It continues in inconsistent amounts during the period of months or years that the cat is asymptomatic. Once clinical signs develop, antibody production and antigen-antibody complexing increases. By the time the cat has been ill for more than 2 weeks, virus shedding generally stops because virtually all the antigen is bound by antibody. Thus, the terminally ill cat is no longer contagious. Frequently, owners of ill cats suspected of having FIP want to know about contagion to their other cats. There is no reason to advise isolation; however, they should be advised that the other cats were probably exposed during the preceding months or years.[10]

Pathophysiology

Following experimental oronasal exposure, the FIPV localizes and replicates in regional lymphoreticular tissue such as the tonsils and submandibular and/or mesenteric lymph nodes.[12,13] A primary viremia occurs within about 1 week, disseminating the FIPV to organs with large populations of macrophages. These organs are primarily the liver, spleen, and lymph nodes.[12,14] During this week, the cat may remain normal or may develop a low-grade fever and mesenteric lymph node enlargement.

At this point one of at least five scenarios may develop, depending on the cat's ability or inability to mount an effective cell-mediated immune response (CMIR).

1. An effective CMIR occurs, and the cat is able to terminate the viremia.
2. The infection proceeds rapidly because the cat has coronaviral antibodies from a previous FECV infection or from an infection by an FIPV of low virulence. Generally the effusive form results within a few weeks.
3. No CMIR occurs. Instead, anti-FIPV antibodies develop that are not virus-neutralizing, so the infection proceeds rapidly with the same results as in no. 2.
4. No CMIR occurs. A strong, nonprotective humoral response occurs resulting in effusive FIP, but often not for months to years.
5. A partial CMIR occurs so that the cat develops noneffusive FIP, but often not for months to years.

Unfortunately, an effective CMIR does not always totally eliminate FIPV from the cat's body. A latent or sequestered form of infection may occur in the gastrointestinal tract or its adjacent lymph nodes.[15] If an immunosuppressive event occurs, such as a feline leukemia virus (FeLV) infection, a feline immunodeficiency virus (FIV) infection, another disease, or advancing age, the latent infection may become activated and result in virus shedding and/or clinical FIP.[13]

FIPV antibodies are the basis of the pathogenesis of FIP rather than the foundation upon which protection is built. Furthermore, FIPV antibodies can increase the infectivity of FIPV for macrophages, the target cell for FIPV replication.[7]

Effusive and Noneffusive Forms

The basic lesion of FIP is disseminated pyogranulomatous (Arthus-type) vasculitis.[4] Because of damage to the vessels, a nonseptic exudate pours through the vessel walls into the surrounding tissues. If this process occurs primarily in the abdominal viscera, ascites develops; if it occurs in the chest, pleural effusion results. This is known as the effusive form, or "wet" FIP. If the vascular damage is contained by a partial CMIR, pyogranulomas develop in various target organs, but no outpouring of fluid; this is known as the noneffusive form or "dry" FIP. Wet FIP occurs about four times more frequently than dry FIP.[3]

Infrequently, a combination of wet and dry FIP results in a fluid collection in one body cavity and dry, granulomatous disease in another. Ocular and neurologic manifestations may occur with or without manifestations in other organs.

Effusive Feline Infectious Peritonitis

Effusive FIP is the more fulminant form, having the more rapid onset and a shorter clinical course until death (averaging 5 to 7 weeks).[4] In the early stages, cats exhibit nonspecific signs such as chronic fluctuating fever, appetite depression to anorexia, lethargy, and gradual weight loss. Anemia and/or icterus may occur, giving the mucous membranes a pale to yellow color. Occasionally, recurrent diarrhea may develop.

Fluid begins to accumulate in the thoracic cavity (25% of the cases)[13] or the abdominal cavity (75% of the cases), or occasionally in both. In the former situation, the cat becomes less active because of pulmonary compromise, then develops dyspnea to the point of open-mouth breathing (Fig. 38–1). In the latter situation, the abdomen becomes distended with fluid. Up to 1 liter of fluid may develop with the following characteristics[4]:

1. Straw-colored, bright yellow, or amber; clear to slightly cloudy.
2. Thick consistency; viscous; often having a sticky feeling.
3. Rich in fibrin.
4. Clotting possible upon exposure to air.
5. High specific gravity (1.018 to 1.050).
6. High protein content (5 to 12 g/dL), which creates a pink, homogeneous background on a stained smear.
7. Low leukocyte count, relative to septic peritonitis.
8. Sterile inflammatory pattern (Fig. 38–2). In acute cases, neutrophils predominate. In chronic cases, mononuclear and mesothelial cells predominate. In contrast to bacterial peritonitis, the neutrophils do not exhibit degenerate or toxic characteristics.
9. Likelihood of indicating FIP if the gamma globulin content is greater than 32% (based on protein electrophoresis). The disease is unlikely to be FIP if the albumin content is greater than 48% or if the albumin-to-globulin (A : G) ratio is greater than 0.81.[16]

In the abdominal form, the peritoneum is covered with white, fibrinous plaques.[17] The mesentery is thickened and often has a watery, gelatinous consistency.[18] The omentum often adheres to itself because of the fibrin present (Fig. 38–3), and the mesenteric lymph nodes are often enlarged. In the thoracic form, the white fibrinous plaques adhere to the visceral pleura and pericardium.[13]

Noneffusive Feline Infectious Peritonitis

The noneffusive form is a more insidious disease than the effusive form. It begins with the same nonspecific clinical signs described for effusive FIP. These signs may last for weeks before more organ-specific signs develop. Abdominal

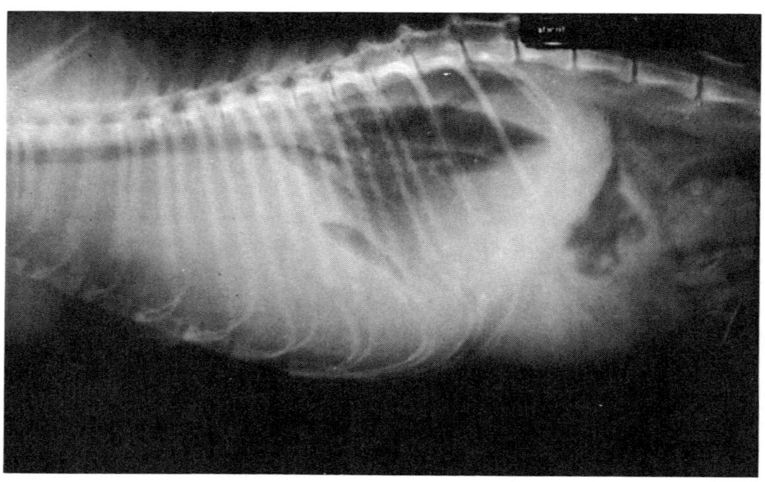

A

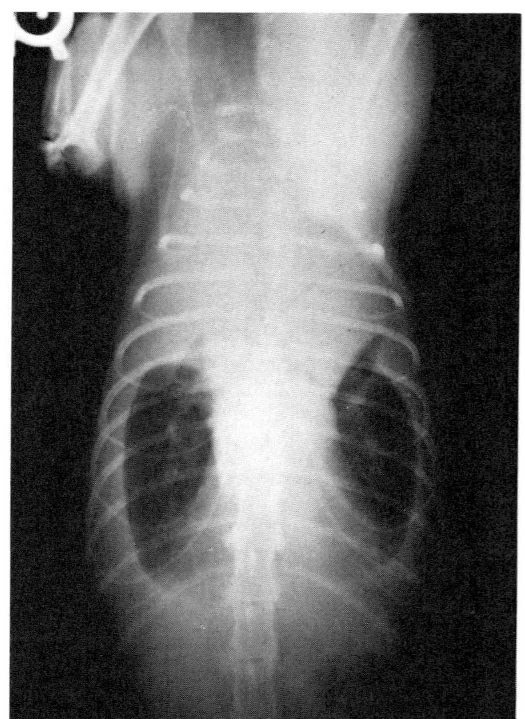

B

Figure 38–1. (*A*) The effusive, or wet, form of FIP that occurs in the thorax produces pleural effusion. On the lateral radiograph this is seen as ventral scalloping of lung borders and obscuring of the cardiac and diaphragmatic silhouettes due to the presence of extrapulmonary fluid. (*B*) The signs of pleural effusion on the ventrodorsal radiographic view include the appearance of fissure lines between the lung lobes, rounding of the lung borders at the costophrenic angles, mediastinal widening, obscuring of the cardiac and diaphragmatic silhouettes, and separation of the lung margins from the thoracic wall.

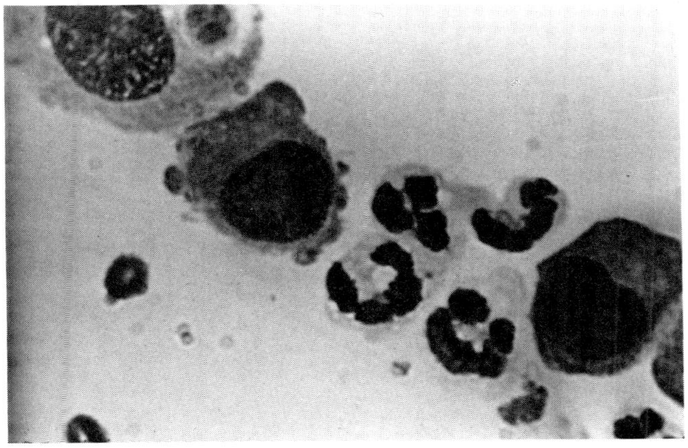

Figure 38–2. FIP-induced fluid recovered from the thorax or abdomen has a sterile inflammatory pattern. In acute cases the predominant cells are neutrophils. In chronic cases, mononuclear and mesothelial cells predominate. The same cytologic pattern is found by aspirating an FIP granuloma in an affected organ.

palpation often reveals mesenteric lymph node enlargement. Pyogranulomas may be palpated as raised nodules on the kidneys (Fig. 38–4) liver (Fig. 38–5), and/or spleen.[19] They may reach 1.5 to 2.0 cm in diameter and account for "lumpy, bumpy kidneys." In the thorax, the various lobes of the lung may become consolidated. They may be seen radiographically as collapsed or adherent to the thoracic wall (Fig. 38–6 *A* and *B*).

The kidneys and liver are the organs most likely to fail, producing early signs of polydipsia and polyuria or icterus, respectively. When advanced organ failure occurs, anorexia, vomiting, and dehydration become terminal events.

The noneffusive form can also have ocular manifestations, which commonly include uveitis, corneal edema, hyphema, and hypopyon. The fundic examination may reveal

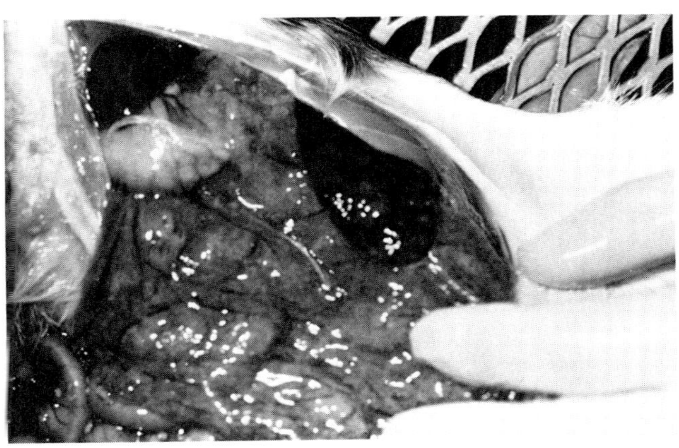

Figure 38–3. In the effusive abdominal form of FIP the abdominal organs or peritoneum is covered with white fibrinous plaques as seen on this spleen. The mesentery is thickened and often has a watery, gelatinous consistency. The omentum is often adherent to itself because of the fibrin present.

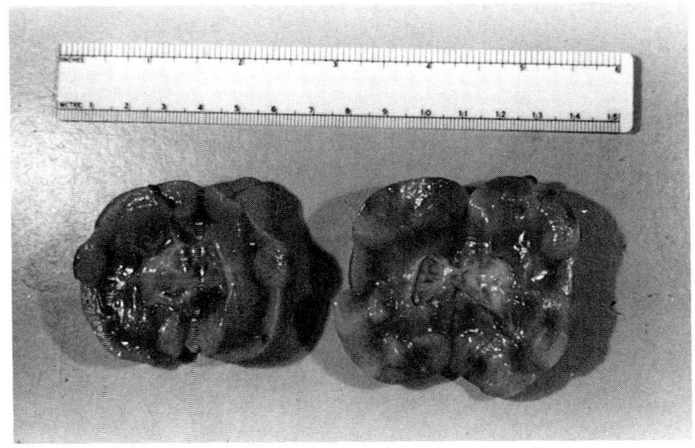

Figure 38–4. Multiple pyogranulomas are seen in these kidneys with noneffusive FIP.

focal areas of retinal hemorrhage due to retinal vasculitis. Affected cats may have ocular signs exclusively or may also have other organ involvement.[20] The central nervous system (CNS) may be involved in noneffusive FIP, resulting in progressive incoordination leading to generalized ataxia, posterior paresis, hyperesthesia, head tilt, convulsions, behavior changes, and urinary incontinence. In many cases histologic lesions exist in the CNS even though the cat never manifests CNS signs prior to death.[21]

Differential Diagnosis

A number of other chronic diseases may have some of the same clinical signs and/or laboratory findings as FIP. These include the following:[3,4,6]

- ***Diseases Causing Dyspnea:*** Lymphosarcoma, pyothorax, chylothorax, cardiomyopathy, diaphragmatic hernia, asthma (see Chapter 18).
- ***Diseases of the Abdomen:*** Lymphosarcoma, visceral malignancies, cholangiohepatitis, pancreatitis, pansteatitis, and bacterial peritonitis.

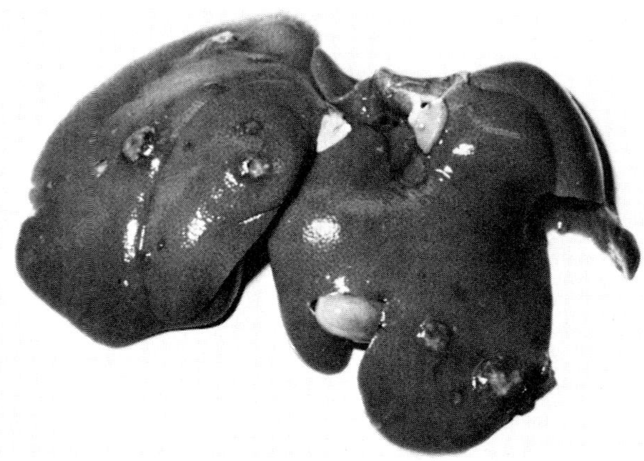

Figure 38–5. Multiple pyogranulomas are seen on the surface of this liver with noneffusive FIP.

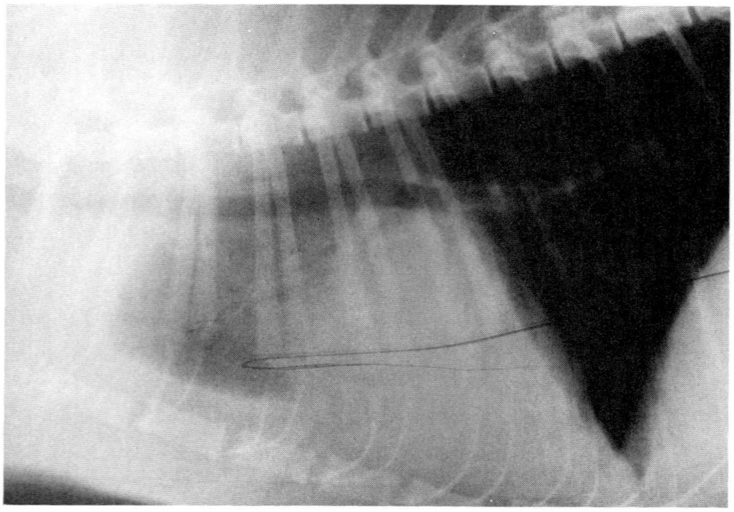

A

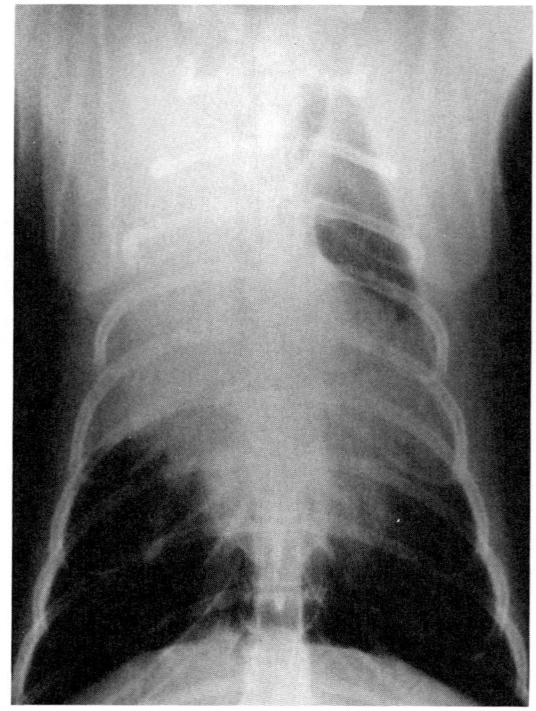

B

Figure 38–6. (*A*) Lateral X-ray of thoracic dry FIP. (*B*) VD view of the same.

- *Systemic Diseases:* Histoplasmosis, cryptococcosis, toxoplasmosis, and, rarely, tuberculosis.
- *Chronic Inflammatory Diseases:* Stomatitis, chronic dermatitis.

Diagnosis

A definitive diagnosis of FIP can be made only by histopathologic examination of an affected organ displaying the typical vasculitis and pyogranuloma formation. The diagnostic lesions include disseminated pyogranulomatous and fibrinonecrotic reactions around small veins.[4] However, organ biopsy is often not feasible in clinical situations, because of either the inaccessibility of the organ involved (e.g., brain, retina) or the condition of the cat. Therefore, a number of tests must be performed in order to make a reasonably firm tentative diagnosis. These are described below in their approximate order of reliability.

Tests of Greater Reliability

Analysis of Effusion Fluid

The mere presence of fluid in the chest or abdomen is not sufficient for a diagnosis of FIP. In addition to looking for the fluid's typical characteristics, one should examine a stained sediment sample. It should have a sterile inflammatory pattern; it should contain neutrophils, lymphocytes, macrophages, and/or plasma cells in relatively low numbers (as compared with a bacterial pleuritis or peritonitis) (see Fig. 38–2). It should not contain bacteria, although the proteinaceous background may have enough granularity to be mistaken for rod-shaped bacteria. It should not contain lymphoblasts or mitotic figures, with the exception of an occasional mesothelial cell undergoing mitosis.

Chylothorax usually occurs secondary to a primary thoracic disease. If the primary disease is FIP, the cellular pattern typical of FIP will be superimposed upon a moderate to large number of very small lymphocytes that have spilled out of the thoracic duct.

Aspiration Cytology of Soft Tissue Masses or Organs

An FIP-affected organ has multiple pyogranulomas containing neutrophils, lymphocytes, macrophages, and plasma cells. Although aspiration recovers these inflammatory cells, their source cannot be identified as a pyogranuloma; the sample is classified as a sterile inflammatory reaction, either subacute or chronic. This finding is not specific for FIP, but it does rule out several other common causes of organomegaly, most notably lymphosarcoma.

Although the pyogranulomas are usually widespread in an affected organ, it is possible to miss them on aspiration. If only normal cells are obtained, another aspiration should be performed.

Serum Protein Analysis

A marked hyperproteinemia is seen in about 50% of cats with effusive FIP and about 70% of cats with noneffusive FIP. This condition is due primarily to an elevation in gamma globulins and, to a lesser degree, beta globulins. Cats so affected have a total serum protein level greater than 7.8 g/dL and an A : G ratio of less than 0.6. Because of the relatively high percentage of noneffusive cases with these findings, serum protein analysis should be one of the primary tests performed. However, the findings are typical of any chronic inflammatory disease and not diagnostic for FIP.[4]

Serum Electrophoresis

If the total serum protein is greater than 7.8 g/dL and the A : G ratio is less than 0.6, serum electrophoresis is indicated. However, FIP is but one of several diseases that produces a polyclonal gammopathy. Others include chronic stomatitis, chronic dermatitis, and systemic fungal diseases; FIP cannot be differentiated from them on the basis of serum electrophoresis.

Serum Fibrinogen

The fibrinogen level can also be helpful for diagnosis. Fibrinogen is an alpha globulin that is elevated above 400 mg/dL in about 45% to 60% of FIP cases.[4]

Tests of Lesser Reliability

Biochemical Testing

Changes found through biochemical testing of serum are not specific for FIP. Rather they reflect the extent of organ involvement due to FIPV. The liver is one of the primary organs involved. Elevations in total bilirubin, with direct bilirubin levels in the 50% to 75% range; elevations of the hepatic enzymes; and the presence of bilirubin in the cat's urine are all common findings.

If the kidneys are involved, the urea nitrogen and creatinine will be increased—to very high levels in terminal cases. High levels of protein are found in the urine.[3]

Hematology

Many cats with FIP, effusive and noneffusive, have normal hemograms. However, some have a marked leukocytosis, with total leukocyte counts exceeding 50,000 cells/mm^3. Some circulating neutrophils may contain inclusion bodies in their cytoplasm. These are thought to be phagocytized antigen-antibody complexes. Some cats, especially those that are terminally ill, have a leukopenia.[4]

About 40% of cats with FIP have a mild to moderate anemia due to chronic bone marrow suppression. It is normocytic and normochromic, showing no evidence of bone marrow response.[4]

In years past, about 50% of FIP cats would be coinfected with the FeLV. However, now the number is approximately 20%, presumably because of the reduction in the incidence of FeLV diseases.[4]

Coronavirus Titers

Presently, the only serologic test for the FIP virus is the test for a coronavirus titer. However, it makes no distinction between FIPV and FECV. In addition, it detects antibodies to TGEV and CCV. Therefore, one must exercise extreme caution in interpreting the test results.

Coronavirus titers are performed by diluting one part of coronavirus with various amounts of a nonreactive component. The dilution is done on a fourfold basis, the first generally being 1 : 25. Subsequent dilutions are 1 : 100, 1 : 400, 1 : 1,600, and 1 : 64,000. Some laboratories interpret their results as "negative" when, in fact, a low positive titer exists. Therefore, one is encouraged to ascertain the laboratory's definition of negative; the most desirable would be a titer in which no detectable antibody exists.

Based on surveys of large numbers of cats, it is assumed that many cats undergo coronavirus seroconversion but never progress to fatal disease. In the general cat population, excluding multiple cat situations, the seropositivity rate is as high as 40%. Therefore, coronavirus seropositivity in a sick cat may be no more than an incidental finding.[4]

The level of the titer can be significant. FECV-induced titers are generally in the low range, 1 : 25 to 1 : 400. They are rarely as high as 1 : 1,600. Titers of 1 : 1,600 or greater are generally indicative of FIP. However, this interpretation should be made only if clinical signs of FIP are present. Cats with FIP may also have titers in the low range that overlap with FECV-induced titers. In addition, some cats with FIP may have no detectable antibody present, i.e., titers that are truly negative. The reason for this is not understood; however, it is thought to result from the formation of immune complexes in cats with terminal illness, from viral serotypic differences, or from inadequacies of the test. If the first theory is correct, the FIPV antibody becomes bound in these complexes and is no longer available for reacting with the test reagents.

False-positive results can also occur. Some cats develop antibodies against the bovine serum components commonly found in feline vaccines. Reactivity to these can be mistaken for coronavirus antibody reactions if proper positive and negative controls are not used in the testing procedure. Bovine serum–stimulated antibody wanes over time and is generally absent within 3 to 4 months following vaccinations. Therefore, a low positive antibody test should be viewed with caution if parenteral vaccines have been administered within the last 3 to 4 months.[4]

Tests of the Future

The ideal test for this disease would be a specific antigen test; however, none are currently available. Several companies are currently developing FIPV tests, including an antiidiotypic FIP antibody test that detects FIPV-specific antibodies in serum. The latter is intended to be specific to virulent strains of FIPV. However, since it will detect antibodies and not virus antigen, it still can be misleading in cats immune to the FIPV but having antibodies. False-negative results can still occur in terminally ill cats when the antibody level falls below detacable levels.[22] Primucell FIP vaccine will likely produce low positive coronavirus titers measured by ELISA tests.[7]

Special Note

The antemortem diagnosis of noneffusive FIP can be one of the most difficult of all diagnoses. The typical cat is a "poor doer," one that may experience months of nonspecific, recurrent illness. Some owners become exasperated because constant testing and treatment produce no answers or results, and seek second and third opinions. Although FIP is suspected, the diagnosis is not confirmed until necropsy.

Clinical Signs

Cats with nonspecific signs of lethargy, poor appetite, weight loss, and recurring, antibiotic-resistant fevers should be suspected of having FIP, although many other diseases can produce these signs. Diagnostic test results must be obtained (the coronavirus titer is not sufficient). Any cat showing the nonspecific signs along with elevated liver enzymes and an elevated serum protein level should be suspected of having FIP.

Treatment

The prognosis of any cat with FIP is poor because there is no known effective treatment. A few effusive FIP cats have spontaneously recovered[3]; however, one should not give the owner unrealistic expectations based on those rare exceptions.

Supportive therapy that includes force feeding (food and fluids) and removing most of the effusion from the thorax and/or abdomen sustains some cats for several weeks.

The most commonly recommended medical treatment regimen includes drugs that suppress the intense immune-mediated response that occurs to FIPV. Some cats respond to drugs such as cyclophosphamide (Cytoxan), azathioprine, and prednisolone, but the results are generally temporary. Aspirin may counteract the inflammatory effects of prostaglandins.

Counseling Owners of FIP Cats

The owner of a clinically ill cat with FIP should be advised to consider euthanasia. If the illness has been protracted and the cat is debilitated, this is usually not difficult to accept. However, if the diagnosis was made quickly and the cat enjoys a reasonable quality of life, the owner may not be ready to accept euthanasia. Prednisolone, azathioprine, cyclophosphamide, or aspirin may provide temporary improvement, providing time for the owner to adjust to the terminal prognosis. The drug's failure to improve the cat's condition would help to convince the owner that treatment will not be successful.

If the owner has other cats, the subject of contagion must be addressed. Assuming a healthy cat was in contact with the sick one, the healthy one is highly likely to test positive for a coronavirus or the FIPV. However, even if the cat is seronegative, contagion could have occurred. If the FIPV test is positive, it has no predictive value for a healthy cat because each cat's immune response determines the outcome of the virus challenge. Therefore, testing the other cats is not recommended. Owners should, however, test any cats they may consider obtaining, especially if they come from a cattery or multi-cat household, to avoid introducing FIPV to the household.

Prevention

Numerous attempts have been made to produce a safe and effective vaccine against the FIPV. These have been derived from killed viruses, other live coronaviruses, avirulent FIPV strains, modified live virulent FIPV strains, and recombinant carrier viruses. Unfortunately, all failed either by providing no immunity or by accelerating the disease compared with the course of unvaccinated controls. Researchers at the Cornell Feline Health Center produced an intranasal vaccine that produced inconsistent results; further research is in progress.

One modified live-virus vaccine, Primucell FIP, is commercially available. It is administered intranasally and contains a temperature-sensitive strain of FIPV. It was derived from a virulent strain of FIPV by serial passage in cell culture, followed by ultraviolet irradiation. The resulting virus replicates well at the cooler temperatures of the oronasal cavity (31°C), but poorly at body temperature (38.5°C), which explains why it is administered intranasally.[7]

The manufacturer of Primucell FIP has conducted extensive safety tests on this vaccine. It appears to be safe when administered parenterally and when given to cats immunosuppressed by steroids and to FeLV-viremic cats. It has passed safety tests in cats with preexisting coronavirus antibodies (FECV or FIPV), in pregnant queens, and in kittens 3 to 8 weeks of age.[7]

An efficacy test conducted by the manufacturer on specific pathogen–free (SPF) cats under experimental conditions has produced a mean efficacy of 69% based on the preventable fraction calculation method. However, field trials in catteries with known losses from FIP have produced results in which the vaccinate and control groups' results were not statistically different. The true efficacy of this or any other vaccine will not be known until thousands of doses are administered under natural conditions to different breeds of cats in different geographic areas.[7]

This vaccine is not approved for use in kittens younger than 16 weeks of age. Since most kittens raised in catteries are exposed to FIPV by then, management practices must prevent exposure of kittens until they are old enough to receive both doses of the vaccine.[7]

Cattery/Multi-Cat Household Situations

The density of the cat population affects the dynamics of disease transmission. The number one cause of epidemics and chronic disease in most catteries and multi-cat households is overcrowding. When a large number of cats interact daily, viruses shed by a few individuals eventually infect almost every cat. In most of these situations, the coronaviral antibody incidence will be either 0% or 80% to 100%.[2,4]

The goal in a cattery should be to eliminate all sources of FIPV. However, this requires that all seropositive cats be eliminated from the colony, which is usually not acceptable to cattery owners. The following recommendations have been made to multi-cat owners, including breeders, to minimize FIP[4]:

- Eliminate FeLV-positive cats.
- Avoid overcrowding (i.e., reduce population).
- Avoid inbreeding.
- Stop breeding particular pairs of cats that produce kittens with FIP.
- Eliminate problem breeding stock.

- Do not allow FIPV antibody–positive cats to enter the population. If a cat tests negative, he or she should not enter the FIPV negative population until a second test is performed 4 to 6 weeks later.
- If some cats are sent out to shows or for breeding, routinely test 10% to 20% (a minimum of three cats) of the population at least every 6 months. Because of the ease of transmission, testing all cats is not necessary.

It has been shown by one study that the FIPV is not transmitted from the queen to kittens vertically. Rather, transmission occurs horizontally after maternal antibodies wane. This occurs at about 7 to 8 weeks of age.[11] Therefore, the following recommendations are also appropriate.

- The queen and her kittens should be isolated from other cats in the household or cattery.
- To prevent infection of the kittens, they should be isolated from FIPV-seropositive cats, including their mother if she is seropositive, after 4 weeks of age.
- To further ensure that the kittens are FIPV-free, they should test seronegative before they are sold.

REFERENCES

1. Scott FW. Update on Feline Infectious Peritonitis. Proceedings, 12th Annual Kal Kan Symposium, Ohio State University, 1988.
2. Saidla JE. FIP: Common questions, current answers. Top Vet Med 1990;2:22.
3. Pedersen NC. Coronavirus Diseases (Coronavirus Enteritis, Feline Infectious Peritonitis). In: Holzworth J, ed. Diseases of the Cat. Philadelphia: WB Saunders, 1987:193.
4. Stoddart CA, Barlough JE. Feline Coronaviruses: Spectrum of Virus Strains and Clinical Manifestations of Infection. In: August JR, ed. Consultations in Feline Internal Medicine. Philadelphia: WB Saunders, 1991:551.
5. Grahn BH. The feline coronavirus infections: Feline infectious peritonitis and feline coronavirus enteritis. Vet Med 1991; 86:376.
6. Barlough JE. Cats, coronaviruses and coronavirus antibody tests. J Sm Anim Pract 1985;26:353.
7. Olsen CW, Scott FW. Feline infectious peritonitis vaccination—past and present. Fel Health Top Vet 1991;6:1.
8. Pedersen NC, Floyd K. Experimental studies with three new strains of feline infectious peritonitis virus: FIPV-UCD2, FIPV-UCD3, and FIPV-UCD4. Compend Cont Ed Pract Vet 1985; 7:1001.
9. Barlough JE. Do feline coronavirus antibody tests provide a conclusive diagnosis? Vet Med/Sm Anim Clin 1984;79:1027.
10. Scott FW. Deadly FIP still mystifies DVMs; research continues on transmission, prognosis, vaccine. DVM Magazine 1990;85:12.
11. Addie DD, Jarrett O. Control of feline coronavirus infection in kittens. Vet Rec 1990;126:164.
12. Weiss RC, Scott FW. Pathogenesis of feline infectious peritonitis: Pathologic changes and immunofluorescence. Am J Vet Res 1981;42:2036.
13. August JR. Feline Viral Diseases. In: Ettinger SJ, ed. Textbook of Veterinary Internal Medicine, 3rd ed. Philadelphia: WB Saunders, 1989:312.
14. Barlough JE, Stoddart CA. Feline Infectious Peritonitis. In: Scott FW, ed. Contemporary Issues in Small Animal Practice. New York: Churchill Livingstone, 1986;3:93.
15. Pedersen NC. Pathogenic differences between various feline coronavirus isolates. Adv Exp Med Biol 1984;173:365.
16. Shelly SM, Scarlett-Kranz J, Blue JT. Protein electrophoresis on effusions from cats as a diagnostic test for feline infectious peritonitis. J Am Anim Hosp Assoc 1988;24:495.
17. Horzinek MC, Osterhaus AD. The virology and pathogenesis of feline infectious peritonitis. Brief review. Arch Virol 1979;59:1.
18. Holmberg CA, Gribble DH. Feline infectious peritonitis: Diagnostic gross and microscopic lesions. Fel Pract 1973;3:11.
19. August JR. Feline infectious peritonitis: An immune-mediated coronaviral vasculitis. Vet Clin North Am (Sm Anim Pract) 1984;14:971
20. Pedersen NC. Feline infectious peritonitis and feline enteric coronavirus infections. Part 2. Feline infectious peritonitis. Fel Pract 1983;13:5.
21. Kornegay JN. Feline infectious peritonitis. The central nervous system form. J Am Anim Hosp Assoc 1978;14:530.
22. Weiss RC. The diagnosis and clinical management of feline infectious peritonitis. Vet Med 1991;86:308.

CHAPTER 39

◇ ◇ ◇

Feline Leukemia Virus Diseases

Gary D. Norsworthy

The feline leukemia virus (FeLV) produces a variety of diseases in the cat. It is the etiologic agent for the most common feline neoplasm, lymphosarcoma, and it is the most common infectious disease agent in the cat. Except for trauma, it is responsible for more feline deaths than any other cause.[1] Because of the wide variety of diseases it causes, it might better be termed the feline catastrophic virus.

The Virus

Historical Perspective

FeLV was first linked to disease in the cat in 1964.[2] The first test for the virus was not developed until 1972,[3] however, and did not become widely available to the practicing veterinarian until 1973. Prior to 1973, lymphosarcoma, several types of leukemia, and nonregenerative anemias were diagnosed frequently but were generally not associated with each other. When Hardy developed the first FeLV test, it led to a new understanding of these diseases. Still, controversy persisted for several years concerning horizontal versus vertical transmission of the virus. Hardy's Test and Removal Program was the first successful means of controlling the transmission of FeLV, and it provided evidence of horizontal transmission.[3] When Norden Laboratory's FeLV vaccine became available in 1985, control of FeLV infection was finally possible on a wide-scale, prophylactic basis.

Virology

FeLV contains complete ribonucleic acid (RNA) and thus is capable of replicating without the aid of a helper virus. This is in contrast to the feline sarcoma virus, which requires the envelope of FeLV for replication. The replication process of FeLV involves the enzyme reverse transcriptase, which copies the RNA of FeLV into complementary deoxyribonucleic acid (DNA). This DNA is inserted into the chromosome of the newly infected cell as a provirus.[4] The provirus begins the process of viral RNA production in the new cell. Eventually, virus particles are produced from the cell membrane of the newly infected cell.

The RNA molecule and reverse transcriptase enzyme are enclosed in a shell of protein containing p27 antigen.[5] The indirect fluorescent antibody (IFA) and enzyme-linked immunosorbent assay (ELISA) tests detect p27 antigen. The feline oncornavirus cell membrane antigen (FOCMA) is a FeLV and feline sarcoma virus–induced antigen found on the cell membranes of FeLV-induced lymphosarcoma, erythroleukemia, and myelogenous leukemia cells. It is also seen on the surface of feline sarcoma virus–induced fibrosarcoma cells. FOCMA is found on the surface of all lymphosarcoma cells, whether the cat tests positive or negative for FeLV. Finding FOCMA antibodies constitutes serologic evidence that FeLV was involved in the development of lymphosarcoma.[4] FOCMA antibodies are considered protective against lymphosarcoma development but not against the development of nonneoplastic FeLV diseases.[3]

There are three subgroups of FeLV designated A, B, and C. The FeLV-A subgroup is found in all viremic cats, and an oncogenic synergism occurs with the FeLV-B subgroup. Subgroups B and C are minimally pathogenic when they occur alone.[6] FeLV-A subgroup is associated with the development of lymphosarcoma and leukemia.[7] FeLV-B subgroup may cause myeloproliferative or myelosuppressive disease and immunosuppression.[4] FeLV-C subgroup, when associated with FeLV-A subgroup, causes erythroblastopenic anemia.[7] Thus, different clinical syndromes occur in the infected cat, depending on the subgroups involved. This helps explain regional differences in disease incidence and presentation that have been reported.

Incidence

One to three percent of the general cat population in the United States are persistently infected with FeLV.[1] A national survey of nearly 28,000 cats that were primarily symptomatic and in at-risk populations found an incidence of 13.3% with FeLV infection.[8] There are three distinct incidence subgroups within the feline population. Free-roaming cats within an urban environment have an incidence of persistent viremia of somewhat higher than 3%. A closed population of cats (household or cattery) with no exposure to FeLV has an incidence of persistent FeLV infection of essentially zero. A closed population of cats with at least one persistently viremic cat has an incidence of persistent viremia of approximately 30%. However, 70% to 100% of this population show serologic evidence of exposure or infection. Cats that show no evidence of exposure or infection are generally the antisocial members of the group that have little interaction with the other cats.

Transmission

FeLV is very unstable in the environment. It is inactivated in a dry environment within 3 to 5 minutes and lives only about 3 days in a moist environment.[9,10] It is easily killed by most common disinfectants and detergents. Therefore, it is unlikely that significant environmental transmission occurs in household or cattery settings, and it is not scientifically tenable to recommend that new cats not be brought into a previously FeLV-infected household for several weeks or months so as to avoid environmental contamination.

The natural reservoir for FeLV is the asymptomatic persistently viremic cat.[11] Such a cat may shed virus for months or years before becoming sick and dying. The highest concentration of FeLV in a persistently viremic cat is found in the saliva. As many as one million viral particles are found in each milliliter of saliva.[11] Therefore, the main means of FeLV transmission is through fight wounds in which significant quantities of virus are literally injected into the bitten cat. Biting also may occur during the mating process. Saliva-assisted transmission may also take place by social means, such as when cats groom one another, eat or drink from common bowls, or use common litter boxes.

The FeLV is also found in many body fluids, including plasma, urine, milk, and tears. However, it has not been found in feces or in fleas removed from viremic cats.[12] Transmammary and transplacental transmission may occur in viremic queens. Kittens that evade these routes of transmission may also be affected horizontally via the queen's saliva.[1] Kittens born to FeLV-infected queens have a very high risk of infection.

FeLV Tests and Testing

Several tests indicate the presence of or past exposure to FeLV. None of these tests should be interpreted as an indication of any FeLV disease. Three tests screen for the presence of the p27 antigen of FeLV. If the results are positive, this is convincing evidence that the FeLV is present in the cat. However, the three tests may produce different findings, depending on the location of the virus within the cat.

The IFA test was the first FeLV test developed. It detects p27 antigen in infected leukocytes and platelets in fixed blood or bone marrow smears. If the findings are positive, FeLV is replicating in the animal's bone marrow.[13] False-negative IFA tests may occur if there is a very low number of circulating neutrophils or platelets.[12] False-positive IFA tests may occur owing to nonspecific immunofluorescence to eosinophils or platelet clumps,[14] thick blood smears, or the use of contaminated microscope slides.

The blood-ELISA test demonstrates the presence of p27 antigen in whole blood, serum, or plasma shown by a color change. Its technology allows in-house testing in any veterinary hospital. Its findings can be positive at an early stage of FeLV infection; therefore it can detect early and transient infections that would normally be missed by the IFA test. It is the test of choice for prevaccination testing; however, a positive test result should not be used to determine prognosis or the need for euthanasia until further testing is performed (see Vaccination: Prevaccination Testing of Healthy Cats).

The tears/saliva–ELISA test detects p27 antigen in saliva and tears. It is more sensitive when testing saliva than when testing tears.[15] It is the last of the p27 antigen–detecting tests to become positive. Therefore, it is not recommended for prevaccination testing. It is best indicated for clinically ill cats. In addition, when the test is performed on saliva, it may also be used to determine the likelihood of contagion, since saliva is the fluid most often involved in transmission.[15] False-positive results may occur if oral debris or pieces of the collecting device are accidentally included in the test sample material.

A positive FOCMA antibody titer indicates that the cat has been infected by FeLV an undefined time in the past. A high titer is considered protective against the formation of lymphosarcoma; however, no protection is conferred against future FeLV infection or against nonneoplastic FeLV degenerative diseases such as nonregenerative anemia.[14]

A positive test for the presence of gp70 antibody indicates that FeLV has infected the cat. This antibody is measured by the serum neutralization test and indicates that the cat has a level of protection against viral infection as a result of a previous successful immune response to viral challenge. This antibody level decreases with time unless a rise in titer occurs owing to subsequent challenge.[14] Therefore, the presence of gp70 antibody is not considered a lifetime immunity. This test is a research instrument that is not currently available to the practicing veterinarian.

The polymerase chain reaction assay is still experimental but promises to be the most sensitive means yet available for detecting the FeLV. If it becomes available to the commercial veterinary laboratory it will provide a practical means for detecting latent carriers of the virus.[15]

Pathway of the Virus in the Cat

There are six stages of an FeLV infection.[16] These are depicted on a time line in Table 39–1 and are as follows:

1. Virus replication occurs in the tonsils and pharyngeal lymph nodes following oronasal exposure. This stage lasts from 2 to 4 days. All FeLV tests given at this time are negative.
2. Small numbers of circulating lymphocytes and monocytes become infected. This stage lasts from 1 to 14 days. Only the blood-ELISA test results are positive.
3. Replication of the virus continues in the spleen, lymph nodes, and gut-associated lymphoid tissue. This stage lasts from 3 to 12 days. Only the blood-ELISA test results are positive.
4. Replication of the virus occurs in the bone marrow in neutrophils and platelets and in the crypt epithelial cells of the intestine. This stage lasts from 7 to 21 days. Only the blood-ELISA test findings are positive.
5. The bone marrow neutrophils and platelets that were

Table 39–1. Time Line for Locations of FeLV During the Six Stages of Infection

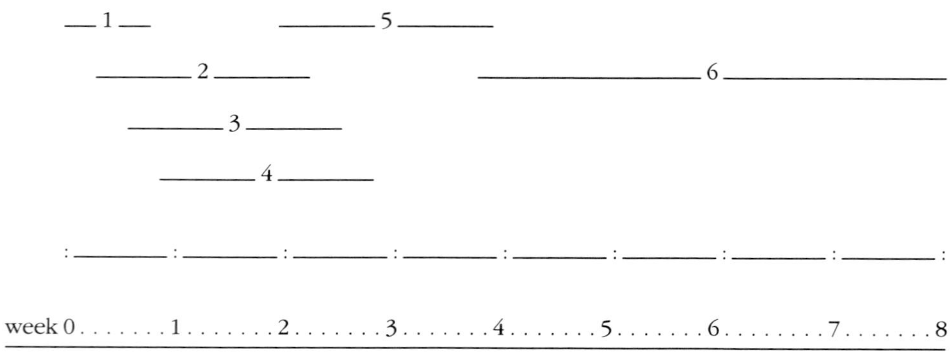

Locations of FeLV (Six Stages of Infection)	Positive Tests
1. Tonsils/pharyngeal lymph nodes	None
2. Circulating lympholysis and monocytis (small numbers)	Blood–ELISA
3. Spleen, lymph nodes, and gut associated lymphoid tissue	Blood–ELISA
4. Bone marrow	Blood–ELISA
5. Systemic circulation	Blood–ELISA/IFA
6. Saliva, tears, and urine	ELISA (Blood, Saliva, and Tears)/IFA

affected in stage 4 become disseminated throughout the body. This stage is termed viremia. It lasts from 14 to 28 days and occurs approximately 2 to 4 weeks from the time of the initial infection. The blood-ELISA and IFA test findings are positive.

6. The virus infects epithelial tissue throughout the body. It is present in saliva and urine. This stage lasts from 28 to 56 days and is approximately 4 to 8 weeks from the time of the initial infection. The blood-ELISA, IFA, and tears/saliva–ELISA test results are positive.

If the cat mounts a successful immune response to the virus, the virus will only pass through Stages 1 and 2 and possibly Stage 3 before being rejected. If the virus reaches Stage 5, the cat becomes persistently viremic, as explained below.

Outcome of FeLV Infection

When most bacteria or viruses infect a host, there are typically only two possible outcomes. Either the recipient's immune system prevails and the infection is aborted accompanied by the development of immunity, or the bacteria or virus prevails and disease occurs. However, there are four possible outcomes of an FeLV infection that are currently recognized (see below).

The outcome of an FeLV infection is influenced by several factors, including the amount of the inoculum, the viral strain, the duration of the exposure, the age of the cat, the status of the cat's immune system, environmental conditions, concurrent infections or diseases, and probably some as yet undetermined genetic elements.[17] The age of the cat is one of the most important factors. Under laboratory conditions, 100 percent of FeLV-infected neonates become persistently viremic compared with 85% of kittens 3 to 6 weeks old and only 15% of kittens over 4 months of age.[18] Thus, catteries or households in which neonates or young kittens are exposed to FeLV and in which cats are kept in crowded conditions generally have very high infection and mortality rates.

Regardless of which of the four possible outcomes occurs, most cats that are FeLV-challenged develop a primary illness identical to that of cats challenged with the feline immunodeficiency virus (FIV). This disease is self-limiting and is characterized by a low-grade fever, leukopenia, listlessness, anorexia, and swollen submandibular lymph nodes. If a biopsy of lymph node tissue is performed, lymphoid hyperplasia, not lymphosarcoma, will be found. This disease generally lasts from 7 to 10 days. The practitioner should be alert to this clinical presentation and, if it is identified, should refrain from administering any drug that would compromise the cat's immune response, such as a corticosteroid.

The first possible outcome of FeLV infection is an *immune response* by the cat that results in neutralization of the virus and the development of immunity.[17] A transient viremia occurs, resulting in the blood-ELISA test becoming positive for up to 8 weeks and then reverting to negative. The IFA and tears/saliva–ELISA tests remain negative. These cats develop protective titers against FOCMA. It is estimated that the immune response is the outcome in about 40% of FeLV-challenged cats.[3]

The second possible outcome is *persistent viremia*.[17] The FeLV reaches the bone marrow and becomes widely disseminated in the cat's tissues and body fluids. The blood-ELISA, IFA, and tears/saliva–ELISA tests are and remain positive. Ninety-seven percent of these cats remain persistently viremic for life.[3] They are highly susceptible to the develop-

Table 39–2. Possibilities for the Outcome of an FeLV Infection

	No Exposure	Initial Infection	Immune Response	Latent Infection	Immune Carrier	Persistent Infection
%	–	–	40	28	2	30
ELISA	–	+	–	–	+	+
IFA	–	–	–	–	–	+
Tears/Saliva	–	–	–	–	–	+
FOCMA	–	+	±	±	+	+
Neutralizing antibody	–	±	±	+	+	+

ment of one or more FeLV diseases, and about 80% die within 3 years.[3] It is estimated that this is the outcome in about 30% of FeLV challenged cats.[3]

The third possible outcome is a period of *viral latency.*[17] In this form, whole virus is not present in the cat; instead, virus-transformed cells are present in the bone marrow and lymph nodes. These transformed cells are capable of being reactivated to produce whole virus, however, resulting in persistent viremia. These cats are not contagious unless reactivation occurs. Reactivation may take place as a result of stress, concurrent bacterial or viral disease, or the administration of high doses of exogenous steroids. These cats typically have FeLV-negative findings on the blood-ELISA, IFA, and tears/saliva–ELISA tests.[19] They produce FOCMA antibodies.[16] Latency lasts an average of 30 months. One study showed that about 50% of latently infected cats are likely to remain in this state, 40% eventually eliminate the virus, and 10% undergo virus activation and become persistently viremic (and FeLV-positive on the IFA and ELISA tests).[20] Latency is the outcome about 30% of the time when cats are FeLV-challenged.

Latency produces a frustrating and sometimes difficult situation for practitioners. If these cats are tested prior to FeLV vaccination, they will test FeLV-negative by any of the three currently available methods. Our best evidence to date is that vaccination does not cause them to clear the virus.[21] Therefore, it they become stressed, develop concurrent disease, or receive a high dose of exogenous corticosteroids, the latent infection may reactivate, the cat will become persistently viremic, and an FeLV disease may develop in spite of a negative prevaccination test and appropriate vaccination with an FeLV vaccine.

The fourth possible outcome of an FeLV infection is that the cat may become an *immune carrier.*[11] Whole virus is present in epithelial tissue, and virus replication occurs in these cats. However, virus does leave the cells because of the presence of antibodies. The cat may remain clinically normal or may experience cyclic episodes of anorexia, listlessness, and neutropenia. The immune carrier is seen 1% to 2% of the time in FeLV-infected cats. During the stage in which the cat is an immune carrier of the virus, the IFA test is FeLV-negative and the blood-ELISA test is FeLV-positive. The cat is not contagious unless virus reactivation occurs. The cat may also revert to a latent infection stage and eventually clear itself of the virus.

These explanations summarize our present understanding of the pathogenesis of FeLV infections. It is not always easy to define which of the possible outcomes has occurred because in a practice setting it is usually not practical to test for the FeLV by both the ELISA and IFA methods and, in addition, to test for FOCMA. However, Table 39–2 summarizes these outcomes based on the results of these tests. It should be noted that the columns marked Initial Infection and Immune Carrier show identical results. However, the Initial Infection category is a very temporary status. After 4 to 8 weeks, either the blood-ELISA test or the IFA test should change as the cat progresses into one of the four outcomes. The columns titled Immune Response and Latent Infection also have identical data, as discussed earlier.

FeLV Test Selection

Since an FeLV infection may have four possible outcomes, the different FeLV tests must be selected based upon specific goals. The tests and their most appropriate uses are listed in Table 39–3.

FeLV Diseases

The diseases caused by the FeLV include several forms of neoplasia. These are classified as proliferative diseases. However, not all of the FeLV diseases are neoplastic in nature. A number of nonneoplastic diseases have been identified and are classified as degenerative diseases (Table 39–4).

Proliferative Diseases

The neoplastic, proliferative FeLV diseases include lymphosarcoma in its many forms and several types of leukemia. These diseases and their treatment are discussed in Chapter 51.

Table 39–3. Selection of FeLV Tests[15]

Goal	Test
Most sensitive test	Blood-ELISA
Determine contagion	Tears/saliva–ELISA
Persistent viremia	IFA
Ease of testing	Tears/saliva–ELISA
Determine latent infection	Polymerase chain reaction assay

Degenerative FeLV Diseases

The most common degenerative disease caused by FeLV is *immunosuppression*. Manifestations of this syndrome occur in adult cats, and it is known as the feline acquired immunodeficiency syndrome (FAIDS).[18] Its name was chosen because the T-lymphocyte disorders and secondary diseases, including an eventual fatal outcome, greatly resemble the human acquired immunodeficiency syndrome.

The primary expression of immunosuppression is an increased susceptibility to pathogens. In clinical terms, this may be seen as nonhealing abscesses caused by cat bites, nonresponsive respiratory infections, bacterial dermatitis, pneumonia, septicemia, or chronic gingivitis. Cats that develop hemobartonellosis, toxoplasmosis, and systemic fungal infections are often concurrently immunosuppressed by FeLV. These cats are clinically identical to cats that are immunosuppressed by the feline immunodeficiency virus (see Chapter 37).

If corticosteroids are administered to immunosuppressed cats, their condition may initially improve, but it will rapidly deteriorate. Corticosteroids depress T-cell function and accelerate virus replication. The more virus that is produced, the greater the degree of immunosuppression.[18]

The only way to reverse immunosuppression is to reverse the viremia. A number of sophisticated methods have been tried, including extracorporeal removal of immune complexes and treatment with staphylococcal protein A, monoclonal antibodies to FeLV, and macrophage stimulants.[18] However, to date, there are no methods that have been successful and that are likely to be economically feasible for veterinary practice.

Thymic atrophy can be induced experimentally by inoculating young kittens with FeLV.[22] Thymic atrophy has been seen in naturally infected kittens born to FeLV-infected queens or infected by contact with other infected cats.[23,24] The T lymphocytes of the thymus and other lymphoid tissue are destroyed by FeLV. A defective cell-mediated immune response results.[22,25] Because of its reduced immune capacity, the kitten is susceptible to secondary infections caused by bacteria, other viruses, or fungi. These kittens typically die within a few weeks of birth from either bronchopneu-

Table 39–4. The FeLV Diseases

Cell Type	Proliferative Diseases (Neoplastic)	Degenerative Diseases (Blastopenic)
Diseases Known to Be Caused by FeLV		
A. Lymphoid cells	Lymphosarcoma Reticulum cell sarcoma	Thymic atrophy (kittens) Immunosuppressive diseases (adults)
B. Bone marrow cells		
Primitive mesenchymal cell	Reticuloendotheliosis	—
Erythroblast	Erythremic myelosis	Erythroblastosis (regenerative anemia)
	Erythroleukemia	Erythroblastopenia (nongenerative anemia) Pancytopenia
Myeloblast	Granulocytic leukemias (neutrophilic and basophilic)	Myeloblastopenia (panleukemia-like syndrome)
Megakaryocyte	Megakaryocytic leukemia	Thrombocytopenia
Fibroblast	Myelofibrosis	—
Osteoblast	Medullary osteosclerosis Osteochondromatosis	—
C. Kidney	—	FeLV immune complex glomerulonephritis
Diseases Thought to Be Caused by FeLV		
A. Placenta and uterus	—	Abortions and resorptions
B. Neural cells	—	Neurologic syndrome
Feline Sarcoma Virus Disease (Feline Sarcoma Virus Derived from Recombination of FeLV and Cat Cellular Genes)		
A. Skin fibroblast	Multicentric fibrosarcoma	—

Used by permission from: Hardy WD, Jr. Feline leukemia virus non-neoplastic diseases. J Am Anim Hosp Assoc 1981;17:941.

monia or enteritis. When necropsy is performed, little or no thymic tissue is found.[22]

Nonregenerative anemia, also known as erythroblastopenia, is a progressive and fatal disease of the erythroid cells. The anemia is normocytic and normochromic. This disease is more common than lymphosarcoma and is probably the most common clinical expression of FeLV. The leukocytes and platelets are not affected and may even be increased in number.[26] These cats may have a packed cell volume as low as 4%. The prognosis is grave even with blood transfusions and chemotherapy.

FeLV *pancytopenia* is also known as aplastic anemia. It is a variation of nonregenerative anemia in which the leukocytes and platelets are also affected. Myelofibrosis may occur prior to death. The prognosis for this disorder is also grave.[26]

FeLV *regenerative anemia* is a form of anemia not as common as the previous two but with just as poor a prognosis. Even though immature erythrocytes are found on the blood smears as a result of extramedullary hematopoiesis in the spleen and liver, these positive signs disappear shortly and most cats soon progress to a nonregenerative anemia and die.[26]

The panleukopenia-like syndrome is known as myeloblastopenia. It is a degenerative disease of the granulocytes that mimics true panleukopenia (feline distemper) hematologically and clinically. These cats often exhibit vomiting, diarrhea, and anorexia. The syndrome may be distinguished from true panleukopenia by a positive blood-ELISA FeLV test (the leukocyte count is usually too low for an accurate IFA test), the presence of anemia, and histopathologic appearance. This syndrome causes erosion of the epithelium of the tips of the intestinal villi, whereas true panleukopenia causes erosion in the crypts of the villi.[26]

Immune complex glomerulonephritis is a fatal kidney disease caused when FeLV antigen-antibody complexes are deposited on the glomerular capillary basement membrane. Complement becomes fixed to the complexes and releases chemotactic factors, which attract granulocytes. Lysosomal enzymes are released by the granulocytes and contribute to the acute inflammatory response. This process probably occurs to some degree in most persistently viremic cats,[26] but some cats have this disease without lymphosarcoma, anemia, or any other FeLV disease.[23]

Some feline *abortions* and *fetal resorptions* are thought to be associated with FeLV because of a significant number of FeLV-positive queens that undergo these events.[27,28] The abortions generally occur in the last 2 weeks of gestation; it is thought that the FeLV damages the placental attachment.

The FeLV *neurologic syndrome* refers to cats with posterior paresis, paralysis, or tetraplegia in which lymphosarcoma cannot be found in the spinal cord or peripheral nerves but which are IFA-positive. These disorders are slowly progressive, leading to eventual paralysis.[26]

It should be reiterated that a positive IFA or ELISA test for the FeLV antigen is not synonymous with the presence of lymphosarcoma or any disease process; nor is it an indication for any type of treatment. Therapy should begin only after sufficient diagnostic procedures have been performed to identify one of the specific FeLV diseases.

Control of FeLV

Test and Removal Program

The first successful method of controlling the spread of the FeLV was the FeLV Immunofluorescent Antibody Test and Removal Program (Table 39–5). This program was based on the IFA test, which was the only test for FeLV available at the time. The Test and Removal Program can now be based on either the IFA or the blood-ELISA test. It should be based on the IFA test if the goal is to eliminate viremic and thus contagious cats. However, if the goal is to increase the chances of eliminating latently infected cats, the blood-ELISA test should be chosen.

Vaccination: Prevaccination Testing of Healthy Cats

Ideally, every cat receiving a FeLV vaccination should be tested previously for the presence of FeLV. Vaccinating an FeLV-infected cat without prior testing could lead to an erroneous conclusion of vaccine failure and possibly subject the veterinarian to negative publicity and/or legal action.

Table 39–5. FeLV Test and Removal Program*

1. Remove all FeLV-infected sick cats from the household.
2. If there are no other cats in the home, wait 10 days before bringing another cat into the household.
3. Immediately test all remaining cats for FeLV.
4. Remove all FeLV-infected healthy cats from the household.
5. Clean all dishes, litter pans, and bedding with detergent.
6. Quarantine all remaining FeLV-uninfected cats in the household.
7. Retest all FeLV uninfected cats 3 months after the first test. The incubation period for FeLV infection can be as long as 3 months.
8. The household can be considered free of FeLV-infected cats only when all cats have tested FeLV-negative in two tests done 3 months apart.
9. Test all new cats for FeLV before they are introduced into the household.

*Use the IFA test if the goal is to eliminate cats that are contagious (viremic). Use the ELISA test if the goal is to maximize the chances of eliminating cats with viral latency.

Adapted from: Hardy WD, Jr. Feline leukemia virus non-neoplastic diseases. J Am Anim Hosp Assoc 1981;17:941.

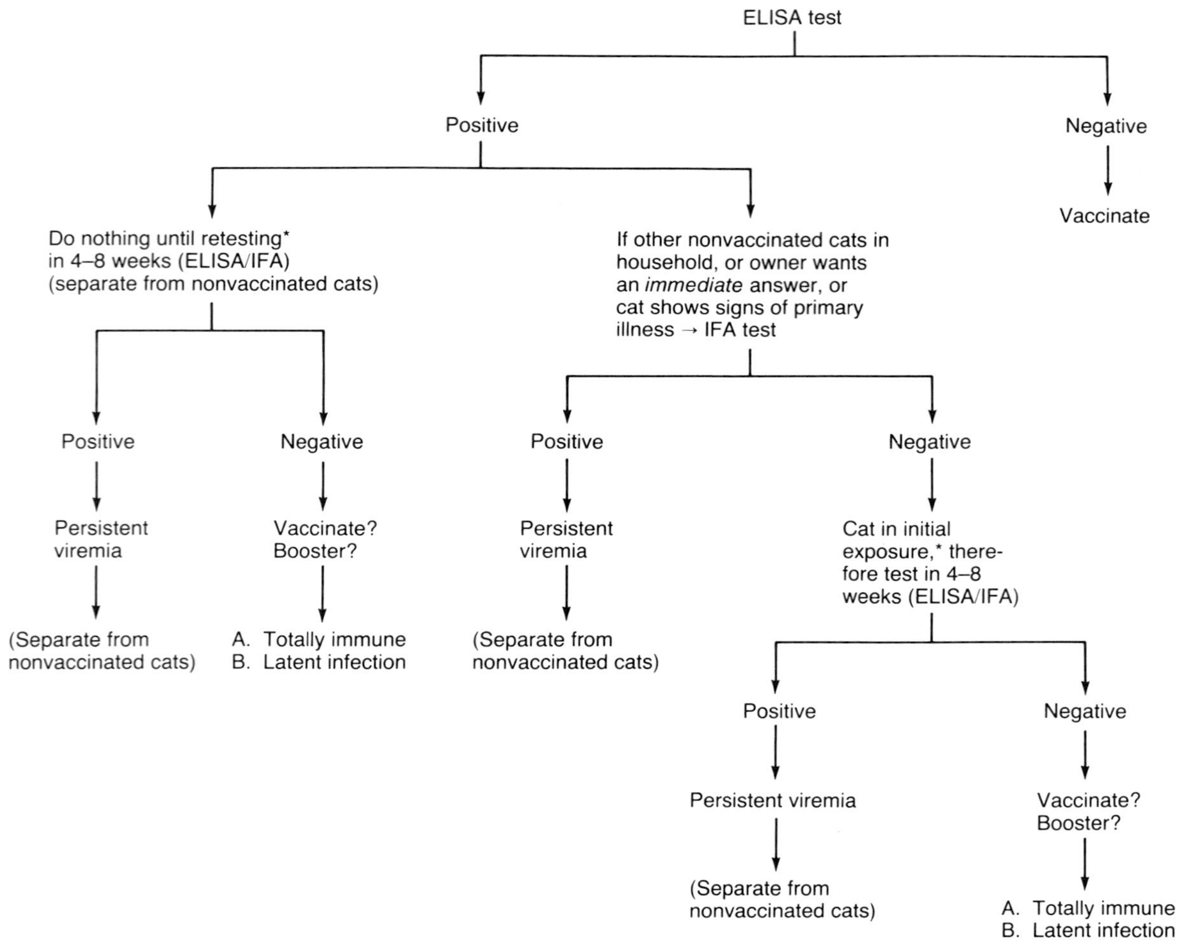

*Do not treat with steroids or other immunosuppressants for 4 weeks. Do not perform euthanasia on this animal.

Figure 39–1. **Flow chart for prevaccination testing of healthy cats.**

However, the economic realities of practice often make this difficult. If the owner is willing to pay for testing, it should be performed. Otherwise, the following groups should be tested prior to vaccination.

1. Cats that the new owner wants tested, regardless of the reason.
2. Cats with known exposure to an FeLV-infected cat, whether the infected cat was healthy or ill.
3. Cats with a history of cat fights or cat fight wounds.
4. Cats with a history of multiple or chronic illnesses, even though they may seem mild or unrelated.
5. Cats with an unknown history, such as cats adopted as strays or from animal shelters.
6. Cats purchased or adopted from multicat environments, such as catteries, animal shelters, multicat households, or "barn cats."

Prevaccination testing should utilize the blood-ELISA test because it will detect the FeLV p27 antigen in the early stages of infection. The other p27 antigen tests may not turn positive for as long as 4 to 8 weeks following initial exposure, whereas the blood-ELISA test may be positive as early as 1 day following exposure.

Figure 39–1 should be utilized to make proper determinations of prevaccination testing of healthy cats based on several possible outcomes. No healthy cat should undergo euthanasia based on one FeLV-positive blood-ELISA test result. It should also be noted that a cat with a latent infection will test FeLV-negative on the blood-ELISA test.

Vaccination: Vaccines

The first FeLV vaccine, Leukocell, was introduced in 1985. It was improved and is currently marketed as Leukocell 2. It contains cell-free multiple subunits of the virus. Since that time several other vaccines have been introduced and some have been removed from the market. The other vaccines currently available include VacSYN/FeLV, which contains inactivated whole virus, Fel-O-Vax, which also contains inactivated whole virus, and GentiVac FeLV, which contains a single subunit, recombinant origin p45 protein consisting of portions of both gp70 and p15E.[15] The efficacy of these vaccines has been a controversial subject, with different studies yielding conflicting results.[29,30] Research is currently ongoing to develop more effective and safer vaccines for the future.

Experimental evidence indicates that the present vaccines do not produce false-positive results on the IFA and ELISA tests for the p27 antigen. However, high FOCMA antibody and serum neutralizing titers result.[21] This should be considered when using Figure 39–1.

It is not recommended that cats with positive IFA tests be vaccinated. Because immunosuppression is likely to occur, no benefit would result. However, there is no evidence that adverse effects are likely to occur.[17,21] There are still a number of unanswered questions concerning the vaccination of cats that have had FeLV-positive ELISA and FOCMA antibody tests. A cat that has gone from blood-ELISA test positive to negative should have developed some degree of immunity. At least one veterinary college suggests that this cat should be vaccine-boostered immediately to further strengthen the immunity and that annual revaccination be given.[17]

Vaccine manufacturers' recommendations should be followed concerning route of administration and frequency of initial injections and boosters. Guidelines are still needed for annual boostering with a different vaccine than the one used by the veterinarian in previous years.

1991 Colloquium on FeLV

On March 1–3, 1991, a colloquium on FeLV and FIV was held in Orlando, Florida. A broad spectrum of issues were discussed relative to these two viruses. The following conclusions and recommendations concerning tests and vaccinations were among those developed by a panel of distinguished veterinary scientists and reported in the *Journal of the American Veterinary Medical Association*.[31]

Concerning Vaccination

1. Only healthy, afebrile cats should be vaccinated; FeLV-infected cats should not be vaccinated.
2. Control of FeLV should involve proper husbandry, in addition to FeLV testing and vaccination. The FeLV-positive cats should not be housed in direct contact with FeLV-negative cats, even when such negative cats have been vaccinated against FeLV.
3. FeLV vaccines attempt to prevent virus infection, or at least persistent viremia if infection does occur. The gp70 virion glycoprotein is the immunogen; immunity against that viral protein prevents infection by virus. Tumor formation can be a consequence of FeLV infection; however, there is no evidence that vaccination, using FOCMA, affords any protection against infection. All FeLV vaccine labels, therefore, should specify "vaccination against feline leukemia virus infection" rather than "vaccination against feline leukemia."
4. The preventive principle of all FeLV vaccines currently available is the same. Although it may be preferable to use the same vaccine for booster vaccinations as originally used (assuming equal efficacy of vaccines), a booster vaccination using a vaccine of a different brand should still stimulate an anamnestic immune response.
5. Testing for FeLV is encouraged prior to primary vaccination for FeLV of all cats whose background or exposure status to FeLV is either at risk or unknown. High-risk situations include shelters, strays, pet cats that roam outdoors daily, multicat households (especially those that take in strays or new cats from nontested catteries), and open catteries. Kittens from a known FeLV-free or low-risk background may not need to be tested for FeLV prior to vaccination.
6. Commercial companies should make only accurate and noninflated claims concerning the efficacy of vaccines. Information concerning the degree of protection or efficacy of the product should include the research data on nonvaccinated controls that are subjected to virus challenge exposure as well as the percentage of vaccinates that remain healthy after virus challenge exposure. The concept of reporting and advertising vaccine efficacy as the preventable fraction is encouraged.
7. Transient viremia develops in many FeLV-vaccinated cats after virus challenge exposure. The aim of FeLV vaccination should be to prevent virus infection entirely (and hence transient viremia), not just persistent viremia.
8. The USDA should proceed with the establishment of a standard requirement for FeLV vaccines without delay, giving consideration to the aforementioned points.
9. There is need for impartial studies on the efficacy of commercial vaccines for companion animals. Almost all evaluations now are either done by the manufacturer or by investigators supported by funding from manufacturers.
10. There is concern about truth in advertising for vaccines and diagnostic tests. There have been recent incidents whereby company claims have exceeded the limit that could be supported by the research from which the claims were derived.
11. Practitioners must evaluate the scientific literature to enable them to choose the best FeLV vaccine and most accurate FeLV and FIV tests. Practitioners should not rely only on information provided by manufacturer's literature or by company salespersons.
12. There is a perception by many within the veterinary profession that more stringent regulations should be established for licensure of veterinary biologics for companion animals . . . The panel recommends the establishment of a blue-ribbon ad hoc committee to review licensure procedures for companion animal biologics to alleviate misconceptions (if they are misconceptions), or to suggest methods for improvement (if any changes should be made).

Concerning Testing

1. The principle of FeLV testing is the detection of p27 core protein or other antigens of the virion. The ELISA test detects p27 antigen in fluids such as serum, plasma, tears, or saliva, whereas the IFA test detects antigens in white blood cells.
2. Vaccination does not interfere with FeLV diagnostic testing. All current FeLV vaccines are either inactivated or subunit; hence, vaccine virus does not replicate within the host after vaccination. The diagnostic tests assay for viral antigens; so, immune response to the vaccine is not detected.
3. Maternal immunity in young kittens does not interfere with FeLV diagnostic tests. Therefore, kittens can be tested as early as deemed necessary by the practitioner.
4. The FeLV ELISA systems are most reliable when serum or plasma is tested, slightly less reliable when blood is tested, and least reliable when saliva and tears are tested.
5. The saliva and tears tests have a disproportionate number of false-positive results. Therefore, if these methods are used, they should be used only as screening tests, and any positive result must be confirmed, using either serum ELISA or IFA testing.
6. After screening by use of any ELISA test, a positive or equivocal result needs to be confirmed by an IFA test. One should always run a confirmatory IFA test on ELISA-positive healthy cats before they are considered persistently viremic.
7. All FeLV-negative exposed cats should be retested at 3-month intervals until all cats within the household or facility test FeLV-negative and the risk of exposure to FeLV infection is past.

Public Health Significance

When the FeLV was discovered in 1964, the only other known leukemia viruses, the avian and the murine viruses, were thought to be spread only vertically.[2] Therefore, there was no concern about any public health consequences for FeLV. However, in 1969 it was reported that natural field isolates of the FeLV could be propagated in human embryonic lung cells.[32] Another study published in 1973 reported that when FeLV was inoculated in newborn puppies, it produced lymphosarcoma, although this did not occur in adult dogs.[33] These findings raised serious concerns among health professionals about risks that humans might be taking when in close proximity to FeLV-infected cats. These concerns led a number of researchers to perform a number of serologic and epidemiologic studies to confirm or deny any cat-to-human transmission.

Several studies of veterinarians, children, and nonveterinarian adults failed to find any epidemiologic link between an increase in human leukemia or lymphoid tumors and exposure to FeLV-infected cats. A large number of veterinarian and nonveterinarian cancer patients were tested for the presence of FeLV antibodies and FeLV antigens. No significant findings occurred.[3] To date, there is no evidence that the FeLV causes or is associated with any disease in humans. However, warnings are still issued against close association with FeLV-infected cats and immunocompromised humans, such as neonates and persons taking immunosuppressive drugs.

REFERENCES

1. August JR. Infectious Diseases. In: Ettinger SJ, ed. Textbook of Veterinary Internal Medicine. 3rd ed. Philadelphia: WB Saunders, 1989:312.
2. Jarrett WFH, Crawford EM, Martin WB, Davie F. A virus-like particle associated with leukemia (lymphosarcoma). Nature 1964;202:567.
3. Hardy WD Jr. The feline leukemia virus. J Am Anim Hosp Assoc 1981;17:951.
4. Hardy WD Jr. Oncogenic Viruses of Cats: The Feline Leukemia and Sarcoma Viruses. In: Holzworth J, ed. Diseases of the Cat. Vol. 1. Philadelphia: WB Saunders, 1987:246.
5. Moennig V. Feline leukemia prophylaxis. J Am Anim Pract 1986;27:344.
6. Lane SB, Kornegay JN. Spinal Lymphosarcoma. In: August JR, ed. Consultations in Feline Internal Medicine. Philadelphia: WB Saunders, 1991:487.
7. Rojko JL. Feline leukemia virus vaccines. Semin Vet Med Surg (Small Animal) 1986;1:61.
8. Verdon D. Largest FIV/FeLV study shows infection greater in neutered animals. DVM Magazine 1991;22(5):36.
9. Hardy WD, Jr. The Virology, Immunology, and Epidemiology of the Feline Leukemia Virus. In: Hardy WD, Jr, Essex M, McClelland AJ, eds. Feline Leukemia Virus. New York: Elsevier/North Holland, 1980:33.
10. Francis DP, Essex M, Gayzagian D. Feline leukemia virus: Survival under home and laboratory conditions. J Clin Microbiol 1979;9:154.
11. Barton CL. The Feline Leukemia Virus: Pathogenesis of Disease. In: Scott FW ed. Contemporary Issues in Small Animal Practice. Vol. 3. New York: Churchill Livingstone, 1986:109.
12. Gerstman BB. The epizootiology of feline leukemia virus infection and its associated diseases. Compend Contin Educ Pract Vet 1985;7:766.
13. Hoover EA, Olsen RG, Mathes LE, Schaller JP. Relationship between feline leukemia virus antigen expression and viral infectivity in blood, bone marrow, and saliva of cats. Cancer Res 1977;37:3707.
14. Kiehl AR, Macy DW. Feline leukemia virus: Testing and prophylaxis. Compend Contin Educ Pract Vet 1985;7:1038.
15. Macy DW. Testing cats for the feline leukemia virus. Vet Med 1991;86:278.
16. Beck ER, Harris CK, Macy DW. Feline leukemia virus: Infection and treatment. Compend Contin Educ Pract Vet 1986;8:567.
17. Cockerell GL. Unifying Concepts of Feline Leukemia Virus Infection. In: Kirk RW, ed. Current Veterinary Therapy IX. Philadelphia: WB Saunders, 1986:1055.
18. Rojko JL, Mathes LE. Feline Acquired Immunodeficiency Syndrome (FAIDS) Induced by the Feline Leukemia Virus. In: Kirk RW, ed. Current Veterinary Therapy IX. Philadelphia: WB Saunders, 1986:436.
19. Olsen RG. Feline Leukemia: The Virus. In: Feline Leukemia: Virus and Vaccine. Lawrenceville: Veterinary Learning Systems, Inc., 1986:7.
20. Jarrett O, Madewell BR, Pacitti A. Latent FeLV infection in the bone marrow of naturally infected cats. Proceedings 4th International FeLV Meeting 1983:74.
21. Kiehl AR, Macy DW. Feline leukemia virus: Testing and prophylaxis. Compend Contin Educ Pract Vet 1985;7:1038.
22. Anderson LJ, Jarrett WFH, Jarrett O, Laird HM. Feline leukemia virus infection of kittens: Mortality associated with atrophy of the thymus and lymphoid depletion. J Natl Cancer Inst 1971; 47:807.
23. Cotter SM, Hardy WD, Jr, Essex M. The association of the feline leukemia virus and lymphosarcoma and other disorders. J Am Vet Med Assoc 1975;166:449.
24. Mackey L. Feline leukemia virus and its clinical effects in cats. Vet Rec 1975;96:5.
25. Mathes LE, Olsen RG, Hebebrand LC. Abrogation of lymphocyte blastogenesis by a feline leukemia virus protein. Nature 1978;274:687.
26. Hardy WD, Jr. Feline leukemia virus non-neoplastic diseases. J Am Anim Hosp Assoc 1981;17:941.
27. Hardy WD, Jr, McClelland AJ. Feline leukemia virus: Its related diseases and control. Vet Clin North Am 1977;7:93.
28. Hardy WD, Jr. Feline Leukemia Virus Diseases. In: Hardy WD, Jr, Essex M, McClelland AJ, eds. Feline Leukemia Virus. New York: Elsevier/North Holland, 1980:3.
29. Pollock RVH, Scarlett JM. Randomized blind trial of a commercial FeLV vaccine. J Am Vet Med Assoc 1990;196:611.
30. Legendre AM, Mitchener KL, Potgieter LND. Efficacy of a feline leukemia virus vaccine in a natural exposure challenge. J Vet Intern Med 1990;4:92.
31. Scott FW, Hancock B, Hardy WD, Jr, et al. Panel Report on the Colloquium on Feline Leukemia Virus/Feline Immunodeficiency Virus: Tests and vaccinations. J Am Vet Med Assoc 1991; 199:1273.
32. Jarrett O, Laird HM, Hay D. Growth of feline leukemia virus in human cells. Nature 1969;224:1208.
33. Rickard CG, Post JE, Noronha F, Barr LM. Interspecies Infection by Feline Leukemia Virus: Serial Cell-Free Transmission in Dogs of Malignant Lymphomas Induced by Feline Leukemia Virus. In: Duthcer RM, Chieco-Bianchi L, eds. Unifying Concepts of Leukemia. Basel: Karger, 1973:102.

CHAPTER 40

◇ ◇ ◇

Feline Urologic Syndrome

Gary D. Norsworthy

Terminology

Scientists who describe medical diseases have been classified as "lumpers" and "splitters." One school of thought, represented by the lumpers, is to collect clinical findings that seem to go together logically into a package and describe them as a "syndrome." This method may, indeed, result in the formation of a group of findings that are etiologically homogeneous, or it may result in the formation of a group that is not justified in being classified as such. The other school of thought, the splitters, is to avoid grouping any set of clinical entities together. This method may create "diseases" that do not exist.

Feline urologic syndrome (FUS) is a term that has gained and lost popularity in the veterinary community in the last few years. It was chosen originally in an attempt to group several related events into an explanatory whole that could be understood by veterinarians and owners alike. Such grouping could be considered the work of lumpers. In reaction to this grouping, the splitters have taken FUS and divided it into a multiplicity of independent "diseases." At present, some veterinarians like the term FUS, whereas others do not.

For the purposes of this discussion, the term FUS is used to describe a disease of currently unknown etiology that affects male and female cats and causes several of the following manifestations:

- Difficulty and/or pain during urination (dysuria)
- Increased frequency of urination (pollakiuria)
- Slow and painful discharge of urine (stranguria)
- Urination in inappropriate places
- Crystalluria (usually struvite)
- Hematuria
- Formation of a mucoid matrix in some male cats resulting in urethral obstruction due to a plug formed (generally) of struvite crystals mixed with the mucoid matrix.

This definition makes this syndrome a "diagnosis of exclusion" and one that is not accepted by all authorities. However, it describes the symptoms of the cat that practitioners frequently see in their offices.

Etiology

The etiology of FUS has eluded serious investigators for over 20 years. Prior to 1970, ingestion of dry cat food containing large amounts of "ash," ingestion of fish-flavored cat foods, neutering at an early age, avitaminosis A, endocrine imbalance, and hyperparathyroidism were considered etiologic factors or at least factors strongly predisposing to FUS.[1] Cat owners with cats with FUS were advised to discontinue feeding them dry and fish-flavored cat foods and encouraged to delay neutering of their male pets until 1 to 2 years of age. It was subsequently shown that the adult penile urethral diameter was not influenced by prepubertal castration.[2]

In 1969, investigators Rich and Fabricant at Cornell University produced urethral obstruction in male cats by injecting them with filtered urine from the bladders of previously obstructed cats.[3] In subsequent studies, these investigators isolated a picornavirus (calicivirus) from the bladder of a naturally obstructed cat and produced obstruction in another cat by inoculating this virus into the susceptible cat's bladder. Further studies concluded that this calicivirus was not the primary etiologic agent but rather acted as a catalyst to activate a latent virus, then considered to be the feline syncytium-forming virus.[4,5] Finally, after further investigations, they concluded that FUS was caused by a cell-associated herpesvirus (CAHV) that acted in association with the calicivirus. On the basis of antigenic and genomic analyses, the CAHV has been reclassified as a member of the bovine herpesvirus 4 (BHV-4) group and is now called the BHV-4 (strain FCAHV).[6]

At that time it appeared that the etiology of FUS was settled. However, other investigators were unable to replicate these studies. They could not produce urethral obstruction by injecting filtered urine from obstructed cats into nonobstructed cats, nor could they isolate the viruses found by Rich and Fabricant. Therefore the debate continued into the 1970s and 1980s.

During the 1970s and 1980s most etiologic investigation of FUS was in two directions—other infectious agents and dietary factors. The results of several studies have shown that bacteria, mycoplasmas, ureaplasmas (urease-producing mycoplasmas), and fungal agents are rarely found in the urine of FUS cats. In one study at the University of Minnesota, only 4 of 143 patients (2.8%) had bacteria in their urine.[7-10]

Concurrent dietary studies looked for minerals and other factors that might cause FUS. Various calculogenic diets were formulated, some of which would produce urethral obstructions, but these diets had few similarities to commercial diets commonly fed household cats. After many research projects, it was concluded that a dietary excess of magnesium would supply the mineral most needed in urine to form struvite (magnesium ammonium phosphate), the crystal type present in the bladders of 80% of FUS cats.[11] However, it was found that for this mineral to be calculogenic, the urine pH must be correct. Struvite is more soluble in acidic than in alkaline urine, and struvite crystals usually do not form as long as the urine pH is below 6.5.[12] Therefore, the two factors that are important in the development of struvite crystals are the dietary (and therefore, urinary) level of magnesium and an alkaline urinary pH.

However, investigators recognize that just the presence of an alkaline urinary pH and a diet high in magnesium does not produce urethral obstruction in a large percentage of cats. If that were the case, the incidence of urinary obstruction would far exceed its present level. Therefore, the current focus of etiologic investigation has returned to the concept of an infectious, contagious agent that produces clinical signs in the presence of elevated urine magnesium and alkaline urine. Once again, the calicivirus and the BHV-4 (strain FCAHV) have engendered renewed interest. Part of this interest is because herpesvirus infections in all species have several general characteristics that seem applicable to cats with FUS.[11]

1. They are usually transmitted by direct contact within the affected species.
2. Not all individuals that are in contact with an infected individual will be infected with the virus.
3. The clinical signs of the initial disease episode are generally severe, with subsequent episodes less severe.
4. Once infected, the host remains infected for long periods of time, even for life.
5. Stress or concurrent disease can exacerbate the clinical signs of the infection.

Another reason for an investigational return to the feline calicivirus and the BHV-4 (strain FCAHV) as causative in FUS is a recognition that previous failures have probably been attributable to technical errors or inadequacies. Osborne has stated: "However, negative findings may be related to the cell-associated nature of some viruses, the virucidal characteristics of feline urine, inappropriate handling of samples, and/or improper selection of cases. Support for the latter statement is derived from the fact that cell-associated herpesvirus has been consistently isolated from the urinary bladders of experimentally infected cats by explantation-cocultivation techniques, even though viruses could not be isolated from their urine. To date, very few cases of naturally occurring lower urinary tract disease have been evaluated by explantation-cocultivation methods."[10] Since writing that statement, Osborne has been a coauthor of several articles concerning various aspects of the CAHV in relation to FUS.[6,13,14] Only time and further investigation will result in our finally understanding the etiology of FUS.

Clinical Signs

Nonobstructed Form

There are two distinct clinical syndromes of FUS, which are distinguished by the presence or absence of urethral obstruction. However, the obstructed form begins with the clinical signs typical of the nonobstructed form, even though this phase may not be observed or properly interpreted by most owners. Instead, most cats with urethral obstruction are brought for examination by owners who think that the obstruction occurred as the first pathologic event.

The clinical signs of the nonobstructed form are caused by inflammation of the urinary bladder and urethra. Once the etiology of this disease is understood, we will be able to explain the nature of this inflammatory process. However, we do know that crystals form in the bladder and mix with an organic matrix that has the consistency of toothpaste (Fig. 40–1).

In 80% of cats with FUS, the crystals that form in the bladder are composed of struvite (magnesium ammonium phosphate). Technically, they are not uroliths. A urolith is an organized, macroscopic concretion composed primarily of organic or inorganic crystals with a small quantity of an organic matrix. The urethral plugs that cause the typical feline urethral obstruction are made up primarily of organic matrix with a relatively small amount of crystalline material. Struvite crystals lack the size and organization of uroliths. Therefore, urolithiasis is not a term that is synonymous with FUS, even though it has been used in that manner.[11,15]

Once the inflammatory process begins, the cystitis and urethritis it causes result in one or more of the following: (1) difficulty and/or pain when urinating (dysuria), (2) increased frequency of urination (pollakiuria), (3) slow and painful discharge of urine (stranguria), and (4) urinating in inappropriate places.

The client frequently tells the veterinarian that the cat is making repeated trips to the litter box as if constipated. The cat may sit in the litter box for long periods of time and only pass a few drops of urine, which in the owner's mind appears to be a problem of constipation. The owner

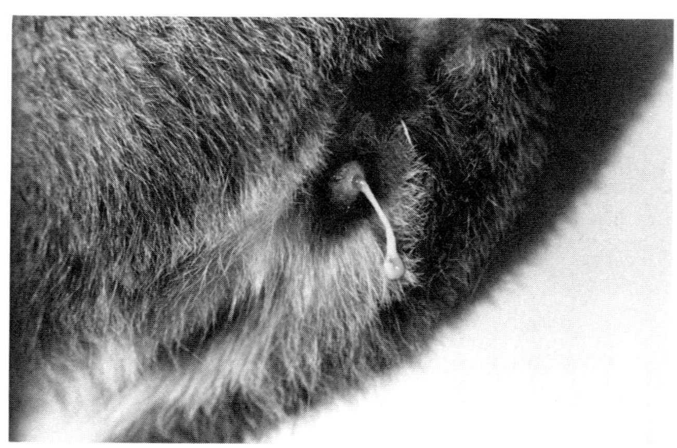

Figure 40–1. **The typical urethral plug contains a large organic matrix and a small amount of crystalline material. It often has the consistency of toothpaste.**

also often states that the cat is urinating on hard surfaces such as a countertop, a tile or hardwood floor, or in a bathtub or sink. When this happens, the owner may be able to detect the presence of hematuria, which generally cannot be seen when the cat is using a litter box. Otherwise, the cat appears to be normal; activity and appetite are not affected and the cat does not have a fever.

Obstructed Form

The nonobstructed form of FUS occurs in both male and female cats. Because of anatomic differences, primarily urethral diameter, the male cat may experience a potentially fatal obstructed form of FUS. When the quantity of struvite and matrix becomes great enough to form a urethral plug, obstruction occurs. Typically, the point of obstruction is in or near the penile urethra as a result of the tapered configuration of the distal urethra. Obstruction of the urethra results in additional clinical signs. This cat also makes repeated trips to the litter box, but now there is no passage of urine. The cat becomes more determined and the condition becomes more painful, resulting in the animal's vocalization while in the litter box. The owner may still interpret this as constipation and often calls the veterinarian asking for a laxative suitable for cats. Veterinarians and their assistants should recognize the significance of this request and ask to see the cat immediately. With the passage of time, attempts at urination become progressively more painful for the cat. If the owner is skeptical about the veterinarian's interpretation of the cat's "constipation," have the owner palpate the animal's abdomen. Most obstructed cats resist abdominal pressure and cry out in pain.

After the urethral obstruction has been present for 1 to 3 days, dehydration, electrolyte imbalances (hyperphosphatemia and hyperkalemia), and metabolic acidosis occur. Vomiting also is seen as these metabolic disturbances develop. Death follows in 3 to 6 days, generally owing to toxemia, not bladder rupture.[10]

Diagnosis

Nonobstructed Form

The diagnosis of the nonobstructed form of FUS is generally based on clinical signs and the results of a urinalysis. The typical urinalysis reveals hematuria, a pH of 7.0 or greater, and crystalluria. However, some cats exhibiting marked dysuria and inappropriate urination have normal urinalysis results. The veterinarian should be alert to the owner's description of the clinical signs and not be misled by a normal urinalysis. If the urinalysis is normal, other lower urinary tract diseases should also be considered. If a diagnosis of FUS is made based solely on clinical signs of dysuria, hematuria, and inappropriate urination and these signs do not resolve within 1 week of treatment, a urine culture and negative, positive, and double-contrast cystograms should be performed. If these are normal and the cat is male, a urethrogram should follow (see Chapter 14).

Because of the constant attempts of the cat to urinate, little urine collects in the bladder. Therefore when the cat with FUS is brought in for examination, he or she will generally have an empty bladder and urine collection is not possible. When this occurs, the cat should be confined to a cage without a litter box for several hours so that urine will accumulate. If several hours of confinement are not possible, the cat may be given intravenous (IV) or subcutaneous (SC) fluids (but not containing glucose). To hasten urine production even more, 12 mg of furosemide (Lasix) may be administered intravenously, intramuscularly, or subcutaneously. If furosemide is given urine will be produced within minutes. Urine produced as a result of furosemide administration has an artificially low specific gravity and a dilutional decrease in crystal, protein, and red blood cell concentrations. The urinalysis findings should be interpreted in light of these changes.

If an owner brings in a cat with a suspected history of hematuria and inappropriate urination but the cat has a full bladder that is easily expressed, the clinician should be suspicious of the owner's observations. It is unusual for a nonobstructed FUS cat to have a full bladder. The owner should be asked if other cats are in the household and if one of them might be responsible for the bloody urine found in inappropriate locations.

Some dysuric, pollakiuric cats have normal urinalysis findings. Even some cats reported by their owners to have hematuria may have a normal urinalysis. If the urine is collected by bladder compression, the bladder may begin to hemorrhage within a few minutes, and the cat may pass frank blood from the urethra before or soon after leaving the hospital, which can be difficult to explain for the veterinarian and quite alarming to the client. The client should be assured that this bleeding would not have happened if the bladder wall had been normal; rather, it is caused by the cystitis, even in the presence of a normal urinalysis. However, also be aware that excessive compression of the bladder can be injurious. It is preferable to collect urine by cystocentesis when possible.

Obstructed Form

The diagnosis of the obstructed form of FUS is based on bladder palpation. By the time most of these cats are seen, the bladder is two to fives times its normal full size, and abdominal palpation causes significant pain for the cat. If the bladder is digitally compressed, urination will not occur. However, this test is not recommended because of friability of the bladder after 1 to 2 days of urine retention.

A patient that is an exception to the digital compression test is the intact tomcat. Many of these cats have enough detrussor muscle tone that they appear obstructed. However, when an anesthetic is administered, catherization does not meet any resistance, and it is obvious that the animal was not experiencing urethral obstruction. The difference between this cat and the obstructed cat is the lack of pain on compression of the bladder and the lack of marked bladder distention.

Treatment

Nonobstructed Form

A number of drugs have been used to treat nonobstructed FUS cats. Although they are quite popular and extensively used, many have been shown to be ineffective. Chlor-Ethamine and vitamin C were once widely used as "effective urinary acidifiers," only to be proved otherwise.[16,17] Various antispasmodics have been used, such as Jenotone, some of which were later removed from the market.

It is now recognized that FUS without obstruction is a self-limiting disorder. The clinical signs frequently subside within 1 week in nonobstructed male or female cats.[9,15,18] Therefore, many forms of therapy that have not been harmful have been interpreted as being effective.

Antibiotics have been used routinely, even though less than 3% of FUS cases have associated bacteriuria. The rationale has generally been that they might be helpful, and they are unlikely to do harm. Urinary tract antiseptics have been used widely in humans and frequently in dogs. Methylene blue–containing compounds were once used extensively in cats for FUS. However, their use has diminished greatly since it was shown that they may cause methemoglobinemia and severe anemia[19] (see Chapter 42). Methenamine in an acidic environment hydrolyzes to form formaldehyde, a powerful antimicrobial. It is marketed as methenamine mandelate and methenamine hippurate. If FUS does, indeed, have a viral etiology, this drug might prove efficacious unless the virus(es) are cell-associated and not found in the urine. However, dosage, efficacy, and toxicity studies with this agent have not been performed on cats.[10]

Urge incontinence is an involuntary loss of urine due to the development of an uncontrollable desire to urinate. It is a frequent component of FUS that is often manifested as inappropriate urination. The cat may suddenly squat and urinate, often appearing surprised at doing so. Logically this condition should be treated with smooth muscle antispasmodics. The commonly used products currently on the market contain atropine, hyoscyamine, or scopolamine. Although they are in widespread use, controlled studies have not been done to demonstrate their efficacy in cats.[10]

Three drugs should be considered for the treatment of urge incontinence. Propantheline (Pro-Banthine) works on the detrussor muscle to minimize the force and frequency of contractions. It is supplied as 7.5- and 15-mg tablets and is dosed at 7.5 mg every 72 hours, that is, every third day. Phenoxybenzamine (Dibenzyline) relaxes urethral striated muscle. It is supplied as 10-mg capsules and dosed at 2.5 mg s.i.d. to t.i.d. Diazepam (Valium) also relaxes urethral striated muscle. It is supplied as 2-, 5-, and 10-mg tablets and dosed at 1 mg t.i.d.[11]

Megestrol acetate (Ovaban) has been found to be effective in relieving dysuria in cats.[20] The author has used this successfully to relieve otherwise intractable dysuria. Its mode of action is probably related to its powerful anti-inflammatory effects. (See Chapter 7 for a discussion on the use and misuse of megestrol.)

Acidification of the urine is needed to dissolve struvite crystals. This may be accomplished by the administration of ammonium chloride (Uroeze) at a dose of 0.8 to 1.0 g/cat/day or 300 mg/kg/day or DL-methionine (Methio-Form) at a dose of 1.0 to 1.5 g/cat/day. However, urine alkalization occurs following a meal; therefore, in order for the acidifier to be effective, it must be given with each meal. Since this is difficult for most cat owners, it is preferable to feed a food that contains an acidifier. A number of foods on the market are formulated for this purpose, including Prescription Diet Feline c/d (Hill's Pet Products, Topeka, KS) and Science Diet Feline Maintenance (Hill's Pet Products, Topeka, KS).

Although struvite crystals have been found in up to 96% of cats with FUS, other types have also been recovered. Calcium oxalate crystals were found in about 2% of cats in one study.[21] Although the incidence of calcium oxalate crystals is small, their presence is significant because they form in acidic, not alkaline, urine.[10] If dietary or pharmacologic acidification occurs in these cats, crystalluria increases rather than decreases. Therefore, the crystal type should be determined.

Cystotomy to lavage and debride the urinary bladder has been recommended for cats with chronic, recurring, nonobstructive FUS. This seems somewhat logical if the bladder can be shown to be very thickened radiographically. However, reports from veterinarians who do this procedure are not consistent; they usually conclude that this technique has little benefit.[10]

Obstructed Form

The self-limiting nature of nonobstructed FUS has confused our understanding of why some cats develop urethral obstructions. A theory that best explains the urethral obstruction phenomenon has been proposed by Osborne.[21] It states that a combination of crystals and a mucoid matrix are essential for the production of a urethral plug. Each of these elements is theorized to be caused by a different virus. If only one virus is present, the cat will experience cystitis, as evidenced by hematuria and dysuria. If both are present, a urethral plug will form, resulting in urethral obstruction. Further research is needed to confirm the validity of this theory.

Regardless of the pathophysiology involved, once the urethra becomes obstructed, certain clinical and biochemical abnormalities develop. These intensify with the passage of time and are as follows:[10]

- Dehydration
- Hyperphosphatemia
- Hyperkalemia
- Metabolic acidosis
- Postrenal azotemia
- Death in 3 to 6 days

Despite the catastrophic results of urethral obstruction, the biochemical abnormalities generally can be reversed with rapidly administered appropriate therapy.

Therapy must begin with removal of urine from the bladder and re-establishment of renal function. This process begins with relief of the urethral obstruction. However, if this cannot be accomplished, two temporary alternatives, cystocentesis and bladder marsupialization, exist and are discussed in the section entitled When Urethral Obstruction Cannot Be Relieved.

Restraint

Some form of physical or chemical restraint is necessary to catheterize a cat with a urethral obstruction. The general rule is to use as little restraint or sedation as needed for the situation. Cats that are critically ill may be catheterized using physical restraint alone; tranquilizers or anesthetics pose greater risk to these patients. Wrapping the cat in a bath towel or placing him in a "cat bag" may be adequate; however, the urethra is often friable and easily damaged by a catheterization attempt on a struggling patient. Therefore, good judgment is essential in selecting the appropriate form of restraint.

Short-acting barbiturates (thiamylal sodium or Bio-Tal) are metabolized by the liver and are therefore suitable agents for restraint. Inhalant anesthetic gases such as halothane (Fluothane) and isoflurane (AErrane) are also good choices for restraint. Ketamine was originally thought to be excreted renally; however, subsequent studies have shown its route of excretion is hepatic.[22] Therefore, ketamine is also an appropriate choice, especially if combined with diazepam and given intravenously (see Chapter 8).

Techniques

A number of techniques have been devised for dislodging urethral plugs. The goal should be to relieve the obstruction without causing further damage to the urethra. The following techniques have both advantages and disadvantages.

Gentle massage of the penis between the thumb and forefinger may be adequate to dislodge a plug in the penile urethra. It should be tried initially with the penis retracted into the prepuce; if unsuccessful, it should be attempted with the penis extended. Although the success rate of this technique is low, it is simple and worth the effort.[10]

Gentle compression of the bladder after penile massage may exert enough pressure to dislodge fragments of urethral plugs. However, if it is not immediately successful, this procedure should be abandoned so as to prevent bladder rupture or retrograding of urine and possibly crystals or microbes into the upper urinary tract.[10]

Performing cystocentesis prior to dislodging the urethral plug may have two advantages. If the urinary bladder is overly distended, cystocentesis relieves some of the pressure on the urethral plug and allows it to be dislodged and expelled more easily. Also, the composition of the urine may be assessed visually. If the urine contains large quantities of visible precipitates, extra time should be spent flushing the bladder and the owner should be warned of an increased likelihood of reobstruction. It should be noted that this procedure carries a small risk of urine leaking into the peritoneal cavity. However, this is generally not clinically significant. If cystocentesis is performed, the bladder should not be totally emptied because of the trauma the needle is likely to cause to the bladder mucosa as the sides of the bladder wall collapse upon one other.[10]

Back flushing of the urethra with sterile saline solution is the method of choice in relieving urethral obstructions. It is important to be gentle when manipulating the catheter and the urethra and to use a catheter that has minimal chance of damaging the urethra.

Various catheters have been used. Since most plugs are in the penile urethra, a 20- to 22-gauge, stiff, open-ended catheter is needed for initial plug breakdown and repulsion. Lacrimal cannulas, blunted stainless steel (nondisposable) hypodermic needles, and commercially marketed urethral catheters (Minnesota Feline Olive Tipped Urethral Catheter, EJAY International, Inc., Glendora, CA) have been used with success (Fig. 40–2). A metal catheter should be inserted no more than 1 cm into the urethra. At that point, a softer, open-ended catheter (Tom Cat Catheter, Sherwood Medical, St. Louis, MO) should be used for further advancement into the urethra.

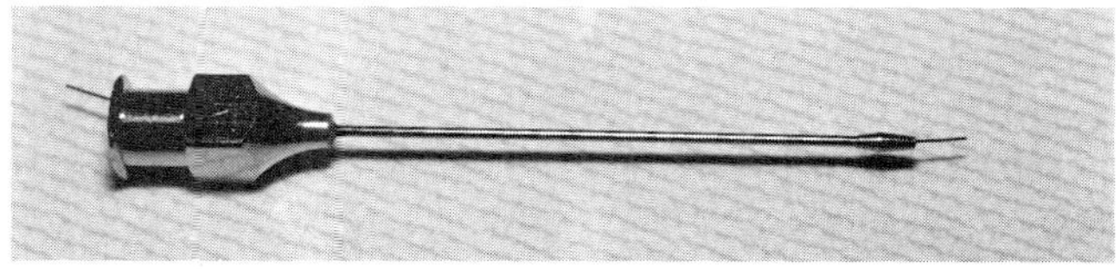

Figure 40–2. **The Minnesota Feline Olive Tipped Urethral Catheter has an olive-shaped tip and a stylet. It can be used in the distal urethra with minimal chance of urethral damage.**

The cat should be restrained physically or chemically and placed in the lateral recumbent position. The operator should face the ventrum of the cat, and a technician should hold the cat so it cannot be pushed away from the operator. The cat's head should be to the left of the right-handed operator; the cat's left rear leg should be raised at a 45-degree angle by the technician (Fig. 40–3). The cat's penis should be extended from the prepuce to straighten the normal curvature of the distal urethra. It should be displaced dorsally so that the long axis of the urethra is parallel to the vertebral column.

The stiff catheter should be advanced no more than 1 cm into the penile urethra. The urethra should not be compressed around the catheter, so that when the obstructing material is dislodged, it will wash out the distal urethra and not back into the bladder. Alternate flushing against the obstructing material with manual compression of the bladder should be performed until the obstruction is relieved. In this manner, the obstructing material is expelled from the urethra and not repelled into the bladder.

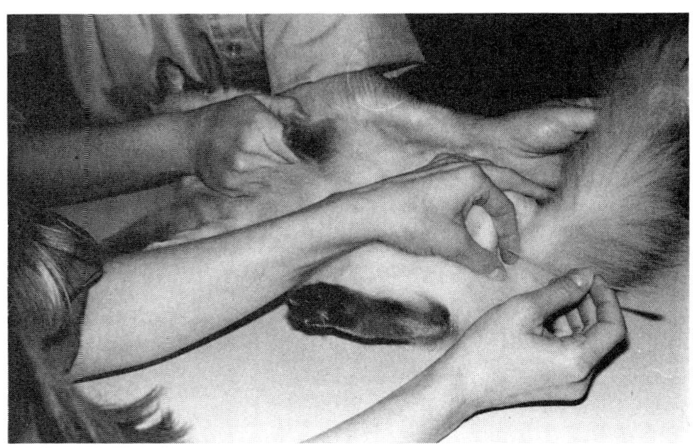

Figure 40–3. **Catheterization should begin with physical or chemical restraint, and the cat in the lateral recumbent position. The operator should face the ventrum of the cat, and a technician should prevent the cat from being pushed away from the operator by holding the animal with his or her left hand.**

If repeated attempts to dislodge the obstruction fail, sterile saline solution from a 12-mL syringe should be forced through the catheter until the plug is pushed back into the bladder. A flexible catheter should be substituted for the rigid one for further advancing and flushing.

Urine should be gently aspirated from the bladder through the catheter. When most urine has been evacuated, the bladder should be flushed with about 100 mL of sterile saline solution in an attempt to remove as much crystalline material as possible. Filling the bladder with saline solution and then shaking the cat to suspend the crystalline material in the fluid will aid in removing the crystalline material from the bladder.[10] If the urine is extremely hemorrhagic, a cold saline flush may help to constrict mucosal vessels and reduce the hemorrhage.

The decision to place an indwelling catheter is controversial. Some authorities discourage it because of the potential for further damage to the urinary tract.[23] The need for an indwelling catheter is lessened if aggressive flushing is used to remove crystalline material from the bladder. However, indwelling catheters have some distinct advantages. They can be attached to an IV set and empty IV fluid bag (or bottle) to allow monitoring of the urine output (Fig. 40–4). They can promote recovery of the detrussor muscle tone by keeping the bladder empty even when large volumes of fluids are administered intravenously or subcutaneously. In addition, they can prevent reobstruction of the urethra.[10] It is the author's practice to place an indwelling catheter for about 24 hours. The cat should wear an Elizabethan collar to prevent premature catheter removal.

When using an indwelling catheter, several steps should be taken to minimize complications. The catheter should be composed of a soft, pliable material that will not further irritate the urethra and be short enough so as not to irritate the bladder wall with the distal end. If the cat is not experiencing bladder atony, the catheter should not extend into the bladder; this lessens the chance of ascending urinary tract infections. Connection of the catheter to a closed drainage system and the administration of a broad-spectrum antibiotic, such as amoxicillin, will also help to minimize ascending urinary tract infections. Catheters should be removed as soon as possible, preferably in no more than 36 hours.[10]

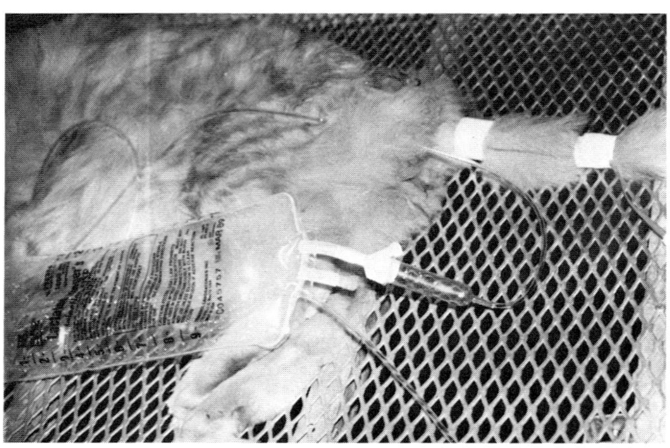

Figure 40–4. **A No. 3.5 French catheter is placed in the bladder of this cat. It is long enough to be secured to the cat's tail so as to prevent it from being dislodged from the bladder. The catheter is attached to an intravenous set and a fluid bag so that urine production can be monitored. This closed system decreases the chances of bacterial infections ascending into the bladder.**

Table 40–1. Proper Administration of Sodium Bicarbonate ($NaHCO_3$)[36]

1. Only administer if the blood pH is below 7.1 or the total CO_2 is less than 10.
2. Use the following formula and give half the calculated amount in the first 6 hours, then the other half in the next 6 hours *if needed.*
3. Amount of $NaHCO_3$ (mEq) $= 0.3 \times$ body weight in kg $\times$ (24 $-$ total CO_2).

The medical treatment of the cat with a urethral obstruction should be tailored to the cat's condition. If an indwelling catheter is used, a broad-spectrum antibiotic, such as amoxicillin, should be given. Dehydration, metabolic acidosis, hyperphosphatemia, and azotemia are corrected in most cats with the IV or SC administration of lactated Ringer's solution; the quantity and route of administration are determined by the severity of the condition. If severe metabolic acidosis is present, judicious use of sodium bicarbonate can be beneficial (Table 40–1). If the cat is hyperkalemic, he will experience generalized muscle weakness, bradycardia, and peripheral vascular collapse. The judicious use of the following drugs is indicated if the electrocardiographic findings indicate severe cardiac effects[24] (Table 40–1 and Fig. 34–2).

Calcium gluconate (10%): 0.5 to 1.0 mL/kg IV over 10 to 15 minutes with cardiac monitoring

Sodium bicarbonate: 0.5 to 1.0 mEq/kg

Glucose: 0.5 g/kg

Regular insulin: 0.25 U/kg

Antispasmodic drugs, such as phenoxybenzamine or diazepam, are indicated because of their effects on the striated muscle of the urethra. Megestrol acetate should not be used in a catheterized cat; because of its steroidlike effect on the immune system, it would be a poor choice in the presence of an infection. Any cat with an indwelling catheter is susceptible to ascending bacterial cystitis.

It is best to use propantheline initially because it affects the detrussor muscle. The potential for bladder atony is always present in an obstructed cat but may not be evident immediately, and this drug is effective for up to 3 days after one dose (7.5 mg p.o.).

IV or SC fluids are indicated for several reasons. Many of these cats are dehydrated on presentation and need to be rehydrated. Following catheterization, many cats experience postobstructive diuresis that causes or further contributes to dehydration. They may also experience metabolic acidosis, which can generally be corrected by administration of lactated Ringer's solution. Sodium bicarbonate may be needed if the acidosis is severe. The kidneys are in varying degrees of dysfunction and are supported with fluids. Creating a large volume of urine also serves to continue the flushing of crystalline material from the bladder.

If bladder atony develops, it generally corrects itself in a few days if the bladder does not redistend with urine. Preventing redistension may be accomplished with an indwelling catheter; however, the longer the catheter remains in place, the greater the chance of the development of ascending bacterial cystitis.[25] An alternative to the indwelling catheter is manual expression of the bladder three to four times per day. This frequency might have to be increased if large volumes of IV or SC fluids are being given. If atony does not resolve in 2 to 3 days, bethanechol (Urecholine) should be considered. It is supplied in 5-, 10-, 25-, and 50-mg tablets and dosed at 1.25 to 2.5 mg b.i.d. to t.i.d.[26] This parasympathomimetic agent causes contraction of all smooth muscle. If given on an empty stomach, it may cause vomiting. Some cats have abdominal pain and gastrointestinal cramping; therefore, this drug should be used judiciously.

Many of these cats are anorectic for several days, which can greatly complicate recovery. If anorexia occurs, the cat should be force fed, as discussed in Chapter 5, beginning on the day following anesthesia and catheterization.

Because of the possibility of reobstruction, it is not wise to send a cat home too early. Reobstruction is especially likely to occur in the 24 hours following removal of an indwelling catheter.

Prescription Diet Feline s/d (Hill's Pet Products, Topeka, KS) should be fed for about 30 days following an obstruction in order to dissolve any remaining crystalline material in the bladder and urethra and to prevent formation of more. After 30 days, the cat should be fed a food that will maintain an acidic urine, such as Prescription Diet Feline c/d (Hill's Pet Products, Topeka, KS). Although an acidified diet is preferable, it is essential that the cat be on a diet that is consumed in sufficient quantity to provide proper nutritional balance. Unfortunately, some cats are very reluctant to change diets or will not eat Prescription Diet Feline s/d or acidified diets. If that occurs, acidifiers in tablet or powder form should be used.

The relationship of dry cat foods to FUS has been debated for many years. Studies done on the effects of dry cat foods on water intake have produced somewhat conflicting results. Three studies have demonstrated a decrease in total water intake by cats fed dry diets.[27-29] Two other studies demonstrated no difference in the influence of dry and canned foods on water intake.[30,31] Still other studies have shown that the method of processing dry foods, i.e., expanded versus nonexpanded, can have an influence on urine output.[27] In light of the lack of unequivocal evidence, it seems prudent to recommend an acidified diet such as Prescription Diet Feline c/d in either the dry or canned form. If the cat is eating the dry form and FUS continues to occur, the canned form should be tried.

When Urethral Obstruction Cannot Be Relieved

Occasionally, it is not possible to relieve a urethral obstruction because an extremely large urethral plug is causing severe urethral spasm, because the urethra has suffered extensive scarring as a result of repeated previous catheterizations, or because of excessive amounts of crystalline material in the urinary bladder (Fig. 40–5). If the obstruction cannot be relieved, it is still essential that urine be removed from the bladder.

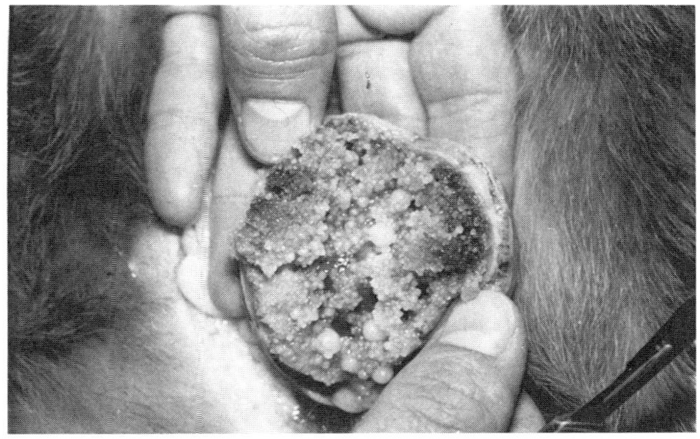

Figure 40–5. **Urethral catheterization was not possible because of the copious amount of mucoid and crystalline material in this cat's bladder.**

Cystocentesis should be performed to reduce pressure on the urethral plug from the urine in the bladder. Care should be taken to cause minimal damage to the bladder wall. A 22-gauge needle and a three-way valve should be attached to a 60-mL syringe so that, ideally, only one puncture is made through the bladder wall. As much urine as possible should be removed without jeopardizing the integrity of the bladder wall with the needle point. One to two mg of diazepam should be administered intramuscularly (not orally) to reduce urethral spasm, but no SC or IV fluids should be given. The cat should be confined to a cage for 1 to 3 hours and then the diazepam repeated intravenously. Catheterization should again be attempted. If catheterization is not successful, the process should be repeated.

If cystocentesis is not successful, bladder marsupialization can be performed (see Chapter 55). As an alternative to bladder marsupialization, a perineal urethrostomy can be performed (see Chapter 55). However, this leaves the cat with a compromised lower urinary tract. This surgery also has the disadvantage of requiring a longer surgical time than bladder marsupialization. It requires neutering an intact tomcat, and if this is a breeding tom, the owner will probably not be enthusiastic about neutering. However, both procedures, bladder marsupialization and perineal urethrostomy, require major surgery on a high-risk surgical candidate and should be considered procedures of last resort.

Vesicourachal Diverticula

The urachus is a fetal structure that allows passage of urine from the fetal bladder to the placenta. At the time of birth, the urachus is nonfunctional and undergoes atrophy. It has been assumed that the presence of a partially patent urachus is the result of a congenital abnormality. However, recent

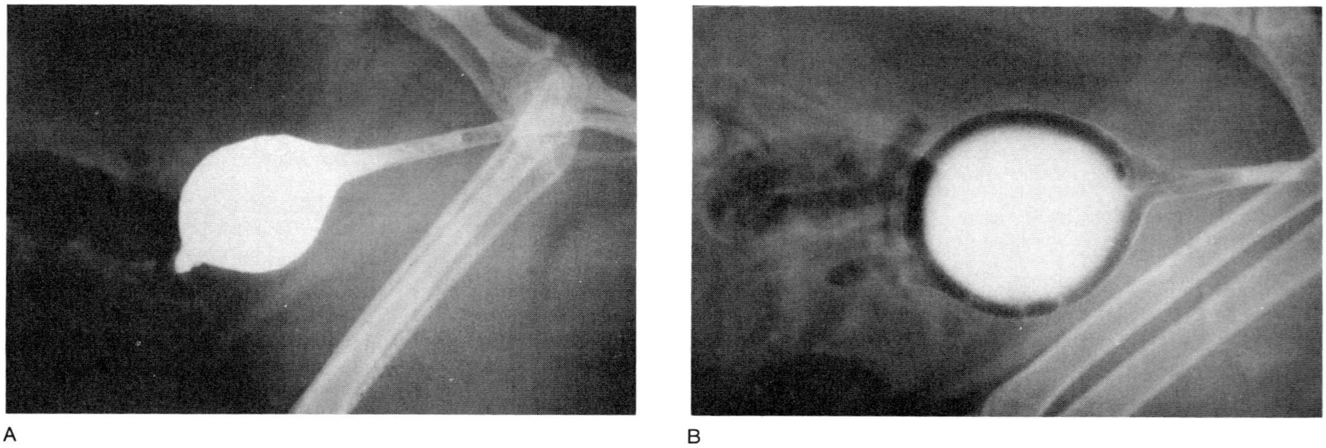

Figure 40–6. (*A*) A positive contrast cystogram clearly delineates the vesicourachal diverticulum at the cranial end of this bladder. (*B*) A double-contrast cystogram also delineates the vesicourachal diverticulum in this bladder, but not as clearly as the positive contrast study.

studies have changed our understanding of the patent urachus.

In the normal cat, there is microscopic evidence of urachal remnants at the vertex of the urinary bladder.[32,33] These are called microscopic diverticula. In contrast, macroscopic diverticula are remnants of the urachus that are large enough to be detected radiographically (Fig. 40–6 *A, B*). In one study these were found in almost one of four adult cats with hematuria, dysuria, and/or urethral obstruction; they were present in males twice as frequently as in females.[32]

Two distinct forms of macroscopic diverticula exist. A presumably congenital form develops prior to or soon after birth and persists for an indefinite period of time. The congenital form is not common; the acquired form is much more common. The acquired form develops from microscopic diverticula caused by increased bladder lumen pressure, generally due to FUS with or without urethral obstruction. These diverticula can be demonstrated radiographically but spontaneously resolve with time. One group observed spontaneous resolution in 15 of 15 adult male cats by serial radiography. It is thought that most diverticula resolve in 2 to 3 weeks following resolution of the cause of increased bladder pressure.[10]

These findings challenge our traditional concept that urachal diverticula must be removed surgically. It now seems prudent not to remove a urachal diverticulum surgically unless it can be shown by serial radiographs to persist for at least 1 month.

Prevention and Home Monitoring

The single most effective form of prevention of FUS is urinary acidification. This is best accomplished by an acidified diet. Minimizing stressful situations is also important, since this disease has a tendency to exacerbate following stress. This plan of prevention includes a good level of nutrition, preventing the onset of other diseases with vaccinations and a controlled environment, and alleviating social overcrowding.

Home monitoring of urine pH and for the presence of blood may be performed with urine dipsticks after urine has been collected from the litter box. This may be accomplished by replacing the normal litter with Non-Absorbable Cat Litter (Veterinary Concepts, Inc., Spring Valley, WI), aquarium gravel, or the perforated strips from computer paper, or by using the Uro-Collect Feline Kit (Jorgensen Laboratories, Loveland, CO). These do not absorb urine; therefore the test strip can be dipped into the urine while it is still in the litter pan. Other alternatives include material that is added to normal litter and reacts to the presence of an alkaline pH or blood (CatScan pH and CatScan B, Health-Check, Buford, GA) and pH-indicating cat litter.

Other Lower Urinary Tract Diseases

Until rather recently, many have believed that the only disease of the lower urinary tract of cats is idiopathic FUS. Based on work by a number of investigators, however, we know that even various forms of urethral obstruction may be caused by diseases that do not fit the description of what we call idiopathic FUS.

The terms urolithiasis and FUS should not be used interchangeably, as has been the convention of the past. A urolith is primarily composed of crystalline material with a minimal amount of matrix holding the crystals together. Urethral plugs are just the opposite, large amounts of matrix with minimal amounts of crystals.

There are some notable differences between canine and feline urolithiasis. Dogs of both genders may have a variety of bladder and urethral stones, but solitary or multiple bladder stones are rare in male cats that have not had a perineal urethrostomy, even though they are fairly common in female cats (Fig. 40–7). The typical female cat with a bladder stone or stones has a history of dysuria, hematuria, and inappropriate urination similar to the signs of FUS. However, the dysuria is often resistant to treatment or it recurs soon after treatment is discontinued. Recurrent hematuria is a consistent finding. These stones may be wa-

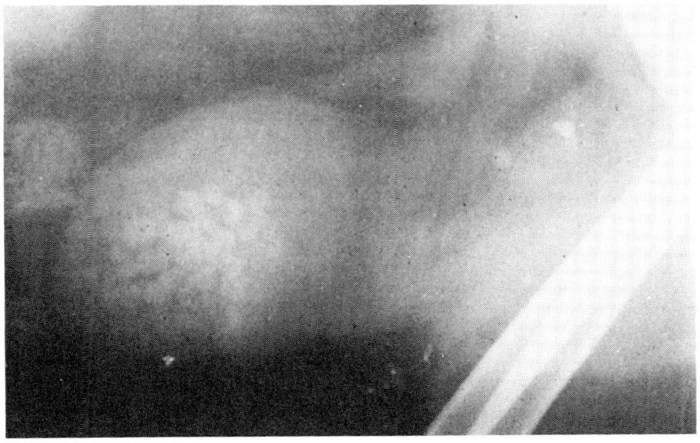

Figure 40–7. **Single or multiple uroliths are not common in male cats unless they have had a perineal urethrostomy, as was the case in this cat.**

ferlike, as much as 1 to 2 cm in diameter but only 1 to 2 mm thick. Positive, negative, and double-contrast cystograms should be performed, since some stones are radiopaque and some are radiolucent (see Chapter 14 for technique).

Dysuria that is nonresponsive to treatment may be caused by strictures in the urethra. Presumably, most of these are the result of urethral damage caused by previous episodes of FUS; however, this is not true in all cases. Such strictures can be demonstrated radiographically with a urethrogram and can generally be relieved surgically with a perineal urethrostomy[34] (see Chapters 14 and 55).

Although it is not common, primary bacterial cystitis does occur in cats. There is a significantly increased incidence in males that have had a perineal urethrostomy.[35]

Bladder and urethral tumors occur in cats, the former being much more frequent than the latter. Most bladder tumors are transitional cell carcinomas, which carry a grave prognosis because of their propensity to be locally invasive and to metastasize.

REFERENCES

1. Whitehead JE. Diseases of the Urogenital System. In: Catcott EJ, ed. Feline Medicine and Surgery. Santa Barbara: American Veterinary Publications, Inc., 1964:255.
2. Herron M. The effect of prepubertal castration on the penile urethra of the cat. J Am Vet Med Assoc 1972;160:208.
3. Rich LJ, Fabricant CG. Urethral obstruction in male cats. Can J Comp Med 1969;33:164.
4. Fabricant CG. Urolithiasis: A review of recent viral studies. Fel Pract 1973;3:22.
5. Fabricant CG. Feline viruses XI. Isolation of a virus similar to myxovirus from cats in which urolithiasis was experimentally induced. Cornell Vet 1969;59:667.
6. Kruger JM, Osborne CA, Whetstone CA, Goyal SM, Semlak RA. Genetic and serologic analysis of feline cell-associated herpesvirus-induced infection of the urinary tract in conventionally reared cats. Am J Vet Res 1989;50:2023.
7. Martens JG, McConnell S, Swanson CL. The role of infectious agents in naturally occurring feline urologic syndrome. Vet Clin North Am (Small Anim Pract) 1984;14:503.
8. Lees GE. Epidemiology of naturally occurring feline bacterial urinary tract infections. Vet Clin North Am (Small Anim Pract) 1984;14:471.
9. Barsanti JA, Finco DR, Shotts EB, Blue J, Ross L. Feline urologic syndrome: Further investigation into etiology. J Am Anim Hosp Assoc 1982;18:391.
10. Osborne CA, Kruger JM, Johnston GR, Polzin DJ. Feline Lower Urinary Tract Disorders. In: Ettinger SJ, ed. Textbook of Veterinary Internal Medicine. 3rd ed. Philadelphia: WB Saunders, 1989:2057.
11. Ross LA. Feline urologic syndrome: Understanding and diagnosing the enigmatic disease. Vet Med 1990;85:1194.
12. Buffington CA, Rogers QR, Morris JG, Cook NE. Feline struvite urolithiasis: Magnesium effect depends on urinary pH. Fel Pract 1985;15:29.
13. Kruger JM, Osborne CA, Goyal SM, O'Brien TD, Pomeroy KA, Semlak RA. Clinicopathologic analysis of herpes-virus-induced urinary tract infection in specific-pathogen-free cats given methylprednisolone. Am J Vet Res 1990;51:878.
14. Kruger JM, Osborne CA, Goyal SM, Pomeroy KA, O'Brien TD. Clinicopathologic and pathologic findings of herpesvirus-induced urinary tract infection in conventionally reared cats. Am J Vet Res 1990;51:1649.
15. Osborne CA, Johnston GR, Polzin DJ, Kruger JM, Poffenbarger EM, Bell FW, Feeney DA, et al. Redefinition of the feline urologic syndrome: Feline lower urinary tract disease with heterogenous causes. Vet Clin North Am (Small Anim Pract) 1984; 14:409.
16. Chow FHC, Taton GF, Lewis LD, Hamar DW. Effect of dietary ammonium chloride, DL-methionine, sodium phosphate, and ascorbic acid on urinary pH and electrolyte concentrations of male cats. Fel Pract 1978;8:29.
17. Hardy RM, Osborne CA. The Use and Misuse of Urinary Acidifiers. Proceedings of 40th Annual Meeting of American Animal Hospital Association 1973:278.
18. Osborne CA. New Insights into the Cause of FUS: The Diagnosis That Never Was. Proceedings 54th Annual Meeting AAHA, 1987:146.
19. Schecter RD. Heinz body hemolytic anemia associated with use of urinary antiseptics containing methylene blue in the cat. J Am Vet Med Assoc 1973;162:37.
20. White SD. Megestrol Acetate: Indications and Effects. In: August JR. Consultations in Feline Internal Medicine. Philadelphia: WB Saunders, 1991:263.
21. Kruger JM, Osborne CA, Sagar MG, Wickstrom MS, Johnston GR, Fletcher TF, Brown PA. Clinical evaluation of cats with lower urinary tract disease. J Am Vet Med Assoc 1991;199:211.
22. Wright M. Pharmacologic effects of ketamine and its use in veterinary medicine. J Am Vet Med Assoc 1982;180:1462.
23. Lees GE, Osborne CA. Use and misuse of indwelling urinary catheters in cats. Vet Clin North Am (Small Anim Pract) 1984;14:599.
24. Frenier SL, Dhein CR. Diagnosis and Management of Acute Renal Failure. In: August JR, ed. Consultations in Feline Internal Medicine. Philadelphia: WB Saunders, 1991:281.
25. Smith CW, Schiller AG, Smith AR, Wells SK, Kissil M. Effects of indwelling urinary catheters in male cats. J Am Anim Hosp Assoc 1981;17:427.
26. Moreau PM. Neurogenic disorders of micturition in the dog and cat. Compend Contin Educ Pract Vet 1982;4:12.
27. Jackson OF, Tovey JD. Water balance studies in domestic cats. Fel Pract 1977;7:30.
28. Jenkins EE, Coulter DB. Effects of diet on water; intake, food intake, and feces production in the cat. Georgia Vet 1981;33:8.

29. Sauer LS, Hamar D, Lewis LD. Effect of diet composition on water intake and excretion by the cat. Fel Pract 1985;15:16.
30. Seefeldt SL, Chapman TC. Body water content and turnover in cats fed dry and canned rations. Am J Vet Res 1979;40:183.
31. Thrall BE, Miller LG. Water turnover in cats fed dry rations. Fel Pract 1976;6:10.
32. Osborne CA, Johnston GR, Kruger JM, O'Brien TD, Lulich JP. Etiopathogenesis and biological behavior of feline vesicourachal diverticula. Vet Clin North Am (Small Anim Pract) 1987;17:697.
33. Wilson GP. The Relationship of Urachal Defects in the Feline Urinary Bladder to Feline Urologic Syndrome. Proceedings 7th Kal Kan Symposium, Kal Kan Foods, Vernon, CA 1983:125.
34. Norsworthy, GD: The steps in performing a urethrogram in male cats. Vet Med 1991;86:110.
35. Gregory CR. The effects of perineal urethrostomy on urethral function in male cats. Compend Contin Educ Pract Vet 1987; 9:895.
36. Garvey MS. Complications of Diabetes Mellitus. In: Viewpoints in Veterinary Medicine: Proceedings of ESVC. ALPO Pet Center, Allentown, PA 1986:3.

CHAPTER 41

◇ ◇ ◇

Heartworm Disease

Gary D. Norsworthy

The cat is an abnormal host for the mosquito-borne heartworm, *Dirofilaria immitis*. However, *D. immitis* does, on occasion, infect the cat and cause heartworm disease (HWD). Its incidence is about 20% of that in dogs, with the male cat being at higher risk.[1]

Feline and Canine Differences

There are several striking differences in the effects of this parasite on the cat compared with the dog. (1) Experimental infections are more difficult to achieve in the cat; less than 25% of third-stage larvae (L_3) reach adulthood. (2) The heartworm burden is significantly lower; the cat is generally infected with fewer than 10 worms, and most have only 2 to 4. (3) About 80% of infected cats have no circulating microfilaria, and the adult worm typically lives less than 2 years, compared with about 5 years in dogs.[2] (4) The effects on the pulmonary arteries are more severe in the cat.[3] Pulmonary enlargement occurs within 1 week of experimental infection. Pulmonary artery hypertension and embolism occur frequently, often resulting in peracute death.[1]

Clinical Signs

There are two distinct clinical presentations for feline HWD. The *acute form* is generally due to worm embolism or thromboembolism within the pulmonary arteries. Owners may report sudden death in apparently healthy cats. Other cats may present with marked salivation, dyspnea, syncope, hemoptysis, ataxia and circling, sudden onset of blindness, dementia, and/or seizures.

The more common form of feline HWD, the *chronic form,* causes anorexia or inappetence, weight loss, lethargy, exercise intolerance, coughing, dyspnea, and/or vomiting. If heart failure occurs, the cat may develop distention of the jugular veins and ascites. Chronic vomiting may be one of the only early clinical signs of feline HWD; since it is common in apparently healthy cats, a history compatible with HWD should also be established. Coughing from heartworms may also be confused with feline asthma. Cats with either disease may have a dry, chronic cough, a peripheral eosinophilia, and tracheal wash findings of a predominance of eosinophils. Cats with both diseases may temporarily respond to antiinflammatory doses of corticosteroids.[4]

Cats with the chronic form of HWD may seem stable during treatment, then experience sudden death, typically caused by pulmonary embolism (Fig. 41–1).

Diagnosis

Abnormalities found on routine laboratory testing are inconsistent. The most common ones are nonregenerative anemia, eosinophilia, basophilia, and hypergammaglobulinemia. The eosinophilia is present in only one third of the cases and tends to be transient. Experimentally, it becomes prominent about 5 months after inoculation and subsides about 4 months later.[5]

The demonstration of microfilaria is diagnostic. However, less than 20% of cats with adult heartworms are microfilaremic. In most cases, therefore, serologic evidence of heartworm antigens is sought. The enzyme-linked immunosorbent assay (ELISA) for heartworm antigens is much more sensitive than the corresponding test for heartworm antibodies. However, even the ELISA test produces an occasional false-negative result due to a low (<5) worm load.[1]

Radiographically, some cats show few signs of cardiac or pulmonary pathology (Fig. 41–2). However, some radiographic findings are typical for feline HWD, although they are significantly different from those in the dog. In the dog, the right ventricle and the pulmonary artery segment are often enlarged to produce the classic "reverse-D" appearance. In the cat, focal or diffuse interstitial infiltrates are often seen in the caudal lung lobes (Fig. 41–3). Some cats experience moderate cardiomegaly (Fig. 41–4). The caudal pulmonary arteries, when viewed on a ventrodorsal (VD) projection, may be enlarged and have poorly defined margins. They tend to end abruptly and have a blunted appearance (Fig. 41–5 *A*). This is usually due to embolic disease. The arterial changes are even more dramatically visualized when a nonselective angiogram is performed (Fig. 41–5 *B*).

Echocardiography can be valuable in diagnosing feline HWD. It consistently reveals right-sided enlargement. Occasionally, the adult heartworms can be visualized in the right

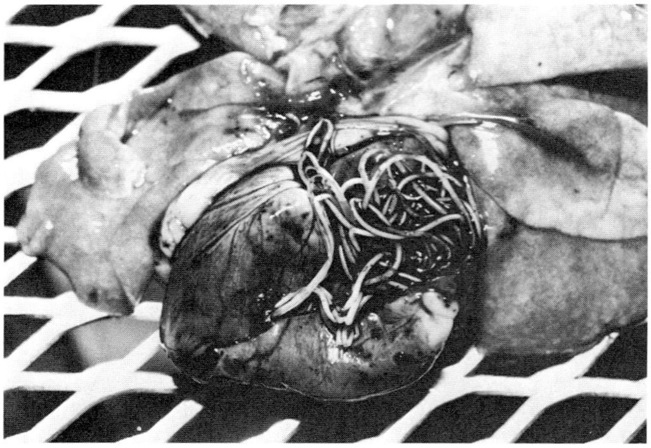

A

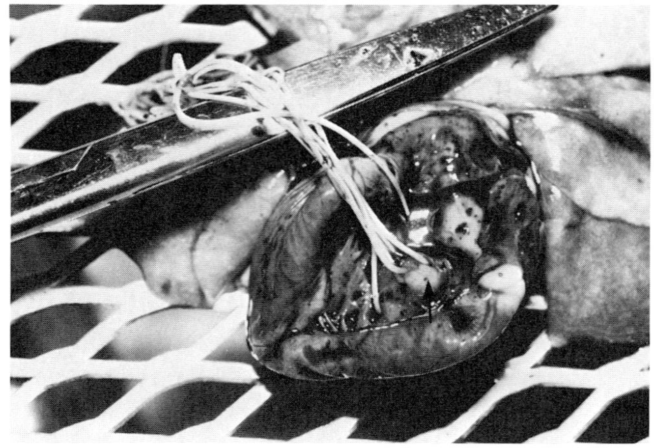

B

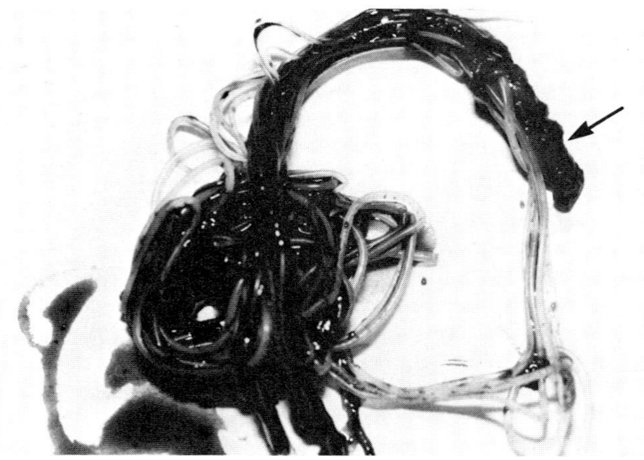

C

Figure 41–1. (*A*) An unusually large number of adult heartworms (15) were found in this cat that was stable but died acutely while boarding. (*B*) The adult heartworms of the cat in *A* were entwined within the papillary muscles (*arrow*). (*C*) Acute death in this cat was due to a large thrombus that occluded the main pulmonary artery (*arrow*). (Courtesy of Dr. Lewis Radicke, San Antonio, TX.)

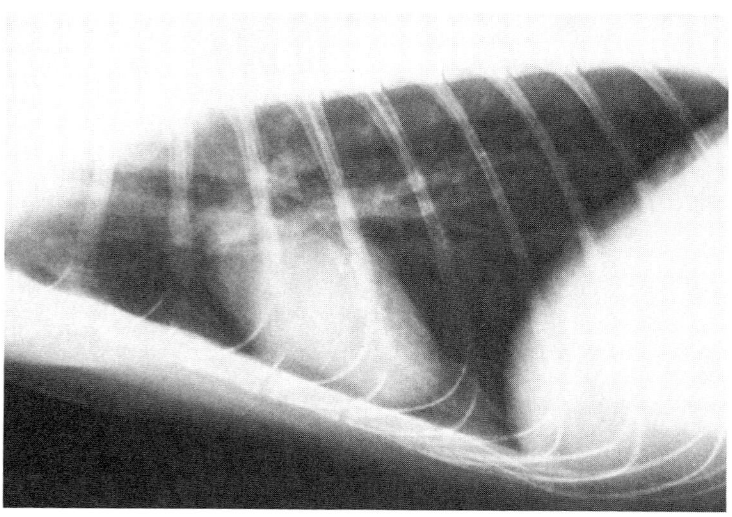

A

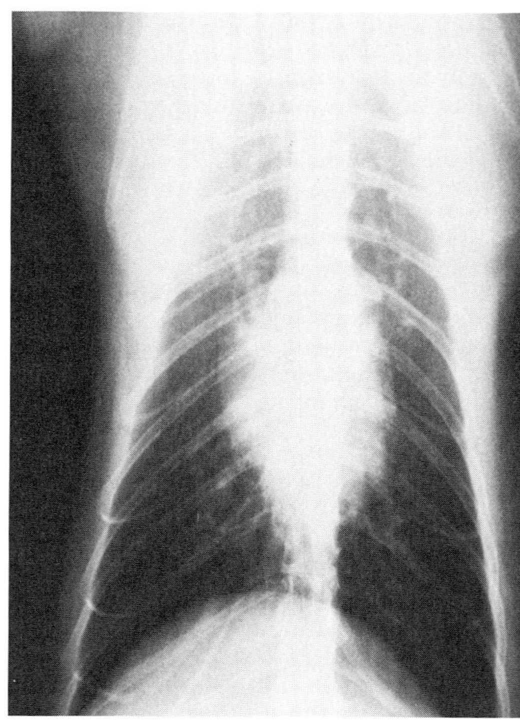

B

Figure 41–2. (*A*) This heartworm-infected cat has a radiographically normal thorax. (*B*) Ventrodorsal (VD) view of the cat in *A*.

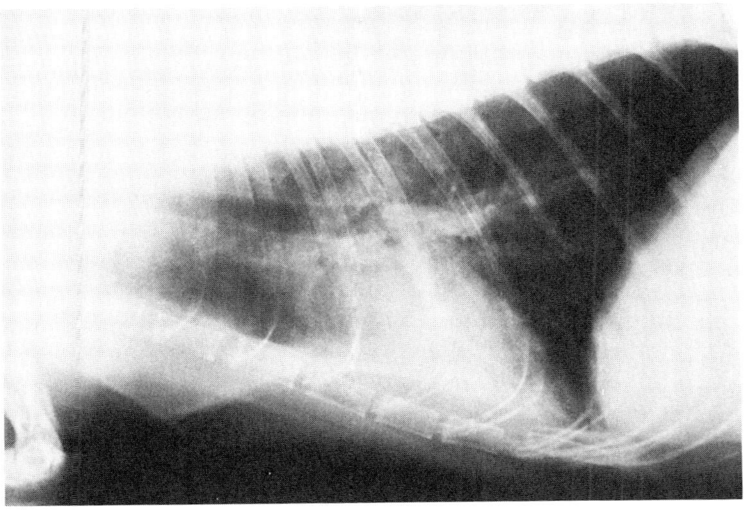

A

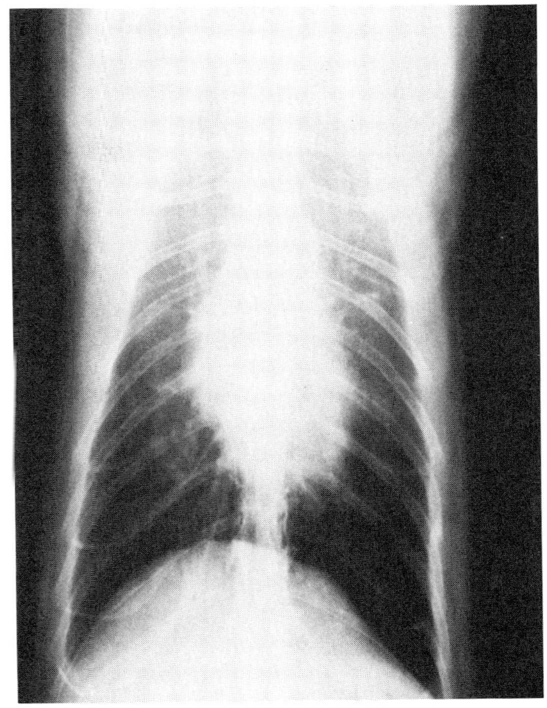

B

Figure 41–3. (*A*) Focal or diffuse interstitial infiltrates are seen in the caudal lung lobes of this heartworm-infected cat. (*B*) VD view of the cat in *A*.

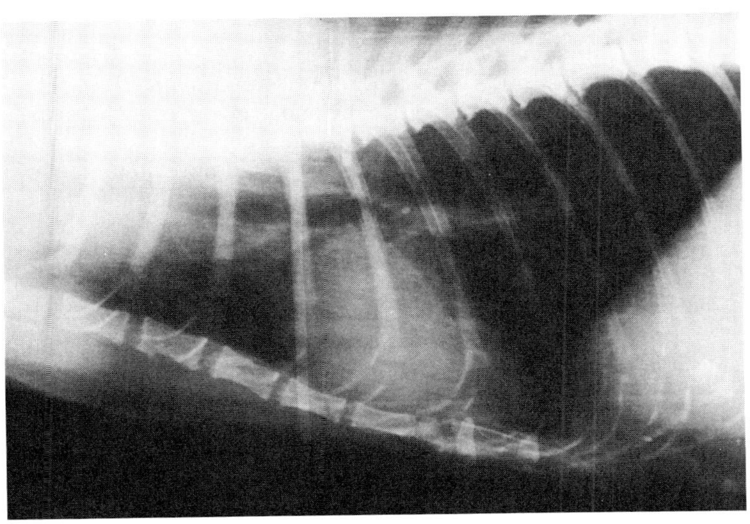

A

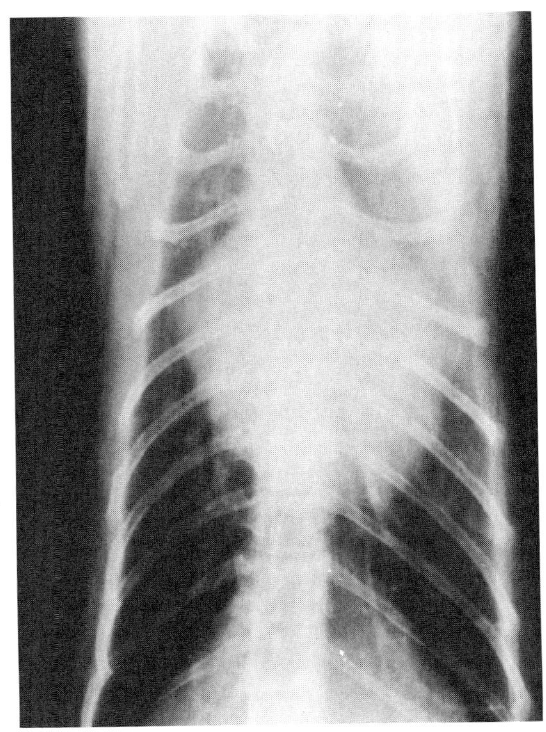

B

Figure 41–4. (*A*) Cats with heavy heartworm burdens may experience moderate cardiomegaly. This cat is the one shown in Figure 41–1. (*B*) VD view of the cat in *A*. (Courtesy of Dr. Lewis Radicke, San Antonio TX.)

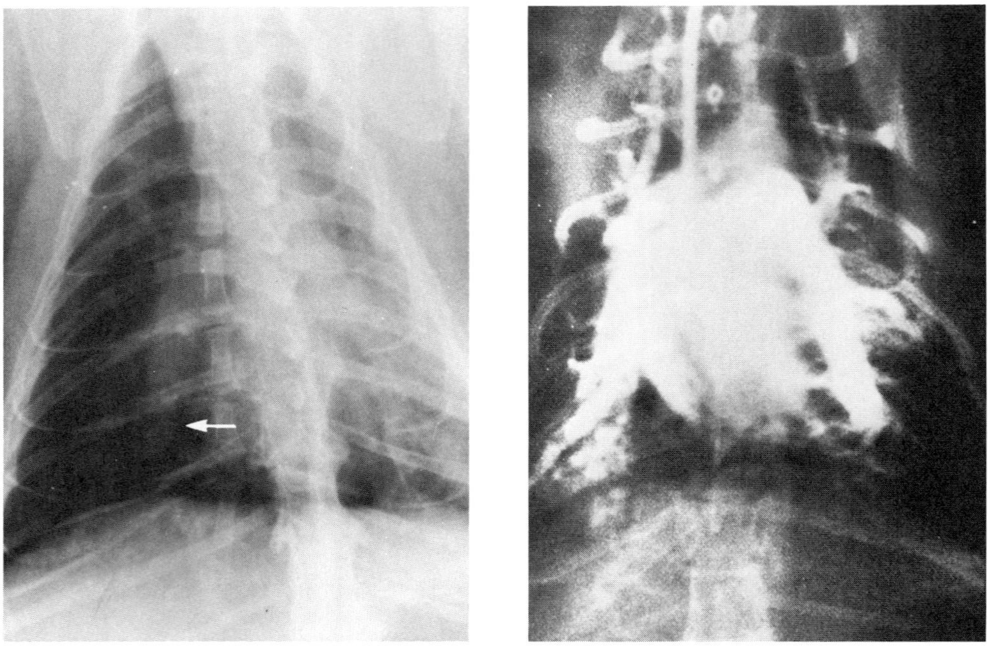

A B

Figure 41–5. (*A*) The most diagnostic radiographic finding in heartworm infected cats is blunting of the caudal pulmonary arteries on a VD view. This slightly obliqued VD view clearly demonstrates an enlarged, blunted pulmonary artery (*arrow*). (*B*) This nonselective angiogram vividly demonstrates arterial blunting due to pulmonary embolism.

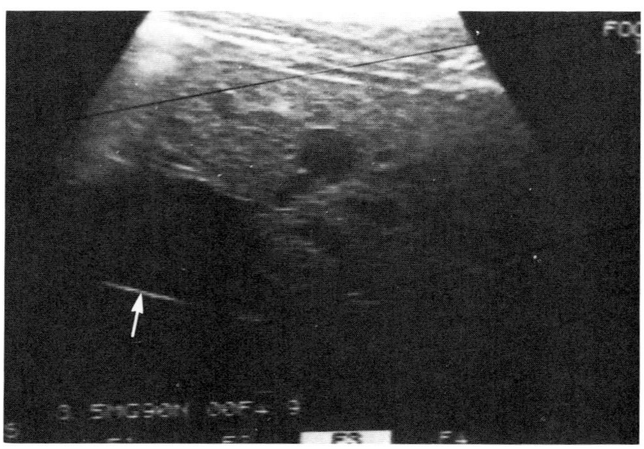

Figure 41–6. Echocardiography may reveal a heartworm in the right ventricle (*arrow*) (same cat as the one shown in Figure 41–1). This finding is inconsistent and is more likely to occur in cats with heavy heartworm burdens. The two oblique, dark lines are artifactual. (Courtesy of Dr. Sherm Mathey, San Antonio, TX.)

ventricle (Fig. 41–6) or the pulmonary outflow tract (Fig. 41–7).

Treatment

Because adult heartworms live less than 2 years, many cats spontaneously recover from a heartworm infection. Undoubtedly, this occurs in many undiagnosed cats. This is the treatment of choice for cats that do not exhibit heart failure, even though the possibility of sudden death due to pulmonary embolism is always present. It is also the treatment of choice for cats whose heart failure can be controlled medically.

Authorities do not agree on the best therapeutic regimen. Some believe that cats with HWD should receive aspirin (12 mg/lb p.o. twice weekly for up to 2 years) to minimize the chance of pulmonary embolism. Others think that prednisolone (0.5 to 1.0 mg/lb b.i.d.) on a p.r.n. basis for 16 to 22 months is the preferred method of managing HWD.

Treatment to control heart failure should be based on clinical, radiographic, and electrocardiographic findings. Although aspirin has been advocated, recent experimental evidence suggests that, even at near-toxic doses, it has little effect on the arteriographic, hemodynamic, and histopathologic abnormalities associated with feline HWD.[6-8] Cats with coughing or dyspnea should be treated with prednisolone (0.5 to 1.0 mg/lb s.i.d. p.o. for up to 2 weeks, then reduced) and aminophylline (3 mg/lb t.i.d. p.o. p.r.n.) and furosemide (0.5 to 1.0 mg/lb p.o. p.r.n.). If possible, these cats should also be confined indoors to limit their activity; this helps to

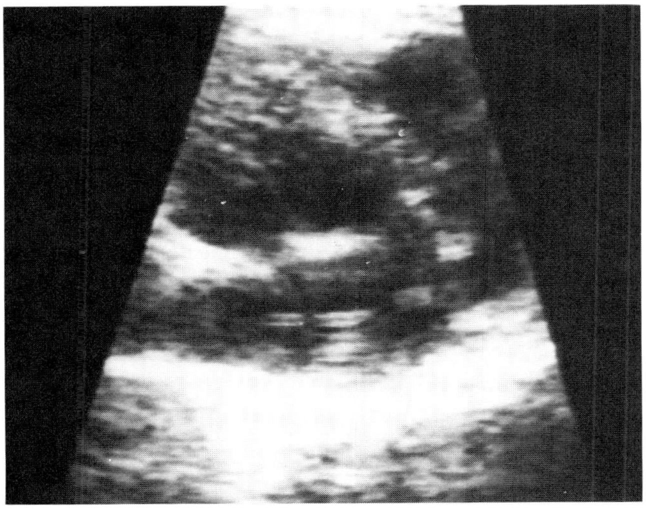

Figure 41–7. **The short, parallel lines in this echocardiogram are heartworms in the pulmonary outflow tract of the cat in Figure 41–1. (Courtesy of Dr. Sherm Mathey, San Antonio, TX.)**

control clinical signs of heart failure and reduce the chance of pulmonary embolism.

Cats whose heart failure cannot be controlled by these methods should be considered for therapy with thiacetarsamide sodium (Caparsolate). This drug is dosed at 1.0 mg/lb b.i.d. intravenously for 2 days.[9] It has several significant side effects in cats that must seriously be considered and discussed with the owner before administration. One study demonstrated a 21% death rate among adult cats given thiacetarsamide, resulting from a fulminating respiratory crisis.[10] However, other authorities report relatively safe use of the drug.[11] Pulmonary embolism may occur 10 to 14 days following treatment, resulting in dyspnea, hemoptysis, and/or sudden death. Cage rest and aspirin for 2 to 3 weeks following treatment is recommended to minimize complications.[4] Some cats develop an eosinophilic pneumonitis that can be treated for 3 to 5 days with prednisolone at a dose of 1 to 2 mg/lb p.o. t.i.d.[1]

Treatment for microfilaria is usually not needed because most cats with HWD are amicrofilaremic. However, if microfilaria are present, two drugs have been recommended. Levamisole hydrochloride (Levasole) has been recommended at a dose of 5 mg/lb s.i.d. for 7 days.[1,4] Ivermectin has also been used at a dose of 0.025 mg/lb p.o. once.

Prevention

Although we do not understand why certain cats are predisposed to *D. immitis* infection, it is reasonable to assume that, with adequate exposure, a cat that has developed heartworms once will do so again. The best means of prevention is restricting exposure; if these cats become indoors-only dwellers, their chances of contracting heartworms again are minimal. However, many cats are accustomed to an outdoor existence. For them, a pharmacologic means of prevention should be considered. Diethylcarbamazine (Difil syrup or tabs; Diro-Form) has been used successfully at a dose of 2.5 mg/lb p.o. s.i.d. Field trials are now in progress to evaluate ivermectin (Heartgard-30) and milbemycin oxime (Interceptor) for this purpose. Initial results for both products have been promising. Preliminary studies suggest that a higher monthly dose than that for dogs will be required in cats for ivermectin[6] and possibly a lower dose for milbemycin oxime.

REFERENCES

1. Atkins CE. Heartworm Disease. In: Allen DG, ed. Small Animal Medicine. Philadelphia: JB Lippincott, 1991:341.
2. Calvert CA, Mandell CP. Diagnosis and management of feline heartworm disease. J Am Vet Med Assoc 1982;180:550.
3. Dillon R. Feline Heartworm Disease. In: Kirk RW, ed. Current Veterinary Therapy IX. Philadelphia: WB Saunders, 1986:420.
4. Center SA, Randolph JF. Eosinophilia. In: August, JR, ed. Consultations in Feline Internal Medicine. Philadelphia: WB Saunders, 1991:349.
5. Donahoe JMR. Kneller SK, Lewis RE. Hematologic and radiographic changes in cats after inoculation with infective larvae of *Dirofilaria immitis*. J Am Vet Med Assoc 1976;168:413.
6. Miller, MW. Feline Heartworm Disease. Proceedings 9th American College of Veterinary Internal Medicine Forum, San Francisco CA, 1991:201.
7. Rawlings CA. Pulmonary arteriography and hemodynamics during feline heartworm disease. J Vet Intern Med 1990;4:285.
8. Rawlings CA, Farrell RI, Mahood RM. Morphologic changes in the lungs of cats experimentally infected with *Dirofilaria immitis*. J Vet Intern Med 1990;4:292.
9. Calvert CA. Feline Heartworm Disease. In: Sherding RG, ed. The Cat: Diseases and Clinical Management. New York: Churchill Livingstone, 1989:495.
10. Turner JL, Lees GE, Brown SA, et al. Thiacetarsamide in healthy cats: Clinical and pathological observations. J Am Anim Hosp Assoc. 1991;27:275.
11. Dillon R. Feline dirofilariasis. Vet Clin N Am (Sm Anim Pract) 1984;14(6):1185.

CHAPTER 42

◇ ◇ ◇

Heinz Body Hemolytic Anemia and Methemoglobinemia

Gary D. Norsworthy

Oxidant agents can affect red blood cells (RBCs) in several ways. The iron found in hemoglobin is normally in the ferrous state. Oxidation to the ferric state produces methemoglobin, which is not capable of oxygen transfer. Oxidation also results in the precipitation of hemoglobin, which coalesces to form inclusion bodies within the RBCs; these are known as Heinz bodies (HB). RBCs that contain HBs have cell membranes of increased rigidity that are susceptible to rupture and entrapment in the spleen. Thus, survival time of these RBCs is shortened. The resultant anemia that develops is called Heinz body hemolytic anemia (HBHA).[1]

The degree of HBHA varies from subclinical to severe. Because the bone marrow is not affected, the anemia is regenerative, and an increase in the number of reticulocytes should occur as seen on a blood sample. The presence of methemoglobinemia is variable. Some oxidants produce methemoglobinemia as the major form of erythrocyte injury, whereas others produce HB formation and hemolysis as the major form.[1]

Clinical Signs

The clinical signs of HBHA are typical of those of cats in an anemic crisis. Because the hemolysis occurs rapidly, these animals become dyspneic and very weak. In addition, the RBCs with HBs do not transport oxygen as efficiently as normal RBCs; therefore the cats can become cyanotic. If methemoglobin is present, the blood appears dark or brown, and the normal red color is not restored when the blood is exposed to air.[1]

Blood Smear Findings

HBs are present in up to 36% of RBCs in cats with certain types of HB anemias.[2] When HBs are properly stained, they are readily visible on the margin of the RBCs (Figs. 42–1, 42–2). However, they should not be confused with erythrocyte refractile bodies, which are found in the blood of some normal cats. When a drop of blood and new methylene blue mixture is examined under a microscope, erythrocyte refractile bodies appear as shiny red to purple inclusions.[3] Their presence is thought to be the result of oxidative denaturation, a process to which the cat has increased susceptibility. Erythrocyte refractile bodies are also known as nonpathologic HBs.[1]

Because HBHAs are regenerative, the characteristics of a regenerative bone marrow response should be seen on the blood smear (Figs. 42–1 and 42–2 and see Chapter 16). If these are not present, further investigation should be carried out to search for another disease process to account for bone marrow suppression.

Specific Oxidants

A number of drugs, agents, and conditions that cause HBHA have been discovered in the last 10 years.

Propylene Glycol

Propylene glycol is a preservative used in soft-moist cat foods in amounts of from 5% to 13%.[4] When kittens were fed a commercial soft-moist diet for 12 weeks, they were found to have HBs on 36% of their RBCs. However, they did not develop anemia or methemoglobinemia. Once induced, the HBs were present for 6 to 8 weeks in the blood of the cats, even when they were no longer ingesting propylene glycol. Although these kittens showed no signs of clinical disease, RBC survival times were decreased by about 33%.[2]

In another study, propylene glycol was fed at commercial cat food concentrations (12% of diet on a dry weight basis) and at a very high level (41% of diet). Twenty-eight and ninety-two percent of RBCs, respectively, contained HBs in those cats eating the 12% and 41% propylene glycol diets. The packed cell volume was not affected by the 12% propylene glycol diet, but cats fed the 41% diet had a mean decrease in packed cell volume of 22%. It was concluded that cats consuming unusually large amounts of propylene glycol, for example lactating queens and possibly their nursing kittens and untreated diabetic or hyperthyroid cats, would be more prone to developing HBHA.[5]

It is likely that the subclinical damage to RBCs caused by propylene glycol sensitizes a cat to further oxidant insult. Although cats eating soft-moist cat foods are unlikely to develop methemoglobinemia or HBHA, if they receive some of the drugs listed below, even in low doses, or if they

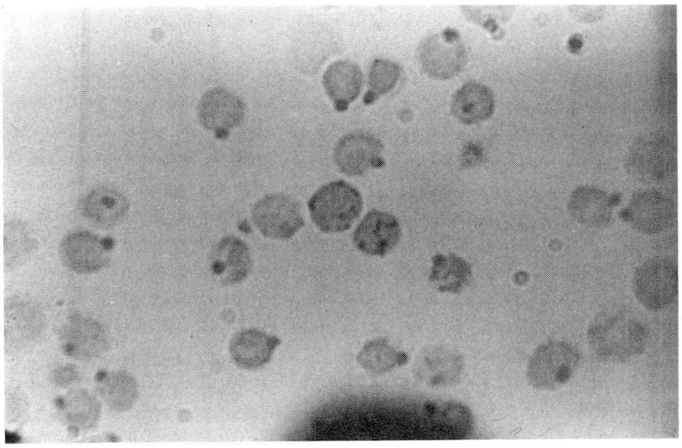

Figure 42–1. **When RBCs are stained with new methylene blue stain, the HBs can be seen prominently as dark protrusions on the cell margins (see Chapter 12). The two cells in the center of the field are reticulocytes and are evidence of a regenerative anemia.**

develop polyphagia, they are much more likely to develop clinical disease. This may account for why the drug methylene blue was used for so many years for cats with lower urinary tract diseases but only sporadic cases of HBHA developed in those cats. Many of these cats were not on a diet of soft-moist food and were not otherwise exposed to propylene glycol.

Methylene Blue

The first identified cause of HBs in the cat was methylene blue.[6,7] This drug has been frequently used for treating feline lower urinary tract diseases, and it was present in a number of veterinary urinary combination products. Cats affected with lower urinary tract diseases who were given methylene blue developed HBHA, and severely affected white-haired cats have been observed to literally develop blue skin.

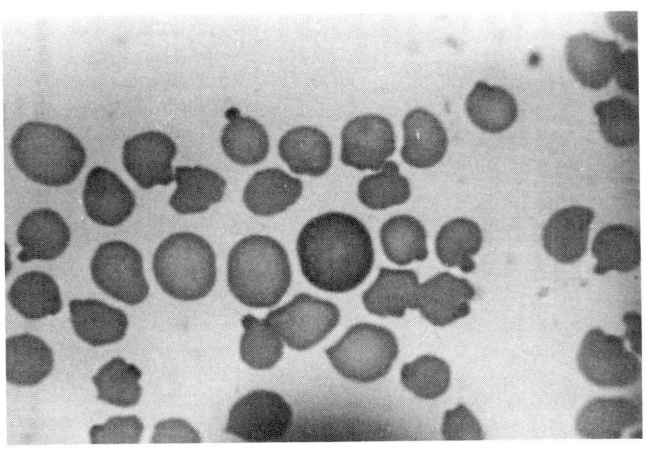

Figure 42–2. When RBCs are stained with Wright's stain, the HBs are also seen prominently as dark protrusions on the cell margins. The large, darkly stained cell in the center of the field is a macrocyte and is evidence of a regenerative anemia.

This author, as well as most veterinarians who practiced veterinary medicine prior to 1975, used this drug extensively but only occasionally observed the subsequent development of HBHA; HBHA is apparently more likely to develop in certain cats, especially those eating semimoist cat foods.

Table 42–1 contains the results of a study conducted by the author in 1975 on eighteen cats who received 5.4 mg of methylene blue (with other drugs in a combination urinary antiseptic agent) twice daily for varying durations of therapy. The following observations and conclusions were arrived at:

1. One cat died after receiving the drug for 3 weeks; all seventeen others did not show *clinical* signs of HBHA, i.e., anorexia, lethargy, and blue color of skin and/or mucus membranes.
2. Sixteen of eighteen (84%) of these animals developed HBs with varying degrees of bone marrow regeneration.
3. Three of eighteen (16%) did not develop HBs or other hematologic signs of toxicity. Their duration of therapy was 7, 10, and 10 days, respectively.
4. In one cat that was followed for 35 days, HBs persisted for 14 days following cessation of the drug.
5. Affected cats frequently showed a moderate to marked increase in eosinophil and/or basophil counts.
6. HBs were more readily seen on Wright's stained blood smears than with new methylene blue stain, with one exception. The cat that was followed for 35 days initially had increased visibility of HBs with Wright's stain but the increased visibility changed to new methylene blue stained blood smears after 10 days.

Acetaminophen

Acetaminophen is commonly found in households and used freely as a pain reliever and antipyretic. Cat owners have used this drug for the same purposes in sick cats without realizing that it causes methemoglobinemia. As little as one oral dose of 143 mg/kg (about one extra-strength tablet per 9 lb of body weight) has been fatal to a cat.[8]

Treatment has been successful with *N*-acetylcysteine (Mucomyst) and sodium sulfate. The latter has been used successfully in experimentally induced acetaminophen toxicosis at a dose of 50 mg/kg intravenously at 4.5, 8.5, and 12.5 hours following toxicosis.[9] The following recommendations are the treatments of choice of the Animal Poison Control Center for acetaminophen toxicosis:[10]

1. If ingestion of acetaminophen has been within 2 hours of presentation, induce vomiting. This may be done with activated charcoal at 2 g/kg of body weight given with a saline cathartic, preferably sodium sulfate (0.5 g/kg of body weight) as a 20% slurry.
2. If cyanosis is present, stress should be minimized and oxygen administered.
3. *N*-acetylcysteine should be given intravenously or orally on the following schedule:
   a. Initial dose: 140 mg/kg
   b. Every 6 hours thereafter: 70 mg/kg
   c. Give a total of seven treatments

Table 42–1. Methylene Blue Study

Name: Owner, Cat	Cat #	Dosage	Duration	PCV	Retic	% HB: 1–4	HJB: 1–4	Macro: 1–4	NRBCs	Miscellaneous
Corrigan, Taffy	1	1 b.i.d.	2 wk		2%	0	+1	0	0	
Corrigan, Taffy	1	1 b.i.d.	3 wk	34%	<1%	0	+1	0	0	2% Basophils
Slane, Pete	2	1 b.i.d.	2 wk		<1%	0	+1	0	1%	
Slane, Pete	2	1 b.i.d.	3 wk	36%	1%	+3	+1	0	0	2% Basophils
Slane, Pete	2			38%	0	0	0	0	0	Pretreatment values
Slane, Pete	2	1 b.i.d.	7 days	37%	3%	+1	+1	+2	+2	Several stimulated lymphocytes
Slane, Pete	2	None for 7 days		40%	1%	+1	+1	0	0	HBs on Wright's stain only
Wertheim, CC	3	1 b.i.d.	3 wk	25%	5%	+4	+2	+3	6%	Stimulated lymphocytes; died
Fajkus, Sam	4	1 b.i.d.	1 wk	34%	<1%	+1	+1	0	0	
Fajkus, Sam	4	1 b.i.d.	2 wk	32%	18%	+1	+1	+2	0	
Wertheim, Afro	5	1 b.i.d.	1 wk	35%	<1%	+1	+1	0	0	HBs on Wright's stain but not on new methylene blue
Nelson, Dinky (fe)	6	1 b.i.d.	1 wk	26%	3%	0	+1	0	0	2% Basophils
Nelson, Dinky (fe)	6	1 b.i.d.	1 wk	26%	4%	+2	+3	+2	2%	1% Basophils
Westberry, Squeeker	7	1 b.i.d.	1 wk	40%	1%	0	0	+1	0	
Westberry, Squeeker	7	1 b.i.d.	2 wk	36%	2%	+1	+1	+1	0	More HBs on Wright's stain
Munson, Pinky	8	1 b.i.d.	1 wk	42%	<1%	+1	0	0	0	HBs on Wright's stain only
Allen, Camino	9	1 b.i.d.	1 wk	–	3%	+2	+2	+1	0	More HBs on Wright's stain
Allen, Camino	9	1 b.i.d.	10 days	37%	1%	+1	0	+1	0	More HBs on Wright's stain
Allen, Camino	9	1 b.i.d.	10 days	37%	1%	+1	0	+1	0	More HBs on Wright's stain
Tyra, Folly (fe)	10	1 b.i.d.	1 wk	31%	2%	+1	+2	+1	0	HBs on Wright's stain only
Tyra, Tang	11	1 b.i.d.	10 days	42%	<1%	0	0	0	0	
McDougall, Paco	12	1 b.i.d.	3 wk	32%	2%	+3	+1	+1	0	1% Basophils
McDougall, Paco	12	None	1 wk	32%	<1%	+1	+1	0	0	
Huckle, Batman	13	1 b.i.d.	10 days	23%	<1%	0	0	0	0	
Baker, Boots	14	1 b.i.d.	1 wk	48%	2%	0	0	0	0	
Norsworthy, Arn	15	1 b.i.d.	10 days	30%	5%	+4	+1	+2	0	1% Basophils, 8% eosinophils
Norsworthy, Arn	15	None for 2 days		25%	5%	+3	+2	+3	0	More HBs on Wright's stain; 1% basophils; 15% eosinophils
Norsworthy, Arn	15	None for 4 days		25%	8%	+2	+1	+3	0	14% Eosinophils
Norsworthy, Arn	15	None for 6 days		25%	6%	+1	+1	+2	0	18% Eosinophils
Norsworthy, Arn	15	None for 8 days		26%	12%	+1	0	+1	0	More HBs on Wright's stain; 2% basophils; 9% eosinophils
Norsworthy, Arn	15	None for 10 days		28%	25%	+1	+2	+3	0	More HBs on Wright's stain; 10% eosinophils
Norsworthy, Arn	15	None for 12 days		30%	20%	+1	+1	+1	0	More HBs on new methylene blue; 1% basophils; 12% eosinophils
Norsworthy, Arn	15	None for 14 days		30%	5%	+1	+1	0	0	More HBs on new methylene blue; 1% basophils; 26% eosinophils
Norsworthy, Arn	15	None for 35 days		39%	<1%	0	0	0	0	22% Eosinophils
Lindsey, Tommy	16	1 b.i.d.	9 days		17%	+4	+2	+2	+1	2% Basophils; 9% eosinophils
Gallagher, Chip	17	1 b.i.d.	1 wk	38%	1%	+1	+1	+1	0	1% Basophils
Anderson, Sonny	18	1 b.i.d.	1 wk	38%	4%	+3	+1	+2	0	

Note: Multiple entries for the same cat indicate different treatment periods with the exception of cat no. 15.

Abbreviations: PCV, packed cell volume; Retic, reticulocytes; HBs, Heinz bodies; HJB, Howell-Jolly bodies; Macro, macrocytes; NRBCs, nucleated red blood cells.

4. Administer ascorbic acid orally or parenterally at a dose of 30 mg/kg with each dose of *N*-acetylcysteine.
5. Administer lactated Ringer's solution to correct acidosis.
6. Do not administer steroids; they may increase the mortality rate.[11]

Phenacetin

The severity of toxicosis of this drug in the cat is similar to that of acetaminophen. It produces intravascular and extravascular hemolysis, methemoglobinemia.[1]

Benzocaine

Benzocaine is a topical anesthetic. It has been used most commonly in cats as a laryngeal spray (Cetacaine) to aid in endotracheal intubation. If it is administered during inhalation, enough can be absorbed from the respiratory tract to induce marked methemoglobinemia and cyanosis, but HBs generally do not form.[1,12] Cetacaine has also been sprayed into the urethra to aid in the relief of urethral obstructions. Krake, Arendy, Teachout, et al. postulate that an inflamed urethral and/or urinary bladder mucosa could permit enough absorption of benzocaine to result in toxicosis.

Benzocaine is also available as a topical cream and sold over-the-counter for use in humans (Lanacaine). It is poorly absorbed through normal skin but rapidly through inflamed skin. It has caused vomiting, open-mouth breathing, and collapse within 15 minutes of application to inflamed feline skin, with severe methemoglobinemia.[13]

Phenazopyridine

This human drug is available individually (Pyridium) and in combination with a urinary sulfa drug (Azo Gantrisin). It is a urinary tract analgesic that is commonly prescribed for human patients. It has also been used frequently to treat feline cystitis.[1] It causes methemoglobinemia and HB formation.

Methionine

Methionine, a urinary acidifier, has been shown to cause HBHA and marked methemoglobinemia in cats given 250 mg/lb or higher. In spite of continued administration past 31 days, recovery from HBHA occurred, indicating that some metabolic adaptation had occurred. This drug is not likely to be a clinical problem because the dose required to induce this toxicosis is considerably higher than the dose generally used to produce urinary acidification.[14]

Onions

The most common cause of HBHA in dogs is the ingestion of onions.[1] This generally occurs when a dog eats onions that have been used in cooking meat. HBHA caused by eating onions is not common in cats but has been documented in three cats.[15]

Endogenous Oxidants

A variety of metabolic and systemic diseases have also been associated with the production of high numbers of HBs.[16] Christopher postulated that metabolic derangements may provide the necessary endogenous oxidants and that the HBs may contribute to the anemias that often accompany chronic systemic or metabolic diseases. High numbers of HBs have been associated with feline abscesses, urologic disease, intestinal obstruction, chronic nephritis, peritonitis, stomatitis, and upper respiratory tract diseases.[17-20] However, the strongest correlation between HBs and disease is with diabetes mellitus, hyperthyroidism, and lymphoma.[16]

It is interesting to note that diabetes mellitus and hyperthyroidism typically cause chronic polyphagia. If cats with these disorders were also fed soft-moist diets, the chances of their developing HBHA could be significantly increased.

Treatment

With the exception of acetaminophen, most causes of HBHA do not have specific antidotes. Therefore, treatment consists primarily of removal of the oxidant. In many cases, this is adequate; however, supportive therapy, consisting of cage rest and oxygen administration, may also be helpful. In cases of severe anemia, the administration of whole blood may be lifesaving. Blood administration may be warranted if more than 20% of the RBCs have HBs, even if the packed cell volume is not severely low, since these damaged RBCs have reduced oxygen-carrying capacity.

Methylene blue is used to treat methemoglobinemia in other species. Obviously it is not indicated in the cat because it, too, is a cause of HBHA and methemoglobinemia.

REFERENCES

1. Blue JT. Anemia in cats (Part II). Feline Health Topics for Veterinarians 1991;6:1.
2. Hickman MA, Rogers QR, Morris JG. Effect of diet on Heinz body formation in kittens. Am J Vet Res 1990;50:475.
3. Schalm OW. Standardization of Nomenclature of Cells and Diseases of the Blood and Blood-Forming Organs. In: Schalm OW, ed. Veterinary Hematology. 2nd ed. Philadelphia: Lea & Febiger, 1970:130.
4. Moser E, Branam JE. Topical issues in feline nutrition. Compend Contin Educ Pract Vet 1990;12:1227.
5. Christopher MM, Perman V, Eaton JW. Contribution of propylene glycol-induced Heinz body formation to anemia in cats. J Am Vet Med Assoc 1989;194:1045.
6. Sodikoff CH. Heinz body anemia in a cat induced by methylene blue. Fel Pract 1973;3:38.
7. Boon GD Rich LJ. Heinz body anemia associated with methylene blue administration in a cat. Fel Pract 1974;4:49.
8. Gaunt SD, Baker DC, Green RA. Clinicopathologic evaluation of *N*-acetylcysteine therapy in acetaminophen toxicosis in the cat. Am J Vet Res 1981;42:1982.
9. Savides MC, Oehme FW, Leipold HW. Effects of various antidotal treatments on acetaminophen toxicosis and biotransformation in cats. Am J Vet Res 1985;46:1485.
10. Cullison RF. Acetaminophen toxicosis in small animals: Clinical signs, mode of action, and treatment. Compend Contin Educ Pract Vet 1984;6:315.

11. Nimmo J, Dixon MF, Prescott LF. Effects of mepyramine, promethazine, and hydrocortisone on paracetamol-induced hepatic necrosis in the rat. Clin Toxicol 1973;6:75.
12. Krake AC, Arendy TD, Teachout DJ, et al. Cetacaine-induced methemoglobinemia in domestic cats. J Am Hosp Assoc 1985;21:527.
13. Wilkie DA, Kirby R. Methemoglobinemia associated with dermal application of benzocaine cream in a cat. J Am Vet Med Assoc 1988;192:85.
14. Maede Y, Hoshino T, Inaba M, Namioka S. Methionine toxicosis in cats. Am J Vet Res 1987;48:289.
15. Kobayashi K. Onion poisoning in the cat. Fel Pract 1981;11:22.
16. Christopher MM. Relation of endogenous Heinz bodies to disease and anemia in cats: 120 cases (1978–1987). J Am Vet Med Assoc 1989;194:1089.
17. Jain NC. Studies on the occurrence and persistence of Heinz bodies in erythrocytes of the cat. Folia Haematol (Leipzig) 1973;99:28.
18. Schalm OW. Heinz body hemolytic anemia in the cat. Fel Pract 1977;7:30.
19. Schalm OW, Smith R. Some unique aspects of feline hematology in disease. Small Anim Clin 1963;3:311.
20. Sedgwick CJ, Simpson JG, Schalm OW. Clinical hematology in zoo animals. I. Hemograms. Am J Vet Clin Pathol 1967;1:105.

CHAPTER 43

◇ ◇ ◇

Hemobartonellosis

Gary D. Norsworthy

Hemobartonella felis (*H. felis*) is an epicellular parasite of feline red blood cells (RBCs) that can cause anemia. The resulting disease is called hemobartonellosis, or feline infectious anemia (FIA).

Historical Perspective

Prior to the discovery of the feline leukemia virus (FeLV), anemia was common among sick cats. Because they were unfamiliar with the association of FeLV and anemia, veterinarians thought that most cases of anemia were either the "acute" or "chronic" form of FIA. If the cat exhibited bone marrow response, the disease was diagnosed as "acute FIA." If the anemia was nonregenerative, it was assumed that bone marrow exhaustion was occurring owing to "chronic FIA."

Incidence

Prior to the availability of FeLV testing, as mentioned, FIA was reported as a very common disease.[1,2] When rigid diagnostic criteria were applied, an incidence of FIA of 3.6% in healthy cats and 7.5% in sick cats was found.[3]

Mechanisms of Anemia

The development of anemia is attributed to two mechanisms. The parasite-damaged RBCs are phagocytized by the spleen.[4] In addition, cold agglutinins are associated with this disease, and most affected cats have a positive response to the Coombs test. Therefore, autoimmune mechanisms are thought to be a factor in the development of anemia.[5] Because neither of these mechanisms adversely affects the bone marrow, it should exhibit a strong response to the anemia.

Experimental hemobartonellosis progresses through four stages. It seems reasonable to assume that the naturally infected cat experiences a similar progression of disease. These four stages[6] are:

1. A *prelatent period* lasting from a few days to a few weeks.
2. An *acute phase* characterized by a fluctuating parasitemia and hematocrit reading.
3. A *recovery phase* in which the parasitemia remains at a low level and the hematocrit rises rapidly.
4. A *carrier phase* characterized by a nearly nonperceptible parasitemia and a normal hematocrit value.

Predisposing Conditions

It has been assumed that the carrier state is activated to full clinical disease by some form of stress. Practitioners have been encouraged to aggressively search for an underlying primary disease.[2,7] However, these assumptions have been challenged by a study in which *H. felis*–infected cats were stressed with (1) cyclophosphamide, (2) 6-mercaptopurine, (3) experimentally induced abscesses, (4) splenectomies, and (5) glucocorticoids. Parasitemias were not observed in the first three groups, moderate parasitemias were observed in the forth group, and parasitemias were irregularly observed in the fifth group. Clinical signs of FIA did not occur in any of the stressed cats.[8] In spite of these findings, recent articles on this disease continue to link FIA and stress.[6]

Several risk factors that predispose a cat to developing FIA have been identified:[3]

1. Other types of anemia
2. A positive FeLV test
3. No prior vaccinations
4. A history of cat bite abscesses
5. An age less than or equal to 3 years
6. An outdoor roaming status.

Other factors that were studied but that did not appear to be significant in the development of FIA were

1. Sex
2. Breed
3. Number of cats in the household
4. Presence of fleas.

It may seem unusual that the presence of fleas was listed as a nonrisk factor. However, the authors point out that nearly all cats in this study were parasitized with fleas and therefore no distinction was possible in this respect between the two groups of cats included.

Clinical Signs and Physical Examination

Cats with hemobartonellosis are generally lethargic and anorectic as a result of the anemia, which may be profound. Many are febrile, icteric, and have palpable splenomegaly.

Diagnosis

Two criteria must be met for a confirmed diagnosis of FIA. The cat must have a regenerative anemia, and *H. felis* must be identified on the cat's RBCs. *H. felis* may appear as coccoids, rings, or rods on the RBC membrane (Fig. 43–1). It is not always possible to fulfill both of these criteria because of the cyclic nature of the parasitemia. In the absence of the parasites, these cats are indistinguishable from cats with autoimmune hemolytic anemia, since both are likely to have positive Coombs' test responses.

When looking for *H. felis,* the practitioner should be aware that false-negative responses to testing may occur because of the cyclic parasitemia that is typical of this disease. In one study in which blood samples were taken frequently from experimentally infected cats, one cat went from a marked level of parasitemia to nonparasitemia within a period of 1.5 hours.[9] This observation is consistent with clinical cases in which multiple blood samples may have to be tested before the organism is identified. Another possible cause of false-negative findings is the effect of ethylenediaminetetra-acetic (EDTA) acid on the parasite. This anticoagulant may dislodge the organisms from the RBCs so they are not found on a stained blood smear. This can be prevented by making a fresh blood smear at the time of blood collection or by using heparin as an anticoagulant. False-positive results may also occur in the identification of *H. felis,* since these organisms can be confused with stain precipitation, nuclear remnants, or debris.[3]

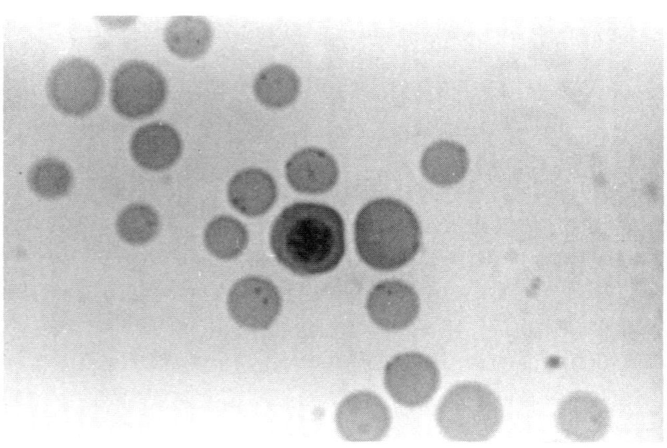

Figure 43–1. **The hematologic signs of FIA are a regenerative anemia and the presence of *H. felis.* The large nucleated cell in the center of this field is a rubricyte (nucleated RBC). The large non-nucleated cell next to it is a macrocyte (reticulocyte). Both are indicators of a regenerative anemia. Several of the surrounding RBCs contain small *H. felis* organisms on the erythrocyte membranes.**

Since autoimmune hemolytic anemia is a rare condition in cats, a cat with a regenerative anemia and a positive Coombs' test should be tentatively diagnosed as having hemobartonellosis until multiple attempts at finding the organisms are unsuccessful or unless some other cause of the regenerative anemia can be confirmed. A positive response to tetracycline therapy is further evidence that the disease is FIA.

Some commercial veterinary laboratories have a specific test for FIA. Generally, however, this test is for the presence of *H. felis* and does not consider the RBC count or the level of bone marrow activity. The laboratory's criteria for positivity should be determined before interpreting a positive response as diagnostic of FIA.

Transmission

The exact mode of natural transmission of *H. felis* is not known. It can be transmitted by blood transfusions;[10] therefore, it is assumed that most means of inoculation of blood from an infected cat to a noninfected cat are potential forms of transmission. Those means of transmission generally cited are insect vectors such as fleas, ticks, and biting flies. However, none of these have been documented.

Treatment

Doxycycline (Vibramycin and Doxy-Tabs), at a dose of 2.3 mg/lb initially, then 1.1 mg/lb 12 hours later, then 1.1 mg/lb every 24 hours by mouth, or tetracycline, at a dose of 15 mg/lb b.i.d. by mouth, or chloramphenicol, at a dose of 7 mg/lb b.i.d. by mouth, are the treatments of choice. These antibiotics are reported to suppress the activity of the organisms, allowing the cat to recover. Duration of therapy should be about 30 days. However, these agents do not rid the cat of *H. felis,* since the carrier state occurs following treatment. Each of these drugs also has adverse side effects. Tetracycline often causes a marked fever, as high as 107°F. In high doses, chloramphenicol causes anorexia and may reduce the bone marrow response.

Thiacetarsamide (Caparsolate) has also been used to treat FIA. It was originally thought to rid the cat of *H. felis* and thus prevent the carrier state.[1] However, it has not been shown to possess that quality. It has also caused as high as a 20% death rate in normal cats because of its ability to produce a fulminating pulmonary crisis when administered at the dose sufficient to kill heartworm.[11] However, the dose for treatment of FIA is considerably lower and considered safe. The currently recommended dose of thiacetarsamide is 0.5 mg/lb given once on days 1 and 3.

Prednisolone, at a dose of 0.25 mg/lb s.i.d. to b.i.d., should be used for its ability to decrease hemolysis, to decrease phagocytosis of RBCs by the reticuloendothelial system, and to stimulate appetite. It should be used for 1 to 2 weeks.

H. felis and Nonregenerative Anemias

Frequently a cat is identified that has *H. felis* on its RBCs and is anemic, but the anemia is nonregenerative. In such cases, FIA is probably a correct diagnosis but not a complete one. Since *H. felis* has no adverse effects on the bone marrow, some other cause must be sought to account for the lack of bone marrow response. FeLV is the most likely cause. FeLV and FIV testing should occur on all cats suspected to have FIA, even those with regenerative anemias. (If the anemia is regenerative and the FeLV test is positive, the short-term prognosis for the anemia will probably be good, but the long-term prognosis will be grave. About 80% of FeLV-positive cats die within 3 years of diagnosis.)[12]

REFERENCES

1. Fishler JJ, Birzele FD. Feline Infectious Anemia. In: Kirk RW, ed. Current Veterinary Therapy V. Philadelphia: WB Saunders Co., 1974:358.
2. Loeb WF. Blood and Blood Forming Organs. In: Catcott EJ, ed. Feline Medicine and Surgery. 2nd ed. Santa Barbara: American Veterinary Publications, Inc., 1975:225.
3. Grindem CB, Corbett WT, Tomkins MT. Risk factors for *Haemobartonella felis* infection in cats. J Am Vet Med Assoc 1990; 196:96.
4. Maede Y. Sequestration and phagocytosis of *Haemobartonella felis* in the spleen. Am J Vet Res 1979;40:691.
5. Zulty JC, Kociba GJ. Cold agglutinins in cats with haemobartonellosis. J Am Vet Med Assoc 1990;196:907.
6. Blue JT. Anemia in cats (Part I). Feline Health Topics 1990;5:3.
7. Schall WD, Perman V. Diseases of the Red Blood Cells. In: Ettinger SJ, ed. Textbook of Veterinary Internal Medicine. Philadelphia: WB Saunders Co., 1975:1581.
8. Harvey JW, Gaskin JM. Feline haemobartonellosis: Attempts to Induce Relapses of Clinical Disease in Chronically Infected Cats. J Am Animal Hosp Assoc 1978;14:453.
9. Harvey JW, Gaskin JM. Experimental feline haemobartonellosis. J Am Anim Hosp Assoc 1977;13:28.
10. Splitter EJ, Castro ER, Kanawyer WL. Feline infectious anemia. Vet Med 1956;51:17.
11. Turner JL, Lees GE, Brown SA, et al. Thiacetarsamide in healthy cats: Clinical and pathological observations. J Am Anim Hosp Assoc 1991;27:275.
12. Hardy WD, Jr. The feline leukemia virus. J Am Anim Hosp Assoc 1981;17:951.

CHAPTER 44

◇ ◇ ◇

High-Rise Syndrome

J. Thomas Ross

Feline high-rise syndrome (HRS) is a collection of injuries sustained by cats that fall from substantial heights, usually from high-rise buildings in large urban areas.[1-4] It is generally diagnosed by a history of a substantial fall accompanied by dyspnea and other typical abnormalities.

Pathophysiology and Clinical Findings

The sensitive vestibular apparatus allows cats to orient themselves quickly to land on all four limbs during a fall. Because of this phenomenon, certain injuries are commonly encountered, including pneumothorax, pulmonary contusions, facial and dental trauma, limb fractures and luxations, pelvic fractures, vertebral fractures, urinary bladder rupture, traumatic pancreatitis, and hemoperitoneum.[1,2] The keen feline vestibular mechanism may also help explain the cat's ability to survive falls from great heights. Because of the cat's upright posture, drag is maximized and a maximum or terminal velocity of approximately 60 mph is attained after the cat falls approximately five stories (60 feet). The greatest rate of injury is seen in cats that fall approximately seven stories because impact occurs just after terminal velocity is reached. Surprisingly, cats that fall from heights greater than seven stories have a lower rate of injury. It is thought that after the cat has reached maximum velocity the vestibular apparatus is no longer stimulated by acceleration, the cat relaxes, and the limbs move into a more horizontal position, evenly distributing impact to the rest of the body.[2]

In a recent report, 90% of 115 cats treated for HRS survived. Thirty-seven percent of the cats required emergency treatment and all that did not survive died within 24 hours of examination, a fact that emphasizes the importance of emergency care.

The HRS patient poses a special challenge to the veterinarian. Many cats suffer respiratory distress because of pneumothorax and pulmonary contusions. Many are in shock and in pain because of multiple injuries sustained in the fall. The combination of dyspnea, shock, and pain in a cat can lead to maniacal thrashing and struggling. This can initiate a vicious cycle of more dyspnea and deeper shock, terminating in respiratory and cardiac arrest. Therefore, the emergency high-rise patient must be treated quickly and efficiently. Injuries must be prioritized to first treat the most life-threatening ones without causing further distress to the patient. If these principles are followed and combined with effective emergency care, successful treatment of HRS can be achieved.

Treatment Principles

Because of the multiple injuries seen with the HRS it is difficult to outline a standard treatment protocol. Each case must be carefully evaluated and treatment individualized. There are, however, important guidelines to follow when treating these cats.

Physical Examination

Treatment of the emergency high-rise patient begins with a brief physical examination concentrating on vital areas that are most often injured in falls. Respiratory patterns are observed before the cat is distressed with any other portion of the examination. For severe dyspnea, the respiratory distress should be relieved before the examination proceeds. If respiratory function is stable enough to allow further examination, the mucous membrane color, capillary refill time, heart rate, pulse quality, and temperature should be determined to evaluate the degree of shock. Cats in severe shock should have appropriate treatment initiated before the examination continues.

Only cats presented in stable cardiovascular and pulmonary condition should have a complete physical examination before treatment is instituted. The mouth should be inspected for dental fractures, a split hard palate, or mandibular fractures. The chest cavity should be auscultated, with special attention for the absence of respiratory sounds in the dorsal and caudal fields, which could indicate pneumothorax. This can be difficult if epistaxis and swollen, fractured nasal turbinates are creating loud upper respiratory tract sounds. The abdominal cavity should be carefully palpated for the presence of an intact urinary bladder, renal and splenic injuries, or free fluid. The spine should be palpated for areas of pain or malposition that might indicate a vertebral fracture or luxation. A brief neurologic examination to determine intact pain sensation and reflexes should be performed if spinal trauma is suspected. All limbs should be palpated to identify fractures or luxations. Inspection

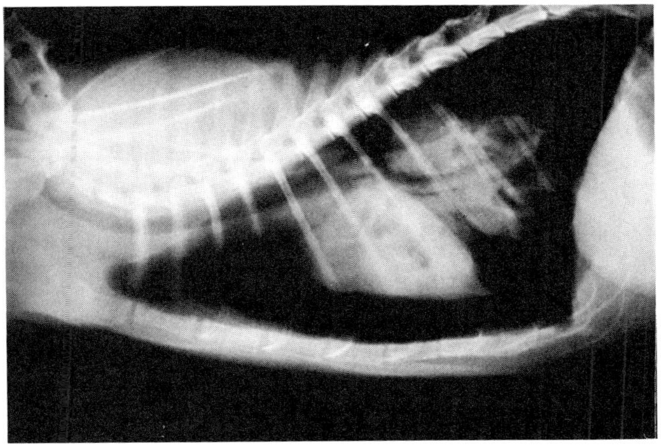

Figure 44–1. **Thoracic radiograph demonstrates pneumothorax with pulmonary atelectasis and elevation of the cardiac silhouette. Notice the intact pulmonary bullae. (Courtesy of Dr. Holly Mullen.)**

for abrasions, lacerations, and penetrating wounds of the abdominal or thoracic cavity completes the examination.

Thoracic Trauma

It has been reported that 90% of cats with HRS sustain pulmonary injuries.[2] Approximately two thirds are affected with pneumothorax, two thirds with pulmonary contusions, and one third with both of these injuries. (Fig. 44–1) Fifty-five percent of the cats in the same study exhibited abnormal respiratory patterns at presentation. Pneumothorax and shock are the most common and most immediately life-threatening and distressing injuries in HRS. Therefore, if a cat is dyspneic, both sides of the chest cavity should be aspirated to remove any free air. A small-gauge butterfly catheter can be placed in the ninth intercostal space approximately 5 to 6 cm ventral to the spine to remove the air from the caudodorsal area. A three-way stopcock can make evacuation of the thoracic cavity faster and easier. In many cases more than 75 mL of air may be removed from both sides of the chest.[2] In most cases a single aspiration will relieve the respiratory distress from the pneumothorax. A chest tube should be placed and secured if repeated aspirations (usually 3 or more) are needed to control dyspnea. However, chest tubes are rarely necessary.[1,2] If a cat is not dyspneic and physical examination or radiographs identify mild pneumothorax, thoracocentesis is not necessary. Pneumothorax of mild degree resolves with time and rest.

An oxygen mask should be placed over or near the mouth and nose of the patient during thoracocentesis, to increase the level of inspired oxygen. If the mask causes distress it should be abandoned. Stabilization in an oxygen cage, when available, is recommended after aspiration.

Although thoracic radiography can demonstrate pneumothorax, the stress of obtaining radiographs can be dangerous to a dyspneic cat. Because pneumothorax is so common in the HRS, it is recommended to attempt thoracocentesis and to stabilize dyspneic patients prior to radiography.[2]

Pulmonary contusions are identified with thoracic radiographs. Rest in a high oxygen tension environment while the alveolar spaces clear is recommended when contusions are severe.

Removing dried blood from around the nostrils may relieve some upper airway obstruction, and this should be done as the cat becomes more comfortable. This procedure should be abandoned if struggling aggravates the respiratory difficulty.

Pain and anxiety can compound the respiratory distress associated with thoracic trauma. Cats that are vocalizing, thrashing, and dyspneic are extremely difficult to treat and examine. The administration of analgesic medication to provide comfort while administering oxygen can calm the distressed cat enough to allow completion of thoracocentesis and effective stabilization of respiration. Butorphanol (Torbugesic) has been shown to be an effective and safe analgesic for cats when administered at doses of 0.1 to 0.2 mg/kg intravenously (IV) or 0.4 mg/kg subcutaneously (SC).[5] The use of analgesics in the management of the extremely frantic HRS patient may make the difference between a successful and an unsuccessful outcome.

Shock

Shock is a frequent finding in HRS. It has been reported to occur in 24% of 132 cats that fell from heights of two stories or more.[2] Shock is identified by pale mucous membranes, prolonged capillary refill time, elevated heart rate, weak peripheral pulses, and hypothermia. Shock should be treated with intravenous fluids and corticosteroids. For a dyspneic cat it is important to delay placement of the intravenous catheter until steps have been taken to relieve the respiratory distress and make the cat more comfortable and manageable. In these cases, thoracocentesis, oxygen, injectable analgesic medication, and rest in a quiet area of the hospital, calms these cats without seriously delaying the treatment of shock. Cats that are weak and recumbent or not suffering serious respiratory distress may undergo intravenous catheterization after examination. Catheters are usually placed in a cephalic or saphenous vein, but with multiple limb fractures placement of a jugular catheter, although usually more stressful, may be necessary.

Lactated Ringer's solution (LRS) is administered at a dose of 15 mL/kg IV in the first hour of treatment to the cat in severe shock. After the first hour of treatment the patient is reassessed and it is determined what additional fluid is needed. In most cases the fluid administration rate should be slowed after the first hour of treatment. Rapid fluid administration may be harmful to patients with severe pulmonary contusions, and fluids should be administered at a rate less than 15 mL/kg/h unless the cat is in severe shock. The total fluid volume administered should be monitored carefully in these patients.[2]

Corticosteroids should be administered in conjunction with intravenous fluids to the patient in shock. A rapidly acting corticosteroid such as prednisolone sodium succinate (Solu-Delta-Cortef) at a dose of 10 to 20 mg/kg is administered IV when the fluid drip is started. A longer-acting corticosteroid effective in treating central nervous system inflammation should be administered to cats that have evidence of more severe head trauma such as multiple facial injuries or abnormal mentation. Dexamethasone may be administered IV or intramuscularly (IM) in a single dose of 1 to 2 mg/kg. Dexamethasone is often continued at a dose of 0.05 mg/kg IM b.i.d. to t.i.d. for 24 to 48 hours to cats with severe head trauma.

In most cases IV fluids and corticosteroid therapy are sufficient treatment for shock in HRS. Occasionally shock from abdominal hemorrhage requires blood transfusion. Feline whole blood or packed red cells should be given IV through a blood administration filter (see Chapter 10). All hypothermic patients should be warmed to elevate the body temperature while the intravenous medications are administered. Lamps and heating pads must be used correctly to avoid burning the patient.

Abdominal Trauma

A significant amount of blunt abdominal trauma occurs with a fall from a substantial height. Abdominal injuries as a result of this trauma are surprisingly uncommon in cats. Rupture of the urinary bladder, rupture of the spleen or a liver lobe, or both, diaphragmatic hernia, and abdominal wall herniation are rare injuries.

Careful abdominal palpation, as the cat's respiratory and circulatory condition permits, is helpful in the identification of abdominal injuries. An intact urinary bladder can be felt to enlarge and fill with urine produced from the initial fluid and corticosteroid administration. If an intact urinary bladder is not palpable after IV fluid and corticosteroid administration, abdominal radiography should be performed if the cat is stable. Radiographs should be used to identify the silhouette of an intact urinary bladder or free abdominal fluid, which might indicate rupture with urine leakage. Abdominocentesis should be performed in all cats that have free abdominal fluid. Urine can be identified and distinguished from nonclotting blood by a high urea nitrogen content as identified by a blood urea nitrogen strip (Azostik, Miles, Inc., Elkhart, IN). A ruptured urinary bladder can be confirmed by a positive contrast cystogram (see Chapter 14). Surgical repair should be performed as soon as the cat's pulmonary and cardiovascular system are stable enough for general anesthesia. If thoracic injuries will not allow surgery, two to four ½-inch Penrose drains may be placed quickly through the caudal ventral abdominal wall to allow drainage of urine for cats that might not survive a more lengthy surgical procedure. These drains are bandaged with sterile, absorbent material and drain for 24 to 48 hours while pneumothorax and contusions resolve. Bandages should be changed two or three times daily. Cats with urinary bladder injuries should be given doses of IV fluids sufficient for diuresis before, during, and after surgery. Some cats have hematuria without a ruptured bladder, presumably the result of renal hemorrhage, bladder wall hemorrhage, or both. In these cases hematuria should resolve spontaneously in a few days.

Urinary bladder ruptures are rare in HRS cats, occurring in only 2% of 132 cats in one report.[2] It is presumed that cats usually urinate while falling and that the bladder is empty when the intraabdominal pressure is increased at impact.

Liver lobe or splenic tears should be suspected in extremely pale patients. Abdominal radiography and abdominocentesis can be used to identify hemoperitoneum. These cats usually respond to IV fluid and corticosteroid administration and rarely require blood transfusion or abdominal surgery to treat the hemorrhage. Abdominal pressure wraps that are sometimes used to treat shock and intra-abdominal hemorrhage should be avoided in HRS patients because of their poor tolerance of bandaging and the interference it creates for diaphragmatic excursions and ventilation.

Penetrating abdominal wall wounds or abdominal wall herniation are ocassionally part of the HRS. These are presumably the result of impalement by sharp objects in the free fall or with the increased abdominal pressure of impact. All wounds should be clipped, cleaned, and inspected after initiating shock treatment. Fresh wounds may be sutured after cleansing and débridement. Highly contaminated or infected wounds should be treated as open wounds and allowed to heal by secondary intention. Penetrating wounds may require exploratory laparatomy to inspect injury to abdominal organs and to facilitate abdominal cavity lavage. Broad-spectrum antibiotics should be administered in all cases. Abdominal wall hernias should be repaired as soon as pulmonary and cardiovascular systems are stable, to avoid possible abdominal organ entrapment and strangulation.

Diaphragmatic hernias are rare, presumably because thoracic and abdominal cavity pressure increase simultaneously with impact. Diaphragmatic hernias should be repaired after treatment of shock and stabilization for 24 hours if the cat's respiration is not severely compromised.

Cats should be placed in a high oxygen tension environment, if one is available. If the stomach is within the thorax, emergency surgery should be performed to reduce and repair the hernia. This is to avoid gastric dilatation with air and fatal respiratory compromise. The combination of pneumothorax and diaphragmatic hernia is usually rapidly fatal.[1]

Traumatic pancreatitis can occasionally be seen after a high-rise fall. It is usually identified a few days after the initial injury by palpation of increasing cranial abdominal fullness and firmness as adhesions form around the pancreas. Affected cats are extremely lethargic and anorectic but rarely vomit. Cats should be supported with intravenous fluids. Oral alimentation should be avoided until the cat's attitude improves and the pancreatic inflammation begins to subside. Bland food is gradually reintroduced at that time. HRS cats with traumatic pancreatitis have a guarded prognosis.

Spinal Injuries

Thoracic and lumbar vertebral fractures occur infrequently in high-rise accidents. Cats must be carefully evaluated to determine the degree of spinal cord trauma secondary to fracture displacement. Fractures should be temporarily stabilized after starting necessary treatment for respiratory distress and shock. It is difficult to make decisions about treatment or base a prognosis on the neurologic examination of a cat affected by shock, pain, or respiratory distress.

A body splint can be made with thick layered cotton bandage material and conforming roll gauze, reinforced with aluminum rod or fiberglass casting material, and secured with tape. Cats object to a full truncal bandage and usually require sedation for splinting. If the body splint causes excessive struggling or respiratory distress it should be quickly removed and the cat should be sedated and kept in a quiet area of the hospital to minimize movement. It is also important to make sure that the splint is immobilizing the fracture but still allows full chest excursions and does not interfere with respirations.

Corticosteroids should be administered to cats with spinal cord trauma. Methyl prednisolone sodium succinate (Solu-Medrol) should be given IV at an initial dose of 30 mg/kg. It is repeated at 2 and 6 hours at 15 mg/kg.

Definitive repair of the vertebral fracture should be based on the fracture type, location, inherent stability, and neurologic signs. Some fractures require internal stabilization, whereas other, more stable fractures may be managed conservatively with external support. Decisions for treatment of spinal trauma should be based on an accurate assessment of the cat's neurologic injuries. Cats that lack deep pain sensation after sufficient treatment of shock have a poor prognosis for walking, and euthanasia should be considered.

Orthopedic Trauma

Orthopedic trauma is common with high-rise falls. In one study of 132 cats, limb fractures occurred in 39%, luxations in 24%, hard palate fractures in 18%, mandibular fractures in 9%, and pelvic fractures in 3%.[2]

It is not the intent of this chapter to describe fracture repair. Numerous other texts are available for that purpose. The intent is to outline an approach to the management of HRS cats with orthopedic trauma and to describe injuries that may be common to HRS cats but are rare injuries from other forms of trauma.

Management Principles

It is essential to treat the most life-threatening problems first in HRS. Only after the initiation of treatment for respiratory distress and shock should a careful orthopedic evaluation be made. Each limb must be carefully palpated to identify fractures or luxations. Multiple long bone fractures or joint injuries of more than one limb are common. These cats are in pain, and inspection of orthopedic injuries may require analgesic medication to identify the extent of orthopedic injuries without causing unnecessary distress. The orthopedic examination should not cause dyspnea. In cats with severe thoracic trauma a thorough orthopedic examination may not be completed for 24 hours or more.

All suspect fractures or luxations should be radiographed when the cat is stabilized. The use of manual restraint, sedation, or general anesthesia to obtain the radiographs should be based on the physical condition and cooperation of the patient and the location and type of fracture.

Many orthopedic injuries require general anesthesia and surgical repair. It is important to allow for improvement of thoracic injuries and shock before attempting a definitive surgical repair. In cases of thoracic trauma, radiographs should be repeated every 24 to 48 hours to monitor improvements in pneumothorax and pulmonary contusions. Most cats benefit much from a 48-hour period of rest and support in the hospital.[1] No cat should be anesthetized or operated on before cardiovascular and pulmonary status are stabilized.

Limb Fractures and Luxations

Fractures or luxations below the elbow or stifle joints should be splinted. The support provides comfort to the patient and reduces the likelihood of further injury. A Robert-Jones bandage or laterally reinforced soft padded bandage is sufficient to immobilize injuries distal to the elbow and stifle while the cat is being stabilized for definitive repair. Fractures of the humerus or femur are rarely splinted, as they are more difficult to immobilize. If open humeral or femoral fractures are present, Schroeder-Thomas splints may be used to provide comfort and protect wounds. Spica splints are sometimes used for open humeral fractures, but they may not be tolerated by cats. For any open fracture the surrounding hair should be clipped and the skin surgically scrubbed. Wounds should be flushed with sterile saline to remove debris and decrease bacterial numbers. Exposed bone should be replaced within the soft tissues, to prevent desiccation and further contamination. Broad-spectrum antibiotics should be administered. Bandages should be changed and wounds should be scrubbed and flushed again at least every 12 to 24 hours until definitive repair is possible. Open fractures should be repaired as soon as the patient can be safely anesthetized.

A combination of ketamine (25 mg/kg) and Valium (1.25 mg/kg) may be mixed in a single syringe and administered IV to effect, to provide safe, short-acting anesthesia for splinting cats that are in pain and in stable cardiovascular condition. As an alternative, butorphanol may be administered IV at a dose of 0.1 to 0.2 mg/kg. This may be combined with a small dose of isoflurane or halothane and oxygen to provide more sedation for cats in serious pain. Cats that are depressed and in severe shock should not be chemically restrained but should have splints placed while their shock is treated.

Single or multiple metacarpal or metatarsal fractures may be repaired with coaptation. The use of a padded Mason metasplint for 4 to 6 weeks works well. Splints are usually changed every 10 to 14 days to avoid bandage complications. Intramedullary pin fixation is sometimes necessary in cases of nonunion.

Unilateral or bilateral carpal hyperextension and luxation is a common injury marked by carpal joint laxity, swelling, and pain with manipulation. Many carpi become stable with approximately 6 weeks of coaptation. The carpus should be maintained in slight flexion with an aluminum rod–reinforced splint or fiberglass cast. Carpal arthrodesis should be considered if laxity is apparent after appropriate splinting.

The radius was the long bone most often fractured in a study of 132 cats. In most cats the ulna also was broken (Fig. 44–2A,B).[2] Bilateral radial and ulnar fractures also occur. Radial fractures from high-rise falls usually occur from the midshaft diaphysis distally to the metaphysis. Midshaft fractures can heal with coaptation, but adequate reduction

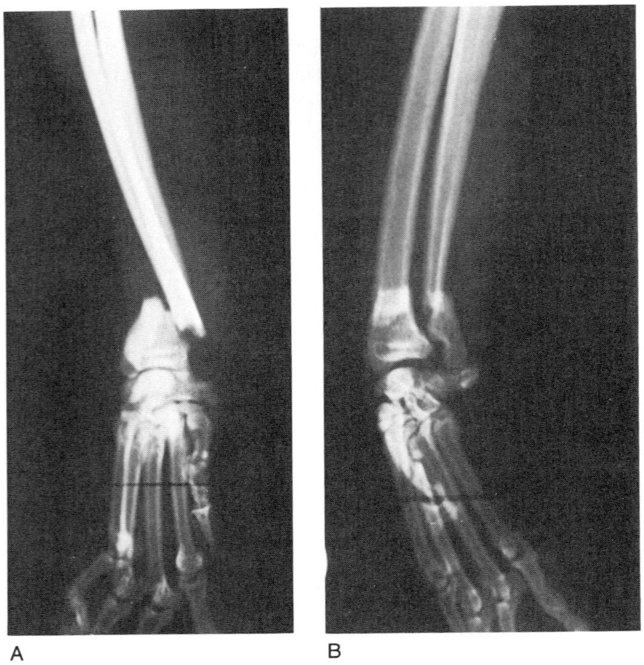

Figure 44–2. **(*A*) A typical distal radial and ulnar fracture. (*B*) Lateral view.**

must be maintained for the application of a cast or rigid splint. If midshaft fractures are not reducible with one third cortical contact or if they are not stable for casting, open reduction and internal fixation is recommended. Distal fractures of the radius require open reduction and internal fixation for best results. The ASIF four-hole mini-T plate for 2.0-mm screws or the six-hole veterinary mini-T plate for 1.5- or 2.0-mm screws (Synthes) provides excellent stability and fits the distal feline radius well.

The humerus is less commonly fractured in falls from high-rise buildings.[2] The distal articular surface can be disrupted by humeral condylar fractures. In most cases the weaker lateral component of the condyle is fractured, but medial condylar and intercondylar Y and T fractures are also seen. As with all articular fractures, open, anatomic reduction and rigid internal fixation provides the most satisfactory results.

Femoral fractures, which are common after high-rise falls, are most often seen in immature cats with open physes. Salter II fractures of the distal physis were the most common femur fracture identified in one report.[2] These fractures can be repaired with various intramedullary pinning techniques. Capital physeal injuries are treated by femoral head and neck excision arthroplasty, with very good results.

Fractures of the tibia and fibula are also common (Fig. 44–3*A,B*). These fractures can often be open, and cats should be carefully inspected for wounds that communicate with the fracture site. All open fractures should be treated appropriately, as described above. Broad-spectrum antibiotics should be administered, and fractures should be repaired as soon as the cat is stable, to lessen the likelihood of osteomyelitis. Open fractures are usually managed with rigid internal fixation or external skeletal fixation devices.

Comminuted fractures of the tarsal bones are seen occasionally. Anatomic reconstruction is usually impossible. External fixation with splints, casts, or external skeletal fixa-

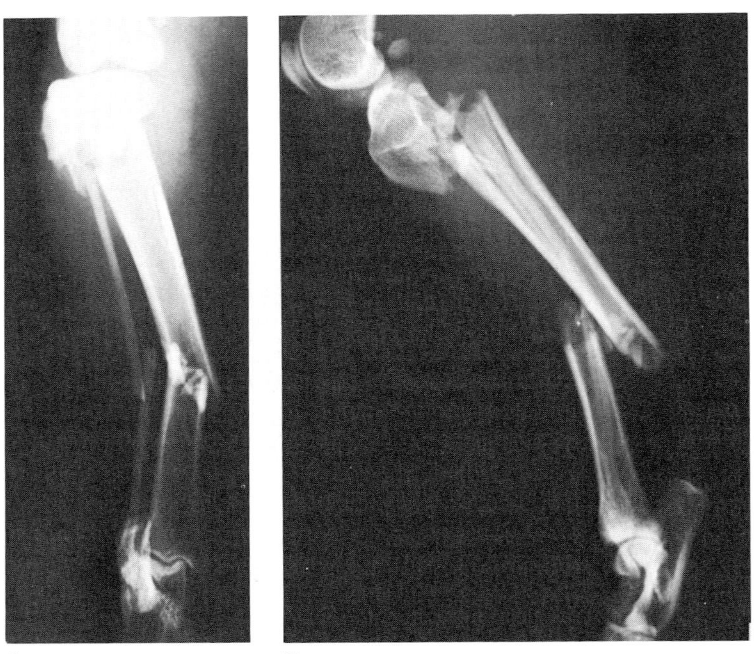

Figure 44–3. **(*A*) An open, severely comminuted, segmental tibial and fibular fracture. (*B*) Lateral view.**

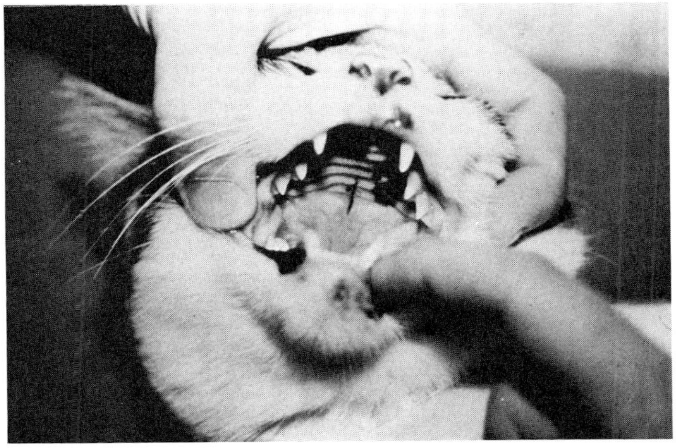

Figure 44–4. This cat suffered a split hard palate. Notice the chin and lip abrasions. (Courtesy of Dr. Holly Mullen.)

tion devices usually allow for healing with some compromise in joint mobility. If fractures are severely comminuted and the tibiotarsal joint surface is severely disrupted, tarsal arthrodesis is recommended.

Facial Trauma

Facial trauma is a common finding in HRS cats. The nasal planum, maxilla, and mandible hit the ground surface as the limbs break the fall. Epistaxis and abrasions of the lips and nose frequently occur. The hard palate is often split longitudinally on the midline (Fig. 44–4). Almost all palate defects heal by granulation and epithelial cell migration while cats are fed soft, canned food. Rarely is surgical intervention required to close oronasal fistulas. At least 1 month of conservative treatment should be attempted before the decision is made for surgical correction of palate defects in HRS.[2]

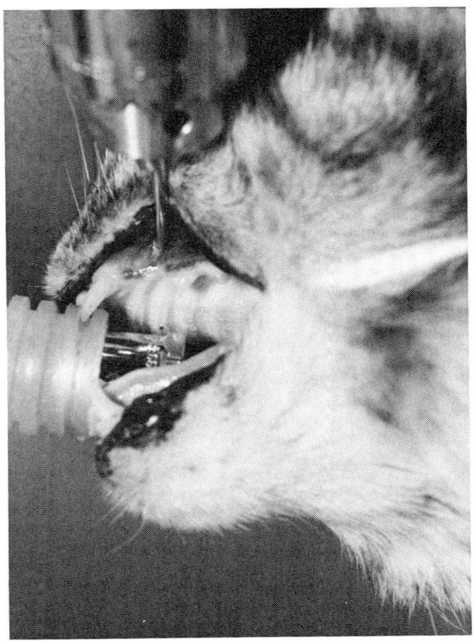

A

Figure 44–5. (*A*) A full maxillary-mandibular cerclage wire is passed to stabilize a temporomandibular luxation or caudal mandibular fractures. A hole is drilled just dorsal to the hard palate and caudal to the root of the canine tooth. (*B*) The Steinmann pin or drill bit exits the maxilla at the same location on the contralateral side. Twenty-gauge orthopedic wire is passed through this hole and placed in the intermandibular space, as for a mandibular cerclage wire. (*C*) The wire is tightened just enough to maintain interdigitation of the canine teeth, but it still allows prehension of food. This acts as an internally positioned muzzle.

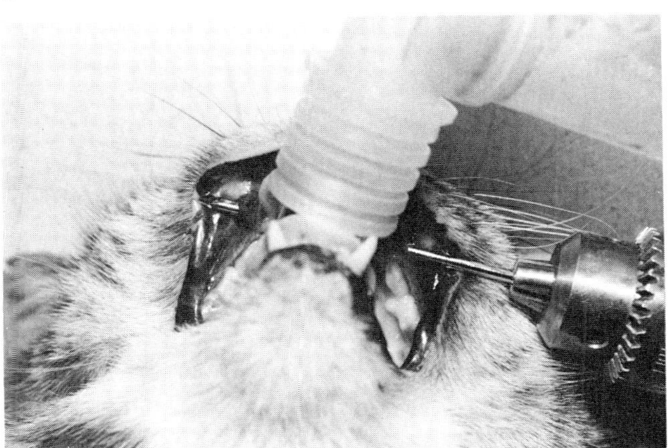

B

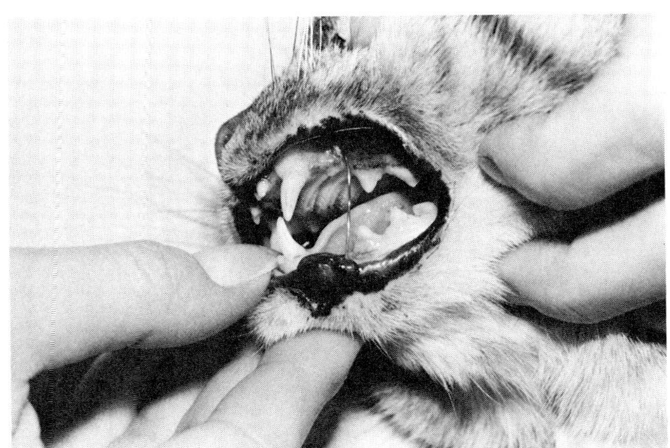

C

Mandibular fractures also occur. Symphyseal separation is common. Symphyseal separation can be easily repaired with a single 20-gauge, full cerclage wire placed subcutaneously around each mandible, caudal to the canine teeth with a twist knot made in the intermandibular space. The wire is left in place approximately 6 weeks. Unilateral and bilateral mandibular body fractures are also seen. Most mandibular body fractures require surgical correction with internal fixation or the use of an external skeletal fixator to maintain normal occlusion. Temporomandibular luxations are usually easy to reduce under general anesthesia with an approximately 5-mm rod (pen or pencil) placed in the caudal aspect of the mouth to act as a fulcrum between the molar teeth. The jaws are closed, causing separation of the temporomandibular joint. This allows the mandibular condyle to fit back into the mandibular fossa of the maxilla. If the mandible reluxates, an 18- or 20-gauge full cerclage wire placed through the maxilla and under the mandible just caudal to the canine teeth prevents the mouth from opening widely and maintains the interdigitation of the canine teeth (Fig. 44–5). Reduction of the temporomandibular joint is maintained by the wire and the interdigitating canine teeth, but the mouth is allowed to open enough for the cat to lap blended food. After approximately 4 weeks the wire is removed. If the cat is unable to eat, an esophagostomy tube may be placed (see Chapter 5).

Teeth should be inspected carefully for fractures. Canine teeth often are broken and the pulp cavity exposed. Any teeth with exposed pulp should be extracted or endodontically treated to prevent root abscess formation. Roots of teeth fractured below the gumline should be extracted[4] (see Chapter 33).

REFERENCES

1. Robinson GW. The high-rise trauma syndrome in cats. Feline Pract 1976;6:40.
2. Whitney WO, Mehlhaff CJ. High-rise syndrome in cats. J Am Vet Med Assoc 1987;191:1399.
3. Diamond JM. Why cats have nine lives. Nature 1988;332:586.
4. Kapatkin AS, Matthiesen DT. Feline high-rise syndrome. Compend Contin Educ, Small Anim Pract 1991;13:1389.
5. Sawyer DC, Rech RH. Analgesia and behavioral effects of butorphanol, nalbuphine, and pentazocine in the cat. J Am Anim Hosp Assoc 1987;23:438.

CHAPTER 45

◇ ◇ ◇

Hyperesthesia Syndrome

James R. Cook, Jr.

Feline hyperesthesia syndrome (also called neurodermatitis) is a relatively rare condition that can affect male and female cats of any age or breed.[1] Siamese cats may be somewhat more predisposed than others.[2]

Since the cause is unknown, numerous empirical treatments have been suggested. Success of therapy is variable.

Clinical Signs

The cat with hyperesthesia syndrome is typically healthy and without overt signs of systemic disease. It may be an excessively nervous or excitable animal, or it may have a recent history of environmental changes that lead to emotional distress.

Manifestations include episodic rippling of the skin over the back, twitching of the tail, and biting, scratching, and licking at the back, flanks, axillae, inguinal regions, and the tailhead. This behavior may be precipitated by petting or stroking. Tail chasing, painful response to stroking, and hallucinatory behavior may also be present. These responses may appear to be compulsive and almost uncontrollable. In severe cases, persistent licking, scratching, and biting may result in alopecia, surface trauma to the skin, and lichenification of the affected areas.

Differential Diagnosis

The differential diagnoses include any conditions that would result in persistent skin irritation, episodic abnormal behavior, back pain, or paresthesia.

Skin irritation and pruritus are common in the cat; ectoparasites, allergic skin disease, infectious diseases (pyodermas), and anal sacculitis should be considered, as well as manifestations of the eosinophilic granuloma complex (see Chapters 56 to 60).

Alterations in behavior that mimic the hyperesthesia syndrome might be produced by psychomotor seizure activity or unusual manifestations of female estrus behavior.

Back pain in cats can be caused by numerous diseases, including meningeal irritation (lymphoma, infectious meningitis), intervertebral disk herniation, discospondylitis, cellulitis or abscesses from bite wounds, and nerve root compression from hypertrophic bone in hypervitaminosis A.

Paresthesia (abnormal or altered sensation resulting in perceived irritation without noxious stimuli) is rare in cats. The most likely organic cause of such a situation would be polyneuritis, which is both rare and poorly characterized in cats.

Diagnosis

Since there is no specific test for the hyperesthesia syndrome, the thrust of diagnostic efforts is directed at eliminating as many disorders in the differential diagnoses as possible while making the best possible case for hyperesthesia syndrome.

The history should be examined for causes of emotional distress, including a new home, new pets or children, or loss of a favorite companion, either human, feline, or canine. The owner should also provide as much dietary information as possible.

The physical examination should be thorough, with special care taken to note the presence of parasites, evidence of allergic skin disease or infectious pyoderma, and the condition of the anal sacs. Fever may indicate an infection. The retinas should be examined closely for inflammatory changes, which would also incriminate an infectious agent.

A complete neurologic examination should also be performed at the initial presentation; localizing neurologic deficits would indicate the presence of a primary nervous system abnormality that might possibly explain the symptoms.

At this point, given an appropriate history and a lack of physical evidence of other disease processes, the hyperesthesia syndrome should be strongly suspected. Ancillary tests to rule out other possibilities would include a complete blood count (CBC), skin biopsy of the affected area, survey radiographs of the spine, and blood or serum tests for feline leukemia virus (FeLV), feline immunodeficiency virus (FIV), feline infectious peritonitis (FIP) virus, cryptococcosis, and toxoplasmosis.

If nothing is found to point toward another primary disease process, treatment should be initiated (see following section). If treatment is unsuccessful, referral to a specialty practice or university teaching hospital should be considered. At these institutions, advanced diagnostic procedures such as nuclear imaging, cerebrospinal fluid (CSF) collection and analysis, myelography, electromyography, and sensory and motor nerve conduction studies can be performed as needed.

Treatment

Since there is not a specific definitive cause for this syndrome, therapy is based on providing the most stable physical and emotional environment possible for the patient and utilizing chemical behavior modification. The following regimen has been recommended,[3] and I have found it to be beneficial in most cases, although it is not considered curative.

- Relieve any obvious emotional frustrations, and try to analyze and solve other behavior problems. Consultation with a veterinary behaviorist may be very helpful.
- Provide a balanced diet that is as free as possible from preservatives and artificial chemicals. Balanced vitamin and mineral supplements may be beneficial, particularly if there is history of poor nutrition.
- Give oral megestrol acetate (5 to 10 mg daily) for 1 week. Then give half the original dose daily for 1 month. Give alternate-day therapy (5 mg) for an additional month, followed by 5 mg every third or fourth day. Permanent intermittent therapy may be needed; however, there is significant risk of diabetes mellitus and malignant mammary neoplasia in cats treated with long-term megestrol acetate. (See Chapter 7 for a detailed discussion of the rational use of megestrol acetate.)

  Alternatively, prednisolone or prednisone may be used in place of megestrol acetate. The dose is 10 mg orally every day for 2 weeks, then 5 mg daily for 2 weeks, followed by 5 mg every 2 to 4 days, as needed.
- Give oral phenobarbital (1 mg per pound twice daily) *or* oral diazepam (2 mg two to four times daily), which may help control emotional distress and modify the undesirable behavior.

Conclusion

While the feline hyperesthesia syndrome is an uncommon entity, the diagnosis is usually easy to make from the history and typical clinical findings. Laboratory tests routinely available to most veterinary practices can eliminate the majority of diseases that may mimic the feline hyperesthesia syndrome. Treatment, although not considered curative, can provide long-term relief of signs.

Veterinarians should keep in mind that since no specific cause has been established for this syndrome it may actually represent several different diseases that have similar manifestations. In some cases the manifestations of feline hyperesthesia might represent the onset or early stage of a condition in the differential diagnosis, before positive reactions develop to routine tests. For this reason serial evaluations or referral to a specialty institution for more exhaustive examination should be considered in difficult cases.

REFERENCES

1. Scott DW. Diseases of the Skin. In: Sherding RG, ed. The Cat: Diseases and Clinical Management. New York: Churchill Livingstone, 1989:1529.
2. Muller GH, Kirk RW. Neurodermatitis (Localized). In: Muller GH, Kirk RW, eds. Small Animal Dermatology. 2nd ed. Philadelphia: WB Saunders, 1976:530.
3. Tuttle J. Feline hyperesthesia syndrome. Vet Professional Topics, Urbana, IL: University of Illinois, 1979:2.

CHAPTER 46

◇ ◇ ◇

Hyperthyroidism

Jane M. Turrel and Gary D. Norsworthy

Hyperthyroidism, the most commonly diagnosed endocrine disease of the cat, was virtually unknown and unrecorded in the veterinary literature before 1980.[1] The recent appearance of this disease has been verified by review of histopathologic preparations of thyroid tissues from cats in the preceding two decades by at least two institutions. This information has initiated a wave of speculation concerning etiology; a dietary factor is the most likely possibility.

In cats, hyperthyroidism is caused by multinodular adenomatous hyperplasia, functional adenomas, or functional carcinomas of thyroid tissue. These three forms are difficult to differentiate histologically. In this chapter only thyroid adenomas and thyroid carcinomas are considered, because adenomatous hyperplasia of the thyroid gland behaves in the same fashion as thyroid adenoma. Thyroid adenomas involve both lobes in 70% of cases and one lobe in 30% of cases.[2] Malignant thyroid tumors (usually involving one lobe) have an estimated prevalence of 3% to 5%.[3,4] Although most cats with hyperthyroidism are elderly (average age, 14 years), treatment to restore a euthyroid state is rewarding and feasible.

Clinical Signs

Although historical and physical findings of feline hyperthyroidism are usually numerous, occasionally only a single sign will be present.[1,2,5,6] Weight loss is the most common finding and may be profound; up to 50% of body weight may be lost in a relatively short time. Weight loss of more than a few ounces in older cats should prompt investigation for this disease. A cat with undiagnosed hyperthyroidism that is placed on a reducing diet for other reasons may not be suspected of having hyperthyroidism until the weight reduction goal has been exceeded. Owners may also believe that weight loss is an expected geriatric characteristic. Typically, a brisk to ravenous appetite is observed in cats that were previously finicky eaters.

Integumentary changes include an unkempt, greasy, easily matted hair coat. Excessive shedding is often noted. The hair coat may change color, typically to reddish or brownish. Hair may be lost in clumps during grooming, although excessive grooming without significant hair loss is more common. Long-haired cats previously easily groomed are commonly seen clinically with heavily matted coats. The ears and feet may feel warm because of peripheral vasodilation.

Vomiting is common and is usually related to hair balls resulting from excessive shedding or grooming, increased intestinal motility, or a voracious appetite that causes gastric overdistention. Stools may have a fetid odor, change to a pale gray color, and become voluminous. The frequency of defecation is increased. In occasional cats the change in stool character may progress to diarrhea.

Polydipsia and polyuria are frequently noted clinical signs. Many cats will double their water consumption and seek unusual sources of water such as bathtub or sink faucets. Owners may notice the need to change the litter pan more frequently because of increased urination.

Behavior and personality changes are seen in 20% to 30% of affected cats. Classic hyperthyroidism is characterized by hyperactivity and restlessness. Most owners reject the concept of hyperactivity until they are reminded that it is unusual for an older cat to be awake for more than a few hours a day. On presentation, hyperthyroid cats are difficult to control because of increased activity. Some cats become aggressive, often attacking and biting. Other cats become more affectionate and seek more attention. Inappropriate defecation or urination have been reported. The owner may report that the cat hides in unusual locations in the house or has become withdrawn. One striking sign associated with hyperthyroidism is increased vocalization, often when the cat is alone in a room. Owners may ascribe this behavior to senility. Some cats will change sleeping locations from sunny or warm areas to cool bare floors or shady areas because of increased peripheral circulation.

A small number of cats have an apathetic form of hyperthyroidism, with clinical signs markedly different from those of typical feline hyperthyroidism.[2,5,6] The predominant signs are poor appetite or anorexia, extreme emaciation, and marked lethargy and weakness. These signs may or may not be preceded by the classic signs of hyperthyroidism. Some cats have congestive heart failure and/or cervical ventroflexion. Apathetic hyperthyroidism is much more serious than the classic form and necessitates immediate definitive treatment as well as good supportive care if the cat is to survive.

Diagnosis

Physical Examination

Palpation of the thyroid gland is an essential part of the physical examination and should be performed on all cats regardless of age. The normal thyroid gland is a bilobed structure, with no connecting isthmus, located on either side of the trachea just caudal to the larynx. The two lobes are not palpable in normal cats. Most cats with overt signs of hyperthyroidism have at least one palpable thyroid lobe. Frequently one lobe is larger than the other; the larger lobe usually gravitates caudally into the ventral cervical region. Markedly enlarged thyroid lobes may be located in the thoracic inlet or even in the cranial mediastinum. The disease is not always bilateral, so both sides of the trachea should be carefully palpated.

To properly palpate the thyroid gland, the examiner places the cat in a standing position with the head and neck extended. The examiner's thumb and index finger are placed on either side of the trachea at the thoracic inlet and gently slid toward the larynx. Enlarged thyroid lobes will slip under the finger or thumb as the hand is advanced cranially. Because the thyroid lobes are usually located on the dorsolateral aspect of the trachea, palpation of the ventral aspect of the trachea may miss a mildly to moderately enlarged lobe.

Thyroid tumors may elude palpation because of their location dorsolateral to the trachea, gravitation of tumors through the thoracic inlet into the cranial mediastinum, or inexperience of the veterinarian. Therefore, hyperthyroidism cannot be ruled out on the basis of palpation alone. Conversely, palpation of one or both thyroid lobes is abnormal and should be investigated further.

Cardiovascular Findings

Hyperthyroid cats have a variety of cardiac abnormalities, including tachycardia, premature beats, gallop rhythm, and systolic murmurs. In one study only 30% of hyperthyroid cats had normal cardiac function.[2] Clinical signs associated with feline hyperthyroidism include tachycardia, dyspnea, and systolic murmurs, but these signs can also be seen with hypertrophic cardiomyopathy. Approximately 50% of cats with hyperthyroidism will have radiographic evidence of cardiomegaly, but echocardiography usually shows hyperdynamic function of the myocardium rather than the findings associated with cardiomyopathy. Cats with concurrent cardiomyopathy and hyperthyroidism may have signs of heart failure, including pleural or pericardial effusion and pulmonary edema.

Recent studies have shown that 80% of hyperthyroid cats are also hypertensive.[7] Clinical signs of hypertension include venous distention, hyperemic pinnae, polyuria, polydipsia, and tachycardia. The kidneys are usually small.

Thyroxine Testing

The most reliable and widely used diagnostic test for feline hyperthyroidism is radioimmunoassay for serum thyroxine (T_4) concentrations. This test is available in commercial veterinary laboratories. Each laboratory has established a normal range for cats for the particular assay used; therefore, blood values are not interchangeable between laboratories. Hyperthyroid cats may have serum T_4 concentrations 30 times higher than normal, or, in older cats, in the high normal reference range. Normal T_4 concentrations in older euthyroid cats are typically near the low end of the normal reference range; a T_4 concentration in the middle or high end of the reference range is atypical. If abnormal T_4 values are found in conjunction with an enlarged thyroid nodule, further diagnostic testing should be performed.

Serum T_4 concentrations fluctuate from day to day and hour to hour, with greater variation over a 15-day period than over a 10-hour period.[8] The degree of fluctuation can result in a normal serum T_4 concentration one day and a high serum T_4 concentration the next. Many nonthyroidal diseases can lower serum T_4 concentrations, but the severity of the depression is directly related to the seriousness of the disease rather than to the disease itself.[9] Lowered serum T_4 concentrations can occur with any disease that causes systemic illness of several days' duration.

Hemolysis of a blood sample will decrease serum T_4 levels because of the presence of thyroxine-binding substances from red blood cells. Therefore, serum T_4 concentrations should be determined on a nonhemolyzed sample.

A test for qualitative determination of serum T_4 concentrations is commercially available for veterinarians to perform in their hospital (CITE Semi-Quant T4 Test Kit, IDEXX Corp, Portland, ME). The results are scored as hypothyroid, euthyroid, or hyperthyroid. This test is adequate as a screening test in highly suspicious cases of hyperthyroidism but is not adequate for assessing response to treatment or for detecting marginally elevated serum T_4 concentrations.

Technetium-99m Pertechnetate Thyroid Scanning

The most reliable procedure for establishing the diagnosis of hyperthyroidism in cats is the technetium-99m (^{99m}Tc) pertechnetate thyroid scan.[2,5,10] The test is simple and easily performed. Approximately 1 to 3 mCi of ^{99m}Tc is injected intravenously (IV). The radioisotope is trapped in the iodine-seeking tissues of the body—the thyroid gland, salivary glands, and gastric mucosa. At 20 to 60 minutes after injection the body is imaged using a radiation-detecting gamma camera. Normal thyroid lobes and the salivary glands should accumulate approximately the same amount of ^{99m}Tc and be approximately the same size and intensity on the scan (Fig. 46–1). Findings typical of hyperthyroidism are (1) increased uptake in the thyroid gland relative to salivary tissue and (2) increased thyroid lobe size.

From the scan images, one can determine unilateral versus bilateral disease, the relative size of the affected thyroid lobes, the presence of functional ectopic thyroid tissue, and the presence of malignancy. If one thyroid lobe is involved, thyroidal uptake of radioisotope will occur on that side; the normal contralateral lobe will be atrophied and will not trap ^{99m}Tc (Fig. 46–2). The vast majority of cats will have bilateral thyroid adenomas; some will have symmetric lobe involvement and others will have asymmetric disease. Ectopic thyroid tissue is rarely seen in hyperthyroid cats

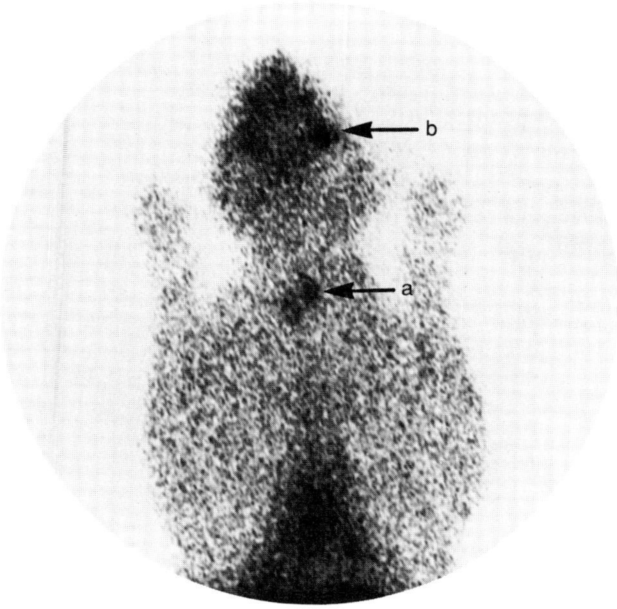

Figure 46–1. Radionuclide scan for diagnosing hyperthyroidism. Normal thyroid lobes (*a*) and the salivary glands (*b*) should accumulate approximately the same amount of ^{99m}Tc and should be approximately the same size and intensity on the scan.

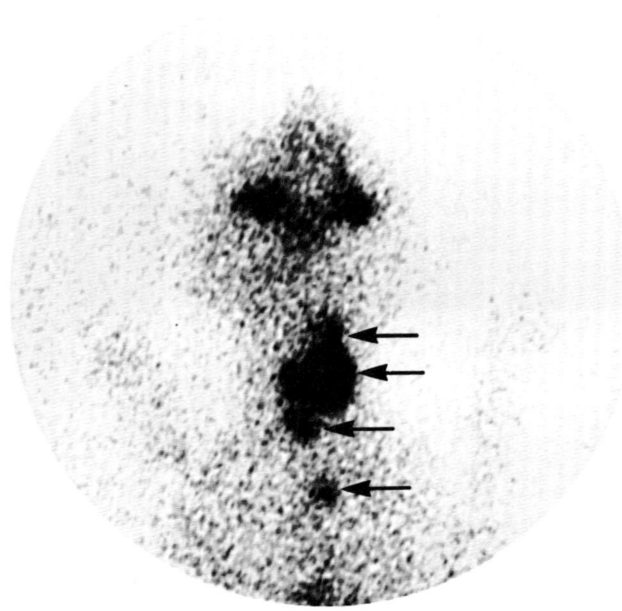

Figure 46–3. Multiple areas of increased radioisotope uptake are seen throughout the cervical region in a cat with confirmed metastatic thyroid carcinoma. Most thyroid carcinomas are functional—that is, capable of producing thyroid hormone—and can readily be identified by thyroid imaging.

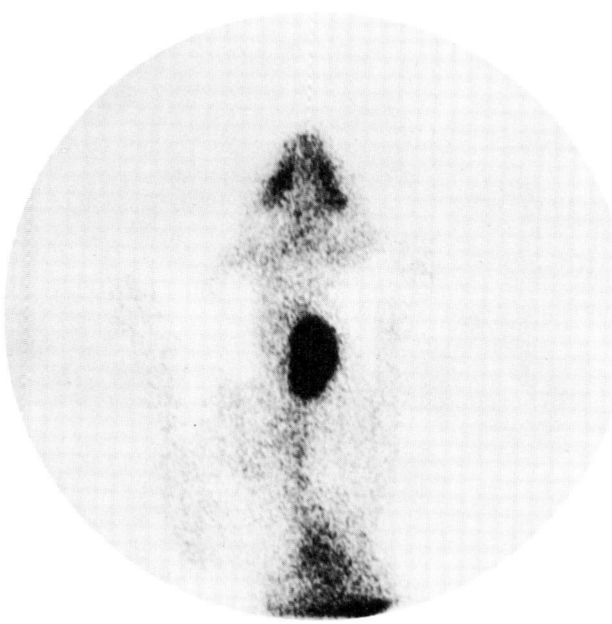

Figure 46–2. ^{99m}Tc scan of a thin, hyperthyroid cat showing a large unilateral thyroid lobe in the left caudal cervical region and cranial mediastinum. No uptake has occurred in the right thyroid region, indicating that all thyroid tissue in this lobe is normal and as a result has atrophied, and will not trap ^{99m}Tc or iodine.

because it will be atrophied unless a functional tumor is also present in the ectopic tissue.

Malignant thyroid tumors have a high rate of metastasis. Metastases appear as multiple nodules distributed throughout the neck and cranial mediastinum (Fig. 46–3). Other common sites of metastases include lung, liver, and bone. Metastatic nodules are usually functional and easily identifiable on the scan. Malignant nonfunctional thyroid tumors are rare and will not trap radioisotope. In some cats, the opposite thyroid lobe may contain a functional benign tumor.

Serum Biochemistry

Although several changes have been noted on serum chemistry profiles of hyperthyroid cats, the only consistent changes are mild to moderate elevations of liver enzymes (serum alkaline phosphatase, serum alanine aminotransferase, serum aspartate aminotransferase).[2,6] These elevations are related to the high metabolic rate of the cat and usually are not caused by pathologic changes in the liver.

Renal disease often occurs simultaneously with hyperthyroidism and may or may not be caused by the hyperthyroidism. Because most cats with hyperthyroidism are older, preexisting renal disease may be exacerbated by the metabolic changes of hyperthyroidism. Some cats will develop renal failure due to renal hypertension. Regardless of the etiology, biochemical changes commonly seen include high normal to elevated blood urea nitrogen levels, high normal to elevated creatinine levels, and elevated serum phosphorus levels. Urinalysis is helpful in detecting early renal disease. A specific gravity of less than 1.035 should increase the index of suspicion and prompt the clinician to recommend further renal testing.

Tests for Borderline Cases

Some cats will have clinical signs of hyperthyroidism before serum T_4 concentrations exceed the normal reference range. Several methods of detecting these small, autonomously functioning thyroid nodules have been advocated. Perhaps the most definitive test is the ^{99m}Tc thyroid scan. Other hormone assays and provocative tests may be helpful when thyroid imaging is unavailable; these are described below.

The triiodothyronine (T_3) suppression test aids in the diagnosis of hyperthyroidism in cats with marginally elevated serum T_4 concentrations.[11,12] Exogenous T_3—liothyronine—administered over a short period of time will suppress normal thyroid hormone production by the negative feedback mechanism from the pituitary gland and hypothalamus. Functioning thyroid tumors are autonomous and therefore are not suppressed.

The T_3 suppression test begins by obtaining and storing serum for baseline T_3 and T_4 concentration determinations. The cat is given 12.5 to 30 μg of liothyronine (Cytobin, Cytomel) orally every 8 hours for seven doses. Approximately 2 to 4 hours after the last dose, a second serum sample is obtained. Both serum samples, which must be nonhemolyzed, are submitted at the same time for T_3 and T_4 concentration determinations. Simultaneous specimen submission eliminates interassay variation.

The results of the T_3 suppression test must be interpreted with care. If the postsuppression T_4 level is greater than 50% of the baseline T_4 level or less than 1.5 μg/dL, the cat is considered normal. If the postsuppression T_4 level is greater than 50% of the baseline T_4 level or greater than 1.5 g/dL, the cat is considered hyperthyroid from autonomously functioning thyroid tissue. Borderline results are not diagnostic of hyperthyroidism. If results are equivocal, the cat should be retested in a month or more, or should undergo a thyroid scan. T_3 concentrations should be greater than baseline values in all cases. If they are not, the exogenous T_3 was not properly administered or absorbed, and the test results are invalid. If concomitant disease is present, T_4 values will be depressed. Therefore, interpretation of the test results should take into account the cat's overall health.

Preliminary work with a thyrotropin-releasing hormone (TRH) stimulation test indicates that this provocative procedure may have some value in detecting hyperthyroidism in cats with marginally high serum T_4 concentrations.[13] Blood is collected for serum T_4 and T_3 concentration determinations before and 4 hours after administration of TRH at a dosage of 0.1 mg/kg IV. Normal cats should have a poststimulation elevation in T_4 concentrations of 60% to 310%. All but one of 21 hyperthyroid cats tested with this method had a T_4 elevation of less than 60%.[13]

The T_3 concentration is rarely elevated when the T_4 concentration is normal, so that routine testing of T_3 is not warranted.[11] A thyroid-stimulating hormone (TSH) response test is useful for evaluating thyroid function in the dog, but TSH is very expensive and only intermittently available. Theoretically, serum TSH concentrations would be undetectable in hyperthyroid cats because of the negative feedback mechanism of T_4 on hypothalamic production of TRH and pituitary production of TSH. However, no standardized testing method has been established for the cat, and no assay for determining feline TSH concentrations exists at this time.

Differential Diagnosis and Concurrent Diseases

Many other diseases produce the signs of hyperthyroidism or can occur simultaneously and be obscured because of the similarity of signs. Diabetes mellitus, mild chronic renal disease, inflammatory bowel disease, and hypertension are the most common diseases producing at least some signs similar to those of feline hyperthyroidism. Most of the signs of these diseases will be exacerbated by even mildly elevated serum T_4 concentrations. Elimination of hyperthyroidism will often facilitate control or cause remission of these concurrent diseases.

Potentially fatal concomitant diseases need to be diagnosed before definitive treatment for hyperthyroidism is undertaken. These diseases may include lymphosarcoma of the abdominal viscera, other neoplasms of the viscera, severe renal disease, and cardiomyopathy. Treatment for hyperthyroidism should not be delayed while the clinician is searching for concomitant disease. If other disease is suspected, antithyroid drugs to temporarily control hyperthyroidism are indicated while further diagnostic testing occurs.

The best strategy for detecting concurrent disease is a complete physical examination that includes examination of the oral cavity for infection, dental disease, and neoplasia, auscultation of the heart and lungs, and thorough palpation of the abdominal cavity. A complete blood cell (CBC) count, serum biochemistry profile, and urinalysis constitute the minimum data base. Abdominal and thoracic radiographs may be indicated based on the physical examination findings. Further testing may include examination of the abdomen and heart by ultrasound or electrocardiography.

Initial Treatment

After the diagnosis of hyperthyroidism has been made, the owner should be advised of treatment options. If the cat is seriously ill from hyperthyroidism or concurrent disease, it should be stabilized before definitive treatment is undertaken. If the cat is asymptomatic or in stable condition, definitive treatment can be instituted immediately.

Antithyroid drugs are indicated for cats seriously ill with hyperthyroidism.[2,5,14] Propylthiouracil and methimazole are commonly used to counteract excess thyroid production. Methimazole is used more frequently because it produces fewer side-effects. Both drugs act by preventing thyroid hormone synthesis and can result in a return to euthyroidism in 1 to 2 weeks. The initial dose of methimazole is 2.5 to 5.0 mg given orally b.i.d. to t.i.d., but is dependent on the T_4 concentration. After 1 to 2 weeks of antithyroid drug therapy, the cat's medical condition should stabilize, and the T_4 concentration should return to the normal range. If it does not, the dose, interval, and duration of methimazole therapy should be adjusted. Cats that are stable after 1 to 2 weeks of therapy should receive radioiodine treatment or should undergo thyroidectomy.

Regardless of treatment modality, if tachycardia or other cardiac arrhythmias are present, propranolol should be given at a dosage of 2.5 to 5.0 mg b.i.d. to t.i.d. Other treatments, including antihypertensive drugs and uremic therapy, may be indicated.

Definitive Treatment

Radioiodine

Radioiodine (^{131}I) treatment is the safest and most effective treatment for feline hyperthyroidism and is the treatment of choice[2,5,15] ^{131}I has a half-life of 8 days and emits a spectrum of beta and gamma radiation. It is actively trapped and incorporated into functional thyroid tumors but does not accumulate in atrophied, normal thyroid tissue. Therefore, normal thyroid tissue, as well as the parathyroid glands and other surrounding tissues, are spared the effects of irradiation.

The dose of ^{131}I activity administered is based on the serum T_4 concentration, the size of the thyroid tumor on palpation and thyroid scan, and the likelihood of malignancy according to the thyroid scan. Activities of ^{131}I administered for benign tumors range from 1 to 15 mCi, and the drug is given IV. The dose of ^{131}I for malignant tumors ranges from 15 to 30 mCi. Antithyroid drugs must be discontinued 5 to 7 days before ^{131}I treatment to prevent lowered uptake and accelerated excretion of ^{131}I. If the cat's condition is so fragile that discontinuation of antithyroid drugs before treatment is not feasible,^{131}I is given at a higher dose to counteract the effects of these drugs.

Many facilities have the expertise, equipment, and radioisotopic license necessary perform ^{131}I treatment safely and effectively. Many hyperthyroid cats can be readily transported to these referral centers. Scanning and treatment takes only a few hours. After treatment, cats quickly show an improvement in clinical condition, followed by a reduction in T_4 production (Fig. 46–4).[16] Cats treated with radioiodine are usually hospitalized for 6 to 21 days, depending on the radiation safety rules of the state in which they are treated, so that radioactive excreta can be collected and disposed of properly. The major disadvantage of ^{131}I treatment is the hospitalization time required. No treatment-specific side-effects occur. Normal thyroid tissue and parathyroid glands are spared, and normal thyroid function returns within 1 month after treatment.

Cats with thyroid carcinoma given therapeutic doses of radioiodine will have complete ablation of all thyroid tissue and will require lifelong thyroid supplementation and frequent monitoring to ensure tumor control. Long-term remission and good quality of life are the usual results; only rarely will such cats die of recurrent or persistent malignancy.[2,3]

Approximately 2% of cats with benign thyroid disease given an individualized dose (i.e., a dose selected for the tumor and the cat) need a second treatment to eliminate the tumor. Another 2% develop hypothyroidism after radioiodine treatment; this is easily treated with T_4 supplementation. Recurrence of hyperthyroidism after successful treatment is rare, occurs 2 to 8 years after initial treatment, and is usually associated with a malignant thyroid tumor.

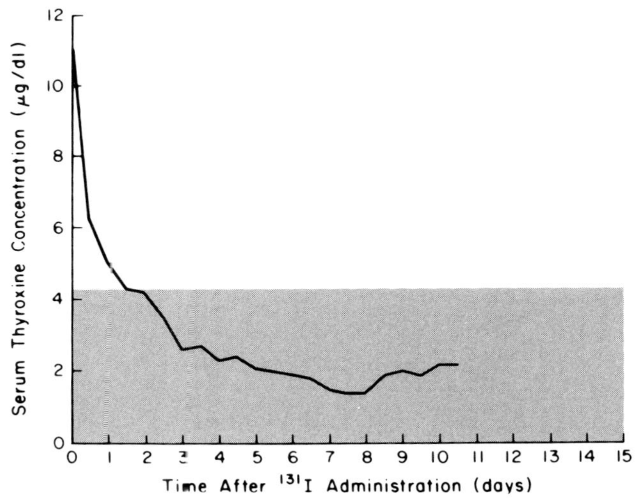

Figure 46–4. **Serum thyroxine concentrations in ten hyperthyroid cats from which blood was collected at 12-hour intervals after ^{131}I administration. Shaded region represents normal reference range (0.4–4.2 µg/dL). (Reproduced with permission from Meric SM, Hawkins EC, Washabau RJ, Turrel JM, Feldman EC. Serum thyroxine concentrations after radioactive iodine therapy in cats with hyperthyroidism. J Am Vet Med Assoc 1986;188(9):1038.)**

Thyroidectomy

Thyroidectomy, another therapeutic option, may be performed by practitioners with reasonable surgical skills. Ideally, a preoperative thyroid scan should be performed to identify which thyroid lobes are involved and the location of all the abnormal tissue. In reality, however, few cats are scanned before thyroidectomy, so the decision to remove one or both lobes is based on the gross appearance of the thyroid lobe(s) at the time of surgery.

The metabolic and cardiovascular effects of hyperthyroidism pose special considerations for surgery; these are listed in Table 46–1.

Surgical thyroidectomy may entail a unilateral thyroidectomy, a bilateral thyroidectomy, or a staged bilateral thyroidectomy.[17,18] Either an extracapsular or intracapsular technique may be used. The intracapsular technique involves peeling the thyroid tissue from the capsule while leaving intact the blood supply to the parathyroid glands. The extracapsular technique involves removing the entire thyroid lobe while leaving the external parathyroid gland (see Chapter 55).

Unilateral thyroidectomy is performed in cats with unilateral thyroid tumors identified on ^{99m}Tc thyroid scan or on inspection of the thyroid lobes at surgery. Because only one lobe is removed, the cat is unlikely to become hypothyroid or hypocalcemic. However, the probability that adenomatous tissue already exists or will develop in the opposite lobe approaches 70%, so a second surgery may be indicated.

Table 46–1. Special Precautions for Surgery on Hyperthyroid Cats

1. Avoid ketamine and xylazine.
2. Preanesthetize with acepromazine or acepromazine-oxymorphone.
3. Avoid anticholinergics. If an anticholinergic must be used, glycopyrrolate is preferred.
4. Induce with a thiobarbiturate.
5. Isoflurane anesthesia is preferred, although halothane is acceptable.
6. If intraoperative tachycardia develops, give propranolol: dilute to 0.1 mg/mL and give 0.1 mL every 2–3 minutes until the heart rate slows to 160 beats/min.
7. Because hyperthyroid cats may maintain a high body temperature, use external heat with caution.

Bilateral thyroidectomy is performed when both lobes are determined to be affected. This surgery can be performed simultaneously or in staged procedures separated by an interval of 3 to 5 weeks. Staged surgical procedures reduce the likelihood of hypoparathyroidism. Theoretically, a minor disruption of the vascular supply to the parathyroid gland on one side will self-correct in the interval between the two operations. One report found no difference in the complication rates between single procedure and a staged procedure.[17] However, staged procedures may be very advantageous to practitioners who perform thyroidectomies infrequently.

Regardless of the surgical procedure used, all tissue should be submitted for histological examination to determine if thyroid tissue was removed (instead of lymph nodes), whether parathyroid glands are present in the sample, and if thyroid tissue is benign or malignant. If malignancy is diagnosed histologically, a thyroid scan should be performed soon after surgery to determine whether the tumor has metastasized to lymph nodes and lungs. If metastases are found, high-dose radioiodine treatment is indicated.

Intraoperative complications include damage to the vagosympathetic trunk, causing Horner's syndrome, damage to the laryngeal nerve, causing laryngeal paralysis, damage to the esophageal nerves, causing megaesophagus, and uncontrolled hemorrhage. Occasionally both thyroid lobes cannot be found despite lengthy dissection. This situation usually results from gravitation of the larger lobe into the thoracic inlet. A few cats will have neoplastic ectopic thyroid tissue in the cranial mediastinum that is difficult to retrieve. In either situation, the cat will remain hyperthyroid after surgery.

The most serious postoperative complication is disruption of the blood supply to the parathyroid glands, resulting in hypocalcemia. This situation is life-threatening and, despite intensive treatment for hypocalcemia, can be fatal. Serum calcium levels should be monitored daily for 4 to 7 days after bilateral thyroidectomy. If the serum calcium concentration falls below 7.0 mg/dL, the cat may show signs of hypocalcemia, including restlessness, facial pruritus, ear twitching, abnormal behavior, muscle tremors, tetany, and convulsions. Calcium gluconate is administered IV slowly to effect, with careful electrocardiographic monitoring for bradycardia or arrhythmias. As soon as the tremors cease, oral vitamin D_3, dihydrotachysterol, should be administered at a dosage of 0.25 mg/cat/day for 2 weeks, and then reduced to 0.25 mg/cat every 3 to 4 days. Oral calcium supplementation of either calcium gluconate (500–700 mg/kg/day divided into three or four doses) or calcium lactate (400–600 mg/kg/day divided into three or four doses) should also be started immediately. Persistence of hypocalcemia is of variable duration. Medication to control serum calcium levels may be needed for a few days or for the remainder of the cat's life. Serum calcium concentrations should be maintained at 8 to 10 mg/dL and should be measured every few weeks.

The other complication of thyroidectomy is deregulation of thyroid hormone concentrations. If unilateral thyroidectomy is performed and the remaining thyroid lobe is normal, serum T_4 concentrations will return to normal in the ensuing month as the atrophied thyroid tissue responds to stimulation by TRH and TSH. After bilateral thyroidectomy the serum T_4 concentration will become subnormal, and the cat should be given T_4 supplementation, 0.1 mg/cat s.i.d. to b.i.d. In the vast majority of cats that have undergone bilateral thyroidectomy, clinical signs of hypothyroidism will not develop, either because the ectopic thyroid tissue is stimulated to produce T_4 or, perhaps more commonly, because of production of thyroid hormones by residual thyroid tumor cells adhering to the thyroid gland capsule. Several months to years postoperatively, these cells may once again produce excessive levels of thyroid hormones. Serum T_4 concentrations should be measured every 6 months in cats that have undergone any thyroidectomy procedure. If a cat becomes hyperthyroid after a total thyroidectomy, radioiodine treatment should be given because the likelihood of hypocalcemia increases greatly with subsequent operations.[19]

Continuous Medical Management

A few hyperthyroid cats are not good candidates for either radioiodine treatment or surgery because of either concurrent disease or advanced geriatric changes. In addition, clients may refuse definitive treatment for a variety of reasons, including stress or risk to the cat and expense. The only treatment alternative to surgery or ^{131}I therapy is continuous medical management with antithyroid drugs. Generally, methimazole is given at a dosage of 5 mg/cat s.i.d. to t.i.d. As the tumor enlarges, the dose of methimazole must be increased. Ultimately, some cats need as much as 20 mg/day.[14] The T_4 concentration and CBC count should be monitored frequently to ensure proper dosage and to detect hematologic abnormalities. If cats are maintained on antithyroid drugs for longer than 6 months, owner compliance with the treatment regimen may falter, and the risk of side-effects may increase.

There are several disadvantages to continuous medical therapy. Antithyroid drugs do not affect the growth of the thyroid tumor, so that increasing amounts of drug must be given. These drugs must be administered up to three times daily for the remainder of the cat's life to control clinical signs. T_4 concentrations and CBC counts should be determined every 2 to 4 weeks for 6 months, then every 4 to 8 weeks, to ensure that the correct dosage of drug is given and that toxic bone marrow effects or autoimmune disorders do not develop. The cost of the drug and of hematologic monitoring may exceed the cost of definitive therapy within 1 to 3 years. Finally, as many as 25% of cats on antithyroid drugs will experience mild to fatal side-effects with an onset as late as 6 months after initiation of therapy. Methimazole is less toxic than propylthiouracil, but both drugs can cause similar side-effects.

Side-effects associated with antithyroid drugs include anorexia, vomiting, dehydration, lethargy, and skin rashes/excoriations or alopecia.[14] More severe side-effects are the hematologic complications, which can be life-threatening. They include the presence of antinuclear antibodies, Coombs-positive hemolytic anemia, thrombocytopenia, neutropenia, and eosinophilia.

Side-effects are more likely to occur in the first 3 months of treatment but can develop at any time. If side-effects occur, the drug should be withdrawn immediately and supportive care provided. The decision to undertake definitive treatment must be reconsidered at this time.

Treatment Sequelae

Cats receiving definitive treatment for hyperthyroidism generally have a dramatic improvement in health and will regain normal behavior, appetite, and physical appearance within 1 to 2 months. However, during the posttreatment recuperative period (i.e., up to 6 weeks), some cats will be sluggish, have a decreased appetite, and appear to sleep more than usual, owing to temporary hypothyroidism. These signs gradually lessen as thyroid hormone concentrations return to normal. In the first few weeks after treatment several important physiological changes occur that need to be identified and monitored. Cardiac changes are dramatic, with return to normal heart rate and rhythm. An important sequel to these cardiac changes is a lowering of blood pressure. Lowered blood pressure results in a reduction of the glomerular filtration rate by approximately 25%. This drop can be significant in cats with early renal disease and can precipitate decompensated renal failure. These cats need to be managed with either oral or subcutaneous fluid supplementation, a low-quantity, high-quality protein diet, calcium supplementation to increase available calcium in the gastrointestinal tract, and other supportive therapy. Intense and aggressive treatment and careful monitoring of these cats must occur until the kidneys have readjusted to the physiological changes.

If a formerly hyperthyroid cat does not return to its weight and predicted good health, an aggressive search for concomitant disease must be undertaken.

REFERENCES

1. Holzworth J, Theran P, Carpenter JL, et al. Hyperthyroidism in the cat: Ten cases. J Am Vet Med Assoc 1980;176:345.
2. Feldman EC, Nelson RW. Hyperthyroidism and Thyroid Tumors. In: Feldman EC, Nelson RW, eds. Canine and Feline Endocrinology and Reproduction. Philadelphia: WB Saunders, 1987:91.
3. Turrel JM, Feldman EC, Nelson RW, Cain G. Thyroid carcinoma causing hyperthyroidism in cats: 14 cases (1981–1986). J Am Vet Med Assoc 1988;193:359.
4. Turrel JM, Broome M. Diagnosis and Radioiodine Treatment of Thyroid Carcinoma in Cats (abstr). In: Proceedings of the 1991 ACVS Veterinary Symposium, 1991:62.
5. Peterson ME, Turrel JM. Feline Hyperthyroidism. In: Kirk RW, ed. Current Veterinary Therapy. Section IX. Philadelphia: WB Saunders, 1986:1026.
6. Peterson ME, Randolph JF. Endocrine Diseases. In: Sherding RG, ed. The Cat: Diseases and Clinical Management. New York: Churchill Livingstone, 1989:1095.
7. Kobayashi DL, Peterson ME, Graves TK, Lesser M, Nichols CE. Hypertension in cats with chronic renal failure or hyperthyroidism. J Vet Intern Med 1990;4:58.
8. Peterson ME Graves TK, Cavanagh PG. Serum thyroid hormone concentrations fluctuate in cats with hyperthyroidism. J Vet Intern Med 1987;1:142.
9. Peterson ME, Gamble DA. Effect of nonthyroidal illness on serum thyroxine concentrations in cats: 494 cases. J Am Vet Med Assoc 1990;197:1203.
10. Peterson ME, Becker DV. Radionuclide thyroid imaging in 135 cats with hyperthyroidism. Vet Radiol 1984;25:23.
11. Graves TK, Peterson ME. Diagnosis of Occult Hyperthyroidism in Cats. In: Nichols R, ed. Problems in Veterinary Medicine: Endocrinology. Philadelphia: JB Lippincott, 1990:683.
12. Peterson ME, Graves TK, Gamble DA. Triiodothyronine (T_3) suppression test: An aid in the diagnosis of mild hyperthyroidism in cats. J Vet Intern Med 1990;5:233.
13. Peterson ME. The use of endocrine testing in the diagnosis and treatment of endocrine disorders. In: Proceedings of the Ninth Annual Veterinary Medical Forum, 1991:112.
14. Peterson ME, Kintzer PP, Hurvitz AI. Methimazole treatment of 262 cats with hyperthyroidism. J Vet Intern Med 1988;2:150.
15. Turrel JM, Feldman EC, Hays M, et al. Radioactive iodine therapy in cats with hyperthyroidism. J Am Vet Med Assoc 1984;184:554.
16. Meric SM, Hawkins EC, Washabau RJ, Turrel JM, Feldman EC. Serum thyroxine concentrations after radioactive iodine therapy in cats with hyperthyroidism. J Am Vet Med Assoc 1986;188:1038.
17. Flanders JA, Harvey HJ, Erb HN. Feline thyroidectomy: A comparison of postoperative hypocalcemia associated with three different surgical techniques. Vet Surg 1987;16:362.
18. Welches CD, Scavelli TD, Mattison DT, Peterson ME. Occurrence of problems after three techniques of bilateral thyroidectomy in cats. Vet Surg 1989;18:392.
19. Birchard SJ, Peterson SJ, Jacobson A. Surgical treatment of feline hyperthyroidism: Results of 85 cases. J Am Anim Hosp Assoc 1984;20:705.

CHAPTER 47

◇ ◇ ◇

Idiopathic Hepatic Lipidosis

Gary D. Norsworthy

Idiopathic hepatic lipidosis in the cat is "an acquired disorder of metabolism resulting in the hepatocellular accumulation of triglycerides in quantities sufficient to be visible by light microscopy."[1] More simply stated, it is an accumulation of fat in the liver to the degree that liver dysfunction or failure results. It is also known as the fatty liver syndrome. In 1984 idiopathic hepatic lipidosis was the most commonly diagnosed liver disease in cats at the Animal Medical Center, New York.[2] At one time it had a very high mortality. With aggressive, prolonged therapy based on force feeding, the mortality is much lower.

Hepatic lipidosis may be associated with diabetes mellitus or the administration of tetracycline.[3] Because the treatment of these forms is the same as for the idiopathic condition, this discussion will focus on the idiopathic disease.

Etiology

Humans develop hepatic lipidosis, and a number of theories regarding the etiology of idiopathic hepatic lipidosis in the cat have been advanced based on what is known about the human disease. The most logical theory extrapolates from the relationship between the human disease and obesity, because obesity predisposes to the development of feline idiopathic hepatic lipidosis. In the final analysis, however, we do not know the cause of this disease and therefore refer to it as idiopathic.

History and Clinical Signs

There are no findings in the history or physical examination that are diagnostic for idiopathic hepatic lipidosis. The typical anamnesis includes obesity followed by a period of anorexia and rapid weight loss. Many cats with idiopathic hepatic lipidosis have a history of fever or diarrhea; however, some will be constipated and have very hard stools. If hepatoencephalopathy occurs, vomiting, salivation, and severe mental depression will occur. Lethargy, dehydration, and icterus are common.[4,5] Icterus may be quite pronounced.

Laboratory Findings

The hematologic findings and biochemical profiles reflect hepatic insufficiency. A study of 73 cats with spontaneous severe idiopathic hepatic lipidosis revealed certain findings that are listed in Table 47–1.[1] The most reliable laboratory indications of this disease are:

- Serum alkaline phosphatase (ALP) increased more than twofold over normal.
- A fold increase in γ-glutamyltransferase exceeding the fold increase in ALP.
- An increase in fasting bile salts.
- An increase in postprandial bile salts.

Diagnosis

A diagnosis of idiopathic hepatic lipidosis cannot be confirmed without evaluating hepatocytes. Hepatocytes may be evaluated in two ways; both are reliable. Histopathology may be performed on a hepatic tissue sample collected either with a percutaneous biopsy needle or at laparotomy. The former is less stressful on the cat but yields a blindly directed sample. However, because idiopathic hepatic lipidosis is a generalized liver disorder, a tissue sample from virtually any part of the liver should be diagnostic. An exploratory laparotomy is less than desirable because of the stress it induces in a seriously ill patient.

The other method of obtaining a diagnostic liver sample is by percutaneous fine-needle aspiration. The sample obtained is prepared for cytologic examination. A very small needle is passed percutaneously into the liver. Anesthesia is not necessary, and the aspiration biopsy is performed much more rapidly than a percutaneous needle biopsy. Because of the small size of the needle, there is significantly less chance of hepatic hemorrhage than when a biopsy needle is used. The samples obtained are usually diagnostic for this disease.

A liver aspirate or biopsy should reveal swollen, lipid-filled hepatocytes without evidence of inflammation (Figs.

Table 47–1. Selected Hematologic and Biochemical Findings in 73 Cats with Spontaneous Severe Idiopathic Hepatic Lipidosis.[8]

Finding	Prevalence (%)
Mild to moderate hyperglycemia	30
Hypercholesterolemia	30
ALP > 2-fold increase	80
ALP > 5-fold increase	50
Fold increase in GGT exceeding fold increase in ALP	0
Hepatic transaminases ≥ 2-fold increase	70
Hepatic transaminases ≥ 5-fold increase	40
Increase in fasting bile acids	75+
Increase in postprandial bile acids	100
Coagulation tests abnormal (generally prothrombin time and fibrinogenemia)	50
Hypokalemia	30
Hyponatremia	25
Decreased serum urea nitrogen (with normal creatinine)	50

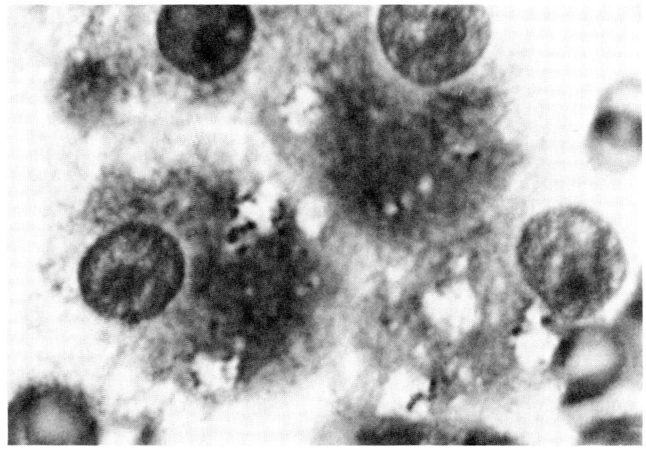

Figure 47–1. Normal hepatocytes obtained by fine-needle aspiration of the liver. Note the absence of fat as compared to Figure 47–2*B*.

47–1 and 47–2). The amount of fat present is generally so profound that there is no question as to the diagnosis. Findings associated with other common feline liver diseases, such as lymphoblasts, mitotic figures, fungal organisms, or marked inflammation, should be absent.

Percutaneous Fine-Needle Aspiration of the Liver

Percutaneous fine-needle aspiration of the liver is performed with the cat in sternal recumbency. The site of needle insertion is determined from radiographs of the abdomen. If radiographs are not available, the following location will generally be acceptable in the vertical plane, at the costochondral junction; in the horizontal plane, between ribs 8 and 9 or 9 and 10.

A small area of skin at the insertion site should be prepared as for surgery. A 25-gauge, 5/8-inch needle attached to a 3- or 6-mL syringe is inserted toward the midline. Because the liver is adjacent to the body wall, a needle of this length is generally adequate. If the cat is very large or obese, a 1-inch needle should be used. Although idiopathic hepatic lipidosis is a generalized hepatic disease, many clinicians prefer to aspirate both the left and right sides of the liver. However, care should be exercised when aspirating from the right side, because the gallbladder may be enlarged in an anorectic cat.

The various stages of fine-needle aspiration are shown in Figure 13–1. The needle is inserted into the liver while vacuum is simultaneously created in the syringe. If the cat struggles, the procedure should be terminated until sedation can be administered, because the liver can be lacerated

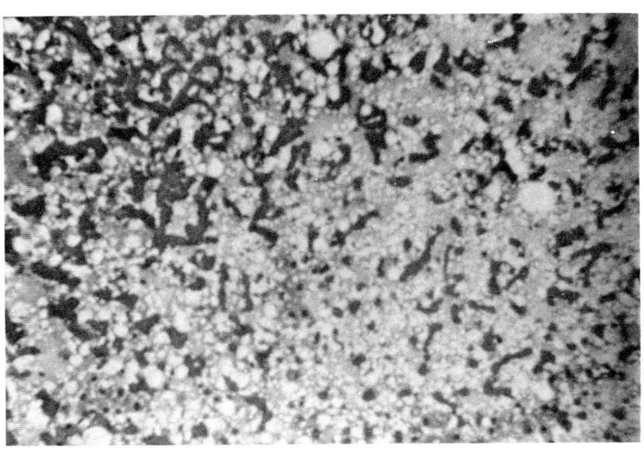

A

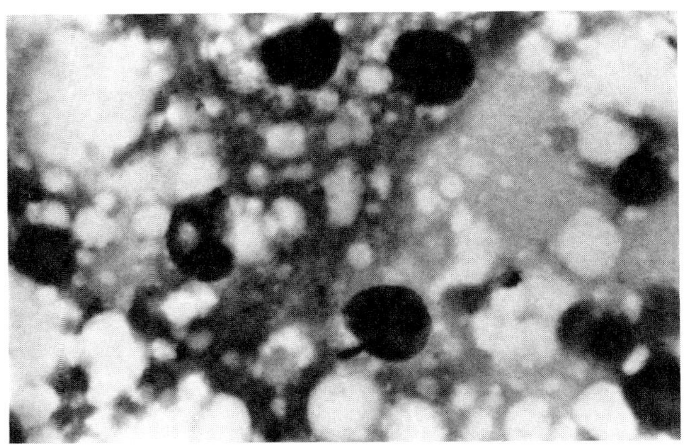

B

Figure 47–2. Liver sample obtained by fine-needle aspiration. (*A*) Low-power magnification. The round white areas are fat globules typical of idiopathic hepatic lipidosis. (*B*) High-power magnification. The fat globules seen intra- and extracellularly are characteristic of hepatic lipidosis.

easily. The vacuum is released, and the needle is withdrawn. The needle is disconnected from the syringe, and the syringe is filled with air. The needle is reconnected to the syringe, and the contents of the needle are forced onto a microscope slide. The hepatic material will look like a tiny drop of blood. This material is spread with the needle or another microscope slide so that a one-celled layer is created. The slide is stained with a modified Wright's stain, generally Diff-Quik, and examined under 100× and 1,000× magnification.

Treatment

Initial Treatment

If the cat is dehydrated, initial treatment entails intravenous administration of an isotonic, balanced electrolyte solution to correct the dehydration. The degree of dehydration, from 4% to 15%, is estimated based on various clinical signs (Table 47–2). The following formula is used to determine the correct amount:

$$\text{Amt of fluid (mL)} = \text{body wt (lb)} \times \text{\% dehydration} \times 500\ \text{mL}$$

For example, in a 10-lb cat with 5% dehydration:

$$10 \times 0.05 \times 500 = 250\ \text{mL}$$

In addition to fluid, B-complex vitamins are given to replenish those lost due to anorexia and fluid therapy. Lipotropic agents containing methionine are contraindicated because methionine is metabolized to encephalopathic toxins in the alimentary tract.

If hepatoencephalopathy is present, as evidenced by vomiting, salivation, and severe mental depression, a warm saline (6.8 mL/lb) enema is administered. Lactulose (Cephulac) is administered orally at a rate of 1 to 2 mL, t.i.d. If diarrhea occurs, the lactulose dose is reduced. Metronidazole (Flagyl, 4.5 mg/lb PO t.i.d.) and/or neomycin (9 mg/lb PO b.i.d.) are administered to further reduce the bacterial population of the colon and to reduce ammonia absorption from the colon.[4]

Certain drugs must be avoided to prevent further complications. These are listed in Table 47–3.

Long-term Therapy

Long-term therapy is based on a balanced, high-protein diet that nourishes the cat and assists in mobilizing the fat trapped in the hepatocytes. (If hepatoencephalopathy is present, a low-protein diet should be used until it resolves, then a high-protein diet introduced.) Because these cats are anorectic, a convenient form of force feeding must be used to allow the owner to feed the cat at home. On average, force feeding is needed for 6 to 7 weeks, but it may be needed for months.[6]

Table 47–2. Degree of Dehydration Based on Clinical Signs[11]

Dehydration	Clinical Signs
4%	Thirst increased
6%	Ocular and oral mucus membranes dry, skin resiliency diminished
8%	Skin inelastic, conjunctiva congested, oral mucosa dry and sticky, eyes sunken and soft, pulse rate elevated
10–12%	All of the above, intensified
15%	Shock begins

Table 47–3. Drugs to Avoid in Cats with Idiopathic Hepatic Lipidosis[8,10]

1. Tetracycline: Inhibits mitochondrial oxidation of fatty acids and therefore may contribute to hepatic lipidosis
2. Chloramphenicol: Dependent on hepatic metabolism and may induce anorexia
3. Trimethoprim-sulfa drugs: May cause cholestasis
4. Anabolic steroids (stanozolol, oxymetholone, nandrolone decanoate): May cause cholestasis
5. Glucocorticoids (prednisolone, dexamethasone, etc.): Promote fatty acid mobilization to the liver
6. Lipotropic agents containing methionine: Methionine is metabolized to encephalopathic toxins in the alimentary tract
7. Benzodiazepine compounds: Require hepatic biotransformation for elimination

Proper Diet

A number of diets have been used in cats with idiopathic hepatic lipidosis. Many of them are concentrated, expensive products made for enteral feeding in humans.[5,6] Some of these have produced diarrhea, vomiting, and hyperglycemia when used in cats.[5]

Carnitine has been proposed as an important dietary component in the treatment of feline hepatic lipidosis, based on its role in the treatment of human hepatic lipidosis.[6] Carnitine is believed to assist in the removal of fat from the liver. However, a study by Jacobs et al. found that the levels of carnitine in the plasma, liver, and skeletal muscles of cats with hepatic lipidosis did not differ significantly from levels in normal cats. They concluded that a carnitine deficiency does not contribute to the pathogenesis of idiopathic hepatic lipidosis and would likely be of no value in its treatment.[7] A number of other dietary additives have been proposed for the treatment of hepatic lipidosis. These are listed in Table 47–4 with their dosages and proposed indications.

A good, blenderized diet is given below; details are given in Chapter 5.

Ingredients:

1 can Feline P/D

+

10 oz water

+

2 oz Wesson Oil

+

5.5 tbsp Casec powder

+

Additives in Table 47–4 (as needed)

Table 47–4. Dietary Additives Recommended for Cats with Idiopathic Hepatic Lipidosis

Additive	Dose	Reason and Reference
Arginine	1 g/cat/d	Many cats with hepatic lipidosis have low serum arginine levels[8]
Taurine	500 mg/cat/d	Many cats with hepatic lipidosis have low serum taurine levels[8]
Carnitine	500 mg/cat/d	Accelerated rate of recovery, according to clinical impressions[8]
Choline	500 mg/cat/d	Accelerated rate of recovery, according to clinical impressions and theory[12]
Citrulline	1 g/cat/d	Accelerated rate of recovery, according to clinical impressions and theory[12]
Vitamin K	5 mg/cat q2–3d	Coagulation tests abnormal in 50% of 73 cats studied[11]
Thiamine	100 mg/cat/d	Improvement in strength and alertness[11]
Multiple vitamins with zinc		Generally deficient in hepatic dysfunction in humans[11]
Potassium	500 mg/cat/d	If hypokalemia is present[11]

Procedure:

Blenderize and pour through kitchen strainer.

Feed a 9-lb cat 200 mL per 24 hours in two to four feedings.

When supplemented with protein as described, this diet has been very successfully used by the author to meet the needs of the cat with idiopathic hepatic lipidosis. If the cat also has hepatoencephalopathy, the diet is appropriate without the protein supplementation. The additives listed in Table 47–4 should be considered until controlled studies have proved or disproved their value.

Feeding Methods

A number of methods have been used for force feeding of anorectic cats with idiopathic hepatic lipidosis. In cats that are eating but have very poor appetites, the benzodiazepine compounds stimulate the appetite to a more normal level.[4] However, they require hepatic biotransformation for elimination, and so are contraindicated in patients with hepatic lipidosis.[8]

Several methods of force feeding with passed or implanted tubes have been used in cats;[9] each has advantages and disadvantages (see Chapter 5). I prefer an esophagostomy tube for long-term feeding. A 12 French feeding tube is inserted percutaneously into the proximal esophagus on the left side of the neck. It is sutured to the skin so that its distal end is in the distal two thirds of the esophagus and its proximal end is behind the right ear (see Chapter 55).

The advantages of the esophagostomy tube are many. Its placement is less stressful than placement of most other surgically implanted tubes and does not require specialized equipment, such as an endoscope. A laparotomy is not needed; the tube may be placed through a stab incision in the skin and esophagus that requires only about 10 minutes of anesthesia. The tube is well tolerated by most cats without the use of an Elizabethan collar, and the cat's swallowing is not affected, as can occur with a pharyngostomy tube. There is little chance of significant postsurgical infection, as has occurred with the use of gastrostomy tubes.[6] Strained, blenderized diets will pass through the tube.

Successful treatment requires force feeding for as long as several months. The method chosen must be suitable for the cat and the owner. The owner must be educated to feed the appropriate food in an appropriate amount until the cat's appetite returns, generally in 6 to 7 weeks.

A Nosocomial Disease

Nosocomial diseases are those acquired in a hospital. Because of its association with anorexia, idiopathic hepatic lipidosis may in some cases be a nosocomial disease. Many cats admitted to the hospital for treatment of a disease have not eaten for several days prior to admission. Many have been anorectic longer than the owners realized. To avoid appearing negligent, owners will often say that the cat has been eating when in fact the cat has not been eating or the owner really does not know. If an anorectic cat is allowed to remain without food for several days in the hospital, idiopathic hepatic lipidosis may be added to the primary disease. The chain of events leading to idiopathic hepatic lipidosis can begin with a few days of anorexia, especially if the cat is obese. Therefore, force feeding of anorectic cats should be a routine part of hospital care (see Chapter 5).

REFERENCES

1. Center SA. Hepatic lipidosis in the cat. Proc 4th Annu ACVIM Vet Forum 1986;2:13.
2. Zawie DA, Garvey MS. Feline hepatic disease. In: August JR, Loar AS, eds. Vet Clin North Am (Small Anim Pract) 1984;14(6):1201.
3. Hardy RM Diseases of the Liver and Their Treatment. In: Ettinger SJ, ed. Textbook of Veterinary Internal Medicine, 3rd ed. Philadelphia: WB Saunders, 1989:1479.

4. Wolf AM. Feline idiopathic hepatic lipidosis. Kal Kan Forum 1990:3.
5. Biourge V, MacDonald MJ, King L. Feline hepatic lipidosis: Pathogenesis and nutritional management. Comp Cont Educ Pract Vet 1990;12:1244.
6. Jacobs G, Cornelius L, Allen S, Greene C. Treatment of idiopathic hepatic lipidosis in cats: 11 cases (1986–1987). J Am Vet Med Assoc 1989;195:635.
7. Jacobs G, Cornelius L, Keene B, Rakich P, Shug A. Comparison of plasma, liver, and skeletal muscle carnitine concentrations in cats with idiopathic hepatic lipidosis and in healthy cats. Am J Vet Res 1990;51:1349.
8. Center SA. Severe hepatic lipidosis in the cat: Clinicopathologic features and management considerations. Proc 9th ACVIM Forum, 1991:519.
9. Crowe D. Nutrition in critical patients: Administering the support therapies. Vet Med 1989;84:152.
10. Center SA. Hepatic Lipidosis. In: August JR, ed. Consultations in Feline Internal Medicine. Philadelphia: WB Saunders, 1991:451.
11. Smith CR. Fluid Therapy. In: Catcott EJ, ed. Canine Medicine. Santa Barbara, Calif: American Veterinary Publications, 1968:67.
12. Biourge V, Pion P, Lewis J, Morris JG, Rogers QR. Dietary management of idiopathic feline hepatic lipidosis with a liquid diet supplemented with citrulline and choline. J Nutr 1991;121: S155.

CHAPTER 48

◇ ◇ ◇

Inflammatory Bowel Disease

Douglas C. Bronstad

Feline inflammatory bowel disease (IBD) is a newly recognized disease and has been cited in several recent papers in the veterinary literature.[1-4] The increased recognition of this unique disease has stimulated clinicians to include it in the differential diagnosis when a cat presents with signs of vomiting, diarrhea, or weight loss. In my experience, it is the most common chronic primary gastrointestinal (GI) disorder of cats.

Etiology

The cause of IBD is unknown, although numerous theories have been proposed. One favored by most academicians is that this disease is an immune-mediated hypersensitivity reaction to indiscriminate antigens, including enteric bacteria and dietary components.[4,5] Response to corticosteroids in the majority of the cases supports assertions of immune-mediated disease. There is no evidence that this disease is heritable.

Pathophysiology and Histopathology

Inflammatory bowel disease is characterized by an infiltration of inflammatory cells in the mucosal lining of the bowel (i.e., stomach, intestines, or colon). Depending on the degree of inflammation and their location within the bowel, these infiltrates can affect the secretions, motility, and absorptive capacity of the bowel, creating an environment in which vomiting and diarrhea may develop.

The inflammatory infiltrates can be quite variable, in terms of severity and cell type. The most common cell types are lymphocytes and plasma cells. When both are present, the infiltrate is termed lymphoplasmacytic). Eosinophilic infiltrates may be seen as the primary infiltrating cell (i.e., eosinophilic gastroenteritis); however, this cell line is more commonly seen as a component in a mixed population of cells that includes lymphocytes and plasma cells. Neutrophils can also be part of a mixed inflammatory response and have been suggested by one author to result from a microbial component of the disorder.[4]

Terms often used by pathologists to describe this disease process include lymphocytic, plasmacytic, lymphoplasmacytic, eosinophilic, suppurative (i.e., predominantly neutrophilic), and commonly, a mixed inflammatory infiltrate. This disease is often segmental, and the degree of infiltrate may vary considerably, depending on the biopsy site.[6] In order to make a definitive diagnosis of IBD, multiple biopsies of the GI tract may be required. The degree of mucosal infiltrate reported may not be a true reflection of the severity of the disease process.

History, Clinical Signs, and Physical Examination

Historical background and clinical signs of IBD can be quite variable and often are vague. The most common clinical signs noted in chronic or refractory cases are vomiting, diarrhea, or both, but anorexia and weight loss may be the sole presenting complaints in some cases. In the author's experience vomiting is the most common clinical sign on presentation. The character of the vomitus can be variable, and hematemesis is occasionally seen. Weight loss is also a variable component of the disease. Many cats have not lost weight at the time of presentation; however others may be severely emaciated owing to the chronicity of the condition and the area of bowel involved, leading to a malabsorption syndrome. Diarrhea is usually present when there is intestinal or colonic involvement, and the character of the diarrhea depends on what area of the bowel is predominantly affected (i.e., small bowel versus large bowel diarrhea). If the mucosal infiltrate is predominantly gastric or duodenal, vomiting is the primary presenting clinical sign and stools may be normal.

An IBD patient can have variable physical findings, depending on a number of factors including chronicity of the disease process and location of the disease in the bowel. The physical findings may be unremarkable in some cases, whereas other affected cats present with more severe changes, such as a thin to emaciated body condition, varying degrees of abdominal tenseness, palpably thickened intestinal loops, mesenteric lymphadenopathy, and various degrees of dehydration. It is very important for the clinician to do a complete organ system review during the physical examination, to rule out concurrent disease processes.

Diagnosis

A minimum data base for all IBD cases should include a fecal examination, complete blood count (CBC), biochemical profile including baseline thyroxine (T4), urinalysis, and survey abdominal radiographs. It is important for the clinician to screen for other disease processes that may be causing the clinical signs (see Chapter 24).

Laboratory findings in cases of IBD can be variable; however, the majority of cases have minimal laboratory changes. The complete blood count often is normal, although mild to moderate leukocytosis may be seen. Eosinophilia is a nonspecific indicator of eosinophilic gastroenteritis.[7] Occasionally, mild elevations in alanine aminotransferase, alkaline phosphatase, amylase, and lipase may be associated with IBD. Urinalysis usually is normal. Survey abdominal radiography is often unremarkable, and barium GI contrast studies may demonstrate normal to irregular mucosal lining abnormalities and thickened intestinal walls. In most cases radiography is unrewarding.

A definitive diagnosis of IBD can be made only by mucosal or full-thickness intestinal biopsy. Gastric, duodenal, or colonic mucosal biopsy can be easily obtained by fiberoptic endoscopic techniques. However, many general practices cannot justify the expense of this equipment and must rely on other techniques to acquire a biopsy or utilize a referral center that has endoscopic capability. Full-thickness intestinal biopsy specimens can be obtained via an exploratory celiotomy. Multiple areas of the bowel (i.e., gastric, duodenal, jejunal, ileal) can be biopsied with this approach. At least two or three specimens should be taken from various areas of the bowel at the time of surgery. Since IBD is predominantly a mucosal disease, the gross appearance of the serosal side of the bowel may be normal. Do not assume that the cat does not have IBD because the gross appearance of the bowel is normal. Full-thickness biopsy specimens have the advantage of histopathologically evaluating both the submucosal and serosal region. Endoscopic biopsy is less invasive but limited to the mucosal side of the bowel and by the inability to reach certain areas of the small intestine (i.e., jejunum).

Treatment

The treatment of choice for most cases of IBD is prednisone or prednisolone. The dosage should be individualized, depending on the severity of clinical signs and the chronicity of the problem. Initially 1.0 to 2.0 mg/lb per day divided in two doses is recommended. Reduction of the dose should be slow and gradual, especially in chronic cases. I typically recommend for an average 10-lb cat 5 mg of prednisolone b.i.d. for 2 weeks, 5 mg s.i.d. for 2 weeks, then 5 mg q.o.d. for 4 weeks or as needed for maintenance therapy. The larger dose (2 mg/lb/day) can be used for severe or refractory cases. The most common mistakes made during treatment of IBD are starting with an insufficient dose of prednisolone and not giving the drug long enough. Parenteral administration (i.e., intramuscular [IM] or subcutaneous [SC] may be necessary for the initial 24 to 48 hours if vomiting precludes absorption of orally administered medication. For fractious animals or ones whose owners have difficulty administering oral medications, methylprednisolone acetate (Depo-Medrol) may be tried; however, response to this varies.

Prophylactic antibiotic therapy may be indicated in cases of IBD. Criteria that determine antibiotic use include the presence of peripheral leukocytosis, elevated hepatic or pancreatic enzymes on the biochemical profile, bleeding from the GI tract, suspected bacterial overgrowth or stagnant loop syndrome, and severe mucosal inflammatory changes with a neutrophilic component. Two antibiotics that are often used in combination with prednisolone therapy are amoxicillin (Amoxi-tabs) and metronidazole (Flagyl). Amoxicillin has both aerobic and anaerobic bactericidal effects and is dosed at 5 to 10 mg/lb b.i.d. for 10 to 14 days or as long as deemed necessary by the clinician. Metronidazole is primarily an anaerobic bactericidal antibiotic and often shows dramatic clinical response in combination with prednisolone therapy in refractory IBD cases. Metronidazole also has an antiprotozoan effect and aids in inhibiting cell-mediated immune responses in the intestinal tract. For IBD therapy metronidazole is typically dosed at 5 to 10 mg/lb twice or thrice daily for 2 to 4 weeks, or as deemed necessary by the clinician. An average cat would receive approximately a quarter to a half of a 250-mg tablet two or three times a day.

Additional immunosuppression may be necessary in cases that are refractory to prednisolone. Azathioprine (Imuran), may be added to the therapeutic regime at 0.14 mg/lb every other day in combination with prednisolone.[4] Azathioprine is available only in a 50-mg tablet; to achieve a small dose the tablet can be crushed and mixed in a palatable liquid (see Chapter 6). I have used a dose of a quarter tablet (12.5 mg) every other day in an average 10-lb cat without severe complications, although this is about ten times the recommended dose. Bone marrow suppression is a potential side effect of azathioprine therapy, and a CBC should be monitored every 2 weeks during the first month, then monthly thereafter. Most cats tolerate the drug well.

If colitis is a predominant part of the IBD, sulfasalazine (Azulfidine) can be added to the regimen. The typical dose is 7 to 10 mg/lb b.i.d. or t.i.d., or approximately a quarter of a 500-mg tablet at each dose for an average 10-lb cat. Potential side effects in cats include anorexia and anemia. This drug must be administered more cautiously to cats than it is to dogs.

If dietary allergens are a possible cause of IBD, a hypoallergenic diet is indicated. Hypoallergenic diets (e.g., lamb and rice) have been discussed in depth in other references, and the reader is referred to these sources for additional information. Long-term dietary management may be necessary in chronic IBD cases. Low-gluten diets that have been suggested include Iams Feline and Science Diet Feline Maintenance. Other recommended diets are Tender Vittles and Prescription Diet Feline c/d. Bran supplementation has also been suggested for colitis.[4] The clinician must use clinical judgment and gauge response to dietary changes via trial and error.

REFERENCES

1. Leib MS. Chronic Vomiting: A Diagnostic Approach. In: August JR, ed. Consultations in Feline Internal Medicine. Philadelphia: WB Saunders, 1991:406.
2. Tams TR. Inflammatory Bowel Disease. In: August JR, ed. Consultations in Feline Internal Medicine. Philadelphia: WB Saunders, 1991:409.
3. Sherding RG. Idiopathic Inflammatory Bowel Diseases. In: Sherding RG, ed. The Cat—Diseases and Clinical Management. New York: Churchill Livingstone, 1989:976.
4. Tams TR. Feline Inflammatory Bowel Disease. In: Kirk RW, ed. Current Veterinary Therapy IX. Philadelphia: WB Saunders, 1991:881.
5. Strombeck DR. Chronic Inflammatory Bowel Disease. In: Strombeck DR, ed. Small Animal Gastroenterology. Davis, CA: Stonegate, 1979:240.
6. Tappe J. Personal communication. Pal Pathology Associates; Dallas, Texas.
7. Center SA, Randolph JF. Eosinophilia. In: August JR, ed. Consultations in Feline Internal Medicine. Philadelphia: WB Saunders, 1991:355.

CHAPTER 49

◇ ◇ ◇

Megacolon

Gary D. Norsworthy

Megacolon is a condition in which the colon dilates, resulting in fecal retention. Affected cats have recurrent and often progressive episodes of constipation. When the hard fecal material can no longer be expelled, the constipation becomes unmanageable and obstipation exists.

Pathophysiology

Most cases of megacolon in cats are idiopathic and occur in adult animals. Although the etiology is unknown, most cases are thought to be related to a defect in colonic innervation.[1] Megacolon may also occur secondary to mechanical obstruction by rectal or colonic neoplasms, strictures, or extraluminal masses, or in the setting of neurologic disease (Manx syndrome) (Fig. 49–1) or endocrine disease (diabetes mellitus).[2,3]

Hirschsprung's disease is a genetic disease of humans in which the caudal part of the colon becomes irreversibly dilated first, and subsequently the cranial part becomes dilated.[4] Although feline idiopathic megacolon has been considered a form of Hirschsprung's disease, it behaves differently. The feline disease does not occur in the distal colon first; it affects the entire colon simultaneously.

History and Clinical Signs

Affected cats have a history of months to years of constipation.[5] They often strain or have pain when defecating (dyschezia) and pass hard, dry fecal masses. As the condition progresses, obstipation may occur, resulting in anorexia and vomiting.[3]

Diagnosis

The diagnosis is based on a history of constipation that often leads to obstipation. A colon that is greatly distended and filled with hard fecal material is palpable within the abdomen. Radiographs show a large, fecal-filled colon with a diameter two times or more the length of the body of the seventh lumbar vertebra (Fig. 49–2). Cats that become obstipated and whose colon has been mechanically emptied usually have a relapse within a few weeks to a few months.

Megacolon should be differentiated from other conditions that cause dyschezia, such as vertebral spondylosis and anal sacculitis. The former usually responds to management with anti-inflammatory drugs, and the latter to medical or surgical therapy. When the primary disease is resolved, constipation should not recur.

Treatment

Conservative treatment of constipation is based on the use of drugs and dietary agents that aid in emptying the colon. These drugs are categorized according to their modes of action or methods of formulation (Table 49–1). Specific drugs are listed in Table 49–2. Dietary agents that aid in the control of constipation are bulk-forming and include Prescription Diet r/d and Prescription Diet w/d (Hill's Pet Products, Topeka, KS).

When obstipation occurs, more aggressive therapy is needed. Mineral oil, 15 to 25 mL, should be administered via orogastric tube. Dehydration must be corrected and hydration maintained with intravenous or subcutaneous fluids. Twelve to twenty-four hours later the cat is anesthetized and enemas are administered until the colon is evacuated. The practitioner must avoid lacerating the colon with an instrument or enema solution.

Subtotal colectomy is the sugical removal of nearly all of the colon (Fig. 49–3). It was performed on cats with megacolon as early as 1968.[6] Its successful use was reported in a total of 42 cats in the mid- to late 1980s.[7,8] However, not until the early 1990s did subtotal colectomy become the treatment of choice for idiopathic megacolon,[1] based on consistently good clinical results and on a study that showed no significant subclinical evidence of abnormal bowel function postoperatively.[9] The procedure is described in Chapter 55.

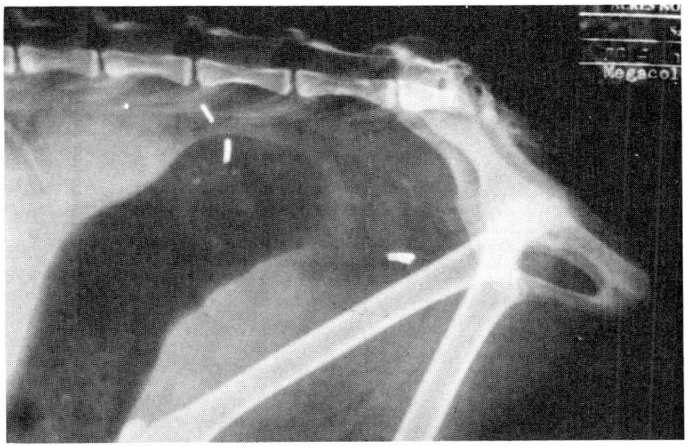

A

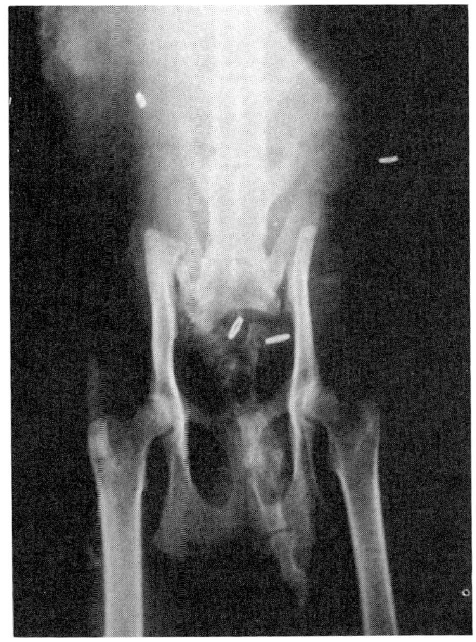

B

Figure 49–1. Radiographs of a Manx cat with a form of secondary megacolon not amenable to surgical treatment. The cat also had fecal incontinence. (*A*) Lateral view, (*B*) ventrodorsal view.

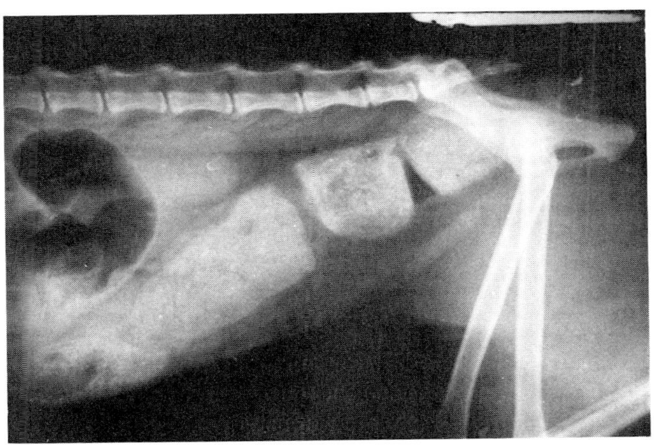

Figure 49–2. The radiographic evidence of megacolon is a fecal-filled colon with a diameter equal to or greater than twice the length of the body of L7.

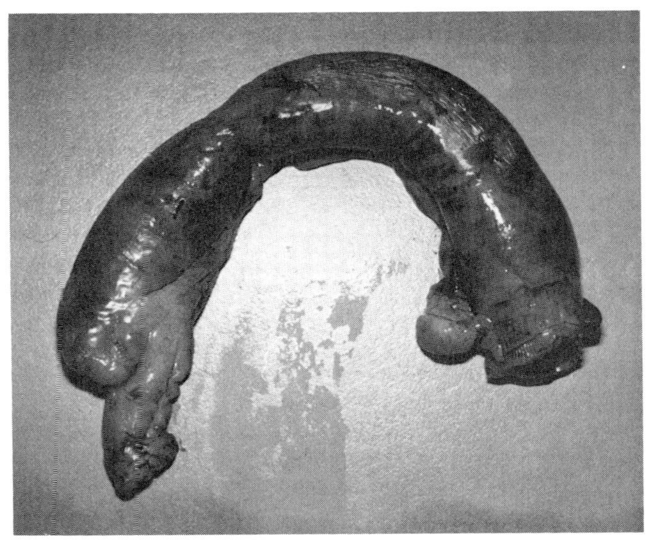

Figure 49–3. Section of colon removed in subtotal colectomy. Subtotal colectomy is the treatment of choice for idiopathic megacolon.

Table 49–1. Categories of Drugs Used to Treat Constipation[1]

Emollients (Wetting Agents or Surfactants)

Actions: Act as detergents to alter surface tension of liquids. Promote emulsification and softening of feces by facilitating the mixture of water and fat.

Examples:
Dioctyl sodium sulfosuccinate (DSS) (Colace, Mead Johnson Laboratories, Evansville, IN)
Dioctyl calcium sulfosuccinate (DCS) (Surfak, Hoechst-Roussel Pharmaceuticals, Somerville, NJ)

Caution: May contribute to or cause dehydration. Only use in hydrated patients. DSS and DCS have very objectionable tastes if the cat bites the capsule. The oral liquid is contraindicated because it has an equally objectionable taste. Some studies question the efficacy of DSS/DCS in humans and dogs. Studies on its efficacy in cats are needed.

Lubricants

Action: Soften feces by coating them, thus preventing absorption of fecal water in the colon.

Examples:
Mineral oil (liquid petrolatum)
Laxatone (Evsco Pharmaceuticals, Buena, NJ) (white petrolatum)

Caution: Mineral oil is tasteless, making aspiration pneumonia possible. It is best administered via an orogastric tube. These drugs inhibit absorption of fat-soluble vitamins and should be administered only between meals.

Bulk-Forming Agents

Actions: Absorb water in the intestinal tract, swell, soften the adjacent feces, normalize the transit time, and provide bulk.

Examples:
Vetasyl (Veterinary Prescription, Harbor City, CA) (psyllium)
Metamucil (Procter & Gamble, Cincinnati, OH) (psyllium)
Bran in many cereals
Canned pumpkin (pumpkin pie filling).

Note: Canned pumpkin mixed with the cat's food can be very effective for long-term control in some cats.

Caution: Bran is not palatable to most cats. Metamucil is somewhat expensive.

Stimulant Laxatives

Actions: Increase peristaltic activity of the intestine by irritating the bowel and stimulating the intramural nerve plexus.

Examples:
Castor oil
Cascara
Senna
Dulcolax (Boehringer-Ingelheim Pharmaceuticals, Inc., Ridgefield, CT) containing bisacodyl

Caution: Long-term use of drugs that stimulate the mesenteric plexus (Dulcolax) may damage the plexus and result in refractory constipation.

Enemas

Actions: Soften feces in the distal colon and rectum. Stimulate colonic motility and the urge to defecate.

Examples:
Tap water
Normal saline
Mineral oil
Soapy water

Note: A warm saline or tap water enema is the preferred treatment for obstipation. A soapy water enema is second choice, a mineral oil enema is the third choice.

Caution: Hexachlorophene soap (pHisoHex, Winthrop Pharmaceuticals, New York, NY) and Fleet Enemas (C.B. Fleet Co, Inc., Lynchburg, VA) are contraindicated in cats.[10,11]

Suppositories

Provide a means of administering the above drugs directly into the rectum and distal colon in a convenient fashion.

Actions: Act by the actions listed above.

Examples:
Glycerin
Bisacodyl
DSS
DCS

Note: Bisacodyl, DSS, and DCS are more effective than glycerin. They may be used in lieu of an enema.

Caution: Only effective for mild to moderate constipation.

Table 49–2. Classification and Properties of Laxatives

Class and Drug	Dosage Form	Dosage/Range	Site of Action	Time Required for Action (hr)
Emollients (Wetting Agents)				
Dioctyl sodium sulfosuccinate (e.g. Colace [Mead Johnson])	50-mg capsules	One 50-mg capsule daily	Small and large intestines	12–72
Dioctyl calcium sulfosuccinate (e.g., Surfak [Hoechst-Roussel])	50-mg capsules	One or two 50-mg tablets daily	Small and large intestines	12–72
Lubricants				
Mineral oil	Liquid (oral)	5–25 mL twice daily	Colon	6–12
White petrolatum (e.g., Laxatone-Evsco)	Paste	1–5 mL daily	Colon	12–24
Bulk-Forming Laxatives				
Psyllium (e.g., Vetasyl [Veterinary Prescription]	Capsule	One 500-mg capsule daily for 7-lb or heavier cat	Colon	12–24
or Metamucil [Searle])	Powder	1–3 tsp mixed with food once or twice daily	Small and large intestine	12–24
Canned pumpkin	Soft paste	1–2 tbsp per can of food	Small and large intestine	12–24
Stimulant Laxatives				
Bisacodyl (e.g., Dulcolax [Boehringer-Ingelheim])	5-mg tablet (suppository)	1 or 2 tablets daily	Colon	6–12

Adapted with permission from Burrows CF. Constipation, obstipation, and megacolon. In: August JR, ed. Consultations in Veterinary Internal Medicine. Philadelphia: WB Saunders Co, 1991:445.

REFERENCES

1. Burrows CF. Constipation, Obstipation, and Megacolon. In: August JR, ed. Consultations in Feline Internal Medicine. Philadelphia: WB Saunders, 1991:445.
2. Burrows CF. Diseases of the Colon, Rectum, and Anus in the Dog and Cat. In: Anderson NV, ed. Veterinary Gastroenterology. Philadelphia: Lea & Febiger, 1980:555, 576.
3. Strombeck DR. Functional Bowel Problems. In: Strombeck DR, ed. Small Animal Gastroenterology. Davis, Calif: Stonegate Publishing, 1979:264.
4. Lynen FK. Motor function of the large bowel in megacolon congenitum. In: Proceedings of the 4th International Symposium on Gastrointestinal Motility. Vancouver: Mitchell Press, 1974:189.
5. Aronsohn M, Johnston DE. Surgical Diseases: Large Intestine. In: Slater DH, ed. Textbook of Small Animal Surgery. Philadelphia: WB Saunders Co, 1985:753.
6. Yoder JJ, Dragsted LR, Starch CJ. Partial colectomy for correction of megacolon in a cat. Vet Med Small Anim Clin 1968; 63:1049.
7. Bright RM, Burrows CF, Goring R, Fox S, Tilmant L. Subtotal colectomy for treatment of acquired megacolon in the dog and cat. J Am Vet Med Assoc 1986;188:1412.
8. Rosin E, Walshaw R, Mehlhaff C, Matthiesen D, Orsher R, Kusba J. Subtotal colectomy for treatment of chronic constipation associated with idiopathic megacolon in cats: 38 cases (1979–1985). J Am Vet Med Assoc 1988;193:850.
9. Gregory CR, Guilford WG, Berry CR, Olsen J, Pedersen NC. Enteric function in cats after subtotal colectomy for treatment of megacolon. Vet Surg 1990;19(3):216.
10. Schaer M, Cavanagh P, Hause W, Wilkins R. Iatrogenic hyperphosphatemia, hypocalcemia and hypernatremia in a cat. J Am Anim Hosp Assoc 1977;13:39.
11. Jorgensen LS, Center SA, Randolph JF, Brum D. Electrolyte abnormalities induced by hypertonic phosphate enemas in two cats. J Am Vet Med Assoc 1985;187:1367.

CHAPTER 50

◇ ◇ ◇

Multicat Facilities: Disease Control

Frederic W. Scott and John E. Saidla

When large numbers of cats are housed together, infectious diseases may reach epidemic proportions. Since cats are plagued by a number of bacteria, viruses, and protozoa the potential for transmission may reach exponential proportions, resulting in mild to serious, or even fatal, infections. Fortunately, our understanding of feline diseases and their pathogens allows us to eliminate many of these problems. Preventive health measures, including vaccinations, coupled with proper management techniques, enhance our efforts in disease control programs. Control of infectious diseases in catteries, shelters, multicat households, and farms is discussed here.

Catteries are facilities where three or more breeding queens are maintained for the purpose of rearing kittens. The cattery is often in a private home, or the cats may be housed in a separate building. There are also several large, commercial catteries, or cat colonies, where hundreds, even thousands, of cats are raised each year.

Shelters are public or private facilities that exist to find homes for unwanted pets. Shelters are often municipal facilities of a city, town, or county. There are numerous private shelters across America, and many individuals have established "shelters" in their homes, in an attempt to find homes for rescued stray cats.

Multicat households are homes that have three or more cats at any given time. In most households the cats have free access to all or most of the house and intermingle at will. In some situations, cats are restricted to individual rooms, a converted garage or barn, or a specially built enclosure. A multicat household differs from a cattery in that cats are usually neutered, or kittens are not raised for sale.

On farms cats have free access to the buildings and land, and they may even be feral. The cats provide rodent control; often they are not neutered. Preventive care and general care may be minimal or nonexistent.

General Principles of Control of Infectious Diseases

Infectious diseases can be transmitted from a diseased or carrier cat to a susceptible one in several ways. The most common method is by direct contact, or nose-to-nose transmission. A second way is by acquiring the infectious agent from contaminated feeding dishes, water bowls, litter pans, floors, resting boards, or furniture. A third way, by which respiratory tract disease is transmitted, is by aerosol transmission: the pathogen is carried through the air on moisture droplets, usually from a sneeze, much as human common cold virus is spread.

The periodic introduction of litters of susceptible kittens presents special problems for control of infectious diseases. Certain feline viruses are transmitted vertically, from a carrier or latently infected queen to her kittens. In special circumstances a virus or other agent may be transmitted from the infected mother to the unborn fetus while the fetus is still in utero.

Cats that are persistently or latently infected with certain agents—feline herpesvirus, feline calicivirus, feline leukemia virus, feline infectious peritonitis virus, and feline immunodeficiency virus—are frequently a source of infection to kittens and other cats. Small quantities of infectious virus or other pathogens are shed in saliva and respiratory secretions, feces, or urine. Viruses may be shed continually, as are feline calicivirus and feline leukemia virus, or intermittently, as is latent feline herpesvirus infection. Once an acute or primary infection occurs, large quantities of virus are shed by the infected cat. The virus then spreads rapidly to other susceptible contact cats, creating an outbreak of disease in the cat population.

Barriers against transmitting infectious agents include distance, physical walls, cages, and fences. The greater the degree of separation, or the better the physical barrier between an infected cat and a susceptible cat, the less the chance that the infectious agent will be transmitted. Separate buildings are better than separate rooms in one building, separate rooms are better than separate cages in the same room, and individual cages in turn are better than having cats in the same run or cage. Wire cages that allow nose-to-nose contact through the wire may prevent diseases that usually are transmitted by biting, such as feline immunodeficiency virus, but such wire cages do little to prevent the rapid transmission of infectious respiratory tract agents such as feline herpesvirus and feline calicivirus.

Transmission of infectious agents by humans is often the weak link in controlling infectious disease in animals. Anyone who works with cats must constantly be aware of

This chapter first appeared in slightly different form in *Feline Information Bulletin No. 11, 1990.* Copyright Cornell Feline Health Center, Ithaca, New York.

the potential for transmission of viruses or other agents from an infected cat to a susceptible cat via contaminated hands, shoes, or clothing. The source of the virus may be an acutely ill cat, an infectious cat during the incubation period, or a healthy-looking chronic carrier cat. Simple procedures, if routinely applied, can greatly reduce the risk of a disease outbreak in a population of cats. These procedures include (1) handling and caring for clean or noninfected cats before caring for infected cats, (2) washing hands thoroughly after handling infected cats, (3) changing shoes or disinfecting footwear as one leaves a contaminated room or building, and (4) changing outer clothing after handling infected cats.

Principles of Disease Control

1. A population of immune cats should be established through an appropriate vaccination program. An acute infection in a population of susceptible cats results in large quantities of virus being shed into the environment, thus contaminating food and water dishes, litter pans, pens or cages, and floors. This contaminated environment, and not just the infected cats, serves as an additional source of virus to infect other cats. Immune cats resist infection and thus aid in blocking the cycle of infection.
2. Infected and susceptible cats should be separated. New cats to be introduced into a group must be isolated or quarantined at least 3 weeks, during which time they should be monitored carefully and tested for infectious disease. Only after they have been shown to be free from infectious disease should they be introduced into the main group of cats. Cats in the population that develop an infectious disease must be immediately isolated from all other cats and then either treated until they are no longer infectious or culled from the population.
3. The number of latently infected and persistently infected cats in the population must be reduced or eliminated. Latent or persistent infection results in a nidus of virus that can serve as a source for an infectious disease outbreak within a population. Efforts must be made to identify "healthy" carrier cats whenever possible and to prevent them from coming in close contact with susceptible cats, especially young unvaccinated kittens.
4. The amount of infectious agent in the environment must be eliminated or reduced. This is done through proper disinfection of floors, cages, resting boards, litter pans, and food and water dishes. Adequate ventilation to remove virus particles from the air is also necessary.

Infectious Diseases

Several infectious diseases of cats are common problems in multicat facilities.

Feline leukemia virus (FeLV) infection is caused by a retrovirus. This virus causes a wide variety of clinical diseases, including tumors (lymphosarcoma), chronic enteritis, anemia, and immunosuppression with increased susceptibility to other pathogens.[1-4] Approximately 30% of exposed cats develop persistent infection[1,3] and continually shed virus in their saliva. These cats can transmit the virus to other cats in close contact (see Chapters 39 and 51).

Feline immunodeficiency virus (FIV), another retrovirus, may produce persistent infection resulting after several months of incubating immunosuppression, and a disease that resembles human acquired immunodeficiency syndrome (AIDS).[2] The infection appears to be transmitted primarily by cat bites (see Chapter 37 and 39).

Feline herpesvirus (FHV) infection, feline viral rhinotracheitis (FVR), or rhino, is a common and serious upper respiratory tract infection of cats.[2,4,7,8] Clinical disease produced by FHV includes sneezing, ocular and nasal discharge, crusty eyes, fever, occasional ulceration of the cornea, and depression. The virus is highly contagious and especially common and troublesome in breeding catteries. Cats recovered from FHV infection are latently infected with the herpesvirus, and, during periods of stress can suffer a recrudescence of infection with shedding of virus. This virus can infect susceptible cats, especially nursing kittens, that come in contact with the carrier cat (see Chapter 63).

Feline calicivirus (FCV) infection may produce one or more of several clinical manifestations, including mild upper respiratory tract infection (ocular and nasal discharge), ulcerations on the tongue, in the mouth, and possibly on the nose, pneumonia (sometimes fatal), acute arthritis with joint pain, high fever, and enteritis.[2,4,7,8] FCV is highly contagious during acute infections, and recovered cats are persistently infected and continually shed small quantities of virus in the saliva (see Chapter 63).

Feline chlamydiosis, or feline pneumonitis, is an upper respiratory tract infection or pneumonia caused by a bacterium. *Chlamydia psittaci.*[4,7,8] Chronic ocular or nasal discharge and signs of chronic bronchitis and pneumonia are frequently seen with this infection after an incubation period of 6 to 10 days. The pathogen is spread by direct contact, by contaminated areas or dishes, and by aerosol transmissions (see Chapter 63).

Feline parvovirus (FPV) infection, or feline panleukopenia (FP) (also known as feline "distemper" or feline infectious enteritis), is a highly contagious viral disease of cats, and is the disease most often fatal to unvaccinated populations of cats. FP is characterized by sudden onset of vomiting, complete inappetence, severe depression, severe dehydration with sunken eyes, and acute diarrhea.[4,9-11] The mortality rate for young kittens during an outbreak in a shelter or on a farm may be 50% to 90%. Fortunately, excellent vaccines for FP are available, and properly vaccinated cats are completely protected against this devastating virus. Transmission is by direct contact of infected and susceptible animals, or by contact with a contaminated environment. This virus is extremely stable and remains infectious for years in a contaminated environment unless it is inactivated with appropriate disinfectants.

Feline rabies is a fatal neurologic disease of cats that is always of serious concern because it is transmissible to humans.[2,12,13] More cases of rabies are now reported in cats than in any other species of domestic animal in the United States. Cats usually acquire the infection through contact with infected wildlife such as a skunk or a raccoon. Any outdoor cat that shows abnormal behavior—either aggressiveness or unusual friendliness—should be handled with extreme caution, immediately isolated, and examined by a veterinarian. Shelter personnel and farm workers, especially in areas where rabies is endemic in wildlife, must be constantly aware of possible rabies in cats and dogs.

Feline infectious peritonitis (FIP) is a common coronavirus infection of cats that often is subclinical but that can develop into a slowly progressive disease that is nearly 100% fatal.[2,5,14-16] Clinical disease is characterized by an incubation period of a few days to 2 or 3 weeks (but is sometimes as long as several months) followed by an insidious onset of clinical signs, including persistent fever and inappetence with progressive weight loss. Some cats have a progressive accumulation of fluid in the abdomen (ascites) or the chest cavity, and some develop neurologic disease, enteric disease, or various other clinical signs. FIP is especially troublesome in breeding catteries, and it is the disease most feared by cattery owners. Currently no effective treatment is available; the only effective measures are vaccination and prevention of exposure. If cats are tested and found to be negative for coronavirus antibodies, strict measures of isolation and vaccination should be established to keep this population free of the FIP virus. Since the virus is not transmitted in utero or in milk, removing 4-week-old kittens from their infected queen or other infected cats in the environment prevents exposure (see Chapter 38).

Types of Facilities

Catteries

Control of infectious diseases in catteries presents special problems associated with the raising of kittens. Latently or persistently infected queens can transmit viruses—FHV, FCV, FeLV, and presumably FIV and FIP—to their kittens. Acute respiratory tract disease frequently occurs in kittens 5 to 8 weeks of age, and FeLV and FIP may occur in kittens several months after they have left the infected cattery as apparently healthy kittens. Kitten mortality complex may occur in certain catteries, the mortality rate ranging from 40% to nearly 100%; many of these kitten losses are due to various infectious diseases.[17]

All cats in a breeding cattery, and any cats introduced into it, should test negative for FeLV and FIV. Because these two viruses must not be present in a breeding cattery the cat population should be screened for FeLV and FIV every 6 to 12 months. In addition, some cattery owners are beginning to test all cats, in an attempt to prevent FIP. Cats that have any coronavirus antibody titer should be isolated from the breeding cattery. This procedure to control FIP is drastic and should be attempted only where there are actual losses caused by FIP.

All cats should be routinely vaccinated against FPV, FHV, and FCV. Depending upon circumstances (e.g., outdoor access) cats should also be vaccinated against feline chlamydiosis, FeLV, FIP, and rabies. When respiratory disease is a problem in the cattery all kittens should be vaccinated against FHV, FCV, and feline chlamydiosis starting at 4 weeks of age and again at 8 and 12 weeks. All cats should be vaccinated annually, and it may be advantageous to revaccinate breeding queens one month before mating, in order to transfer as much passive immunity as possible to the kittens through the colostrum or early milk.[4]

Breeding catteries have five distinct populations that should be housed in separate rooms or facilities: (1) the main cattery, (2) a "maternity ward" for pregnant queens and queens with nursing kittens, (3) a "nursery" for weaned kittens, (4) a quarantine room for incoming cats, and (5) an isolation room for infected cats.[18,19]

Shelters

Adoption shelters run the complete spectrum from the small, private shelter in a home run by a single person to the very large corporate shelter with numerous personnel and large facilities. The degree and quality of control of infectious diseases, unfortunately, also runs the complete spectrum from almost nonexistent to very effective. People who operate small, private shelters with inadequate facilities and financial resources, however noble their intentions, may do more harm than good for the cat population in the neighborhood. We have interacted with numerous persons who are attempting to run a private adoption shelter from their home, and who, unfortunately, end up with 40 or 50 cats living in circumstances of no vaccination or disease-control program. The most effective disease control these people could establish would be to reduce the cat population to a reasonable number for their facilities and financial resources and to refrain from taking in additional strays.

Shelters with multiple personnel should establish a written policy or procedure for operation of the shelter that includes detailed procedures aimed at control of infectious disease. No shelter controls and prevents infectious disease all the time, but the best workable procedures possible should be clearly established, given the limitations of facilities, monies, and personnel. The director of each facility should critically evaluate the operations of the facility, monthly or every few months, to see if shortcuts have crept into the operation that will compromise the control of infectious disease. Accurate records should be kept of the number and type of infectious diseases encountered each month in the facility.

Each shelter should have a minimum of three rooms or areas for housing cats. The main room or rooms house healthy kittens and adult cats that are ready for adoption. If possible, this adoptable population should be divided into units of no more than ten cats per run or room. The second area, the quarantine room, should be as isolated as possible and should contain only healthy-looking cats that are entering the facility. Cats in the quarantine room should be caged individually or as litters of kittens. Cats entering the facility should be examined as soon as possible, tested for FeLV and FIV, vaccinated, and placed in recently disinfected cages. New cats should remain in the quarantine area as long as possible—at least 14 days is recommended, although not always possible in public shelters—before entering the main adoption facility. The shorter the quarantine period, the poorer the disease control in the facility; vaccinated cats will not have time to develop the full degree of immunity from the vaccine, and some cats will be incubating disease when they enter, though it may not be evident for several days. The third necessary area is an isolation room for housing sick cats. The isolation room must not be used as the quarantine room for entering healthy cats, a procedure mistakenly used in some shelters. Sick cats should be treated and held in isolation until they are judged healthy and ready for adoption, when they may be returned to the main adoption area. Incurably ill cats and those judged to be persistently positive for FeLV should be humanely euthanized.

Multicat Households

Homes that have three or more cats but no active breeding program classify as multicat households. In these homes infectious diseases are not as prevalent as in the other multicat facilities, as long as the cat population is stable. When problems occur it is usually because a stray cat is introduced into the household, often without proper quarantine and testing for infectious diseases like FeLV. This Good Samaritan syndrome is all too familiar to veterinarians: an owner with three or four cats states emphatically that she or he will not be adopting another cat, but a stray, pathetic kitten appears on the doorstep. The kitten then "adopts" this household and in the process can expose the rest of the cats to FeLV, respiratory tract viruses, or even FIP or FIV. Prevention of infectious disease in a multicat household should be aimed at maintaining a properly vaccinated group of cats and introducing new cats only after they have been isolated in quarantine at least 4 weeks and have tested negative for FeLV, FIV, and FIP.

Farms

Farms present a unique set of disease-control difficulties. Cats on farms are outdoors and free roaming and therefore readily come in contact with other outdoor cats and wild animals. Prevention of infectious diseases on farms generally is limited to establishing at least a minimal vaccination program against FPV, FHV, and FCV in kittens at 8 and 12 weeks of age. All kittens should be vaccinated for rabies at 12 to 16 weeks. Above this minimal program, one should consider annual revaccinations, FeLV testing, and vaccination. Population control—a spay and neuter program—often is necessary.

Vaccinations

An appropriate vaccination program diligently carried out is an absolute necessity for any multicat facility. Vaccination recommendations can be found in various publications.[2,4,20,21] Table 50–1 gives general recommendations for vaccination of cats.

All cats must be vaccinated against FPV, FHV, and FCV.[7,10,20,22] Kittens should be vaccinated at 8 to 10 weeks of age and again at 12 weeks or older and revaccinated annually. In breeding catteries where respiratory tract disease is endemic, vaccination of kittens should begin at age 4 weeks, with repeat vaccinations at 8 and 12 weeks. In shelters or other facilities where there is a rapid influx of cats, modified live-virus vaccines give faster protection and, so, are preferred over inactivated vaccines.

Additionally, cats can be vaccinated for feline chlamydia, feline leukemia, feline infectious peritonitis, and rabies if conditions warrant. Cats that may be exposed to wildlife, including all farm cats and all outdoor cats, should be vaccinated against rabies.[4,20,21,23] Some states require rabies vaccinations for all cats, regardless of circumstances.

Disinfection

Proper daily disinfection of areas frequented by cats is essential to control infectious disease in facilities where many cats are housed together. Each type of facility varies in the amount and type of disinfection possible, but as much as practical all areas should be disinfected daily.

The type of disinfectant used should be selected carefully.[24] Not all disinfectants that are sold as virucidal inacti-

Table 50–1. Recommendations for Feline Vaccination

Disease	Vaccine Type	Route of Administration	Age at First Vaccination (wk)	Age at Second Vaccination (wk)	Revaccination Intervals (mo)
Panleukemia	MLV	SC or IM	8–10	12–16	12
	Inactivated	SC or IM	8–10	12–16	12
	MLV-IN	IN	8–10	12–16	12
Viral rhinotracheitis	MLV	SC or IM	8–10†	12–16	12
	Inactivated	SC or IM	8–10	12–16	12
	MLV-IN	IN	8–10	12–16	12
Calicivirus disease	MLV	SC or IM	8–10†	12–16	12
	Inactivated	SC or IM	8–10	12–16	12
	MLV-IN	IN	8–10	12–16	12
Pneumonitis (chlamydiosis)	MLV	SC or IM	8–10	12–16	12
Rabies*	Inactivated	IM	12	64	12 or 36
Feline leukemia	Inactivated	SC or IM	9	12	12
Feline infectious peritonitis	MLV-IN	IN	16	20	12

MLV = modified live virus; SC, subcutaneously; IM, intramuscular; IN, intranasal.
*For more details see the 1990 compendium of animal rabies control. J Am Vet Med Assoc 1990;196:36.
†May be performed earlier but at the risk of increased maternal antibody interference.
Modified from Canine and feline immunization guidelines. J Am Vet Med Assoc 1989;195:314.

vate or kill all viruses. FPV and FCV are particularly difficult to inactivate, while some viruses (FHV) are easily inactivated by almost any disinfectant. The most practical and effective disinfectant is ordinary household bleach diluted 1 : 32 in water (4 ounces per gallon). A cleaning solution or other disinfectant or soap preparation may be carefully added to the bleach solution just before use.

All food and water dishes should be washed, soaked for 5 to 10 minutes in the bleach solution, and then thoroughly rinsed in clear water before being reused. Litter pans should be cleaned and disinfected daily or as often as practical, and the litter should be disposed of properly.

Hard surfaces such as cages, floors, and exposed walls should be disinfected daily. Towels, rugs, and pads should be frequently washed in hot water. Rugs and upholstered furniture cannot be adequately disinfected, however. In such situations, where routine disinfection cannot be done, the degree of control of infectious diseases will be compromised.

Summary

Feline infectious diseases caused by viruses and other pathogens are serious and common problems in facilities where multiple cats are housed, especially ones that have a rapid turnover or breeding catteries raising kittens. The incidence of infectious disease outbreaks can be much reduced by exercising basic knowledge of controlling infectious diseases, a dedicated protocol for operation of the facility, and a stringent vaccination program.

REFERENCES

1. Hardy WD Jr. Oncogenic Viruses of Cats: The Feline Leukemia and Sarcoma Viruses. In: Holzworth J, ed. Diseases of the Cat. Philadelphia: WB Saunders, 1987:246.
2. Pedersen NC. Feline Infectious Diseases. Goleta, CA: American Veterinary Publications, 1988:1.
3. Rojko JL, Hardy WD Jr. Feline Leukemia Virus and Other Retroviruses. In: Sherding RG, ed. The Cat: Diseases and Clinical Management. New York: Churchill Livingstone, 1989:229.
4. Scott FW, Barlough JE, Barr M. Feline Viral Diseases. In: M. Siegal, ed. The Cornell Book of Cats. New York: Willard Books, 1989:254;371.
5. Ishida T, Washizu T, Toriyabe K, et al. Feline immunodeficiency virus infection in cats of Japan. J Am Vet Assoc 1989;194:221.
6. Yamamoto JK, Hansen H, Ho EW, et al. Epidemiology and clinical aspects of feline immunodeficiency virus infection in cats from the continental United States and Canada and possible mode of trasmission. J Am Vet Med Assoc 1989;194:213.
7. Ford RB. Infectious Diseases of the Respiratory Tract. In: Sherding RG, ed. The Cat: Diseases and Clinical Management. New York: Churchill Livingstone, 1989:367.
8. Hoover EA. Viral Respiratory Diseases and Chlamydiosis. In: Holzworth J, ed. Diseases of the Cat. Philadelphia: WB Saunders, 1987:214.
9. Pollock RVH. Feline Panleukopenia and Other Enteric Viral Diseases. In: Sherding RG, ed. The Cat: Diseases and Clinical Management. New York: Churchill Livingstone, 1989:357.
10. Scott FW. Panleukopenia. In: Holzworth J, ed. Diseases of the Cat. Philadelphia: WB Saunders Co, 1987:182.
11. Scott FW. Feline Parvovirus Infection. In: Tiussen P, ed. Handbook of Parvoviruses. Vol. II. Boca Raton, FL: CRC Press, 1990:103.
12. Abelseth MK. Rabies. In: Holzworth J, ed. Diseases of the Cat. Philadelphia: WB Saunders, 1987:238.
13. Hand PJ. Rabies and Other Viral Diseases of the Nervous System. In: Sherding RG, ed. The Cat: Diseases and Clinical Management. New York: Churchill Livingstone, 1989:379.
14. Pedersen NC. Coronavirus Diseases (Coronavirus Enteritis, Feline Infectious Peritonitis). In: Holzworth J, ed. Diseases of the Cat. Philadelphia: WB Saunders, 1987:193.
15. Scott FW. Update on FIP. In: Johnson SE, ed. Feline Medicine. Kal Kan Symposium for the Treatment of Small Animal Disease. Lawrenceville, NJ: Veterinary Learning Systems, 1989:43.
16. Weiss RC. Feline Infectious Peritonitis and Other Coronaviruses. In: Sherding RG, ed. The Cat: Diseases and Clinical Management. New York: Churchill Livingstone, 1989:333.
17. Scott FW, Weiss RC, Post JE, et al. Kitten mortality complex (neonatal FIP). Feline Pract 1979;9:44.
18. August JR. Preventive Health Care and Infectious Disease Control. In: Sherding RG, ed. The Cat: Diseases and Management. New York: Churchill Livingstone, 1988:391.
19. August JR. Maintaining a healthy cattery. Kal Kan Forum 1988; 12:49.
20. Canine and feline immunization guidelines. J Am Vet Med Assoc 1989;195:314.
21. Jenkins SR, Clark KA, Currier RW, et al. Compendium of animal rabies control. J Am Vet Med Assoc 1990;196:36.
22. Scott FW. Evaluation of a feline viral rhinotracheitis–feline calicivirus disease vaccine. Am J Vet Res 1977;38:229.
23. Raef TA. AVMA encourages mandatory rabies vaccinations for cats. J Am Vet Med Assoc 1990;196:528.
24. Scott FW. Virucidal disinfectants and feline viruses. Am J Vet Res 1980;41:410.

CHAPTER 51

◇ ◇ ◇

Neoplastic Diseases

Steven J. Susaneck

The increased popularity of cats, combined with improvements in nutrition and control of infectious disease, has led to an increased number of geriatric cats in veterinary practice. In recent years we have become acutely aware of many differences between canine and feline diseases. Much of our knowledge of oncology in domestic animals has been derived from dogs. We are now learning that many neoplastic conditions may differ significantly in the two species, as, indeed, do many of the principles of therapy.

Advances in diagnostic techniques and better understanding of tumor biology and therapeutic modalities have led to an increase in the number of feline tumors that are diagnosed and treated. In this chapter I concentrate on the major tumor types seen in cats, with emphasis on diagnosis, treatment, and prognosis. Other discussions of feline neoplasms are found in Chapters 39, 52, and 59.

The incidence of tumors in cats varies between 158 and 470 per 100,000 cats at risk.[1-3] Unlike dogs, cats have a much higher rate of malignant tumors (70%) than benign ones.[1-3] The most common organ systems involved are the hematopoietic system and the skin.[1-3] With the exception of lymphosarcoma, most tumors affect older animals.[1-4]

Diagnosis

The single most important step in the management of cancer in cats is making the correct diagnosis. The greatest advance in the control of neoplasia is the ability to detect and treat it in its earliest stages. The clinical signs associated with many tumors are nonspecific; they include weight loss, anorexia, depression, vomiting, diarrhea, chronic nonhealing lesions, halitosis, and palpable masses.

The first step in the diagnosis of cancer is a thorough physical examination. Most abdominal organs can be palpated externally if the cat is not obese. Abnormalities in the shape or size of an organ should be investigated. Often a presumptive diagnosis can be based on the physical findings. Routine laboratory tests should include a complete blood count (CBC), serum biochemistries, urinalysis, and feline leukemia virus (FeLV)/feline immunodeficiency virus (FIV) tests. Survey radiographs of the affected area, lungs, and internal lymph nodes are indicated to determine the presence of metastasis.

Although a presumptive diagnosis can be made from history, physical examination, and radiographs, a definitive diagnosis requires confirmation. This may be accomplished through cytologic or histopathologic examination of a tissue sample. Biopsy is the single most important step in the diagnosis of cancer in animals. Many more animals have died because a biopsy was not performed than because one was performed. Far too many times I have been told by referring veterinarians that the owner did not want a biopsy performed. We must educate the pet-owning public that this is not acceptable. Several forms of biopsy are available, including fine-needle aspiration, large-bore needle biopsy, incisional biopsy, and excisional biopsy. The most important rules to remember are these:

1. When in doubt perform a biopsy.
2. Any mass worth removing merits a biopsy.

A biopsy is one of the most important steps in the proper planning of cancer treatment. The major objectives of a biopsy are to (1) diagnose disease, (2) monitor response to therapy, (3) stage disease, (4) plan future therapy, and (5) determine prognosis. Much information can be gained from a properly obtained and properly handled biopsy specimen. The evaluation of a biopsy is only as good as the sample being evaluated, and this should be a cooperative effort between the pathologist and the clinician.

Aspiration Biopsy. The simplest form of biopsy is fine-needle aspiration. This technique allows rapid interpretation of the sample and differentiates tumors and inflammatory lesions. It is ideally suited for the preoperative evaluation of cutaneous masses. Major advantages include speed, lack of expense, and most can be performed without anesthesia. The major disadvantages are the small sample size and the expertise needed to differentiate certain lesions (see Chapter 13).

Needle Punch Biopsy. The needle punch biopsy utilizes a variety of needle core instruments. These include the Tru-Cut Biopsy Needle and the Bauer Temno Biopsy Needle. These instruments obtain a sample 1.0 to 1.5 cm long and approximately 1 to 2 mm in diameter. A good sample provides the pathologist a diagnostic section of tissue. Virtually any palpable mass of adequate size can be sampled with this method. A major advantage is that in most cases no anesthetic is needed. Many biopsies can be obtained on an outpatient basis.

The most common use of the needle biopsy is for externally palpable masses. Deep organs, such as the liver and kidney, lend themselves well to this technique; lymph nodes and highly inflamed masses do not.

Incisional Biopsy. An incisional biopsy is one in which a small sample is taken from the lesion. This technique is utilized when cytologic examination and needle biopsy have failed to yield diagnostic results or when a tumor is associated with necrosis or ulceration. The biopsy should be taken from an area in which the biopsy tract can later be completely excised. Large scars or open wounds that might interfere with subsequent therapy should be avoided.

Marginal Biopsy. A marginal biopsy is a technique in which a section is removed from the tumor bed after the tumor is removed. In cases of large tumors it may be of value to excise a small section of tissue that appears to be normal for evaluation of microscopic tumor infiltration. This technique allows exact determination of tissue margins.

Excisional Biopsy. When a mass has been surgically excised it should be submitted for histopathologic examination. The pathologist should be able to identify the tumor type and to determine if there is normal tissue on all margins. The latter information is vital for determining that all local tumor tissue has been removed.

Interpretation of Results. Once the specimen has been obtained it must be properly prepared and interpreted. It is important to understand that a pathologist may render an opinion on the sample that is equivocal. There are several steps that can facilitate the interpretative process.

- Avoid biopsy specimens that contain ulcerated or inflamed areas.
- Provide the pathologist adequate tissue: the more samples the better.
- Take care not to unduly deform the sample.
- Identify margins.
- Properly fix samples with one part tissue to ten parts of 10% formalin. Tissue sections should not be thicker than 1 cm.
- Provide a detailed history.
- Develop a good working relationship with your pathologist. The results are only as good as the sample and the pathologist. Pathologists are not infallible. If the diagnosis does not seem appropriate, ask for another reading of the sample.

Treatment Modalities

When the tumor has been diagnosed and staged, treatment can begin. The major treatment modalities are surgery, chemotherapy, radiation, and immunotherapy.

Surgery

Surgery is the most common, and in many cases the most effective, treatment for nonhematopoietic cancers. Many advances have been made in surgical oncology over the past few years, including partial mandibulectomy and maxillectomy and hemipelvectomy.[5-8] Some of these procedures should be performed by specialists, but it is important for every veterinarian to be cognizant of them so they may be offered to clients. In addition, cytoreductive surgery allows the surgeon to reduce the tumor volume so that other modalities may be more effective.

Several good reviews of veterinary surgical oncology have been written[4-6]; it is beyond the scope of this chapter to cover all aspects of surgical oncology. Several important points are pertinent. Surgical removal of a tumor is most effectively accomplished when the surgeon knows what tumor type is being removed. Since different tumors have different local growth patterns, presurgical biopsy will allow more effective planning. It is impossible to assess thoroughness of surgery by viewing a gross sample; postsurgical histopathologic examination of the surgical margins is required. It is important to thoroughly stage the disease prior to surgery, to ensure that the tumor has not advanced beyond the surgical field.

Chemotherapy

The use of chemotherapy has expanded greatly in the past 10 years, owing principally to a better understanding of the drugs and their benefits and wider client acceptance. The greatest single problem with client acceptance is a negative bias due to misinformation about human experience with chemotherapy. In human chemotherapy, a high priority is placed on aggressive treatment to achieve cure; this results in high morbidity. In cats, the focus is less on cure and more on maintaining disease-free remission while maintaining a high quality of life.

Several important issues must be addressed before chemotherapy commences. Does the cat have a chemotherapy sensitive tumor? Is the cat's overall health good enough to allow it to tolerate therapy? Can the owners cope with the expense and possible side effects of chemotherapy? When all three of these questions have been answered in the affirmative, a chemotherapy plan can be formulated. Every protocol for a particular tumor type is not the correct one for every cat; each must be developed for the individual cat based on tumor type, ability of the cat to handle a particular drug, expense, and logistics.

The single most important concern of most owners and veterinarians is toxicity. Toxicity must be acceptable to the owner, the cat, and the treating veterinarian. The major toxicities involve the bone marrow and the gastrointestinal (GI) tract.[9,10]

The bone marrow is a major site of chemotherapy-induced toxicity owing to the rapid turnover of cells.[9,10] The most important cytopenias involve the leukocytes and the thrombocytes.[9,10] These are most commonly seen 5 to 10 days after administration of the drug and are followed by return to normal values in 2 to 4 days. Neutropenia may

Table 51–1. Anticancer Drugs Commonly Used in Cats

Drug	Route	Dose	Toxicity
Alkylating agents			
Cyclophosphamide	PO	50 mg/m^2 q48hr	GI/M
	IV	100–200 mg/m^2 q7d *or* 250 mg/m^2 q3wk	BM/S
Chlorambucil	PO	2 mg/m^2 q48hr	BM/M
Antimetabolites			
L-Asparaginase	SC	400 IU/kg q1–3wk *or*	GI/R
	IM	10,000 IU/m^2 q1–3wk	BM/R
Methotrexate	PO	2.5–5.0 mg/m^2 2–3×/wk	GI/M
	IV	10–15 mg/m^2 q1–3wk	GI/M
Cytosine arabinoside	IV, SC	100 mg/m^2 q over 24 hr s.i.d. for 2–4 d *or* 10 mg/m^2 q24hr for 2 wk	BM/S
Antibiotics			
Doxorubicin	IV	20–30 mg/m^2 q3–5wk	BM/S
Antimitotics			
Vincristine	IV	0.5–0.75 mg/m^2 q7d to q3wk	BM/M

IV, intravenous; SC, subcutaneous; IM, intramuscular; GI, gastrointestinal; BM, bone marrow; S, severe; M, mild; R, rare

place the cat at increased risk of infection.[10-12] Clinical signs associated with neutropenia include anorexia, nausea, vomiting, lethargy, and fever. Neutropenic febrile cats should be treated with broad-spectrum bacteriocidal antibiotics.[9-11]

The GI tract is also a common site of toxicity.[9,13] GI toxicities include nausea, vomiting, diarrhea, and anorexia. The drugs most often associated with GI side effects are doxorubicin and cyclophosphamide. Doxorubicin has also been shown to cause profound anorexia in some cats.[14]

Table 51–1 lists the commonly used anticancer drugs and their indications.

Hemolymphatic Neoplasms

Feline hemolymphatic neoplasms account for 35 to 40% of all feline tumors.[1-4,15-17] Cats have the highest incidence of hemolymphatic tumors of any species, and lymphosarcoma accounts for 90% of hemolymphatic tumors.[1-4,15-17] The high incidence of hemolymphatic neoplasia is directly related to the FeLV.[15] Feline hemolymphatic diseases affect between 41 and 200 cats per 100,000 in the population, depending on the geographic location and the characteristics of the local feline population.[15] Most cats (70%) with lymphosarcoma and bone marrow suppression have FeLV antigen, while a variable percentage (10% to 30%), depending on the tumor location, have no detectable FeLV antigens or infectious virus in any tissue.[15] However, most FeLV-negative cats with lymphosarcoma display the feline oncornavirus–associated cell membrane antigen (FOCMA) on neoplastic cells, indicating that the FeLV is also a cause of lymphosarcoma in these cats.[15]

Lymphosarcoma

Lymphosarcoma affects primarily solid lymphoid tissues such as lymph nodes, spleen, or liver. Because lymphosarcoma can arise from any organ that contains lymphatic tissue, it has been reported in a number of organs. Lymphoid leukemia arises from lymphocytes of the bone marrow.

Classification

Clinically, feline lymphosarcoma is classified according to anatomic location: alimentary, mediastinal, multicentric, and miscellaneous. The frequency of the various anatomic forms varies with geography.[15,17-23] These discrepancies in tumor type frequency apparently represent inconsistent geographic distribution of different FeLV strains of varying pathogenic potentials. The most commonly reported form is the mediastinal form, followed by alimentary, multicentric, and miscellaneous forms.[15,17-23]

The average age of cats affected with lymphosarcoma is 5 to 6 years but the age varies considerably with the form. The mediastinal form generally affects young cats; the gastrointestinal form most commonly affects older ones.

The mediastinal form of lymphosarcoma, also referred to as thymic lymphosarcoma, arises primarily from the anterior and posterior mediastinal lymph nodes.[24] This form is seen primarily in young cats (average 2.5 years), and 80% of affected cats test positive for FeLV.[15,19]

The most common presenting complaint of cats with mediastinal lymphosarcoma is dyspnea characterized by open-mouthed breathing. Other common presenting signs include tachypnea, orthopnea, cyanosis, dysphagia, regurgitation, and weight loss. Physical examination often reveals muffled and caudally displaced heart sounds, a noncompressible anterior chest wall, absence of bronchovesicular sounds, dyspnea, and cyanosis.[19]

Thoracic radiographs vary, depending on the amount of pleural fluid. Commonly, radiographs reveal bilateral pleural effusion with caudal displacement of the heart and lungs and dorsal displacement of the trachea. These radiographic findings are highly suggestive of an anterior mediastinal mass. When minimal pleural effusion is present or after thoracocentesis, masses in the anterior and posterior mediastinum can be visualized[19] (see Chapter 18).

Confirmation of lymphosarcoma can be made by cytologic examination of cells from both the fluid and mass (see Chapter 13). In some cases the masses can be quite large and can safely be aspirated using a 23- to 25-gauge needle.

When severe dyspnea is associated with the presence of large volumes of fluid, therapeutic thoracocentesis should be performed before further diagnostics or handling of the cat.

The alimentary form of lymphosarcoma is characterized by neoplastic infiltration at any site in the gastrointestinal tract or mesenteric lymph nodes.[17-19,25] The tumor may be a single mass, multiple masses, or a diffuse infiltration of the intestinal wall. The mesenteric lymph nodes may or may not be involved. Renal and hepatic LSA has been included in the GI form by some authors[17,18] and in the miscellaneous form by others.[13] The average age of cats with alimentary lymphosarcoma is older (8 years) than for other forms, and the percentage of cats positive for FeLV antigens is lower (30%).[15]

Clinical signs often include weight loss, anorexia, vomiting, diarrhea, and constipation. In some cases of colonic involvement, tenesmus and frank blood may be associated with diarrhea. The duration of clinical signs is variable but often is prolonged owing to the chronic nature of this disease. When diffuse small intestinal involvement is present, severe wasting and protein-losing enteropathy can occur. This can present clinical signs of polyphagia (instead of anorexia) and weight loss, which may be confused with diabetes mellitus or hyperthyroidism. Anemia is uncommon in alimentary lymphosarcoma, and when present is usually associated with blood loss or anemia of chronic disease.

Physical examination may reveal an abdominal mass, thickened bowel, and enlarged mesenteric lymph nodes. Survey radiographs often are normal unless there are signs of obstruction or large abdominal masses. Positive-contrast radiographs can be helpful in diagnosing mass lesions and obstruction.

A presumptive diagnosis can sometimes be made on the basis of cytologic examination of enlarged mesenteric lymph nodes or an abdominal mass. Care should be taken in interpreting such preparations because there may be overlap of inflammatory hyperplasia and neoplasia. A definitive diagnosis should be made by histopathologic examination of an endoscopic biopsy or laparotomy specimen. Endoscopic biopsy specimens of upper and lower GI lesions are generally diagnostic; however, caution should be exerted when interpreting endoscopic biopsy tissue that is negative for neoplasia. Lymphosarcoma may be limited to the submucosa or serosa and thus be missed on mucosal biopsy. Cases of lymphocytic-plasmacytic and lymphocytic gastroenteritis may be associated with early lymphosarcoma, regional involvement of lymphosarcoma, and submucosal or serosal involvement. If a case of lymphocytic-plasmacytic enteritis fails to respond to therapy, full-thickness biopsy is indicated.

The multicentric form of lymphosarcoma is characterized by primary involvement of most lymphoid tissues of the body and secondary involvement of other structures such as liver, bone marrow, kidney, and lungs. Cats with primary bone marrow involvement should be classified as having lymphoid leukemia. The average cat with multicentric lymphosarcoma is 4 years old; 80% are FeLV positive.[15,17,18,22-24]

Presenting signs and physical findings are variable and depend on the location and volume of the tumor. Enlarged painless peripheral lymph nodes may be palpated. Internal lymph nodes, liver, and spleen may also be enlarged. In addition, extranodal sites such as the eye, kidney, and the central nervous system (CNS) may be involved. Anemia is a common finding with this type of lymphosarcoma and is often nonregenerative and normocytic, normochromic.[13,17]

Confirmatory diagnosis can often be made through cytologic examination of lymph nodes, liver, spleen, or an extranodal lesion. In some cases of well-differentiated lymphosarcoma, a definitive cytologic diagnosis may be difficult and surgical biopsy indicated. Generalized lymphosarcoma must be differentiated from nonmalignant lymphadenopathy resulting from primary FeLV or FIV infection. Other items in the differential diagnosis include granulomatous diseases, systemic viral infections, and other primary and secondary neoplasms (see Chapter 21).

The treatment of multicentric lymphosarcoma is chemotherapy. All cats with generalized lymph node enlargement should be tested for FeLV antigens and FIV antibodies. In cases of suspected lymphosarcoma bone marrow biopsy may be beneficial.

The miscellaneous form of lymphosarcoma, the least common form, accounts for fewer than 10% of all cases. The lesions in this form generally affect extranodal tissues, including the eyes, skin, kidney, nose, CNS, or any other nonlymphoid tissues. Since this form of lymphosarcoma affects extranodal tissues, some authors prefer the term "extranodal lymphoma."

Involvement of the CNS with lymphosarcoma has been reported: it is the second most common CNS tumor.[26] The most common clinical signs are secondary to spinal cord compression. Peripheral nerve involvement and brain involvement have also been reported.[26] The differential diagnosis for CNS disease includes feline infectious peritonitis (FIP), toxoplasmosis, intervertebral disk disease, other primary or metastatic vertebral tumors, meningioma, FIV, and FeLV-associated nonneoplastic neuropathy.

CNS metastasis has been reported in cats with renal lymphosarcoma that have achieved complete remission of their primary tumor.[27] For cats with CNS lymphosarcoma the prognosis for return to normal function is poor.

Renal lymphosarcoma may be concurrent with other forms of lymphosarcoma or may exist as a primary disease. It is considered to be a primary disease when one or both kidneys are involved with no other organ involvement. Cats with renal lymphosarcoma often present with a palpable abdominal mass or signs referable to renal failure. Physical examination usually reveals unilateral or bilateral renomegaly. Diagnosis is made by percutaneous fine-needle aspiration or percutaneous biopsy. The differential diagnosis includes FIP, polycystic kidney disease, renal pseudocyst, hydronephrosis, and other primary renal tumors.

Other less common sites of involvement are the skin, eye, nasal cavity, and oral cavity.

Treatment

Since in most cases lymphosarcoma is a systemic disease, chemotherapy is the treatment of choice. In selected cases other therapies may also be indicated, including radiation and surgery plus various forms of supportive therapy. Client education is extremely important in the management of cats with lymphosarcoma. Clients must understand that even with treatment lymphosarcoma is a fatal disease and that the goal of therapy is not cure. The objective in successful management is to attain a prolonged remission with minimal side effects. Since most cats with lymphosarcoma have FeLV antigens, the possible ramifications of the virus for other cats must be explained to the owner. The owner must be aware that even when the tumor is controlled, other effects of the virus can be lethal (see Chapter 39).

Multiple drugs have been used in the treatment of lymphosarcoma. What specific combination of drugs is used in any particular case varies depending on several factors: anatomic location of the tumor, disposition of the cat, general health of the cat, cost, potential side effects, and logistics.

Multiple drug combinations appear to be more effective than single-drug treatments. Chemotherapy is generally divided into three phases: induction, maintenance, and rescue. The goal of induction is to cause a complete remission and to render the cat free of detectable disease. The goal of maintenance is to prolong the remission as long as possible. Some cats never attain a complete remission but may attain a partial one. For them and for cats that have come out of remission, a rescue drug may be indicated. Several different protocols have been published and evaluated (Table 51–2). The most successful protocols include cyclophosphamide, Oncovin, cytosine arabinoside, and prednisolone (COAP); cyclophosphamide, Oncovin, and prednisolone (COP); and sequential multiagent chemotherapy.

The median remission time for all forms of lymphosarcoma that respond to cytotoxic chemotherapy varies from 4 to 28 months, depending on the stage of the disease.[24] Occasional animals survived longer than 4 years. In cats with mediastinal lymphosarcoma, complete response rates of 90% have been attained with a median survival time of 6 to 7 months.[13,28,29] Fifteen to twenty percent of the animals in these two studies lived longer than a year.[13,27] The prognosis is much worse when the initial response is less than a 5% reduction in tumor mass.[13,27]

Cats with alimentary tract lymphosarcoma treated with chemotherapy have been reported to have a median survival

Table 51–2. Chemotherapy Protocols for Lymphosarcoma

Cotter's COP Protocol[13]

Week 1: Vincristine, 0.75 mg/m² IV
Cyclophosphamide, 200 mg/m² PO
Week 2: Vincristine, 0.75 mg/m² IV
Week 3: Vincristine, 0.75 mg/m² IV
Week 4: Vincristine, 0.75 mg/m² IV
Cyclophosphamide, 200 mg/m² PO

After 4 weeks, vincristine and cyclophosphamide are given every 3 weeks until 1 year or relapse. Prednisone is given at 2 mg/kg/day.

MacEwen's Protocol[21]

Week 1: Vincristine, 0.025 mg/kg IV
L-Asparaginase, 400 IU/kg IM
Prednisone, 2 mg/kg/day PO
Week 2: Cyclophosphamide, 10 mg/kg IV
Week 3: Vincristine, 0.025 mg/kg IV
Week 4: Methotrexate, 0.8 mg/kg IV*

Repeat treatments on a weekly basis for another four cycles (except L-asparaginase). Then continue on an every 2 weeks basis.

COAP[17]

Cyclophosphamide, 50 mg/m² 4 days a week
Vincristine, 0.5 mg/m²/week
Cytosine arabinoside, 100 mg/m² SC for 2 days
Prednisone, 40 mg/m²/day PO for 1 week then 20 mg/m² every other day

The protocol is administered weekly for 6 weeks.

After 6 weeks the drugs are administered every other week for six treatments, then every third week for six treatments, then monthly.

*Doxorubicin can be substituted for methotrexate at a dose of 25 mg/m² IV. When substituting doxorubicin, wait 14 days before the next vincristine injection.

time of 4 to 5 months.[13,28,29] The median survival time for cats with multicentric lymphosarcoma is also approximately 5 months. Cats with only peripheral node involvement may have a better prognosis.[13]

Without chemotherapy the prognosis for any cat with lymphosarcoma is grave. The disease is usually rapidly progressive and death occurs within 30 to 45 days.

Radiation therapy may be utilized to treat mediastinal lymphosarcoma, localized lymphosarcoma of the nervous system, or lymphosarcoma of the nasal cavity. Because lymphosarcoma cells are very sensitive to radiation, large tumors can be shrunk rapidly with radiation. Radiation is best used in combination with chemotherapy.

Leukemias

Most leukemias are lymphoid in origin; they represent 7% to 30% of all lymphoid neoplasms.[13,15,30,31] In some cases it is difficult to identify the exact cell line of origin without special staining procedures available at most commercial laboratories. Leukemias can arise from lymphoid, myeloid, or erythroid cell lines. The treatment of most feline leukemias is unrewarding, and the prognosis for any cat with leukemia is poor.

The clinician is reminded that the term "leukemia" is not synonymous with a positive FeLV test. No veterinarian should say, "Your cat has leukemia" on the basis of this test alone.

Mammary Tumors

Incidence

Mammary tumors are the third most common tumor of cats.[1-4,32,33] The overall risk is 25.4 per 100,000 female cats.[4] The age range is 2.5 to 19 years, and 70% occur between age 9 and 13 years; the average age is 10.8 to 11.5 years, depending on the study cited.[1-4,34] Several reports cite overrepresentation of Siamese cats.[1-4,34] In rare instances intact and neutered male cats develop mammary carcinomas.[32,33]

One study showed a sevenfold greater incidence of mammary carcinoma in intact cats than in spayed ones. Other surveys have also demonstrated that mammary carcinomas are more common in intact females than in ovariohysterectomized ones, but to a lesser extent.[35-37] In one survey only 8% of 221 cats with mammary gland carcinomas had been ovariohysterectomized before age 1 year.[3] Performing ovariohysterectomy before 1 year does not eliminate the possibility of mammary tumors as it does in dogs, but it does appear to have some sparing effect.[3,22,33]

It has been observed that long-term progestational hormone therapy (i.e., megestrol acetate) in cats may be associated with an increased incidence of mammary tumors as well as other mammary disease (see Chapter 7).[34,38,39]

Pathology

One study found 86% of feline mammary tumors to be malignant.[34] Of the malignant tumors, adenocarcinoma is the predominant type[34]; it takes tubular, papillary, and solid forms.[4,32,33] Other more rarely reported mammary tumors include sarcomas,[4,33] myoepitheliomas,[4,33] comedocarcinomas,[4] and squamous cell carcinomas.[4] Benign mammary tumors are uncommon, accounting for only about 14% of feline mammary tumors.[4,34]

Mammary carcinomas have been further classified by (1) cellular differentiation and the degree of tubule formation, (2) nuclear pleomorphism, and (3) frequency of mitosis. By these criteria, cats with well-differentiated tumors appear to survive longer than those with poorly differentiated tumors.[33]

History and Clinical Signs

Most mammary tumors are diagnosed because the owner or veterinarian notices a mass or masses in the mammary chain. Most cats do not exhibit any other signs at the time of presentation. In some advanced cases the cat may be presented for weight loss or dyspnea due to metastatic disease.

Feline mammary tumors tend to grow rapidly. The average historical duration of the tumor at time of diagnosis is 5 months.[3] The size of the tumor varies (mean diameter of 3 cm); tumors are rarely larger than 6 cm in diameter. The tumors usually lie in the subcutaneous tissue adjacent to the nipple and adhere to the overlying skin. Local invasion into underlying musculature is common. About 15% to 25% are ulcerated at the time of diagnosis. Ulcerated tumors are often necrotic and draining at the time of diagnosis.[3]

Multiple-gland involvement is common (40% to 66%).[3,23] Several reports indicate that the cranial glands may be affected more frequently.[3] In some cases, beadlike chains of tiny nodules may be palpated, suggesting venous or lymphatic invasion. Metastasis is common with mammary carcinomas; the most common sites of metastasis are regional lymph nodes, lungs, pleura, and liver.

Diagnosis

A presumptive diagnosis of mammary gland tumor can be based on the presence of a mass lesion in the breast tissue. Definitive diagnosis can be made only by surgical biopsy, although fine-needle aspiration can be highly suggestive. Owing to the high metastatic potential of feline mammary gland tumors, a thoracic radiograph should be performed prior to surgery; however, the absence of detectable metastatic lesions at the time of diagnosis does not guarantee that metastasis has not already occurred.

Treatment

The treatment of choice should be removal en bloc of all glands on the affected side. Bilateral mastectomy should be performed when both sides are involved. In some cases both sides can be removed at one time; in other cases two operations should be employed. When only one chain is clinically involved, removal of the opposite chain should be considered, owing to the possibility of microscopic metastasis and of multicentric origin. All regional lymph nodes should be palpated and removed for histologic examination.[21]

To date nonsurgical therapies have not proven to have

significant clinical value. Chemotherapy with adriamycin and cytoxan has shown some effectiveness in advanced cases.[38] Chemotherapy using mitoxantrone is presently being investigated.

Prognosis

The overall prognosis is poor owing to the high rate of malignancy.[40] The median survival time for cats treated with surgery alone is 10 to 14 months.[34] Tumor volume seems to be the most prognostic clinical factor. Cats with a total tumor volume of 8 cm had a median survival time of 4½ years; cats with a volume of 9 to 17 cm had a medium survival of 2 years.[3] Cats with a tumor greater than 27 cm had a medium survival of 6 months.[3] The type of surgery, conservative versus aggressive, affected the disease-free interval but not the survival time.[41]

Digestive Tract Neoplasms

Tumors of the digestive system, including oral tumors, are common. Patnaik reported that during an 11-year period at The Animal Medical Center, GI tumors were the most common nonhematopoietic tumor found in cats at necropsy.[32] Engle reported that GI tumors were the second most common nonhematopoietic tumor seen at the University of Pennsylvania Diagnostic Laboratory.[16]

The most common sites are the mouth, pharynx, and small intestine. The most common histologic types are squamous cell carcinoma (SCC; oral cavity) and adenocarcinoma (small intestine). The vast majority of feline GI tumors are malignant.

Oral Tumors

The most frequent sites of oral tumors are the gingiva and the tongue.[3,42-44] Oral cancer risk is greatest for older cats (mean age 10 to 11 years).[3,42,43] The most common tumor type is SCC.[3,42,43] Oral SCCs are characterized by local invasion and extension; ulceration and secondary infection are common sequelae. The morbidity associated with oral tumors is usually due to local disease rather than metastasis. Metastasis, when it occurs, usually develops late in the course of disease to cervical lymph nodes and the lungs.

Fibrosarcoma (FSA) is the second most common tumor of the oral cavity, accounting for about 15% to 20% of feline oral neoplasms. Oral FSA generally affects the gingiva. Other tumors rarely identified in the mouth include undifferentiated sarcoma, hemangiosarcoma, hemangioma, melanoma, lymphosarcoma, adamantinoma, salivary gland carcinoma, and oncocytoma.

History and Physical Examination

The history often includes dysphagia, halitosis, salivation, and weight loss. Physical examination often reveals a proliferative, ulcerated, often necrotic mass involving the tongue or gingiva. Lingual SCCs tend to involve the underside and lateral margins of the tongue. In most cases the tumor extends deep into the base of the tongue. In prolonged cases involving the gingiva, radiographs may reveal bony destruction, and enlarged lymph nodes may be palpable. All ulcerated oral lesions of older cats should be investigated by examining a biopsy specimen. Multiple adjacent loose teeth may be seen with SCC. The differential diagnosis includes ulcerative stomatitis, eosinophilic granuloma complex, chronic granuloma, and lymphocytic-plasmacytic stomatitis.

Treatment

Most oral tumors of cats are diagnosed too late to be completely surgically resected; however, when possible surgical resection is the treatment of choice. Aggressive surgical procedures are necessary, since SCC and FSA are extremely locally invasive. These procedures often include partial mandibulectomy and maxillectomy. Unfortunately, the visualized portion of the tumor may be only a small part of the overall malignancy. When an oral tumor is excised it is extremely important to submit the entire mass for histopathologic examination and to have the surgical margins evaluated. Cryosurgery may be beneficial for small oral tumors; radiation alone has not proven very effective. Combinations of radiation and chemotherapy have been reported to be of some benefit. In general, oral tumors carry an extremely poor prognosis (see Chapter 52).

Intestinal Tumors

Lymphosarcoma and mast cell tumors are the most common tumors of the gastrointestinal tract.[43] The small intestine is the most common site of nonlymphoid GI neoplasia outside the oral cavity.[3,42,44,45] Lymphosarcoma is the most common tumor involving the intestine, but since it is often multicentric and classified with the hematopoietic system, the true prevalence of GI lymphosarcoma is difficult to establish. Other intestinal tumors reported are SCC of the small intestine and rectum,[44] leiomyosarcoma,[16,44] and sarcomas.[36]

Adenocarcinoma is the most common nonlymphoid neoplasm of the intestinal tract.[42,46,47] Although adenocarcinomas may occur anywhere in the intestinal tract, the majority occur in the jejunum, ileum, or ileocecal junction.[42,46,47] Grossly, adenocarcinomas often appear as firm, white, annular masses or mural thickening.[56,57] Intestinal strictures as a result of this tumor are common. Adenocarcinomas are highly malignant and at the time of diagnosis often have metastasized to regional lymph nodes and the omentum.[42,46,47] Other less common tumors that have been reported in the feline intestine are fibrosarcomas, leiomyosarcomas, and carcinoids.[36,42,44]

Siamese cats are at increased risk for developing small intestinal carcinomas, but large intestinal carcinomas are the most common type in all domestic cats.[44,46,47] The mean age of cats with small intestinal adenocarcinoma is 10.6 years, and males may be affected more often than females.[42,44,45,47]

The most common clinical signs associated with intestinal adenocarcinoma are weight loss, vomiting, and anorexia. Signs are often present for many months before diagnosis. Less common signs are constipation, tenesmus, diarrhea, and ascites. Constipation or tenesmus is typically associated with colon tumors.

Intestinal neoplasia should be suspected if an older cat exhibits chronic weight loss or gastrointestinal signs that are unresponsive to symptomatic therapy. In some cases an intestinal mass can be palpated. A thorough physical examination, CBC, serum biochemistry profile, FeLV/FIV test, and urinalysis should be performed to rule out metabolic disease. Plain radiographs of the abdomen are commonly not diagnostic, and contrast radiographic studies are needed. In general, carcinomas encircle the lumen (apple core sign), causing narrowing of the lumen with an irregular surface. This may also occur with lymphosarcoma; however carcinomas may also appear as an irregular, ragged filling defect or as multiple nodular defects causing scalloping of the bowel wall. Surgical biopsy is required to confirm a neoplasm. If abdominal fluid is present, cytologic analysis may reveal exfoliated tumor cells, which may be diagnostic. These cells must be differentiated from reactive mesothelial cells.

Surgical resection is the treatment of choice for all nonlymphoid intestinal neoplasms. Wide surgical margins should be obtained, and affected lymph nodes should be removed and evaluated. Normal-looking lymph nodes and lymph nodes that are not removed should also be evaluated. Enlarged lymph nodes may be only reactive; therefore, they, too, should be evaluated. To date, chemotherapy has not been effective in treating these tumors.

The prognosis for malignant intestinal tumors is poor. Unfortunately, most cats are presented late in the course of the disease, when metastasis has already occurred. Common metastatic sites include lymph nodes, spleen, lungs, and kidney as well as local extension into the mesentery.[4,46,48] Although the mean survival time for cats treated surgically is 4 to 6 months, a significant number of cats survive several years. The prognosis is better for cats that do not have metastasis to lymph nodes at the time of surgery.[4,46,48]

Hepatobiliary Tumors

Primary hepatic neoplasms are uncommon: the prevalence is between 0.5% and 1.5% of all feline tumors, excluding myeloproliferative tumors.[4,16,32,36] Bile duct carcinoma (BDC) is probably the most common hepatic tumor. In general, hepatic tumors are most common in older cats.

The majority of liver tumors are malignant.[4,16,32,36] The most common tumor types are BDC and hepatocellular carcinoma. Other tumors that can arise in the liver are hepatocellular adenoma, cystadenoma, hemangiosarcoma, hemangioma, fibrosarcoma, and mast cell tumor.

BDCs are malignant tumors that arise from the biliary system, either from intrahepatic or extrahepatic bile ducts or the gallbladder. Intrahepatic BDCs are more common than those arising from the extrahepatic bile duct or gallbladder. BDCs tend to metastasize along the portal lymphatics to regional lymph nodes. Carcinomatosis frequently occurs due to transcelomic metastasis. Hepatocellular carcinoma is a malignant tumor of hepatocytes. Grossly the tumor may be nodular, diffuse, or massive.[4]

The clinical signs of hepatic neoplasia are often nonspecific. History often includes progressive anorexia, weight loss, vomition, lethargy, icterus, and ascites. Hepatomegaly is usually present as the disease progresses. Other less common signs are polyuria, polydipsia, diarrhea, and ataxia.

Physical examination often reveals hepatomegaly or a large anterior abdominal mass that may be visible radiographically. Serum biochemical abnormalities are of little value in differentiating primary neoplasms from secondary ones, inflammation, or hepatic lipidosis. The most consistent finding is an elevated serum alkaline phosphatase value. Other findings may include elevated levels of alanine aminotransferase, aspartate aminotransferase, and anemia. The total bilirubin level is variable, depending on the amount of biliary obstruction. Definitive diagnosis requires a tissue biopsy specimen, although cytologic examination can often be very helpful in obtaining a presumptive diagnosis. Biopsy specimens can be obtained through blind percutaneous liver biopsy, laparoscopy, ultrasound-guided biopsy, and laparotomy.

The treatment of choice is surgical removal of the tumor, though in most cases of hepatic neoplasia the tumor is inoperable at the time of diagnosis. Chemotherapy has not proven to be of value. The prognosis for malignant hepatic tumors is grave.

Other sites of GI tumors that have been reported are the salivary gland, esophagus, and stomach. Salivary gland tumors are very uncommon but usually highly malignant. The gland affected most often is the mandibular salivary gland, and the tumor type is usually adenocarcinoma. Esophageal tumors are also very rare. Nonhematopoietic tumors of the stomach are rare; the most such tumors are gastric polyps and leiomyomas.

Bone Tumors

Both primary and secondary bone tumors are rare. The incidence rate for feline bone tumors was determined to be 3.1 per 100,000, as compared to 7.9 per 100,000 for dogs.[1] Bone tumors can arise in cats of any age but most often occur in middle-aged to older domestic shorthaired cats.[1,4,49]

Osteosarcoma

Osteosarcoma, the most common bone tumor, accounts for about 70% of all feline bone tumors.[4,44,49-52] The average age of cats with osteosarcoma is 10.2 years.[4,49] The long bones are most often affected, especially the distal femur, proximal humerus, and proximal tibia. One study reported that the appendicular skeleton was affected 2.4 times more frequently than the axial skeleton[49]; another reports an appendicular-to-axial skeleton ratio of 1.4 : 1.[4] The hindlimbs were affected more frequently than the forelimbs.[4,49]

Clinical signs include lameness and/or the presence of a large, firm mass tightly adherent to bone. The average time from the onset of signs to presentation is 2 to 3 months.[4,49] The severity of clinical signs varies with the size and location of the tumors. Tumors on the head are often presented for facial deformity.

Radiographic features of osteosarcoma are those of an aggressive bone lesion.[49] Tumor margins are indistinct. Radiographic appearance varies from osteolysis to a large radiodensity extending into soft tissue. Although clinical signs, history, and radiographs may be suggestive of an osteosarcoma, histopathologic examination is needed for confirmation.

The recommended treatment for feline osteosarcoma is surgical removal. In most cases this requires amputation of the involved limb. Several authors feel that feline osteosarcomas are less metastatic than their canine counterparts.[49,51,53] In one report of five cases treated with surgery, one cat developed metastasis after 5 months and the other four were alive up to 26 months after surgery.[51] In another study of three cats treated with amputation and doxorubicin, the mean survival time was approximately 8 months.[53]

Parosteal Osteosarcoma

Parosteal osteosarcomas arise from the periosteum and have a histologic pattern composed of well-differentiated fibrous, osseous, and chondroid components.[50] They are usually slow-growing tumors and are often associated with protracted clinical courses of lameness or palpable firm swellings. (Note: This is explained in the next paragraph.) One report of four cases suggested a predilection for the head,[51] and another report of two cases involved long bones.[49]

Clinically, the cat may be presented with a hard mass that is firmly attached to bone. In appendicular parosteal osteosarcomas, lameness and locomotor difficulty may be presenting complaints. Radiographically they appear as irregular, poorly defined masses of variable density attached to the cortex.[49] Definitive diagnosis requires tissue biopsy. The treatment of choice is wide surgical excision or amputation. With complete surgical removal the prognosis is good, owing to the apparently low metastatic rate.

Chondrosarcoma

Chondrosarcomas, malignant tumors of cartilage, represent fewer than 10% of feline bone neoplasms.[49] The average age is 8 to 9 years, and males may outnumber females. There appears to be a predilection for the scapula and humerus. Clinical signs often include a firm, fixed, rapidly growing mass that causes lameness and pain on palpation. The duration of signs ranges from 4 months to 6 years (median 6 months).[49]

Radiographically, chondrosarcomas appear as lobulated radiopaque masses that are primarily osteoblastic. Often there is minimal cortical or periosteal response, and they have a more organized tumor matrix appearance than osteosarcomas. The treatment of choice for chondrosarcomas is wide surgical excision or amputation. Owing to the limited number of documented treatments with follow-up, accurate prognosis is not possible, but chrondrosarcomas do not appear to be highly metastatic.

Osteochondromatosis

Osteochondromatosis in cats differs from osteochondromatosis (multiple cartilaginous exostoses) in dogs, humans, and horses, in which it is thought to be a skeletal dysplasia rather than a true tumor. Growth in these species is often progressive until skeletal maturity is achieved.

Feline osteochondromatosis occurs principally in young adult cats (mean age 3.2 years). The tumors preferentially originate in the perichondrium of the flat or irregular bones (vertebrae, skull, and scapula). Unlike in dogs, the masses appear after skeletal maturity and continue to grow, often resulting in functional impairment.[4,54,55]

Although the origin of this condition has not been proven, it is felt to result from infection with the FeLV, because most cats with this disease test positive for FeLV antigen. In at least seven cases virus particles have been identified in the cartilaginous cap.[4,54,55]

Radiographically this disease presents as multiple ovoid or spherical masses protruding from the surface of the flat bones. The masses are usually well-organized and have smooth borders. Presently, no proven treatment exists. Masses often recur following surgical removal, or new masses appear. Any cat suspected to have osteochondromatosis should be tested for the FeLV; the prognosis is poor.

Fibrosarcoma

Primary fibrosarcomas of the bone arise from the fibrous component of the medulla. In one study primary fibrosarcomas ranked as the second most common bone tumor.[51] Six of eleven tumors in the study involved the head. No metastasis was seen in ten of the eleven cats for which autopsy data were available. The treatment of choice is surgical excision.

Rare Primary Tumors Involving Bone

The giant cell tumor is a rare tumor involving bone or periarticular soft tissue. Giant cell tumors arise from giant cells within the bone and possess varying degrees of aggressiveness. Too few cases have been evaluated to establish patterns of biologic activity. Of the tumors reported, radiographic findings were of intramedullary origin with marked lysis of the cortex.

Ossifying fibromas and osteomas are rare benign tumors of bone most commonly found in the skull.[49] An osteoma is typically a benign solitary growth with a sessile base that arises from the surface of intramembranous bone. An ossifying fibroma is a tumorlike growth that produces an expansile lesion of the fibro-osseous tissue replacing alveolar and cortical bone. Osteomas and ossifying fibromas can cause pressure damage or can be clinically silent.[49] The treatment is surgery, and the prognosis is good.

Other rare tumors that have been reported to involve bone are hemangiosarcomas[52] and chondromas.[44]

Secondary Bone Tumors

Secondary bone tumors are periosseous soft tissue or metastatic tumors that invade adjacent bone. The most common secondary bone tumors are fibrosarcomas and squamous cell carcinomas. Many of these involve bones of the head. Other soft tissue tumors reported to invade bones are lymphosarcoma, rhabdomyosarcoma, malignant melanoma, hemangiosarcoma, reticulum cell sarcoma, and meningioma. These tumors are best treated with surgery; radiation therapy has also proven successful in treating meningiomas.

Intranasal, Nasal, and Paranasal Sinus Tumors

Nasal tumors, excluding tumors of the nasal planum, are rare. More than 90% of feline nasal tumors are malignant.[4,36,44] SCCs and adenocarcinomas are, most commonly reported tumor types, account for approximately 65% of all feline nasal tumors.[3,6,44] Other tumors reported include lymphoreticular tumors, fibroma, fibrosarcoma, osteosarcoma, adenoma, fibropapilloma, and undifferentiated sarcoma and carcinoma.[4,36,44]

The mean age of cats with nasal tumors is 8 to 10 years.[4] Sneezing and nasal discharge are the most prominent clinical signs. In the initial stage nasal tumors may mimic chronic upper respiratory tract infections. Chronic nasal discharge unresponsive to initial therapy warrants further diagnostic studies (see Chapter 30). Other signs are distortion of the nasal bone, exophthalmos, epistaxis, and chronic epiphora. As the tumor progresses obstruction of the nasal cavity may result in noisy respiration.

The major considerations in the differential diagnosis for feline nasal tumors are chronic rhinitis as a sequela of viral respiratory tract diseases, cryptococcoid rhinitis, and nasopharyngeal polyps.[56] Radiography, rhinoscopy, and biopsy should be employed diagnostically (see Chapter 30). For radiography of the nose and frontal sinus the animal should be under general anesthesia. Radiographic changes associated with nasal tumors include nasal turbinate destruction, erosion of the vomer bone, and destruction of the maxilla, frontal bone, palate, or zygoma. In some cases the only radiographic sign is diffuse soft tissue density in the nasal sinus with loss of definition of the turbinates, which can be radiographically identical to chronic infection. Although radiographs may suggest a tumor, definitive diagnosis can only be made by histopathologic examination.

Tissue for histologic examination can be obtained through the nasal bone if bone erosion is present. If there is no erosion through the nasal bone, tissue can be obtained through the nares. The most effective treatments for nasal tumors are radiation therapy and surgical excision via rhinotomy.

Mast Cell Tumors

There appear to be three forms of feline mast cell tumors (MCT): (1) generalized mastocytosis, (2) cutaneous mastocytoma, with or without visceral involvement, and (3) intestinal MCT. In this section I deal only with the generalized forms; see Chapter 59 for a discussion of cutaneous forms.

Visceral MCTs are uncommon and originate most often in spleen.[4,58-61] Other organs commonly affected include the liver, lymph nodes, and peripheral blood.[4,59-61] Bone marrow involvement is noted in many of these cases.

The history and clinical signs that accompany visceral mastocytoma are variable; emesis is the most common finding. Other reported clinical signs include depression, weight loss, anorexia, abdominal distention, and diarrhea. Mast cells contain large amounts of histamine, serotonin, and prostaglandin. These may result in direct irritation of the gastric mucosa and vasoconstriction causing vomiturition and even ulceration. Although vomiting is common, ulceration is not.

Physical examination often reveals a spleen that is massively enlarged; it may be nodular or smooth. The spleen is only rarely palpable in a normal cat, but it is easily palpated in a cat with MCT. Other physical findings may include hepatomegaly, lymphadenopathy, mucous membrane pallor, and peritoneal or pleural effusion.

A CBC with buffy coat evaluation (see Chapter 12) and a biochemical profile should be performed to help rule out other causes of vomiting and splenomegaly. A radiographic or ultrasonographic examination of the abdomen should be performed to detect splenic and hepatic enlargement when signs are suggestive of a MCT or when an unspecified abdominal mass is palpated. Bone marrow biopsy is indicated in any case of suspected MCT, mast cell leukemia, or nonregenerative anemia (see Chapter 12). However, nests of mast cells may be found in a cat with a nonregenerative anemia but without mast cell leukemia.

Presurgical diagnosis can often be made by cytologic examination of a specimen obtained by fine-needle aspiration of the spleen. Mast cells are large (20 to 30 μm), round or oval cells with slightly eccentric rounded nucleoli. The cytoplasm contains variable numbers of granules, which may stain blue with Diff-Quik stain (AHS). In isolated cases of highly undifferentiated, MCT special stains, such as toluidine blue or Giemsa, might be needed. Definitive diagnosis and clinical staging may require surgical exploration, splenectomy, and histologic examination.

When possible, the treatment of choice for cats with systemic MCT is splenectomy. Circulating blood and bone marrow mast cells often disappear following splenectomy but may reappear if the tumor recurs. When hepatic or lymph node involvement is present or in cases unresponsive to splenectomy, systemic prednisone (20 to 40 mg/m^2 s.i.d.) as well as an H2 antihistamine (cimetidine, 5 mg/kg by mouth [PO], t.i.d. or famotidine, 1–2 mg/cat PO, s.i.d.) is indicated. These help reduce the clinical signs that result from vasoactive amine production.

The prognosis for cats with systemic mastocytosis should be considered fair to good. Here are several reports of cats living 1 to 3 years postoperatively.[4,59,60]

Intestinal MCT is the third most common tumor involving the feline intestine,[4] and it is most common in the small intestine. The clinical signs of intestinal MCT are similar to those of other intestinal tumors. Most intestinal MCTs have achieved widespread local invasiveness or have metastasized.[4] The treatment of choice for isolated nonmetastatic disease is surgical removal. The prognosis is generally poor.

Respiratory Tract Tumors*

Feline primary lung tumors are uncommon but may account for 1% of all feline neoplasms. Few benign lung tumors are reported; the vast majority are malignant.[3] Adenocarcinoma is the most common histologic type (prevalence approximately 75%). Adenocarcinoma of the bronchial gland is much less common (15%), and SCC is approximately half that prevalence. No species or sex predeliction is noted; the average age of affected cats is 12 years (range 2 to 18 years). Typical historical findings are either respiratory tract signs (cough, polypnea, and dyspnea) or generalized signs of weakness, anorexia, and lethargy.[3,62-65] Lameness, ataxia,

*Portions of this material were contributed by Jane M. Turrel, DVM, MS, Pacifica, CA.

pain, or paralysis is associated with more than 25% of primary lung tumors and is related to metastatic disease in muscle and bone. Digital metastases (mistakenly diagnosed as bite wound abscesses, fungal infections, and other paronychial disorders) is a frequent presentation for cats with lung tumors.

Clinical findings are usually present only a short time (less than 2 weeks) before presentation.[3] Although dyspnea, polypnea, cough, and hemoptysis are expected signs from a pulmonary tumor, they were seen in only slightly more than half the cats in one study. Clear evidence demonstrates that these tumors metastasize by arterial emboli and thus can cause signs that are generally associated with cardiomyopathy, including weak femoral pulses or a brain infarct. Metastasis to muscle and bone causes digital swelling, firm palpable masses in the muscles and soft tissue, and severe weakness and pain. A unique clinical finding is the presence of digital metastases, which are seen in almost 25% of the cats and produce swollen digits, with or without bone destruction, and the loss of the nail. Several cases have been reported in which treatment for the lameness (amputation) or another predominant clinical sign was performed only to discover that the cause was metastasis from a primary lung tumor. Vomiting is unusual; it results from tumor invasion into the esophageal wall.

Radiographic examination of the thorax of cats with pulmonary carcinoma shows solitary or multiple focal masses in approximately 50%, localized lesions in 20%, and diffuse lesions in 25%.[66] Generally, primary lung tumors are equally distributed between the right and left lung lobes. The caudal lobes are most affected with equal distribution to right and left sides. Lesions may be cavitated or calcified and are found in the peripheral or middle portion of the lung. Hilar or mediastinal lymphadenopathy is a feature of approximately one third of cases. Pleural thickening and pleural fluid may develop when pleural metastases are present.

Other radiographic findings include destructive and proliferative bony lesions with attendant soft tissue swelling. Tissues of the appendicular skeleton are most frequently involved: the digits typically, but also long and flat bones. Hypertrophic pulmonary osteopathy has been reported in at least one cat.

Metastases are common; regional lymph nodes and other lung lobes are most often affected.[3] Other sites include mediastinum, pleura, heart, kidney, bladder, spleen, adrenal glands, esophagus, and intestines. Unique metastatic sites are those of the skeletal muscle, appendicular and axial skeleton, and soft tissues of the digits and subcutis. Most cats with digital metastases have lung tumors arising from squamous cell carcinomas.

Treatment for primary lung tumor has been attempted in a few cats.[3,62-65] If no metastatic disease is present surgical resection of the lung tumor should be curative. In most cases, however, signs of metastatic disease either prompted examination or were present when the lung tumor was found. Chemotherapy would be the only logical treatment modality, and it has been attempted in a few cases, but results have been poor. Unfortunately, in the remainder of the cats, where treatment was attempted it was directed toward elimination of overt metastatic disease, and the pulmonary mass was believed to be inconsequential. Pulmonary tumors progress rapidly, and all but a few cats are euthanized shortly after diagnosis.

It is critical that cats with multiple soft tissue masses have thoracic radiographs as part of the diagnostic work-up. Once a pulmonary mass is identified diagnosis can be made by fine-needle aspiration biopsy of the pulmonary mass or cytologic examination of pleural fluid. Cells retrieved from the lung or pleural fluid should be compared with those obtained from more accessible soft tissue masses. The differential diagnosis of pulmonary lesions includes abscess, infarct, granuloma, hematoma, cyst, other neoplasms, and pneumonia.

Urinary Tract Tumors

Lymphosarcoma is the most common renal tumor. Other tumors of the kidneys are rare, and most are malignant. The most common nonlymphatic tumor affecting the kidneys is adenocarcinoma.[4,36,44] Most kidney tumors are metastatic or have infiltrated into the surrounding tissue by the time of diagnosis. If the tumor is diagnosed early, the treatment of choice is nephrectomy. Excretory urography verifies prior to surgery that the remaining kidney is functional (see Chapter 14).

The most common tumor of the feline urinary bladder is transitional cell carcinoma. Cats with transitional cell carcinoma usually present for stranguria and hematuria that is not responsive to antibiotics or antispasmodics. In some cases transient improvement may be seen initially in response to medical treatment. Diagnosis is made using contrast cystography and biopsy (see Chapter 14). Transitional cell carcinomas appear to be highly metastatic.[57] The treatment of choice is complete surgical removal. However, owing to the invasive nature of these tumors and their location, complete surgical removal usually is not possible. The prognosis in most cases is poor because of metastasis.[4,56]

REFERENCES

1. Dorn CR, Taylor DON, Schneider R, et al. Survey of animal neoplasms in Alameda and Contra Costa counties, California. II. Cancer morbidity in dogs and cats in Alameda county. J Natl Cancer Inst 1960;40:307.
2. MacVean DW, Monlux AW, Anderson PS Jr, et al. Frequency of canine and feline tumors in a defined population. Vet Pathol 1978;15:367.
3. Carpenter JL, Andrews LK, Holzworth J. Tumors and Tumor-like Lesions. In: Holzworth J, ed. Diseases of the Cat. Philadelphia: WB Saunders, 1987:406.
4. Priester WA, Mantel N. Occurrence of tumors in domestic animals. Data from 12 United States and Canadian colleges of veterinary medicine. J Natl Cancer Inst 1971;41:1333.
5. Winthrow SJ. Surgical oncology: Old and new ideas. Semin Vet Med Surg (Small Anim) 1986;1:17.
6. Winthrow SJ. Surgical Oncology. In: Winthrow SJ, ed. Clinical Veterinary Oncology. Philadelphia: JB Lippincott, 1989:58.
7. Bradley RL, MacEwen EG, Loar AS. Mandibular resection for removal of oral tumors in 30 dogs and 6 cats. J Am Vet Med Assoc 1984;184:160.

8. MacEwen EG. Cancer Chemotherapy. In: Kirk RW, ed. Current Veterinary Therapy VII. Philadelphia: WB Saunders, 1980:586.
9. Cuoto CG. Principles of Chemotherapy. In: Proceedings of the Tenth Kal Kan Symposium. Ventura CA: Kal Kan Foods, 1987:29.
10. Cuoto CG. Toxicity of Anticancer Chemotherapy. In: Proceedings of the Tenth Kal Kan Symposium. Ventura, CA: Kal Kan Foods, 1987:37.
11. Giger U, Gorman NT. Acute Complications of Cancer and Cancer Therapy. In: Gorman, NT, ed. Oncology. New York: Churchill Livingstone, 1986:645.
12. Madewell BR. Adverse Effects of Chemotherapy. In: Kirk RE, ed. Current Veterinary Therapy VIII. Philadelphia: WB Saunders, 1983:269.
13. Cotter SM. Treatment of lymphosarcoma and leukemia with cyclophosphamide, vincristine, and prednisone II. Treatment of cats. J Am Anim Hosp Assoc 1983;19:166.
14. O'Keefe D. Doxorubicin therapy in the cat. In: Proceedings of the 9th Annual Forum of the American College of Veterinary Internal Medicine. Madison, WI: Omnipress, 1991:711.
15. Hardy WD. Hematopoietic tumors of cats. J Am Anim Hosp Assoc 1981;17:921.
16. Engle GC, Brody RS. A retrospective study of 395 feline neoplasms. J Am Vet Med Assoc 1969;21:155.
17. Theilen GH, Madewell BR. Leukemia-Sarcoma Disease Complex. In: Theilen GH, Madewell BR, eds. Veterinary Cancer Medicine. 2nd ed. Philadelphia: Lea & Febiger, 1986:403.
18. Meincke JE, Hobbie WV, Hardy WD Jr. Lymphoreticular malignancies in the cat: Clinical findings. J Am Vet Med Assoc 1972;160:1093.
19. Takahashi R, Goto N, Ishii H, et al. Pathological observations of natural causes of feline lymphosarcomatosis. Jpn J Vet Sci 1974;36:163.
20. Gruffy DD, Jones TJ, and Gaskell CJ. Clinical and radiological features of anterior mediastinal lymphosarcoma in the cat: A review of 30 cases. Vet Rec 1979;104:304.
21. MacEwen EG, Mooney S, Brown NO, et al. Treatment of Feline Tumors. In: Holzworth J, ed. Diseases of the Cat. Philadelphia: WB Saunders, 1987:459.
22. Mackey LJ. Feline leukemia virus and its effects in cats. Vet Rec 1975;96:5.
23. Cotter SM, Hardy WD Jr, Essex M. Association of feline leukemia virus with lymphosarcoma and other disorders in the cat. J Am Vet Med Assoc 1975;166:449.
24. Loar AS. The management of feline lymphosarcoma. Vet Clin North Am, Small Anim Pract 1984;14:1299.
25. Crighton GW. Feline Leukemia (lymphosarcoma) symposium I. The diagnosis of leukemia in the cat. J Small Anim Pract 1969;10:571.
26. Cotter SM. Feline Lymphoid Hyperplasia. In: Kirk RW, ed. Current Veterinary Therapy X. Philadelphia: WB Saunders, 1989:535.
27. Zaki FA, Hurvitz AI. Spontaneous neoplasias of the central nervous system of the cat. J Small Anim Pract 1976;17:773.
28. MacEwen EG, Mooney S, Hayes AA, et al. Combination Chemotherapy of Natural Occurring Feline Lymphosarcoma. In: Advances in Medical Oncology, Research Education. Proceedings of the International Cancer Congress II. Oxford: Pergamon Press, 1979.
29. Holzworth J. Leukemia and related neoplasms in the cat. I. Lymphoid malignancies. J Am Vet Med Assoc 1960;47:136.
30. Couto CG. Clinicopathological aspects of acute leukemias in the dog. J Am Vet Med Assoc 1985;186:681.
31. Thrall MA. Lymphoproliferative disorders. Lymphocytic leukemia and plasma cell myeloma. Vet Clin North Am, Small Anim Pract 1981:321.
32. Patnaik AK, Liu SK, Hurvitz AI. Nonhematopoietic neoplasms in cats. J Natl Cancer Inst 1975;54:855.
33. Weijer K, Head KW, Misdrop W, Hampe JF. Feline malignant mammary tumors. I. Morphology and biology: Some comparison with human and canine mammary carcinomas. J Natl Cancer Inst 1972;49:1697.
34. Hayes AA, Mooney SF. Feline mammary tumors. Vet Clin North Am, Small Anim Pract 1985:513.
35. Hayes HM, Priester WA, Pendergrass TW. Epidemiological features of feline mammary carcinoma. Vet Rec 1981;108:476.
36. Cotchin E. Neoplasia in the cat. Vet Rec 1957;69:425.
37. Hayden DW, Neilson SW. Feline mammary tumors. J Small Anim Pract 1971;12:687.
38. Jeglum KA, de Guzman E, Young KM. Chemotherapy of advanced mammary carcinoma in 14 cats. J Am Vet Med Assoc 1985;187:157.
39. Hinton M, Gaskell H. Non-neoplastic mammary hypertrophy in the cat associated with either pregnancy or with oral progestogen therapy. Vet Rec 1977;100:277.
40. Weiger K, Hart AAM. Prognostic factors in feline mammary carcinoma. J Natl Cancer Inst 1983;70:709.
41. MacEwen EG, Hayes AA, Harvey HJ, et al. Prognostic factors for feline mammary tumors. J Am Vet Med Assoc 1984;185:201.
42. Brody RS. Alimentary tract neoplasms in the cat: A clinicopathological survey of 46 cases. Am J Vet Res 1967;27:116.
43. Dorn CR, Priester WA. Epidemiological analysis of oral and pharyngeal cancer in dogs, cats, horses and cattle. J Am Vet Med Assoc 1976;169:1202.
44. Turk MA, Gallina MA, Russell TS. Nonhematopoietic gastrointestinal neoplasia in cats: A retrospective of 44 cases. Vet Pathol 1981;18:614.
45. Lingeman CH, Garner FM. Comparative study of intestinal adenocarcinomas of animals and man. J Natl Cancer Inst 1972; 48:325.
46. Kosovsky JE, Mathiesen DT, Patnaik AK. Small intestinal carcinoma in cats: 32 cases (1978–1985). J Am Vet Med Assoc 1988; 192:233.
47. Patnaik AK, Liu S-K, Johnson GF. Feline intestinal carcinoma: A clinicopathological study of 22 cases. Vet Pathol 1976;13:1.
48. Patnaik AK, Johnson GF, Green RW, et al. Surgical Resection of intestinal adenocarcinoma in a cat with a survival of 28 months. J Am Vet Med Assoc 1981;178:479.
49. Turrel JM, Pool RR. Primary bone tumors in the cat: A retrospective study of 15 cats and a literature review. Vet Radiol 1982; 23:152.
50. Misdrop W, VanederHuel RO. Tumors of bones and joints. Bulletin WHO 1976;53:265.
51. Liu S-K, Dorfman H, Patnaik AK. Primary and secondary bone tumors in the cat. J Small Anim Pract 1974;15:141.
52. Quigley PJ, Leedale AH. Tumors involving bone in the domestic cat: A review of 58 cases. Vet Pathol 1983;20:670.
53. Madewell BR, Leighten RL, Theilen GH. Amputation and doxorubicin for treatment of canine and feline osteogenic sarcoma. Eur J Cancer 1978;14:287.
54. Pool RR, Carrig CB. Multiple cartilaginous exostosis in a cat. Vet Pathol 1972;9:350.
55. Pool RR, Harris JM. Feline osteochondromatosis. Feline Pract 1975;5:24.
56. Bradley RL. Selected oral, pharyngeal and upper respiratory conditions in the cat. Oral tumors, nasopharyngeal and middle ear polyps and chronic rhinitis and sinusitis. Vet Clin North Am, Small Anim Pract 1984:1173.
57. Schwarz PD, Greene RW, Patnaik AK. Urinary bladder tumors in the cat: A review of 27 cases. J Am Anim Hosp Assoc 1985;21:237.
58. Allard AW. Splenic mastocytosis. Feline Pract 1979;9:21.
59. Confer AW, Langloss JM, Cashel IG. Long-term survival of 2 cats with mastocytosis. J Am Vet Med Assoc 1978;172:160.
60. Liska WD, MacEwen EG, Zaki FA, Garvey M. Feline systemic

mastocytosis: A review and results of splenectomy in seven cases. J Am Anim Hosp Assoc 1979;15:579.

61. Nielsen SW, Howard EB, Walke RE. Feline Mastocytosis. In: Clarke WI, Howard E, Hackett PL, eds. Myeloproliferative Disorders of Animals and Man. Oak Ridge, TN: US Atomic Energy Commission, 1970:359.
62. Pool RR, Bodle JE, Mantos JJ, Ticer JW. Primary lung carcinoma with skeletal metastasis in the cat. Feline Pract 1974;4(4):36.
63. Schmitz JA, Bailey DE, Bailey RB Bronchogenic carcinoma in a cat presenting as rear leg lameness. Feline Pract 1978;8:18.
64. May C, Newsholme SJ. Metastasis of feline pulmonary carcinoma presenting as multiple digital swelling. J Small Anim Pract 1989;30:302.
65. Moore AS, Middleton DJ. Pulmonary adenocarcinoma in three cats with non-respiratory signs only. J Small Anim Pract 1982; 23:501.
66. Koblik PD. Radiographic appearance of primary lung tumors in cats. Vet Radiol 1986;27:66.

CHAPTER 52

◇ ◇ ◇

Oral Diseases

Robert B. Wiggs and Heidi B. Lobprise

After covering specific diseases of tooth structure in Chapter 33, this chapter is devoted to problems associated with extradental oral tissues. Diseases of the periodontium or supportive tissues, such as periodontal disease, feline plasmacytic-lymphocytic stomatitis, neoplasms, and eosinophilic granuloma complex are the majority of lesions seen in domestic felines. Traumatic injuries to both soft and hard support tissues in the oral cavity include fractures, avulsions, burns, lacerations, and foreign bodies. Congenital defects of the palate are also discussed.

Periodontal Disease

Periodontal disease, the most common oral disease of cats, ranges from simple subclinical gingivitis to advanced, more progressive forms. In general, the presence of bacteria attached to the tooth surface starts an inflammatory response that in early stages can be reversible, depending on the commitment to treatment and care as well as the animal's immune status.

Plaque accumulation, especially in the absence of regular home care, can elicit changes in relatively young cats, and by age 6 years it is estimated that up to 85% of felines have Stage 2 periodontal disease or worse that would benefit from treatment.[1] The impact of good oral health on overall health cannot be overemphasized, not merely from the standpoint of the mouth being the opening to the digestive tract, but also the fact that advanced dental disease can cause chronic bacteremia, poor grooming habits, and general demise, in addition to anorexia.

Pathology

Early signs of periodontal disease are often discovered by the clinician on routine physical examination, even before any clinical symptoms such as halitosis or reluctance to eat are noticed by the owner. The presence and accumulation of oral bacteria and their byproducts in the gingival sulcus stimulate an immune response within 2 days, initially increased vascularity and capillary permeability, leading to the deposition of neutrophils and exudates.[2,3] At this stage the inflammation is still reversible, but with an impaired immune response or persistent challenge this can develop into a more chronic condition marked by increased sulcular exudate and a change to a plasmacytic-lymphocytic infiltrate. The bacterial flora also generally changes from gram-positive, aerobic, immotile cocci, to gram-negative, anaerobic, motile rods. Both the exogenous and endogenous byproducts and metabolite toxins affect the integrity of the epithelial attachment and connective tissue of the gingiva, which can eventually lead to inflammation and injury to the periodontal ligament.[2] As these deeper periodontal structures are affected, teeth can become loose and ultimately are lost. Since the supporting alveolar bone is structurally very thin in cats, even mild cases may be associated with tooth loss earlier in life, particularly incisors.[4]

Throughout the process of bacterial plaque accumulation and periodontal disease the soft plaque can be mineralized to form calculus, which is found most often on the buccal (cheek) surfaces of the upper third and fourth premolars, close to the site of major salivary gland duct openings.[4-6] It is the plaque that is the most active in continuing the inflammatory process; in fact, the inflammation usually precedes the mineralization process.[7]

Infectious viral agents have a probable, yet indistinct association with the pathogenesis of many forms of oral disease.[8] Feline calicivirus (FCV) has been isolated frequently from cats with moderate to severe ulcerative periodontitis, and gingivitis or stomatitis is a frequent finding in cats affected by feline leukemia virus (FeLV) or the feline immunodeficiency virus (FIV)[9-12] probably because of their immunosuppressive effects.[12] But an exact cause and effect relationship has not been accurately established for FCV alone, and the role of any two or all three seems to be a synergistic influence on the severity of the disease, rather than an absolute increase in prevalence as compared to "virus-negative" cats.[13] Future studies will likely clarify the role of viruses in peridontal disease.

Nutritional factors, principally deficiencies, may also affect gingival health.[2] Vitamin A and nicotinic acid are involved in sustaining proper bacterial resistance of buccal epithelium and ulcers due to bacterial infections. Severe vitamin B deficiencies (especially niacin functioning with folic acid) usually are associated with other deficiencies, and more pronounced cases may exhibit general reddening of the oral mucosa, vermilion bands on the upper lips, and persistent diarrhea. In chronic cases supplementation may be warranted. Vitamin C is instrumental in forming and maintaining intracellular collagen and epithelial cement substance of capillaries, but it normally can be synthesized by cats

Clinical Signs

Inflammation is a consistent finding—simple marginal gingivitis caused by the presence of bacterial plaque on the tooth surface.[3] Gingival bleeding on probing may be one of the earliest symptoms[14] and can be quite variable, depending on severity (Fig. 52–1). Ruling out coagulation abnormalities would help determine whether the bleeding is purely inflammatory. Gingival color may change from coral pink to red and even reddish-blue, and gingival bleeding may have marginal, focal or generalized manifestations.[2] Systemic disease (e.g., cholestasis, anemia) must be ruled out before dental factors are assessed. Edema may be slight or marked as inflammation increases, and it should not be confused with true gingival hyperplasia, an uncommon finding in cats unless they are taking diphenylhydantoin.[15]

As the disease progresses, clinical signs become more apparent: slight halitosis without discomfort progresses to increased plaque and calculus buildup, gingival edema and color change, pocket formation, and loosening of teeth, then to even heavier accumulations of calculus, gingival recession exposed roots, gingival hyperemia and edema, and deposition of purulent material and debris.[3] The patient with signs of chronic disease—ulcerations, discomfort, drooling, and loss of appetite—often has complicating factors of cervical line lesions, immunosuppressive symptoms, or possibly plasmacytic-lymphocytic stomatitis (see below).

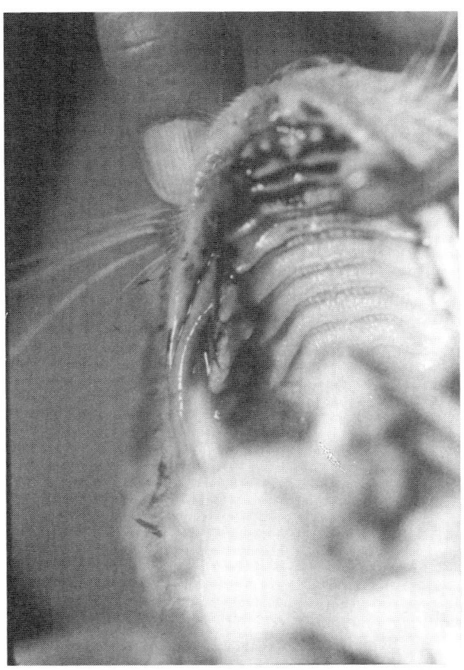

Figure 52–1. **Extensive periodontal disease with spontaneous gingival bleeding.**

Diagnosis

Diagnosis of most uncomplicated forms of periodontal disease is relatively straightforward, relying on visual and tactile inspection and assessment of ongoing disease. Even in refractory cases results of bacteriologic studies are often confusing and not entirely useful, owing to the ever-changing picture of incriminating flora.[16] The increased presence of anaerobic bacteria in later stages would indicate the use of appropriate antibiotics, but specific culture and sensitivity assays are warranted only in certain cases. Biopsy and histopathologic examination usually are reserved for unresponsive or unusual presentations.[16] Thorough physical examination and routine lab work for a minimum data base are always helpful, especially for preanesthesia evaluation and to rule out ulcerative uremic gingivitis and other systemic diseases that have oral signs. Determination of FeLV, FIV, thyroid, and autoimmune status gives the clinician a more complete impression of the cat's condition.[17]

Although it can be relatively uncomplicated, assessment of periodontal disease should not be taken lightly. Meticulous examination of all areas of the dentition is necessary for accurate recording, determination of treatment, and evaluation of response to therapy. The clinician should perform a systematic, thorough inspection of the gingival tissue, tooth structure, and periodontal structures of each tooth and record the findings. This is best done with the animal under general anesthesia, often during dental prophylaxis. Before any manipulation, the condition of the gingiva should be scrutinized for bleeding, color changes, presence of edema, or any changes in position or contour of the margins.

One of the most important single pieces of equipment in oral diagnostics is the periodontal explorer and probe. The probe end, calibrated in millimeter increments, can be gently inserted into the gingival sulcus to check for bleeding, and, more important, to measure the depth of the pocket. Normal sulcus depth should not exceed 0.5 mm (as compared to 1 to 3 mm in dogs), but often it is almost negligible in cats. Deep gingival pockets are less common in cats than in dogs and should alert the practitioner to possibly severe disease.

Stages

The common method of staging periodontal disease is extrapolated from human and canine dentistry, but caution should be used in applying it to cats, because the relative depths of periodontal pockets require adjustment for the cat's smaller oral structures. We have devised a staging system based on human and canine values and modified according to clinical impressions (Table 52–1). The importance of staging lesions is the same as throughout veterinary medicine: to evaluate lesions, to group treatment plans, and to evaluate therapeutic response.

Stage I periodontal disease describes conditions of subclinical to more advanced gingivitis with minimal inflammatory changes and minimal or no changes in normal sulcus depth. In Stage I disease the probe occasionally can be introduced 0.5 mm into the crevice, but this is usually due to slight inflammation or edema of the gingival margin. Gin-

Table 52–1. Staging of Feline Periodontal Disease

Stage
Stage I: Gingivitis
Pocket depth less than 0.5 mm
Gingival inflammation
On probing, slight bleeding or none
Slight erythema
No loss of supporting structure
Stage II: Early periodontitis
Pocket depth or root exposure less than 1 mm
Inflammation of periodontal ligament
Bleeding with probing with periodontal probe
Mild color change and edema
Minor attachment loss (periodontal ligament)
Crestal bone loss
No tooth mobility
Satisfactory gingival topography
Stage III: Moderate periodontitis
Pocket depth or root exposure less than 2.0 mm
Moderate attachment loss (periodontal ligament)
Marked bleeding on probing with periodontal probe
30–50% loss of support bone
Slight tooth mobility
Unsatisfactory gingival topography
Stage IV: Advanced periodontitis
Pocket depth or root exposure 2 mm or more
Advanced attachment loss (periodontal ligament)
Spontaneous bleeding, extreme color change, and edema
Greater than 50% loss of support bone
Moderate or severe tooth mobility

Table 52–2. Gingivitis Index*

Grade
Grade I: Mild gingivitis
Mild inflammation
Slight color change
Slight edema
No bleeding on probing with periodontal probe
Grade II: Moderate gingivitis
Moderate inflammation
Slight redness
Moderate edema
Very slight bleeding on probing with periodontal probe
Grade III: Severe gingivitis
Severe inflammation
Marked redness
Marked edema
Ulceration
Slight bleeding on probing with periodontal probe

*Various grades of gingivitis can be associated with the various stages of periodontal disease.

givitis can be indexed into three grades (see Table 52–2). In Stage II, inflammation of the periodontal ligament and crestal bone loss is initiated. Pocket depth may increase, but instead of pocket formation cats may start to develop areas of exposed root structure due to gingival recession. Another indication of inflammatory disease is root exposure uncovering cementum surfaces that are often more sensitive to pain and possibly more susceptible to pathologic changes. The sulcus depth or amount of root exposure is still close to the normal range (less than 1.0 mm), and the gingiva is more hyperemic with an increase in sulcus fluid. In Stage III, peridontal ligament inflammation leads to a moderate loss of attachment (less than 2 mm), evident as increased sulcus pocket depth, root exposures, or a combination of the two. Concurrent loss of 30% to 50% of the bony support may result in slight tooth mobility. Gingival recession is often more noticeable with advanced lesions, and radiographs are helpful for monitoring bone loss. Stage IV periodontal disease presents with multiple signs of varying degrees of deep pockets or root exposure (theoretically 2 mm or more, which would be difficult to attain in some teeth of the cat due to their small size), significant alveolar bone loss (50% or more), and moderate to severe tooth mobility. Root exposure can be quite extensive, particularly in cuspids, where more than half the root structure may eventually be uncovered. Comparatively, in humans and dogs normal pocket depth is 2 to 3 mm and a pocket depth of 4 to 5 mm is substantial, because that is the subgingival depth standard periodontal instruments can reach without creating extensive flaps or advanced procedures.[18]

In addition to pocket depth and root exposure indices, evaluating inflammatory signs such as gingival bleeding, color change, edema, and position of the margins allows more complete assessment. Basically, lesions of Stage I disease exhibit slight bleeding, if any, on probing and slight, if any, color change or edema. Bleeding on probing and color change with mild edema that does not necessarily encompass the tooth is typical of Stage II lesions, whereas Stage III would have marked bleeding on probing and color changes with moderate edema encircling the tooth. The most extreme changes—spontaneous bleeding, extreme color change, and severe edema—alert the clinician to a Stage IV process and one with a much poorer prognosis.

Throughout the prophylaxis and examination, indications of cervical line lesions (CLL) may be detectable: hyperplastic gingiva or calculus trying to fill in the defect, involuntary twitching when the sensitive lesion is touched, and "hooking" of the pointed explorer end in the concave defect itself (see CLL, in Chapter 33). The explorer should be used with great care, so as not to damage soft tissue, including the epithelial attachment at the depth of the sulcus. This curved, sharp-pointed end is a very tactile instrument and can also be used to detect soft, carious lesions (uncommon in cats and dogs) and subgingival deposits of calculus.

Radiography, another important diagnostic tool, is used to detect alveolar bone loss, tooth or root resorption, and fractures. Intraoral films are extremely useful in examining cats and are relatively easy and inexpensive to use (see Radiographs, Tooth Fractures, in Chapter 33). Loss of crestal bone is the first radiographic sign of periodontal disease. Further alveolar bone loss can be either horizontal, extending along the plane of the maxilla or mandible involving several teeth to a similar depth, or vertical, involving a single area with deeper bone loss extending apically.[3] In our experience alveolar bone resorption surrounding the distal (caudal) root of the mandibular molar is common.

There often seems to be a greater degree of bone resorption at the cuspid and incisor area, even with minimal plaque and calculus.[3] Reactive bone lesions resulting from periodontitis have also been reported,[19] and they must be differentiated from neoplasms by biopsy, especially if radiographic changes look suspicious.

Treatment

The basic goals of treatment for periodontal disease rely initially on prevention (prophylaxis), but if regular professional and home care have not been provided treatment often necessitates salvage procedures. Exceptions may include immunocompromised cats, which can fail to respond to even conscientious treatment plans. The purpose of dental care is to maintain the teeth and associated structures in a normal, functional state, hopefully before any disease processes have irreversibly altered their structure. More than 35% of patients older than 6 years have Stage II or worse periodontal disease and would benefit much from proper prophylaxis and home care.

Concentrating on the specific phases of treatment, primarily in the steps of a complete prophylactic treatment, is where practitioners can make a significant difference in the oral health of their patients. Complete prophylaxis involves much more than removing the visible supragingival calculus (Table 52–3). An important part of dental disease is under the gum line (subgingival), and adequate treatment cannot be performed on an awake cat. In addition, using an endotracheal tube with inflated cuff is highly recommended to prevent aspiration of fluids, calculus, and aerosolized bacteria. It is imperative for the clinician or technician performing the prophylaxis to wear a mask to protect against inhalation of the aerosolized bacteria and gloves to protect the hands. Eye protection is also recommended.

The primary goal of dental prophylaxis is the removal of plaque, calculus, and associated bacteria. The first step involves gross removal of plaque and calculus, most of which is supragingival. Several different methods of scaling are available, including hand, sonic, ultrasonic, and high-speed rotary. These are listed in order, from the least traumatic, slowest method (hand) to the fastest, more traumatic (rotary). For cats, the sonic scaler used on a high-speed handpiece outlet is an extremely efficient method of cleaning without excessive risk of direct dental or thermal periodontal or pulp damage. The clinician or technician should always keep in mind the diminutive structure of feline teeth and the fact that all scaling methods can cause some etching or damage to the enamel, specifically if used improperly. In particular, neither the ultrasonic handpiece nor the rotary scaler should remain on any one tooth more than 12 to 15 seconds at a time, lest there be hyperthermic damage to the pulp. Owing to the potential for damage to the epithelial attachment, an ultrasonic scaler that is not specifically designed to be used subgingivally should not be introduced into the sulcus; in addition, the side should be utilized, and not the tip, which vibrates in a jack-hammer fashion and could damage teeth. Although they are slower and require more skilled technique, hand instruments are gentler on the enamel surfaces; a large variety of instruments are available for specific uses. In general, scalers have working heads that are crescentic or triangular in cross section, with sharply pointed ends. The opposite working heads are mirror images of each other, to be used on opposing sides of the teeth, but not to be used subgingivally, owing to the damage the sharp point could do to the epithelial attachment. Curettes, on the other hand, have a crescentic cross section with a rounded toe that can be used gently in subgingival areas. The proper cleaning of sub- and supragingival surfaces should result in a glassy smooth texture, and is the key to a successful prophylactic procedure.

Table 52–3. The Complete Oral Prophylactic Procedure

Gross removal of supragingival plaque and calculus
Subgingival calculus scaling
Root planing*
Subgingival curettage*
Radiography*
Polishing
Sulcus irrigation
Fluoride treatment
Periodontal probing and charting
Home care instruction

*Part of a complete prophy in advanced stages of periodontal disease.

At this point the problem areas of deeper pockets, exposed roots, or even cervical line lesions need to be addressed. The deeper exposed surfaces also need to be glassy smooth, and root planing is the method of choice, using the curette in repeated overlapping strokes to remove all calculus deposits and necrotic cementum. At the time of closed root planing the curette can be angled to lightly engage the subgingival soft tissue and gently pulled against soft external digital pressure to skim away debris and diseased tissue. If the pocket is deeper than 2 or 3 mm (unusual in a cat unless the disease is severe and the tooth unsalvageable) a gingival flap may be necessary to expose the area to be treated. By making releasing incisions at the rostral and caudal (mesial and distal) aspect of the lesion and using a periosteal elevator (such as a No. 2 Molt) to raise the flap, adequate exposure is usually obtained. Simple interrupted sutures of small (3-0 to 4-0) absorbable suture material are usually adequate for flap closure.

Occasionally, owing to the effects of more severe periodontal disease, an oronasal fistula (ONF) may occur, generally associated with the maxillary cuspids. This condition is much less common in cats than in dogs.[20] Our clinical impression has been that the underlying infective process, by the time of detection sometimes severe or even progressing to extensive osteomyelitis, gives any corrective procedure a more guarded prognosis in certain instances. In uncomplicated cases a mucoperiosteal flap, with mesial and distal diverging releasing incisions, is usually adequate to cover the defect. A No. 2 or No. 4 Molt periosteal elevator works extremely well to undermine the tissues. The periosteal attachment of the flap must be severed at its stalk in order to release the flap enough to slide it over the defect. The surface around the defect should be débrided adequately to avoid placing suture lines directly over the defect. Good surgical technique—large bites of tissue and absolutely no tension on the suture line—is imperative for ONF lesions. Owners should be cautioned not to handle the site and that follow-up procedures are sometimes necessary to close difficult areas.

Once the steps of gross calculus removal and subgingival scaling are complete the surfaces should be examined for residual calculus deposits. The teeth need to be polished with an appropriate prophylaxis paste and polishing unit to remove the etching defects made by the scalers. Without proper polishing, the tooth surfaces remain roughened, which increases the rate of plaque adhesion.[21] Using inadequate amounts of prophylaxis paste, polishing speeds greater than 3000 rpm, excessive pressure, or remaining more than 15 seconds on a tooth at one time may cause thermal damage, so caution is warranted. A thorough flushing of the sulcal areas with a dilute chlorhexidine (1% to 2%) or stannous fluoride product flushes debris and calculus from the pockets. A gel, foam, or varnish fluoride treatment at this point helps inhibit plaque formation, aids in desensitizing exposed dentin (including shallow cervical line lesions), and strengthens tooth structure.[22]

Throughout the prophylaxis the operator observes structures and problems, but it is very important to systematically and correctly note all pertinent data on the patient's record. Radiographs assist in diagnosis of some lesions and are necessary for all cervical line lesions or fractures, in order to determine the correct treatment, including extraction. Depending on the conditions found during the prophylaxis and examination additional therapy with antibiotics, antiinflammatory drugs, and other drugs should be instituted on an individual basis (see Plasmacytic-Lymphocytic Stomatitis below).

Home Care

Once the professional prophylaxis is completed education of the client in the importance of home care and regular checkups is essential. Some patients are poor candidates for daily brushing, and others with severe ulcerative lesions would benefit from having the inflammation reduced first. But by starting out slowly and progressing step by step, a significant number of cats can enjoy the benefits of oral care. After getting the cat more accustomed to having its face and lips gently handled and caressed, a disposable foam brush or gauze pad wrapped around a finger and dipped in the liquid from tuna fish packed in water can be used to carefully touch the buccal tooth surfaces. Keeping the mouth closed with one hand over the head while brushing with the other can facilitate the procedure. Some patients then allow the owner to begin to use a small cat toothbrush; it is directed at a 45-degree angle into the sulcus, and brushing proceeds coronally with a flavored enzyme toothpaste. Daily brushing is ideal, but at least 2 or 3 times weekly is suggested. One study indicates that "cats that brush" 1 or 2 times per week showed 95% less calculus than the control group, and those that were brushed once a week had 76% less.[23] Oral rinses, including dilute chlorhexidine or zinc ascorbate combinations, may be used in conjunction with brushing, or alone if the cat cannot tolerate brushing. Weekly stannous fluoride applications is beneficial to arrest plaque development. This is especially important for cats with a history of cervical line lesions. Owners need to be informed of the potential toxic effects of excess amounts of ingested fluoride; the products should be used judiciously, in small amounts, on a weekly basis. An added benefit of regular home care is the early detection and increased owner awareness of oral lesions.[21] Lesions such as those of recurrent periodontal disease, fractured teeth, erosions, and oral tumors might be discovered in early stages, increasing the probability of successful treatment. An educated client also realizes the importance of regular professional checkups and prophylaxis, recommended at intervals from 3 to 18 months, depending on the extent of problems. Pets with more severe periodontal disease require diligent care on all fronts to maintain dental health and save as many teeth as possible. A total oral health program will have a positive influence on the patient's health, the client's education, and the veterinarian's practice.

Plasmacytic-Lymphocytic Stomatitis

Beyond the scope of "routine" periodontal disease lies a realm of chronic, unresponsive oral disease usually characterized by a distinct infiltrate of plasma cells and lymphocytes. The exact cause is still unknown, but various infectious (bacterial, viral) and immune-mediated factors have all been implicated. An unfortunate manifestation of this syndrome is the lack of permanent response to conventional oral hygiene, antibiotics, antiinflammatory agents, and immune modulators.[3,24-26] Often, refractory cases require eventual extraction of at least the caudal (premolars and molars), if not the entire, dentition.

Pathology

The hallmark of this form of inflammation is evident in the name. Plasma cells, the first line in the humoral immune response,[27] are seen in varying proportions with lymphocytes.[3] This, usually along with polyclonal gammopathy,[3,28-31] lends credence to the supposition that the syndrome has an immune basis. It is presumed that the patient is predisposed to respond in excess to polyclonal B-cell activators in oral bacteria.[32] The antibodies to specific antigens of plaque bacteria correspond to those seen in other species (dogs, humans); antibodies reacting to *Actinobacillus* and *Bacteroides species,* and certain strains of black-pigmented *Bacteroides* have been isolated in affected cats.[33-35] The similarities in bacterial type (anaerobic and aerobic) involved and colony percentage to dogs and humans with similar symptoms may lead to studies that could benefit all species.[33] However, the severity and prevalence of the disease in cats suggests possible involvement of cofactors such as viruses or flagellate bacteria. Viruses have been implicated: one study notes a high prevalence of FCV in affected cats,[8,36] but there is no hard evidence of a direct cause-and-effect relationship. Immunosuppression from FeLV and FIV infections could lead to unresponsive infections[37,38] that would mimic the syndrome.[40] But most patients with distinct plasmacytic stomatitis are not infected with them. Those that are infected require special considerations when determining treatment, especially in avoiding corticosteroids.

Although some authors have seen no breed, sex, or age predilection in the classic presentation,[17] some indicate that certain breeds (e.g., Siamese, Abyssinian, Persian, Himalayan, Burmese)[3,39] tend to have more severe disease, indicating a possible genetic diathesis tendency.[17,40] A somewhat distinct syndrome, juvenile-onset periodontitis, has been reported.[40] It starts before 9 months of age and is prevalent in Siamese, Maine Coon Cats, and some domestic shorthaired cats. It causes abundant plaque and calculus, resulting in inflammation that causes anatomic changes of bone loss, gingival resorption, pocket formation, and furcation exposure. This is sometimes further differentiated from a hyperplastic response seen in some young cats termed feline juvenile gingivitis.[40] For the latter cats aggressive early gingivectomy, prophylaxis (even though minimal plaque is usually present), and meticulous home care in the first 2 years may help minimize initial anatomic changes. At that point these patients often "mature" into a more normal state.[3] It has been suggested that the inflammation associated with the plaque bacteria can extend from the gingival margins to the other areas by physical contact, leading to pharyngitis and glossitis with acute pain, particularly if untreated.[37]

In general, plasmacytic-lymphocytic stomatitis does not appear to be a distinct disease entity; rather, it is an out-of-control or excessive immune inflammatory response that indicates a disturbance of the oral environment.[37,41] In light of this, treatment to prevent or control it seems a logical course of action.

Clinical Signs

Common presenting complaints of plasmacytic-lymphocytic stomatitis include ptyalism, halitosis, dysphagia, anorexia (notably reluctance to eat hard foods), and weight loss.[3,4,28,38,42] A classic picture of a hyperemic, proliferative (though sometimes recessing), ulcerative mucosa with a raspberry or cobblestone appearance is often seen.[3,17,29,43,44] This, of course, represents cases that have progressed beyond the initial marginal gingivitis, as the commissures, glossopharyngeal arches, and palate become increasingly involved (Fig. 52–2).

Diagnosis

Diagnosis can tentatively be made on the basis of clinical features and failure to respond to conventional oral hygiene techniques; however, biopsy is sometimes necessary to rule out neoplasia[2,3,4,28,37,38,43-45] and eosinophilic granulomas, or possibility to assess the severity. Histopathologic examination usually reveals an ulcerative mucosa with a dense submucosal infiltrate. This infiltrate consists of heavy sheets of plasma cells,[3,42] but it also contains some lymphocytes and neutrophils.[38]

Routine lab work, including a minimum data base, FeLV and FIV testing, and bacterial culture and sensitivity, will enhance the veterinarian's overall assessment, but with few exceptions tests typically fail to reveal any pertinent information. Autoimmune mechanisms might be suspected in unusual cases with lip ulceration, and hypothyroidism in humans has been implicated in some similar syndromes.[46] Bilateral proliferative commissure ulceration may or may not be present in plasma cell pododermatitis, a rare disease of possible immune origin also represented by an ulcerative granulomatous soft swelling of the footpads.[17,47]

Treatment

Current recommendations for treatment of feline plasmacytic-lymphocytic stomatitis concentrate on elimination or control of the excessive inflammatory response described earlier.[37] Yet, even intensive efforts at oral hygiene to control plaque, antibiotics to fight the bacteria, and anti-inflammatory drugs fail to elicit an acceptable response in most cases.

Frequent professional prophylaxis and additional treatments (i.e., root planing, treating cervical line lesions, resecting proliferative gingiva, and selective extractions) combined with vigorous home care are the first steps. The ideal—no plaque—is virtually unattainable, even for patients that tolerate home care daily or after each meal. The next line of defense in the clinician's arsenal, appropriate antibiotic therapy, is employed frequently. An initial re-

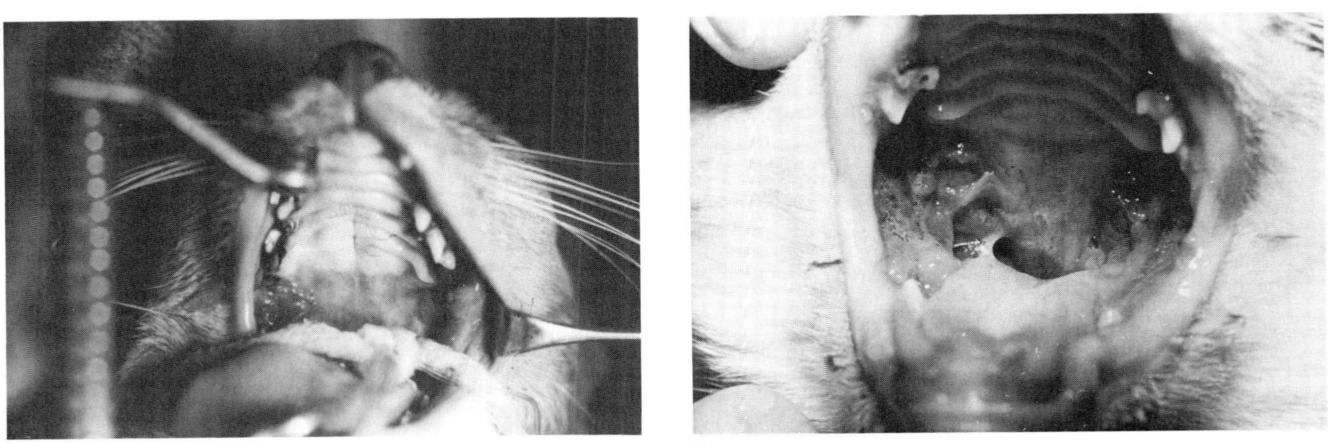

A B

Figure 52–2. (*A*) "Red line" lesion across the hard palate is common in plasmacytic-lymphocytic stomatitis and is probably an extension of the severe periodontitis. (*B*) Cobblestone-type lesion of plasmacytic-lymphocytic stomatitis at the angle of the jaw.

sponse is the rule, but it usually decreases in time, even with protracted treatment.[34,43]

Since the primary pathogens tend to be anaerobic, metronidazole is frequently prescribed. Published doses vary from 30 to 60 mg/kg, daily or in divided doses twice daily, for 5 to 10 days,[2,3,42,45] to a maximum of 250 mg twice daily.[43] One regimen suggests that, after the initial 5 to 10 days, one third of the dose be administered every 2 or 3 days for long periods.[37] Topical metronidazole solution may have local activity.[34] Clindamycin, at a dose of 5 mg/kg every 12 hours for as long as 3 to 4 weeks, may be an alternative.[2,45]

If the patient does not respond well to prophylaxis, home care, and antibiotics, or if the owners are less likely to comply with home care instructions, immunosuppressive doses of anti-inflammatory drugs may be required (as long as FeLV and FIV tests are negative). Initial doses of prednisolone should be administered at 2 to 4 mg/kg one or two times a day. Dosing should be decreased to every other day as the patient responds.[2,3,34,37,43] If oral administration is difficult, 20 mg of longer-acting methyl prednisolone acetate can be given every 2 weeks for three to six treatments, and then as needed.[2,42] Intralesional injections are also possible in anesthetized cats, utilizing triamcinolone to a maximum dose of 10 mg.[37] The progestin, megestrol acetate, has both direct and indirect antiinflammatory effects[34] at a level of 2.5 mg daily for 7 days, then weekly,[43] or 5 mg for 3 days, then 5 mg twice weekly.[34] Owners should be informed about the possible side effects, and this drug should probably be used only when absolutely necessary (see Chapter 7).[37] Other treatments have been attempted with variable results, including gold salts (1 to 2 mg weekly for 8 weeks, then monthly),[3,43] levamisole (2 to 5 mg/kg or 30 mg three times weekly),[3,44] azathioprine,[2] lactobacillus,[19] laser therapy,[48] and sodium salicylate (25 mg/kg once daily for 4 weeks). The latter drug has no gastric side effects, as aspirin does, and produces no toxicity if given every 3 days long term. The immunostimulant ImmunoRegulin has been used with some success in doses of 0.5 mL twice weekly for 3 weeks then tapered to a maintenance dose every 2 to 4 weeks. Vitamin supplementation, especially vitamins A, C, B complex, and E, and zinc may be given to help maintain oral soft tissue health.[3,38,42] In this practice, mixed results have been seen utilizing human orthodontic topical anesthetics to alleviate pain of ulcerative lesions, the goal being to increase appetite. These are often impossible to apply owing to patient resistance because of the pain.

Throughout the course of treatments teeth that are unsalvageable should be extracted with meticulous care, removing all root structure and débriding reactive bone tissue. In severe or chronic cases, often the only course of action that will help resolve the inflammation is extraction of the caudal teeth (premolars and molars), or in some cases the entire dentition.[3,28,38,43] The discomfort and inflammation frequently subsides after extraction and the partial or complete loss of teeth typically has little negative effect on the cat's ability to eat.

Home Care

In mild to moderate cases a strong commitment to home care is essential to provide the best chance of saving the teeth. Removing plaque daily, or even after every meal, can be facilitated with chlorhexidine, oral hygiene rinses, fluoride, and others (see Periodontal Disease, Home Care, above). Additional care should be taken with more severe cases, as oral discomfort may make oral cleaning and even medication administration more difficult. Often waiting a week or two after a dental cleaning for the inflammation to subside makes things relatively easier.

Acute Necrotizing Ulcerative Gingivitis

Another syndrome, acute necrotizing ulcerative gingivitis (trench mouth, Vincent's stomatitis), is usually associated with stress, especially in conjunction with compromised health or immune status (FeLV or FIV infections), and is caused by fusiform bacteria and spirochetes.[40] A mass of gray, necrotic debris covers the ulcerative lesion, causing bleeding and discomfort. Dealing with the underlying cause, cleaning, extracting, and antibiotics are the treatments of choice.

Autoimmune Diseases

Autoimmune disease involving the oral cavity is not common, but it should be considered as a differential diagnosis if lesions resemble chronic ulcerations of the oral mucosa, lips, or philtrum.[17] Pemphigus vulgaris is the only form typically seen; affected cats have vesiculobullous involvement and almost half have initial sites in the mouth.[38]

Diagnosis is made by biopsy with special handling techniques, using Michel's medium. Treatment is aimed at immunosuppression with large doses of corticosteroids (prednisolone, 1 to 3 mg/lb daily),[45] azathioprine,[38] cyclophosphamide,[49] or gold (aurothioglucose, 1 to 2 mg weekly).

Neoplasms

The oral cavity is the fourth most common site of neoplasms of cats,[3,50-53] and the great majority of oral tumors are malignant.[54] Squamous cell carcinoma (SCC) is seen most frequently, followed in order of prevalence by fibrosarcoma[3] and melanosarcoma. Both are relatively rare.[53,54] Odontogenic tumors and benign growths are uncommon in cats,[3,42,54-57] and all forms of questionable lesions should be biopsied to accurately differentiate them from other conditions that may be present in the oral cavity.[42] Owners are usually alerted to a problem by signs of halitosis, bleeding, dysphagia, anorexia ulceration, or dental disease.[3] For the majority of neoplastic lesions in the oropharyngeal region simple excision usually is inadequate, owing to the locally aggressive nature of these tumors and the likelihood of metastasis.[54]

Squamous Cell Carcinoma

In felines, nontonsillar SCC is the most frequent neoplasm of the oral cavity. It usually occurs in cats older than 10 years and exhibits no sex predilection.[42,54,57] Initially the lesion may resemble gingivitis or look like a white or

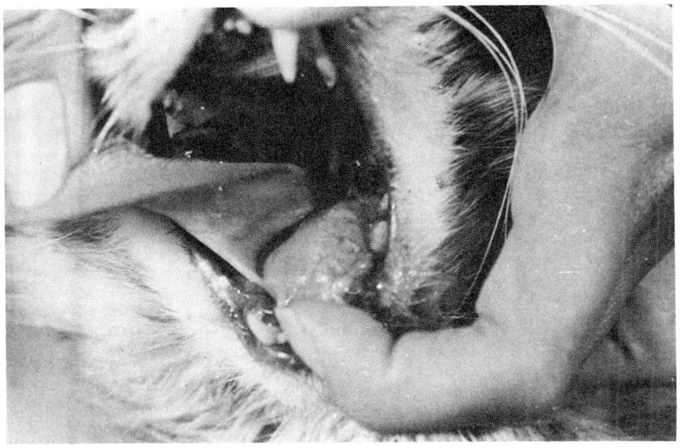

Figure 52–3. Lesion adjacent to the tongue is squamous cell carcinoma.

pink nodule associated with progressively more mobile teeth.[3,17,55] These lesions are seen primarily in the ventrolateral tongue region or frenulum (Fig. 52–3) and sometimes in the gingiva (especially mandibular) occasionally with ulceration and proliferation.[17,55] Often there are already radiographic bony changes at the time of presentation, varying from proliferation to lysis, or possibly resembling a primary bone tumor or chronic osteomyelitis.[58] Metastasis to distant sites is not a significant problem with nontonsillar SCC in cats,[57] as aggressive local invasiveness causes the majority of pathologic changes.[42,54]

Wide surgical resection—sometimes requiring mandibulectomy or maxillectomy—is effective only for early lesions, owing to the rate of local recurrence.[42,54] Typically, lesions are not discovered until they have progressed beyond that point. The use of intraoral radiography, before and even during excision, is essential to determine the amount of bony involvement, in order to remove enough tissue to obtain a 1-cm margin of normal tissue. Prognosis is poor: only half live longer than 1 year.[42] Tonsillar SCC carries an even poorer prognosis owing to its highly aggressive, extremely early metastasis.[58] Excision of lesions under or involving the tongue can also be difficult, because unlike dogs, cats function less well in eating or grooming when part of the tongue is excised.[30]

Other Oral Tumors

Fibrosarcoma, the second most common oral neoplasm of cats,[3,58] is usually found on the gingiva, palate, or mucosal surfaces.[58,59] It is also characterized by highly destructive local invasion and frequent local recurrence and late metastasis.[42] An early lesion, firm, fleshy, red or pink, may be pedunculated at the gingivopalatal margin, even resembling a benign growth.[1] But even aggressive resection, as for SCC, is frequently unsuccessful for all but the earliest lesions, owing to eventual recurrence. The poor prognosis reflects the fact that fewer than 20% live longer than 1 year.[42]

Malignant melanoma is very rare in cats[58] but tends to act as malignantly as tumors in dogs.[42] By the time of detection, no matter how small the initial mass, it can be assumed that distant metastasis has already occurred, as well as significant local destruction.[54] Surgical excision is usually only palliative; the average survival time is 65 days.[54]

Tumors of the dental laminar epithelium arising from dental primordium are also rare, ameloblastoma being the most common one.[56,57,58] Typically seen in middle-aged to older cats, it is a slow-growing, rounded to lobulated, firm, rubbery projection from the gum.[55] Radiographically, multiple radiolucent areas may be present, and some resorption of tooth roots.[55] A variation, the inductive fibroameloblastoma, is found only in young (average age 18 months) cats, usually at the rostral maxilla.[54,57] The term "inductive" refers to the relationship between the ameloblastic epithelial cells and the dental pulp–like stoma.[55,58]

Benign growths, including epulides,[55,57] are uncommon in cats,[42] but fibromas,[52,58-61] odontomas, papillomas,[55] and others have been reported. Treatment of the benign lesions, including those of odontogenic origin, is usually excision and extraction of involved teeth.

Eosinophilic Granuloma Complex

A suspicious oral lesion requires biopsy to definitively identify it. Sometimes a suspected neoplasm may be of the granulomatous group, and the converse may also be true. Much has been written about the eosinophilic granuloma complex (EGC), a wide variety of syndromes encompassing indolent (rodent) ulcers, eosinophilic plaques, and linear granulomas.[62,63] Of the three, indolent ulcers are most frequently found in the oral region of the lips, followed in rate of incidence by linear granulomas. Eosinophilic plaques are rarely associated with oral manifestations.[3] Due to probable immune-related causes, treatment generally entails the use of corticosteroids or progesterone compounds.[3,6,7,17,47,58,64-66]

Clinical Signs

Indolent ulcers, also referred to as eosinophilic or rodent ulcers, are well-circumscribed, ulcerative, red or brown lesions found usually on the upper lip (80%), either bilaterally or unilaterally,[64] at the philtrum or by the maxillary cuspid teeth.[6] Females are two to three times more likely than males to have the lesions, and cases from patients aged 9 months to 9 years have been reported; the incidence is higher in the middle to older age range.[38,42] The exact cause is unknown, but it is thought to be inflammatory, in response to irritation (e.g., trauma from a tooth, excessive grooming) or as a result of allergies.[17,47,67] Tissue eosinophilia is an inconsistent finding.[64] The possibility that this could be a precancerous lesion (SCC) has been suggested,[17,68] so early diagnosis and treatment are essential.

Linear granulomas, the only true granulomas in the group, exhibit degenerative collagen with a granulomatous inflammatory response and tissue eosinophilia[38] found in the deeper dermal areas.[64] Occasionally an indolent ulcer also exhibits these collagen changes, especially if present with an intraoral linear granuloma.[64] Typical signs include linear bands on the caudal legs of young cats.[64] Oral lesions are smooth or nodular,[17,38] sometimes ulcerated,[66] and frequently lie on the tongue, lips, or gingiva, or in the pharynx.[64] Peripheral eosinophilia should alert the practitioner to make a more guarded prognosis, and the possibility of long-term therapy is likely.[17,47]

Eosinophilic plaques, found on the abdomen and medial thigh, are often red and ulcerated, probably from the repeated trauma of licking.[47,64] These plaques are less likely to be found in the oral cavity,[17,62] and allergies are also implicated as a possible cause.

Diagnosis of these lesions often relies on the clinical presentation and a positive response to appropriate treatment;[66] however, in order to have a definitive diagnosis or in cases that are refractory to typical therapy, biopsy is recommended.[3] With any suspicious oral lesion it is never too early to obtain a histopathologic evaluation in order to rule out a neoplasm.[3,58]

Treatment

For all three forms of the EGC the treatment of choice often is an adequate amount of corticosteroids in the early stages,[47] since the EGC is likely to be a manifestation of hypersensitivity.[64] Immunosuppressive doses of prednisolone (1 to 2 mg/kg b.i.d.,[3,58] for up to 4 or 5 weeks),[6] occasional intralesional administration of triamcinolone (3 mg weekly),[3,6,58] or injections of methylprednisolone (20 mg every 2 weeks for at least 3 doses)[36,58] are some proposed protocols. Hormone therapy, in the form of oral megestrol acetate (2.5 to 5 mg every other day),[36,69] progesterone (2 to 20 mg/kg), or medroxyprogesterone (50 to 175 mg every 2 weeks)[58] may also be used, but the owner should be cautioned about potential side effects.[38] Recent responses to antibiotic therapy alone indicate the need to further explore this avenue of treatment.[6,67] Radiation treatment, cryotherapy, immune modulators, hypoallergenic diets, topical erythromycin, aurothioglucose, and even topical cyclosporine have been suggested as possible remedies.[6,7,37,70,71] Frequently, cases have recurrences and require long-term (even lifelong) therapy.[3,17,58] Treatment of insufficient duration with inadequate doses is particularly prone to failure, and concurrent diseases (i.e., diabetes mellitus, Cushing's disease, recurring pancreatitis) that contraindicate corticosteroids or progesterones make the prognosis even poorer.

Salivary Gland Disease

Salivary gland disease is rare in cats, but neoplasms, mucoceles, and infarctions have been reported.[72,73] Malignancies are more typically seen in older cats, usually in the mandibular glands, but any gland may be affected. Surgical resection may be sufficient if the lesion is localized to that gland, but local infiltration[72] and metastasis to the lymph nodes and lungs is possible.[30] Benign growths have been seen in cats.[72]

Salivary mucoceles are most likely caused by trauma to the gland, resulting in saliva leakage with accumulation of salivary fluid in the tissues.[30,73] The sublingual gland and submandibular-mandibular gland complex are most often affected, and surgical removal of the gland and the defect usually is curative.[74] Pharyngeal mucoceles are less common, but rapid accumulation of saliva in such lesions can lead to pain and even pharyngeal obstruction.[73]

Though it is not widely reported, salivary gland infarction can occur in cats. The active coagulative necrosis of acinar tissues, usually in a mandibular salivary gland, may result in a firm swelling with associated fever and an increased white blood cell count, which usually resolves in 7 to 10 days.[72]

Oral Trauma

Trauma to the oral cavity and associated structures is a prevalent injury in domestic cats.[75] In the maxillary region fractures and avulsed teeth are sometimes seen. Both soft and hard tissue separation of the palate can occur. In the mandible, lip avulsions, fractures, symphyseal separations, and temporomandibular joint (TMJ) fractures and luxations are of primary concern. Separation of the mandibular symphysis is currently the most common oral injury of cats.[30] In addition, oral burns (electrical or chemical), lacerations, and foreign bodies are seen sporadically.

Clinical Signs

The clinical signs of oral trauma vary with the type, location, and severity of the lesion. The signs of lip avulsion are obvious; fractures and dislocations typically present as an open mouth or dropped jaw. Characteristic, nonspecific signs may include halitosis, ptyalism, dysphagia, and pawing at the mouth.

Tooth Avulsion

The teeth most often involved in partial or complete avulsion are the maxillary cuspids (canine teeth). Although avulsion of incisors, premolars, and molars occurs, treatment is usually exodontia (extraction) with symptomatic care of the wound.

Treatment of partially avulsed teeth is based on underlying disease, and the condition of the alveolar socket and the tooth. Teeth compromised by cervical line lesions or loss of supporting tissues due to periodontal or other disease are poor candidates for replantation, even when only partly avulsed. The treatment of choice in these areas consists of complete exodontia and treatment of the wound.

Teeth completely avulsed for less than 30 minutes often can be replanted if the tooth has been kept moist with saline or milk. After 30 minutes the prognosis quickly becomes worse, but success has been achieved even after several hours.[76] When replanting teeth removal of debris and blood is imperative to success. Saline solutions may be used to gently flush and cleanse the alveolus and the tooth, but these structures are not scrubbed lest remaining attachment tissues be damaged. In partial avulsions gentle pressure usually replaces the tooth and associated buccal cortical bone plate if it has been pushed out of place. Stabilization can be obtained by suturing soft tissue tears and using figure-of-eight wiring to the contralateral cuspid. For the wire to be secure, the teeth may have to be notched slightly with a high-speed dental handpiece and bur or anchored with composite bonded to the teeth. Wires can usually be removed in 3 to 6 weeks.

With complete avulsion (and some partial avulsions) it must always be understood that the endodontic vitality of

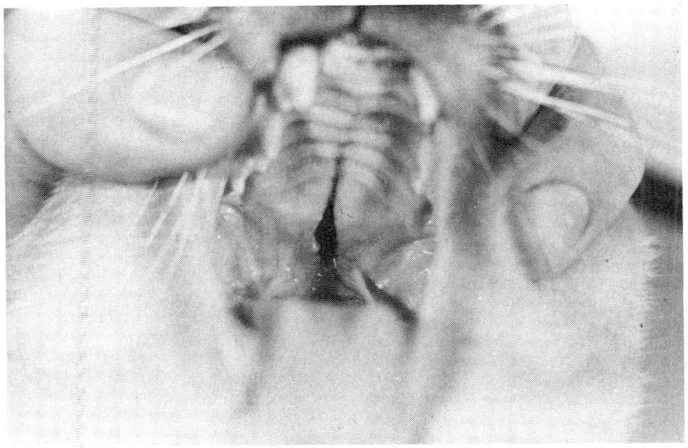

A

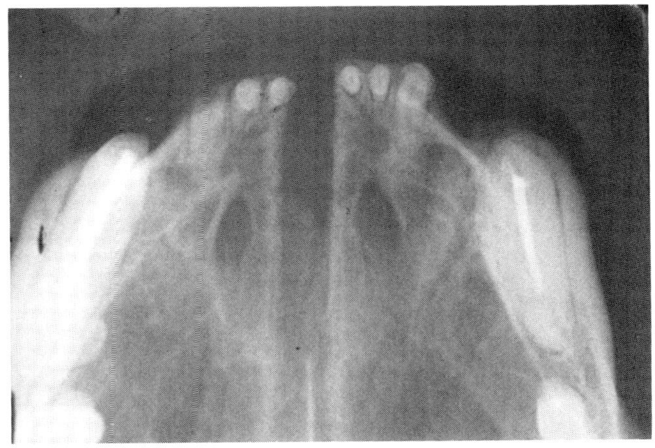

B

Figure 52–4. (*A*) Hard palate separation (courtesy of Dr. Gary D. Norsworthy). (*B*) Radiograph of maxillary midline fracture shows hard palate separation.

the tooth has been endangered by the interruption of circulation through the apical delta or foramen. It is best to consider all avulsed teeth to be endodontically compromised, because apical disease and tooth loss may occur several months after replantation. These teeth must have complete endodontic (root canal) therapy to avoid this complication (see root canal therapy in Chapter 33). Teeth can be endodontically treated at the time of replantation or, if kept on antibiotics, in 3 to 5 weeks if the cat is maintained on antibiotics during that time. The decision is a clinical one; the majority of cases in our practice are treated endodontically at the time of replantation.

Lip Avulsion

Lip avulsion is typically seen with mandibular trauma, and the first step of treatment is thorough cleansing and débridement. The subcutaneous tissue can usually be reattached at the midline to the fascia under the symphysis with absorbable suture material.[77] If sufficient soft tissue remains the lip may be replaced using a mattress suture pattern. In cases where there is excessive tension, a more extensive suture pattern is required.[77] Braided wire placed through the buccal mucosa at the level of and slightly behind the cuspids is passed subcutaneously around through the lip to the canine of the opposite side. The two ends of the wire are passed through a small-gauge tube immediately behind the canine teeth and tightened until the tissues are restored to approximately normal position. Once this has been attained the wire may be tied in a knot and the tubing slid over the knot. The suture should be left in place until healing is adequate, usually 3 weeks.

Hard Palate Separations

Hard palate separations are common in high-rise fall injuries[78] and in head injuries from car accidents (Fig. 52–4). Most soft tissue separations can be easily repaired with a mattress suture pattern using absorbable suture material. If the separation is extensive, with involvement of the palatal midline bones, intraarcade wiring may be required to reestablish proper occlusion.[78] Small holes are placed through the gingiva and interproximal bone mesial and distal to the upper fourth premolars. A wire is placed in a figure-of-eight configuration around the two upper fourth premolars. Gentle tightening usually brings the separation back into alignment. In more complicated presentations, where the upper fourth premolars have been damaged, avulsed, or are absent owing to a cervical line lesion or periodontal disease, an alternate wiring technique is required. The fracture is compressed with digital pressure. A transverse pin is passed across the fracture line dorsal to the bone of the hard palate at the approximate level of the third or fourth premolar. Both ends should extend a short distance from either side of the arcade. A figure-of-eight wiring technique is applied, looping over the exposed ends of the pin and across the hard palate, and the wires are tightened. Acrylic may be applied to the ends of the exposed pin, or orthodontic wax dispensed to the client for application at home, if needed to reduce buccal lip trauma. The soft tissue separation is sutured together in a mattress pattern with absorbable suture material. In a healthy adult the wires can generally be removed in 2 to 3 weeks. In young, developing cats, interdental wires should be adjusted or loosened every 7 to 14 days until removed, to prevent malocclusion. If the wires are left unsupervised by the clinician, malocclusion may ensue, resulting in early contact, open bite, or an anterior cross bite. Gingival inflammation due to trauma associated with the wire usually heals rapidly in the healthy patient once the wire is removed. Placement of tubing over the wire knot, as described previously, might also be recommended.

Unless compression is a problem most other maxillary fractures are treated conservatively. Fractures of the zygomatic arch are treated in similar fashion. If there is any pressure on the ocular tissues an incision is made and the fragment can be retracted laterally and stabilized.[78] Transverse fractures of the maxillae are very uncommon, but they can be treated with interdental figure-of-eight or Ivy loop wiring, extending from the maxillary canine tooth to the ipsilateral upper fourth premolar.

Oral Burns

Burns involving the oral cavity are usually electrical: often a cat chews on an electrical cord. Lesions are typically distinctive; they are generally well-circumscribed and grayish to tan. The commissures of the lips, roof of the mouth, and the tongue are the most frequently affected sites. The lesions are the result of heat coagulation of the proteins in tissues. Additionally, the electrophysiologic activity can result in muscle spasms, ventricular fibrillation, unconsciousness, and respiratory distress due to pulmonary edema.[79]

Immediate treatment is symptomatic; furosemide is used to treat pulmonary edema, if needed. Bleeding and other symptoms are customarily treated conservatively.[79] Topical orthodontic local anesthetics are applied occasionally to ease inappetence resulting from oral discomfort.

Severe burns involving the tongue may heal locally, but if any degree of tongue structure is lost, particularly the tip, the cat usually does very poorly, not eating well and unable to properly groom itself.[30] Some palatal lesions may require reconstructive surgery, particularly if any defects exend into the nasal cavity.

Oral injury from direct ingestion of chemicals and caustic agents is less likely in cats than in dogs, owing to their more discriminating eating habits. Cats, however, may get mild to severe ulcers of the tongue when such agents are contacted through grooming of exposed surfaces of the fur or feet. Symptomatic treatment of the oral cavity is recommended, in addition to washing off any residual chemicals from the fur.

Mandibular Trauma

Trauma and fractures of the jaws are common; 6% of all feline fractures involve the mandible.[80] These may be symphyseal separations (Fig. 52–5), fractures (vertical ramus, horizontal ramus, or condyle), or luxations of the TMJs.

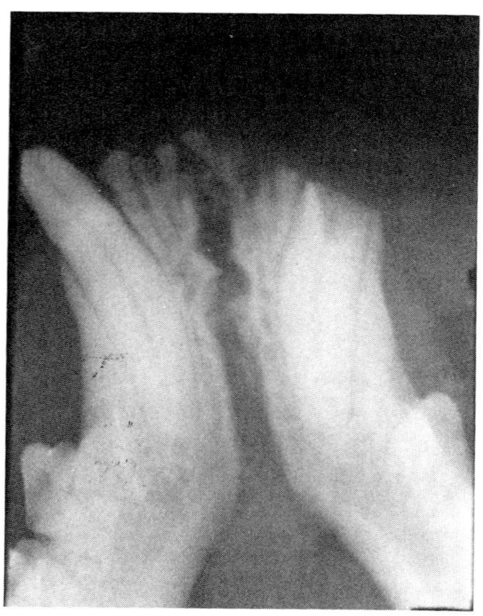

Figure 52–5. **Mandibular trauma with resulting symphyseal separation (Type III) and fractured lower cuspid and incisors.**

Table 52–4. Symphyseal Injury Classification[81]

Type I:	Separation with no break in soft tissue
Type II:	Separation with break in soft tissue
Type III:	Separation with torn intraoral soft tissues and comminution of bone; broken teeth

Separation of the mandibular symphysis is the most common traumatic oral lesion of cats.[30] Midbody fractures of the horizontal ramus are not common, whereas injury or luxations of the TMJs are occasionally seen. Fractures as a result of underlying disease, such as advanced periodontal disease or endocrine disorders, or those located distal to the first molar on the horizontal ramus, can be difficult to treat.

Clinical Signs

Clinical signs vary with the location and severity of the disease. Inappetence, ptyalism, dysphagia, the appearance of a dropped jaw, and malocclusion are some common presenting signs.

Symphyseal Separations and Fractures

Symphyseal separations are normally presented with an anterior malocclusion that may interfere with mastication. A drop at the midline of the incisors resulting in an uneven or stair-step appearance of these teeth is typical. Should the soft tissue be torn, drooling and bleeding from the mouth may occur. Table 52–4 describes a commonly used classification system for symphyseal injuries.[81]

Simple circummandibular wiring may be effective therapy for uncomplicated Type I and II injuries.[82] This procedure is described and illustrated in Chapter 55. In Type III conditions, where mildly comminuted fractures are present, circummandibular wiring aided by a submandibular figure-of-eight wiring around the canine teeth is generally necessary. The two wire patterns are tightened or adjusted individually until the fracture is stable and occlusion is acceptable. For severely comminuted rostral injuries where the canine teeth are intact, Zetner has indicated[30] that placing dentinal pins in all four canine teeth and bonding adjacent cuspids together with composite between the pins can maintain normal occlusion during the 2 to 4 weeks required to initiate the healing process. This type of treatment renders the cat unable to open the mouth, so feeding by esophagostomy or gastrostomy tube is typically required (see Chapter 55).[30] Intraoral radiographs to delineate the extent of the pulp cavity and avoidance of the cavity during pin placement are imperative.

Fractures of the Horizontal Ramus

Most fractures of the midbody of the ramus can be treated with an open front muzzle that fits loosely enough to allow eating and drinking but keeps the canine teeth in proper occlusion interlock at all times for the 2- to 4-week recovery period. Muzzles may be difficult to maintain on some cats. For these and more complicated fractures, interarcade wiring of the jaws to keep them closed may facilitate healing. Placement of a wire through the maxilla rostral to the third premolar, through the mandible rostral to the premolars (using radiographs to avoid the mandibular canal and root structures), or around the mandible can stabilize the fracture site sufficiently. Directing the wire around the mandible on one side can be helped by using a large-bore needle to guide it and a notch placed on the ventral mandible to prevent movement. Other authors have described passing a wire through holes predrilled apically to the furcations of the maxillary fourth premolar and mandibular first molar.[83] In all cases, the wires are tightened adequately to reduce the fracture while maintaining proper occlusion (see Chapter 44). Alternatively, TMS (Thread Mate System) dentinal pins can be placed in the canine teeth and the adjacent canines bonded together with composite as discussed earlier. These authors have found that passing a small wire between the pins to reinforce the composite is useful in some cases. Some cases benefit from bonding of additional teeth farther caudad in the arcade. These latter procedures require tube feeding. Complicated fractures that are bilateral, severely comminuted, and associated with missing teeth or segments of bone may require a more extensive treatment plan. External fixation combining the use of multiple orthopedic pins and an open-ended muzzle would be helpful. Pins can be placed transversely across the rostral and caudal segments of the mandible, while avoiding tooth roots and slightly altering the transverse angle of each pin. The excess pin length is cut approximately 1 cm from the skin surface. Methyl methacrylate (acrylic) is injected into an appropriate-sized tubing, impaled on the pin segments, and allowed to harden, forming an external oral splint.[77] A loose-fitting open-ended muzzle aids in maintaining occlusion while allowing the cat to eat and drink.

Fractures of the Vertical Ramus

Uncomplicated fractures of the vertical ramus frequently require no specific treatment, as the encompassing muscle mass holds most of the segments in satisfactory alignment (see TMJ, for vertical ramus fractures involving the TMJ).

Temporomandibular Joint Injuries

Details of TMJ injuries, notably fractures, can be difficult to discern clearly on radiographs.[84] A ventrodorsal radiograph taken 20 degrees lateral-oblique provides suitable detail in some cases.[84] The normal TMJ is seen in Figure 52–6 (see Chapter 14).

Acute uncomplicated luxations of the TMJ are relatively easy to replace, and affected cats typically have a dropped jaw appearance (Fig. 52–7 *A*). A wood or plastic dowel (wooden pencil, plastic toothbrush) should be placed between the upper and lower carnassial teeth of the affected jaw (Fig. 52–7 *B*). The nose and rostral mandible are gently pressed together.[77] As the jaws are allowed to close the mandible can be pulled forward if luxated caudad or pushed back if luxated rostrad (Fig. 52–7 *C*). If the jaws seem unstable, a loose-fitting open-ended muzzle should be applied for approximately a week. If there is difficulty in pressing the jaws together with the dowel pin in place, the affected

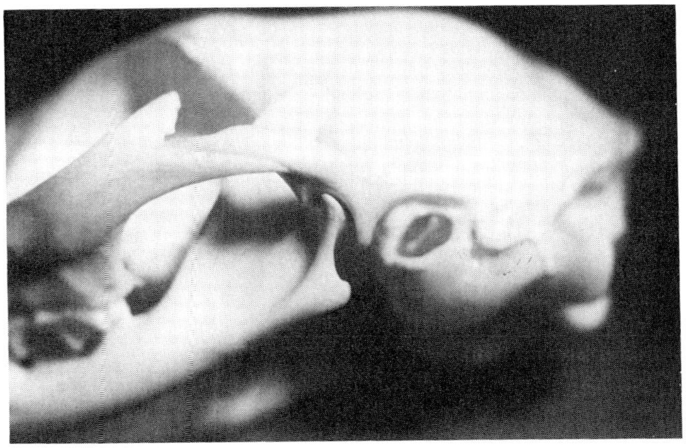

Figure 52–6. Normal orientation of the TMJ.

side should be palpated in the area of the zygomatic arch. If a lateral bulge is felt, the vertical ramus is flared laterally to the zygomatic arch and locked, thus preventing the bite from closing. If the mouth is opened wide while gentle pressure is placed on the area of the bulge, the mouth usually closes easily as the ramus returns to a medial position. In these cases muzzling is highly recommended because recurrence is more likely. We have found these patients frequently have some form of TMJ disease or dysplasia, which may eventually require condylectomy or resection of a portion of the ventral zygomatic arch to prevent repeated episodes of locking.

Fractures of the vertical ramus involving the TMJ, fractures of the TMJ, and chronic luxations may result in dysphagia, ankylosis, or pain in the joint. Mandibular condylectomy is frequently the treatment of choice in these cases.[85,86] A ventrocaudal approach to the zygomatic arch through the masseter muscle, avoiding facial nerve branches and the parotid duct, provides the best access. After severing the TMJ lateral ligament, the articular condyle—and even the articular disk, if injured—are removed with rongeurs. Suturing the masseter aponeurosis, subcutis, and skin completes the procedure, which sometimes results in only minor changes in occlusion.

Palate Defects

Defects in the palates, soft and hard, have been described in domestic cats but are not common.[30,87] They are usually of two general categories, congenital and acquired. Congenital defects may be hereditary or the result of fetal maldevelopment.[87] Acquired defects are most notably the consequence of severe chronic infection (Stage IV periodontal disease), trauma (electrical cord burns, head trauma), or surgery (aggressive tumor removal),[87] acquired conditions discussed earlier in this chapter.

Clinical Signs

Congenital abnormalities may be manifested as two distinct classifications, primary palate and secondary (hard and soft) palate. The first, primary palate defect, may externally ap-

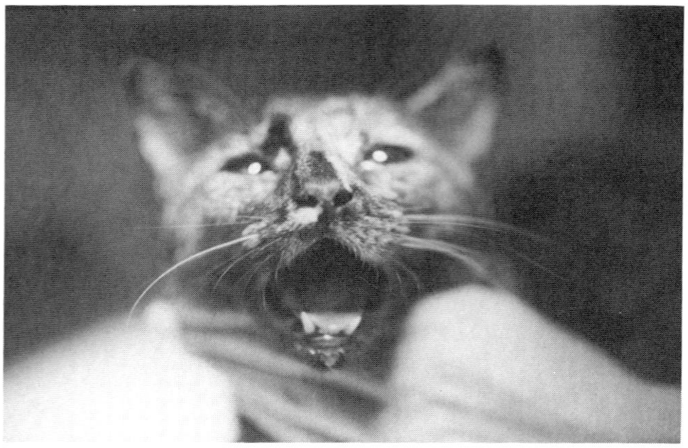

A

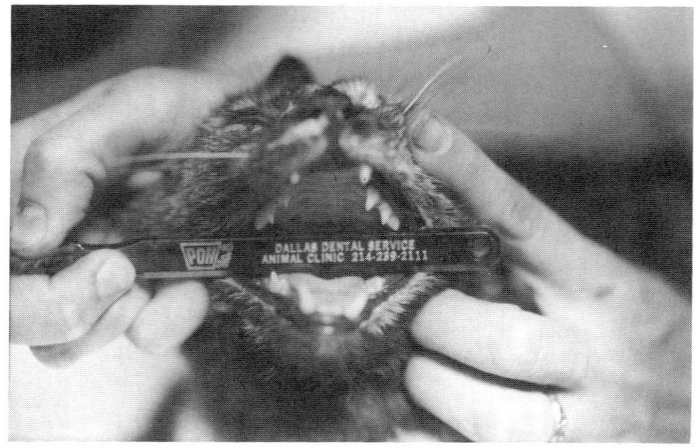

B

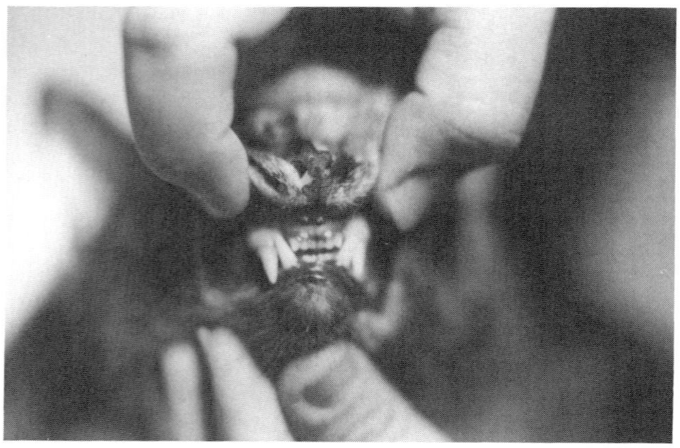

C

Figure 52–7. (*A*) Open-mouthed presentation of patient with TMJ joint luxation. (*B*) Use of toothbrush as fulcrum to correct TMJ luxation (notice incline of mandible). (*C*) Proper closure of mouth with luxation reduced.

pear as harelip (Fig. 52–8). The palatal defect is located just distal to the upper third incisor, and if it communicates with the nasal cavity lingually it can contribute to chronic rhinitis infections if left untreated. If located on the buccal gingival surface alone, minimal side effects occur. Secondary palate lesions affect the midline of the palate and are often found in very young kittens on initial oral examination or when nursing abnormalities (milk coming out of the nose) are suspected (Fig. 52–9). These carry a more serious prognosis because of the risks of aspiration infections. Additionally, primary and secondary defects may combine to produce a more complicated harelip and midline palatal abnormality. Soft palate defects may or may not be associated with intercurrent hard palate abnormalities and can occur on or just lateral to the midline.[87]

Treatment

With uncomplicated cases of primary buccal disorders corrective surgery of the harelip is generally done for aesthetic purposes. Simple sliding flaps have poor connective tissue support and are not consistently successful.[88] Lingual lesions or deeper buccal lesions that extend into the nasal cavity should be corrected to close the oronasal fistula that can constantly introduce bacteria and food particles into the nasal cavity. Basic rules for gingival and palate surgery apply here. The flap should be large, to minimize tension; epithelial edges should have a fresh surface; suture lines should not overlie the defect; and tissues should be handled gently, using large bites of tissue and preserving the blood supply.[87] Using an adequate mucoperiosteal flap and removing any remaining teeth that might interfere with the healing process will increase the chance of success.

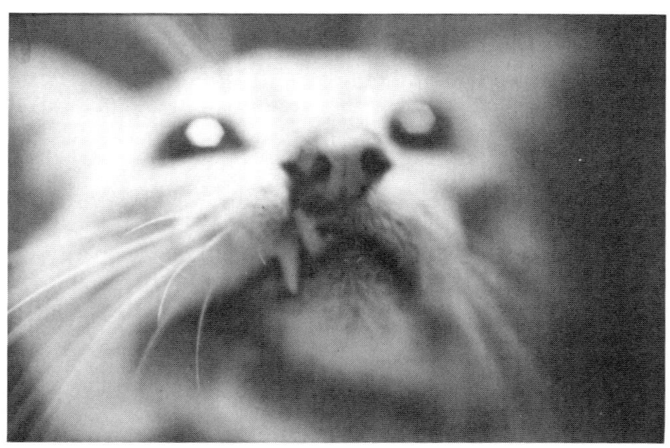

Figure 52–8. Primary cleft palate with cleft lip (harelip).

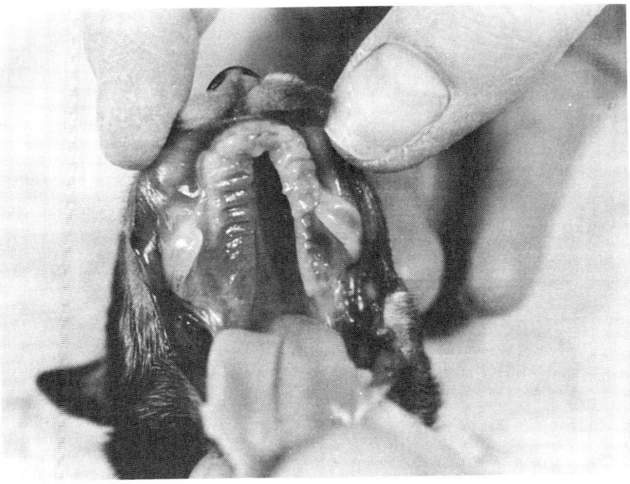

Figure 52–9. **Extensive congenital palate defect (Courtesy of Dr. Gary D. Norsworthy).**

Secondary hard palate defects are often more critical, particularly in young kittens. Tube feeding to avoid aspiration and to support growth until age 2 to 4 months is often necessary. An overlapping flap is harvested from one side of the defect, with the releasing incision made far enough laterally to provide a generous amount of tissue for the flap, sometimes near the dental arcade. Care must be taken to avoid the palatine arteries. The flap is left intact and hinged at the margin of the defect, then flipped so the mucosa is facing the nasal cavity. The harvest site must be treated gently, as this tissue is much thinner and more delicate than in dogs. This is sutured (horizontal mattress) to the underside of the contralateral oral mucosal tissue that has been incised and elevated from the bone along the edge of the defect.[87] Alternatively, releasing incisions may be made close to the arcades and the two flaps elevated to bring them together centrally,[89] but tension is a potential problem. Extensive defects seen in acquired lesions often require creative corrections that still rely on the basic principles.

Midline soft palate lesions are managed with a double-flap technique.[30] The medial margins of both sides of the edge of the soft palate defect are incised. These are separated by blunt dissection until dorsal and ventral flaps are fabricated. The dorsal flaps are sutured with an absorbable suture material in a simple interrupted pattern to produce an epithelial floor on the nasal side. The ventral flaps are closed similarly to provide an epithelial roof to the oral cavity. The caudal extent of the soft palate should extend just to the level of the caudal extent of the tonsils.

REFERENCES

1. Tholan M, Hoyt RF. Oral Pathology. In: Bojrab MJ, Tholen M, eds. Small Animal Oral Medicine and Surgery. Philadelphia: Lea & Febiger, 1990:42.
2. Lyon KF. The differential diagnosis and treatment of gingivitis in the cat. Am Vet Dent Soc Proceedings; Apr 1991:47.
3. Frost P, Williams CA. Feline Dental Disease. Vet Clin North Am (Small Anim Pract) 1986;16:851.
4. Frost P. Feline Dentistry. In: Frost P, ed. Canine Dentistry. 3rd ed. Philadelphia: WB Saunders, 1990:56.
5. Reichert PA, Durr UM, Triadan H, Vickendey G. Periodontal disease in the domestic cat. J Periodont Res 1984;54:67.
6. Gruffydd-Jones TJ, Evan RJ, Gaskell CJ. The Alimentary System. In: Pratt PW, ed. Feline Medicine. Santa Barbara, CA: Am Vet Publ, 1983:201.
7. Reed JH. The Digestive System: Diseases of the Mouth. In: Feline Medicine and Surgery. 2nd ed. Santa Barbara, CA: Am Vet Publ, 1979:154.
8. Thompson RR, Wilcox GE, Clark WT, Jansen KL. Association of calicivirus infection with chronic gingivitis and pharyngitis in cats. J Small Anim Pract 1984;25:207.
9. Loar AS. Feline Retrovirus. In: Dallas County Veterinary Medical Association Proceedings, August 1990.
10. Barr MC, Barlough JE. Feline immunodeficiency virus. Cornell Feline Health Ctr Bull 1989;10:2.
11. Gardner SA. Current concepts of FIV infection. Vet Med 1991;86:300.
12. Sparger EE. Feline T-lymphotrophic lentivirus infection. In: Feline Medicine IV. Eastern States Veterinary Conference. January, 1988 9.
13. Tenorio AP, Franti CE, Madewell BR, Pedersen NC. The relationships of chronic oral infections of cats to persistent oral carriage of Feline calici-, immunodeficiency, and leukemia viruses. Am Vet Dent College/Acad Vet Dent Proc 1990:47.
14. Meitner SW. Identification of inflamed gingival surfaces. J Clin Periodontal 1979;6:93.
15. Ishikawa J, Glickman I. Gingival response to the systemic administration of sodium diphenylhydantoin in cats. J Periodontal 1961;32:149.
16. Holmstrom SE. Treatment and management of feline stomatitis. Acad Vet Dent Proc 1988:11, .
17. Lyon KF. Approach to feline oral disease. J Vet Dent 1988;5:11.
18. Emily P, Tholen M. Periodontal Therapy. In: Bojrab MJ, Tholen M, eds. Small Animal Oral Medicine and Surgery. Philadelphia: Lea & Febiger, 1990:121.
19. Eisner E. A case of reactive bone secondary to periodontal disease in a 14-year-old cat. J Vet Dent 1990;7:16.
20. Manfra-Marretta S. The diagnosis and treatment of oronasal fistula in three cats. J Vet Dent 1988;5:8.
21. Emily P, Penman S. Handbook of Small Animal Dentistry. Oxford: Pergamon Press, 1990.
22. Hawkins BJ. Cervical line lesions (neck lesions) in the cat. Acad Vet Dent Proc 1987:6.
23. Richardson R. Dental calculus accumulation in the cat. J Small Anim Pract 1965;6:475.
24. Harvey CE, Shofer F, Venner M, Haskins M. Results Following Conservative Treatment of Gingivitis/Stomatitis in Cats. Philadelphia: University of Pennsylvania School of Veterinary Medicine, 1988.
25. Harvey CE, Shofer F, Venner M, Haskins M. Clinical features and periodontal indices in cats with chronic gingivitis/stomatitis. Philadelphia: University of Pennsylvania School of Veterinary Medicine, 1989.
26. Lyon K. Spring feline focus: An approach to feline dental disease. Ithaca, NY: Cornell Fel Hlth Ctr, 1990;12:493.
27. Joachim F, Barber F, Newman HN, Osborn J. The plasma cell at the advancing front of the lesion in chronic periodontitis. J Periodont Res 1990;60:25.
28. Pope WT. Plasma cell gingivitis-pharyngitis in a cat. J Am Assoc Feline Pract 1988;1:6.
29. Johnesse JF, Hurvitz A. Feline plasma cell gingivitis/pharyngitis. J Am Anim Hosp Assoc 1983;19:179.
30. Sams DL, Harvey CE. Oral and Dental Diseases. In: Sherding

RG, ed. The Cat: Diseases and Clinical Management. New York: Churchill Livingstone, 1989:889.

31. Zetner VK, Kampher P, Lutz H, Harvey CE. Vergleichende immunologische und virologische Untersuchungen von Katzen mit chronischen oralen Erkrankungen. Wien Tierarztl Monatsschr 1989:303.
32. Smith S, Pick PH, Miller GA, et al. Polyclonal B-cell activation: Severe periodontal disease in young adults. Clin Immunol Immunopathol 1980;16:354.
33. Sims TJ, Moncla BJ, Page RC. Serum antibody response to antigens of oral gram-negative bacteria by cats with plasma-cell gingivitis-pharyngitis. J Dent Res 1990;69(3):877.
34. Gruffydd-Jones TJ. Gingivitis and Stomatitis. In: August JR, ed. Consultations in Feline Internal Medicine. Philadelphia: WB Saunders, 1991:307.
35. Harvey CE. Bacteriology of oral inflammatory diseases in cats. Am Vet Dent College/Acad Vet Dent Proc 1990:45.
36. Fiske R. Plasma cell stomatitis. J Texas Vet Med Assoc 1985; 47:20.
37. Harvey CE. Stomatitis-gingivitis in the cat. Western States Vet Conf, Las Vegas, NV, 1991.
38. Burrows CF, Miller WF, Harvey CE. Oral Medicine. In: Harvey, CE. Veterinary Dentistry. Philadelphia: WB Saunders, 1985:34.
39. Beard G, Emily P, Mulligan T, Williams C. Cervical Line Lesions: Gingivitis/Stomatitis complex. CE Seminars 1988:43.
40. Williams CA, Aller MS. Feline stomatology. Am Vet Dent College/Acad Vet Dent 1991:101.
41. Nisengard R, Newman MG, Sanz M. The Host Response: Basic Concepts. In: Glickman, ed. Clinical Periodontology. 7th ed. Philadelphia: WB Saunders, 1990.
42. Manfra-Marretta S, Matheissen D, Matus R, Patniak A. Surgical Management of Oral Neoplasia. In: Bojrab MJ, Tholen M, eds. Small Animal Oral Medicine and Surgery. Philadelphia: Lea & Febiger, 1990:108.
43. Holmstrom SE. Feline dentristry. Am Anim Hosp Assoc Proc 1989;16:12.
44. Eisenmenger E, Zetner K. Veterinary Dentistry. Philadelphia: WB Saunders, 1985.
45. Lyons KF. An approach to feline dentistry. Comp Contin Educ 1990;12:493.
46. Goldstein G. Some new thoughts on feline stomatitis/gingivitis complex. J Vet Dent 1988;5:8.
47. Stover GC. A Differential for Oral Ulcers in Cats. Feline Health Topics—Cornell. Ithaca, NY: Cornell Hlth Ctr, 1987;2(2):1.
48. Lyons KF. The effect of gallium-arsenide laser application on feline lympho-plasmacytic gingivitis/stomatitis in eight cats. World Dent 1990;12:29.
49. Withrow SJ, Holmberg DL. Mandibulectomy in the treatment of oral cancer. J Am Anim Hosp Assoc 1983;19:273.
50. Dorn CR, Taylor DON, Frye FL, Hibbard HH. Survey of animal neoplasms in Alameda-Contra Costa Counties, California. I. Methodology and description of cases. J Natl Cancer Inst 1968;40:295.
51. Dorn CR, Taylor DON, Schneider R, Hibbard HH. Survey of animal neoplasms in Alameda-Contra Costa Counties, California. II. Cancer morbidity in dogs and cats from Alameda County. J Natl Cancer Inst 1968;40:307.
52. Dorn CR, Priester WA. Epidemiological analysis of oral and pharyngeal cancer in dogs, cats, horses and cattle. J Am Vet Med Assoc 1976;169:802.
53. Priester WA, McKay FW. The occurrence of tumors in domestic animals. [NIH Publ No. 80-2046] Bethesda, MD, National Cancer Institute, 1980.
54. Cotter SM. Oral-pharyngeal neoplasms in the cat. J Am Anim Hosp Assoc 1981;17:917.
55. Carpenter JL, Andrews JK, Holzworth J, et al. Tumors and Tumorlike Lesions. In: Holzworth J, ed. Diseases of the Cat. Vol. 1. Philadelphia: WB Saunders, 1987:431.
56. Dubielzig RR, Goldschmidt MH, Brodey RS. The nomenclature of periodontal epulides in dogs. Vet Pathol 1979;16:209.
57. Dubielzig RR. Proliferative dental and gingival disease of dogs and cats. J Am Anim Hosp Assoc 1982;18:577.
58. Withrow ST, Norris AM, Dubielzig RR. Oropharyngeal Neoplasms. In: Harvey CE, ed. Veterinary Dentistry. Philadelphia: WB Saunders, 1985:123.
59. Gilmore CE. Tumors of the Gastrointestinal Tract of Cats. In: Kirk RW, ed. Current Veterinary Therapy V. Philadelphia: WB Saunders, 1974:736.
60. Gorlin RJ, Peterson WC. Oral disease in man and animals. Arch Dermatol 1967;96:390.
61. Brodey RS. Alimentary tract neoplasms in the cat: A clinicopathologic study of 46 cats. Am J Vet Res 1966;27:74.
62. Scott DW. Observations on the eosinophilic granuloma complex in cats. J Am Anim Hosp Assoc 1975;1:261.
63. Rosenkratz W. Eosinophilic granuloma confusion. DVM Spring Skin Seminar. May 1988.
64. Kunkle GA. Update on the feline eosinophilic granuloma complex. J Am Assoc Feline Pract 1989;1:6.
65. Freiman HS. Protocol for treating feline indolent ulcers: A lip tip. Vet Forum 1991;9:96.
66. Juliff WR, Helman RG. Linear granuloma involving the tongue of a cat. Feline Pract 1984;14:39.
67. Reedy LM. Results of allergy testing and hyposensitization in selected feline skin diseases. J Am Anim Hosp Assoc 1982; 18:618.
68. Wiggs RB. Latest practical advances in veterinary dentistry. Dallas County Vet Med Assoc Proc 1991;1:1.
69. Theilen GH, Hills D. Comparative aspects of cancer immunotherapy: Immunologic methods used for treatment of spontaneous cancer in animals. J Am Vet Med Assoc 1982;181:1134.
70. Hess PW, MacEwen EG. Feline Eosinophilic Granuloma. In: Kirk R, ed. Current Veterinary Therapy. Philadelphia: WB Saunders, 1977:534.
71. Willemese A, Lubberink AAMF. Eosinophilic ulcers in cats. Trjdschr Diergen 1978;103:1052.
72. Spangler WL, Culbertson MR. Salivary gland diseases in dogs and cats: 254 cases. J Am Vet Med Assoc 1991;198:465.
73. Feinman JM. Pharyngeal mucocele and respiratory distress in a cat. J Am Vet Med Assoc 1990;197:1179.
74. Wallace LJ, Guffy MM, Gray AP, Clifford JH. Anterior cervical sialocele (salivary cyst) in a domestic cat. J Am Anim Hosp Assoc 1972;8:74.
75. Weigel JP, Dorn AS. Diseases of the Jaw and Abnormal Occlusion. In: Harvey CE. Veterinary Dentistry. Philadelphia: WB Saunders, 1985:106.
76. Rossman LE, Garber DA, Harvey CE. Disorders of the Teeth. In: Harvey CE, ed. Veterinary Dentistry. Philadelphia: WB Saunders, 1985:79.
77. Todoroff RJ, Pavletic MM. Soft Tissue Surgery—Oral Cavity and Pharynx. In: Holzworth J, ed. Diseases of the Cat. Philadelphia: WB Saunders, 1987:75.
78. Leighton RL, Robinson GW. Orthopedic Surgery—Maxilla and Mandible. In: Holzworth J, ed. Diseases of the Cat. Philadelphia: WB Saunders, 1987:133.
79. Kolata RJ, Burrows CF. The clinical features of injury by chewing electric cords in dogs and cats. J Am Anim Hosp Assoc 1981;17:219.
80. Salisbury SK, Cantwell HD. Conservative management of fractures of mandibular condyloid process in three cats. J Am Vet Med Assoc 1989;194:85.
81. Weigel JP. Trauma to Oral Structures. In: Harvey CE, ed. Veterinary Dentistry. Philadelphia: WB Saunders, 1985:140.

82. Schrader S. Dental Orthopedics. In: Bojrab MJ, Tholen M, eds. Small Animal Oral Medicine and Surgery. Philadelphia: Lea & Febiger, 1990:254.
83. Umphlet RC. Interarcade wiring: A method for stabilization of caudal mandibular fractures and temporomandibular joint luxations in the cat. Companion Anim Pract 1987;1:16.
84. Ticer JW, Spencer CP. Injury of the feline temporomandibular joint: Radiographic signs. Vet Radiol 1978;19:146.
85. Lantz GC. Temporomandibular joint ankylosis: Surgical correction of three cases. J Am Anim Hosp Assoc 1985;2:173.
86. Harvey CE. Oral and dental disease in cats. Am Anim Hosp Assoc Proc 1985;27:148.
87. Harvey CE. Oral Surgery. In: Harvey CE, ed. Veterinary Dentistry. Philadelphia: WB Saunders, 1985:167.
88. Howard DR, Merkley DF, Lammerding JJ, et al. Primary cleft palate and closure repair in puppies. J Am Anim Hosp Assoc 1976;12:636.
89. Long DA. Surgical repair of cleft palate. Vet Med Small Anim Clin 1975;70:434.

CHAPTER 53

◇ ◇ ◇

Pyothorax

Gary D. Norsworthy

Pyothorax is the accumulation of purulent material in the pleural space. The pleural effusion is composed of cellular debris, neutrophils, fibrin, and bacteria. When a large amount of pus is present, the condition is often referred to as *empyema*.

Infectious agents may reach the pleural space by three routes:[1]

1. Septicemia resulting in lymphatic or hematogenous spread to the pleural space
2. Bacteria originating from adjacent structures (lungs, esophagus, mediastinum) that rupture or fistulate
3. Bacteria introduced directly into the pleural space by penetrating wounds, thoracocentesis, or surgery

Pathogenesis

As a result of pressures within the systemic circulation, the pulmonary circulation, and the intrapleural space, a gradient of approximately 9 cm of H_2O exists between the parietal pleura and the pleural space. This gradient favors the movement of fluid from the parietal pleura into the pleural space. However, a gradient of approximately 10 cm of H_2O moves fluid from the pleural space into the visceral pleura's circulation. The net effect of these forces is to move fluid from the parietal pleura to the visceral pleura's circulation. If the delicate balance of these forces is interrupted, fluid will collect in the pleural space. The balance of forces can be altered by changes in systemic or pulmonary capillary pressure, in the competence of the lymphatics, in the permeability of the local capillaries, or in the effective surface area. To some degree, all of these changes occur in pyothorax, owing to the severe inflammation that accompanies infection in the pleural space.[1]

Clinical Presentation

Cats with pyothorax exhibit signs of progressive decline over a period of several days to a few weeks. These signs include weight loss, lethargy, inappetence, exercise intolerance, and dyspnea; fever may or may not be present. Dyspnea may begin as rapid, shallow breathing and progress to open-mouth breathing. Owners often do not seek veterinary care until the dyspnea is obvious, and then report it as having an acute onset. The report of an "acute onset" generally reflects the ability of the cat to conceal illness until a crisis develops, rather than lack of responsibility on the part of the owner.

One study revealed that domestic short- and long-haired cats are primarily affected. Affected cats had a mean age of 5.6 years, and there was no sex predisposition.[1] None of the cats had a history of a previous debilitating disease such as neoplasia, immunologic disorders, or chronic pulmonary disease.

Many cats have a borderline normocytic, normochromic anemia, with a reported mean of 26%, as is typical of cats with any chronic disease. The leukocyte count is generally elevated, with a reported mean of 27,000 cells/mm^3. However, some affected cats have a normal or low leukocyte count that does not necessarily correlate with disease severity or prognosis. Cats with overwhelming sepsis will be neutropenic. The typical biochemical profile and urinalysis results are normal. A mild prerenal azotemia may occur if the cat is dehydrated.[1]

Pyothorax is not typically associated with the immunosuppressive effects of feline leukemia virus (FeLV) infection or feline immunodeficiency virus (FIV) infection. However, the cat should be tested for both. If either test is positive, the prognosis is significantly worse because the cat's immune system will be severely challenged during the course of pyothorax and its treatment.

Diagnosis

The diagnosis of pyothorax is suspected on the finding of pleural effusion on a thoracic radiograph (Fig. 53–1). The effusion may be unilateral but is usually bilateral. The diagnosis is confirmed by a cytologic examination of the effusion revealing copious mature and degenerative neutrophils and bacteria, without neoplastic cells (Fig. 53–2). However, inability to see bacteria on a cytologic prep does not rule out pyothorax. Degenerative cellular debris, reactive mesothelial cells, macrophages, and fibrin are also frequently present.

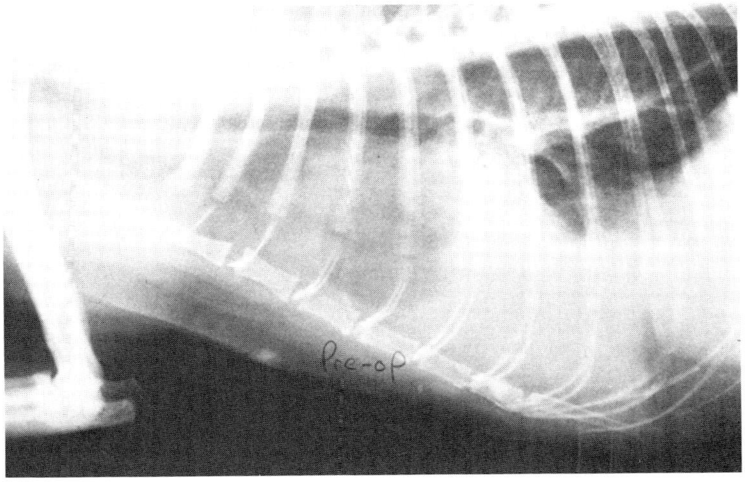

A

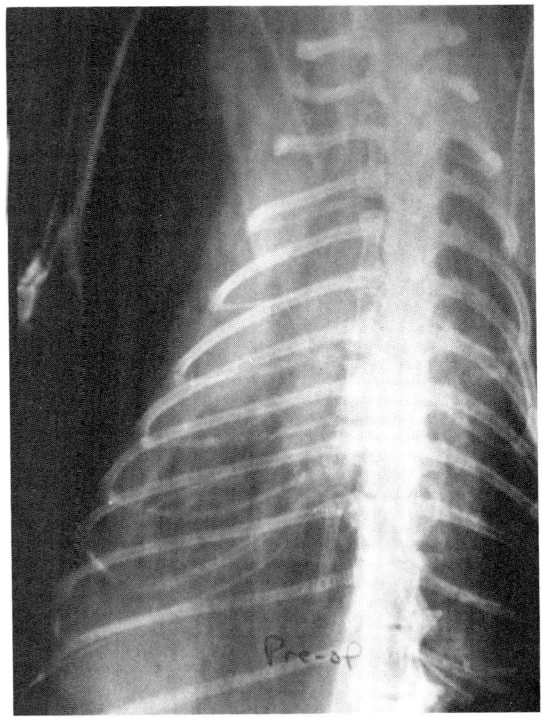

B

Figure 53–1. Radiographs of a cat with pyothorax, showing signs characteristic of pleural effusion. (*A*) Lateral view. The trachea is generally not elevated as would occur with an anterior thoracic mass. (*B*) Ventrodorsal view.

Microbiology

A rapid assessment of the microorganisms may be made with a Gram stain or a modified Wright's stain (Diff-Quik, AHS del Caribe, Inc., Aguada, Puerto Rico). Culture is necessary to properly identify the organism; however, one should be aware of the most common organisms associated with this disease (Table 53–1).

Because a large percentage of cats will have an anaerobic infection, it is essential that both aerobic and anaerobic cultures be performed. Some cats will have both aerobic and anaerboic infections.[2] Certain characteristics are helpful in making a tentative diagnosis of an anaerobic infection (Table 53–2), which will aid in the selection of an initial antibiotic regimen before culture results become available.

Because most obligate anaerobes can withstand exposure to atmospheric oxygen for only a few minutes, effusive fluid must be collected and transported in a manner that will optimize their growth.[3,4] In addition, facultative bacteria generally grow faster than obligate anaerobes, so that delays in culturing may result in their overgrowth. Aspirated fluid

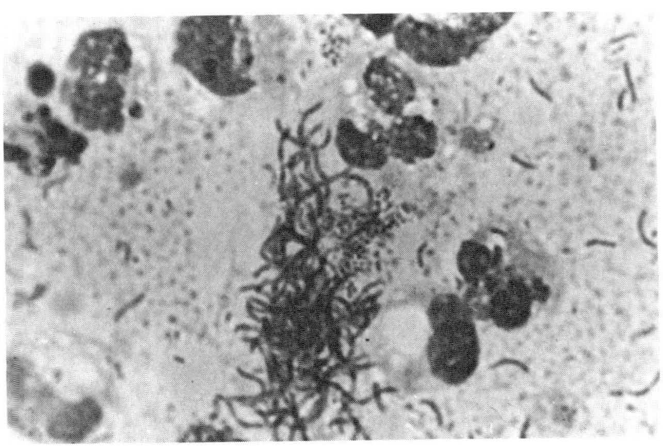

Figure 53–2. Cytologic preparation of the pleural effusion of a cat (radiographs shown in Fig. 53–1) reveals degenerate neutrophils and a large number of bacteria.

Table 53–1. Common Pathogens of the Feline Pyothorax[1,2,3]

Aerobic
Pasteurella multocida (most common)
β-hemolytic *Streptococcus* spp.
Staphylococcus spp.
Klebsiella spp.
Escherichia coli
Pseudomonas spp.
Proteus spp.
Enterobacter spp.
Corynebacterium spp.
Anaerobic
Bacteroides spp.
Peptostreptococcus
Fusobacterium
Mycoplasma
Actinomycetes

Table 53–2. Common Characteristics of Anaerobic Infections[5]

1. Foul-smelling exudate
2. History of bite wound
3. History of penetrating foreign body
4. Bacteria seen on Gram stain or modified Wright's stain that fail to grow on aerobic media
5. Black discoloration of the exudate
6. Sulfur granules in the exudate
7. Infection unresponsive to aminoglycosides, polymyxins, and sulfonamides
8. Infection characterized by a very high fever and/or a very high leukocyte count

that will be inoculated onto media within a few hours may be transported in a capped syringe from which the air has been expelled, or in a red-top blood collection tube from which air has been aspirated. However, if more than several hours will elapse before the material is inoculated, a sterile cotton-tipped applicator should be soaked with the collected material and the applicator placed in a commercially available semisolid transport medium (Port-A-Cul Tubes, BBL Microbiology Systems, Becton Dickenson, Rutherford, NJ). This will keep the culture viable for up to 72 hours at 25°C (77°F).[5]

Treatment

Initial treatment should focus on relieving life-threatening clinical signs. If severe dyspnea is present, thoracentesis performed using a butterfly catheter, three-way stopcock, and syringe, with aspiration of 50 to 100 mL (or more) of pleural effusion, can be lifesaving. Confining the cat to an oxygen cage may also be advantageous. Fluids should be administered intravenously (IV) or subcutaneously (SC) to correct dehydration. However, care should be exercised to prevent overstressing the cat with IV catheterization and with rapid administration of IV fluids. If the cat is very dyspneic or fractious, SC fluids may be preferred.

An antibiotic regimen should be started before culture and sensitivity results are available. If the cat's signs strongly suggest an anaerobic infection (see Table 53–2), penicillin G, amoxicillin (Amoxi-Tabs), ampicillin (Polyflex), amoxicillin/clavulanic acid (Clavamox), or clindamycin (Antirobe) are the initial drugs of choice. Aminoglycosides, polymyxins, and sulfonamides are not good choices to use alone because they lack a significant anaerobic spectrum of activity. The combination of an aminoglycoside such as gentamicin (Gentocin) or amikacin (Amiglyde) with a penicillin derivative is appropriate because the common anaerobes and aerobes generally show sensitivity to one or both of these drugs. Enrofloxacin (Baytril) is another good choice until culture and sensitivity results are available. Because antibiotic treatment should continue for 2 to 3 months,[5] it is essential that a quantitative culture and sensitivity be performed so that correct choices of antibiotics can be made. Because of potential side-effects, it is not good practice to use an aminoglycoside for 2 to 3 months.

The pleural space must be continuously drained for the treatment to be effective. Drainage is best achieved with an indwelling thoracostomy tube and intermittent drainage. Generally, a single tube will adequately drain both sides of the chest; however, postsurgical radiographs should be obtained to confirm drainage. If adequate bilateral drainage is not achieved with a single tube, a second tube should be placed (see Chapter 55 for a description of thoracostomy tube placement). Lavage of the pleural space should occur twice daily. Fluid should be aspirated from the chest. Warm saline should be infused at the rate of 2.5 mL/lb of body weight, with care taken not to induce dyspnea. If labored breathing occurs, the infusion should be stopped, regardless of how little fluid has been infused. When the infusion is completed, the cat should be gently rolled to disperse the fluid into all aspects of the chest, then the fluid should be removed. On average, 75% of the amount of fluid infused is recovered.

During early treatment, the cat should be monitored radiographically and by cytologic examination of lavage fluid every 48 hours. Improvement should be seen within the first 48 hours, with a significant reduction in bacterial concentration. If the results are equivocal, another quantitative culture can be performed. Marked clinical improvement should occur within 4 days (Fig. 53–3). The average time of therapy with the thoracostomy tube in place is 5 to 7 days.[6] As long as the thoracostomy tube is in place, there is a constant risk of loss of serum proteins and electrolytes (especially potassium) and of the introduction of new bacteria into the chest. The finding of new types of bacteria on cytologic examination is an unfavorable sign.

When the lavage fluid becomes clear, free of bacteria, and of minimal quantity, the thoracostomy tube is removed.[2] Antibiotics should be continued for up to 3 months.

If after 4 to 6 days of treatment with the thoracostomy tube in place there is not obvious improvement radiographically, cytologically, and on culture results, two options should be considered: changing antibiotics, or performing a thoracotomy. A thoracotomy is undertaken to look for a foreign body. It also affords the surgeon the opportunity to break down adhesions and remove proliferative fibrotic tissue.

Although most cats will recover completely (Fig. 53–4), there are a few potential sequelae. These include constrictive pleuritis, pleural adhesions, and pulmonary abscessation. If present, these will result in reduced pulmonary capacity and function.

Some have advocated repeated thoracentesis without the use of a thoracostomy tube. This form of therapy increases the chances of lung laceration and bacterial contamination; it is also painful for the cat.

Prognosis

Reported mortality rates have ranged from 42% to 80% when therapy consisted of repeated thoracentesis and antibiotic therapy alone.[1] In one study, almost 50% of 20 cats with pyothorax died or were euthanized during the first 3 days after presentation.[7] In another study involving 42 dogs and cats, there was only one canine fatality and no feline fatalities.[1] The author of that study concluded that pyothorax is a very treatable disease if the patient is immunocompetent and if aggressive therapy is begun early.

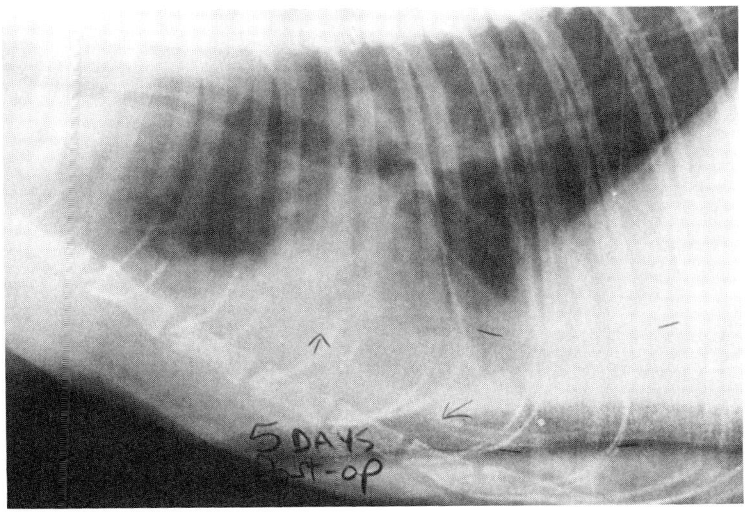

A

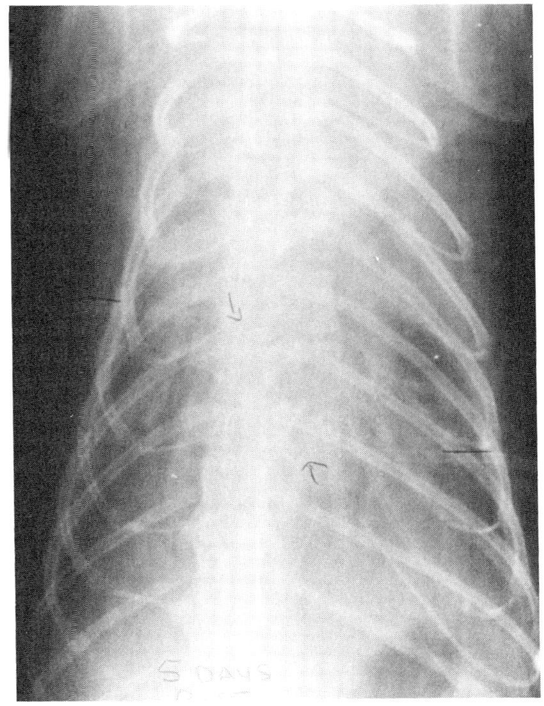

B

Figure 53–3. Radiographs made after thoracostomy tubes had been in place for 5 days, same cat as in Figure 53–1. Marked improvement is evident. The ends of the two tubes are faintly visible at the *arrows.* (*A*) Lateral view; (*B*) ventrodorsal view.

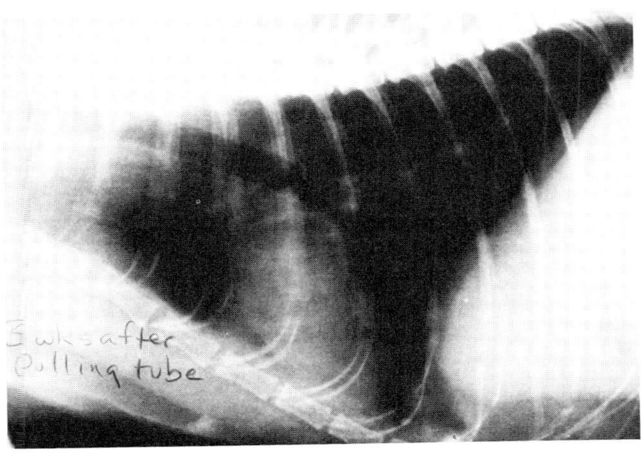

Figure 53–4. Three weeks after the thoracostomy tubes were removed, the cat in Figure 53–1 is clinically and radiographically normal.

REFERENCES

1. Bauer T. Pyothorax. In: Kirk RW, ed. Current Veterinary Therapy IX. Philadelphia: WB Saunders, 1986:292.
2. Sherding RG. Pyothorax in the cat. Comp Cont Educ Pract Vet 1979;1:247.
3. Gorbach SL, Bartlett JG. Anaerobic infections [3 parts]. N Engl J Med 1974;290:1177, 1237, 1289.
4. Sheperd WE, ed. Cumitech 5: Practical Anaerobic Bacteriology. Washington, DC: American Society for Microbiology, 1977.
5. Dow SW, Jones RL. Anaerobic infections. Part II. Diagnosis and treatment. Comp Cont Educ Pract Vet 1987;9:827.
6. Ware WA. Dyspnea: Diagnosis and Management. In: August JR, ed. Consultations in Feline Internal Medicine. Philadelphia: WB Saunders, 1991:147.
7. Jonas LD. Feline pyothorax: A retrospective study of twenty cases. J Am Anim Hosp Assoc 1983;19:865.
8. Suter PF, Head JR. Mediastinal, Pleural, and Extrapleural Diseases. In: Ettinger SJ, ed. Textbook of Veterinary Internal Medicine, 1st ed. Philadelphia: WB Saunders, 1975:767.

CHAPTER 54

◇ ◇ ◇

Reproductive Disorders

Bruce E. Eilts, Dale L. Paccamonti, and Robert Causey

While the cat shares individual aspects of its reproductive physiology with other domestic species, in combination they set the cat apart as unusual. Like the mare, the queen is seasonally polyestrous and responsive to photoperiod. Like the bitch, the queen is unusual in maintaining sexual receptivity for some days after ovulation, while the corpus luteum is forming. Most importantly from a clinical standpoint, the queen is an induced ovulator, like the rabbit and ferret, requiring a copulatory stimulus or exogenous hormones for ovulation and corpus luteum formation. Veterinarians need to understand the normal reproductive physiology of the cat in order to accurately diagnose and treat reproductive disorders and complications that may arise in breeding management.

Seasonality

Puberty in the cat usually occurs at 9 to 10 months of age.[1] Puberty may occur as early as 4 months or as late as 2 years[2]; however, because cats are seasonal breeders, the season in which the kitten was born influences the age at which puberty occurs. Kittens born early in the year may be too young to reach puberty before the onset of seasonal anestrus. With the onset of cyclicity the following year, they would be older than kittens born after them in the previous year who would be entering puberty with them. Cyclicity of the cat has been determined to be dependent on the photoperiod. Cats are "long-day breeders" and require 12 hours or more of light to maintain normal cyclicity. Normal polyestrous behavior can be induced by controlling exposure to light.[3] Cyclicity stopped abruptly and folliculogenesis was inhibited in queens exposed to less than 8 hours of light.[4] Cyclicity in the cats resumed at an average of 16 days after returning to a 14-hour photoperiod.[4] Seasonality is more pronounced in cats subjected to natural lighting,[1] especially at higher latitudes. Long-haired breeds tend to be more seasonal than short-haired breeds, with 90% of long-haired cats experiencing a period of anestrus compared with only 39% of short-haired cats.[1] In an extensive survey of 168 queens, approximately 50% of cats cycled year-round, while the remainder experienced a period of anestrus from September to the end of January.[1]

Stages of the Estrous Cycle

The phases of the feline estrous cycle are identified as proestrus, estrus, interestrus, diestrus or pseudopregnancy, and anestrus. *Proestrus,* the period preceding estrus, lasts 1 to 2 days.[5] This phase is seen in only 16% of estrous cycles according to one report.[5] During this time, the female is attractive to but not willing to accept the male. The queen may rub against objects, vocalize, and assume a lordotic posture. In the "dragster posture," she will place her front quarters on the ground, elevate her hind quarters and lift her tail to one side. When the dorsal caudal area is stroked, she will tread with her hind legs.

Estrus is the period of sexual receptivity, which lasts 3 to 16 days (average of 7)[5,6] and then subsides for 3 to 14 days (average of 9).[5] Behavioral changes are more pronounced in estrus than in proestrus; however, no conspicuous changes in the appearance or size of the external genitalia are evident.[5] The length of estrus is not affected by breeding or ovulation.[7,8] Inducing ovulation in a queen in an effort to abruptly terminate objectionable estrous behavior will not shorten the duration of estrus for that cycle. However, it will prolong the interestrual interval and delay the return of the undesirable behavior. The period following estrus is affected by ovulation induced by either copulation or exogenous hormones.

Interestrus is the period between successive estrus periods if ovulation does not occur. If the queen is not bred, she will cycle into estrus on an average of every 2 to 3 weeks.[3,7] If the queen ovulates, corpora lutea are formed and secrete progesterone. Elevated progesterone levels are the hallmark of *diestrus.* If the queen is not pregnant, diestrus is also termed pseudopregnancy and lasts for 35 to 40 days.[6] *Anestrus* is the seasonal period when the cat does not cycle.

Queens are induced ovulators, ovulating in response to vaginal/cervical stimulation from copulation. Following proestrus and estrus, there are three alternatives in the feline: (1) ovulation does not occur, resulting in a return to estrus in 4 to 22 days (average 9 days)[5]; (2) ovulation occurs without fertilization, resulting in pseudopregnancy lasting 35 to 40 days and a return to estrus in an additional 1 to

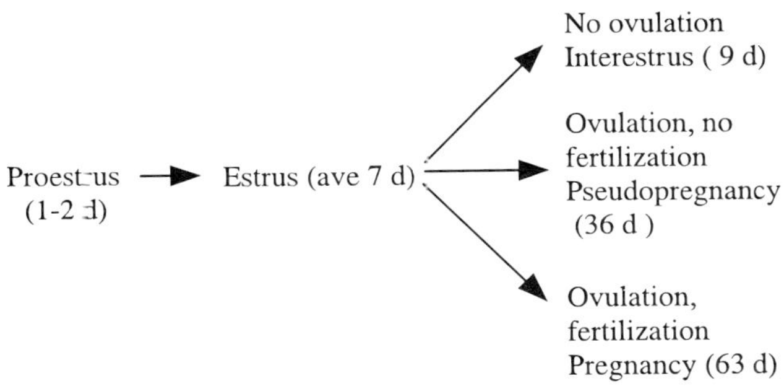

Figure 54–1. **Possible outcomes of estrus in the queen.**

10 days[33,35]; or (3) ovulation occurs and ova are fertilized, followed by pregnancy (Fig. 54–1).

Vaginal Cytology

Because of several factors, such as the relatively short length of proestrus, the ability to induce ovulation by mechanical stimulation of the vagina, and the less dramatic changes observed in the queen, vaginal cytology is not as useful as it is in the bitch. It may provide information, though, in some cases of infertility or problem breeders. Because of the size of the reproductive tract and the possibility of inducing ovulation with a swab, a cytologic sample is best obtained using a pipette or eyedropper and a small amount of saline. The saline is infused into the vagina and retrieved by aspiration. The sample is placed on a microscope slide and stained with a modified Wright's stain (Diff-Quik). Clearing of the background is the earliest sign of follicular activity.[5] Progressive cornification, the cornerstone of vaginal cytologic interpretation in the bitch, cannot be relied upon to predict estrus in the queen, since one third of queens in one report exhibited estrus before cornification was evident.[5] Some inconsistency exists in the nomenclature of cells obtained with vaginal cytologic techniques.[5,9] Cornified cells are characterized by pyknotic or faded nuclei, while noncornified cells have nuclei with a normal mottled appearance. Parabasal and intermediate cells are considered noncornified, while superficial and anuclear cells are cornified. Parabasal cells are small and rounded with normal nuclei and a low cytoplasm-to-nucleus ratio. Compared with parabasal cells, intermediate cells have an increased cytoplasm-to-nucleus ratio with increased angularity of the cell, even though the nucleus is not yet pyknotic. Superficial cells are similar to intermediate cells but with increased angularity of the cytoplasm and a pyknotic nucleus. Anuclear cells are superficial cells with a nucleus that does not take up stain. The overall trend seen, along with a clearing of the background on the slide, is for an increase in cornification as the queen progresses from proestrus through estrus (Fig. 54–2). Using these criteria, parabasal cells are low throughout the cycle and rare during estrus.[5] Superficial cells show a slight increase from 40% to 50% prior to estrus to 50% to 60% during estrus.[5] Changes are most notable in anuclear and intermediate cells. Intermediate cells decrease markedly, from 45% to less than 10%, as proestrus and estrus advance, while anuclear cells increase from approximately 5% during early proestrus to 40% during estrus. Red blood

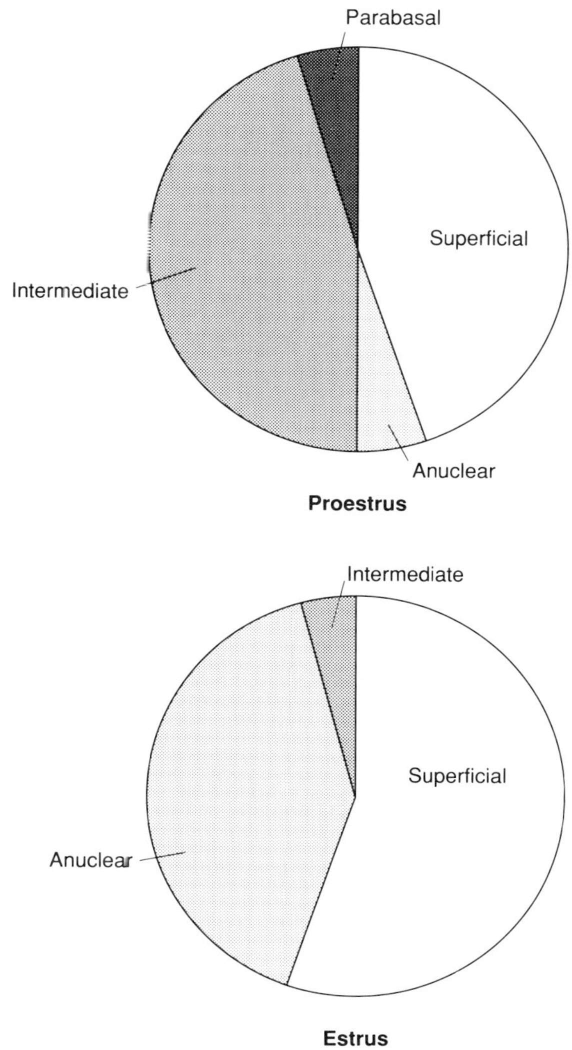

Figure 54–2. **Percent cornified (superficial and anuclear) and noncornified (intermediate and parabasal) cells seen with vaginal cytology during proestrus and estrus in the queen.**

cells, characteristic of proestrus in the bitch, are normally absent during proestrus and estrus in the queen.

Ovulation

Reports have verified that spontaneous ovulation does not occur in the queen.[8,10] Ovulation is triggered by copulation or mechanical stimulation of the vagina and cervix. Stimulation of nerves in the cervix and vagina causes a reflex stimulation of the hypothalamus via pathways in the spinal cord. The hypothalamus releases gonadotropin-releasing hormone (GnRH), which acts on the anterior pituitary resulting, in turn, in a release of luteinizing hormone (LH). LH, then, stimulates ovulation and the development of corpora lutea. A recent report indicates that other forms of stimulation, for example stroking, may occasionally be responsible for ovulation. Active corpora lutea were found in cats unexposed to males or artificial coital stimuli. Whether they had

Table 54–1. Hormone Levels Associated with Reproduction

Testosterone in males
Normal = 1,000 pg/mL
Progesterone in females
Normal (anestrus) = 0.5 ng/mL
Ovulation ≥ 1 ng/mL
Progesterone in pregnancy
Basal level (anestrus) = 0.5 ng/mL
21 days postovulation = 30–40 ng/mL (peak)
Adequate production by placenta by Day 50 to maintain pregnancy (ovaries no longer needed)
Progesterone in pseudopregnancy
Basal level (anestrus) = 0.5 ng/mL
5 days postovulation = 8 ng/mL
18–25 days postovulation = 16–17 ng/mL (peak)
40 days postovulation = 0.5 ng/mL

ovulated spontaneously or in response to some unknown stimuli could not be determined.[143]

Ovulation depends on adequate LH release. Both the peak concentration and the duration of elevation of LH are important in determining whether ovulation takes place.[10-12] Insufficient copulatory stimuli will fail to induce the release of enough LH to cause ovulation. LH release occurs within minutes of coitus[7,11,13,14] and peaks about 1 to 2 hours later.[11] Release of LH by the pituitary appears to be, in part, dependent on the duration of its prior exposure to estrogen.[7,11] The LH response to copulation, therefore, may vary depending on the day of estrus on which coitus occurs. Multiple copulations result in higher levels of LH in plasma[10,12,15] and are more likely to result in ovulation than single matings.[7,10,12] The duration of elevated LH in plasma also determines whether ovulation occurs.[10,16] According to one report, LH decreased to baseline values within 12 to 24 hours after a single mating or after multiple matings at less than a 2-hour interval. However, LH remained elevated up to 38 hours after multiple mating intervals of every 3 hours.[7] Therefore, to achieve sufficient LH release, repeated breeding at a reasonable interval should be encouraged. The LH response to a single mating can vary substantially,[13] and neither single nor multiple copulations can ensure ovulation.[8] *To increase the likelihood of ovulation, breeders should try to maximize the number of matings and breed on successive days of estrus.*

Ovulation reportedly occurs 24 to 60 hours postcoitus and may vary depending on the mating pattern.[8,14] Progesterone levels in the blood can be used to verify ovulation (Table 54–1). Concentrations greater than 1 ng/mL are considered indicative of ovulation.[7] Peak levels of 35 ng/mL in the pregnant queen and 24 ng/mL in the pseudopregnant queen are observed at approximately Day 21 postcoitus.[3]

Control of the Estrous Cycle

Induction of Ovulation

Ovulation can also be induced with exogenous hormones.[7,16,17] Administration of GnRH (Cystorellin) or an LH-like hormone, human chorionic gonadotropin (HCG) (Follutein), after mating can be used to increase the likelihood of ovulation. Both stimulate ovulation by bypassing the vaginal/cervical-hypothalamic neural pathway. According to one report, administration of 25 μg of GnRH on the second day of estrus resulted in all mature follicles ovulating in all queens treated.[16] Two reports found an efficacious dose of HCG to be 500 IU on Day 1 or Days 1 and 2 of estrus.[7,17] With lower doses, all queens ovulated but ovulation rates per queen were less than 100%.[17] HCG, administered at a dose of 250 IU on Days 2 and 3 of estrus, and coupled with mating three times per day at 3-hour intervals for the first 3 days of estrus resulted in a doubling in the number of corpora lutea formed.[7] Unlike HCG, GnRH administered in conjunction with natural mating did not enhance ovulation.[7,18] HCG administration may be useful when the male has a low libido and when a sufficient number of copulatory stimuli are not achieved.

Mismating

The length of time the embryo spends in the oviduct is critical. A prolonged period in the oviduct is associated with increased early embryonic death. Embryos arrive in the uterus after 4 to 5 days of oviductal transport.[19] When estradiol cypionate (ECP) is administered shortly after ovulation, embryo transport in the oviduct is retarded, negatively affecting viability.[19] Pregnancy can be successfully prevented by administration of 250 μg ECP intramuscularly (IM), 36 to 48 hours after coitus.[19] ECP at a dose of 125 to 250 μg/cat is also effective in preventing pregnancy when given up to 6 days after the end of estrus.[20] During this time frame, ECP is apparently either directly embryotoxic or blocks implantation.[20] ECP has potentially serious side effects in the queen, such as pyometra or aplastic anemia due to bone marrow suppression, but the incidence is apparently less than in the bitch. Prostaglandins (PGs) are ineffective for mismating when administered in the early luteal phase. Doses sufficiently high to approach toxicity, given on Days 4 and 5 or Days 12 and 13, had no effect on progesterone concentrations.[21]

Induction of Estrus

Estrus can be induced in the queen using follicle-stimulating hormone (FSH-P)[7,22] or pregnant mare serum gonadotropin (PMSG).[22,23] Currently, PMSG is commercially available in the United States only in combination with HCG (P.G.600). The effect of using HCG combined with PMSG in an estrus induction scheme is unknown. The most successful protocol for induction of estrus using currently available products administers 2.0 mg FSH IM daily until estrus, but for not more than 5 days.[22] With this protocol, normal fertility was observed in mated queens after estrus induction.[22] Prolonged administration of FSH resulted in follicular ovarian cysts that subsequently failed to rupture.[22] Although they stimulated mature follicular development, higher doses of FSH given as a single injection resulted in inconsistent sexual receptivity.[22] Some queens, especially those under 1 year of age, appear to be sensitive to ovarian hyperstimulation by exogenous gonadotropins.[7,22,24] Queens experiencing an induced estrus may have an increased number of both unovulated follicles and corpora lutea than queens having a natural estrus.[18]

Estrus Prevention or Suppression

Practitioners are at times asked to prevent or suppress estrus in the queen. No approved drugs exist for this purpose. Cases of pyometra and cystic endometrial hyperplasia associated with the use of progestogens in queens have been reported.[25] These side effects, however, are less common in queens than in bitches.[25] Megestrol acetate (Ovaban), although not approved for use in cats, has been used for both estrus prevention and suppression. When begun during seasonal anestrus, 2.5 mg/wk for up to 18 months prevented a return to estrus.[26] During the breeding season, 2.5 mg/day begun during the interestrus interval and continued for up to 60 days similarly delayed a return to estrus.[26] When suppression of estrus is desired, a dosage of 5 mg/day for 3 days,[27] or until signs of estrus ceases,[26] should be given. In this case, therapy is continued at a dose of 5 mg/wk for 10 weeks[26,27] or 2.5 mg/day for 60 days.[26]

The return of estrus was successfully delayed during treatment and for 1 to 3 months after cessation of treatment.[26,27] Other than weight gain, no serious side effects of megestrol acetate were observed.[27] More recently, significant adrenal cortical suppression has been reported with the use of megestrol acetate (see Chapter 7).[28] The queen should be allowed to have a normal estrus without hormonal manipulation before retreatment.[26]

Mibolerone, an androgenic steroid, is effective in preventing estrus in queens.[29] Serious side effects, however, preclude its use in cats. Possibly fatal hepatic disease; changes in thyroid function, serum cholesterol, thyroid histology, and weight; and slight masculinization, noted by clitoral hypertrophy and thickening of the cervical dermis, were observed.[26,29]

Although not currently available in the United States, delmadinone acetate (DMA) offers promise for estrus control in the queen. It was found to be safe and effective when administered for up to 36 months.[30] For estrus prevention, DMA can be administered orally once a week or injected subcutaneously (SC) every 6 months.[30] For estrus suppression, DMA is administered orally once daily for 6 days or injected SC once or twice in a 24-hour period.[30] No short- or long-term side effects were noted with use of DMA in cats.[30]

Permanent estrus prevention is best achieved by ovariohysterectomy. No undesirable side effects, other than possible weight gain if fed ad libitum, have been associated with ovariohysterectomy in queens.[31] Recent studies indicate ovariohysterectomy may be performed on prepubertal puppies as young as 7 weeks of age.[32] At this age, the procedure is relatively simple and recovery is rapid, compared with its effect on older animals. Similar results may be expected in prepubertal female kittens. Neutering male puppies at a similar age results in a smaller penis in the adult dog. Similar results in toms would be undesirable considering the incidence of lower urinary tract disease.

Normal Events of the Luteal Period

Physiology of Pseudopregnancy

Pseudopregnancy results when ovulation and corpora lutea formation occur, but pregnancy does not result. The corpora lutea produce progesterone, which rises rapidly from basal concentrations (0.5 ng/mL) to 8.0 ng/mL 5 days after ovulation to a peak of 16 to 17 ng/mL 18 to 25 days postovulation.[6,33] Following the peak, progesterone concentrations decline to basal values at approximately 40 days postovulation.[3,33] The normal duration of pseudopregnancy has been observed to be from 35 to 40 days, with an average of 36.5 days.[6] The corpora lutea appear to have a preprogrammed finite lifespan in that they are not subject to regression from uterine sources of PGs, as is the case with cattle and horses.[34] The corpora lutea also have been shown to be resistant to multiple luteolytic doses of PGs through Days 11 to 25 postovulation,[33] indicating that it is clinically difficult to shorten the time interval from the onset of pseudopregnancy to the subsequent estrus. This interestrus interval normally lasts 30 to 50 days and includes a luteal phase lasting around 35 days followed by a short, 1- to 10-day, anestrus phase.[33,35] This anestrus phase may last several months if the queen is entering seasonal anestrus at the end of the pseudopregnant luteal period. It is rare for the queen to have the overt signs of lactation (pseudogenetra) at the end of pseudopregnancy that are seen in the bitch.[35]

Pregnancy

Assuming successful induction of ovulation has occurred, fertilization can occur if viable sperm meet viable ova. Sperm cells undergo capacitation in vitro in approximately 1 hour.[36]

Fertilization probably occurs at the ampulla-isthmic junction, and the embryos move into the uterine lumen 4 to 5 days postcoitus.[19] Upon entry into the uterus, the embryos migrate for 6 to 8 days then spread out so that each embryo has an equal share of the uterus.[37] As the number of ovulations increases to greater than five, the percentage of embryos that implant at 12 to 13 days diminishes from 90% for five ovulations to around 53% for 9 to 11 ovulations. This overcrowding phenomenon results in an observed average litter size of 4 to 4.5 kittens, with the largest litters averaging 6.6 kittens from eight ovulations.[37] The fecundity of queens, therefore, appears limited by ovulation rates and uterine spacing.

Four known proteins have been shown to be produced de novo by the feline conceptus. These are retinol-binding protein, alpha-fetoprotein, albumin, and transferrin.[38] Retinol-binding protein, probably needed for retinoid (vitamin A analogs) transport, is present from Days 10 to 36.[38] Alpha-fetoprotein, possibly having an immunosuppressive role, is secreted from Days 5 to 50, and transferrin, needed for iron transport, is secreted from Days 15 to 30.[38] Other novel proteins have also been identified as secretions from the feline conceptus.[38]

Hormones of Pregnancy

In the pregnant queen, progesterone, secreted by the corpora lutea, rises rapidly after ovulation and peaks at a concentration of 30 to 40 ng/mL on Day 21, which is very similar to that of the pseudopregnant queen[3] (Table 54–1). The concentration of progesterone then gradually falls to basal concentrations through the remainder of gestation.[3] Unlike in the pseudopregnant queen, the corpora lutea may not regress.[3] In the pregnant queen, the placenta produces the enzyme needed for progesterone production starting around Days 28 to 32[39] of gestation, and the ovaries are not needed to maintain pregnancy after Day 50 to term.[40]

Prolactin from the anterior pituitary increases at Day 35 and peaks about Day 50 of gestation.[35] Prolactin appears to be needed for pregnancy maintenance. When a prolactin inhibitor, cabergoline, is administered after Day 42, abortion results.[41]

Relaxin, from the fetal-placental unit, is detectable after 25 days of gestation, remains elevated from Day 30 to term, and declines abruptly at parturition.[42,43] Laboratory tests using relaxin to diagnose pregnancy are being considered for the commercial market.

Superfetation

During pregnancy, the queen has been reported to continue to mate, and ovulations at Days 10 to 14 of pregnancy have been reported to result in a younger, secondary litter.[40,44] This ovulation and secondary pregnancy is referred to as superfetation. However, reports on superfetation are mostly nonscientific and anecdotal, and the phenomenon may not truly exist.

Diagnosis of Pregnancy

Pregnancy diagnosis in the queen is easily determined by abdominal palpation. Discrete swellings in the uterus, which are the evenly spaced fetal-placental units, can be palpated as early as Day 16 postcoitus in some queens until approximately Day 30. After Day 30, the fetal-placental units converge so that the discrete swellings become confluent. Radiography can be used to diagnose pregnancy after fetal mineralization occurs at about Day 43 postcoitus.[45] At this stage, counting the number of conceptuses radiographically is easily performed. Ultrasound can be used to determine pregnancy as early as Days 14 to 15 postcoitus.[46,47] The gestational sac appears as a round, nonechogenic (black) structure located within a hyperechoic (white) uterus. Heartbeats are visible in the fetus starting around Day 20.[46,47] Although it is difficult to count the number of conceptuses accurately using ultrasound, the presence of fetal heartbeats gives an absolute indication of fetal life. The determination of fetal life is important in establishing when and if an early embryonic death occurs.

Care During Pregnancy

Care of the pregnant queen should include adequate nutrition, adequate exercise, isolation from potentially infectious diseases, and restraint from administration of vaccines or medications, if at all possible. Queens eat more as gestation progresses.[48] In one report, individual queens ate an average of 178 g of canned food during the first week of pregnancy, 267 g during Week 7 and 256 g during Week 8, an approximate increase of 50%.[48] Queens with larger litters tended to gain more weight than those with smaller litters,[48] with an average gain of about 900 g (2.0 lb).[48] The caloric requirement for pregnant queens is 100 kcal/kg of body weight.[49] The ration must be balanced and specifically designed for cats. Vitamin A is essential in the queen's diet. Taurine deficiency may result in abortion or small kittens.[50,51] Lack of adequate vitamin A can also cause early embryonic death and abortions.[49]

Gestation length in the cat is 63 to 66 days when measured from a fertile mating.[52] Because kittens born before 60 days of gestation have little chance of survival, it is important that gestation progress to 63 days for maximum kitten viability.[52,53]

Abnormal Events of the Luteal Period

Pyometra

Pyometra is a common disorder associated with the luteal period. Its pathogenesis is probably not rooted in the luteal phase but in the multiple exposures to estrogen when the queen is cycling frequently and not induced to ovulate. This repeated exposure to estrogen results in endometrial hyperplasia. Endometrial hyperplasia predisposes queens to pyometra when a luteal phase occurs. [54] In one study, almost all queens greater than 5 years old (the mean age being 6.3 years) had evidence of endometrial hyperplasia.[54] The mean age of queens with pyometra is 7.2 to 7.6 years.[54,55]

The primary clinical signs of pyometra include abdominal distension, vaginal discharge, anorexia, weight change, and lethargy (Fig. 54–3).[54,55] Queens with corpora lutea on the ovaries have a neutrophilic lymphocytosis with a total white blood cell (WBC) count averaging 57,000/μL, whereas those without corpora lutea have a WBC count averaging 25,000/μL.[54] Abdominal radiographs or ultrasound will help in determining if the uterus is enlarged. Only about 20% of queens with pyometra have bacteriologic growth from the pyometra fluid.[55] The most commonly isolated organism is *Escherichia coli*.[55]

Treatments for pyometra include ovariohysterectomy, PGs, and surgical uterine lavage. Ovariohysterectomy is the treatment of choice for queens not intended for breeding; however, care should be exercised in handling the uterus,

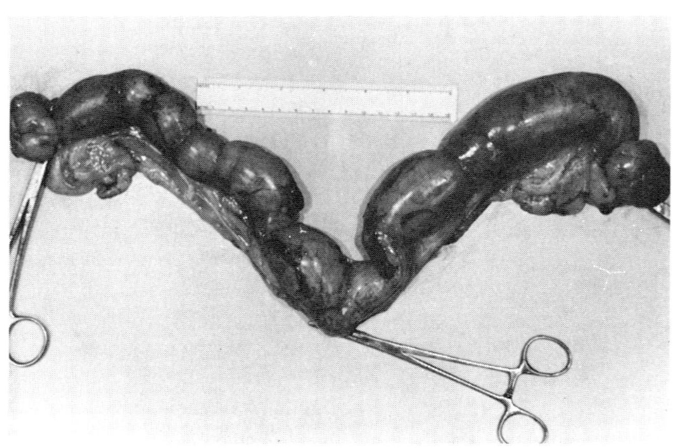

Figure 54–3. **Pyometra causes a significant enlargement of the uterus (and abdomen) due to a collection of pus within this organ. (Courtesy of Dr. Gary D. Norsworthy, San Antonio, TX.)**

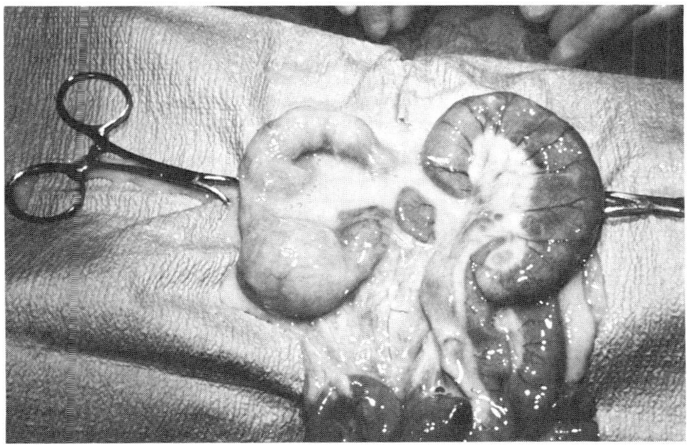

Figure 54–4. During pyometra the uterus may become friable and rupture either before or during surgery. (Courtesy of Dr. Gary D. Norsworthy, San Antonio, TX.)

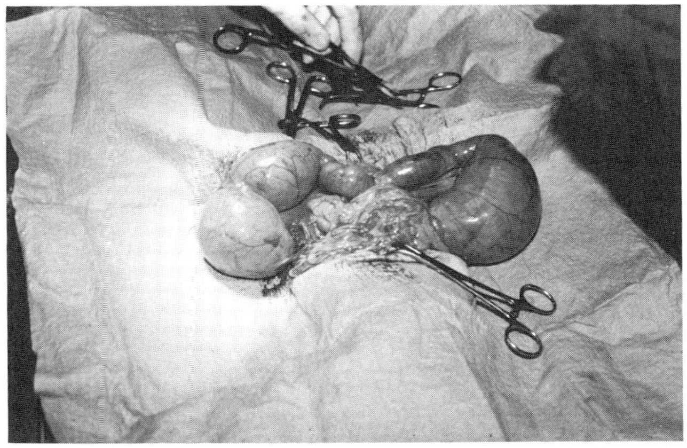

Figure 54–5. Hydrometra is a collection of nonpurulent fluid within the uterus. (Courtesy of Dr. Gary D. Norsworthy, San Antonio, TX.)

which may be very friable and subject to rupture (Fig. 54–4). For queens with breeding potential, medical treatment with PGs is preferred[56-58] Prostaglandin $F_{2\alpha}$ ($PGF_{2\alpha}$) (Lutalyse) at a dosage of 200 μg/kg/day IM for 2 days followed by 500 μg/kg/day for 3 days combined with a broad-spectrum antibiotic is an effective treatment and can restore fertility.[56-58] An increase in vaginal discharge is often noted within 15 minutes to 3 hours after treatment.[57,58] Transient side effects with PG treatment include defecation and vomiting.[57,58] Relative circulatory hypovolemia, as seen in the dog following PG therapy, has not been reported in the cat. The side effects and vaginal discharge usually diminish with each subsequent treatment. Because of the reported success of PG therapy for pyometra, treatment by surgical uterine lavage may only be warranted in cases refractory to PG treatment.

Prevention of pyometra includes strategies to minimize the number of exposures to estrogen dominance. These strategies include inducing ovulation, breeding at estrus to keep the queen pregnant or in pseudopregnancy, manipulating lighting so the queen will remain in anestrus, or preventing estrus pharmacologically.

Other diseases seen during the luteal phase include endometritis and hydrometra. Endometritis may be an early stage in the development of pyometra, since clinical signs may be similar, but the uterine pathology is not as severe. Hydrometra is a collection of nonpurulent fluid in the uterus (Fig. 54–5). These two conditions are treated in the same manner as pyometra.

Fibroadenometous Mammary Hyperplasia

Fibroadenometous mammary hyperplasia is characterized by the enlargement of the mammary glands resulting from the progesterone phase in young queens (pregnancy or pseudopregnancy) and exogenous progestagens in older queens[59] and occasionally in the male cat. The enlarged mammary glands are very firm and may succumb to secondary mastitis or traumatic ulceration. Regression has been reported following pregnancy and lactation.[60] Since this condition is associated with progesterone domination, the treatment of choice, ovariohysterectomy, or cessation of treatment with a progestational drug should eliminate the progesterone source. Surgery during the acute phase is usually not warranted, as the condition normally will subside spontaneously.[60] However, extremely rapid growth of a mammary gland may result in necrosis or infection and necessitate mastectomy. Administration of progestational hormones should be avoided.

Induction of Abortion

$PGF_{2\alpha}$ given at a dosage of 500 μg/kg IM daily for 2 days after Day 40 of gestation can induce abortion within 8 to 48 hours after administration.[61] Whether $PGF_{2\alpha}$ treatment produces abortion of dead kittens or the birth of live, viable kittens is dependent upon the duration of gestation.[61]

Parturition

Normal Parturition

Relaxin is thought to be important in relaxation of the soft tissues around the pelvis. Detectable after 25 days of gestation, relaxin from the fetal-placental unit declines abruptly at parturition.[42,43] Prolactin from the anterior pituitary increases at Day 35 and peaks from about Day 50 of gestation to term.[35] Prolactin is important for mammary development, evident around 24 to 48 hours before parturition, and for subsequent lactation. Estradiol concentrations are variable during pregnancy, but the concentration surges about 9 days before parturition.[62] It is theorized that initiation of parturition in the queen is similar to that documented in the ewe. An initial fetal cortisol rise alters placental progesterone production into estrogen. The estrogen causes a release of prepartum PG. The PG, or the abrupt decline in progesterone, may have a hypothermic effect on the queen, an effect observed as a drop of the rectal temperature of the queen during the first stage of labor.[63] Since the queen can control parturition to some extent, it is important that she be in a secluded, comfortable area for queening. Provision of a queening or nesting box 7 days prepartum will give the queen familiar surroundings for parturition. She may be placed in total isolation, in a prepared queening box, in an area of her choosing, or in the company of a trusted human companion. Parturition may last as long as 24 to 36 hours, but kittens are usually expelled after a mild labor of 30 to 60 minutes and a 5- to 10-minute period of intense labor. After the birth of a single kitten, the queen may not exhibit signs of labor for 0.5 to 2 hours. Usually a placenta is passed after each kitten, or it may be passed after a subsequent kitten. The queen commonly ingests the placenta and then cleans the kittens.

Abnormal Parturition (Dystocia)

Dystocia is not normally a problem in the healthy, physically conditioned queen. It is most commonly associated with the birth of the first kitten. After delivery of the first kitten, parturition usually proceeds normally. Diagnosis of dystocia can be based upon any of the following observations during queening: (1) 20 minutes of intense labor without a kitten being delivered, (2) 10 minutes of intense labor when a kitten is visible in the birth canal, (3) acute depression, (4) elevation of body temperature, or (5) the presence of fresh blood for more than 10 minutes.

When dystocia is diagnosed, it is important to differentiate between a fetal and maternal dystocia in order to proceed with the correct therapeutic measures. Fetal dystocias are caused by oversized or malpositioned fetuses in the uterus or birth canal (Fig. 54–6 *A* to *C*). Maternal dystocias are caused by failure of the queen to pass normal-sized kittens. Maternal dystocias include uterine inertia, small pelvic diameter, uterine torsion, uterine rupture, and ectopic pregnancy (Fig. 54–7). Fetal dystocia can usually be corrected if the kitten can be palpated per vaginum by liberally applying lubricant and allowing the queen to continue with parturition. Cleanliness is essential because introduction of bacteria into the uterus during manipulations can be a major cause of postparturient metritis. If the kitten cannot be palpated per vaginum, it is best to radiograph the queen to determine the kittens' positions and relative sizes. Very small litters tend to have larger, oversized kittens that cause dystocia. In these cases, cesarean section is the preferred method to correct the dystocia, since excessive manipulation or use of instruments harms the kittens and queen.

Maternal dystocias are most commonly caused by uterine inertia. This occurs when the birth process has exhausted the uterine musculature, making contractions impossible or nonrhythmic (secondary uterine inertia). It can also occur when the uterine musculature has insufficient uterotonic stimulation from oxytocin (primary uterine inertia). Uterine inertia can be treated by administration of oxytocin at a dosage of 2 to 4 IU IM every 20 minutes. If two or three injections of oxytocin fail, 1 to 2 mL of 10% calcium gluconate solution should be administered slowly intravenously (IV) followed by oxytocin. Cesarean section should be considered the best option for saving the litter if two doses of the combination of both drugs fail. Determining exactly when a queen is experiencing dystocia may be difficult because the duration of normal parturition may be up to 24 hours. Therefore, a secluded queening area may be the best option for both queen and client. The queen can voluntarily control parturition, so excessive intervention by humans can actually prolong its length or delay its onset.

If the queen has signs of acute depression, elevation of

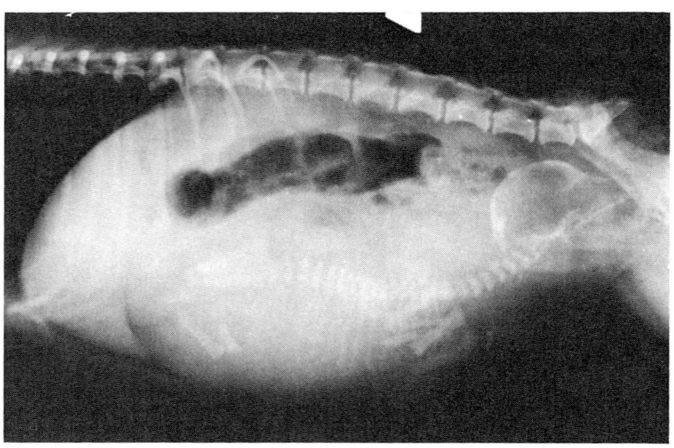

A

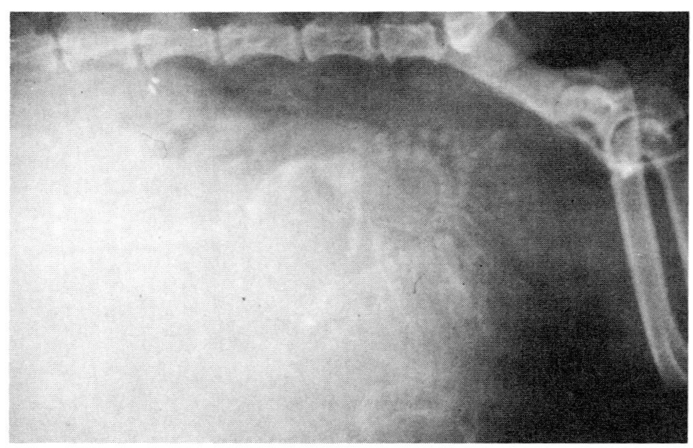

B

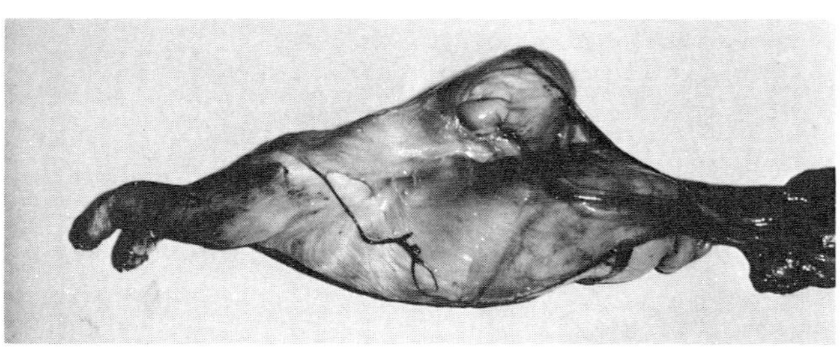

C

Figure 54–6. (*A*) One of the causes of fetal dystocia occurs when the head is too large to pass through the birth canal. (*B*) Fetal dystocia may also be caused by the fetus' head being reflected as shown in this radiograph. (*C*) Dystocia due to fetal head reflection. (Courtesy of Dr. Gary D. Norsworthy, San Antonio, TX.)

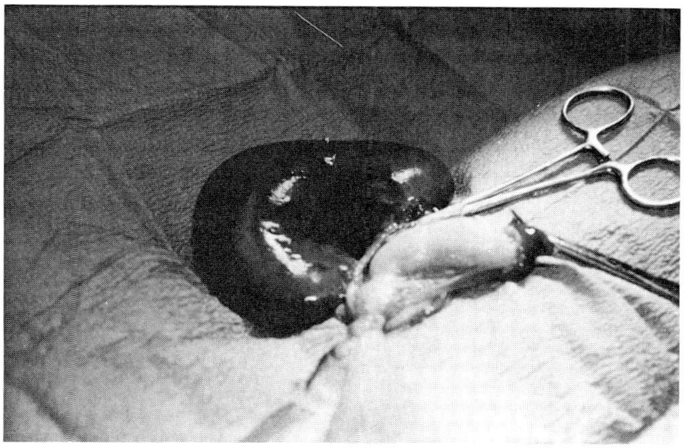

Figure 54–7. **One of the causes of maternal dystocia is rotation of one uterine horn. (Courtesy of Dr. Gary D. Norsworthy, San Antonio, TX.)**

body temperature, or fresh blood coming from the vagina, then uterine torsion, uterine rupture, or ectopic pregnancies should be considered. Although these are uncommon signs, upon seeing them, the dystocia is best handled via laparotomy to maximize the queen's chances for survival.

If a cesarean section is performed, the owner should be given detailed instruction on what to do and signs of impending problems (see Chapter 4).

The Postpartum Period

The Normal Postpartum Period

Involution of the uterus is accompanied by the discharge of lochia from the vulva for up to 3 weeks. Normally, the discharge is nonodorous and red to black. The queen should show no signs of fever, depression, or anorexia if involution is normal. Should the discharge persist more than 3 weeks and/or the queen appear ill, metritis, rupture/torsion of the uterus, or mastitis should be considered possible causes. Kittens should gain weight; they should double their weight in the first 2 weeks.

The owners should be counseled concerning the importance of proper nursing (or bottle feeding) and prevention of chilling (see Chapter 4).

Return to estrus is reported to be inhibited by lactation and results in an anestrus period lasting 2 to 8 weeks postweaning.[64] However, it is not uncommon clinically to find queens 2 to 4 weeks pregnant when performing ovariohysterectomies shortly after a normal weaning. Current data have indicated that recently weaned queens have spontaneously ovulated; therefore, lactation may not inhibit return to estrus.[143] To avoid lactational anestrus, early weaning at 3 days postpartum can hasten the onset of estrus to around 7 days postweaning.[64] Abortion without an ensuing lactation also results in a return to estrus within around 7 days.[64]

Abnormal Events of the Postpartum Period

Retained placentas may not be a problem unless they result in secondary metritis, but secondary metritis is an infrequent sequel to retained placentas.[47] Unless the queen shows signs of metritis, retained placentas need not be a cause for immediate concern.

Postparturient *metritis,* although not common, is seen as early as 1 day to as late as 10 days postpartum. It is most commonly seen in queens experiencing dystocia, but it can occur in any postpartum queen. Queens suffering from this condition generally show depression, pyrexia, anorexia, and a vulvar discharge. The kittens may also become sick secondary to the metritis.

Diagnosis of postparturient metritis is based upon clinical signs, leukocytosis, and cytology of the vaginal discharge. Cytologically, the discharge will have a large number of bacteria (Fig. 54–8). (The normal postpartum vaginal discharge contains red blood cells and degenerating inflammatory cells but very few bacteria.) Therapy should include the administration of supportive fluids and systemic antibiotics based on culture results. PGs have been reported to be effective in successfully treating postparturient metritis.[47] Ovariohysterectomy may be advised for queens with refractory cases.

Uterine prolapse has been described in the postparturient queen.[53,65] Manual reduction under general anesthesia (in conjunction with laparotomy when needed) is generally successful. Ovariohysterectomy is indicated in cases of severe uterine damage. Pregnancy subsequent to treatment of uterine prolapse has been reported.[145]

Mastitis is also seen during the postparturient period.[66,67] The clinical signs include swollen, painful mammary glands that cause the queen to show discomfort when nursing, anorexia, pyrexia, and depression. Kitten mortality from ingestion of septic milk may also be an early indicator of mastitis.[66,67] The most common organisms isolated from mastitis are *Streptococcus* spp., *Staphylococcus* spp. and *E. coli.*[53,66] Treatment should include supportive care of the queen along with the administration of broad-spectrum antibiotics until a specific organism can be isolated. Gangrenous mastitis is best treated with hot packs followed by lancing, debriding, and draining the affected gland(s) if needed[67]; surgical removal may be necessary. If kitten mortality oc-

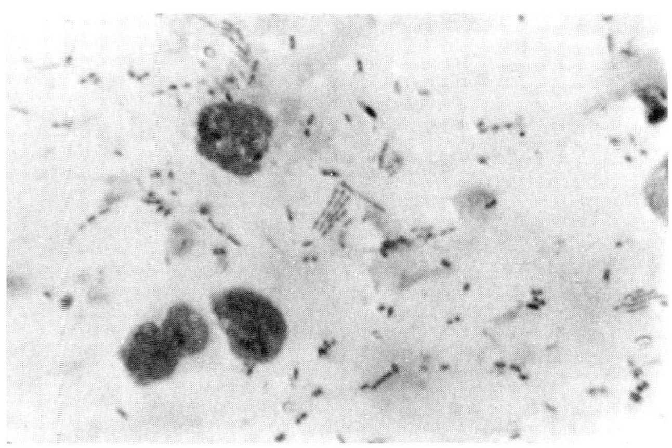

Figure 54–8. **The large number of bacteria in the vaginal discharge indicate the presence of postpartum metritis. Diff-Quik stain, 1000×. (Courtesy of Dr. Gary D. Norsworthy, San Antonio, TX.)**

curs, the remaining kittens should be removed from the queen and raised as orphans or placed on another queen, if feasible.[67]

Fading Kittens

Death of neonatal kittens from birth to 3 days of age is common. One survey[144] found an incidence of 10.2% to be stillborn and another 10.5% dead by Day 2. Death may result from trauma, maternal neglect or inexperience, immaturity, anoxia, or sepsis. Bacterial sepsis is generally a sequel to metritis or mastitis; therefore, the queen of fading kittens should be examined. Since an entire litter may be lost within a few days, prompt therapeutic intervention is essential.

Therapy for neonatal bacterial sepsis is based on antibiotic administration and treating or preventing dehydration, malnutrition, and hypothermia. Kittens should be maintained at environmental temperatures between 85° and 90° F. The use of injectable antibiotics is preferred since the gastrointestinal tract may not permit adequate absorption of orally administered therapeutic agents. Antibiotic choice should be based on culture and sensitivity of infected milk or the vaginal discharge. Initial therapy with gentamicin, enrofloxicin, or potentiated sulfas is recommended at doses based on body weight. Isotonic fluids may be administered subcutaneously to correct dehydration. Orogastric tube feeding (every 2 to 4 hours) with *warm* commercially prepared milk replacers is essential since most of these kittens will continue to receive bacterial exposure if they continue to nurse or remain with their queen. If they are capable of nursing, the use of an adoptive, lactating queen is an alternative.

Male Reproduction

Normal Breeding

Puberty in the male (tom) is reached at approximately nine months or 3.5 kg.[1] Breeding is most likely to occur in the male's home breeding territory during the nocturnal period.[68,69] The copulatory act of the male and queen has been described in detail.[69] Mounting the queen and firmly grasping the neck with his teeth, the male positions himself for insertion of the penis into the vagina. After successful breeding, the queen emits a scream and strikes at the male while he rapidly retreats. During the queen's period of sexual receptivity, the tom may breed the queen eight times in 20 minutes and then repeatedly during a day.[70-72] In natural breeding situations, a tom may breed until he either loses interest or is physically exhausted.[70,71] Multiple matings over a 24-hour period are conducive to fertilization because this enhances the chance that the queen will ovulate.[10,13] Although repeated matings occur over a short time period, only one report shows the effect of multiple semen collections on tomcat semen characteristics.[73] Most published data available on tomcat semen characteristics report only single collections taken daily, every other day, or weekly.[74-76] In the report that collected multiple ejaculates, electroejaculation was used on anesthetized toms to collect four consecutive semen samples at weekly intervals. There were more sperm cells in the second ejaculate than in the first, third, or fourth ejaculates. Electroejaculation, however, has been shown to produce larger volumes of semen with fewer total cells than collections using an artificial vagina.[74] Using current information, it is therefore commonly advised to breed a tom in one of two ways: three times a week (every other day) or once daily for a short time.[68] Multiple breedings each day for 1 to 3 days, however, are preferred for maximum fertility.[75] Despite the preference for multiple matings, no convincing research exists that suggests the effect of continual repeated mating on tomcat semen characteristics. Current information does not reveal whether the multiple matings by the tom are primarily for deposition of more semen, to enhance successful induction of ovulation, or a combination of both.

Breeding Soundness Examination

Collecting an ejaculate from the tom can be performed using an artificial vagina[76,77] or an electroejaculator.[77] An artificial vagina has been described by Sojka and consists of a test tube on a rubber pipettte bulb inserted into the mouth of a small plastic bottle.[76] A daily training period of 2 to 3 weeks is needed before the tom will become accustomed to an artificial vagina.[76,77] Since 30% to 40% of toms cannot be trained to use an artificial vagina, it is not a procedure commonly performed in veterinary practice. A normal ejaculate should contain 21.5 to 117.0 $\times$ 10^6 cells in 0.03 to 0.09 mL.[78] Motility should be approximately 40% to 80%, and 50% to 70% of the cells should be morphologically normal.[78]

An electroejaculator can be used on the anesthetized tom to collect an ejaculate.[78] A special probe and instrumentation are needed to do so. A semen sample collected by this means should have a volume of 0.11 to 0.49 mL and contain 11.1 to 65.9 $\times$ 10^6 cells.[78] Motility should be approximately 50% to 70%, and 40% to 80% of the cells should be morphologically normal.[78]

A more practical method to prove the existence of spermatogenesis is the recovery of sperm cells from the vagina immediately after natural mating. Sperm cells can be collected from the vagina using a cotton swab or flushed out using a pipette and observed under a microscope. An alternative method of proof is to recover sperm cells from the bladder of the tom after mating. Retrograde flow of the tom's ejaculate into the bladder normally occurs when ejaculates are induced by natural mating, an artificial vagina, or an electroejaculator.[79] In one report, 9 to 45 $\times$ 10^6 sperm cells were recovered from the bladder after the tom ejaculated into an artificial vagina. Retrograde flow into the bladder was calculated to be 14% to 90% of the total ejaculate. Clinically, the urine in the bladder collected by cystocentesis immediately after natural mating can be conservatively assumed to contain about 20% of the total number of the cells in the ejaculate. Counting the total number of cells in the bladder postcoitus, and multiplying by five can be used to estimate the total number in the ejaculate.

Artificial Insemination

Artificial insemination (AI) can be performed in the queen using semen collected with an electroejaculator or an artificial vagina. A 3.5 French catheter can be used to inseminate the ejaculate into the queen. Following AI, the queen needs the appropriate stimulus to induce ovulation. Results of artificial insemination have yielded pregnancy rates of 75% using fresh semen[76] and 10% using frozen semen.[74] If the tom has very poor semen or the queen is chronically infertile, surgical insemination via a laparotomy and deposition of the semen directly into the uterine lumen using a needle may improve chances of conception.

Male Infertility

Infertility in the tom can be broken down into three categories: (1) failure to show sexual interest, (2) failure to breed successfully, and (3) failure to impregnate queens after successful breeding. Failure to show sexual interest can arise when the tom is placed in strange surroundings to breed (see Failure to Copulate). Some toms have poor libido, which may be a primary problem of the tom or may result from a queen's dominance in the social order. No hormonal therapy is recommended for toms that show no sexual interest. If testosterone concentrations are normal (1,000 pg/mL), testosterone therapy will not enhance libido and will probably decrease sperm production. Artificial insemination may be considered.

When a tom shows good libido but fails to breed successfully, dental and penile problems should be considered (see Failure to Copulate). The failure to impregnate queens after successful matings that induce ovulation should alert the clinician to the possibility of congenital or acquired azoospermia, which can be detected by performing a breeding soundness examination. Cryptorchid toms should not be used for breeding because of the hereditary potential of the problem.

Reproductive Failure

Although reproductive failure is a rare complaint in the individual cat, it is a common problem in multiple cat households, catteries, and breeding colonies.[80,81] Due to a wide range of factors, varying from social and environmental stress to nutritional and infectious disease, cats can be difficult to propagate under intensive conditions.[82] Reproductive failure, whether it be a problem in an individual cat or a widespread problem of the cattery, is best handled by initially defining at which point in the reproductive cycle the problem lies.

Failure to Exhibit Estrus

Failure of a queen to exhibit estrus must first be differentiated from inadequate estrus detection. The signs of estrus (increased vocalization, rubbing, lordosis, and treading of the hind legs when exposed to a male) should be reviewed with the client to establish that estrus can be detected when it occurs.

Ovarian activity should then be investigated in the queen who genuinely fails to exhibit estrus. It should be verified that general conditions necessary for ovarian activity are met: the cat should be of at least pubertal age, sexually intact, healthy, and exposed to adequate light. Since cats can show pubertal estrus from 4 to 21 months of age, failure to show pubertal estrus by 24 months is necessary to diagnose primary anestrus.[2] Ovarian activity can be most conveniently detected by demonstrating the effects of circulating estrogen on vaginal cytology.[5] Since the follicular phase lasts about a week in the cat,[5] vaginal smears twice a week can detect cyclic changes in vaginal cytology.

If vaginal cytologic changes suggest normal ovarian activity, the inhibition of behavioral estrus may be due to social or psychological factors.[5,83] Inexperienced queens or queens low in a social hierarchy of other females may not exhibit estrus.[53] While some queens show distinct male preferences,[84] others are inhibited in unfamiliar surroundings or in the presence of people.[47,53] To promote behavioral estrus, the queen should be kept at home until she is obviously cycling before introducing her to the male's territory. She should be periodically introduced to the breeding area by herself to familiarize her with the surroundings.[47] If possible, a gentle but experienced male should be used for breeding. If estrus behavior does not appear and the client insists on breeding, artificial insemination can be attempted during cytologic estrus.[76]

Absence of ovarian activity can be detected by an absence of cyclic changes in vaginal cytology.[5] To be convincing, vaginal cytology should be performed twice a week for about 3 months. An alternative, and perhaps more convenient approach, is to test for the presence of functioning ovaries by pharmacologic induction of estrus.[85] A minimum data base should be assembled including a complete medical history and physical examination, complete blood count, serum chemistry, urinalysis, abdominal and thoracic radiographs and feline leukemia virus (FeLV) test.[47] T_4 levels should be assessed if the cat is underweight[47] or overweight.

Normal ovarian activity may be inhibited due to environmental stress, chronic disease, cystic ovarian degeneration, administration of pharmacologic agents, or abnormal gonadal development. Environmental stresses include poor nutrition, overcrowding, temperature, subclinical disease, extensive showing, and traveling.[86] The stress of any chronic infectious, metabolic, or neoplastic condition can disrupt normal ovarian function. Commonly administered steroids, such as progestogens, and glucocorticoids may also inhibit gonadotropin release.[47]

Failure to exhibit pubertal estrus by 2 years of age indicates primary anestrus and premature gonadal failure, discussed in detail in the section on abnormal sexual development.[2] Diagnostic evaluation of the patient suspected of abnormal sexual development should include determination of karyotype, gonadal histology, and gross appearance of the reproductive tract at laparotomy.[2] While XO monosomy will cause premature gonadal failure and primary anestrus, other cases of abnormal phenotypic or genetic sex may be accompanied by normal cyclic activity[87] and even normal fertility.[88,89]

One can attempt to induce fertile estrus in the anestrous queen pharmacologically, as described earlier in this chapter, by housing the anestrus queen with cycling queens[86] or changing light exposure to 8 hours of light (natural or artificial) for 1 week and then increasing to 14 hours of light for several weeks.[47]

Persistent or Prolonged Estrus

Persistent or prolonged estrus (greater than 1 week) may be due to individual variations of cyclic activity[5,53] or hormonally active pathologic conditions of the ovary.[90,91]

Individual variations of cyclic activity in cats include persistent behavioral estrus during an endocrinologically normal estrous cycle,[5] slightly elevated estrogen levels during the interestrous period due to overlapping follicular waves,[5] and estrous behavior during diestrus.[5] The above conditions are characterized by a cyclic and seasonal pattern to the periods of estrus.[53] In the first two cases, ovulation might bring the cat into diestrus and eliminate estrous behavior. This could be attempted by repeated vaginal and cervical stimulation during the estrous period or by pharmacologic induction of ovulation as described above.

Estrus that is prolonged or persistent but not seasonal is commonly due to cystic ovarian follicles (Fig. 54–9)[40,49,53] or, rarely, due to neoplasia of the ovary.[90,91] Cystic ovarian follicles are commonly found at routine ovariohysterectomy and tend to occur in older, nulliparous queens, many of which have concurrent cystic endometrial hyperplasia.[40] Queens with cystic ovarian follicles may exhibit signs of hyperestrogenism, such as persistent estrous behavior, nymphomania, and aggression to the point of becoming unsuitable as pets.[92] The treatment of choice is ovariohysterectomy.[49] In those queens required for breeding purposes, prognosis for fertility is low.[92] Medical rupture of the follicles can be attempted using 250 IU of HCG IM once daily for 2 days,[47] although its efficacy is controversial.[92] Alternatively, laparotomy and manual rupture of the cystic follicles may be attempted.[49] On the subsequent estrus after either treatment, the queen should be bred to an aggressive tom to prevent recurrence of the problem.[49] Not all cystic structures of the ovary are follicular cysts, however. Cysts of the rete ovarii may be found at routine ovariohysterectomy without any particular clinical signs observed prior to surgery.[93] The clinical and functional significance of these cysts is not yet known. Parovarian cysts may also be incidental findings in the mesovarium at routine ovariohysterectomy.[90]

Tumors of the feline ovaries occur rarely, and are unlikely causes of persistent estrus in cats.[49] However, granulosa cell tumors are frequently accompanied by signs of hyperestrogenism and account for half of all feline ovarian tumors.[90,91] A Sertoli-Leydig–like tumor has been associated with what appeared to be estrogen-induced endometrial hyperplasia in a cat.[94] Estrus-like behavior was reported in a Siamese cat with a dysgerminoma,[95] although this tumor is otherwise considered to have minimal endocrine activity.[90] Malignancy is reported in both granulosa cell tumors[91] and a proportion (16%) of dysgerminomas,[95,96] metastasis being to other abdominal viscera. Ovariohysterectomy should be considered in intact females that show persistent, nonseasonal estrus. Such females are predisposed to cystic endometrial hyperplasia and pyometra due to the prolonged effect of estrogen on the endometrium.[97]

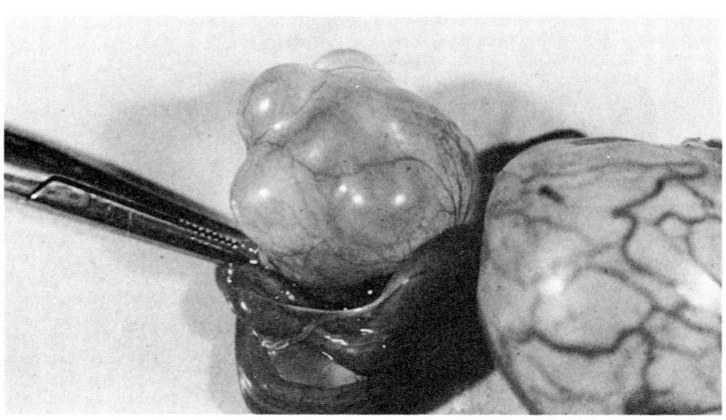

Figure 54–9. **Cystic ovaries. (Courtesy of Dr. Gary D. Norsworthy, San Antonio, TX.)**

Failure to Copulate

When the estrous female is introduced to the male for breeding, copulation may not occur or it may be unsuccessful. Either may occur due to behavioral or physical abnormalities.[47,98]

Behavioral failure of copulation may result primarily from an inappropriate social setting. Breeding should take place in territory where the male is dominant, and at night because cats are nocturnal breeders. Copulation may fail when a shy male is introduced to a dominant female, or if the pair are members of the same household where the female has a higher social position. Additionally, an experienced male may be required to achieve coitus in an inexperienced female and vice versa. Finally, the female needs to exhibit adequate behavioral estrus. The queen in proestrus usually does not accept the male, and receptive behavior during estrus may by suppressed owing to shyness, social stress, or male preferences.

Physical incompatibility or abnormalities in both the male and female can prevent successful coitus. Male difficulties may include dental problems that prevent the male from establishing an adequate grip on the female, hair rings around the penis, or penile injury or abnormality preventing extension and intromission. Body size differences between male and female may also prevent normal intromission.[98] The female with stricture, aplasia, inflammation, infection, or neoplasia of the vagina or vestibule may not allow breeding. A limited vaginal speculum examination can be achieved under sedation using an otoscope with a sterile cone and may allow detection of mechanical obstructions.[40] High numbers of neutrophils in the vaginal smear can indicate a vaginitis, but the possibility of purulent endometritis or pyometra should not be ignored. Owing to the likelihood of contamination, positive vaginal cultures by themselves do not indicate vaginitis, but must be interpreted in conjunction with cytology and otoscopic examination to confirm inflammation.

Repeated Breeding: Ovulation Failure

A queen that continues to show heat every 2 to 3 weeks despite repeated breeding is probably failing to ovulate. This can be diagnosed by progesterone levels less than 2 ng/mL from Day 7 postestrus to Day 40.[43,47] Ovulation can fail if coital stimulation is inadequate or mistimed or if a primary dysfunction of the neuroendocrine reflex exists. Infectious infertility is unlikely to be a cause of repeated breeding in the cat, because of its unique estrous cycle with the requirement for induced ovulation.

Inadequate coital stimulation may result from unsuccessful or too-few attempts. Unsuccessful coitus (absence of both a copulatory cry and postcoital reaction), if documented should be analyzed as a failure to copulate. Too-few mountings may also result in a failure of the LH spike necessary for ovulation. Ideally, the female is left with the male for at least three or four breedings and is bred on more than 1 day during estrus. Only one mount may be necessary if the follicles are mature.[53]

If coitus occurs too early in estrus, the follicles are not yet mature; if too late, the follicles may have undergone regression. Before Day 2 of estrus, breeding may fail to result in ovulation. Optimal response to vaginal stimulation usually occurs on Day 3 of estrus and shortly thereafter.[53]

Failure of the neuroendocrine reflex is most likely associated with cystic follicles. Treatment may be 250 IU HCG IM daily for 2 days[47] at the time the queen is bred; however, its success is controversial.[49] Additionally, any number of neurologic, endocrine, or developmental abnormalities could lead to a failure of the neuroendocrine reflex.

A cat with spinal neurologic disease might have difficulty transmitting sensory information to the hypothalamus. Neuroendocrine disease may prevent GnRH or LH release. Gonadal abnormalities may prevent ovulation. An apparently normal queen that showed cyclic estrous behavior, but upon ovariohysterectomy revealed enlarged gonads with testicular morphology,[87] would not have been expected to undergo normal ovulation postcoitus. To improve current diagnosis and therapy, ovulation failure in the cat needs further research.

Nonpregnancy or Loss of an Undetected Pregnancy

When examination reveals a cat not to be pregnant, a minimum data base should be performed to determine if she is healthy, if appropriate breeding practices were followed using a fertile male, if she ovulated after breeding, and if primary reproductive disease is present. Possible causes of infertility in the queen who ovulates when bred to a fertile male are failure of sperm to reach the egg, failure of fertilization, and undetected death of the developing embryo.

The minimum data base for the queen who is nonpregnant at pregnancy examination should include history, physical, serum progesterone, abdominal radiographs, complete blood count, chemistry panel, urinalysis, FeLV antigen test, and depending on the presence of a vaginal discharge, vaginal cytology, culture, and vaginoscopy. T_4 levels should be run if the cat is thin[47] or obese. The clinician should attempt to detect abnormalities in the queen's cycling behavior that may indicate a failure to exhibit normal estrus (frequency and duration of estrous periods) or a failure to ovulate (success, number and timing of copulations, repeated breeding every 2 to 3 weeks). Inquiries should be made into the general hygiene, nutrition, and environment in the cattery. Problems with the male should be ruled out either by confirming recent siring of litters or by results of recent semen evaluations. The physical examination should include determination of the presence of a vaginal discharge, abdominal palpation to detect uterine or ovarian enlargement, and an ophthalmic examination to detect retinal degeneration due to taurine deficiency.[50,51] Routine blood work and urinalysis are performed to detect any chronic underlying disease that may prevent normal cycling or predispose to reproductive failure. A progesterone level greater than 2 ng/mL before Day 40 of gestation indicates that ovulation has occurred. A uterus visible on abdominal radiograph suggests abnormal uterine enlargement and requires further investigation (see below). Vaginal cytology, culture, and vaginoscopy help determine the nature and source (uterus or vagina) of a vaginal discharge.

Failure of sperm to reach the egg may be due to blockage of the cervix, uterus, or oviducts. Assessing the patency of these structures can be attempted at laparotomy by infusing sterile saline into the uterine horn using a small-gauge needle[47] and milking fluid through the oviducts, both horns, or retrograde through the cervix. Owing to the risk of peritonitis, this procedure is contraindicated if the uterus appears infected or if free fluid is detected in the uterine lumen before infusion. Since semen traverses the oviduct during estrus, this is the appropriate time to perform the procedure.

Failure of fertilization is not yet commonly evaluated in practice. However, new developments in feline oocyte collection, in vitro fertilization, and embryo transfer suggest that oocyte evaluation may soon be possible, perhaps in the clinical setting. It is now possible to obtain oocytes by laparoscopic aspiration of follicles for in vitro fertilization studies.[36] Fertilized embryos and unfertilized oocytes have been obtained 7 days after the first breeding from the uterine lumen by placing a flanged tomcat catheter in the caudal terminus of the uterine lumen, 2 to 3 cm cranial to the uterine bifurcation, and flushing 25 to 30 mL of culture media in a cranial-to-caudal direction through a 17-gauge catheter placed near the uterotubular junction.[99] The fluid is collected into gridded petri dishes and searched with a stereomicroscope. If fertilized embryos can be collected from the queen that consistently fails to become pregnant, one can establish that the entire reproductive tract is patent, that fertilization took place, and that infertility is likely due to loss of the undetected pregnancy.

Likely causes of undetected pregnancy loss include cystic endometrial hyperplasia and endometritis (see also Confirmed Pregnancy Loss). Cystic endometrial hyperplasia and endometritis are presumptively diagnosed by detecting a radiographically visible uterus. Definitive diagnosis requires exploratory surgery accompanied by uterine biopsy and culture of the uterine lumen. Cystic endometrial hyperplasia is thought to result from prolonged exposure to estrogen in an aged, nonpregnant queen or in one that develops cystic follicles. The treatment of choice is ovariohysterectomy. Endometritis can result from cystic endometrial hyperplasia aggravated by bacterial contamination, persistence of mummified or incompletely resorbed fetuses, retained fetal membranes, or postpartum metritis following a previous pregnancy. If culture of the endometritic uterus is successful, one can institute specific antibiotic therapy. Vaginal cultures are of value if the endometritis is of sufficient magnitude to cause a vaginal discharge and if surgical culture is not an option. PG therapy[56,100] at a dose of 0.2 mg/kg

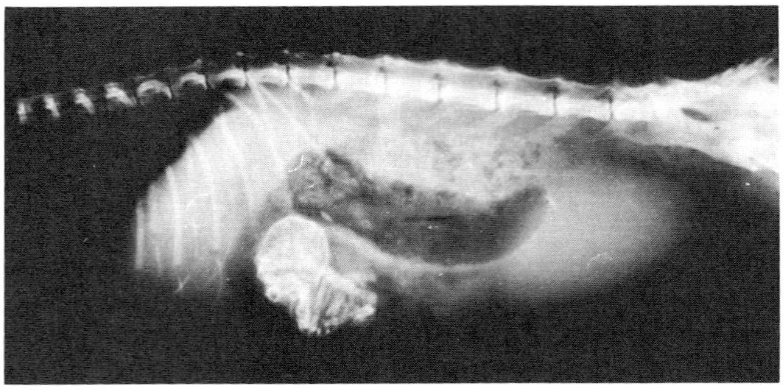

A

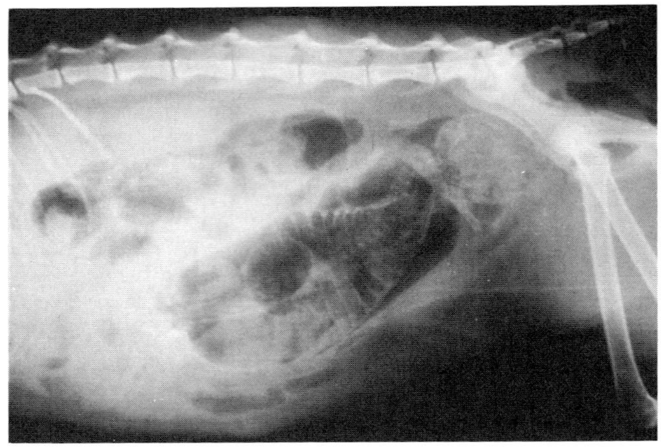

B

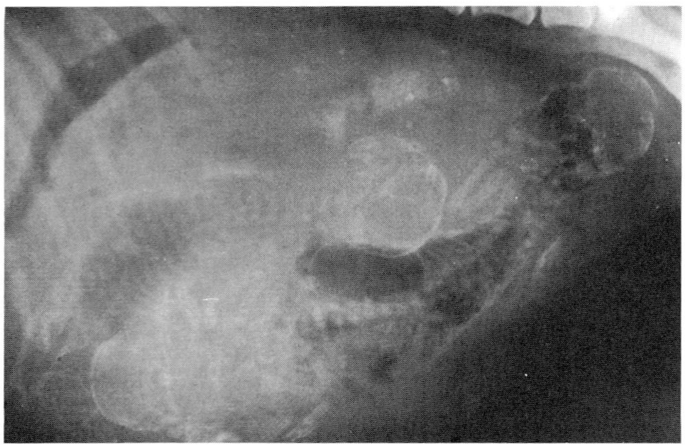

C

Figure 54–10. (*A*) A mummified fetus can be seen in this radiograph. (*B*) The large amount of gas around this fetus indicates fetal degeneration and death. (*C*) Fetal death can also be diagnosed by finding destruction (collapsing) of the calvarium as in the fetus on the right. (Courtesy of Dr. Gary D. Norsworthy, San Antonio, TX.)

subcutaneously once daily for 2 days followed by 0.5 mg/kg for 3 days, in conjunction with broad-spectrum antibiotics, has been successful in treating pyometra (see Pyometra) with good subsequent fertility. A similar protocol may be appropriate in cases of presumptively or definitively diagnosed endometritis in the cat. PGs have been used successfully to treat endometritis in the dog.[100] If abdominal radiography suggests that fetal remnants are present in the uterus, surgical removal of fetal remains may be necessary.

Confirmed Pregnancy Loss

Viable fetuses that die may be resorbed, mummify, or degenerate and abort (Fig. 54–10 *A* to *C*). When a confirmed pregnancy is lost, either by observed abortion or failure to queen, a minimum data base should include clinical evaluation of the queen and postmortem examination of fetus and placenta, if available. Likely causes for loss of a detected pregnancy include systemic viral or bacterial disease, ascending bacterial infection, nutritional deficiency, exposure to fetotoxic or abortogenic agents, hypoluteoidism, and lethal genetic defects.

Clinical evaluation of the queen should include a history to detect signs of concurrent illness, particularly upper respiratory disease. Physical examination should include abdominal palpation and fundoscopic examination of the retina. Abdominal radiography should be performed to detect retained fetuses, ectopic pregnancies, or evidence of uterine rupture. A CBC, chemistry panel, urinalysis, and FeLV antigen test (ELISA) should be performed. Acute serum, to be paired with convalescent serum 2 weeks later, should be submitted. Paired serology is of uncertain value in the face of an abortion because of the variable time delay between infection and abortion. However, if the cat aborts during an acute viral infection, paired serum samples may be able to detect a diagnostic rise in antibody titer. Feline panleukopenia virus and feline herpesvirus are two organisms that may show meaningful rises in titers. If the queen is showing signs of upper respiratory infection, ocular, nasal, and oropharyngeal swabs should be submitted for viral, chlamydial, and mycoplasmal isolation, and impression smears of the conjunctiva should be submitted for detection of *Chlamydia* (see Chapter 35 for illustration). The chilled fetuses and frozen and formalin-fixed samples of placenta should also be submitted, if available. The receiving diagnostic laboratory should be contacted for preferred methods of collecting and transporting specimens.

Systemic Infectious Agents

Systemic infectious agents that are considered potential causative agents of abortion include FeLV, feline panleukopenia virus (FPV), feline infectious peritonitis (FIP) virus, feline herpesvirus (FHV), *Chlamydia, Mycoplasma, Ureaplasma,* and *Toxoplasma.*

The effect of FeLV on reproduction depends upon whether the queen is viremic. In viremic queens (positive ELISA or indirect fluorescent antibody [IFA]), FeLV appears to cause pregnancy loss. In a report describing 10 IFA-positive cats, four underwent unsuccessful breeding, two became pregnant but resorbed the fetus, three aborted, and one developed purulent endometritis with several degenerating fetuses.[101] A pregnant cat with lymphosarcoma was also reported to resorb fetuses at 5 weeks of gestation.[101] Another author has reported a pattern of fetal resorption in FeLV-infected queens[102] and the virus has been isolated from litters of unborn fetuses, newborn kittens, and the uterus of viremic, pregnant queens.[103] While it appears that pregnancy loss is due to direct fetal infection, it is also suggested that the virus disrupts the endometrium at the sites of placental attachment.[102,104] However, further study is necessary to accurately define the occurrence and pathogenesis of abortion in FeLV-infected queens.

Nonviremic queens (ELISA- or IFA-negative), which have overcome the initial infection but are latently infected in the bone marrow, can reproduce normally and do not appear to have a significantly increased risk of pregnancy loss.[105] However, the virus may be passed to the occasional kitten, who may then infect the litter mates. In a study of six latently infected queens (identified by reactivation of the virus from bone marrow aspirates), none experienced any reproductive problems over multiple pregnancies,[105] nor did they revert to viremia during pregnancy or lactation. One of 30 kittens studied was viremic at 2 weeks of age, and nonviremic litter mates subsequently developed viremia at 10 weeks postpartum. Possible routes of infection in the viremic kitten may have been transplacental or via ingestion of milk. Latent infection was not detected in any kittens born to these latently infected queens. Evidence of milk-borne transmission was presented in another study[106] in which transmission of virus from a supposedly latently infected queen to a suckling kitten occurred, and the milk cultured positive for the virus. This queen was periodically viremic, however. Although direct infection of fetuses with FeLV has been achieved in latently infected queens,[107] the queens were reinoculated with live virus intraperitoneally during gestation. Consequently, this particular model of fetal infection does not apply to the latently infected queen.

Control of FeLV in the cattery is achieved by removing all ELISA-positive cats from the cattery, and retesting all negative cats in 90 days.[108] Cats that test positive then subsequently negative should also be eliminated because many of these will be latently infected and may become viremic at a later date (see Chapter 39).

FPV is a hardy parvovirus with a predilection for mitotic tissue. It has been shown to cause in utero infection, leading to cerebellar hypoplasia and ataxia in kittens. The cerebellar external granule cell layer is highly mitotic in the perinatal period, and ataxia is manifested when the infected kittens first become mobile.[111,112] However, earlier in gestation, tissues located in the kidney and gut are mitotically active and serve as sites of viral replication.[112] Consequently, although neonatal ataxia indicates in utero infection late in gestation, infection earlier in gestation can lead to abortion or fetal resorption. Similar mitogenic viruses have been shown to cause abortion and fetal resorption in rats.[113] Although dams infected during gestation seroconvert, they usually do not show clinical signs.[114] Diagnosis of fetal infection due to FPV may be confirmed by isolation of virus from fetuses or neonates submitted to necropsy, by documenting a seroconversion in the dam, or, clinically, by characteristic ataxia observed in the neonates. However, it should be noted that cerebellar dysfunction can also occur in kittens born to queens fed taurine deficient diets.[50] Vaccination of queens against FPV prior to breeding is recommended.[108]

FIP, once believed to be a major cause of pregnancy loss and kitten mortality in catteries,[80,81] is currently an unproven cause of abortion. FIP does cause fatal neonatal infection, however. The initial association of FIP with poor reproductive performance came from observations of high coronavirus titers in catteries with reproductive problems.[80] With the discovery of the widespread nature of feline enteric coronavirus,[115] which cross-reacts with FIP in serologic tests,[116,117] and similar reproductive problems occurring in specific pathogen-free (SPF) catteries free of coronavirus,[118] the role of FIP as a cause of pregnancy loss has become unclear.[117] It is established, however, that FIP causes disease in the neonate, and that kittens born to infected mothers are at particular risk.[119-122] While milk born transmission is a possibility,[122] transplacental transmission cannot be ruled out. Lesions that could only have been caused in utero have been attributed to a feline coronavirus,[123] and the possibility of dual infection of FIP and FPV has been suggested.[123,124] Since FeLV is a major potentiator of FIP, control of FIP is augmented by elimination of FeLV-infected animals from the cattery. A recently licensed vaccine for FIP is now commercially available in the United States (Primucell FIP). In clinical trials using a highly virulent challenging strain of FIP, 100% of nonvaccinated controls became ill, 83% of which died. Among the vaccinated animals, 85% survived the challenge and exhibited substantially reduced clinical signs compared with the surviving nonvaccinates.[125] However, information concerning safety and efficacy in large trials is not yet available. The vaccine is composed of a temperature-sensitive mutant virus, which grows at 31°C but is inhibited at 37°C. When administered intranasally, the virus replicates in the respiratory tract at the reduced temperature and provides protective cell-mediated and local immunity. Temperature sensitivity prevents systemic spread. Because it is a modified live preparation, its use in pregnant queens is contraindicated. Because vaccinates may experience seroconversion, testing of kittens should occur prior to vaccination. A serologic test by which FIP latently infected animals can be removed from the cattery does not currently exist.[117]

FHV appears to cause abortion because of the debilitating effect of upper respiratory infections in queens. The virus frequently infects kittens in the neonatal period. In utero transmission has not been shown to occur except under certain experimental conditions. In one study,[126] pregnant queens infected intranasally aborted following severe upper respiratory disease. However, no virus was isolated from the uterus, fetus or placenta, nor were any histologic lesions seen. When pregnant cats were infected intravenously,[126] abortions occurred after the queens showed minimal signs of illness. Virus was isolated from uterus and placenta of these queens, and both organs showed histologic lesions. This intravenous inoculation of the virus probably does not represent a true clinical picture of an upper respiratory pathogen. Because approximately 80% of cats infected with the virus become latently infected and shed virus during periods of stress,[127,128] the neonatal kitten is susceptible to infection from the queen who sheds virus during lactation. Although shedders can be detected by isolation of the virus from cats treated with corticosteroids,[129] control of the disease focuses on protecting the neonatal kitten[108] by ensuring adequate colostral protection, preventing exposure to shedding cats, and vaccinating as maternal antibody wanes at 6 to 12 weeks.[108] Chronic FHV infections are one of the most common and most difficult problems faced by cat breeders. (See Chapter 63 for vaccination strategies in catteries.)

Chlamydia psittaci, a causative agent of upper respiratory infection and feline pneumonitis, has been implicated as a cause of reproductive failure and in utero infection. Two queens from a cattery in England had kittens that experienced upper respiratory infection due to *Chlamydia.* Both queens had experienced problems with abortions and failure to conceive. One treated with tetracycline subsequently had two healthy litters.[130] Another report describes a fatal pneumonitis in a litter of kittens infected from birth; the survivors were afflicted with mucopurulent ocular discharge. *Chlamydia psittaci* was isolated from the lung of a dead kitten. Abortions were also reported in this cattery.[125] Diagnosis of chlamydial infection may be made by demonstration of organisms in conjunctival scrapings[131] or by culture of ocular or nasal swabs. *Mycoplasma* and *Ureaplasma* have also been suggested to be causative agents of abortion among cats.[132] Diagnosis is also made by isolation of the organisms from ocular or nasal swabs. Tetracycline is the treatment of choice for *Mycoplasma, Ureaplasma,* and *Chlamydia* and may be warranted when outbreaks occur among nonpregnant animals housed with pregnant queens.[130] The drug should not be administered to pregnant animals, however, since it causes bone and teeth malformation in the developing fetus.[133] Further research is necessary to elucidate the role of these intracellular bacteria in feline abortion and infertility.

Protozoal infections are unlikely causes of reproductive failure. Attempts to transmit *Toxoplasma gondii* from pregnant queens to their fetuses have not been successful.[134] However, one case of neonatal infection characterized by pneumonitis, myocarditis, encephalitis, and retinitis in a 2-week-old kitten is thought to have originated in utero since encysted organisms were found that would have normally taken 4 weeks to develop.[135] Ascending bacterial agents that may cause abortion include coliforms, *Staphylococcus* sp., *Streptococcus* sp., *Salmonella* sp., and *Mycobacteria.*[136] It is felt that bacteria rarely cause abortion unless nonhygienic conditions prevail in the cattery.[136] Bacteria are thought to migrate from the heavily contaminated vagina into the uterus where infection leads to fetal infection and death. Bacterial contamination commonly occurs at parturition, but abortion is more likely to result from contamination at breeding.[136] The cat aborting because of bacterial infection may show signs of systemic illness including fever, malaise, anorexia, abdominal straining, and vaginal discharge.[136] Recommended treatment includes appropriate supportive and antibiotic therapy for 2 to 3 weeks after the abortion. In addition, uterine evacuation can be attempted using PG $F_{2\alpha}$.[47,56,136]

Miscellaneous Causes

Nutritional deficiency should be considered as a possible cause of pregnancy loss if the queen is not fed a commercial, balanced diet. This situation often occurs in catteries. Special attention should be paid to vitamin A and taurine. Vitamin A found in high levels in raw liver, has been associated with reproductive failures such as anestrus, failure to conceive, early embryonic death, abortion, and congenital defects.[49] Queens fed a taurine deficient diet can appear clinically normal yet suffer from reproductive failure. Of 18 queens fed a taurine-deficient diet, only six carried pregnancy to full term.[51] Clinical findings included abortions, early embryonic death, and malformations in the neonates. Mothers were clinically normal except for retinal degeneration detected by fundoscopic examination.[51] Interestingly, affected neonates suffered from cerebellar dysfunction due to a persistence of mitotic activity in the external granule cell layer of the cerebellum. While the histopathologic lesions were thus different from those seen with FPV infection, the clinical signs were similarly indicative of cerebellar dysfunction.[50] The kittens tended to be paretic in the hind legs, which frequently splay outward.

Hypoluteoidism, failure of the corpus luteum or placenta to secrete sufficient progesterone to maintain pregnancy, has not been definitively documented as a cause of pregnancy loss in the cat, although it is suspected in cats that habitually abort around Day 50 to 58 of pregnancy.[47,53,98] The suggested treatment is to administer injections of progesterone in oil to cats at a dose of 1 to 2 mg/kg weekly beginning 1 week prior to the anticipated abortion date, and to discontinue treatment 1 week prior to parturition.[53,98] There is concern that administration of sex steroids during pregnancy can lead to gonadal dysgenesis of the fetus in utero.[137]

Fetal injury due to administration of fetotoxic drugs during pregnancy should also be considered as a potential source of fetal death. The specific drugs below are known to cause fetal injury and should not be administered during pregnancy[133]: antibiotics (quinolones and tetracyclines), antifungals (griseofulvin), anti-inflammatories (dimethyl sulfoxide), anesthetics (pentobarbital), gastrointestinal drugs (misoprostol), anticonvulsants (phenytoin), steroids (testosterone and estrogen analogs), vitamin A analogs (isotretinoin), and mitotane (o,p′-DDD). Organophosphate insecticides, anticancer drugs, corticosteroids, and vaccination with modified live vaccines (e.g., FPL vaccine) should be avoided in pregnant queens. Care should be taken to avoid excessive levels of vitamin A during pregnancy (e.g., from feeding raw liver), since this can be embryotoxic.[49]

Genetic defects tend to occur when close inbreeding takes place. While cats may have many genetic abnormalities, the Manx syndrome is of interest. Breeders of Manx cats find that genetic fetal defects associated with incomplete formation of the spinal cord and fetal death occur in some litters.[138] Some cats are born with a tendency to acquire megacolon or urinary incontinence due to incomplete innervation of the pelvic viscera.[139] Analysis of aborted fetuses or stillborns for genetic defects such as spina bifida or sacral dysgenesis should be considered when one or both parents are of Manx breeding.

Abnormal Sexual Development

Failure of normal development of the gonads is termed premature gonadal failure. A common clinical sign is absence of pubertal estrus by 2 years of age.[2] Diagnostic evaluation of the patient suspected of abnormal gonadal development should include determination of karyotype, levels of plasma LH and FSH, gonadal histology, and gross appearance of the reproductive tract at laparotomy.[2] In the cat, the XO chromosomal abnormality, while uncommon, causes gonadal dysgenesis.[2,140,141] Clinical signs reported include decreased size as compared with litter mates and lack of pubertal estrus by 2.5 years of age; otherwise, the cats are of outwardly normal appearance.[140] The reproductive tract is apparently normal early in life[141] but undergoes ovarian atresia as the animal matures.[2,140] The XO condition can be predicted in some situations if one knows the coat color of the parents. The alleles for orange and black are carried on the X chromosome. Females born to a black female (homozygous for the black allele) by a ginger tom (single orange allele on the single X chromosome) should carry a black gene from the mother and an orange gene from the father. Such a female kitten would be tortoiseshell (heterozygous for orange and black). If black, however, she would probably have failed to receive the X chromosome with an orange gene from the father, and would carry only the X chromosome with its black gene from the mother, making her XO.[141] Similar reasoning is used to predict the likelihood of Klinefelter's syndrome (XXY) and hence sterility in tortoiseshell toms.[89,142]

The presence of abnormal sexual development, however, does not rule out the possibility of cyclic estrous behavior or even normal pregnancy. At routine ovariohysterectomy of an outwardly normal female with normal cyclic behavior, abdominal testes have been reported in the place of ovaries.[87] This male pseudohermaphrodite (male because she had testes, pseudohermaphrodite because gonads of only one sex were present) had essentially normal external genitalia, except that the vulva was slightly smaller than usual, and the clitoris was somewhat enlarged. Normal pregnancies have been reported in two cats with unilateral ovarian dysgenesis, also detected at routine ovariohysterectomy. Both cats exhibited sex chromosome mosaicism in cultured lymphocytes, one X/XXY, the other X/XX, and both cats were pregnant with fetuses of normal gonadal development and genetic sex, occupying both horns of the uterus. While each had a small nodule in place of one ovary, the contralateral ovary was normal. A condition equivalent to Klinefelter's syndrome (XXY) has been described in male blue cream burmese, tortoiseshell, and calico cats.[89,142] Such cats can be recognized as unusual since a normal male (XY) has only one X chromosome. Blue cream, tortoiseshell, and calico indicate heterozygosity (two X chromosomes) at the sex-linked locus for coat color, indicating the XXY genotype in males or a mosaic consisting of two cell populations with different X chromosomes. XXY males have slower-than-average development of external genitalia and libido, but are still within the normal range. No pregnancies have been reported, however, after apparently normal matings using strictly XXY males,[142] although mosaics and chimeras at this locus (e.g., XY/XXY, XX/XY) have been reported to be fertile,[89] as have X chromosome mosaic females.[88]

REFERENCES

1. Jemmett JE, Evans JM. A survey of sexual behavior and reproduction of female cats. J Sm Anim Pract 1977;18:31.
2. Johnston SD. Premature gonadal failure in female dogs and cats. J Reprod Fert 1989;Suppl 39:65.
3. Verhage HG, Beamer NB, Brenner RM. Plasma levels of estradiol and progesterone in the cat during polyestrus, pregnancy and pseudopregnancy. Biol Reprod 1976;14:579.
4. Leyva H, Madley T, Stabenfeldt GH. Effect of light manipulation on ovarian activity and melatonin and prolactin secretion in the domestic cat. J Reprod Fert 1989;Suppl 39:125.
5. Shille VM, Lundstrom KE, Stabenfeldt GH. Follicular function in the domestic cat as determined by estradiol-17B concentrations in plasma: Relation to estrous behavior and cornification of exfoliated epithelium. Biol Reprod 1979;21:953.
6. Paape SR, Shille VM, Seto H, Stabenfeldt GH. Luteal activity in the pseudopregnant cat. Biol Reprod 1975;13:470.
7. Goodrowe KL, Howard JG, Schmidt PM, Wildt DE. Reproductive biology of the domestic cat with special reference to endocrinology, sperm function and *in-vitro* fertilization. J Reprod Fert 1989;Suppl 39:73.
8. Wildt DE, Chan SYW, Seager SWJ, Chakraborty PK. Ovarian activity, circulating hormones, and sexual behavior in the cat. 1. Relationships during the coitus-induced luteal phase and the estrous period without mating. Biol Reprod 1981;25:15.
9. Herron MA. Feline vaginal cytologic examination. Fel Pract 1977;7:36.
10. Concannon P, Hodgson B, Lein D. Reflex LH release in estrous cats following single and multiple copulations. Biol Reprod 1980;23:111.
11. Banks DH, Stabenfeldt G. Luteinizing hormone release in the cat in response to coitus on consecutive days of estrus. Biol Reprod 1982;26:603.
12. Wildt DE, Seager SWJ, Chakraborty PK. Effect of copulatory stimuli on incidence of ovulation and on serum luteinizing hormone in the cat. Endocrinology 1980;107:1212.
13. Johnson LM, Gay VL. Luteinizing hormone in the cat. II. Mating-induced secretion. Endocrinology 1981;109:247.
14. Shille VM, Munro C, Farmer SW, et al. Ovarian and endocrine responses in the cat after coitus. J Reprod Fert 1983;69:29.
15. Concannon P, Lein D, Hodgson B. Sexual behavior and self-limiting reflex LH release during extended periods of ad libitum copulatory activity in domestic cats. J Anim Sci 1982;55 (Suppl 1):344.
16. Chakraborty PK, Wildt DE, Seager SWJ. Serum luteinizing hormone and ovulatory response to luteinizing hormone-releasing hormone in the estrous and anestrous domestic cat. Lab Anim Sci 1979;29:338.
17. Wildt DE, Seager SWJ. Ovarian response in the estrual cat receiving varying dosages of HCG. Horm Res 1978;9:144.
18. Goodrowe KL, Wildt DE. Ovarian response to human chorionic gonadotropin or gonadotropin releasing hormone in cats in natural or induced estrus. Theriogenology 1987;27:811.
19. Herron MA, Sis RF. Ovum transport in the cat and the effect of estrogen administration. Am J Vet Res 1974;35:1277.

20. Concannon PW, Meyers-Wallen VN. Current and proposed methods for contraception and termination of pregnancy in dogs and cats. J Am Vet Med Assoc 1991;198:1214.
21. Wildt DE, Panko WB, Seager SWJ. Effect of prostaglandin $F_{2\alpha}$ on endocrine-ovarian function in the domestic cat. Prostaglandins 1979;18:883.
22. Wildt DE, Kinney GM, Seager SWJ. Gonadotropin induced reproductive cyclicity in the domestic cat. Lab Anim Sci 1978; 28:301.
23. Cline EM, Jennings LL, Sojka NJ. Breeding laboratory cats during artificially induced estrus. Lab Anim Sci 1980;30:1003.
24. Colby ED. Induced estrus and timed pregnancies in cats. Lab Anim Care 1970;20:1075.
25. Wildt DE, Kinney GM, Seager SWJ. Reproduction control in the dog and cat: An examination and evaluation of current and proposed methods. J Am Anim Hosp Assoc 1977;13:223.
26. Burke TJ. Pharmacologic control of estrus in the bitch and queen. Vet Clin N Am, Sm Anim Pract 1982;12:79.
27. Houdeshell JW, Hennessey PW. Megestrol acetate for control of estrus in the cat. Vet Med Sm Anim Clin 1977;72:1013.
28. Middleton DJ, Watson ADJ, Howe CJ, Caterson ID. Suppression of cortisol responses to exogenous adrenocorticotrophic hormone, and the occurrence of side effects attributable to glucocorticoid excess, in cats during therapy with megestrol acetate and prednisolone. Can J Vet Res 1987;51:60.
29. Burke TJ, Reynolds HA, Sokolowski JH. A 180-day tolerance-efficacy study with mibolerone for suppression of estrus in the cat. Am J Vet Res 1977;38:469.
30. Gerber HA, Jochle W, Sulman FG. Control of reproduction and of undesirable social and sexual behavior in dogs and cats. J Sm Anim Pract 1973;14:151.
31. Johnston SD. Questions and answers on the effects of surgically neutering dogs and cats. J Am Vet Med Assoc 1991; 198:1206.
32. Salmeri KR, Bloomberg MS, Scruggs SL, Shille V. Gonadectomy in immature dogs: Effects on skeletal, physical, and behavioral development. J Am Vet Med Assoc 1991;198:1193.
33. Shille VM, Stabenfeldt GH. Luteal function in the domestic cat during pseudopregnancy and after treatment with prostaglandin $F_{2\alpha}$. Biol Reprod 1979;21:1217.
34. Wheeler AG, Walker M, Lean J. Function of hormonally-induced corpora lutera in the domestic cat. Theriogenology 1988;29:971.
35. Banks DH, Paape SR, Stabenfeldt GH. Prolactin in the cat: I. Pseudopregnancy, pregnancy and lactation. Biol Reprod 1982;28:923.
36. Goodrowe KL, Wall RJ, O'Brien SJ, et al. Developmental competence of domestic cat follicular oocytes after fertilization *in vitro*. Biol Reprod 1988;39:355.
37. Tsutsui T, Amano T, Shimizu T, et al. Evidence for transuterine migration of embryos in the domestic cat. Jpn J Vet Sci 1989;51:613.
38. Thatcher MD, Shille VM, Fliss MF, et al. Characterization of feline conceptus proteins during pregnancy. Biol Reprod 1991;44:108.
39. Malassine A, Ferre F. Delta 5, 3 beta hydroxysteroid dehydrogenase activity in cat placental labyrinth: Evolution during pregnancy, subcellular distribution. Biol Reprod 1979;21:965.
40. Lein DH, Concannon PW. Infertility and Fertility Treatments and Management in the Queen and Tom Cat. In: Kirk RW, ed. Current Veterinary Therapy VIII. Philadelphia: WB Saunders, 1983:936.
41. Jochle W, Arbeiter K, Post K, et al. Effects on pseudopregnancy, pregnancy and interoestrous intervals of pharmacological suppression of prolactin secretion in female dogs and cats. J Reprod Fert 1989;Suppl 39:199.
42. Addiego LA, Tsutsui T, Stewart DR, Stabenfeldt GH. Determination of the source of immunoreactive relaxin in the cat. Biol Reprod 1987;37:1165.
43. Stewart DR, Stabenfeldt GH. Relaxin activity in the pregnant cat. Biol Reprod 1985;32:848.
44. Scott PP. Cats. In: Hafez ESE, ed. Reproduction and Breeding Techniques for Laboratory Animals. Philadelphia: Lea & Febiger, 1970:192–208.
45. Boyd JS. The radiographic identification of the various stages of pregnancy in the domestic cat. J Sm Anim Pract 1971;12:501.
46. Davidson AP, Nyland G, Tsutsui T. Pregnancy diagnosis with ultrasound in the domestic cat. Vet Radiol 1986;27:109.
47. Feldman EC, Nelson RW. Feline Reproduction. In: Canine and Feline Endocrinology and Reproduction. Philadelphia: WB Saunders, 1987:525–548.
48. Kane E, Allard RL, Douglass GM. The influence of litter size on weight change during feline gestation and lactation. Fel Pract 1990;18:6.
49. Herron MA. Infertility from Noninfectious Causes. In: Morrow DA, ed. Current Therapy in Theriogenology 2. Philadelphia: WB Saunders, 1986:829–834.
50. Sturman JA, Moretz RC, French JH, Wisniewski HM. Taurine deficiency in the developing cat: Persistence of the cerebellar external granule cell layer. J Neurosci Res 1985;13:405.
51. Sturman JA, Gargano AD, Messing JM, Imaki H. Feline maternal taurine deficiency: Effect on mother and offspring. J Nutr 1986;116:655.
52. Prescott CW. Reproduction patterns in the domestic cat. Aust Vet J 1973;49:126.
53. Stabenfeldt GH, Pedersen NC. Reproduction and Reproductive Disorders. In: Pedersen NC, ed. Feline Husbandry: Diseases and Management in the Multiple-Cat Environment. Goleta, CA: American Veterinary Publications, 1991:129.
54. Potter K, Hancock DH, Gallina AM. Clinical and pathologic features of endometrial hyperplasia, pyometra, and endometritis in cats: 79 cases (1980–1985). J Am Vet Med Assoc 1991;198:1427.
55. Kenny KJ, Matthiesen DT, Brown NO, Bradley RL. Pyometra in cats: 183 cases (1979–1984). J Am Vet Med Assoc 1987; 191:1130.
56. Johnson CA, Wasserfal JL. Prostaglandin therapy in feline pyometra. J Am Anim Hosp Assoc 1984;20:247.
57. Wiessing HG, Thompson KS. Treatment of feline pyometra with dinoprost. NZ Vet J 1980;28:112.
58. Paradis M. Therapeutic uses of $PGF_{2\alpha}$ in the queen. J Am Assoc Fel Pract 1984;2:6.
59. Hayden DH, Johnston SD, Kiang DT, et al. Feline mammary hypertrophy/fibroadenoma complex: Clinical and hormonal aspects. Am J Vet Res 1981;42:1699.
60. Center SA, Randolph JF. Lactation and spontaneous remission of feline mammary hyperplasia following pregnancy. J Am Anim Hosp Assoc 1985;21:56.
61. Nachreiner RF, Marple DN. Termination of pregnancy in cats with prostaglandin $F_{2\alpha}$. Prostaglandins 1974;7:303.
62. Schmidt PM, Chakraborty PK, Wildt DE. Ovarian activity, circulating hormones and sexual behavior in the cat. II. Relationships during pregnancy, parturition, lactation and the postpartum estrus. Biol Reprod 1983;28:657.
63. Lein DH. Female Reproduction. In: Sherding RG, ed. The Cat: Diseases and Clinical Management. New York: Churchill Livingstone, 1989:1479–1497.
64. Concannon PW, Lein DH. Feline Reproduction. In: Kirk RW, ed. Current Veterinary Therapy VIII. Philadelphia: WB Saunders, 1983:932.
65. Herbert CR. Prolapsed uterus in the cat. Vet Rec 1979;104:42.
66. Gruffydd-Jones TJ. Acute mastitis in a cat. Fel Pract 1980;10:41.
67. Roudebush P, Wheeler KG. Peracute gangrenous mastitis in the cat. Fel Pract 1979;9:35.

68. Heron M. Feline reproduction. Vet Clin North Am 1977;7:715.
69. Voith VL. Male Reproductive Behavior. In: Morrow DA, ed. Current Therapy in Theriogenology. Philadelphia: WB Saunders, 1980:845.
70. Beadle M. Sex and Reproduction. In: The Cat: History, Biology, and Behavior. New York: Simon and Schuster, 1977:112.
71. Burke TJ. Feline reproduction. Vet Clin North Am 1976;6:317.
72. Robinson R. Reproduction and Development. In: Genetics for Cat Breeders. New York: Pergamon Press, 1977:12.
73. Pineda MH, Dooley MP, Martin PA. Long-term study on the effects of electroejaculation on seminal characteristics of the domestic cat. Am J Vet Res 1984;45:1038.
74. Platz CC, Wildt DW, Seager SWJ. Pregnancy in the domestic cat after artificial insemination with previously frozen spermatozoa. J Reprod Fert 1978;52:279.
75. Sojka NJ, Jennings L. Collection and utilization of cat semen for artificial insemination. J Am Vet Med Assoc 1970;156:1250.
76. Sojka NJ, Jennings L, Hammer C. Artificial insemination in the cat (*Felis catus*). Lab Anim Care 1970;20:198.
77. Platz CC, Follis T, Demorest N, Seager S. Semen collection, freezing and insemination in the domestic cat. VIII International Congress on Animal Reproduction and Artificial Insemination. Crakow, 1976:1053.
78. Dooley MP, Pineda MH. Effect of method of collection on seminal characteristics of the domestic cat. Am J Vet Res 1986; 47:286.
79. Dooley MP, Pineda MH, Hopper JG, Hsu WH. Retrograde flow of spermatozoa into the urinary bladder of cats during electroejaculation, collection of semen with an artificial vagina, and mating. Am J Vet Res 1991;52:687.
80. Scott FW, Weiss RC, Post JE, et al. Kitten mortality complex (neonatal FIP?). Fel Pract 1979;9:44.
81. Norsworthy GD. Kitten mortality complex. Fel Pract 1979;9:57.
82. Pedersen NC, ed. Feline Husbandry: Diseases and Management in the Multiple Cat Environment. Goleta, CA: American Veterinary Publications, 1991.
83. Shille VM, Stabenfeldt GH. Current concepts in reproduction of the dog and cat. Adv Vet Sci Comp Med 1980;24:211.
84. Voith VL. Female Reproductive Behavior. In: Morrow D, ed. Current Therapy in Theriogenology, 1st ed. Philadelphia: WB Saunders, 1980:839.
85. Shille VM, Massey RE, Chavatte P. Testing endocrine function of gonads. Proc Am Mtg Soc Theriogenology 1991:240.
86. Christiansen IJ. Reproduction in the Dog and Cat. London: Ballière Tindall, 1984.
87 Herron MA, Boehringer BT. Male pseudohermaphroditism in a cat. Fel Pract 1975;5:30.
88. Thomsen PD, Byskov AG, Basse A. Fertility in two cats with X-chromosome mosaicism and unilateral ovarian dysgenesis. J Reprod Fert 1987;80:43.
89. Centerwall WR, Benirschke K. An animal model for the XXY Klinefelter's syndrome in man: Tortoise shell and male calico cats. Am J Vet Res 1975;26:1275.
90. Carpenter JL, Andrews LK, Holzworth J. Tumors and tumorlike lesions. In: Holzworth J, ed. Diseases of the Cat: Medicine and Surgery. Philadelphia: WB Saunders, 1987;1:406.
91. Norris HB, Garner FM, Taylor HB. Pathology of feline ovarian neoplasms. J Pathol 1969;97:138.
92. Herron MA, Stein B. Prognosis and Management of Feline Infertility. In: Kirk RW, ed. Current Veterinary Therapy VII. Philadelphia: WB Saunders, 1980.
93. Gelberg HB, McEntee K, Heath EH. Feline cystic rete ovarii. Vet Pathol 1984;21:304.
94. Hofmann W, Arbiter D, Scheele D. Sex cord stromal tumor of the cat: So-called androblastoma with Sertoli-Leydig cell pattern. Vet Pathol 1980;17:508.
95. Andrews EJ, Stookey JL, Helland DR, Slaughter LJ. A histopathological study of canine and feline ovarian dysgerminomas. Can J Comp Med 1974:85.
96. Dehner LP, Norris HJ, Garner FM, Taylor HB. Comparative pathology of ovarian neoplasms III. Germ cell tumours of canine, bovine, feline, rodent and human species. J Comp Pathol 1970;80:299.
97. Dow C. The cystic hyperplasia-pyometra complex in the cat. Vet Rec 1962;74:141.
98. Wolf AM. Feline infertility. Proc Ann Mtg Soc Theriogenology 1987:273.
99. Goodrowe KL, Howard JG, Wildt DE. Comparison of embryo recovery, embryo quality, oestradiol-17B and progesterone profiles in domestic cats (*Felis catus*) at natural or induced oestrus. J Reprod Fert 1988;82:553.
100. Nelson RW, Feldman EC, Stabenfeldt GH. Treatment of canine pyometra and endometritis with prostaglandin F2 alpha. J Am Vet Med Assoc 1982;181:899.
101. Cotter SM, Hardy WD, Essex M. Association of feline leukemia virus with lymphosarcoma and other disorders in the cat. J Am Vet Med Assoc 1975;166:449.
102. Hardy RM, Osborne CA. Canine pyometra: Pathophysiology, diagnosis and treatment of uterine and extrauterine lesions. J Am Anim Hosp Assoc 1974;10:245.
103. Hardy WD. The Virology, Immunology, and Epidemiology of the Feline Leukemia Viruses. In: Hardy WD, Essex M, McClelland AJ, eds. Feline Leukemia Virus. New York, New York: Elsevier/North-Holland Inc, 1980:33–78.
104. Chapman AL, Weitlauf HM, Bopp W. Brief communication: Effect of feline leukemia virus on transferred hamster fetuses. J Natl Cancer Inst 1974;52:583.
105. Pedersen NC, Meric SM, Ho E, et al. The clinical significance of latent feline leukemia virus infection in cats. Fel Pract 1984;14:32.
106. Pacitti AM, Jarrett O, Hay D. Transmission of feline leukaemia virus in the milk of a non-viraemic cat. Vet Rec 1986;118:381.
107. Rojko JL, Hoover EA, Quackenbush SL, Olsen RG. Reactivation of latent feline leukemia virus infection. Nature 1982;298:385.
108. Shille VM, Thomas PGA, Massey R. Viral causes of pregnancy loss in the multiple cat household. Proc Ann Mtg Soc Theriogenology 1990:275.
109. Ishida T, Washizu T, Toriyabe K, et al. Feline immunodeficiency virus infection in cats of Japan. J Am Vet Med Assoc 1989;194:221.
110. Yamamoto JK, Hansen J, Ho EW, et al. Epidemiologic and clinical aspects of feline immunodeficiency virus infection in cats from the continental United States and Canada and possible mode of transmission. J Am Vet Med Assoc 1989;194:213.
111. Johnson RH, Margolis G, Kilham L. Identity of feline ataxia virus with feline panleukopenia virus. Nature 1967;214:175.
112. Kilham L, Margolis G, Colby ED. Congenital infections of cats and ferrets by feline panleukopenia virus manifested by cerebellar hypoplasia. Lab Invest 1967;17:465.
113. Kilham L, Margolis G. Viral etiology of spontaneous ataxia of cats. Am J Pathol 1966;48:991.
114. Csiza CK, Scott FW, DeLahunta A, Gillespie JH. Feline viruses XIV. Transplacental infections in spontaneous panleukopenia of cats. Cornell Vet 1971;61:423.
115. Pedersen NC. Feline infectious peritonitis and feline enteric coronavirus infections. Part 1: Feline enteric coronavirus. Fel Pract 1983;13:13.
116. Barlough JE, Jacobson RH, Scott FW. Feline coronaviral serology. Fel Pract 1983;13:25.
117. Barlough JE. Cats, coronaviruses and coronavirus antibody tests. J Sm Anim Pract 1985;26:353.
118. Pedersen NC. Feline infectious peritonitis, and feline enteric coronavirus infections. Part 2: feline infectious peritonitis. Fel Pract 1983;13:5.

119. Pedersen NC. Feline infectious peritonitis: Something old, something new. Fel Pract 1976;6:42.
120. Norsworthy GD. Neonatal feline infectious peritonitis. Fel Pract 1974;4:34.
121. Pastoret PP, Henroteaux M. Epigenetic transmission of feline infectious peritonitis. Comp Immun Microbiol Infect Dis 1978;1:67.
122. Hagashi T, Watabe Y, Takenouchi T, Fujiwara K. Role of circulating antibodies in feline infectious peritonitis after oral infection. Jpn J Vet Sci 1983;45:487.
123. McKeirnan AJ, Evermann JF, Hargis A, et al. Isolation of feline coronaviruses from two cats with diverse disease manifestations. Fel Pract 1981;11:16.
124. Bittle JL, Emery JB, York CJ, McMillen JK. Comparative study of feline cytopathogenic viruses and feline panleukopenia virus. Am J Vet Res 1961;22:374.
125. Gerber JD, Ingersoll JD, Gast AM, et al. Protection against feline infectious peritonitis by intranasal inoculation of a temperature-sensitive FIPV vaccine. Vaccine 1990;8:536.
126. Hoover EA, Griesemer RA. Experimental feline herpesvirus infection in the pregnant cat. Am J Pathol 1971;65:173.
127. Gaskell RM, Povey RC. Experimental induction of feline viral rhinotracheitis virus re-excretion in FVR-recovered cats. Vet Rec 1977;100:128.
128. Gaskell RM, Povey RC. Transmission of feline viral rhinotracheitis. Vet Rec 1982;111:359.
129. Gaskell RM, Povey RC. Reexcretion of feline viral rhinotracheitis virus following corticosteroid treatment. Vet Rec 1973;93:204.
130. Wills J, Gruffydd-Jones TJ, Richmond S, Paul ID. Isolation of *Chlamydia psittaci* from cases of conjunctivitis in a colony of cats. Vet Rec 1984;114:344.
131. Cello RM. Clue to differential diagnosis of feline respiratory infections. J Am Vet Med Assoc 1971;158:968.
132. Pedersen NC. Common Infectious Diseases of Multiple Cat Environments. In: Pedersen NC, ed. Feline Husbandry: Diseases and Management in the Multiple-Cat Environment. Goleta, CA: American Veterinary Publications, 1991:163–288.
133. Papich MG. Pharmacologic considerations during pregnancy in small animals. Proc Ann Mtg Soc Theriogenology 1990:224.
134. Dubey JP, Hoover EA. Attempted transmission of *Toxoplasma gondii* infection from pregnant cats to their kittens. J Am Vet Med Assoc 1970;170:538.
135. Dubey JP, Johnstone I. Fatal neonatal toxoplasmosis in cats. J Am Anim Hosp Assoc 1982;18:461.
136. Troy GC, Herron MA. Infectious Causes of Infertility, Abortion and Stillbirths in Cats. In: Morrow DA, ed. Current Therapy in Theriogenology 2. Philadelphia: WB Saunders, 1986:834.
137. Johnston SD. Management of Pregnancy Disorders in the Bitch and Queen. In: Current Veterinary Therapy VIII. Philadelphia: WB Saunders, 1983:952.
138. Kitchen H, Murray RE, Cockrell BY. Spinal bifida, sacral dysgenesis and myelocele. Am J Pathol 1972;68:203.
139. DeForest ME, Basrur PK. Malformations and the Manx syndrome in cats. Can Vet J 1979;20:304.
140. Johnston SD, Buoen LC, Madl JE, et al. X Chromosome monosomy (37, XO) in a Burmese cat with gonadal dysgenesis. J Am Vet Med Assoc 1983;182:986.
141. Long SE, Berepubo NA. A 37 XO chromosome complement in a kitten. J Sm Anim Pract 1980;21:627.
142. Nicholas FW, Muir P, Toll GL. An XXY male Burmese cat. J Heredity 1980;71:52.
143. Lawler DF, Evans RH, Reimers TJ, et al. Histopathologic features, environmental factors, and serum estrogen, progesterone, and prolactin values associated with ovarian phase and inflammatory uterine disease in cats. Am J Vet Res 1991; 52:1747.
144. Scott FW, Geissinger C, Peltz R. Kitten mortality survey. Fel Pract 1978;8:31.
145. Wallace LJ, Henry JD, Clifford JH. Manual reduction of uterine prolapse in a domestic cat. Vet Med Sm Anim Pract 1970; 65:595.

CHAPTER 55

◇ ◇ ◇

Selected Surgical Procedures

Gary D. Norsworthy

This chapter reviews selected surgical procedures that are unique to the cat or that differ significantly from similar procedures performed on other species. Most of these procedures can be performed successfully with several variations in technique; however, the specific techniques presented here have worked well for this author.

Intravenous Catheterization

The placement and maintenance of intravenous (IV) catheters can be frustrating because of the size of feline veins. Proper catheter selection and placement are essential in minimizing problems.

Types of Catheters

There are three styles of IV catheters: butterfly, short, and long. Each has its particular advantages and disadvantages, so the practitioner should be familiar with the indications and placement techniques for each style.

The *butterfly catheter* is an indwelling metal catheter with plastic "butterfly wings" designed for securing the catheter to the skin. The indwelling catheter is generally 1 inch or less in length and is available in several sizes ranging from 18 to 25 gauge. Originally designed for use in the scalp veins of humans, especially infants, the butterfly catheter is commonly called a scalp vein set. These catheters may be placed quickly and easily and are indicated for short-term use (a few hours). Their main disadvantage is that they are easily dislodged from the vein. Additionally, because they are made of metal (stainless steel), they may cause significant trauma to the vein if the cat moves the catheterized leg.

Short catheters are those measuring up to 5 inches in length and having a diameter ranging from 16 to 22 gauge. They consist of a cannula and a stylet and are used for supplying IV fluids and medications for up to 48 hours. Their main advantages are their ease of use and speed of placement, as compared to so-called long catheters. They are the catheter of choice for administering shock doses of fluids because fluids can be administered faster through short catheters than through long catheters of the same diameter. Their disadvantages include irritation of the venous endothelium, a predisposition to phlebitis, and an inability to obtain blood samples with them. Short catheters made of stiff polyvinyl chloride are more irritating than those made of more flexible Teflon. Common brands of short catheters include Sovereign and Medicut (Sherwood Medical Co., St. Louis, MO), Angiocath (Becton Dickinson Deseret Medical, Inc., Sandy, UT), and Abbocath (Abbott Hospitals Inc., N. Chicago, IL).[1]

Long catheters are more than 10 inches long and are available in diameters ranging from 14 to 20 gauge. They are typically passed through a larger-diameter needle to gain access to the vein's lumen. They are indicated for long-term fluid therapy, central venous pressure (CVP) measurement, and administration of hyperosmolar fluids. They are less irritating to the endothelium than are short catheters, so they may be left in place longer. They are also suitable for drawing blood samples. Their main disadvantage is their difficulty of placement.[1] Commonly used long catheters include the Venocath (Abbott Laboratories, Abbott Park, IL) and Intracath (Becton Dickinson Deseret Medical, Inc., Sandy, UT).

Placement Sites

There are three veins suitable for catheter placement in cats: jugular, cephalic, and medial saphenous. The main factors in site selection are ease of catheter placement for the practitioner or technician, stress to the cat, and the likelihood of catheter displacement by the cat. The first factor—ease of placement—is governed by personal choice and practice; many practitioners prefer the cephalic vein for this reason alone. The cat's stress level during placement favors the use of the cephalic vein, whereas the cat's stress level during catheter use often favors the jugular vein.

Catheter Placement

Butterfly Catheters

Butterfly catheters are best placed in the cephalic vein, as they are not long enough for maintenance in the jugular vein, and the medial saphenous vein becomes too tortuous when the cat walks. To place a butterfly catheter, a tourniquet is first applied above the elbow. The hair over the cephalic vein is clipped and the skin is prepped. The catheter is then inserted into the vein just proximal to the cephalic bifurcation, which is just proximal to the carpus. A piece of adhesive tape is used to secure the plastic wings to the leg. At this point, the tourniquet should be released. If a second piece of adhesive tape is placed over the area of the indwelling metal catheter, there is less likelihood of venous laceration.

Short Catheters

Short catheters are best suited for the cephalic vein, but are also suitable for the medial saphenous vein. For placement of this type of catheter, the hair is clipped and the skin is prepped over the distal cephalic or medial saphenous vein. A tourniquet is then applied above the elbow; alternatively, an assistant may occlude the proximal medial saphenous vein. The vein will be least likely to roll away from the needle if the carpus is flexed. The rubber cap or infusion plug is then removed so that the practitioner/technician can quickly determine when blood backflows into the catheter. The metal needle/stylet is then inserted through the skin and into the vein. It may be threaded up the vein its entire distance, or it may be backed out of the polypropylene or Teflon cannula and the cannula advanced up the vein. Because the metal stylet is more likely to repenetrate the vein, the author recommends threading the vein with the more flexible cannula, especially if the medial saphenous vein is being utilized. When the catheter has been threaded to the desired depth into the vein, the tourniquet is released. The catheter is then taped securely to the leg.

If the distal end of the catheter is seated too close to the elbow when one is using the cephalic vein, the catheter will become occluded when the cat flexes the elbow. This may be minimized by using a 1.25-inch catheter instead of a 2-inch catheter. Other strategies may also be employed to avoid this complication. For instance, the catheter's site of entry into the vein should be as distal on the leg as possible so that the catheter's tip is placed about the area of the midshaft of the radius and ulna. This requires a venipuncture just proximal to the carpus. Another strategy is to apply a splint-like device to the leg to keep it from bending at the elbow (Fig. 55–1). A modified Thomas splint or a splint made of Orthoplast (Johnson & Johnson Products, Inc., New Brunswick, NJ) has been used successfully for this purpose.[2] There are several commercial splints designed for this purpose, including the Cochran IV Splint (Jorgensen Laboratories Inc., Loveland, CO) and the Carlin IV Feeding Splint (Carlin Enterprises, Tulsa, OK).

Long Catheters[1]

Long catheters may be placed in the jugular, cephalic, or medial saphenous vein. However, in terms of practicality, the jugular vein is clearly the preferred site in the cat. Because these catheters are often left in place for extended periods of time, they are associated with an increased incidence of catheter-related infections, making preparation of the venipuncture site critical. Hair over the jugular furrow should be clipped liberally and the skin should receive a 2-minute scrub. After the venipuncture site has been prepared, it should not be touched except with sterile gloves.

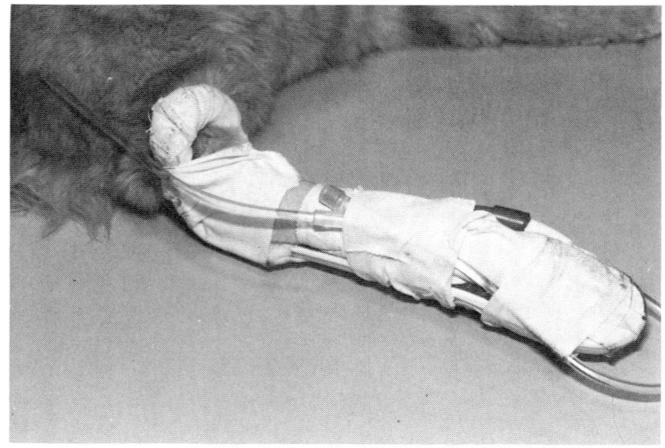

Figure 55–1. **When a catheter is placed in the cephalic vein, a plastic splint can be adapted to prevent the cat from flexing the elbow and disrupting the flow of fluids. (Courtesy of Dr. Eric Lange, San Antonio, TX.)**

The following procedure describes jugular placement of the Venocath.

- Grasp the Venocath in one hand so that the clear ring at the top of the blue needle guard column can be pulled downward toward the base of the column. When the wings over the needle are opened, the needle will be exposed. Be sure the catheter does not extend past the bevel of the needle.
- Occlude the jugular vein by applying pressure across the entire lateral aspect of the neck.
- Select the venipuncture site (proximal to midcervical region), stabilizing the vein by extending the cat's head dorsally and the front legs caudally. The needle should enter the vein at about a 30° angle.
- When blood is seen to enter the catheter, decrease the angle of the needle as the catheter is advanced into the vein.
- Discontinue occlusion of the jugular vein.
- Stabilize the blue portion of the Venocath catheter with one hand while using the other hand to thread the catheter into the vein by pinching it out of the plastic sleeve.
- Continue to feed the catheter into the vein until the white hub end of the catheter is seated into the base of the blue column.
- Withdraw the needle from the vein and subcutaneous tissue. The blue protective wings should be closed over the needle. The guard will stay securely closed when the plastic ring is positioned over the wings.
- Remove the plastic sleeve and withdraw the stylet from the catheter.
- Flush the catheter with heparinized saline.
- If a 10-inch catheter is used, only about 4 inches should be indwelling within the jugular vein. With the several inches of catheter that remain outside the skin, make a ventrally directed, U-shaped loop.
- Securely tape the remainder of the catheter and the blue column/white hub assembly to the neck so that

the cat cannot dislodge it. Avoid wrapping the neck too tightly so as to prevent discomfort or facial swelling.

Abscess Drainage

The fighting style of a cat is different from that of a dog. Typically, a dog will bite into a victim, clamp its jaws tightly, and shake its head. This frequently results in a deep laceration. By contrast, the cat bites quickly and releases, leaving puncture wounds. Oral bacteria are thus deposited in the tissues of the victim, where they incubate for 2 to 4 days before resulting in a clinical infection. By that time, the puncture wounds may be healed or well-hidden in the hair, masking any obvious evidence of the bite.

If the bite occurs in an area where the skin tightly adheres to the underlying tissue, such as the distal extremities, cellulitis will cause tissue swelling as the infection spreads dorsally and ventrally along the tissue planes. Surgical incision of the area will generally not result in drainage of purulent material, so surgery is not indicated. However, if the bite occurs in an area of loose skin, an abscess will develop. If the abscess does not rupture spontaneously (Fig. 55–2), surgical drainage is indicated to enhance healing.

Surgical Technique

The procedure for abscess drainage is as follows:

- Tranquilize or anesthetize the cat unless septicemia has caused depression.
- Determine the proper location for the incision(s) by considering two factors. A mature abscess generally will develop a soft spot, the location of which will generally be near the center of the abscess, producing good drainage. The other factor to be considered is the effect of gravity. If the soft spot of a mature abscess is at the dorsal aspect of the abscess, it will be difficult for drainage to continue for several days. In that situation, a second incision should be made at the ventral aspect of the abscess. The placement of a drain tube is optional.

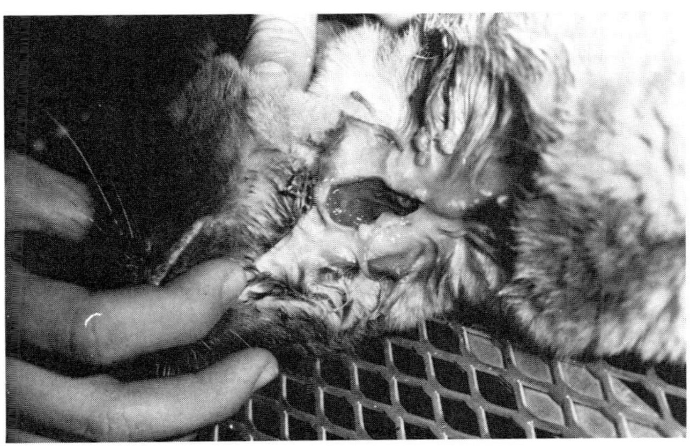

Figure 55–2. Surgically opening an abscess, such as this one in the submaxillary area, will result in drainage of purulent material and promotion of healing. To achieve maximal drainage, the incision should be made in the ventral-most location.

- After the abscess has been surgically opened, flush the wound with an antibacterial agent. This serves to remove purulent and necrotic tissue and initiates the bactericidal process.

Postoperative Care

The cat should be maintained on systemic antibiotics for 5 to 10 days, depending on the severity of the infection. Because most infections secondary to cat fights are caused by *Pasteurella multocida,* β-hemolytic streptococci, anaerobic Fusiformis species, and *Escherichia coli,*[3] penicillin therapy is generally effective. Amoxicillin (Amoxi-tabs) or amoxicillin-clavulanic acid (Clavamox), available in convenient tablet sizes, is generally effective. Local treatment with an antibiotic ointment or solution is optional. Most abscesses will granulate closed in 2 to 4 days and require no suturing; however, extensive sloughing of tissue may necessitate some suturing after the infection has been treated.

Because the feline leukemia virus (FeLV) and the feline immunodeficiency virus (FIV) are transmitted through cat bites, the implications of these infections should be discussed with the owner, including the desirability of FeLV vaccinations (see Chapters 37 and 39).

Bladder Marsupialization

Urethral obstructions which are common in cats with the feline urological syndrome (FUS), are generally relieved quickly by the urethral flushing techniques described in Chapter 40. Occasionally, however, a cat will have such a severe obstruction that urethral flushing and cystocentesis are unsuccessful. At that point, there are two options: perineal urethrostomy, which will not only relieve the obstruction but will also prevent future obstructions, or temporary bladder marsupialization.[4] If the patient is a prized breeding tom, perineal urethrostomy will be unacceptable because it requires that the cat also be neutered.

Surgical Technique

Bladder marsupialization involves the following steps:

- After anesthetizing the cat, drain the bladder as completely as possible by cystocentesis, then prep the ventral abdomen.
- Using a routine surgical approach, exteriorize the bladder.
- Make a 2-cm cystotomy incision on the ventral midline and remove any remaining urine and crystalline debris (Fig. 55–3*A*). At this point, any attempts made to pass a urinary catheter from either direction are generally unsuccessful.
- Suture the bladder wall directly to the abdominal muscles or to the skin (Fig. 55–3*B*); either method is generally successful.
- Close the remaining skin incision so that the bladder remains open to the skin (Fig. 55–3*C*).
- Initiate treatment with broad-spectrum antibiotics and keep the cat in a cage with a slotted floor and without a litter box. Treat the cat's ventral abdominal wall once

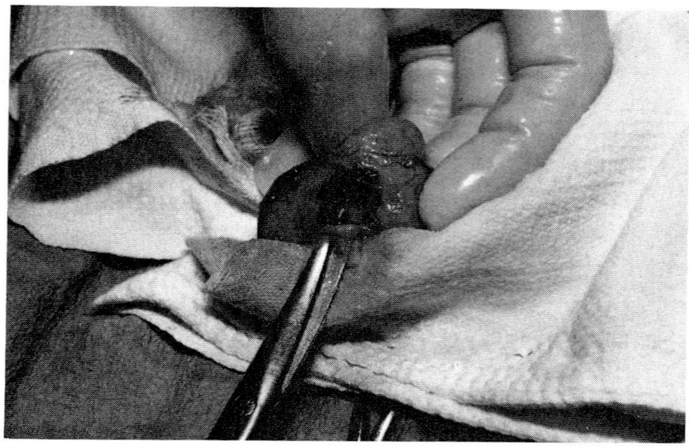

A

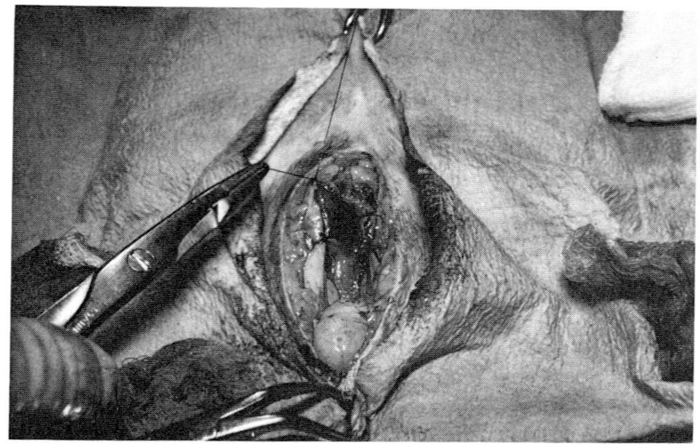

B

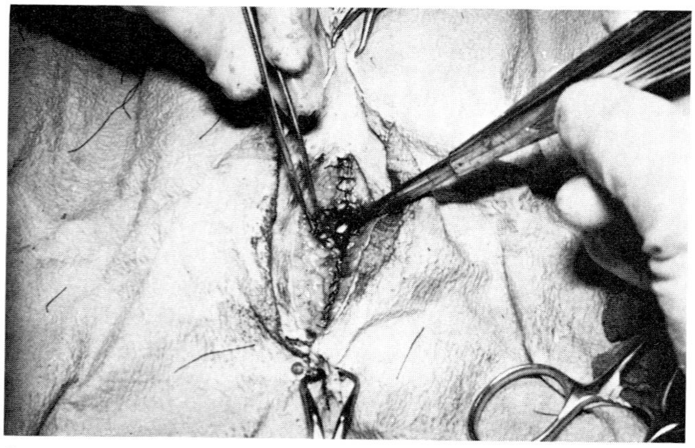

C

Figure 55–3. (*A*) A large amount of mucoid-crystalline material is removed from the bladder. This material had created a urethral obstruction that could not be relieved by backflushing. (*B*) The bladder wall is sutured to the abdominal musculature with a series of interrupted sutures. Alternatively, the bladder wall may be sutured directly to the skin. (*C*) When suturing is completed, the bladder will open directly through the abdominal muscle wall and skin. (Used by permission of Veterinary Practice Publishing Co., Santa Barbara, CA.)

or twice daily with a skin protectant, such as Derma Shield (Benchmark Enterprises, Salt Lake City, UT).

Results

Bladder marsupialization effectively relieves feline urinary obstruction. Because pressure is no longer exerted against the obstructing material, the urethral mucosal inflammation and swelling gradually subside. Repeated attempts are made to catheterize the urethra until it can be performed successfully. Because these attempts require sedation or anesthesia, they are done on an every-other-day or every-third-day basis. Once catheterization is successful, the cat is returned to surgery for bladder closure and replacement into the abdomen.

This procedure is rarely needed, but it can be very rewarding when dealing with a prized breeding tom. As FUS is a recurrent disease, aggressive dietary measures should be instituted to prevent future episodes (see Chapter 40).

Colectomy (Subtotal)

Idiopathic megacolon is occasionally seen in cats. Traditionally, these conditions have been managed medically with various laxatives and stool softeners (see Chapter 49). Medical treatment is generally successful for several months, or even a few years. However, a point may be reached when medical therapy is no longer feasible or successful. At that point, several surgeons have recommended subtotal colectomy.[5,6] Although the typical first reaction of most veterinarians to subtotal colectomy is shock and disbelief, this procedure has proven to be very successful in the management of this condition. Indeed, it is now considered the treatment of choice.[7]

*Surgical Technique**

All of the colon, except the distal portion, is excised for subtotal colectomy. Enough of the distal colon is left to allow attachment to the distal ileum. End-to-end and end-to-side anastomoses have been utilized by various surgeons. The technique described here is relatively simple and has been consistently successful.

- Prepare the cat for colon surgery by withholding food and by administering amoxicillin (Amoxi-tabs) and metronidazole (Flagyl) orally for 24 to 48 hours.
- Administer 25 mL of mineral oil via an orogastric tube 12–24 hours before surgery.
- Once the cat is anesthetized for surgery, cleanse the colon with warm water enemas; manual extraction of stool may be performed if needed.

*Developed by Don C. Miller, DVM, San Antonio, TX.

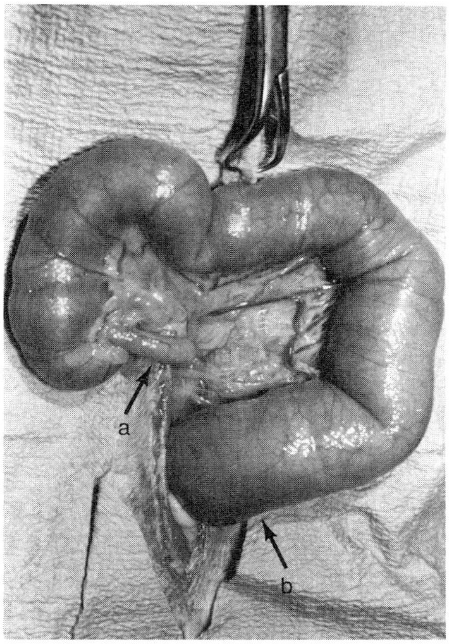

Figure 55–4. The enlarged colon is removed from the abdomen. Its diameter should be compared with that of the ileum (*a*). The ileum is transected at least 2 to 3 cm proximal to its junction with the colon in order to preserve its vasculature. The colon is transected as caudally as possible (*b*) so that enough tissue remains for handling and suturing.

- Approach the caudal abdomen through a routine midline incision.
- Retract the colon and caudal ileum from the abdomen (Fig. 55–4) and pack off with surgical towels.
- Clamp the ileum and transect it about 2 to 3 cm proximal to the cecum so that the vasculature is preserved proximal to the transection (see Fig. 55–4).
- Following this initial transection, transect the ileum again at a 45° angle, keeping the longer ileac border on the mesenteric side.
- Likewise, clamp the colon and transect it 2 to 3 cm cranial to the pelvic inlet, retaining enough colon to permit anastomosis.
- Suture the ileum to the colon, beginning at the mesenteric border. A soft, 4-0 absorbable material, such as Vicryl (Ethicon, Somerville, NJ), is preferred. When completed approximately one-half of the open colonic end will remain unattached to the ileum.
- Make a 45° incision on the antimesenteric side of the colon, beginning at the antimesenteric point of attachment of the ileum.
- Suture the cut margins of the colon together (see Fig. 55–5).
- Test the suture lines by injecting sterile saline into the intestinal tract and observing it for leaks. A mesenteric patch is optional, but encouraged.
- Close the abdomen in a routine fashion.
- Withhold oral food and water for 48 hours; IV fluids may be administered.
- Reinstitute feeding of solids in 2 to 3 days.

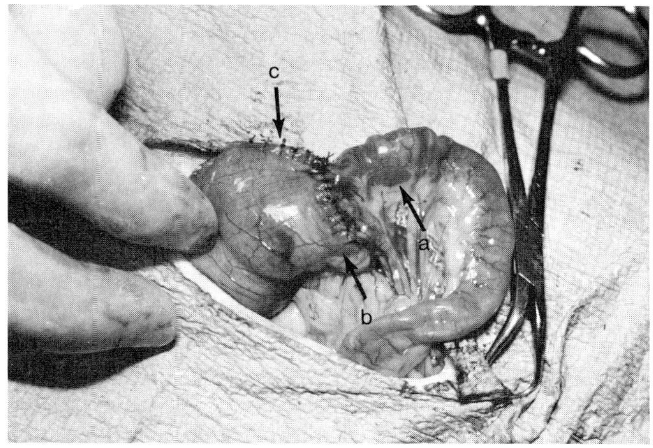

Figure 55–5. The ileum (*a*) is attached to the colon (*b*). The unused portion of the colon is cut at a 45° angle and the edges sutured (*c*).

Results

Because about 80% to 90% of the colon is removed with this procedure, most cats will have soft to watery diarrhea initially with two to five bowel movements each day. Fecal continence will, however, be retained. Within a few weeks, the stool typically becomes firm and the number of bowel movements decreases to one to two per day.

Comminuted Femoral Fracture Repair*

A severely comminuted femoral fracture may occasionally be seen in cats (Fig. 55–6). Repair of this type of fracture may be accomplished using several very expensive and complicated ways, or, alternatively, a single, large intramedullary pin can be placed permanently.[8] For this procedure to be successful, the largest intramedullary pin that will fit the medullary cavity should be used. Moreover, wire, or heavy, slowly dissolving suture material should be used to secure the autogenous bone fragments as close to the pin as possible.

Surgical Technique

A comminuted femoral fracture may be repaired using the following procedure:

- Determine the correct length for the pin by obtaining a radiograph of the normal femur. Making the pin an incorrect length will create a leg that is either too long or too short.
- Do not run the pin through the trochanteric fossa; rather, position it in a retrograde fashion from midshaft, inserting it into the proximal and distal fragments. Place the blunt end of the pin distally. Alternatively, a pin with two blunt ends can be used.

*Developed simultaneously by Don C. Miller, DVM, San Antonio, TX, and R. H. Stine and J. G. Mueller.[8]

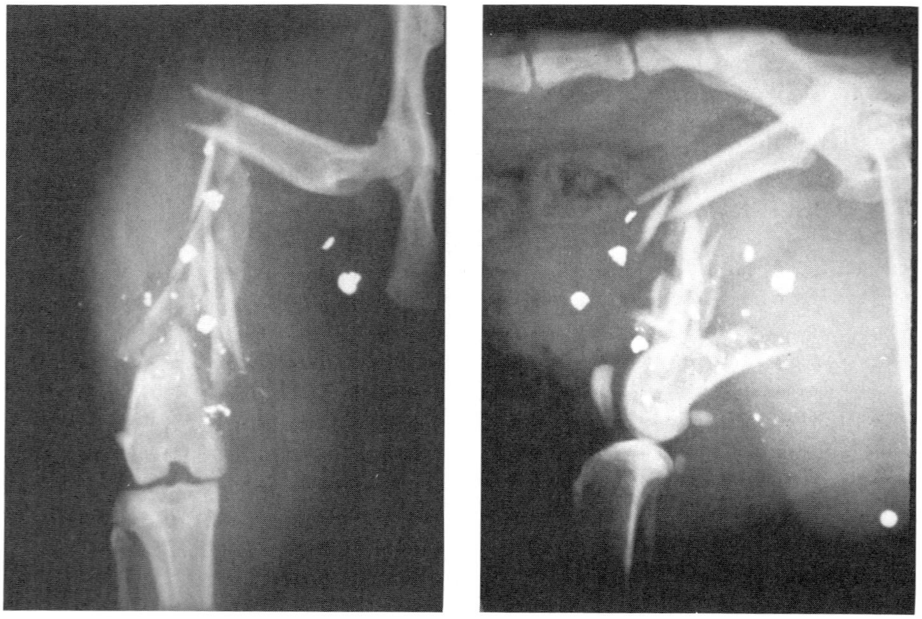

A B

Figure 55–6. (*A*) This comminuted midshaft fracture of the right femur was caused by a gunshot wound. (*B*) Lateral view of the same leg.

- Place the fragments in the gap and secure with wire or suture material (Fig. 55–7, *A* and *B*).

Following surgery, no external fixation should be used. However, the cat should be confined to its cage for 7 to 10 days postoperatively, and should remain indoors for another 2 weeks.

Results

Within 2 to 3 weeks, cats undergoing this surgery should be able to bear weight. By 6 to 8 weeks postoperatively, most such cats will have no noticeable limp. Following complete healing, these cats typically regain full use of their leg and have a normal gait.

Deep Digital Flexor Tendonectomy

Some cat owners have an aversion to declawing their cats. However, they also may not be pleased with the damage being done by their cats to drapes, furniture, and the like. Deep digital flexor tendonectomy offers these clients an alternative (see Fig. 55–8).[9]

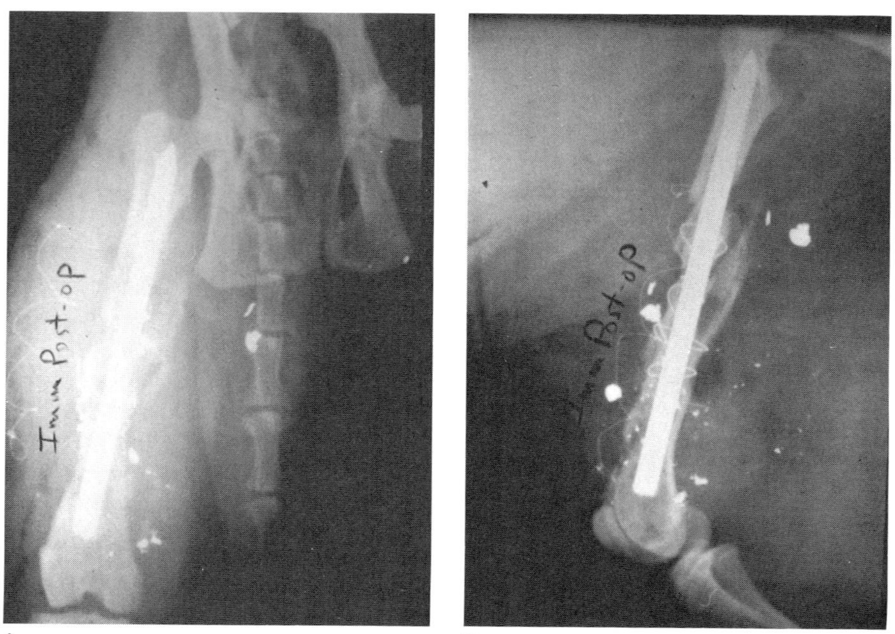

A B

Figure 55–7. (*A*) a stainless steel pin implanted in the femur shown in Figure 55–6. The fragments are approximated in their normal position using several lengths of small-gauge stainless steel wire. (*B*) Lateral view of the same fracture repair.

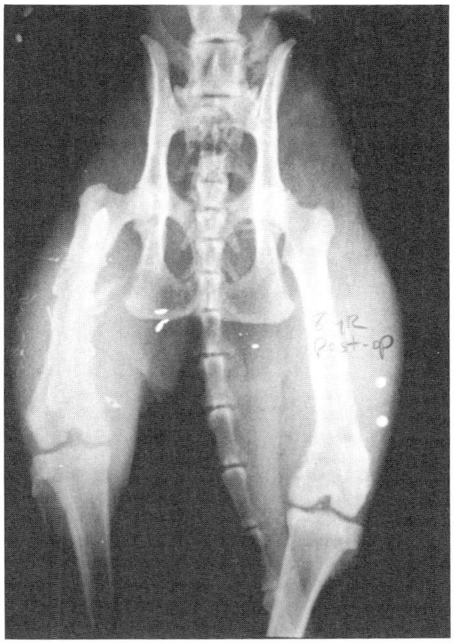

A

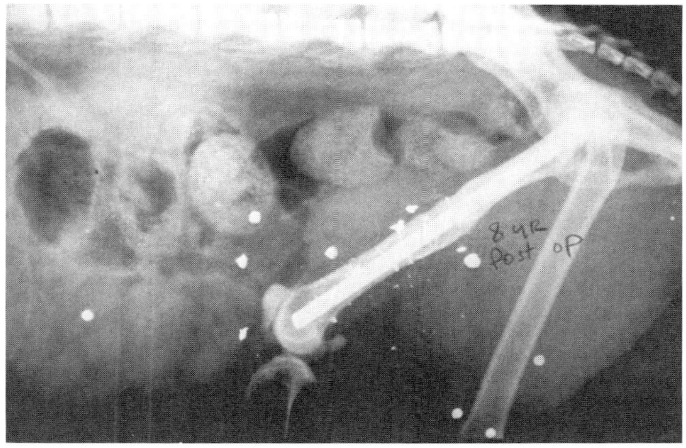

B

Figure 55–8. (*A*) Following healing, the cat had a normal gait. This radiograph was obtained 8 years postoperatively. (*B*) Lateral view of the same leg.

Surgical Technique

The procedure for deep digital flexor tendonectomy is as follows:

- Clip and prep the cat's feet for sterile surgery.
- Make an incision over the deep digital flexor tendon just proximal to the digital pad.
- Expose the tendon by blunt dissection (Fig. 55–9*A*).
- Clamp a straight Halstead hemostat across the tendon (Fig. 55–9*B*).
- Transect the tendon on both sides of the hemostat (Fig. 55–9*C*) to allow removal of a small section, thereby preventing subsequent reattachment.
- Close the skin incision with 4-0 or 5-0 dissolvable suture material.

The other front toes are operated in a similar fashion. It is important that the procedure performed be a tendon*ectomy* and not a tendon*otomy*.

Results

Following surgery, the cat will be unable to sharpen its claws normally. As a result, the owner will need to trim the nails on a regular basis.

Ear Trim

Cats in southern climates frequently develop squamous cell carcinoma on the tips of the pinnae (Fig. 55–10). This neoplasm rarely metastasizes, but it is locally invasive and may eventually involve most of the pinna. Local treatment involves cosmetic, surgical removal of the neoplastic tissue, the procedure for which is as follows:

- Clip and surgically prep the cat's pinnae.
- Excise the distal pinna to remove the neoplastic tissue. Remove sufficient tissue to leave a clean margin without disfiguring the cat.
- Place skin-to-skin sutures so the cartilage is not exposed. The preferred suture material is 5-0 dissolvable suture.

If both ears are affected, the one requiring the greatest amount of resection is operated on first. The other ear is then operated on to match in order to provide the best cosmetic results (Fig. 55–11).

Esophagostomy Tube Placement

Placement of an esophagostomy tube permits long-term feeding of the anorectic cat. No specialized equipment is needed for placement, a very brief period of anesthesia is required, and the tube is generally well tolerated by the patient.[10]

Surgical Technique

The following equipment is needed for placement of an esophagostomy tube:

- Scalpel
- Pair of 5-inch curved hemostatic forceps
- 12-French feeding tube

The procedure for esophagostomy tube placement is as follows:

- Determine the point on the tube where it should enter the skin by placing the tube beside the cat so that the distal end is at the level of the mid to caudal one third of the esophagus. Place a mark on the tube at that point (Fig. 55–12*A*).

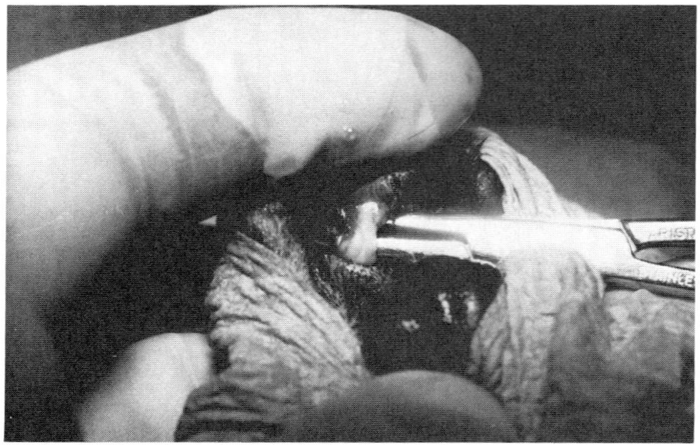

A

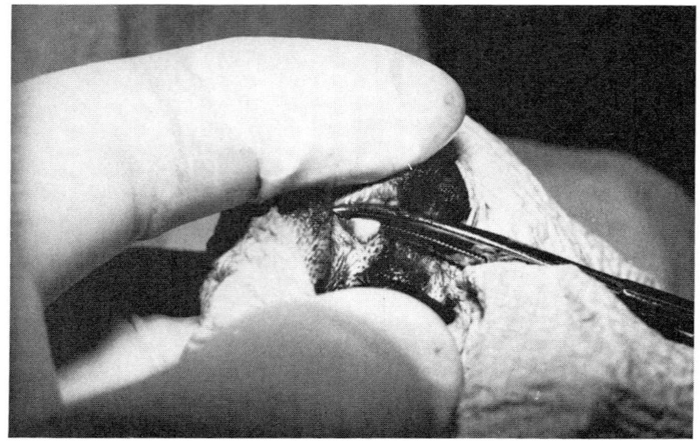

B

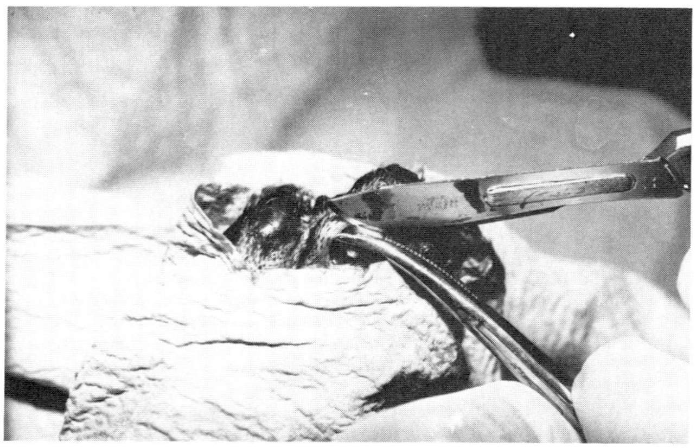

C

Figure 55–9. (*A*) The deep digital flexor tendon is isolated with a pair of hemostats. (*B*) The hemostats are clamped across the tendon. (*C*) The tendon is transected on both sides so that a partial tendonotomy (not a tendonectomy) is performed.

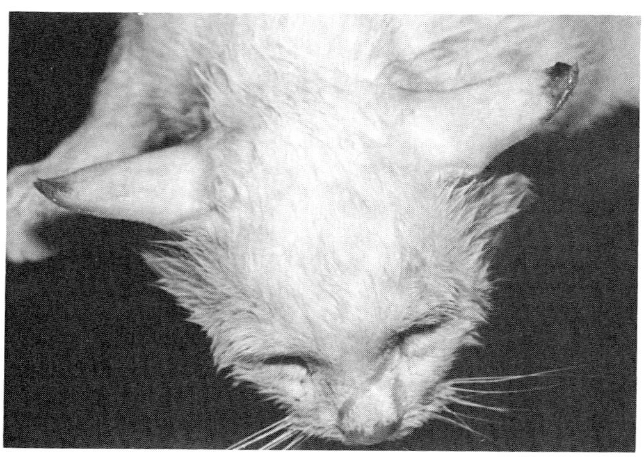

Figure 55–10. Both ear tips are affected by squamous cell carcinoma.

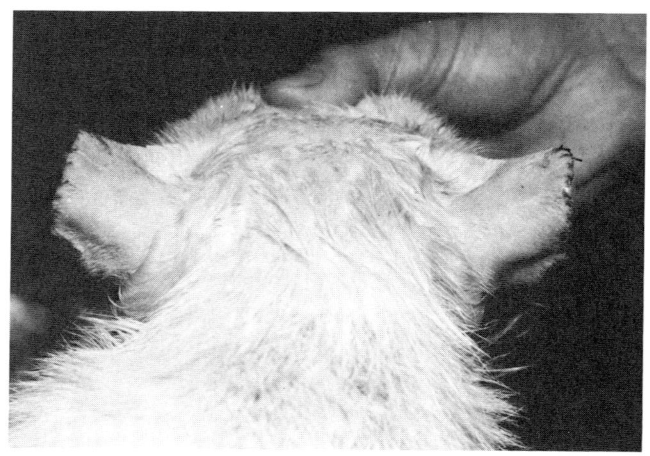

Figure 55–11. The affected tissue has been removed surgically from both ears, as seen in this posterior view. The ears are made as symmetrical as possible to achieve the best cosmetic result.

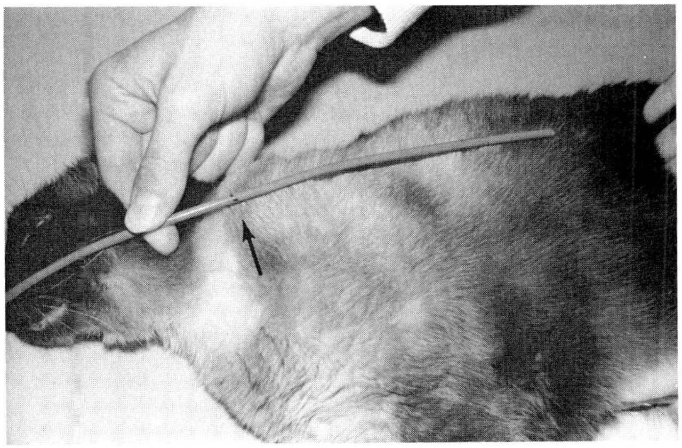

A

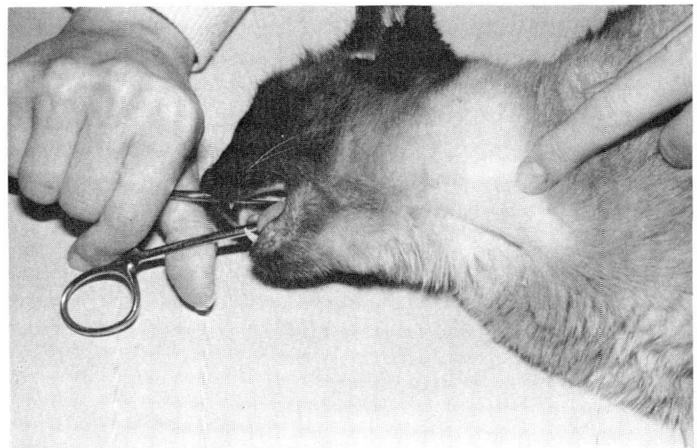

B

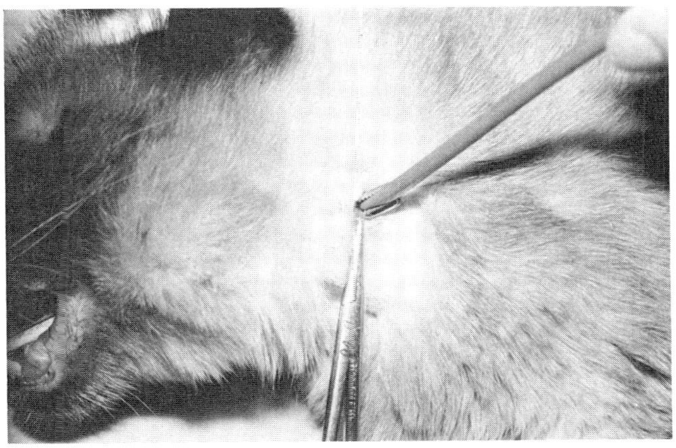

C

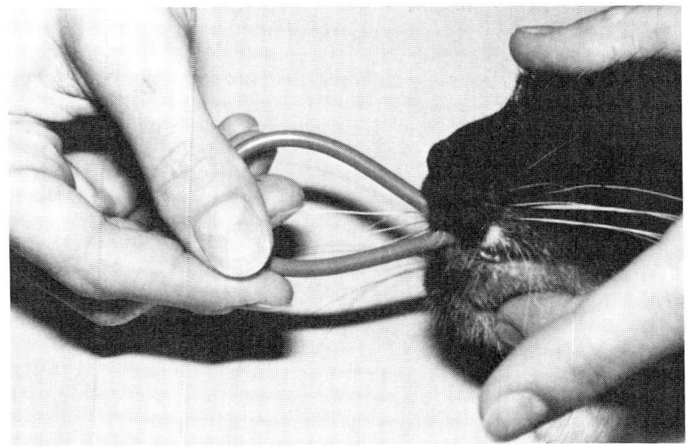

D

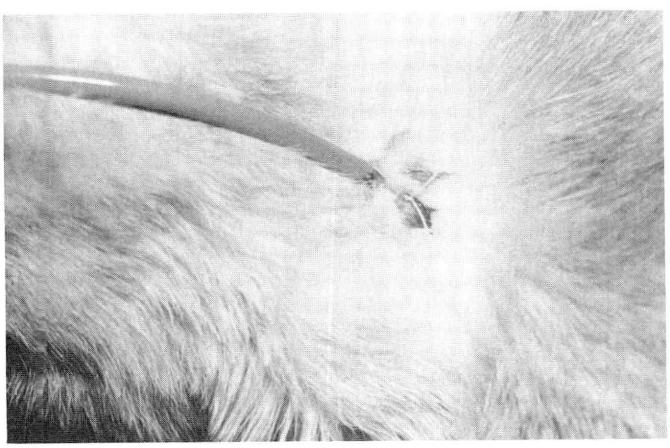

E

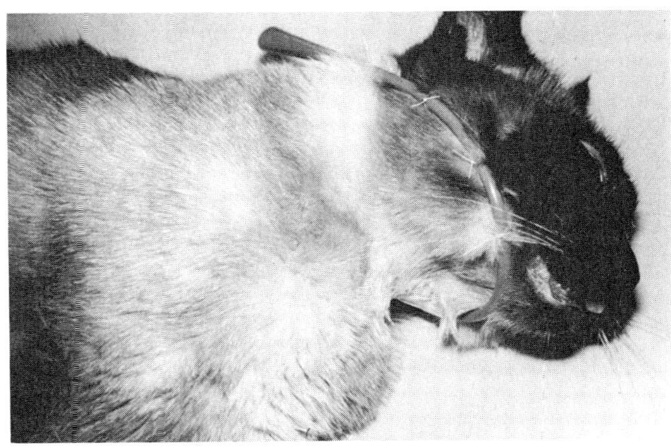

F

Figure 55–12. (*A*) Before placement of an esophagostomy tube, a mark is made on the tube (*arrow*) to identify the point at which it should enter the skin. The location of the caudal end of the tube should be in the mid to caudal third of the esophagus. The fingers seen on the right side of this picture are adjacent to the last ribs. (*B*) A curved 5-inch hemostat is passed through the pharynx and down the esophagus. The surgeon in this picture is pointing to its tips, which are directed laterally in the left cervical esophagus. (*C*) A nick incision is made in the skin and esophagus over the tip of the hemostat. The tips of the hemostat are forced through the incisions and are used to grasp the distal end of the tube. (*D*) The tube exits the mouth, is turned 180°, and is passed down the esophagus. (*E*) A pursestring suture is placed around the tube at the point where it enters the skin. Note the previously placed mark on the tube. (*F*) The tube is sutured to the skin in several places as it passes under the chin and behind the right ear. (*A–F* used by permission of Veterinary Medicine Publishing Co., Lenexa, KS.)

- After anesthetizing the cat, insert the hemostat through the mouth into the cranial esophagus. Push the tips of the hemostat laterally to the left to identify the point of insertion of the feeding tube (Fig. 55–12*B*).
- Make a nick incision in the skin and the esophagus over the point of the forceps.
- Push the forceps through the skin incision and use the instrument to grasp the distal end of the feeding tube (Fig. 55–12*C*).
- Pull the distal end of the tube out of the mouth, cut off the distal end to remove the side ports, and turn it 180° (Fig. 55–12*D*).
- Push the distal end of the tube back through the oral cavity into the esophagus and pass the distal one third of it according to the mark on the tube. Do not place it in the stomach.
- Place a pursestring suture around the tube at the point where it enters the skin (Fig. 55–12*E*).
- Pass the proximal end of the feeding tube under the chin, up the right side of the face, and behind the right ear.
- Secure the tube to the skin at several points along the tube's path using individual nonabsorbable sutures (Fig. 55–12*F*).
- Further secure the tube to the cat by placing a bandage around the neck.
- When the tube is not being used for feeding, place a plug from an IV catheter in the proximal end of the tube.

Removal of the esophagostomy tube begins with the removal of the bandage and sutures. The tube is then pulled out of the esophagus and the opening is allowed to granulate. Esophageal stricture has not been a complication.[11]

Results

Placement of an esophageal tube allows periodic administration of a strained, blenderized diet which, as described in Chapter 5, is formulated to meet an individual cat's nutritional requirements. Following feeding, the tube should be flushed with 5 to 10 mL of water so that it does not become obstructed. This tube does not interfere with the cat's ability to eat, so the point at which the cat's appetite returns will be readily evident and the tube can be removed at that time.

Frontal Sinus Obliteration

Various procedures have been used to treat chronic infection of the frontal sinuses. Trephining the sinuses and flushing them with antibacterial solutions, either with or without the aid of surgically implanted drainage tubes, have been attempted, but have produced poor results.[12] By contrast, obliteration of the frontal sinuses with an autogenous fat graft has proven effective in the hands of some surgeons.[13] Other researchers have added an ethmoid turbinectomy to this procedure, also with reportedly good results.[14] A modification of the sinus obliteration procedure has been used successfully by this author. This procedure is technically easier to perform than the others mentioned because the frontal sinuses are filled with self-curing polymethyl methacrylate bone cement (PMMA) (Kerr Formatray, Sybron/Kerr, Romulus, MI). An antibiotic that has been added to the PMMA is slowly released for as long as 2 years following surgery as a form of continuous medical therapy[15] (see Chapter 30).

Surgical Technique

The modified sinus obliteration procedure is performed as follows:

- Administer a combination of ketamine and diazepam or an ultra–short-acting barbiturate to induce anesthesia. The anesthetic effect is then maintained with isoflurane (AErrane) or halothane (Fluothane) through a non-rebreathing system.
- Clip and prep the dorsal surface of the head for aseptic surgery.
- Place the cat in sternal recumbency with its head resting on a folded towel or sandbag; secure the head in position by taping it to the surgery table.
- Make a skin incision on a line 2 to 3 cm caudal and parallel to a line drawn between the lateral canthi of the eyes. The skin is then undermined and retracted cranially and caudally to expose the underlying bone.
- Incise the periosteum and retract it as far cranially and caudally as possible in the same plane as the skin incision.
- Drill into the left frontal sinus a 16-gauge bone marrow biopsy needle with stylet or, alternatively, an intramedullary pin (1/16 inch in diameter) in a pin chuck. Insert it just off the midline, midway between the medial canthus of the left eye and the medial attachment of the left pinna.
- Drill a second hole immediately adjacent to and lateral to the first.
- Using a fine-tipped Lempert rongeur, open the left frontal sinus. Take small "bites" of bone until almost all of the roof of the sinus is removed (Fig. 55–13*A*). A small lip of bone is left to contain the implant so that it cannot be displaced from the sinus. No attempt is made to preserve a bone flap for reattachment.
- Collect purulent material from the sinus on a sterile cotton-tipped applicator for bacterial culture (Fig. 55–13*B*). (No antibiotics should be administered for at least 3 days prior to surgery so that culture results will be accurate.) Hemostatic forceps, cotton-tipped applicators, and thumb forceps may be used for removal of the purulent material from the sinus.
- The mucoperiosteal lining of the sinus is removed by scraping it with cotton-tipped applicators, gauze sponges grasped with hemostats, and/or a small bone curette. Additionally, a light liquid nitrogen spray can be used to remove the sinus lining. No attempt is made to remove the inner cortical layer of bone, as is done in the fat graft procedure.
- Pack the sinus temporarily with gauze to control hemorrhage (Fig. 55–13*C*).
- Open, clean, and strip the right frontal sinus in a similar fashion. It, too, is then temporarily packed with gauze.
- When both sinuses are thus prepared, instruct a techni-

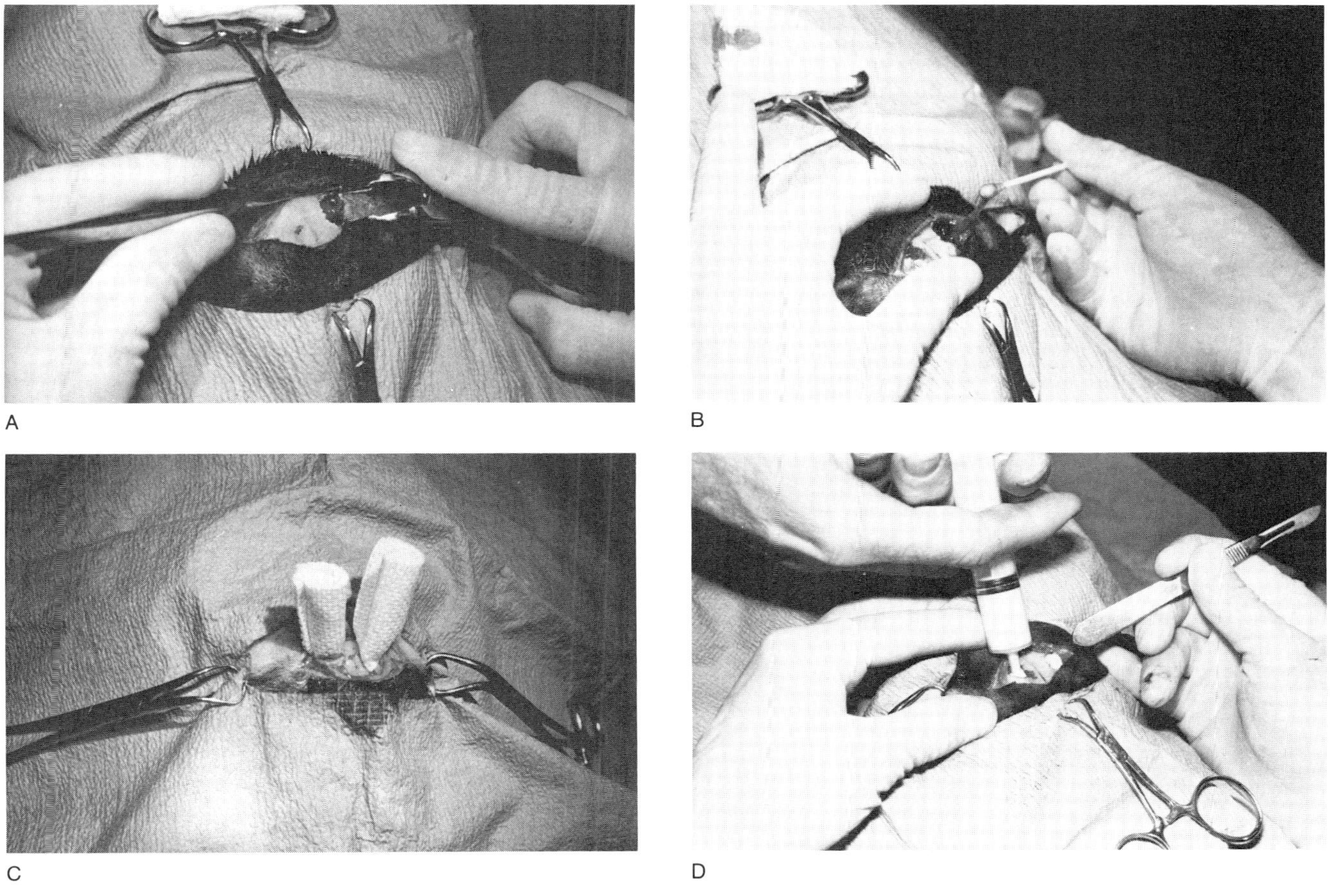

Figure 55–13. (*A*) In frontal sinus obliteration, after the initial holes are made with a 16-gauge bone marrow biopsy needle or a 1/16-inch intramedullary pin, rongeurs are used to remove the bone from the dorsal surface of the frontal sinus. (*B*) Material is collected from the frontal sinus for culture and sensitivity studies. The remainder of the purulent material is removed with cotton-tipped applicators and gauze. (*C*) Rolls of gauze are packed in the frontal sinuses while the PMMA is being prepared. (*D*) The frontal sinuses are filled with PMMA. Care is taken to make the dorsal surface of the PMMA conform to the normal contour of the cat's skull. The handle of a scalpel can be useful in accomplishing this.

cian to prepare PMMA for instillation in the sinuses. Gentamicin (Gentocin) is mixed with the PMMA at a ratio of 1 g of gentamicin to 40 g of PMMA polymer.[16] Gentocin (325 mg) is added to the PMMA powder (polymer) and mixed. (A 12-mL syringe case can be used to measure the correct amount of powder. Two inches of powder in the closed end of the syringe case are approximately 13 g. To this is added the 325 mg of Gentocin.) The PMMA liquid is then added to make a thick paste. The paste is then placed in a 12-mL syringe.

- Remove the packing material from the left sinus and fill the sinus with PMMA, taking care to fill all the crevices in the sinus (Fig. 55–13*D*). Be sure to make the dorsal surface of the PMMA conform smoothly to the contour of the skull. (Because of the viscosity of the PMMA, it is unlikely that a significant amount will pass through the nasofrontal opening into the nasal cavity.)
- Fill the right frontal sinus with PMMA using a similar technique.
- Once the PMMA hardens, pull as much periosteum as possible over it. Make a similar attempt to close a layer of subcutaneous tissue.
- Close the skin with 4-0 absorbable suture material using a subcuticular pattern.

Results

An antibiotic effective against *Pseudomonas aeruginosa,* such as gentamicin or enrofloxacin (Baytril), should be administered to the cat immediately following surgery and until the bacterial culture results are known. The cat should be interested in eating within 12 to 48 hours following surgery, and should be ready for discharge at that time. Subcutaneous emphysema should not be a problem owing to the closure of the frontal sinuses with PMMA. An appropriate antibiotic should be administered for 2 weeks following surgery. Because the gentamicin that leaches from the PMMA will also drain through the nasal turbinates, this procedure may eliminate the need for nasal surgery. However, if the nasal discharge continues, turbinectomy should be considered. Alternatively, both procedures may be performed at the same time.

The only significant complication that has been reported has been a draining fistula over the PMMA implant. This has occurred 2 weeks to 6 months postoperatively. Bacterial cultures have either been negative or have revealed organisms not recovered from the sinuses. The discharge generally lasts 1 to 2 weeks before stopping spontaneously. There have been no long-term sequelae associated with such fistulas.

Ischiocavernosus Myectomy

Spraying by neutered male cats can be a very frustrating problem. Although some of these cats can be managed by behavior modification techniques or progesterone compounds, others cannot and often are euthanatized. Ischiocavernosus myectomy offers another alternative.[17]

Spraying must be differentiated from inappropriate urination. Spraying means that urine is squirted horizontally, generally on a vertical object, such as a wall. Inappropriate urination means that the cat is squatting and urinating vertically onto a horizontal surface, generally a floor. This procedure is not indicated for inappropriate urination.

Surgical Technique

The procedure for an ischiocavernosus myectomy involves the following steps:

- Make a 2- to 3-cm vertical skin incision 1 cm lateral to the scrotum. The center of the incision should be at the level of the dorsum of the scrotum..
- Expose the ischiocavernosus muscle by blunt dissection and clamp two straight Halstead hemostats across the muscle.
- After allowing a few minutes for hemostasis, transect the muscle in two places between the hemostats so that a small section can be removed. This prevents subsequent reattachment.
- Close the dead space with a few sutures and then close the incision using two layers of sutures, one in the subcutaneous tissue and one in the skin.
- Repeat the procedure on the contralateral side.

Results

In the author's experience, the cats undergoing this operation have not stopped spraying completely. However, in all cases, the owner has reported a 90+% reduction in spraying activity by the cat. Even though this procedure is not 100% effective, it is an alternative that should be offered, especially in light of the alternatives, which often includes euthanasia.

Repair of Mandibular Symphysis Separation

One of the most common head injuries suffered by cats is a separation of the mandibular symphysis. This frequently occurs without concomitant fractures.

Surgical Technique

Several methods of repair have been used by veterinary surgeons to correct a separation of the mandibular symphysis,[18] including the use of an encircling nylon band.[19] This author prefers using an encircling stainless steel orthopedic wire to achieve the desired result. The procedure for the latter is as follows:

- Administer anesthesia to the cat.
- Thread 12 to 18 inches of 20-gauge stainless steel into a No. 10 or No. 12 cutting edge needle, placing the middle of the suture material at the level of the eye of the needle.
- Insert the needle into the gingiva immediately lateral to the left lower canine tooth (Fig. 55–14*A*). It should be passed as close to the mandible as possible so that it goes ventral to the left mandible and ventral to the right mandible, exiting lateral to the right lower canine tooth (Fig. 55–14*B*).
- Cut the suture at the eye of the needle to create two individual sutures (Fig. 55–14*C*).
- Reduce the mandibular symphysis separation. Tighten one suture by twisting the wire just caudal to the right lower canine tooth; the other is then tightened in a similar fashion near the left lower canine tooth (Fig. 55–14*D*).
- Cut short the ends of the sutures and bend them in a position that minimizes the risk of lacerating the tongue and lips (Fig. 55–14*E*).
- Remove the wire in 3 to 4 weeks.
- If adequate stabilization is not achieved with this method, place a stainless steel pin across the symphysis.

Nylon Bands for Ligation or Fracture Fixation

Self-locking nylon bands provide a rapid and secure means of ligating tissues[20] or fixating selected fractures. The bands have an integral locking clasp and are available in several lengths. They are marketed for a number of nonmedical uses; indeed, they are often sold at electronic stores as cable ties. As long as the bands are 100% nylon, they should be nonreactive to tissue. Some brands have a small piece of metal in the latch; these are not acceptable. Over the last 12 years, the author and his associates have used more than 10,000 of the bands marketed by Radio Shack (Nylon Wire Ties, 4.1 inches, Tandy Corporation, Ft. Worth, TX) in his practice with no incidences of local or systemic reactions.

The bands are placed around the affected tissues, the latch is engaged, and the band is tightened with forceps or a needle holder. The excess band is cut as close to the latch as possible. The bands should not be used on individual

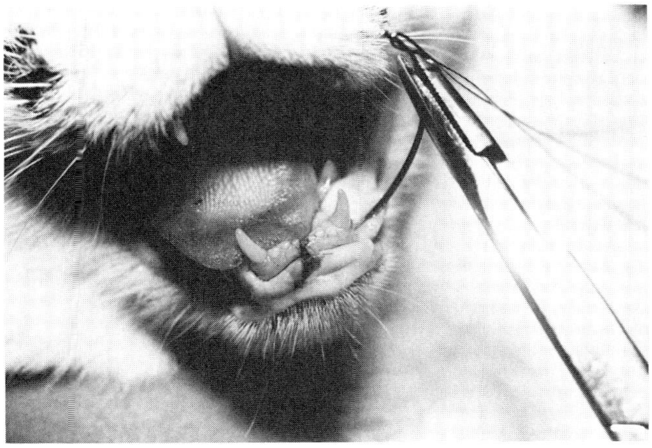

A

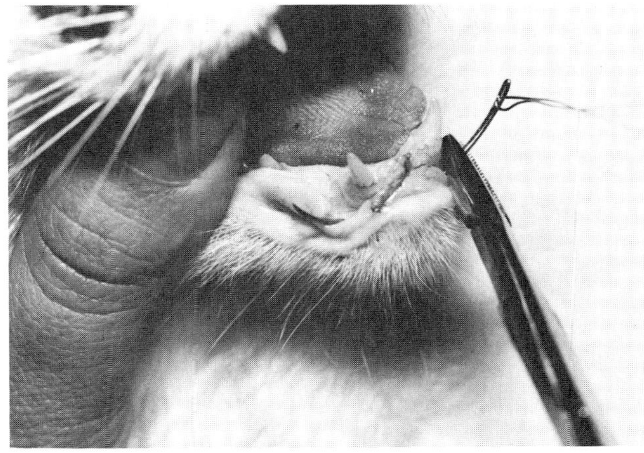

B

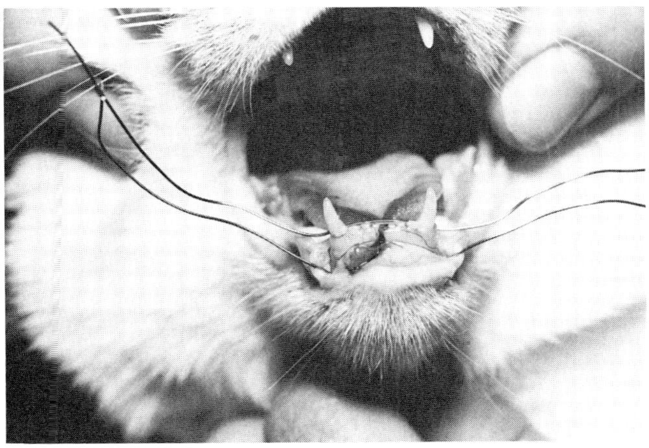

C

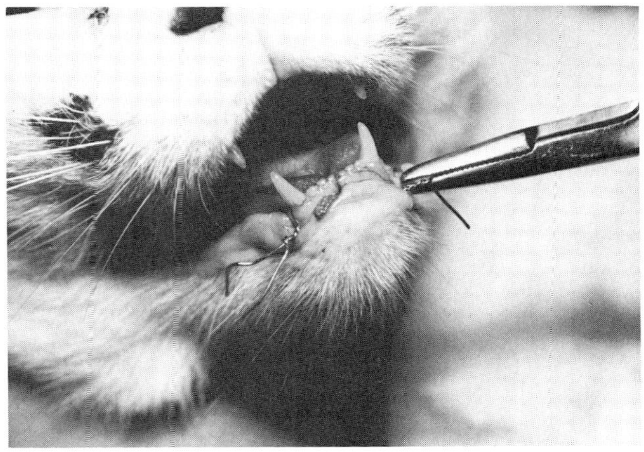

D

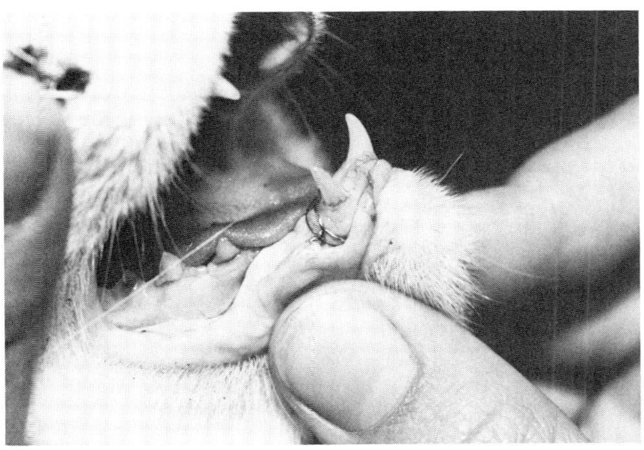

E

Figure 55–14. (*A*) Repair of a separated mandibular symphysis using a No. 10 or No. 12 cutting edge needle and 20-gauge stainless steel wire. The needle should penetrate the gingiva immediately lateral to the left lower canine tooth. (*B*) The needle is passed as close to the mandible as possible so that it goes ventral to the left mandible and ventral to the right mandible, exiting near the right lower canine tooth. (*C*) The suture is cut at the eye of the needle to create two individual sutures. The dorsal wire has encircled the mandible and its ends are crossed behind the incisors. (*D*) The separation of the mandibular symphysis has been reduced. One suture is tightened by twisting the wire just caudal to the right lower canine tooth; the other is similarly tightened near the left lower canine tooth. (*E*) The ends of the sutures are cut short and bent in a position that minimizes the risk of lacerating the tongue and lips.

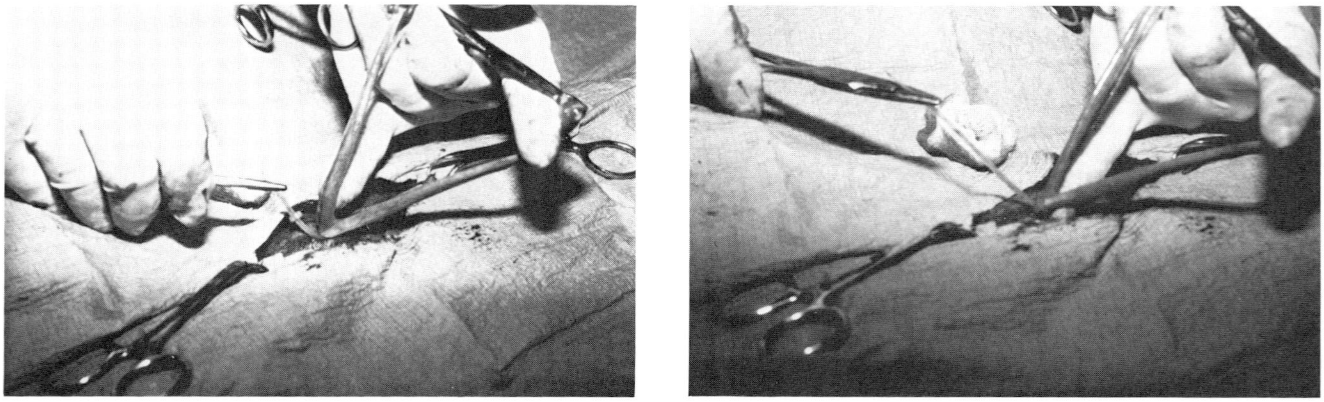

A B

Figure 55–15. (*A*) The nylon band is placed around the uterine stump and the clamp enlarged. (*B*) The nylon is pulled tightly around the uterine stump. Care is taken to prevent cutting through the tissue.

vessels. Their greatest holding power occurs when adjacent soft tissue is included.

Indications

The author has used these bands in the following situations:

- Ligation of the uterine stump for routine ovariohysterectomy (OHE) or ovariohysterectomy in pregnant cats (Fig. 55–15, *A* and *B*)
- Ligation of the uterine stump for pyometra (in which case the cut end of the uterine stump should be sutured closed)
- Mass ligation of the splenic vasculature for splenectomy
- Hepatic lobectomy
- Pulmonary lobectomy
- Selected fracture repair
- Rib apposition for thoracic closure

Adverse Reactions and Complications

There are two potential complications that should be noted. If the bands are applied too tightly, the tissue may be lacerated. This is especially true in tissues that are inherently friable (e.g., liver tissue) or tissues that are friable as a result of disease (e.g., the uterus when pyometra is present). Second, if the band is applied too close to the point of transection, the band is likely to slip off the tissue. This occurs most frequently when tissues, such as the uterine stump, are involved.

There has been one report of band migration into the retroperitoneal space resulting in a granuloma.[21] This is apparently a very unusual occurrence, and probably would not have occurred if the band had been applied properly.

When these bands have been used in fracture repair, there has been concern about possible adverse effects to the periosteum and its vasculature. One physician developed a band with an irregular inner surface so that contact with the periosteum would be limited. When tested against smooth bands, it was found that neither caused periosteal problems. Additionally it was found that the smooth bands stretch enough to prevent damage.[22]

Because of the size of the clasp, it is best not to apply the bands close to the skin, as might be likely when the bands are used for long bone fracture repair. Either the clasp should be placed near a soft tissue mass, such as a muscle belly, or another form of immobilization should be chosen.

The bands are autoclavable. They may be autoclaved several times without losing strength, although they may become slightly discolored. The author's general surgery packs contain several. Any that are not used remain in the pack when it is autoclaved for future use.

Onychectomy (Declawing)

Surgical onychectomy is commonly performed to minimize the damage done by cats to furniture, drapes, and the like. Although many breeders and cat fanciers are philosophically opposed to this procedure for a variety of reasons, one report has demonstrated no adverse behavioral effects in cats undergoing this surgery.[23]

Surgical Technique

This procedure has been performed in a variety of ways by various veterinary surgeons. The views concerning the following issues are likely to differ from one surgeon to the next:

1. Placement of the tourniquet (above or below the elbow or just above the carpus)
2. Degree of presurgical prepping of the feet (ranging from clipping and full prep to no preparation)
3. Type of cutting instrument (scalpel, scissor-type nail trimmer, or guillotine-type nail trimmer)
4. Removal of the dorsal lip of the ungual crest of P3
5. Skin closure (several interrupted sutures per toe versus no sutures versus closure with surgical glue)
6. Duration of bandaging (18 hours to 3 days)
7. Bandaging pattern and materials

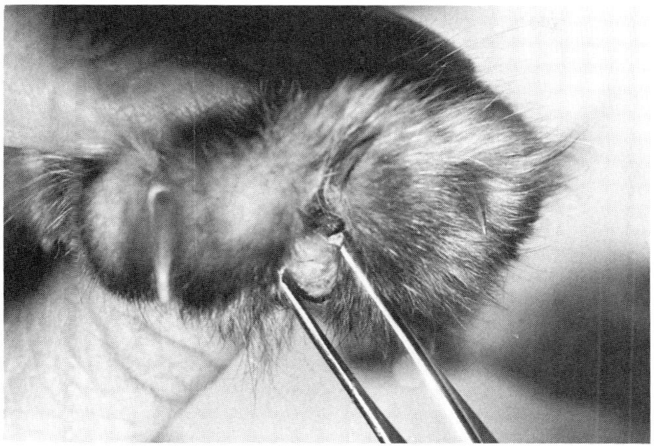

Figure 55–16. In onychectomy, the trimmers are used to cut P3 in such a way as to leave the dorsal lip of the ungual crest intact and to expose the distal end of P2, located between the tips of the forceps. Failure to remove any less than this often results in regrowth of the nail.

The following is the procedure that has been used by the author for many years:

- Anesthetize the cat.
- Apply a rubber band/hemostat tourniquet just below the elbow or just above the carpus.
- Cut the nail to about ½ its length with sterile, scissor-type nail trimmers.
- Extend the nail by applying dorsally directed pressure on the digital pad.
- Use the trimmers to cut P3 in such a way as to leave the dorsal lip of the ungual crest intact and to expose the distal end of P2 (Fig. 55–16). Failure to remove any less than this will often result in regrowth of the nail. Care should be taken to ensure that no part of the digital pad is cut. If this occurs, postoperative pain will persist for several days.
- For adult cats, place a single 4-0 absorbable suture in the skin; kittens younger than 6 months of age are not sutured.
- Apply a bandage so that pressure is directed ventrally over the ends of the toes (Fig. 55–17). The bandage is composed of a layer of soft roll gauze over which a stretchy material (Vet Wrap, Animal Care Products/3M, St. Paul, MN), and adhesive tape are applied. Leave the bandage in place for 18 to 24 hours.
- When the bandage is removed, observe the cat for bleeding for a period of 3 to 6 hours. If bleeding occurs, rebandage the feet for another 18 to 24 hours. The cat may be discharged when no bleeding occurs for 3 to 6 hours following bandage removal.

The owner should be instructed to place strips of newspaper or aquarium gravel in the litter box for 2 to 3 days. These cats should be, or should become, indoor-only pets; however, if they do go outside, their ability to climb trees is not significantly impaired, although they may have difficulty descending gracefully.

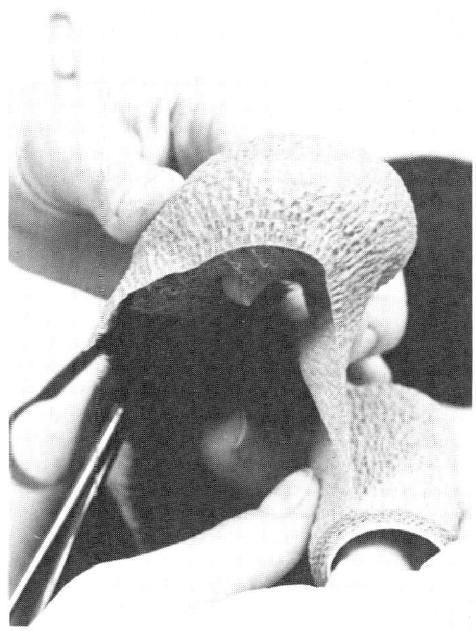

Figure 55–17. When a bandage is applied, its pressure should be directed ventrally, over the end of the toes, to minimize hemorrhage.

Perineal Urethrostomy

Prior to the discovery of effective urinary acidifiers and the development of acidified diets, a large number of cats experienced repeated urethral obstructions. Indeed, in the author's first practice experience in 1972—a feline-only practice—cats with FUS were treated almost every hour of the day. Many of these cats experienced as many as eight urethral obstructions. When a successful perineal urethrostomy technique was developed,[24,25] the author and associates began operating on these repeatedly obstructed cats. For more than 1 year, the author averaged two perineal urethrostomies per week. Because of this extensive experience with this surgical procedure, the author has a perspective not shared by most surgeons trained following the advent of effective acidifiers and prophylactic diets.

Surgical Technique

The purpose of perineal urethrostomy is to remove the narrowed, distal urethra, thereby eliminating the bottleneck at which almost all urethral plugs lodge. If properly performed, the cat should not experience another urethral obstruction except under exceptional circumstances. In order to remove the distal urethra and attach the urethra to the skin so that it functions properly, the entire lower urinary tract should be transplanted about 1 to 2 cm caudally. This requires freeing the structures that support the entire length of the urethra, as a failure to do so may result in several postoperative complications. Following surgery, the new urethral opening will be located 1 to 2 cm dorsal to the original opening. Once healed, the cat should have a large-diameter stream of urine.

The steps involved in this surgical procedure are as follows:

- Anesthetize the cat and prep the perineal area. If the cat is long-haired, the hair on the ventral surface of the tail that may come in contact with the incision postoperatively is also clipped.
- Place the cat in ventral recumbency with its tail pulled cranially out of the surgical field. Some surgeons prefer to position the cat in dorsal recumbency. This is a matter of personal choice; this author has tried both and prefers ventral recumbency.
- Place a pursestring suture around the anus.
- Place a urinary catheter (Sovereign 3.5-French Tom Cat Catheter, Sherwood Medical, St. Louis, MO) in the urethra so that the urethra can be identified when it is split.
- Make an elliptical incision beginning just below the anus to include the scrotum and prepuce (Fig. 55–18, *A* and *B*). The lateral aspects of the incision should be about 0.5 cm from the scrotum and prepuce. (The importance of this will be discussed in the section entitled Complications.)
- Bluntly dissect the tissues connected to the urethra and transect them free.
- Identify the retractor penis muscle on the dorsal surface of the urethra and transect it (Fig. 55–18*C*).
- Expose the ischiocavernosus muscles as they attach to the urethra just caudal to the bulbourethral glands (Fig. 55–18*D*).
- Force one blade of a small hemostatic forceps ventral to the muscle belly, and place the other blade dorsal to the muscle (Fig. 55–18*E*)
- Close the blades of the hemostatic forceps.
- Place another forceps parallel to the first and close it.
- After 1 minute of pressure from the forceps, transect the muscle between the two forceps. Leave the medial forceps in place for about 5 minutes to prevent bleeding from the vessels within the muscle belly.
- Crush and transect the other ischiocavernosus muscle in a similar manner.
- With the ischiocavernosus muscles transected, additional periurethral blunt dissection is possible. When further tissue dissection lateral and dorsal to the urethra is completed, lift the distal urethra dorsally. This will allow you to place the index finger ventral to the urethra and force the finger cranially along the pubic symphysis (Fig. 55–18*F*).
- With the urethra free of its ventral attachments, complete the dissection of the dorsal and lateral attachments. This dissection frees the urethra from its intrapelvic attachments and allows the urethra and bladder to be transplanted caudally about 1 to 2 cm.
- Dissect the scrotum and prepuce away from the penile urethra.
- Grasp the penis with a forceps. Note the relation of the dorsal aspect of the urethra to the forceps, as this orientation is essential to splitting the urethra on its dorsal midline.
- Insert a sharp-pointed (No. 11) scalpel blade into the penile urethra lateral to the catheter, with the sharp side of the blade directed dorsally (Fig. 55–18*G*). Advance the scalpel blade into the urethra so that the urethra is split dorsally (Fig. 55–18*H*). (Note: Some surgeons prefer to use iris scissors instead of the scalpel blade.)
- When the urethra has been split approximately 2 cm, replace the urethral catheter with a similar catheter that is only 4 to 5 cm long (Fig. 55–18*I*). (A catheter is cut to the desired length. After being cut, the distal end is passed through a flame so any sharp edges are rounded.)
- Continue the incision in the urethra until an increased urethral diameter is encountered. One can determine this when the urethral diameter is about equal to the largest diameter of the catheter, although this point is generally at or just cranial to the level of the bulbourethral glands (Fig. 55–18, *J* and *K*). If adequate dissection of the urethra has been achieved, it will be possible to align the point of increased urethral diameter with the normal skin contour without significant cranial traction on the urethra. This is essential in preventing one of the causes of postoperative invagination of the urethra opening and the surrounding skin.
- The first three sutures are the most critical in facilitating proper healing of the urethral : skin junction. Place the first suture, composed of a soft suture material, such as 4-0 or 5-0 Vicryl (Ethicon, Inc. Somerville, NJ), so that it joins the skin immediately dorsal to the new urethral opening (Fig. 55–18*L*). This location should align horizontally with the pubic symphysis. Place the second and third sutures so they attach the urethral mucosa (only) to the skin at the 1:00 and 11:00 positions (Fig. 55–18 *M* and *N*). Place the subsequent sutures ventral to the second and third ones, alternating between the sides of the urethra. Care should be taken to suture the urethral mucosa, without adjacent tissue, to the skin to ensure first intention healing (Fig. 55–18*O*).
- When about a 2-cm section of urethra has been attached to the skin, transect the urethra.
- Suture the skin edges ventral to that point (Fig. 55–18*P*) and dorsal to the new urethral opening (Fig. 55–18*Q*).
- Place one-fourth of a piece of Surgicel (Johnson and Johnson Products, Inc., New Brunswick, NJ) over the exposed urethra to encourage hemostasis.
- Remove the pursestring suture from the anus.
- Place an Elizabethan collar on the cat for 3 days.

Complications

A number of complications have been noted to be associated with perineal urethrostomy.[26] These include immediate postoperative hemorrhage and subcutaneous urine leakage, wound dehiscence, urinary and fecal incontinence, perineal hernia, dysuria and hematuria, urinary tract infection, and future obstructions secondary to strictures or calculi. This author has never encountered most of these; some are described by various authors as rare or transient. The results of a recent study on intrapelvic dissection techniques revealed that extensive blunt intrapelvic dissection had no effect on urinary incontinence and that identification of the

(*Text continues on page 496*)

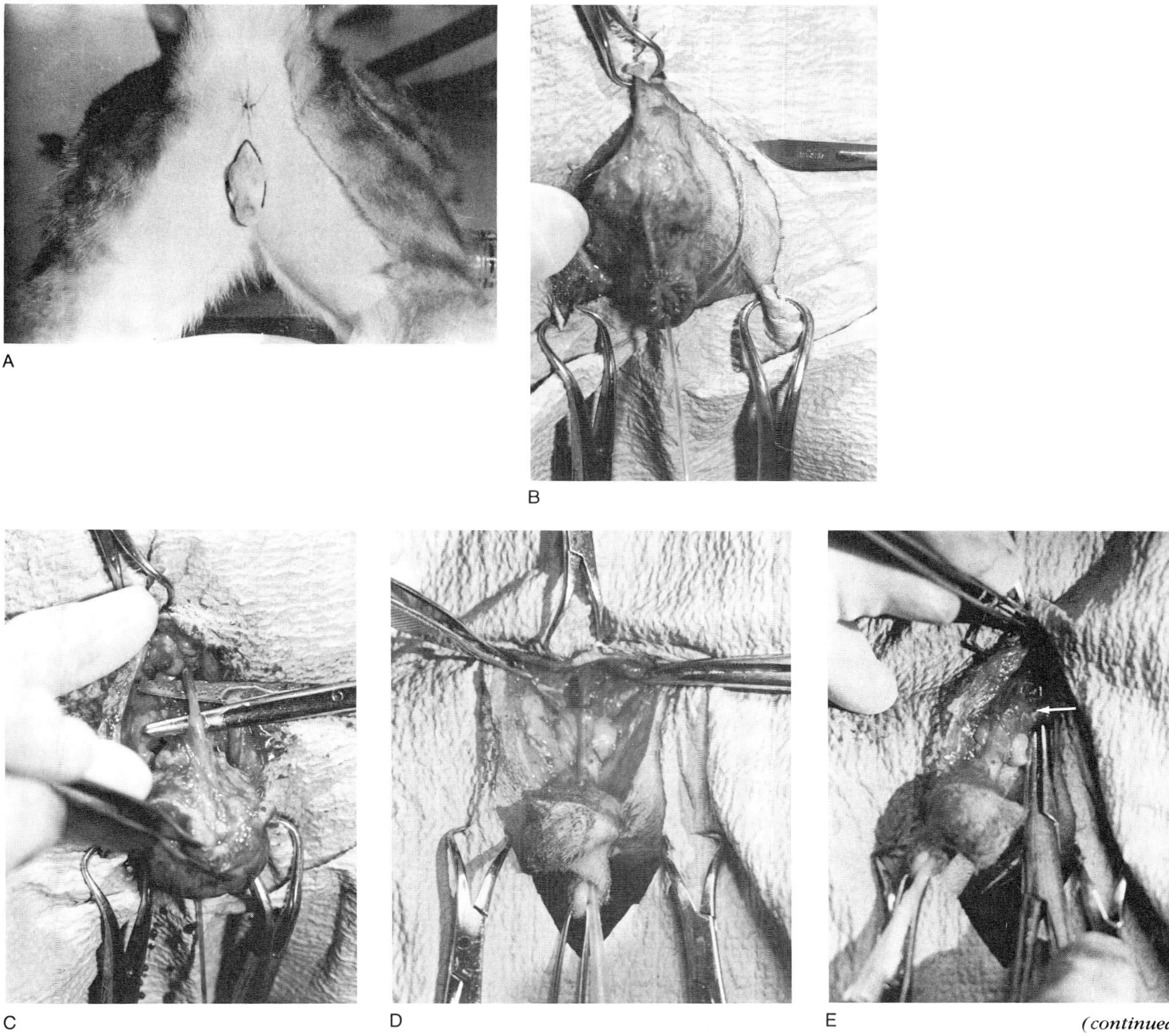

(continued)

Figure 55–18. (*A*) In a perineal urethrostomy, a pursestring suture closes the anus so that fecal material will not contaminate the surgical site. The incision should be made lateral to the dark line around the scrotum and prepuce. (*B*) The skin incision is made 1 to 2 mm lateral to the scrotum and prepuce. If this incision were made along the lines seen in Figure 55–15*A*, postoperative invagination of the urethral opening would be likely to occur. (*C*) The retractor penis muscle, which lies on the dorsal surface of the urethra, should be isolated and transected. (*D*) The isochiocavernosus muscles (*arrows*) should be identified and isolated. (*E*) A small hemostat is forced ventral to the ischiocavernosus muscle belly (*arrow*). This frees the muscle from its ventral attachments and allows the surgeon to clamp the blades of the hemostat across the muscle belly.

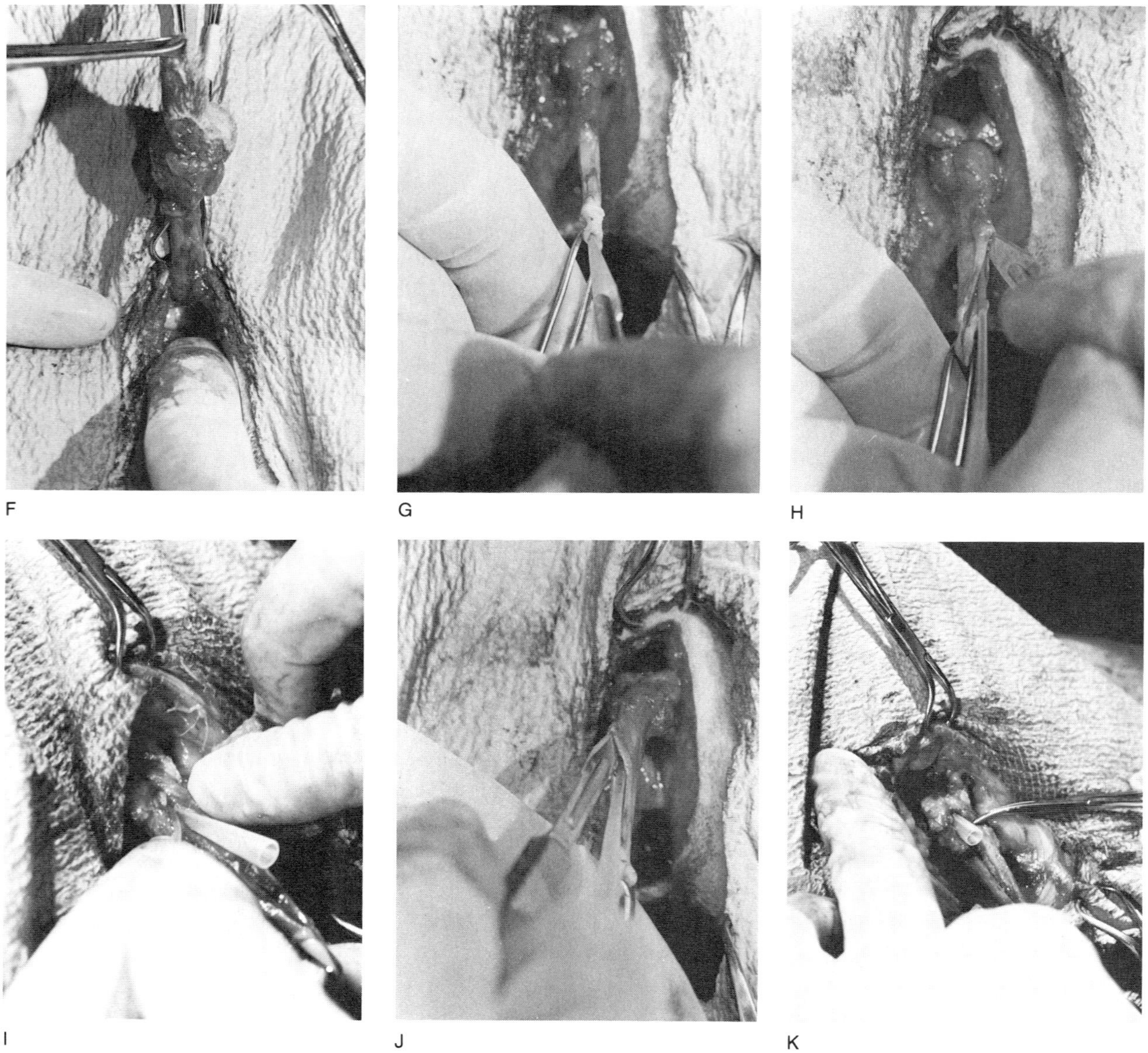

Figure 55–18 (continued). (*F*) The distal urethra is lifted dorsally. This allows the surgeon to place the index finger ventral to the urethra and force the finger cranially along the pubic symphysis, thereby freeing the urethra from its ventral attachments. (*G*) The scrotum and prepuce are dissected away from the penile urethra. The ventral surface of the penis is grasped with a hemostat. A sharp-pointed No. 11 scalpel blade is inserted into the penile urethra lateral to the catheter, with the cutting edge of the blade directed dorsally. (*H*) The scalpel blade is advanced into the urethra so that the urethra is split dorsally. (*I*) When the urethra has been split approximately 2 cm, the urethral catheter is replaced with a similar catheter that is only 4–5 cm long. The short catheter is placed in the urethra before the long one is removed. (*J*) The incision is continued on the midline over the short catheter. (*K*) The urethral incision is continued until an increased urethral diameter is encountered. The incision is completed when the urethral diameter is about equal to the largest diameter of the catheter. This point is generally at or just cranial to the level of the bulbourethral glands.

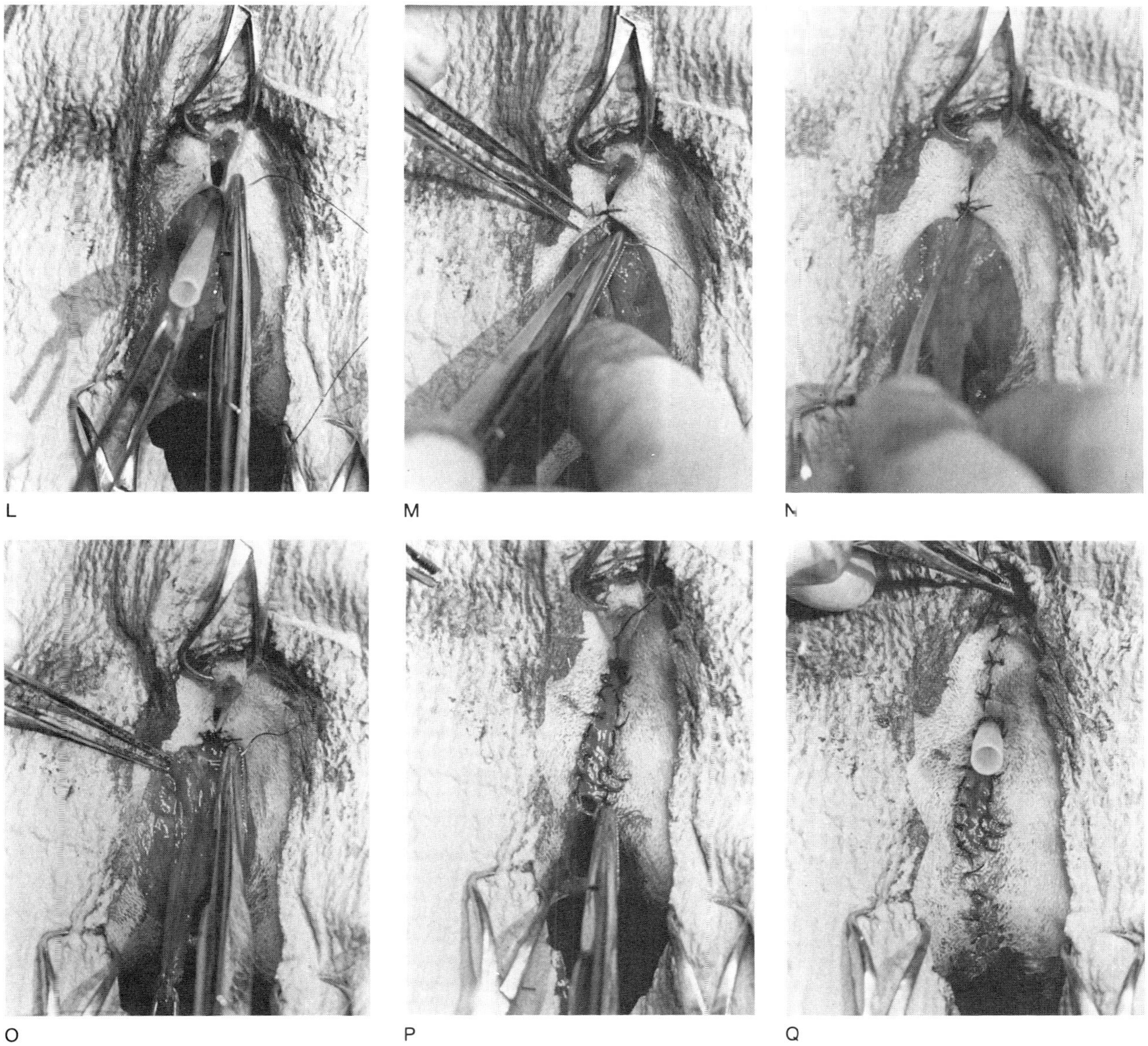

Figure 55–18 (continued). (*L*) The first suture should join the skin (only) immediately dorsal to the new urethral opening. This location should align horizontally with the pubic symphysis. (*M*) The second suture should attach the urethral mucosa to the skin at the 1:00 or 11:00 position. The needle is passed through the urethral mucosa, but not through the musculature surrounding it. (*N*) The first three sutures have been placed. Their proper placement is critical in preventing stricturing of the new urethral opening. (*O*) Subsequent sutures should be placed ventral to the second and third ones, alternating between the sides of the urethra. Only the urethral mucosa, without adjacent tissue, is grasped with the needle. (*P*) After suturing about 2 cm of the urethra to the skin, the urethra is transected horizontally. The skin is joined ventral to that point. Some surgeons advocate including the distal end of the urethra in this suture, closing the cavernous tissue and thus making it less likely to bleed postoperatively. (*Q*) The skin is sutured ventral and dorsal to the new urethral opening. If the flared end of a urethral catheter can be inserted into the new urethral opening and if minimal tension is exerted on the urethra proximally, the surgery should prove successful.

pudendal nerve branches during surgery was not required so long as there was not extensive dissection near the neck of the bladder.[27]

There are two complications, however—bacterial cystitis and urolithiasis—that are significant and need to be addressed. Normally, cats are extremely resistant to bacterial cystitis. This resistance is undoubtedly attributable to several factors, including an effective set of host defenses associated with the curvilinear and tapered urethra. Removal of the curved, tapered part of the urethra compromises some of the urethra's bacteria-resistant properties. Therefore, cats undergoing perineal urethrostomy have a significant incidence of bacterial cystitis. One study found that 23% of cats having a perineal urethrostomy had positive urine cultures within 2 years of surgery.[28] This incidence far exceeds that found in cats with FUS that have not undergone a perineal urethrostomy (3%). Many of these cats also have a very alkaline urine and tend to lick the perineal urethrostomy site intensely. The exposed part of the urethra may experience urine scalding, accounting for the intense pain and subsequent licking. (Interestingly, another study confirmed the increased incidence of bacterial cystitis in cats with a history of FUS and perineal urethrostomy but no such incidence in cats with no history of FUS.[29])

It is rare for the male cat to develop the large uroliths occasionally seen in female cats. However, this resistance, too, is decreased in some cats undergoing perineal urethrostomy. Most of these uroliths are associated with bacterial infections, especially those attributable to *Staphylococcus* species.

Some of the complications associated with perineal urethrostomy are technique-related. The author offers the following suggestions to the surgeon:

1. One of the reasons for postoperative hemorrhage is failure to provide adequate hemostasis where the ischiocavernosus muscles are transected from the urethra. This can be accomplished without ligatures if a small hemostat is left on the muscle belly several minutes prior to transection, and on the medial muscle stump for several minutes thereafter.

   Another cause of hemorrhage is failure to ligate the subcutaneous vessels supplying the scrotum and prepuce. Although proper hemostasis is important, some cats may experience substantial postoperative bleeding; in the author's experience, however, no cat has had bleeding which became more than a cosmetic problem for 1 to 2 days. If hemorrhage occurs, one should not be too hasty in removing the clots that form; rather, it is best to leave them for a few days and let the cat remove them.
2. The use of an Elizabethan collar for 3 days postoperatively is essential. If the cat licks the area of the incision during that time, he can do major damage. On the third postoperative day, remove the collar and allow the cat to clean the area. Most will do so, then discontinue licking. However, the cat must be monitored for several hours to be sure that he does not inflict damage. The cat should be sent home that day without the collàr if no damage has been done, and with the collar if the cat has demonstrated a tendency for excessive licking or if there is uncertainty about what the animal will do. The routine use of a collar for 1 to 2 weeks is neither necessary nor desirable.
3. One of the reasons for stricture development is invagination of the skin from each rear leg over the new urethral opening. This may be prevented by making a wide elliptical incision around the prepuce and scrotum. When the skin is sutured to the exposed urethra, there should be enough tension to prevent invagination.
4. A second reason for stricture development is undue tension on the urethra. This can be prevented by adequately dissecting the urethra free of supporting tissue. All tissue that connects to the urethra from all directions should be bluntly removed. This will free the urethra so that it and the bladder can be transplanted caudally about 1 to 2 cm. Unless this is done, the tension will be so great that the urethra will cause invagination of the skin of the perineum. Damage to the pelvic and pudendal nerves, resulting in urinary incontinence, has been reported. Such damage has been attributed to excessive surgical dissection in the area of the neck and lateral ligaments of the bladder.[30] However, the author has not experienced this complication using the described dissection technique.
5. A third cause of stricture development is failure to split the urethra past the narrowed portion. As mentioned earlier, the narrowed portion generally ends at the level of the bulbourethral glands, but not in all cats. The only way to know where the urethral lumen enlarges is to pass a catheter so that the large part of the catheter (that part which is attached to a syringe) can be inserted into the urethral lumen. It is unusual for even a relatively small male cat to have a urethral luminal diameter much smaller than the large part of a catheter. Once the urethra is split adequately, it must be attached to the skin without being subjected to cranially directed tension. Proper dissection, as described above, is the key.
6. A fourth cause of stricture development is failure to properly place the initial sutures at the new urethral opening, which will result in a smaller opening than desired. The operative description should be read and adhered to strictly.
7. Failure to split the urethra exactly on the dorsal midline will result in a twist in the urethra as it is sutured to the skin. This is most likely to happen if the urethra is not oriented in its normal position, (i.e., twisted).

Results

Cats that have undergone perineal urethrostomy should no longer have urethral obstructions; however, episodes of hematuria and dysuria are possible because of the recurrent nature of FUS. When hematuria or dysuria occurs, one should be aware of the increased incidence of bacterial cystitis and uroliths in cats that have had this surgery. If the urine becomes very acidic, urine scalding at the new urethral opening is likely, and will be manifested by intense licking by the cat.

Placement of a Thoracostomy Tube

Closed chest drainage is indicated when fluids (owing to chylothorax or pyothorax) or air (resulting from pneumothorax) fill the pleural space. A thoracostomy tube permits either continuous or intermittent drainage. Tube placement on one side is adequate in most situations; however, it is advisable to obtain chest radiographs to determine whether a second tube is necessary for proper drainage.

Surgical Technique

The technique for placement of a thoracostomy tube is as follows:

- To minimize dyspnea, drain the pleural space of fluid or air using a syringe and needle prior to anesthetizing the cat.
- Anesthetize the cat, minimizing the amount of stress endured by the cat. Halothane or isoflurane, administered using an induction chamber, is preferred. The use of an induction mask is not advisable owing to the amount of struggling that may occur.
- After placing a pursestring suture around the incision site, make a stab incision in the skin at the level of the costochondral junction at the 10th intercostal space.
- Use a curved Carmalt or Kelley forceps to tunnel under the skin to the level of the 7th intercostal space.
- Place a 12-French soft catheter (Feeding Tube & Urethral Catheter, Monoject, Division of Sherwood Medical, St. Louis, MO) for drainage. Cut one or two extra side ports in the tube to ensure proper drainage. The most proximal port should not be more than 2 inches from the distal end of the tube.
- Grasp the distal end of the catheter by the forceps as the forceps is passed. When the forceps is being passed, the curved end should be pointed away from the body wall.
- At the level of the 7th intercostal space, turn the curved end of the forceps perpendicular to the chest wall. With firm, rapid thrust, penetrate the intercostal musculature and force the forceps and tube into the pleural space.
- Release the forceps' hold on the tube and advance the tube cranially into the chest cavity 2.5 to 4 inches, depending on the size of the cat (Fig. 55–19).
- Rapidly close the pursestring suture, wrapping the end of it around the tube several times before suturing the tube to the skin. Place a tape butterfly suture around the tube and suture it to the skin to prevent tube migration.
- Attach the proximal end of the tube to the body wall with a bandage that encircles the chest. The tube should be capped or clamped when not in use. The use of a one-way flutter valve is generally not successful in cats because the pleural pressures and tidal volumes are not sufficient to adequately expel air through the valve. Likewise, they are not successful for evacuating fluids.[31]
- Aspirate air or fluid frequently. The exact frequency will vary depending upon the specific disease and the rapidity of air/fluid buildup. (The irritation caused by the tube will result in the production of 1 mL of fluid per pound of body weight per day.)
- When chest drainage has been completed, remove the bandage and sutures and pull out the tube. Placement of an encircling pressure bandage, as well as confinement of the cat to its cage, is advisable for the first 24 hours after tube removal. The skin incision should be allowed to granulate.
- Obtain radiographs 24 hours and 2 to 3 weeks following tube removal to monitor the cat's progress (Fig. 55–20).

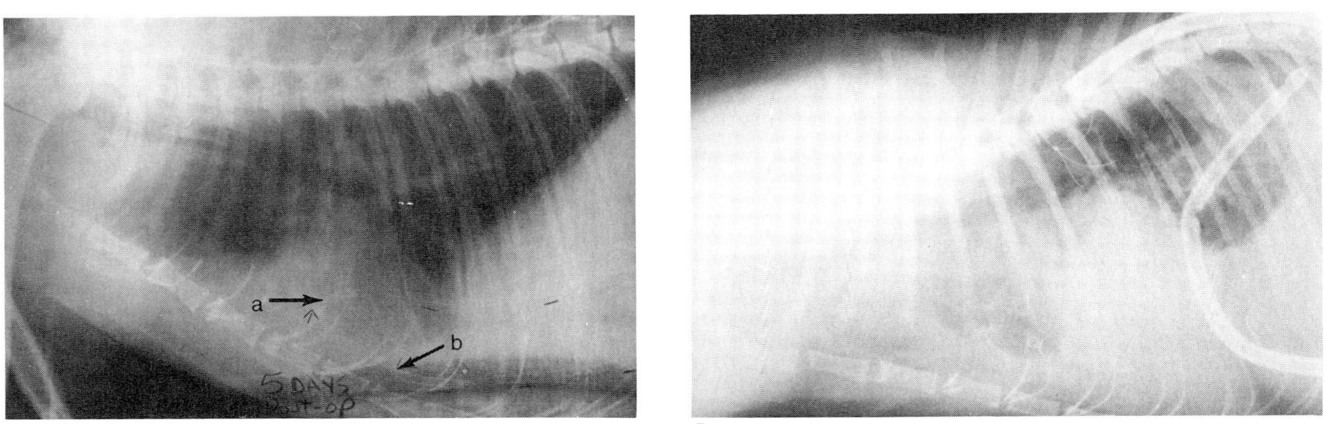

A B

Figure 55–19. Proper placement of the tube positions the distal end of the tube in the ventral cranial or mid-thoracic region. This cat has two implanted tubes. The end of the tube in the right side of the chest (*a*) is properly located in the mid-thoracic region. The end of the other tube (*b*) is too far caudal.

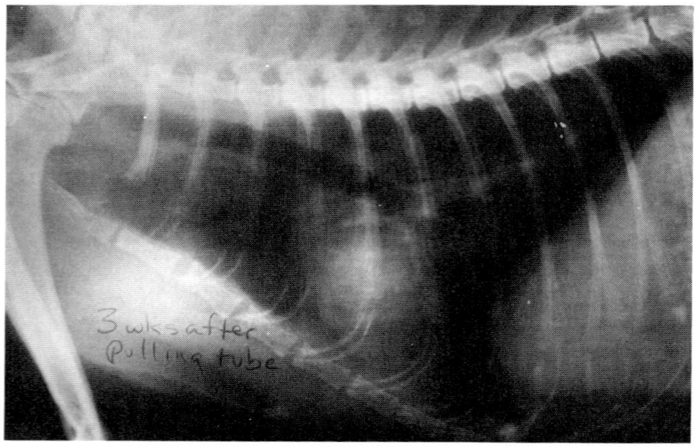

Figure 55–20. Radiographs were obtained 24 hours and 2 to 3 weeks following removal of a thoracostomy tube in order to confirm a resolution of pyothorax.

Thyroidectomy

Thyroidectomy is a procedure that may be performed successfully by most practitioners with reasonable surgical skills; however, there are some complications that may accompany this procedure, the most significant of which is hypocalcemia secondary to dysfunction of both lobes of the external parathyroid gland. Even if a lobe of the external parathyroid gland is not removed, bruising during surgical manipulation may cause a temporary loss of function. Other possible complications include Horner's syndrome and laryngeal paralysis secondary to damage to the vagosympathetic trunk. Careful, blunt dissection and the avoidance of tissue retractors are generally sufficient to prevent the latter two problems.

Anatomic Considerations

There is only one thyroid gland; it has two lobes. Each lobe lies adjacent to the trachea 1 to 3 cm caudal to the larynx. Normal thyroid lobes may lie lateral or dorsolateral to the trachea. Enlarged thyroid lobes are often ventrolateral or ventral to the trachea and in a more caudal location, even at the thoracic inlet. The lobes of the external parathyroid gland are usually located on or near the cranial pole of the thyroid lobes. However, they may also be found in the midthyroid area or near the caudal thyroid poles. The primary blood supply to the thyroid and parathyroid lobes enters from the cranial pole, although there are also vessels at the caudal pole.

Surgical Options

There are three surgical options: partial thyroid lobectomy for unilateral disease, total thyroid lobectomy for either unilateral or bilateral disease, and staged total thyroid lobectomy for unilateral or bilateral disease.

Hyperthyroidism is a unilateral disease 30% of the time. Partial thyroid lobectomy is recommended when only one lobe of the gland is affected, as determined by a technetium 99M scan or by visualization at the time of surgery. The latter is a judgment call based on a visual comparison of the two lobes of the thryoid gland.

If hyperthyroidism is bilateral, removal of both lobes of the gland is mandatory. Some veterinary surgeons recommend this procedure even if one lobe appears grossly normal; this recommendation is based on the theory that eventually, the normal lobe will become affected. When both lobes are removed, studies have shown that about 15% of normal-appearing lobes are found to contain adenomatous tissue.[32] This procedure carries the distinct risk of removing or damaging the parathyroid gland, resulting in severe or even fatal hypocalcemia.

The third option is to perform a total thyroid lobectomy in a staged procedure, whereby the second lobe is removed 30 days following the first.[33] If a parathyroid lobe is traumatized or its vasculature is compromised as a result of the first surgical procedure, the 30-day period will allow for recovery and return of function. This process requires two surgical procedures but greatly decreases the risk of inducing hypoparathyroidism and hypocalcemia. If hypocalcemia develops, the ensuing treatment regimen is usually more stressful for the cat and more expensive than the two staged surgical procedures would have been. This staged approach is the preferred procedure for those practitioners who perform this surgery infrequently.

Anesthetic Precautions

Because of the systemic effects of hyperthyroidism, especially with regard to cardiac function, certain anesthetic precautions are in order. Creating a euthyroid state with methimazole (Tapazole) will greatly diminish the likelihood of complications; surgery should not be performed without doing this unless the side effects of the drug become life-threatening (see Chapter 46). Pay careful attention to the heart rate because tachycardia is a common component of hyperthyroidism. To ensure complication-free anesthesia, the following guidelines should be followed:

1. Avoid using ketamine (Ketaset) or xylazine (Rompum 20).
2. Preanesthetize the cat with acepromazine or acepromazine-oxymorphone.
3. Avoid using anticholinergics. If one must be used, glycopyrrolate (Robinul-V) is preferred.
4. Induce anesthesia with a thiobarbiturate, such as Bio-Tal (Bio-Ceutic).
5. Isoflurane (AErrane) is the preferred anesthetic, although halothane (Fluothane) is an acceptable alternative.
6. If intraoperative tachycardia develops, administer propranolol (Inderal). (Dilute to 0.1 mg/mL and administer at a rate of 0.1 mL every 2 to 3 minutes until the heart rate slows to 160 beats/minute.)
7. Because hyperthyroid cats may maintain a high body temperature, use external heat with caution.

Surgical Techniques

There are two surgical techniques for thyroidectomy: an intracapsular technique, in which the thyroid capsule is incised, and an extracapsular technique, in which the thyroid capsule is left intact. The original versions of both techniques have been modified to preserve a small portion of the thyroid capsule. By removing most of the thyroid capsule, the chance of regrowth of adenomatous thyroid tissue is minimized.

Both procedures involve the following steps:

- Prep a liberal amount of the skin in the ventral cervical area. Because the thyroid lobes are likely to migrate toward or through the thoracic inlet, enough skin should be prepped to allow extension of the incision to the thoracic inlet. Thyroid migration is more likely to occur when the lobes become greatly enlarged. Marked clinical signs and thyroxine (T_4) levels exceeding 10 μg/dL will generally accompany such an enlargement.
- Make a skin incision on the midline adjacent to the thyroid lobe(s).
- Bluntly separate the sternohyoideus and sternothyroideus muscles on the midline and gently retract them.
- Expose the trachea, allowing access to the adherent thyroid lobes.
- Assess both lobes visually to confirm or rule out bilateral disease and to determine which lobe (the largest) should be removed first in the event that a staged procedure is to be performed.
- Handle the lobe(s) gently once they are exposed, being careful not to disrupt the primary blood supply to the thyroid and parathyroid lobes, which enters cranially.

Modified Intracapsular Technique

In the modified intracapsular technique, the following steps apply:

- Split the thyroid capsule in an avascular area using a small scalpel blade or iris scissors.
- Reflect the capsule away from the thyroid lobe; then dissect the thyroid lobe free of the capsule using a cotton-tipped applicator or splinter forceps and remove it.
- Remove as much of the thyroid capsule as possible so that the external parathyroid lobe and its vasculature remain undisturbed.[34]

Modified Extracapsular Technique

The modified extracapsular technique should be performed as follows:

- Cauterize the thyroid capsule 2 mm from the external parathyroid lobe using bipolar cautery forceps, taking care not to disturb the cranial vasculature to the parathyroid lobe. If bipolar cautery is not available, excise the capsule, using a small scalpel blade to incise around the caudal half of the external parathyroid lobe (Figs. 55–21 and 55–22).
- Incise the capsule on the cautery line using iris scissors.

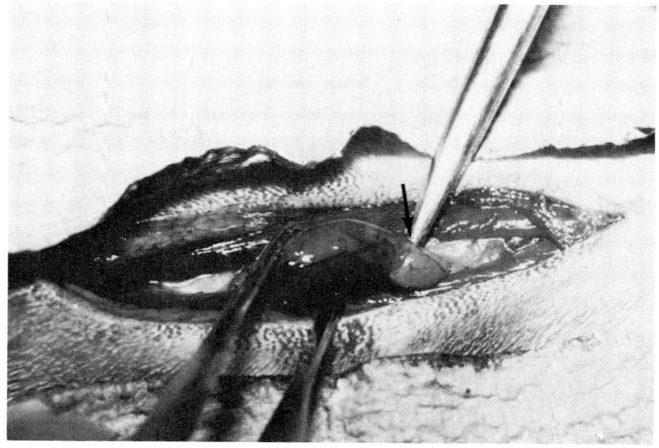

Figure 55–21. The external lobe of the pararthyroid gland is identified (*arrow*).

- Dissect free from the thyroid lobe the external parathyroid lobe, a small portion of the thyroid capsule, and the associated vessels using a cotton-tipped applicator or fine-tipped instruments, such as splinter forceps and iris scissors. These structures should remain in the cat while the thyroid lobe and the remainder of the thyroid capsule are removed (Fig. 55–23).

This technique has a slightly lower rate of postoperative hypocalcemia than does the intracapsular technique.[34]

Although the external parathyroid lobes are generally located on the cranial pole of the thyroid lobes, they may occasionally be located in the center of the thyroids or near the caudal poles. This may complicate dissection and retention of the blood supply. If a parathyroid lobe is inadvertently removed without its vasculature, it should be transplanted into an adjacent muscle belly in the likelihood that it will revascularize and become functional.

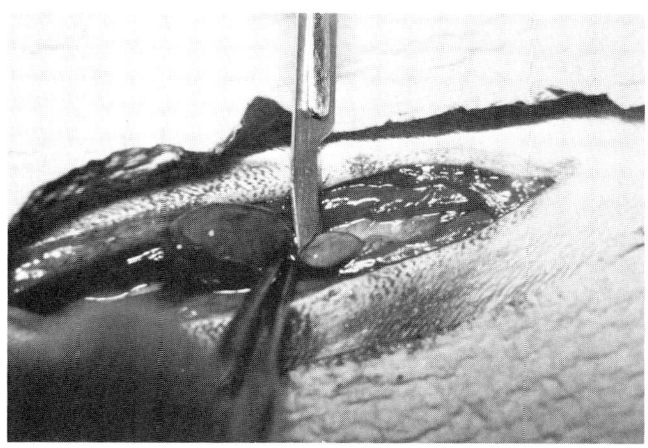

Figure 55–22. A No. 15 scalpel blade is used to dissect the parathyroid lobe from its thyroid lobe.

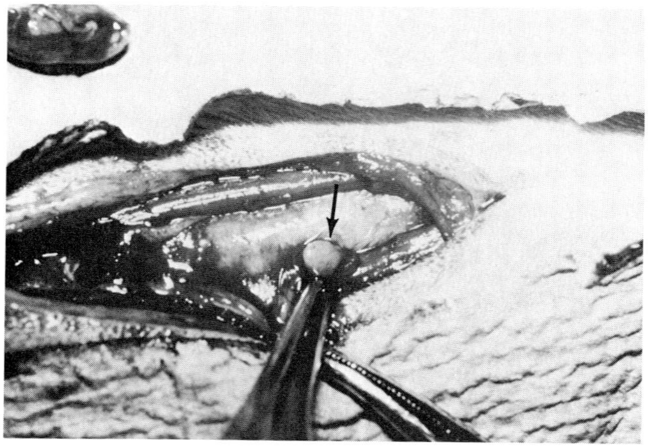

Figure 55–23. The parathyroid lobe (*arrow*) is positioned within the cervical tissues prior to closure of the incision.

Turbinectomy

When chronic bacterial rhinitis exists, medical treatment fails because of the anatomy of the nasal cavity. The intricate pattern of interlocking bones in the maxillary and ethmoid regions of the nasal cavity allows entrapment of bacteria and purulent material, preventing adequate drainage of the area. If frontal sinusitis exists, constant drainage of purulent material through the nasal cavity perpetuates the infection. Cats with a draining frontal sinusitis will invariably have concomitant rhinitis. If sinusitis exists, it must be treated surgically before the rhinitis can be treated successfully. It is the author's preference to surgically treat both conditions simultaneously.

Surgical Technique

The following are the steps involved in performing turbinectomy:

- Induce anesthesia with a combination of ketamine and diazepam (Valium), or with an ultra–short-acting barbiturate. Anesthesia can then be maintained using halothane or isoflurane through a non-rebreathing system.
- Make an incision in the skin of the nose on the midline.
- Retract the soft tissue, including the periosteum, laterally so that the nasal and frontal bones are exposed.
- Make a slot measuring 1 to 2 mm × 1.5 cm in the left nasal and frontal bones using an electric drill (Dremel Moto-tool, Emerson Electric Co., Racine, WI). Remove and discard the bone from the slot. Make a similar slot in the right nasal and frontal bones (Fig. 55–24, *A* and *B*).
- Using a small bone curette and a curved pair of Halstead mosquito hemostatic forceps, remove the maxillary and ethmoid turbinates. Take care to remove all of the turbinate bones, as well as any purulent material. Flush the cavity with saline solution to remove any remaining pus or osseous debris.
- Control hemorrhage by applying direct pressure with a gauze square that has been forced into the nasal cavity. (Unlike in the dog, hemorrhage is not usually a serious problem in the cat.)
- Close the incision in two layers—the periosteum and the skin. Make no attempt to close the bony defect with soft tissue or bone graft.
- Submit some of the turbinate bones that have been removed for histopathologic examination to detect fungal infection or neoplasia.

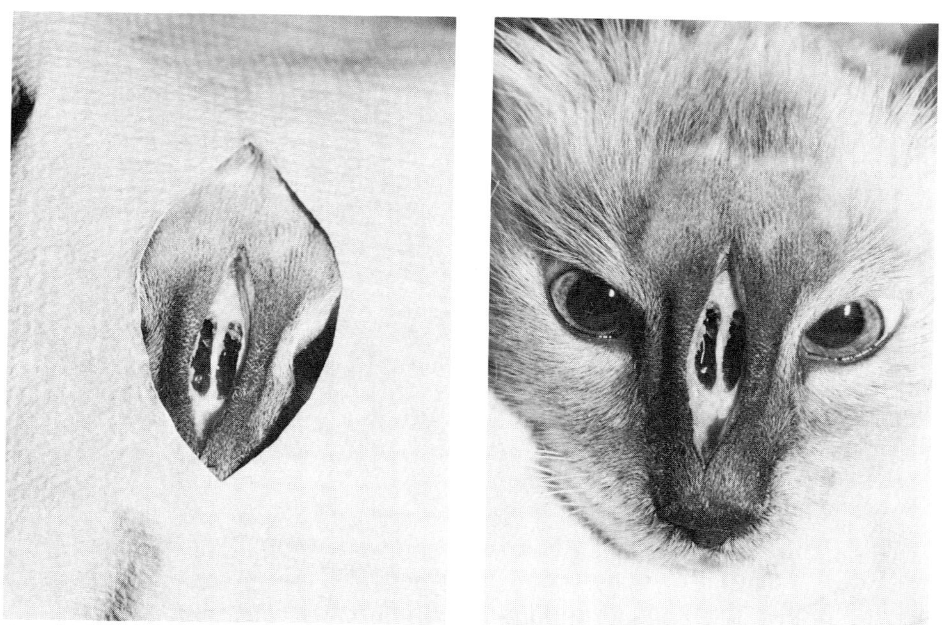

A B

Figure 55–24. (*A*) A slot measuring 1 to 2 mm × 1.5 cm is made in each of the nasal and frontal bones. The bone from the slots is then removed and discarded. (*B*) The surgical drape is removed for orientation of the reader.

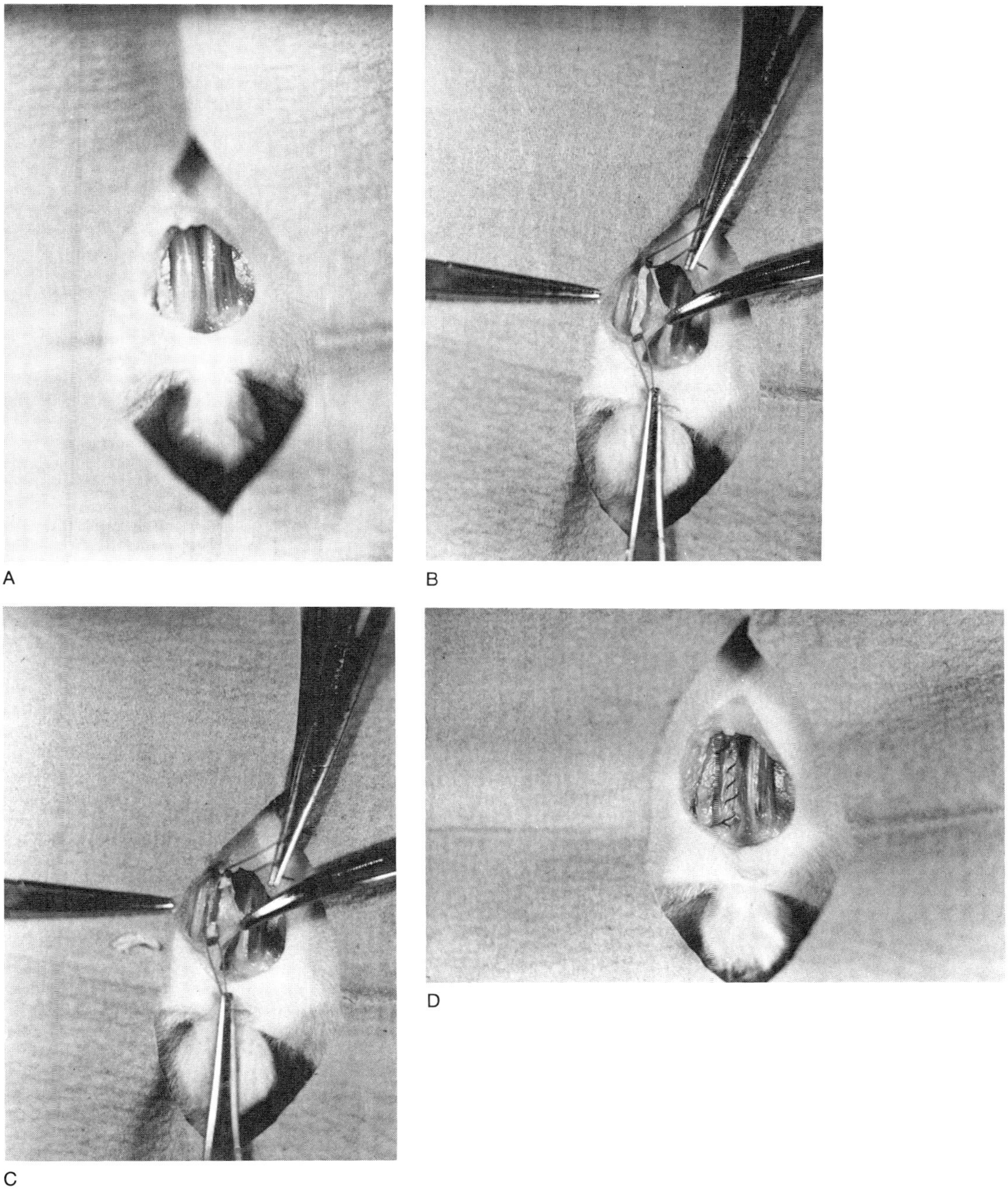

Figure 55–25. (*A*) When the skin incisions are made for a vasectomy, the spermatic cords are encountered almost immediately, although they are often surrounded by adipose tissue. (*B*) One of the spermatic cords is split longitudinally. The vas deferens is identified, separated from the testicular artery and vein, and double-ligated about 0.5 cm apart. (*C*) The vas deferens is transected in two places between the ligatures, and the excised portion is removed. (*D*) The spermatic cord is sutured with 4-0 or 5-0 dissolvable suture material. (Used by permission of Veterinary Practice Publishing Co., Santa Barbara, CA.)

Results

A small amount of epistaxis and sneezing can be expected for about 3 to 5 days, although it is generally not severe enough to warrant treatment. The cat will typically be anorectic for about 24 hours, but the appetite should return on the second postoperative day. An antibiotic, such as gentamicin, should be administered immediately following surgery and every 12 hours thereafter until culture results are available. From that time, treatment is based on the culture results; it should be continued for 2 to 3 weeks depending on the organism, the amount of growth, and the duration of disease before surgery. Subcutaneous emphysema should not occur because the skin is taut over the slot in the bone and because the external nasal opening is not blocked.

If the etiology of the problem is bacterial, the amount of sneezing and nasal discharge should diminish significantly or should stop altogether. If the cat has a chronic feline herpesvirus (rhinotracheitis) or calicivirus infection, improvement should be noted, but it will not be as dramatic as if the rhinitis were bacterial in origin. If *Cryptococcus neoformans* or *Histoplasma capsulatum* organisms are present, the prognosis is much worse. Aggressive therapy with ketoconazole (Nizoral) and/or amphotericin-B (Fungizone) must follow surgery. (See Chapter 61.)

Vasectomy

Indication

Cat breeders often want to control the time of breeding of queens; however, because queens continue to cycle in and out of estrus, their estrus-induced behavior can become quite annoying. Some breeders have found that inducing ovulation can be quite beneficial. This may be accomplished by manual cervical stimulation or by use of a vasectomized tom.[35]

Surgical Technique

The procedure for vasectomy is as follows:

- Induce anesthesia and clip and prep the skin in the groin area.
- Make a midline incision ventral to pubic symphysis.
- Because the spermatic cords lie ventral to the pelvis, they are encountered almost immediately, although they are often surrounded by adipose tissue (Fig. 55–25*A*). Split one of the spermatic cords longitudinally.
- Identify the vas deferens, separate it from the testicular artery and vein, and then double-ligate it about 0.5 cm apart (Fig. 55–25*B*).
- Transect the vas deferens in two places between the ligatures, and remove the excised part (Fig. 55–25*C*).
- Suture the spermatic cord with 4-0 or 5-0 dissolvable suture material (Fig. 55–25*D*).
- Repeat the procedure on the contralateral spermatic cord through the same incision.
- Close the incision with two layers of sutures—one in the subcutaneous tissue and one in the skin.

REFERENCES

1. Wheeler SL, Quirk P. Indwelling intravenous catheters in cats and dogs—Catheter selection and placement. Vet Pract Staff 1991;3(20):1.
2. Stein BS. A method of continuous intravenous fluid therapy in a cat. Feline Pract 1974;4(4):12.
3. Rosser EJ, Ihrke PJ. The Skin. In: Pratt PW ed. Feline Medicine, 1st ed. Santa Barbara: American Veterinary Publications, Inc. 1983:555.
4. Norsworthy GD. Urinary bladder marsupialization. Feline Pract 1984;14(5):43.
5. Bright RM, Burrows CF, Goring R, Fox S, Tilmant L. Subtotal colectomy for treatment of acquired megacolon in the dog and cat. J Am Vet Med Assoc 1986;188:1412.
6. Rosin E, Walshaw R, Mehlhaff C, Matthiesen D, Orsher R, Kusba J. Subtotal colectomy for treatment of chronic constipation associated with diopathic megacolon in cats: 38 cases (1979–1985). J Am Vet Med Assoc 1988;193:850.
7. Burrows CF. Constipation, Obstipation, and Megacolon. In: August JR, ed. Consultations in Feline Internal Medicine. Philadelphia: WB Saunders, 1991:445.
8. Stine RH, Mueller JG. Femoral fracture repair using the slip cap method. Feline Pract 1984;14(6):8.
9. Rife JN. Deep digital flexor tendonectomy—An alternative to amputation onychectomy for declawing cats. J Am Anim Hosp Assoc 1988;24:73.
10. Crowe DT. Nutritional support for the hospitalized patient: An introduction to tube feeding. Compend Contin Educ Pract Vet 1990;12:1711.
11. Crowe DT. Nutrition in critical patients: Administering the support therapies. Vet Med 1989;84:152.
12. Bright RM. Nasal Foreign Bodies, Tumors, and Rhinitis/Sinusitis. In: Bojrab MJ, ed. Pathophysiology in Small Animal Surgery. Philadelphia: Lea & Febiger, 1981:335.
13. Tomlinson MJ, Schenc NL. Autogenous fat implantation as a treatment for chronic frontal sinusitis in a cat. J Am Vet Med Assoc 1975;167:927.
14. Anderson GI. The treatment of chronic sinusitis in six cats by ethmoid conical curettage and autogenous fat graft sinus ablation. Vet Surg 1987;16:131.
15. Norsworthy GD. Surgical treatment of chronic nasal discharge. Vet Med 1993;88(6):526.
16. Lindberg L. Infection and Antibiotics in Relation to Bone Cement. In: Williams E, ed. The Biocompatibility of Orthopedic Implants. Boca Raton, FL: CRC Press, 1982:25.
17. Komtebedde J, Hauptman J. Bilateral ischiocavernosus myectomy for chronic urine spraying in castrated male cats. Vet Surg 1990;19:283.
18. Grandage J. The Oral Cavity and Pharynx. In: Slatter DH, ed. Textbook of Small Animal Surgery. Philadelphia: WB Saunders, 1985:606.
19. Zagraniski MJ. Reduction of a mandiubular symphyseal fracture with nylon cable tie bands. Feline Pract 1980;10:45.
20. Zagraniski MJ. Ovariohysterectomy of the estrous queen utilizing nylon cable tie bands. Feline Pract 1987;8(4):47.
21. Johnston DE, Christie BA. The retroperitoneum in dogs: Anatomy and clinical significance. Compend Contin Educ Pract Vet 1990;12:1027.
22. Rhinelander FW, Oxon MA, Stewart CL. Experimental Fixation of Femoral Osteotomies by Cerclage with Nylon Straps. In: Urist MR, ed. Clinical Orthopaedics and Related Research. Philadelphia: JB Lippincott, 1983:298.
23. Bennett M, Houpt KA, Erb HN. Effects of declawing on feline behavior. Feline Pract 1988;2(12):7.
24. Wilson GP, Harrison JW. Perineal urethrostomy in the cat. J Am Vet Med Assoc 1971;169:1789.

25. Rickard DA. Feline perineal urethrostomy: "The Cleveland Technique." Feline Pract 1974;4:41.
26. Dieringer TM, Lees GE. The Role of Perineal Urethrostomy in the Management of Lower Urinary Tract Obstruction. In: August JR, ed. Consultations in Feline Internal Medicine. Philadelphia: WB Saunders, 1991:327.
27. Sackman JE, Sims MH, Krahwinkel DJ. Urodynamic evaluation of lower urinary tract function in cats after perineal urethrostomy with minimal and extensive dissection. Vet Surg 1991; 20:55.
28. Gregory CR, Vasseur PB. Long-term examination of cats with perineal urethrostomy. Vet Surg 1983;12:210.
29. Griffin DW. Prevalence of bacterial urinary tract infection after perineal urethrostomy in cats. J Am Vet Med Assoc 1992;200:681.
30. Gregory CR. The effects of perineal urethrostomy on urethral function in male cats. Compend Contin Educ Pract Vet 1987; 9:895.
31. Caywood DD, Lipowitz AJ. Surgical approaches and techniques for pulmonary disease. Vet Clin North Am (Small Anim Pract) 1987;17:449.
32. Peterson ME, Becker DV. Radionuclide thyroid imaging in 135 cats with hyperthyroidism. Vet Radiol 1984;25:23.
33. Flanders JA, Harvey HJ, Erb HN. Feline thyroidectomy: A comparison of postoperative hypocalcemia associated with three different surgical techniques. Vet Surg 1987;16:362.
34. Peterson ME, Randolph JF. Endocrine Diseases. In: Sherding RG, ed. The Cat: Diseases and Clinical Management. New York: Churchill Livingstone, 1989:463.
35. Norsworthy GD. Alternative surgical procedures for feline birth control: Tubal ligation and vasectomy. Feline Pract 1975;5(1): 24.

CHAPTER 56

◇ ◇ ◇

The Skin: Fungal Diseases

Sandra R. Merchant

Superficial Fungal Infections: Dermatophytosis

Dermatophytosis in small animals is most commonly caused by one of three species of fungi: *Microsporum canis, Microsporum gypseum,* and *Trichophyton mentagrophytes. Microsporum canis* is responsible for 95% to 98% of the cases of dermatophytosis in the cat, and so will be the focus of this discussion. However, 20 other species of keratinophilic fungi have been documented in cases of ringworm and in surveys of asymptomatic animals.[1]

M. canis is classified as a zoophilic fungus; the cat is considered its natural host. However, surveys of healthy cats have yielded variable numbers positive for *M. canis.*[2] *T. mentagrophytes* is another zoophilic fungus with the rodent as its natural host. *M. gypseum* is classified as a geophilic fungus since the soil is the natural habitat. It is important to classify the type of dermatophyte causing infection, so that the source can be identified and treated or avoided.

Pathophysiology

Many animals are exposed to ringworm fungi, but few develop clinical disease. As the fungus contacts the skin, it may be removed mechanically, may be prevented from invading the skin due to host immunity, may invade the skin but not produce disease, or may invade the skin and produce disease.[3] Conditions that encourage colonization by a fungus include a naive immune system in a young animal, trauma, poor nutritional status, contaminated environmental conditions, or a depressed immune system (old age, poor health, immunosuppressive drug therapy).[4]

Dermatophytes can only survive in keratinized structures that include the horny layer (stratum corneum) of the epidermis, the hair, and the nails. They cannot penetrate living tissue. In addition, dermatophytes can only persist in the anagen, or growing, stage. The classic ring-shaped, alopecic, spreading lesion of dermatophytosis is the result of the fungal invasion of the hair shaft (Fig. 56–1). The fungal invasion weakens the shaft, so it is more susceptible to breakage. When the hair shaft stops growing, the dermatophyte infection in those follicles quickly ends. New growth spreads peripherally to adjacent follicles, giving the lesion its expanding circular appearance. The fungus releases toxins and potential allergens that penetrate the dermis and cause an inflammatory response. Inflammation in infected hair follicles also brings an end to the dermatophyte infection in those follicles. Inflammation may lead to increased scaling, which also aids in spreading of the dermatophyte.

If inflammation is severe, the infection is brought under control without intervention. However, *M. canis* is relatively host-adapted in the cat and may cause very little inflammatory skin disease. Thus a relatively tolerant cat with host-adapted *M. canis* often develops a persistent mild or asymptomatic infection. If left untreated, the *M. canis* infection eventually resolves. This can take anywhere from 18 months to 4 years.[2] However, the human health hazard and risk to other animals strongly warrants therapy. Sixty-nine percent of households with *M. canis*-positive cats have at least one person affected with ringworm.

Clinical Signs

The lesions of dermatophytosis are highly variable and depend upon the nature of the host-fungus interaction. The lesions are often localized, but may be multifocal to generalized. The cutaneous signs of feline dermatophytosis may include any of the following: (1) "classic ringworm," the most common, which is one or more patches of alopecia with some degree of scaling associated with the hair loss with or without pruritus; (2) patchy alopecia, erythema, pruritus, and excoriations (Fig. 56–2); (3) a localized or generalized miliary dermatitis with or without significant alopecia; (4) pigmentary disturbances of hair and/or skin; (5) large areas of papules, pustules, vesicles, and alopecia, with or without pruritus; (6) small to large areas of alopecia and/or broken hairs; (7) firm or fluctuant nodules, which frequently ulcerate and develop draining tracts and are frequently painful and/or pruritic (pseudomycetoma); (8) multifocal or generalized seborrhea sicca; (9) focal or multifocal papules and pustules, with hairs emerging from the centers of these lesions with or without significant alopecia and pruritus; (10) paronychia and/or onychomycosis (discolored, misshapen, crumbly, split, or sloughing nails); and (11) the asymptomatic carrier.[5] Less common clinical

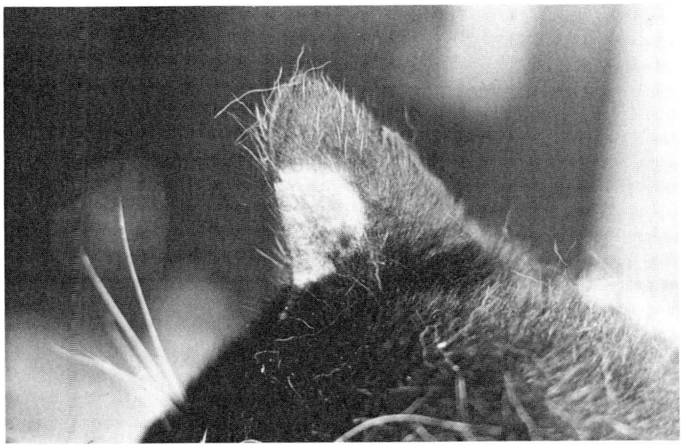

Figure 56–1. Circular, alopecic, scaling lesion of *M. canis* on the ear of a cat.

presentations of *M. canis* infections include recurrent feline chin acne, feline endocrine alopecia, chronic blepharitis (due to infection of the periocular hairs and cornea) and pseudomycetomas.[2] Therefore, dermatophytosis is difficult to diagnose by clinical signs alone. *A dermatophyte infection should be listed in the differential diagnosis of any feline skin disease because of the highly variable clinical signs of the disease in the cat.*

Diagnosis

Dermatophyte infections can be definitively diagnosed by fungal culture of the hair. The fungal culture not only confirms the presence of the fungus, but allows the causative agent to be definitively identified. Wood's lamp examination, microscopic examination of hair and scale, and histologic examination of a skin biopsy specimen can be helpful adjunctive diagnostic tests.

Fungal Culture

The correct method for collecting hairs and interpreting results of a dermatophyte culture must be followed and will

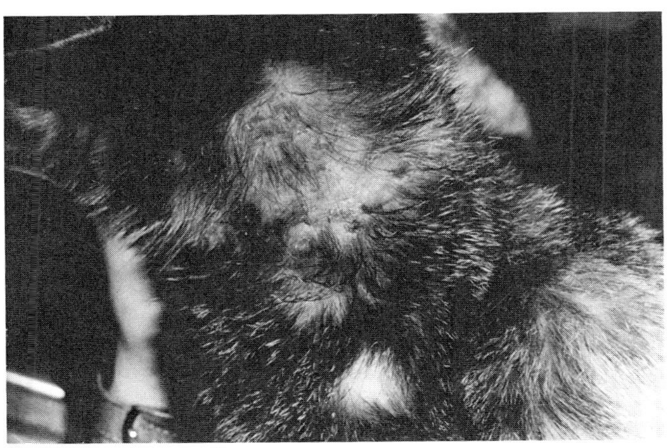

Figure 56–2. Extremely pruritic, excoriated lesion of *M. canis* on the dorsal cervical region of a cat.

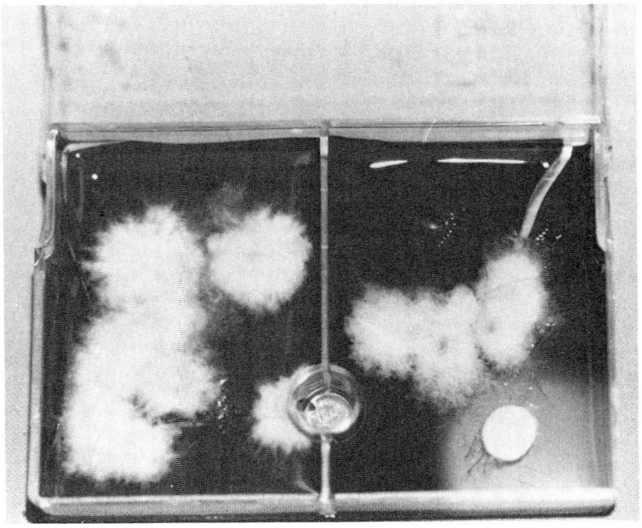

Figure 56–3. Fluffy white colony growth of *M. canis* on DTM test media.

lessen the possibility of both false-positive and false-negative findings.

Dermatophyte test media (DTM) is the most commonly used fungal culture medium. Initially the medium is amber, and as the dermatophyte grows, it produces alkaline metabolites that cause the phenol red indicator dye in the medium to turn red (Fig. 56–3). This usually occurs within 10 to 14 days, although for asymptomatic cats it may take 14 to 21 days. Contaminant fungi use carbohydrates in the medium first and then the protein, turning the medium red only after prolonged incubation (usually longer than 10 to 14 days). However, certain contaminating fungi can mimic pathogens and turn the medium red in 7 to 10 days. It is important to note a color change *at* the first signs of fungal growth, not *after* it has begun to grow.

Dermatophyte test medium is available commercially in glass screw-cap containers (Fungassay, Pitman-Moore, Inc, Mundelein, IL) or in dual compartment plates (Sab-Duets, BactiLabs, Mountain View, CA) with DTM on one side and plain Sabouraud's dextrose agar on the other. The DTM may suppress the development of macroconidia and also makes examination of the gross colonial morphology (the lemon yellow reverse pigment of *M. canis*) difficult to see. This can hinder identification of the colony. The dual compartment plates will obviate the need to subculture to obtain diagnostic macroconidia and will allow for observing the gross colony morphology on the plain Sabouraud's dextrose agar side.

The lesions to be cultured should be clipped and cleaned to reduce the contaminant growth on the DTM agar. The hair should be clipped to 0.5 cm, gently swabbed with alcohol, and dried. The hairs for culture should be grasped with a hemostat and rolled in the direction of the hair growth to aid in including the intrafollicular portion of the hair shaft. Chosen hairs should be broken and near active inflammatory lesions, usually at the periphery of the lesion. The hairs should be placed on the surface of the DTM me-

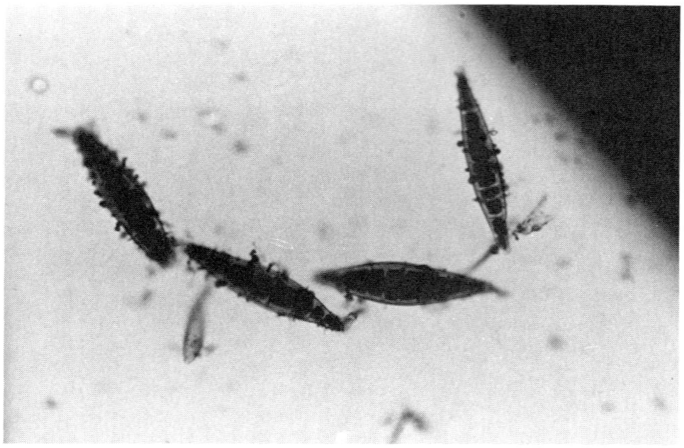

Figure 56–4. Thick, spiny-walled macroconidia of *M. canis.*

dium (not imbedded within). Wood's lamp–positive hairs, if seen, should always be chosen for culture.

If the cat is completely asymptomatic, one can briskly brush the cat with a new toothbrush and then touch the bristles lightly to the surface of the medium. This is the MacKenzie brush technique. Leave the DTM loosely capped (if screw-top bottle) at room temperature and sheltered from ultraviolet light. The DTM samples should be inspected daily. The color change should occur simultaneously with lightly pigmented fungal growth. Any colony that is heavily pigmented is a contaminant and should be discarded.

After 7 to 10 days a macroconidia preparation can be made for positive identification of the dermatophyte. This is the only way to definitively identify and interpret colony growth on DTM. The preparation consists of obtaining a small amount of the growth and placing it on a glass slide with lactophenol cotton blue mounting medium for microscopic examination. This growth can be obtained by the use of transparent tape applied to the top of the colony or by a blunt instrument that can remove growth from the top of the colony.

Macroconidia of *M. canis* are spindle-shaped with thick spiny walls. The spines are more pronounced at the terminal end, which often forms a knob. The macroconidia are usually composed of six or more cells (Fig. 56–4).

Wood's Light Examination

Wood's light examination may be used to screen for dermatophytes that fluoresce. *M. canis* is the only common veterinary dermatophyte that causes fluorescence. Infections with this fungus fluoresce only 50% of the time. A positive test is bright apple-green fluorescence of the hair shaft. Many topical ointments, shampoos, and solutions may destroy the fluorescence or produce a false-positive result. In addition, bacterial infections will produce a bluish-white glow and scale will also fluoresce positive. Positive fluorescence is only suggestive of a *M. canis* infection, whereas negative fluorescence is nondiagnostic. The Wood's lamp examination is best used as an aid in choosing potentially infected hairs for microscopic examination and culture.

Microscopic Examination of Hair and Scale

Another diagnostic method is microscopic examination of hair and scale to identify ectothrix spores and hyphae. This is not commonly performed in general veterinary practices because of the time involved and the low yield. When viewed by an experienced technician, a diagnosis can be made in 10% to 50% of confirmed cases. The inexperienced may find it difficult to distinguish spores from pigment and hyphae from keratin strands. The selection of hairs is critical, and the test is most rewarding if hairs are examined that are Wood's light–positive. There are several compounds available as clearing agents to enhance the possiblity of finding spores. Five clearing agents are utilized: (1) 10% to 20% potassium hydroxide (KOH); (2) KOH and dimethyl sulfoxide (DMSO); (3) KOH and India ink; (4) chlorphenolac; and (5) KOH, DMSO, and chlorazol fungal stain. (Recipes for the last two are included in Table 56–1.)

Hairs and scale or nails are collected and deposited on a slide. Several drops of the chosen clearing agent are applied to the slide, and a coverslip is added. With the plain KOH solution, the slide can be gently heated for 15 seconds and read or the preparation can be allowed to stand for 30 minutes to 24 hours and then read. The KOH and DMSO have the advantage of immediate clearing without heat fixing. Addition of India ink may aid in interpretation of the KOH preparation by staining the hyphae and macroconidia. The chlorphenolac preparation provides immediate clearing without heat fixing and does not produce artifact, even if the microscope slide is not examined for as long as 25 hours.[2] With the chlorazol fungal stain, the hyphae stain green against a gray background.

The cleared specimen is scanned under low power to look for hairs that appear pale, swollen, and filamentous. Once a suspect hair is found, higher magnification is needed. Ectothrix spores appear as round to oval beads surrounding the hairshaft (Fig. 56–5).

Occasionally, ringworm is diagnosed from a skin biopsy. The typical histologic pattern is one of perifolliculitis, folliculitis, and furunculoses, with fungal elements within hair follicles, around hairs, and in the stratum corneum. Visualization of the organism is facilitated with periodic acid–Schiff (PAS) or acid orcein Giemsa (AOG) staining. Biopsy will be most helpful when the dermatophyte is presented as a nodule (kerion) or pseudomycetoma in which the fungus is imbedded in "grains" deep in the dermis and panniculus.

Table 56–1. Recipes for Clearing Agents

Chlorphenolac Formulation
Dissolve 50 g chloral hydrate, 25 mL liquid phenol, and 225 mL liquid lactic acid and mixed together. Several days may pass before the crystal goes into solution.
KOH, DMSO and Chlorazol Fungal Stain
Dissolve 100 mg chlorazol black E dye in 10 mL DMSO and add 90 mL water containing 5 g KOH. This can also be purchased commercially (Dermatologic Lab and Supply)

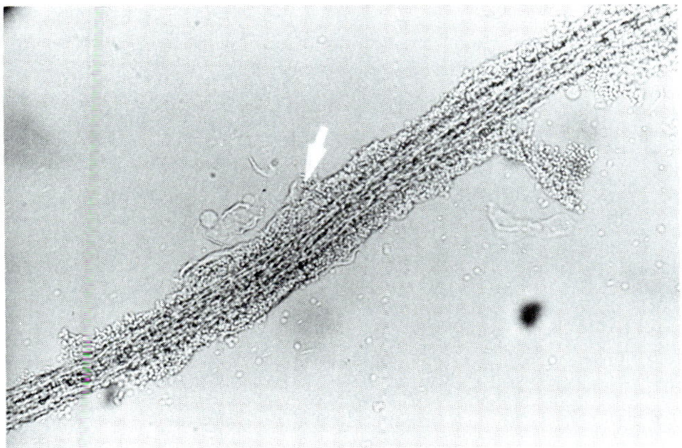

Figure 56–5. **Chlorphenolac prep showing small round ectothrix spores (*arrow*) from a hair sample positive for *M. canis*.**

Antifungal Therapy

Treatment of dermatophytosis includes disinfecting the environment, preventing recontamination of the environment, and using topical fungicides. Systemic fungicides should be utilized when appropriate.

Environmental decontamination is essential, since many fungi may persist in the environment for over 1 year. All grooming equipment should be destroyed or disinfected with a dilute solution of bleach or tamed iodine. All bedding should be laundered, and carpets and furniture thoroughly vacuumed. Prevention of recontamination can be aided by vacuuming and disinfecting the environment frequently (including vents), and isolating the animal to an area with a washable surface during treatment.

Some form of topical therapy, such as miconazole (Conofite), is always indicated in the cat. Clipping of the affected areas (whole body if necessary) and application of topical treatment reduce the potential for spread of the infection (Table 56–2). Treatment for localized infections may involve trimming the area and applying a suitable antifungal cream or ointment. Dips or shampoos are useful for treatment of extensive lesions or generalized infections but are less likely to produce a mycologic cure than are creams or lotions containing antimycotic antibiotics.[1] However, they are very important in preventing environmental contamination and recontamination of the affected cat.

Griseofulvin is the systemic treatment of choice for generalized dermatophytosis and any type of infection in long-haired cats or immunocompromised patients. Some resistance of ringworm isolates to this drug has been documented, but this is rare in veterinary medicine. Treatment failures are more often due to erratic drug absorption, underdosing, lack of environmental decontamination, or failure to identify the source of the infection.

Griseofulvin is supplied in two forms. Microsize griseofulvin is available in tablet formation (Fulvicin, 250-mg tablets) or a pediatric suspension labeled for human use (Grifulvin V, 125 mg/mL). Ultramicrosize griseofulvin is available in tablet formation (Gris-PEG). Published dose ranges vary widely. The dose recommended by the author is 20 to 100 mg/kg divided b.i.d. for the microsize formulations and 5 to 10 mg/kg divided b.i.d. for the ultramicrosize in PEG. Absorption of the microsize griseofulvin from the gastrointestinal tract can be enhanced by administering this formulation with a fatty meal. This is not necessary with the ultramicrosize formulation. Therapy should be continued

Table 56–2. Topical Therapy in Dermatophytosis

Therapy	Product	Brand Name*	Recommended Administration
Local	Miconazole	Conofite cream or lotion (Pitman Moore)	To lesion b.i.d.
	Clotrimazole	Veltrim (Haver Lockhart) Lotrimin (Schering)	To lesion b.i.d.
	Iodine	Xenodine (Solvay)	To lesion b.i.d.
	Thiabendazole	Tresaderm (Merck)	To lesion b.i.d.
Whole body	Lime-sulfur	Lym Dyp (DVM)	2% solution every 5–7 days
	Captan	Orthocide spray (Chevron chemical)	2% solution every 5–7 days
	Chlorhexidine	Nolvasan solution (Fort Dodge)	2% solution every 5–7 days
	Chlorhexidine	Nolvasan shampoo (Fort Dodge)	Every 5–7 days
		Chlorhexiderm shampoo (DVM)	Every 5–7 days

*Companies: Pitman Moore, Mundelein, IL; Haver Lockhart, Mobay Shawnee, KS; Schering, Liberty Corner, NJ; Solvay, Princeton, NJ; Merck Sharpe and Dohme, West Point, PA; DVM, Miami, FL; Chevron, San Ramon, CA; Fort Dodge, Fort Dodge, IA.

until the patient is symptom-free *and* culture-negative. This usually requires 4 to 6 weeks of therapy.

Recognition of griseofulvin toxicity is increasing. These reactions appear to be idiosyncratic and not related to doses given in the suggested range. Side effects include gastrointestinal disturbance, drug eruption, lethargy, pyrexia, anorexia, icterus, ataxia, angioedema, hepatotoxicity, and bone marrow suppression. Pure-bred cats may be more sensitive to the side effects of griseofulvin. Cats with feline immunodeficiency virus infections appear to be at increased risk for griseofulvin-associated neutropenia.[6] Griseofulvin is also teratogenic, and when it is used in a cattery situation, breeding must be suspended until the drug is discontinued. A pretreatment complete blood count (CBC) is warranted, and the clients should be alerted to signs of potential toxicity. The drug should be discontinued and the animal re-evaluated if side effects are seen. If no problems occur, a routine physical examination and hematologic test should be performed every 2 weeks until mycologic cure.

Ketoconazole (Nizoral) is a broad-spectrum fungistatic synthetic imidazole antibiotic. Its use should be limited to griseofulvin-resistant isolates, since ketoconazole-resistant *M. canis* strains have been identified. The recommended does is 10 mg/kg once daily. Side effects seen in the cat include fever, depression, gastrointestinal disease, and neurologic abnormalities.

Management of Dermatophytosis in Catteries

Once dermatophytosis has been diagnosed in one member of a multicat household or cattery, all cats in the household must be suspected as carriers until proven otherwise. A toothbrush culture should be performed on each cat. The culture-positive cats should be separated from the culture-negative cats. The negative cats should be cultured a second time. The cattery should be isolated and no cats should be sold, shown, or sent to breed. New members should not be added, and breeding programs should be interrupted. All affected cats should have a total body clip, and the hair coat should remain short. Therapy should include both topical and systemic treatment and should be continued until each cat is culture-negative. Griseofulvin should be given to all affected nonpregnant queens and kittens over 12 weeks of age.

Environmental decontamination is extremely important. All surfaces should be disinfected (cages daily) and thoroughly vacuumed daily. (See discussion of this topic under Antifungal Therapy.) Air filters should be changed and there should be no unfiltered airflow from affected to unaffected areas. To prevent a colony from becoming reinfected, all cats entering or re-entering the cattery should be cultured and kept in isolation until results are obtained. Visitation to the cattery should be minimized.

Intermediate Fungal Infections

Sporotrichosis

Sporotrichium schenkii is a dimorphic fungus found worldwide. It is found in rich organic debris. It exists as a saprophytic mycelial fungus in the soil and a yeast in tissue or at 36°C in culture. In humans, the disease is considered to be an occupational hazard, most frequently affecting laborers, farmers, and florists.

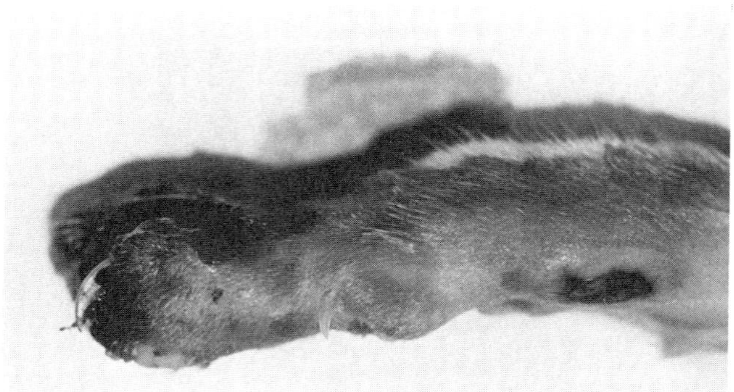

Figure 56–6. **Ulcerative lesions of sporotrichosis on the front leg of a cat. The original lesion is on the paw with a satellite lesion proximal to the original lesion.**

Contact with draining and ulcerated lesions in cats offers the potential for human infection; no penetrating injury is required.[7]

Clinical Signs

Three clinical forms of sporotrichosis have been described. The first and most common is the primary cutaneous form, in which lesions occur at the site of inoculation. These lesions are alopecic, crusted, nonpainful nodules, and ulcers. Satellite lesions may develop near the original site (Fig. 56–6). Lesions may also spread by the grooming behavior of the cat. The cutaneolymphatic form is the formation of nodules at the site of entry and the spread along the lymphatics. Lesions are most commonly seen on the distal extremities. The third form is the disseminated form, which is rare. It is usually an extension of cutaneous inoculation but can be a primary respiratory infection.

Diagnosis

Diagnosis is by identification of the organism by direct smear, fungal culture, or skin biopsy. A greater zoonotic threat is seen in cases where organisms are abundant on cytologic examination. The organism is pleomorphic, oval to cigar-shaped, approximately 2 to 6 μm long, and found primarily in the macrophage (Fig. 56–7). The organism can be cultured on Sabouraud's dextrose agar. Since this organism is a saprophyte, it is important to attempt to demonstrate the tissue form of the fungus. A granulomatous to pyogranulomatous reaction is seen histopathologically, and special stains may be needed to demonstrate the organism. A direct fluorescent antibody test is also available to use on the biopsy specimen.[1]

Therapy

Recommended treatment of the cutaneous or lymphocutaneous form is with a 20% aqueous solution of sodium iodide given at 0.5 mL/5 kg (22 mg/kg) twice daily. The IV preparation is administered orally; it may be mixed with cream or milk to increase palatability. Administration should

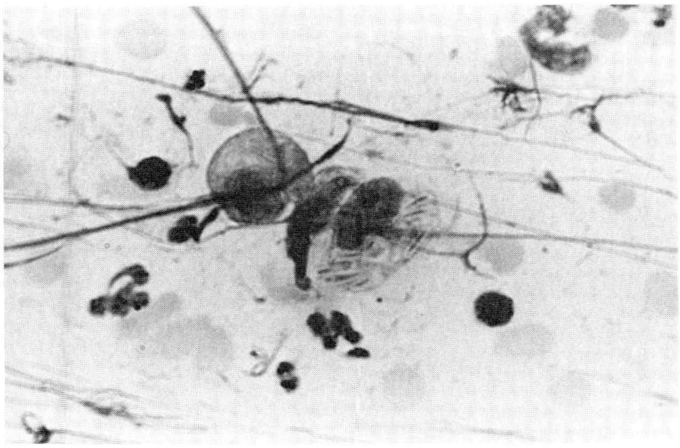

Figure 56–7. **Cigar-shaped and oval organisms of *Sporotrichium schenkii* in a macrophage from an impression smear of the lesion in Figure 56–6.**

be continued 4 weeks beyond clinical remission. Side effects seen in the cat include pyrexia, anorexia, nausea, salivation, lacrimation, sneezing, dry scaly skin, oral ulceration, and reversible cardiomyopathy.[8] Ketoconazole has also been used successfully.

Mycetoma

Mycetomas are caused by saprophytes that are ubiquitous in nature. Infection usually occurs via wound contamination or traumatic implantation. Eumycotic mycetomas are caused by several different fungi that enter the body through wounds. These fungi include *Curvularia* sp., *Allescheria* sp., and *Brachicladium* sp.[5] Actinomycotic mycetomas are caused by *Actinomyces* sp., *Nocardia* sp., and *Streptomyces* sp.[5]

Clinical Signs

Mycetomas are localized granulomatous swellings of subcutaneous tissue and sometimes adjacent bone. They are more commonly seen on the extremities. Fistulous tract formation and grain production are characteristic findings. The grains are fungal colonies coated with fibrin and immunoglobulin. The infections are chronic, fibrosing, and locally invasive.

Diagnosis

Diagnosis is by direct smear, culture of the tissue grains on Sabouraud's dextrose agar, and skin biopsy. A Gram stain of the grains will reveal gram-positive filaments of an actinomycotic mycetoma or hyphae and chlamydospores of eumycotic mycetomas. Culture of the tissue will enable definitive diagnosis of the infection.

Therapy

Therapy is total surgical excision of a eumycotic and actinomycotic mycetoma with addition of penicillin for actinomycosis and sulfonamides for nocardiosis. Therapy should be continued for 2 to 8 months.

Phaeohyphomycosis

Cutaneous phaeohyphomycosis is a nodular disease caused by a saprophytic dematiaceous (darkly pigmented) fungus that forms pigmented septate hyphae in host tissue. These fungi include *Dreschlera* sp., *Phialophora* sp., *Cladosporium* sp., *Exophiala* sp., and *Moniliella* sp. Infection is by wound contamination or traumatic transplantation.

Clinical Signs

Clinical signs can be localized to the skin or subcutaneous tissue or can be systemic with or without cutaneous lesions. The cutaneous lesions are usually solitary nodules that may later ulcerate and form fistulas. Distribution of lesions on the body is variable.

Diagnosis

Diagnosis is made by direct examination of the exudate in 10% to 20% KOH solution, revealing black, septate hyphae or culture on Sabouraud's dextrose agar or biopsy.

Therapy

The only truly effective therapy is complete surgical excision. In systemic disease or unresectable disease, amphotericin B, flucytosine, and ketoconazole have been used with limited success.

Pythiosis

Pythium is a dimorphic flagellate protozoan, not a true fungus. The infective agent is an aquatic flagellated zoospore. The organisms are parasites of aquatic plants, and the habitat is stagnant water with high organic content.[1]

Clinical Signs

Pythium in the cat has not been reported in the literature, but two cases have been seen at Louisiana State University School of Veterinary Medicine, and two others have been diagnosed by biopsies received at the Louisiana Veterinary Medical Diagnostic Laboratory. The clinical signs are nod-

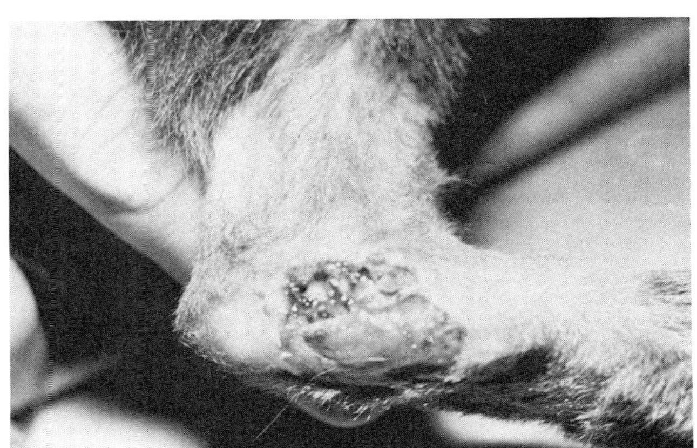

Figure 56–8. **Pythiosis on the hock of a cat. (Courtesy of Dr. Michele Brignac, Baton Rouge, LA.)**

ules with draining tracts (Fig. 56–8). The lesions are singular.

Diagnosis

Diagnosis is by fungal culture on Sabouraud's dextrose agar and histopathology. The histopathologic pattern is pyogranulomatous with organism more prominent in the center of the granulomatous foci. Special stains are often needed, as the organism is difficult to visualize on routine stains.

Therapy

The only effective therapy to date is total surgical excision. Pythium is not susceptible to antifungal agents. An autogenous vaccine has met with limited success in other species.

Deep (Systemic) Fungal Infections

Several systemic fungal infections affect the cat. Although the internal organs are the principal sites of infection, dermatologic manifestations may also occur. These are discussed in Chapter 61.

REFERENCES

1. Foil CS. Cutaneous Fungal Diseases. In: Nesbitt GH, ed. Contemporary Issues in Small Animal Practice: Dermatology. New York: Churchill Livingstone, 1987:123.
2. Moriello KA. Management of dermatophyte infections in catteries and multiple-cat households. Vet Clin N Am, Sm Anim Pract 1990;20:1457.
3. Nesbitt GH. Canine and Feline Dermatology: A Systematic Approach. Philadelphia: Lea & Febiger, 1983:89.
4. Ackerman LJ. Practical Feline Dermatology, 2nd ed. Goleta, CA: American Veterinary Publications, Inc, 1989:64.
5. Scott DW. Feline dermatology 1900–1978: A monograph. J Am Anim Hosp Assoc 1980;16:349.
6. Shelton GH, Grant CK, Linenberger ML, et al. Severe neutropenia associated with griseofulvin therapy in cats with feline immunodeficiency virus infection. J Vet Internal Med 1990;4:317.
7. Dunstan RW, Langham RF, Reimann KA, et al. Feline sporotrichosis: A report of five cases with transmission to humans. J Am Acad Dermatol 1986;15:37.
8. Burke MJ, Grauer GF, Macy DW. Successful treatment of cutaneolymphatic sporotrichosis in a cat with ketoconazole and sodium iodide. J Am Anim Hosp Assoc 1984;19:542.

CHAPTER 57

◇ ◇ ◇

The Skin: Parasitic Diseases

Sandra R. Merchant

Ectoparasitism is one of the most common causes of skin disease in the cat. Its prevalence is most closely correlated with the animal's environmental conditions (indoor vs. outdoor, cattery vs. single-cat household, rural vs. urban, and geographic region of the country). Most feline parasitic dermatoses are manifested clinically as miliary dermatitis, facial dermatitis, alopecia, or exfoliative dermatitis.[1] A varying degree of pruritus is associated with the infestation. Some cats may be nonpruritic and display minimal clinical signs. These cats serve as asymptomatic carriers and a source of infection for other in-contact animals. The common parasites are discussed in this chapter; the most common parasitic disease, flea allergy, is discussed in Chapter 58 under Hypersensitivity Disorders.

Otodectic Mange

Otodectic mange (otoacariasis, ear mites) is caused by the psoroptid mite *Otodectes cynotis*. It is the most common cause of otitis externa and an occasional cause of skin disease in the cat.

Etiology and Pathogenesis

O. cynotis lives on the surface of the skin. Adult mites are large, white, and freely moving. The anus is terminal, they have four pairs of legs, and all, except the rudimentary fourth pair of the female, extend beyond the body margin. The first two pairs of legs of the female and all four legs of the male bear short, unjointed stalks with suckers (Fig. 57–1). The life cycle is completed in 3 weeks primarily in the ear canal where the mites live on blood and lymph. However, they can infest other areas of the body. They are usually thought to live off the host for only a few days,[2] but have been reported to live for months in the environment.[3]

Most ear mite infections are seen in young kittens, because adult cats are much less prone to them. An immune response appears to develop after initial infestation, which helps prevent further disease.[4] Ear mites are highly contagious among cats, rabbits, and dogs. People may be transiently affected with a papular eruption of the arms and trunk.

Clinical Signs

Otodectes may account for up to 84% of otitis externa problems in cats. The mite causes variable degrees of pruritus and irritation due both to mechanical injury of the ear canal and to the hypersensitivity reaction from the mite saliva. Many cats tolerate large numbers of mites with minimal signs of discomfort, while others have extreme pruritus from small numbers. Common clinical signs include head shaking, scratching, rubbing, and ear twitching. Aural hematomas may be seen as a consequence of head shaking. Excoriations of the neck and anteriorly to the nose may be secondary to otoacariasis. The classic otic exudate is a thick reddish brown crust or a black coffee ground–like exudate (Fig. 57–2). Secondary bacterial and yeast infections may alter this classic exudate. Otitis media and interna rarely result from otoacariasis. Occasionally, ectopic infestations are seen on other parts of the body, especially the neck, rump, and tail. Lesions seen in association with this ectopic infestation are miliary dermatitis and diffuse alopecia associated with pruritus.

Diagnosis

The diagnosis is based upon clinical signs and finding the mites on otoscopic examination or from a superficial skin scraping. A large amount of exudate should be placed on a glass slide and examined for mites. Unfortunately, in the very inflamed ear or ear with a secondary bacterial or yeast infection, the mite may be difficult to find. Treatment of the bacterial or yeast infection may kill all or most of the adult ear mites but not their eggs. Within a few weeks of treatment, adult ear mites are likely to recur. Thus, a follow-up examination 4–6 weeks following treatment with an acaricide is warranted (see below).

Therapy

Since otoacariasis is very common in cats, otitis externa should initially be considered secondary to *O. cynotis* if the exudate is suggestive, even if the mite is not identified. Treatment consists of in-hospital application of a cerumino-

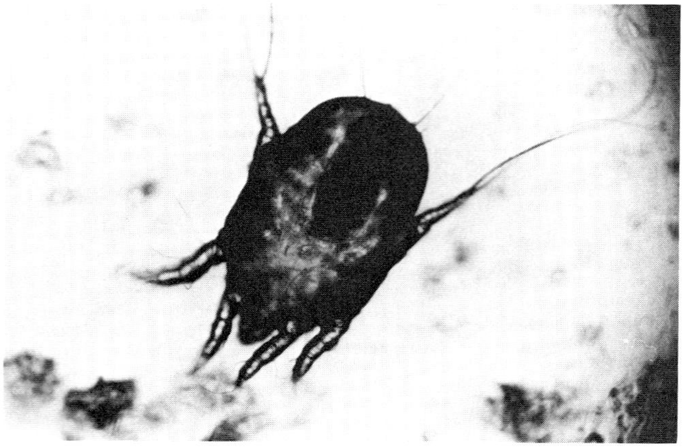

Figure 57–1. Microscopic picture of *O. cynotis* from an ear swab of a cat.

lytic agent to solubilize the cerumen followed by a detergent flushing agent to cleanse the ear of the ceruminolytic agent and debris. An ear-cleaning agent and a topical acaricide should then be used twice weekly for a minimum of 3 weeks. If the canal is severely inflamed, a combination acaricide and steroid is appropriate. If the canal has a significant bacterial or yeast infection, a topical antibiotic or antimycotic agent in combination with an acaricide is helpful. A topical insecticide shampoo, powder, or spray should be used a few times weekly to treat any mites living outside the ears. All other in-contact animals should be treated, even in the absence of clinical signs. Ivermectin has been utilized in the treatment of otoacariasis with good success. Dosages between 200 and 400 μg/kg SC or 500 μg/ear (1 drop) have been used.[6] The routine regimen has been two treatments of ivermectin 2 weeks apart. However, in a recent study an average of 4.2 treatments with 300 μg/kg subcutaneously at 1 to 2 week intervals was needed for complete cure, and 5.4 treatments, on average, of the 500 μg/ear were needed for complete cure.[6] The product is not approved for use in small animals at this dose. Since the mites may live off the animal for a period of time, the environment should be thoroughly cleaned and treated with an insecticide as for flea control.

Notoedric Mange

Notoedric mange is caused by the sarcoptid mite *Notoedres cati.* This is an uncommon external parasite of the cat in most areas of the United States but is endemic and common in a few locales.

Etiology and Pathogenesis

N. cati belongs to family Sarcoptidae and is very similar to the canine scabies mite. The fertilized female burrows through the horny layer of the skin and lays eggs in the tunnel. The life cycle is approximately 3 weeks from egg to adult. Adult mites are small, oval, and white with two pairs of short legs anteriorly, which bear medium length unjointed stalks with suckers, and two pairs of rudimentary posterior legs that do not extend beyond the border of the body (Fig. 57–3). The posterior legs of the females have bristles, while the third pair of legs of the males have bristles and the fourth pair has suckers. The anus is dorsally located.

This mite can infect foxes, dogs, rabbits, and humans, but the infection is self-limiting, and the disease resolves once the source of infection has been treated.[7] Transmission of *N. cati* is by direct contact or by means of fomites.

Clinical Signs

The primary lesion is an erythematous papule that typically first appears at the proximal edge of the pinna of the ear and rapidly spreads to the rest of the face and neck. Because of the intense pruritus, the affected area soon becomes thick, crusted, alopecic, and excoriated (Fig. 57–4). If untreated, lesions may spread to other areas of the body. A secondary bacterial infection is common.

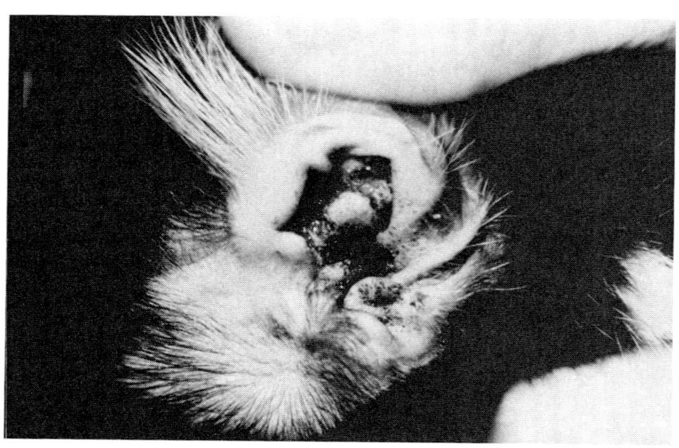

Figure 57–2. Black, granular exudate secondary to *O. cynotis* infestation.

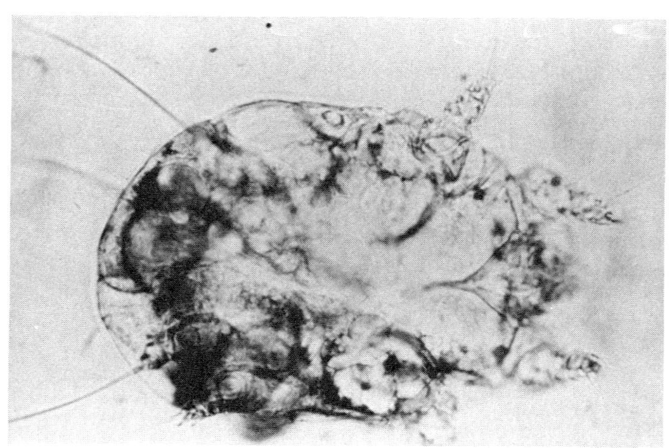

Figure 57–3. Microscopic picture of *N. cati.* (Courtesy of Dr. T. Bonner Stewart, Louisiana State University, Baton Rouge, LA.)

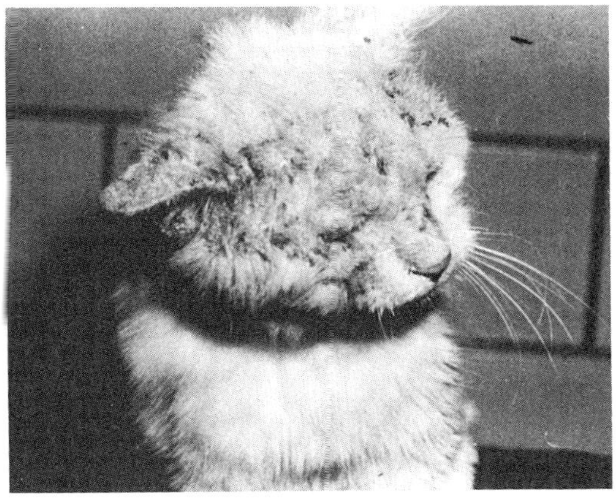

Figure 57–4. Crusts, excoriations and alopecia on the head of a cat infected with *N. cati.* (Courtesy of Dr. Thomas Hribernik, Louisiana State University, Baton Rouge, LA.)

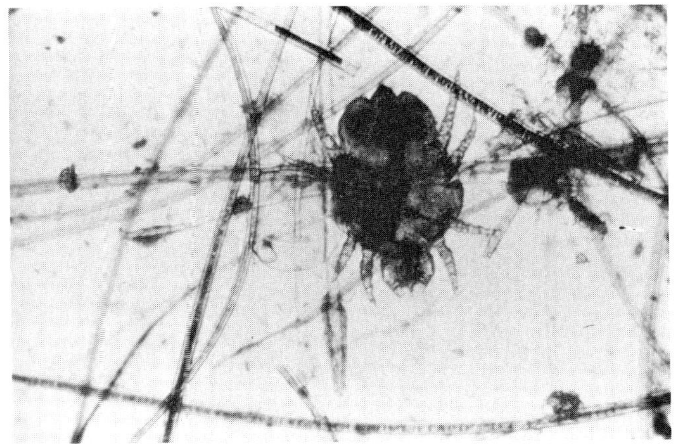

Figure 57–5. Microscopic picture of *Cheyletiella spp.* from a skin scraping. (Courtesy of Dr. Gail Kunkle, University of Florida, Gainesville, FL.)

Diagnosis

N. cati, unlike *Sarcoptes scabiei* in the dog, is usually seen by microscopic examination of scale and debris gathered from several broad superficial skin scrapings. Mites or ova are occasionally found by fecal flotation. Skin biopsy should not be needed to diagnose this parasite, since skin scrapings are usually positive.

Therapy

Several parasiticidal agents are effective against *N. cati.* The safest agent is a 2% lime sulfur (LymDyp) solution. It is the treatment of choice in young, pregnant, or debilitated adults. The organophosphates that are labeled for use in the cat are also effective in treatment of this parasite. These dips should be used every 5 days for a total of six to eight treatments. Amitraz (Mitaban) is also scabicidal but is not currently approved for use in cats.[1] Ivermectin at 200 to 300 µg/kg SC twice at a 2-week interval has proven effective but is also not approved for use in cats. All in-contact animals should be treated. The environment should also be treated, since mites can live off of the host, under certain conditions, for a number of days.[7]

Cheyletiellosis

Cheyletiella dermatitis in the cat is primarily caused by *Cheyletiella blakei.* However, there are two other species of clinical importance, *Cheyletiella yasguri,* primarily parasitizing dogs, and *Cheyletiella parasitivorax,* primarily parasitizing rabbits. These mites can be freely transmitted to other hosts including humans.

Etiology and Pathogenesis

Cheyletiella mites are large (385 µm) and have four pairs of legs bearing combs instead of claws. The most prominent feature of *Cheyletiella* spp. is the accessory mouthparts that terminate in prominent hooks (Fig. 57–5). These mites are surface dwellers and do not burrow into the keratin layer of the epidermis. The parasites spend their entire life cycle on the host. Oval-shaped eggs are laid at the base of the hair follicle and are attached to the hair by a fine fibrillar strand at one end. The eggs develop to mature adults in approximately 3 weeks. Adult females can live apart from the host for as long as 10 days.[8] Mites have been seen crawling in and out of the nostrils of cats.[9] Severe infestations can occur in litters, catteries, and pet shops. Transmission is by direct contact or by means of fomites. The disease has zoonotic potential but is self-limiting in humans. The infection spontaneously clears once the source of the infestation is treated.

Clinical Signs

Clinical signs are variable. Many infested cats are clinically normal. Some patients present with slightly oily coats and increased scaling. The dorsum of the patient is the most commonly affected region. More diffuse, total body involvement occasionally occurs. Pruritus is highly variable; patients can be totally asymptomatic or moderately pruritic. The skin can be completely unaffected or display an erythematous papular eruption.

Diagnosis

Diagnosis is made by careful inspection of the scaly skin surface of the cat. Evidence of mites or eggs can be obtained by wide superficial skin scrapings, cellophane-tape impression smears of the scales, flea-combing the epidermal debris onto dark paper, or gathering and clearing the epidermal debris with potassium hydroxide (KOH), all with examination of the material under the microscope. With a magnifying glass, the mites may be observed moving around on the skin and hair, hence the name "walking dandruff." Trimming the hair from affected areas facilitates better sample collection. The flea comb and KOH technique appears to be the most reliable test for the diagnosis for cheyletiellosis.[10] Eggs and adult mites are occasionally demonstrated by fecal flotation. In some cases, the mites cannot be demonstrated, and thus diagnosis depends on response to therapy.[11]

Therapy

Cheyletiellosis is readily cured by most forms of parasiticidal therapy. Pyrethrins, carbaryl, rotenone powder, and lime sulfur dips can be used. Insecticides should be applied three times at 1-week intervals. In highly contaminated or endemic situations, dips may be used for a total of 6 to 8 weeks.[1] Amitraz and ivermectin are also effective but not approved for this use. Dosages and schedules recommended for ivermectin include 200 to 300 μg/kg SC and repeated in 2 weeks[12] and 300 μg/kg SC and repeated in 5 weeks.[13] All in-contact animals should be treated. The premises should be cleaned and treated with a residual insecticide.

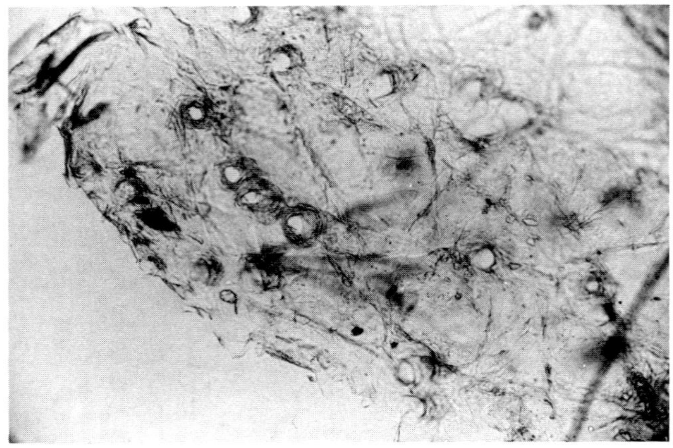

Figure 57–7. **Epidermal pits in stratum corneum cells from a cat with superficial demodicosis.**

Demodectic Mange

Demodectic mange is caused by *Demodex cati* and another as yet unnamed species of *Demodex*. It is rare in cats and less severe than in dogs.

Etiology and Pathogenesis

The demodectic mite is a normal resident in small numbers on the skin of cats. The life cycle and immunopathology of the feline *Demodex* mites are unknown but are reported to be similar to *D. canis* in the dog. *D. cati,* morphologically similar to *D. canis,* resides in the hair follicle. The unnamed species of *Demodex* in comparison, has a broad, blunted abdomen (Fig. 57–6). It is morphologically similar to *Demodex criceti* of the hamster. This mite is believed to live in the superficial stratum corneum and not in the hair follicle.[5] The author has seen this mite associated with pits in stratum corneum cells (Fig. 57–7).

Demodicosis is not considered contagious. Since most cases reported in the literature occurred in adult cats who developed demodicosis as a result of an underlying disease, the pathogenicity has been proposed to be related to endogenous and/or exogenous immunosuppression.[2] Generalized demodicosis has been seen in cats with diabetes mellitus, respiratory infection, feline leukemia virus (FeLV) infection, systemic lupus erythematosus, toxoplasmosis, feline endocrine alopecia, feline immunodeficiency virus (FIV) infection, and hyperadrenocorticism.[2,14-19]

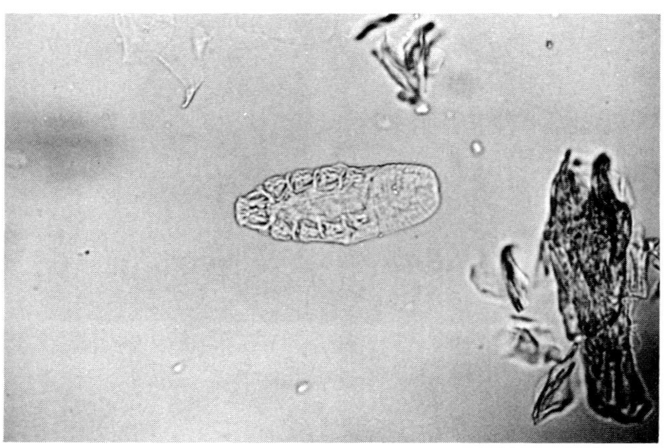

Figure 57–6. **Microscopic picture of the unnamed *Demodex* mite of the cat.**

Clinical Signs

Clinical signs of demodicosis are highly variable, and cases can be localized or generalized. Localized *Demodex* has been seen as a single area of alopecia and scaling of the eyelids, periocular area, head, and neck. A localized ceruminous demodectic otitis externa has also been described.[2] In generalized cases, signs include multifocal to generalized patches of alopecia with variable scaling, macules, papules, erythema, hyperpigmentation, crusting, and symmetric alopecia of the head, neck, legs, and trunk. Pruritus, when present, is either intermittent or mild. Clinical signs associated with the unnamed species of *Demodex* include more severe pruritus, mild erythema, broken hairs, and alopecia of the hindlimbs, flank, and ventral abdomen (Fig. 57–8). In some cats, mild clinical signs and patterns of involvement have been such that the condition could mimic psychogenic alopecia.[2]

Diagnosis

Diagnosis is by broad superficial and concentrated deep skin scrapings from affected areas. Because clinical signs are variable, skin scrapings should be performed routinely on all cats with skin lesions. If mites are found in only one location, further scrapings of the facial region and nonlesional skin are indicated to determine the true extent of the disease. The mites may also be detected on skin biopsy from hair follicles (*D. cati*) or in the stratum corneum (unnamed species).[20,21] A thorough search for an underlying disease should be undertaken in cats with generalized demodicosis.

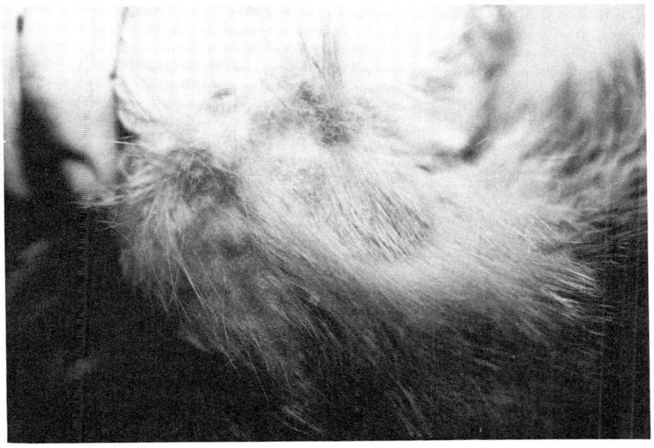

Figure 57–8. **Erythema, alopecia, crusting, and excoriation on the dorsal cervical region of a cat with superficial demodicosis (unnamed species).**

Appropriate tests include a complete blood count, chemistry profile, urinalysis, FeLV and FIV test.

Therapy

Several treatment regimens have been proposed for demodicosis in the cat; however, none is widely recognized as successful. As in the dog, localized forms are usually self-limiting. Topical rotenone and topical amitraz locally applied have been used with success. Generalized demodicosis has been treated successfully with weekly dips of lime sulfur, phosmet, fenchlorphos,[18] 0.0125% amitraz (1/2 strength),[22] carbaryl shampoos, malathion dips, and one part rotenone in three parts mineral oil for the ears.[9] Topical therapy is continued weekly until negative scrapings are achieved. Amitraz and fenchlorphos are not approved for use in the cat. Anorexia, depression, diarrhea, hypersalivation, and hiding under furniture have been seen with the use of amitraz in the cat.[22,25] Generalized demodicosis in cats seems to be much more responsive to therapy compared with the disease in dogs. This may be a reflection of the more superficial location of the mites in many cases. The author suggests use of lime sulfur dips first since they have the least potential for side effects, and many cats clear with this therapy.

Miscellaneous Parasites

Pediculosis (Lice)

Lice are wingless insects that are host-specific and do not survive well off of that host. Infestations are uncommon but are more likely to be seen in young animals. The cat louse, *Felicola subrostratus,* is a biting louse (Fig. 57–9). Infestation is usually associated with debilitation and unsanitary conditions.

Pediculosis is contagious with transmission by direct contact or fomite. Infestation seems to occur more commonly in the winter, when animals have longer hair coats and closer contact. Clinical signs are variable and include seborrhea sicca, miliary dermatitis, mild to severe pruritus, and an unkempt hair coat. Asymptomatic carriers may also be seen. The diagnosis may often be made by physical examination or by acetate tape impressions of the hair coat. Both lice and nits are visible with the naked eye. The eggs are larger than the *Cheyletiella* eggs and are attached to the hair along most of the length of the egg. Pyrethrin or carbamate shampoos have been used with success. This treatment should be repeated within 10 to 14 days to kill any nits that hatched after the first treatment. Two percent lime sulfur dips are also effective. All in-contact animals should be treated. Pediculosis is a self-limiting zoonotic disease after the source of the infestation has been treated.

Trombiculidiasis (Chiggers)

Trombiculidiasis in the cat is caused by the parasitic larval stage of many species of chiggers including *Eutrombicula alfreddugesi, Eutrombicula autumnalis,* and *Walchia americana* among others. Cats, dogs, and humans will become infested through direct contact with the larva-infested foliage in fields and forests. This usually occurs during the late summer and fall. The bite usually produces severe irritation and an intensely pruritic papular and crusting eruption, but it may also cause nonpruritic pustules and crusts. Lesions are most commonly seen on the head, ears, and feet. The small (0.2 to 0.4 mm) orange-colored larvae may be seen associated with the papules early in the course of the disease. Diagnosis is made by skin scrapings to find the six-legged larvae. Because the larvae only attach to the host for a few days, they may be gone by the time of examination. Treatment involves one to two parasiticidal dips with a pyrethrin product or lime sulfur. Tresaderm has been effective for treatment of chigger-induced otitis externa.[24]

Cat Fur Mite

Lynxacarus radovsky, the cat fur mite is an unusual parasitic infection. Cases have been reported from Australia, Fiji, Flor-

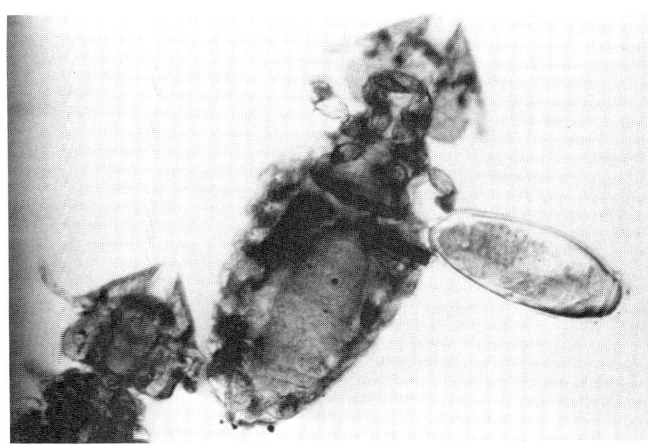

Figure 57–9. **Microscopic picture of *Felicola subrostratus* and egg. (Courtesy of the late Dr. R. R. Bell, Texas A&M University.)**

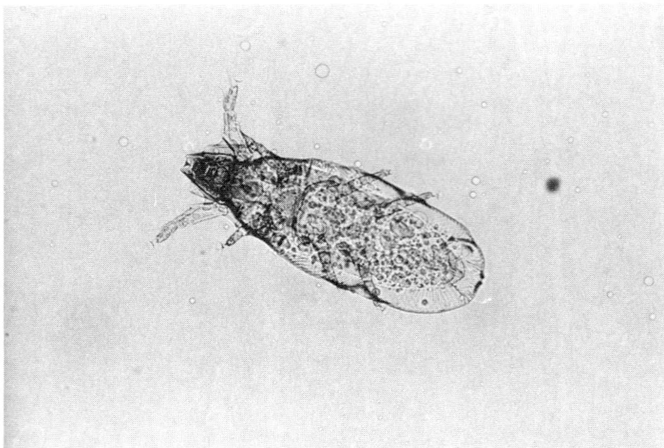

Figure 57–10. Microscopic picture of *Lynxacarus radovsky.* (Courtesy of Dr. E. Greiner, University of Florida, Gainesville, FL.)

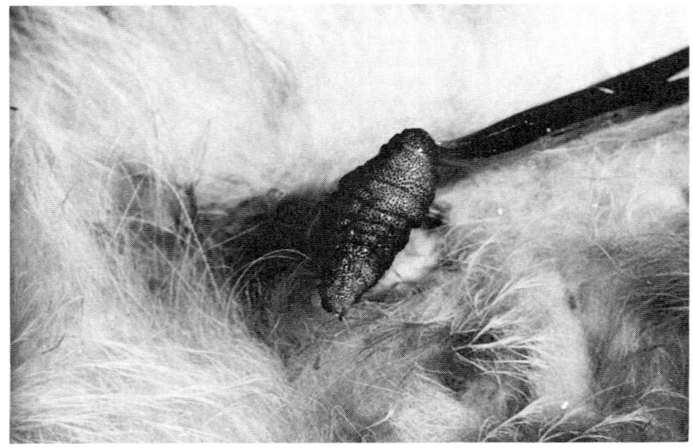

Figure 57–12. Cuterebra larva extracted from its subcutaneous nodule. (Courtesy of Dr. Gary Norsworthy, San Antonio, TX.)

ida, Hawaii, and Puerto Rico.[5] These mites have elongated bodies and flaplike sternal extensions (Fig. 57–10). The extensions contain the first two legs, which grasp the hair of the host. All the legs have terminal suckers. Hair coats of cats infested with these mites have a dull, dry appearance and epilate easily. A heavy infestation may give a light hair coat a "salt and pepper" appearance.[2,5] Other lesions seen are patchy alopecia, seborrhea sicca, and miliary dermatitis. The dorsal aspect of the trunk is most commonly affected. Diagnosis is made by skin scraping or acetate tape impression to isolate the mites. Therapy consists of 0.5% malathion dips, 2.0% lime sulfur dips, and 5.0% carbaryl powder administered weekly for 3 to 4 weeks.[25-27]

Cuterebra

Although rabbits and rodents are considered the primary hosts for *Cuterebra* spp., cats that are near rodent or rabbit burrows are occasionally affected. The adult female *Cuterebra* lays its eggs in soil. The larvae hatch, penetrate the skin of the host, develop in subcutaneous nodules, create a breathing pore, and eventually emerge and pupate on the ground. These subcutaneous nodules are seen most often around the head region (Fig. 57–11). Treatment is gentle removal of the larva with forceps after enlarging the breathing pore (Fig. 57–12). Rupture of the larva should be avoided since anaphylactoid reactions have been reported.[9,24] The lesion should be treated as an open wound.

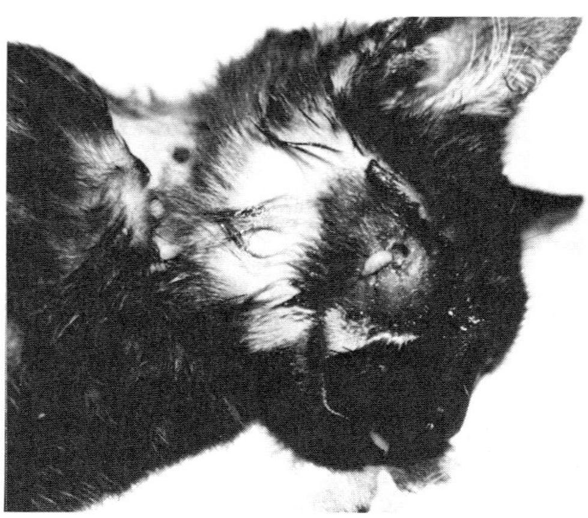

Figure 57–11. Nodule on the head of a cat with the *Cuterebra* larva extruded from the breathing pore. (Courtesy of Dr. Carol Foil, Louisiana State University, Baton Rouge, LA.)

REFERENCES

1. Scheidt VJ. Common feline ectoparasites part 1: Clinical syndromes. Comp Anim Pract 1987;1:6.
2. Scott DW. Feline dermatology 1900–1978: A monograph. J Am Anim Hosp Assoc 1980;16:365.
3. Larkin AD, Gaillard GE. Mites in cat ears, a source of cross antigenicity with house dust mites. Preliminary report. An Allergy 1981;46:301.
4. Weisbroth SH, Powell MB, Roth L, et al. Immunopathology of naturally occurring otodectic otoacariasis in the domestic cat. J Am Vet Med Assoc 1974;165:1088.
5. Kwochka KW. Mites and Related Disease. Vet Clin N Am, Sm Anim Pract 1987;17:1263.
6. Graham D. Treatment of ear mites (*Otodectes cynotis*) in cats: Comparison of subcutaneous and topical ivermectin. 7th Proc Ann Memb Meeting AAVD & ACVD, Scottsdale, AZ, 1991:26.
7. Merchant SR. Zoonotic disease with cutaneous manifestations. Part I. Compend Cont Educ Pract Vet 1990;12:371.
8. Foxx TS, Ewing SA. Morphologic features, behavior, and life history of *Cheyletiella yasguri.* Am J Vet Res 1969;30:269.
9. Muller GH, Kirk RW, Scott DW. Small Animal Dermatology. Philadelphia: WB Saunders, 1989;365.
10. Paradis M, Villeneuve A. Efficacy of ivermectin against *Cheyletiella yasguri* infestation in dogs. Can Vet J 1988;29:633.
11. McKeever PJ, Allen SK. Dermatosis associated with *Cheyletiella* infestation in cats. J Am Vet Med Assoc 1979;174:718.

12. Pulkay BP. Cheyletiellosis. In: August JR, ed. Consultations in Feline Internal Medicine. Philadelphia: WB Saunders, 1991:137.
13. Paradis M, Scott D, Villeneuve A. Efficacy of ivermectin against *Cheyletiella blakei* infestation in cats. J Am Anim Hosp Assoc 1990;26:125.
14. Chalmer S, Schick RO, Jeffers J. Demodicosis in two cats seropositive for feline immunodeficiency virus. J Am Vet Med Assoc 1989;194:256.
15. Bailey RG, Thompson RCA. Demodectic mange in a cat. Aust Vet J 1981;57:49.
16. White SD, Carpenter JL, Moore FM, et al. Generalized demodicosis associated with diabetes mellitus in two cats. J Am Vet Med Assoc 1987;191:448.
17. Stogdale L, Moore DJ. Feline demodicosis. J Am Anim Hosp Assoc 1982;18:427.
18. Medleau L, Brown CA, Brown SA, et al. Demodicosis in cats. J Am Anim Hosp Assoc 1988;24:85.
19. Zerbe CA, Nachreiner RF, Dunstan RW, et al. Hyperadrenocorticism in a cat. J Am Vet Med Assoc 1987;190:559.
20. Conroy JD, Healey MC, Bane AG. New *Demodex* sp. infesting a cat: A case report. J Am Anim Hosp Assoc 1982;18:405.
21. McDougal BJ, Novak CP. Feline demodicosis caused by an unnamed *Demodex* mite. Compend Cont Ed Pract Vet 1986; 8:820.
22. Cowan LA, Campbell K. Generalized demodicosis in a cat responsive to amitraz. J Am Vet Med Assoc 1988;192:1442.
23. Gunaratnam P, Wilkinson GT, Seawright AA. A study of amitraz toxicity in cats. Aust Vet J 1983;60:278.
24. Fadok VA. Miscellaneous parasites of the skin. Part II. Compend Cont Ed Pract Vet 1980;2:782.
25. Bowman WL. The cat fur mite (*Lynxacarus radovsky*) in Australia. Aust Vet J 1978;54:403.
26. Munro R, Munro HMC. Lynxacarus on cats in Fiji. Aust Vet J 1979;55:90.
27. Utteridge T. Cat Fur Mite (*Lynxacarus radovsky*) in South Australia. University of Sydney Post Grad Committee Veterinary Science Control and Therapy No. 1364, 1982.

CHAPTER 58

◇ ◇ ◇

The Skin: Hypersensitivity Diseases

Sandra R. Merchant

Hypersensitivity reactions are the result of an exaggerated immune response that produces undesirable side effects. These hypersensitivity reactions involve basic immune mechanisms that are important for protection against foreign antigens. Unfortunately, because of the exaggerated response, greater damage is induced by response to the antigen than would be caused by the antigen alone. Hypersensitivity reactions have been classified into four basic types by Gell and Coombs. Types I, II, and III each involve an antibody-dependent mechanism, whereas a Type IV response is cell-mediated and involves soluble factors other than antibody.[1]

A detailed understanding of the immune system is not essential to diagnosis of a hypersensitivity reaction, but a basic understanding is helpful in ascertaining the best method for diagnosis of each hypersensitivity disease and what medical intervention is appropriate in each type of hypersensitivity state.

Flea Allergic Dermatitis

Flea allergic dermatitis is the most common allergic skin disorder in cats and may be the most common overall disease problem of pet animals.[2] Each year, in excess of a billion dollars is spent on flea control. Flea-related diseases may account for over 50% of dermatologic cases presented to veterinarians and in excess of 35% of the total small animal veterinary effort.[3]

Etiology and Pathogenesis

Ctenocephalides felis, the cat flea, is the most common flea affecting cats *and* dogs in the United States. Other fleas reported to infest cats include *C. canis, Pulex irritans,* and *Echidnophaga gallinacea.* These ectoparasites lack host specificity. The majority of their life cycle is spent off the host and in the environment. The life span of the flea is influenced by environmental factors but usually ranges from 6 to 12 months. Its life cycle includes an egg, three larval stages, pupae, and adult. The egg and the pupa stages are quite resistant to most insecticides and environmental conditions. Eggs hatch within 2 to 12 days, and the larvae feed on organic debris and flea excrement while molting through three larval stages in 9 to 20 days.

Following a decrease in the production of juvenile hormone, the third larval form spins a cocoon. In several days to months, upon stimulation by the presence of a host, the pupae emerge as adult fleas. Ideal conditions for flea larvae survival are temperatures between 65°F and 85°F and a relative humidity of 75 to 85%. Under ideal conditions, the flea life cycle can be completed in 16 days, or it can take as long as a year to complete under less favorable conditions, including the absence of host activation. A dry climate, extreme cold, or high altitude threatens flea survival.

Flea saliva contains substances that have irritant and pruritogenic properties. The reaction of the host to a flea bite varies from mild irritation in an unsensitized animal to severe pruritus in an animal that is allergic to the flea's saliva. In the development of flea allergy, immediate (Type I) and delayed (Type IV) hypersensitivity reactions have been shown in the dog. The delayed Type IV reaction is questionable in the cat.

Clinical Signs

The most common clinical sign associated with flea allergy is a crusting, erythematous, papular eruption or miliary dermatitis with pruritus. The distribution of these lesions is variable and not as distinctive as in the flea-allergic dog. Distribution patterns range from a "classic" caudodorsal tailhead (Fig. 58–1), medial thigh, or groin distribution to "ring around the collar" only, or generalized miliary dermatitis. A small percentage of flea-allergic cats have miliary dermatitis *without* pruritus. Many allergic cats have no skin lesions but lick excessively, chew, and pull out large tufts of hair. This hair loss can be patchy to diffuse and at times is quite symmetric and bilateral in distribution, mimicking an endocrine pattern of hair loss (Fig. 58–2). The "bald-belly" cat can be an example of an animal with flea allergic dermatitis. Other less common patterns of flea allergy in the cat include facial pruritus and exfoliative dermatitis.

Additional clinical signs seen in the cat with flea-allergic dermatitis may include tapeworms in the stool, hairballs in the stool or vomitus, and peripheral eosinophilia. In severe

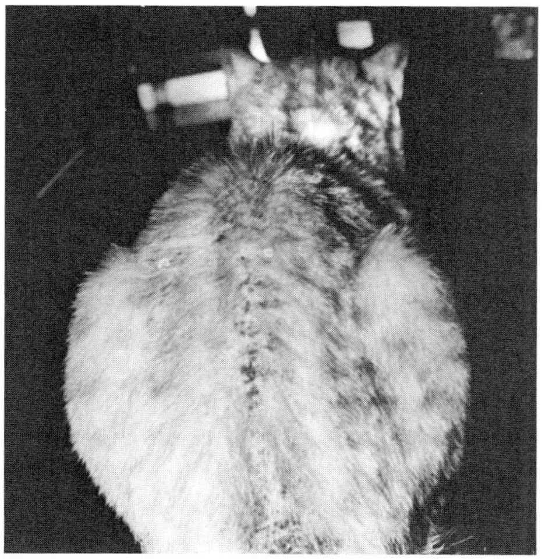

Figure 58–1. **"Racing stripe" of erythema, crust, and alopecia in a cat with flea allergic dermatitis. (Courtesy of Dr. Carol Foil, Louisiana State University, Baton Rouge, LA.)**

infestations, anemia and personality change, e.g., irritability, may be seen. When questioned about any pruritus associated with hair loss or skin lesions in their cats, many owners respond negatively. This may mean that the cat is truly nonpruritic (rare), or that the question was not worded correctly ("Does your cat itch?" versus "Does your cat bite, scratch, chew, or excessively groom?"), or that the cat is a closet groomer. It is important not to let this negative response from the owner decrease your clinical suspicion of flea allergy. In the majority of cases, the hair loss is self-induced.

Diagnosis

Historical information, in addition to clinical signs and evidence of fleas or flea excreta, is helpful in making the diagnosis of flea allergy dermatitis. However, such information may be lacking ("My cat is not itching and has never had fleas!"), the clinical signs can deviate from the "classic" ones, and evidence of fleas or flea excreta on the animal may be lacking or difficult to find. This may reflect the fastidious grooming habits of the cat, a recent bath, or low numbers of fleas in the environment. A fine-toothed flea comb can help pick flea or flea excreta particles out of the coat.

The use of intradermal skin testing with an aqueous flea antigen is important for the diagnostic value of the test as well as an excellent tool for client education. Skin testing is more difficult in the cat than in the dog. The injections are more difficult to place intradermally, and the interpretation of the response is also more problematic. A small area on the lateral thorax is gently clipped, and 0.05 to 0.1 mL of a phosphate buffered saline, 1:100,000 weight/volume (w/v) histamine phosphate, and 1:1000 w/v aqueous flea antigen are injected *intradermally*. It is important to use aqueous extracts because glycerinated extracts can act as primary irritants and cause false-positive reactions.[4]

It is important to keep the cat as calm as possible. Some cats object to being placed in the lateral recumbency position for this test and do better if allowed to stay in sternal recumbency. Only a few cats need to be given a sedative to accomplish flea allergy testing. Phenothiazine and barbiturate drugs should be avoided. The author prefers a combination of ketamine and diazepam given intravenously for this procedure if necessary.

False-negative results can also occur if the cat has recently been treated with systemic glucocorticoids, antihistamines, or tranquilizers. As a rule, oral glucocorticoids should be discontinued a minimum of 2 to 4 weeks prior to testing, injectable reposital glucocorticoids for 8 to 14 weeks prior to testing, and antihistamines for 10 to 14 days prior to testing. A positive response to the skin test can be subtle in a cat and may consist of slight erythema without induration or well-demarcated borders (Fig. 58–3). A positive reaction may be evident within a few minutes and may have faded by 15 minutes. Thus it is important to watch the

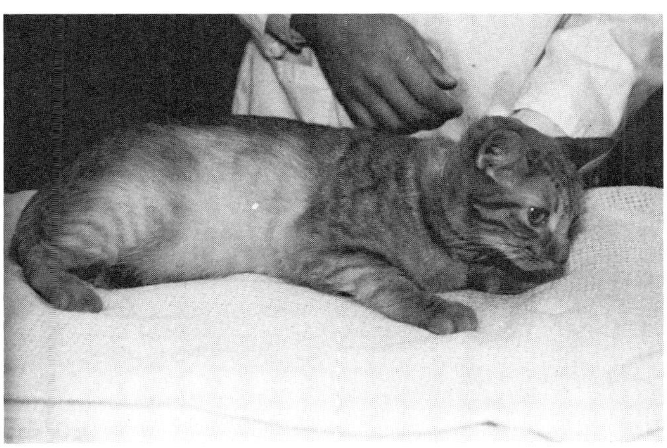

Figure 58–2. Self-induced symmetric hair loss in a cat with flea allergic dermatitis. (Courtesy of Dr. Joy Barbet, Gainesville, FL.)

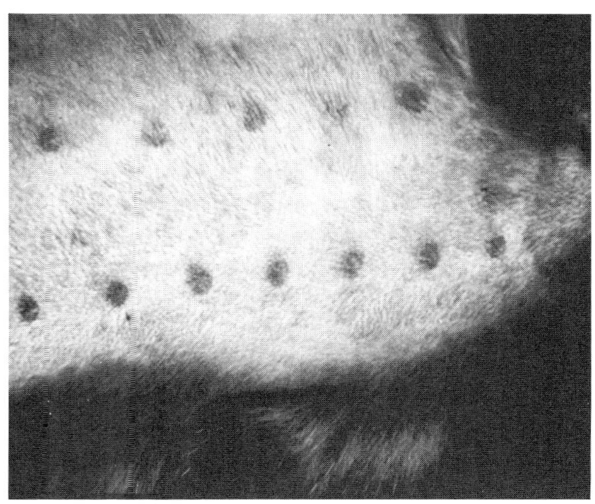

Figure 58–3. A positive flea test response in a cat. Note the circular erythema under dots 4 and 5 in the upper row. (Courtesy of Dr. Carol Foil, Louisiana State University, Baton Rouge, LA.)

test site for the full 15 minutes and record the response at the height of the reaction. A positive skin test alone, without corresponding compatible clinical signs, does not justify a diagnosis of flea allergic dermatitis. Conversely, a negative skin test in a patient with supportive clinical signs warrants a 1-month trial of flea control measures before the flea allergic diagnosis is dismissed.

Therapy

Effective flea control requires elimination of fleas from all in-contact animals and flea eradication in the environment. Total flea control for a cat that lives in a population of exclusively indoor pets is relatively easy, whereas total flea control for an outdoor, free-roaming cat is virtually impossible.

Flea Control on the Animal

It is important that flea control be practiced on all animals in the household. Dips are an effective way to kill adult fleas, but those labeled for use on cats may not continue to kill newly emerging fleas that jump on the animal. Dips are classified into three categories, based upon the active ingredient: dips with organic insecticides, dips with synthetic pyrethroids, and dips with organophosphates or carbamates. All of these can be utilized on in-contact dogs. Package instructions should be followed as to dipping interval. Dips utilized for cats are primarily organic insecticides, with a few in the synthetic pyrethroid and organophosphate/carbamate category. Since most cats object strenuously to dipping, other therapies are preferred by the author; powders and sprays can take the place of dips. In general, powders can be divided into three categories, depending on the active ingredient: powders with pyrethrins, powders with carbamate insecticides (no more than 5% for a cat), and powders with organophosphate insecticides. The last category is rarely used in the cat. Powders should be used several times a week to be effective. They must be applied very thoroughly and worked well into the animal's coat.

Sprays are similar to powders in use and active ingredients. Water- and alcohol-based sprays are available. The author prefers the use of a water-based spray, since many cats salivate excessively with an alcohol-based spray. Microencapsulation of these products provides residual activity and decreases toxicity. For cats that object to the "hissing" sound of the spray, a microencapsulated pyrethrin foam is available (Sectrol Flea Foam, Animal Care Products/3 M, St. Paul, MN). Shampoos and sprays are rarely effective as the sole method of flea control because they provide no residual protection. Flea collars have shown little efficacy against fleas on pets. Ultrasonic flea collars have been found to be ineffective against fleas (personal communication, Dr. R.E.W. Halliwell). Avon Skin-So-Soft (Avon Products Inc., New York, NY) has been reported to have some repellent activity when used as a rinse on dogs.[5]

A flea comb is an important tool in assessing flea control. Owners should be instructed to flea comb the cat a few times weekly. In a controlled environment, after environmental flea control is achieved, no fleas should be found on flea combing.

Flea Control in the Environment

Environmental control is the key to a successful flea control program. A client handout should be prepared, detailing the recommendations for environmental treatment. Thorough cleaning of the home, including mopping and vacuuming, is necessary prior to delivery of insecticides. A professional exterminator can be employed, but the service must follow the same general principles outlined below.

All pets and children should be removed from the environment for several hours after treatment. When traditional insecticides are used, the house (and yard) should be thoroughly treated every 2 weeks for three treatments, with monthly treatment thereafter. The most commonly used insecticides are malathion, chlorpyrifos, and carbaryl. This treatment can be reduced in the winter, especially in areas experiencing freezing temperatures. Sprays are the treatment of choice of the author. Foggers can be utilized for indoor treatment but are not extremely penetrating in a thick rug, under furniture, or around walls. Therefore, one fogger needs to be used per room, and areas not penetrated by the fogger need to be sprayed.

A relatively new environmental flea control product is an insect growth regulator (IGR). Two products are currently available, methoprene and fenoxycarb. The former is inactivated by sunlight and can only be used indoors, but the latter can be used both indoors and outdoors. These products prevent the larvae from reaching the pupa stage, decrease the fecundity of the female, and decrease the viability of the eggs. These IGRs have a residual activity of 90 days. The author recommends use of these products every 60 days.

Another relatively new commercially available environmental flea control product is sodium polyborate (Rx for Fleas, Fleabuster, Ft. Lauderdale, FL). This product acts as a flea irritant and desiccant. The author has received positive response from clients utilizing this product.

Complete environmental control can be achieved by following the above recommendations if all animals are confined to this controlled environment. Unfortunately, many cats are both indoor/outdoor or are completely outdoor and roam freely. In these cases, a topical microencapsulated product with residual activity is advised. Environmental treatment is still extremely important to stop the flea life cycle from being re-established when the cat brings fleas back into the environment. Unfortunately, complete resolution of clinical signs may not be achieved in this situation.

Glucocorticoids may be necessary to control pruritus in the flea allergic cat when environmental control is being initiated or when complete control cannot be achieved. Oral, short-acting glucocorticoids such as prednisone, prednisolone, or methylprednisolone, should be utilized on an alternative-day basis at 0.25 mg/lb if chronic glucocorticoid administration is necessary. For initial control of the very pruritic cat, 0.5 to 1.0 mg/lb may be needed on a daily basis for 7 to 10 days. Unfortunately, many cats cannot be given or do not respond to oral glucocorticoids. Only in these cases should the longer acting repositol glucocorticoids be considered, and they should be used as sparingly as possible and no more often than every 90 days. Antihistamines are relatively ineffective in controlling pruritus associated with flea allergic dermatitis, but they can be tried. The author uses chlorpheniramine maleate at 2.0 mg b.i.d. per cat.

Food Allergic Dermatitis

The immune system of the gastrointestinal tract is almost continually confronted with antigens from food sources. A well-developed barrier system prevents foreign proteins from entering the body via the gastrointestinal tract and eliciting an immunoglobulin response. Despite this barrier system, some food proteins gain access to the systemic circulation and an immune response ensues.

Pathogenesis

The exact pathogenesis of food hypersensitivity has not been defined in the dog or cat. Types I and III hypersensitivities have been proposed to occur.[6-8] The integumentary, gastrointestinal, respiratory, neurologic, and urinary systems can be involved in food hypersensitivity. Dermatologic disease is the most common manifestation of food hypersensitivity, with gastrointestinal disturbance being the second most common effect. No breed or sex predilection has been reported in the cat with food hypersensitivity. This dermatosis is seen almost exclusively in adult cats.[9] Reactions may develop either suddenly or slowly, and age of onset is variable.

Cutaneous Signs

Pruritus is the most common clinical presentation of food allergic dermatitis. Primary lesions can be papular, urticarial, or absent. Food hypersensitivity may manifest as miliary dermatitis, eosinophilic plaques or ulcers, asymmetric to symmetric alopecia, pruritic angioedema (urticaria), and otitis externa.[10] Skin lesions secondary to self-trauma include alopecia, erythema, lichenification, excoriation, ulcer, scale, and crust. A predilection for the head and neck is often seen (Fig. 58–4), although signs may become generalized.

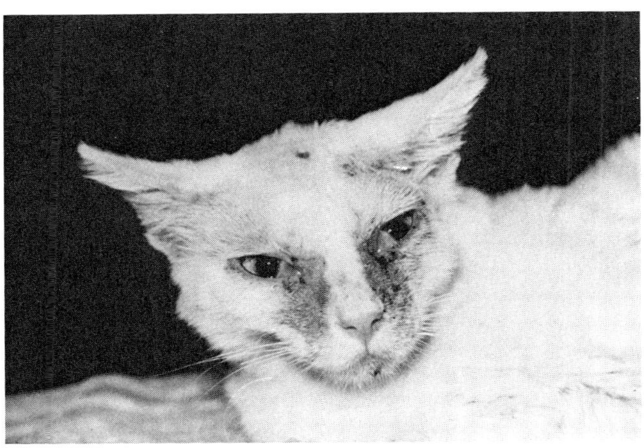

Figure 58–4. Erythema, alopecia, and excoriations on the face of a cat secondary to food allergy. (Courtesy of Dr. Thomas Hribernik, Louisiana State University, Baton Rouge, LA.)

Diagnosis

Diagnosis of food hypersensitivity can only be made by feeding the cat an elimination diet consisting of foods to which he or she has not been previously exposed. The foodstuffs most often recommended by members of the American Academy of Veterinary Dermatology for use in food trials are lamb, fish, venison, rabbit, or tofu as protein sources, mixed with rice or potatoes as a carbohydrate source.[11] The author's preference is lamb baby food. The cat should not be given any treats, table food, or objects that can be chewed. The cat's diet does not need to be supplemented with taurine because the duration of dietary restriction is short.[12] The test diet should be fed for a minimum of 8–10 weeks, at which time clinical re-evaluation should take place.

Therapy

If improvement in symptoms is noted after the diet trial, the cat should be rechallenged with the orginal diet in order to substaniate the diagnosis. Relapse of clinical signs usually occurs within 7 days after reintroduction of the original diet. The owner may then elect to identify the offending antigen by adding one new foodstuff to the diet every 5 to 7 days or may decide to find a commercial diet that the cat can tolerate. Many new "hypoallergenic" diets are now available and can be recommended once the diagnosis has been made. Prescription Diet Feline d/d (Hill's Pet Products, Topeka, KS) is balanced for cats and contains an adequate quantity of taurine.[13]

Unfortunately, symptomatic control of food hypersensitivity is difficult because the pruritis is only partially responsive to corticosteroids and establishing a safe, low, alternate-day dosage may be difficult.

Allergic Inhalant Dermatitis (Atopy)

Atopy is probably underdiagnosed in the cat since skin testing is not performed as often in cats as in dogs. It is still the second most common hypersensitivity disorder of the cat, probably accounting for 8 to 10% of skin disorders seen.[14]

Pathogenesis

The term atopy is used to describe a hereditary hypersensitivity state that is mediated by IgE antibodies formed following contact with an allergen. Although the association of IgE with human and canine atopy has been well documented, the presence of feline IgE has not been proved.

When an antigen contacts the mast cell–bound antibody (primarily IgE), it causes degranulation of the mast cell with release of histamine, serotonin, proteases, thromboxanes, prostaglandins, leukotrienes, and other substances. Many of these substances are ultimately pruritogenic in the skin.

Clinical Signs

The primary clinical sign associated with atopy in the cat is pruritus. However, pruritus may be difficult to diagnose in the cat, as previously mentioned. The cat may be brought

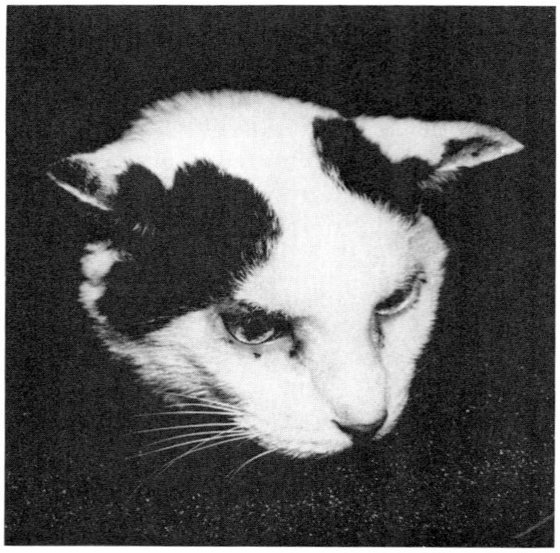

Figure 58–5. **Erythema, alopecia, and crusting on the ears and periocular region of a cat with atopy. An Elizabethan collar was needed to control the self-trauma. (Courtesy of Dr. Carol Foil, Louisiana State University, Baton Rouge, LA.)**

for examination for symmetric hair loss, which is most often secondary to excessive licking and grooming. Cats with atopy may also have miliary dermatitis, "psychogenic" alopecia, eosinophilic ulcers, eosinophilic plaques, or linear granulomas.[15] In many cases the pruritus is concentrated around the head and neck region (Figs. 58–5 and 58–6).

Diagnosis

Diagnosis of allergic inhalant dermatitis is by intradermal skin testing on the lateral thoracic area with aqueous allergen extracts. Antigens are generally used for skin testing at 1000 protein nitrogen units per mL or 1:1000 w/v. House dust is best used at 250 protein nitrogen units per mL. There may be a number of specific allergens in a pollen, and it is important to use extracts from a reliable manufacturer. Most manufacturers supply all the important allergens for a particular region, materials with which to perform the skin test, and the individualized hyposensitization vaccine. In some cases, intradermal skin testing can be performed with minimal restraint, allowing the cat to sit or recline in a normal sternal position. However, many cats tend to resist the physical restraint necessary for skin testing and are also sensitive to the noise of the electric clippers used to shave the test site. In these cats, the use of ketamine intramuscularly, xylazine subcutaneously, or a ketamine-diazepam combination intravenously provides needed sedation and does not block the formation of diagnostic positive wheals.

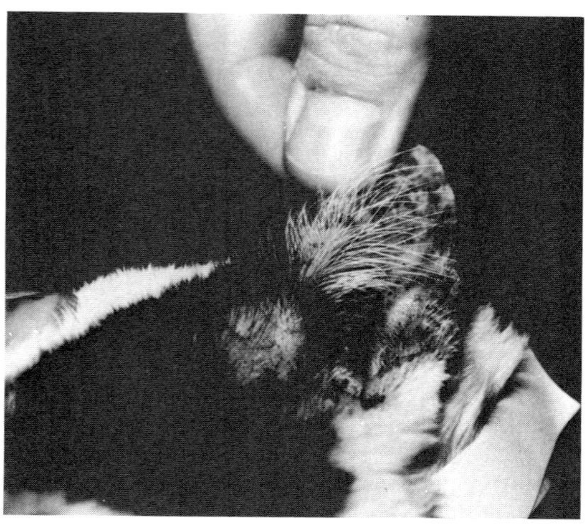

Figure 58–6. **Close-up view of the ear of the cat in Figure 58–5. Note erythema and bloody crusts. (Courtesy of Dr. Carol Foil, Louisiana State University, Baton Rouge, LA.)**

A small bleb of approximately 0.03 to 0.05 mL of each antigen is injected intradermally. The interpretation of a feline skin test is slightly more subjective than that of a canine test in that the feline wheal is smaller and less obvious and the wheals appear and fade more quickly than do those in the dog. Each test site should be watched closely and the site read at the height of the reaction, which may be as early as 5 minutes or as late as 15 minutes after the antigen is administered. Reactions may be subjectively graded from 0 (equal to the saline or negative control) to 4 (equal to the histamine or positive control) or measured with a millimeter ruler or calipers. It is much more difficult to measure the wheal response in the cat; therefore, in the author's opinion, subjective grading is better.

In vitro diagnostic tests are relatively new for diagnosing feline inhalant allergic dermatitis. Until more studies are undertaken to prove the validity of these tests, the author recommends only skin testing for the diagnosis of feline inhalant allergic dermatitis.

Therapy

Avoidance of the offending allergen is the most successful therapy. However, this is impractical in many cases. Medical therapy consists of one or a combination of the following: corticosteroids, antihistamines, fatty acid supplements, or hyposensitization.

Atopy is a very corticosteroid-responsive disease. However, long-term use of corticosteroids may result in unwanted side effects, although less often in cats than in dogs. Short-acting oral corticosteroids given on an every other day protocol for a few months of the year minimize the side effects of this drug in most animals.

Antihistamines may control the pruritus associated with inhalant allergic dermatitis. A recent study of the use of chlorpheniramine showed 73% success rate in controlling pruritus that was presumably associated with food allergy or atopy.[16] This was an open, nonplacebo, controlled study. This success rate is far superior to the response seen in dogs administered antihistamines and to the results seen by the author. However, since antihistamines have miminal side effects compared with corticosteroids, a clinical trial of chlorpheniramine at 2 mg orally b.i.d. for a few weeks is recommended. Other antihistamines are used less often in the cat.

Preparations containing fatty acids (Derm Caps, Efa Vet, and Efa Vet-Z) have been used successfully in dogs for the treatment of canine inhalant allergic skin disease. Currently,

Table 58–1. Immunotherapy Schedule for Atopy

Injection Number	Day Number	Vial #1 (1–200 PNU*/mL)	Vial #2 (1–2000 PNU/mL)	Vial #3 (10–20,000 PNU/mL)
1	0	0.1 mL		
2	3	0.2 mL		
3	6	0.4 mL		
4	9	0.8 mL		
5	12		0.1 mL	
6	15		0.2 mL	
7	18		0.4 mL	
8	21		0.8 mL	
9	24			0.1 mL
10	27			0.2 mL
11	30			0.4 mL
12	33			0.8 mL
13	36			1.0 mL
14	46			1.0 mL
15	66			1.0 mL†

*PNU, protein nitrogen unit.
†Give 1.0 ml of vial #3 subcutaneously every 20 days for maintenance.

there is no information available on their efficacy for this purpose in the cat. Progestational compounds have been used to relieve pruritus in cats. However, the harmful side effects of these drugs often outweigh their therapeutic benefits, and their use is not recommended (see Chapter 7).

Hyposensitization has proved to be a successful method of treatment of atopy in the cat.[17,18] Because improvement with immunotherapy is slow, injections should be continued for at least a year. If improvement is noted, maintenance injections should be continued for life. A sample therapy schedule is found in Table 58–1.

Contact Allergic Dermatitis

Contact allergic dermatitis is rare in cats.[19] It is diagnosed infrequently in veterinary medicine in general because of the protection from environmental contactants in cats and dogs provided by the haircoat.

Pathogenesis

Allergic contact dermatitis is a delayed type, cell-mediated, hypersensitivity reaction. Most allergens are haptens and must be combined with epidermal proteins before an immunologic reaction can be initiated. Sensitization proceeds in two phases, induction and elicitation. The induction phase is the period during which the cat is exposed to the hapten and T-cells are activated. Usually the induction phase occurs over a period of 6 months or longer. The elicitation phase occurs when the cat is re-exposed to the antigen and primed T-memory cells begin the cascade of events leading to inflammation and the delayed hypersensitivity reaction.

Clinical Signs

Contact allergic dermatitis can affect any region of the body, depending on the etiologic agent, but the ventral and nonhairy portions of the body are most frequently affected. Preexisting skin disorders (parasitic or bacterial infections), any other damage to the epidermal barrier, and overhydration of the skin may enhance the passage of the hapten through the epidermis.

Clinical signs vary from mild erythema with or without pruritus to severe pruritus with an outburst of papules and vesicles. Chronic exposure to the allergen results in lesions generated by self-trauma (e.g., crust, alopecia, lichenification, and hyperpigmentation). Substances implicated in causing allergic contact dermatitis include deodorized cat litter, neomycin, propylene glycol, plants, fibers (wool, synthetics), leather, disinfectants and other cleaning agents, fertilizers, insecticides, rubber and plastic products, flea collars (Fig. 58–7), topical sprays, powders, dips, shampoos, and grooming products. The clinical history of a cat with suspected allergic contact dermatitis is very important. New substances in the environment should not be implicated because of the long sensitization period necessary for the development of contact allergic dermatits.

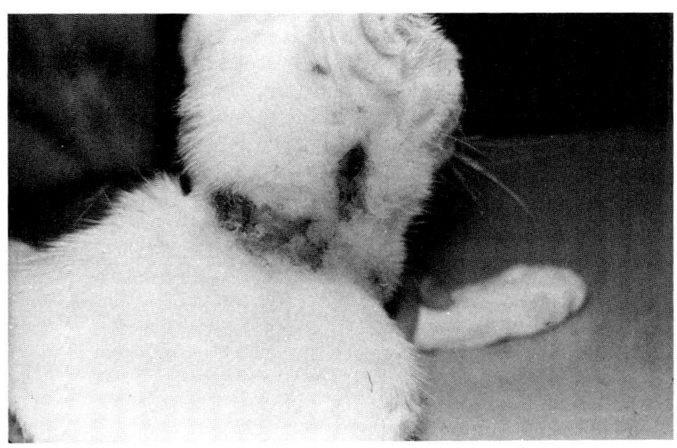

Figure 58–7. **Local dermatitis caused by a reaction to a flea collar. (Courtesy of Dr. Gary Norsworthy, San Antonio, TX.)**

Diagnosis

A complete history, physical examination, and elimination of other more common dermatoses is important because of the rare nature of allergic contact dermatitis and the difficulty in diagnosing it.

If the lesions are confined to one area of the body and their appearance can be correlated with the time a treatment or product was used, the offending substances can be removed for 10 to 14 days. A rechallenge with the agent should lead to the return of the dermatitis in 24 to 72 hours. If the lesions are generalized, removal of the cat from its usual environment for this period is most easily accomplished by boarding. The cat should be kept on the same diet to eliminate this variable, and untreated clay litter or sand should be substituted for the previously used litter. Boarding may be unacceptable to some clients, and confining the cat to a tiled room or large crate may be an alternative. Once the lesions are cleared, rechallenge and identification of the problem are accomplished by returning the animal to the normal, home environment.

Definitive diagnosis can be achieved by patch testing or reintroducing one product or area of the house at a time. If there is a high index of suspicion for a specific item, the cat may remain boarded and the suspected item may be introduced at the boarding place.

Patch testing is not frequently used in veterinary medicine because of the lack of standardized testing and the difficulty in applying the suspected products. Ideally, a normal control animal should be tested under the same conditions as the affected cat in order to separate irritant from allergic reactions. An open patch test can accommodate only liquid allergens. Approximately 0.1 to 2.0 mL of the product is rubbed into a clipped area of skin. The area is left unprotected for 3 to 5 days before it is examined for the presence of inflammation.[20] Self-trauma is commonly associated with this form of testing and can alter the test site. The closed patch test is used more often. In this test, the hair is clipped from the lateral thorax, and the suspected allergen is applied to this area under an occlusive dressing (petrolatum on dry gauze). The area is then wrapped to prevent traumatic removal of the dressing and the allergen by the cat and to stabilize the allergen to this one area. A positive response may be noted in 24 to 48 hours. If no dermatitis appears in this time interval, the test site should be examined again in 72 to 96 hours. A positive response consists of erythema, papules, and macules with or without swelling. Vesiculation may occur in severe allergic reactions.[21]

Therapy

The best therapy for allergic contact dermatitis is avoidance of the offending allergen if it can be definitively identified. If the allergen cannot be identified or avoidance is impossible, topical or systemic corticosteroid therapy may temporarily be effective. If there is continued exposure to the offending substance, the reaction worsens with time in most cases. Mechanical barries to the causative allergen, such as a kitty tee shirt or a stockinette, may be useful, as may frequent washing of the contactant areas.

Drug Eruption (Drug Allergy)

A drug eruption is defined as a cutaneous or mucocutaneous reaction to the administration of a drug. These drugs may be administered orally, topically, or by injection or inhalation. Only a few cases of drug eruption have been reported in cats.[19]

Pathogenesis

Types I, II, III and IV hypersensitivity have been implicated in allergic drug reactions. Drug eruptions in cats have been reported following the administration of sulfisoxazole, ampicillin, hetacillin, penicillin, tetracycline, neomycin, miconazole nitrate, panleukopenia vaccine, and otic preparations and following the use of dichlorvos collars.[7] Since drug eruption is an allergic reaction, there is a lag phase of at least 5 days before antibodies are formed or tissue lymphocytes become sensitized.

Clinical Signs

There are no characteristic clinical lesions associated with a drug-induced allergic dermatitis. Reported lesions seen in the cat include miliary dermatitis, urticaria and angioedema, contact dermatitis, and variable degrees of alopecia and pruritus (Fig. 58–8).

Diagnosis

The diagnosis of a drug eruption is based on the history of exposure to a drug and negative findings on other diagnostic tests that should identify other primary causes. Improvement in clinical signs is usually seen within 7 to 14 days following discontinuation of the drug. Provocative exposure for diagnosis is not recommended.

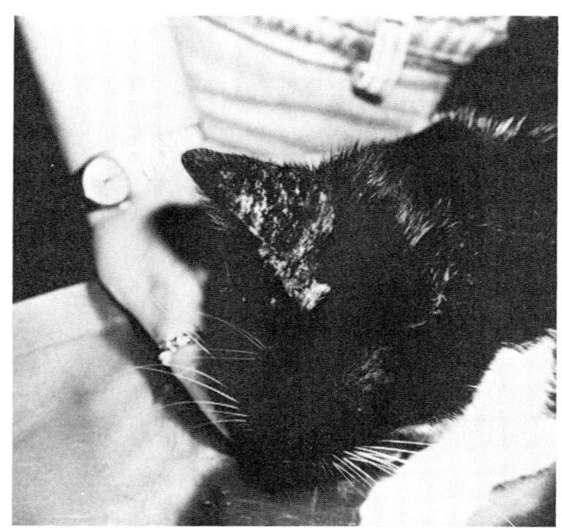

Figure 58–8. **Alopecia and crusting on the ear of a cat secondary to hypersensitivity to miconazole. (Courtesy of Dr. Carol Foil, Louisiana State University, Baton Rouge, LA.)**

Therapy

Therapy consists of discontinuing the drug and symptomatic treatment of the clinical signs. When urticaria or angioedema is present, antihistamines and epinephrine may be needed to treat symptoms. If pruritus occurs, oral short-acting glucocorticoids can be employed. If the damage to the epidermis is severe, use of topical and systemic antimicrobial therapy is warranted. Avoidance of drugs chemically related to the drug causing the reaction is important.

REFERENCES

1. Coombs RRA, Gell PGH. Classification of Allergic Reactions Responsible for Clinical Hypersensitivity and Disease. In: Gell PGH, Coombs RRA, Lachman LB, eds. Clinical Aspects of Immunology. 3rd ed. Oxford: Blackwell Scientific, 1975:761.
2. Halliwell REW. Flea Allergy Dermatitis. In: Kirk RW, ed. Current Veterinary Therapy VIII. Philadelphia: WB Saunders Co., 1983: 496.
3. Halliwell REW. Flea bite dermatitis. Compend Contin Educ Pract Vet 1979;1:367.
4. Scheidt VJ. Flea allergy dermatitis. Vet Clin North Am (Small Anim Pract) 1988;19(5):1023.
5. Fehrer SL, Halliwell REW. Effectiveness of Avon's Skin-So-Soft as a flea repellent on dogs. J Am Anim Hosp Assoc 1987;23:217.
6. Walton GS. Allergic Responses to Ingested Allergens. In Kirk RW, ed. Current Veterinary Therapy VI. Philadelphia: WB Saunders Co., 1977:576.
7. Nesbitt GH. Canine and Feline Dermatology: A Systemic Approach. Philadelphia: Lea & Febiger, 1983:47.
8. August JR. Dietary hypersensitivity in dogs: Cutaneous manifestations, diagnosis and management. Compend Contin Educ Pract Vet 1985;7 469.
9. Foil CS. The Skin. In: Hoskins JD, ed. Veterinary Pediatrics. Dogs and Cats from Birth to Six Months. Philadelphia: WB Saunders Co., 1990:369.
10. Merchant SR, Taboada J. Food allergy and immunologic diseases of the gastrointestinal tract. Semin Vet Med Surg 1991; 6:316.
11. Roudebush P. Results of a Hypoallergenic Diet Survey of AAVD Members. Seventh Proceeding of the Annual Meeting of AAVD and ACVD. Scottsdale, AZ 1991:96.
12. Pion PD, Power HT, Rogers QR, et al. Taurine for cats. J Am Vet Med Assoc 1989;194:1005.
13. Codner EC, Thatcher CD. The role of nutrition in the management of dermatosis. Semin Vet Med Surg 1990;5:167.
14. Muller GH, Kirk RW, Scott DW. Small Animal Dermatology. 4th ed. Philadelphia: WB Saunders Co., 1989:427.
15. Sousa CA. Atopic dermatitis. Vet Clin North Am (Small Anim Pract) 1988;19(5):1049.
16. Miller WH, Scott DW. Efficacy of chlorpheniramine maleate for management of pruritus in cats. J Am Vet Med Assoc 1990;197: 67.
17. Reedy LM. Results of allergy testing and hyposensitization in selected feline skin diseases. J Am Anim Hosp Assoc 1982;18: 618.
18. McDougal BJ. Allergy testing and hyposensitization for 3 common feline dermatoses. Mod Vet Pract 1986;60:629.
19. Scott DW. Feline dermatology 1900–1978: A monograph. J Am Anim Hosp Assoc 1980;16:377.
20. White PD. Contact dermatitis in the dog and cat. Semin Vet Med Surg 1991;6:303.
21. Kunkle GA. Contact dermatitis. Vet Clin North Am (Small Anim Pract) 1988;18:1061.

CHAPTER 59

◇ ◇ ◇

The Skin: Neoplastic Diseases

Sandra R. Merchant

The skin is the second most common site of occurrence of neoplasms in the cat, accounting for 15 to 21% of feline tumors.[1] The most common skin tumor varies from report to report. The four most common skin tumor types are basal cell, mast cell, squamous cell, and fibrosarcoma. The peak period for tumor occurrence is from 6 to 14 years of age, and the median age of occurrence is 12 years. There appears to be no breed predilection for neoplasia in the cat, except for the "histiocytic" form of mast cell tumors seen almost exclusively in Siamese cats less than 4 years of age.[2] Only the most common and clinically relevant tumors are discussed here. Table 59–1 provides a list of skin neoplasms and other references covering uncommon neoplasms in the cat.[1,3–6]

Examination

In evaluating a skin mass on the cat, a thorough physical examination should be performed. Special attention should be given to examination of the lymph nodes, lungs, and hematopoietic system as areas for potential metastasis. Initially, fine-needle aspiration of the mass and any enlarged regional lymph nodes should be performed, as the results may aid in the planning of therapy. Most tumors need to be surgically removed.

Histologic examination of the biopsy specimen is important for two reasons. First, it allows definitive diagnosis of the tumor and the degree of malignancy. Second, it indicates whether the mass was completely removed by surgery. Armed with this information, the clinician can then institute any additional appropriate therapy.

Epithelial Tumors

Squamous Cell Carcinoma: Classic Form

Squamous cell carcinoma is a common malignant neoplasm of the cat. These tumors are found most often in unpigmented or lightly pigmented skin of the nose, eyelids, lips, and pinnae. The pinna is most commonly affected.[7]

Biologic Behavior

Squamous cell carcinomas are locally invasive but appear to have a low metastatic potential. Metastasis to the regional lymph nodes usually occurs late in the disease. Squamous cell carcinoma of the nail bed epithelium, although unusual, is highly aggressive and rapidly spreads to regional lymph nodes and contiguous bone. One case of metastatic squamous cell carcinoma affecting multiple digits in a cat has been recorded.[8] There appears to be a strong correlation between the development of squamous cell carcinomas, exposure to ultraviolet light, and lack of pigmentation. White cats develop squamous cell carcinoma 13 times more frequently than other cats.[9]

Clinical Signs

Squamous cell carcinomas are usually solitary and may be proliferative, erosive, or both (Figs. 59–1 and 59–2). Initially, the affected areas may be erythematous and contain scale and crust, resembling an inflammatory lesion. The proliferative type tends to be verrucous or cauliflower-like in appearance, and the surface tends to ulcerate and bleed easily. The ulcerative or erosive type begins as a shallow, crusted ulcer that slowly deepens. Squamous cell carcinoma of the digit may manifest as a chronic paronychia or as osteomyelitis that is unresponsive to antibiotic therapy.

Treatment

The initial treatment of choice for squamous cell carcinoma in the cat is radical surgery with at least a 1-cm margin of healthy tissue. For tumors involving the ear, resection of the pinna is indicated (see Chapter 55). The prognosis for cure is good after complete surgical excision of the lesion if there is no evidence of metastasis. For tumors involving the pinna, lid margins, or nasal planum, cryosurgery has been used successfully.[10] For digital squamous cell carcinomas, the prognosis becomes more guarded. Local current field radiofrequency hyperthermia has been a rapid and economic treatment method for squamous cell carcinomas that are not deeper than 2 to 3 mm.[11,12] For large, unresectable or deeply invasive tumors, radiation therapy may be used.[13] The deeper the disease, the less likely the cure. However, even though many of these cats cannot be cured, after therapy the lesions are reduced in size and a comfortable life can be extended for more than one year.[1,2] A list of centers that perform radiotherapy can be found in Adams, Veteri-

Table 59–1. Cutaneous Neoplasms in the Cat

Tumor	Relative Incidence	Biologic Behavior	Treatment
Apocrine gland adenoma	U-R	A	F, G, H, K, M
Apocrine gland adenocarcinoma	U-R	B, E	H, I, J
Basal cell tumor	C	A	F, G, H, I, K
Ceruminous gland adenoma	U	A	G
Ceruminous gland adenocarcinoma	U	D	H, I, J
Dilated pore of Winer	R	A	F, G
Eccrine gland adenoma	R	N	F, G, K, M
Eccrine gland adenocarcinoma	R	N	N
Epithelioid sarcoma	R	D	H
Fibroma	U	A	F, G, K, M
Fibrosarcoma	C	D	H, I, J, K
Fibrous histiocytoma	R	B	H, I
Malignant fibrous histiocytoma	R	E	H
Hemangioma	U-R	A	F, G, K, M
Hemangiosarcoma	U-R	E	H, I
Hemangiopericytoma	R	A	H
Histiocytoma	R	N	F, G, K, M
Leiomyoma	U-R	A	G
Leiomyosarcoma	U-R	E	G
Lipoma	U-R	A	F, G
Liposarcoma	U-R	E	H
Lymphangioma	R	A	G
Lymphangiosarcoma	R	N	N
Cutaneous lymphosarcoma* (nonepitheliotrophic)	R	D	I
Mast cell tumor	C	†	†
Melanoma	U-R	A, E	H
Mycosis fungoides*	R	D	I
Myxoma	R	A	H
Myxosarcoma	R	E	H
Neurofibroma	R	N	N
Nodular fasciitis	R	A	G
Papilloma	R	A	F, G, K, M
Pilomatricoma	R	A	F, G, K
Plasmacytoma	R	N	N
Osteoma	R	A	H
Osteosarcoma	R	E	H
Sebaceous gland adenoma	U-R	A	F, G, K
Sebaceous gland adenocarcinoma	U-R	B, E	H, K, M
Schwannoma	R	E	H
Squamous cell carcinoma	C	B	H, I, J, K, L, M
Spindle-cell sarcoma (undifferentiated sarcoma)	R	D	H
Trichoepithelioma	U-R	A	F, G, K, M

This table is an accumulation of information from the following references: 1, 3, 5, 6, 14, 24, and 25. The most common response for incidence and biologic behavior is recorded. All treatments found in the sources are listed in the table. Information concerning incidence is as follows: The source stated common/frequent, uncommon/infrequent, or rare or the incidence was reported as a percentage and converted: common (C) = greater than 10%, uncommon (U) = between 1 and 10%, rare (R) = less than 1% of skin tumors.

*Therapy only palliative.

†See text.

Abbreviations: C, common; U, uncommon; R, rare; A, benign; B, locally invasive, local metastasis; D, malignant; E, malignant, no metastasis; F, no treatment, observation; G, surgery; H, surgery, excision with wide margins; I, surgery ± chemotherapy; J, surgery ± radiotherapy; K, cryotherapy; L, surgery ± hyperthermia; M, electrosurgery; N, not enough information because of case numbers reported, or not reported.

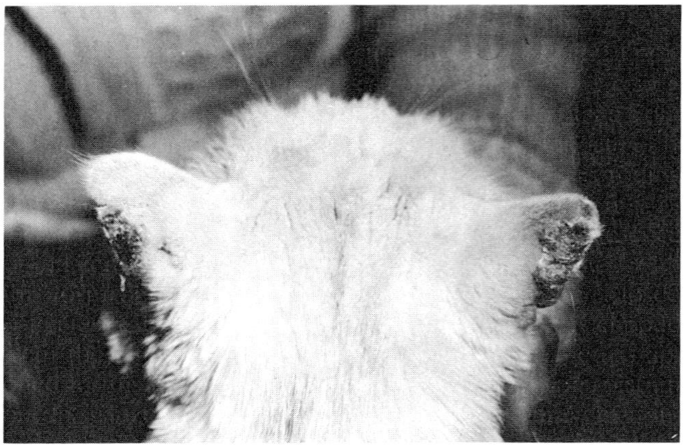

Figure 59–1. Ulcerative, crusting, multifocal squamous cell carcinoma on the pinna of a white cat. (Courtesy of Dr. Gary Norsworthy, San Antonio, TX.)

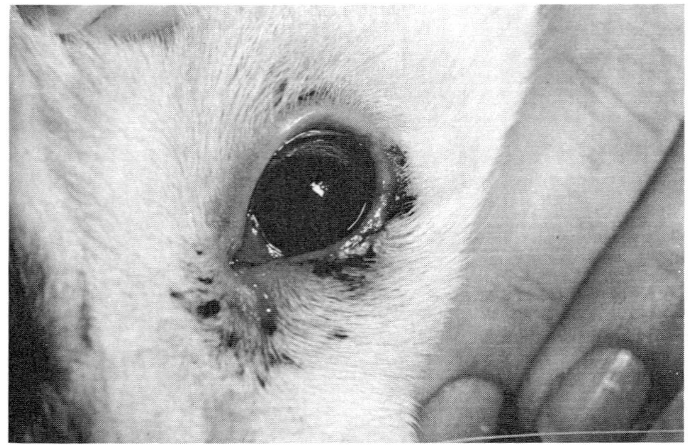

Figure 59–2. Crusting on the upper and lower lid margins caused by squamous cell carcinoma. (Courtesy of Dr. Gary Norsworthy, San Antonio, TX.)

nary Radiation Therapy.[15] Protecting white cats from sunlight may aid in the prevention of primary or recurrent tumors.

Squamous Cell Carcinoma: Bowen's Disease*

Multicentric squamous cell carcinoma in situ (Bowen's disease) has been reported in 15 domestic cats:[14] four long haired, one medium haired, and ten short haired, ranging in age from 7 to 21 years (median, 11.5 years). Ten had pigmented coats, and only one was solid white. Most had had limited exposure to sunlight. Four were neutered males and eleven were spayed females.

Clinical Signs

This form of squamous cell carcinoma begins as skin lesions located predominantly on the head, digits, neck, thorax, shoulders, and ventral abdomen. Lesions on the head are found on the pinnae and external ear canal, preauricular region, eyelids, face, lips, oral mucosa, and chin. Number of tumors may range from 2 to more than 30. As the lesions enlarge, they often coalesce with adjacent lesions.

These lesions differ from those of classic squamous cell carcinoma. Typically, the skin becomes pigmented and then ulcerates. A scab usually forms over the ulcerated area. Removal of the scab is painful, and hair over the lesions epilates easily.

Biologic Behavior

Although the lesions are large and grow in an outward direction, they do not penetrate the basement membrane into the surrounding dermis; thus their name of carcinoma in situ.

Treatment

Several forms of therapy have been attempted for cats with Bowen's disease. Corticosteroids, progesterone, antibiotics, and alkylating agents were found to be ineffective in five cats. Radiation therapy with strontium 90 was effective in healing the lesions in eight cats. Each lesion received a total dose of approximately 150 Gy. The irradiated sites healed in 4 to 6 weeks, and there were no recurrences[14] (Fig. 59–3 *A–C*).

*This section was contributed by Jane M. Turrell, D.V.M., M.S., Pacifica, CA.

Basal Cell Tumors

Basal cell tumors are common in cats. They can occur anywhere on the body but show a predilection for the head and neck areas and are usually found in cats at an average of 9 years of age. These tumors are the most common melanotic feline skin neoplasm, but not all basal cell tumors are pigmented.[1]

Biologic Behavior

Basal cell tumors are usually benign and slow growing, and they rarely metastasize. Most masses are freely movable and firmly fixed to the overlying skin and rarely invade underlying fascia.

Clinical Signs

Basal cell tumors are solitary, well-circumscribed, firm, hairless, dome-shaped, elevated masses varying from 0.5 to 10.0 cm in diameter but usually less than 2.5 cm (Fig. 59–4). Multicentric basal cell tumors have been reported.[16] Feline basal cell tumors may be heavily pigmented and cystic and may ulcerate.

Treatment

The treatment of choice for basal cell tumors is surgical excision. If surgery cannot be performed, radiation therapy or observation without treatment may be elected.

Cerumen Gland Tumors

The ceruminous glands of the external ear canal are modified apocrine sweat glands. Tumors arising from these glands occur more often in cats than in other domestic spe-

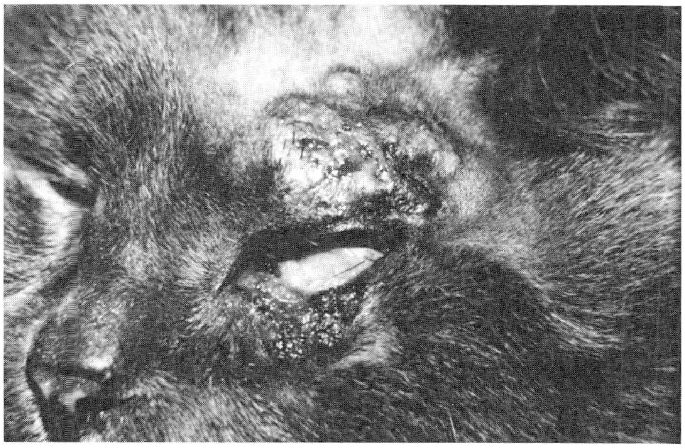

A

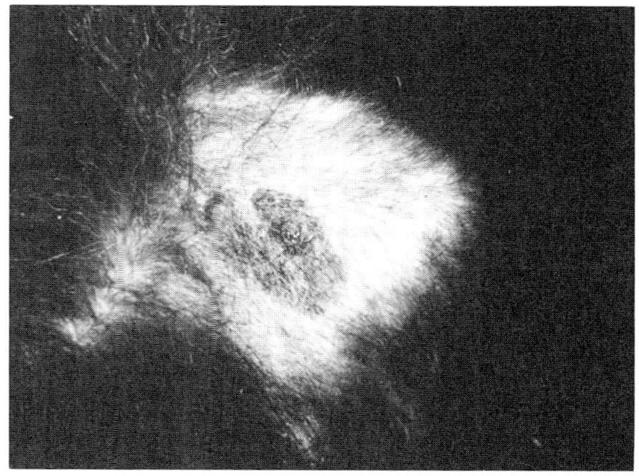

B

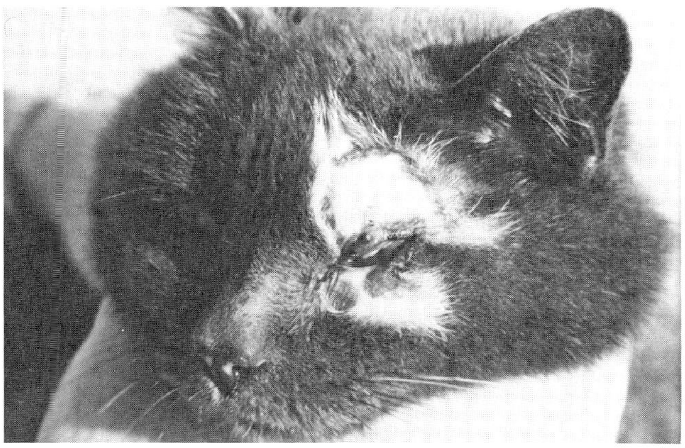

C

Figure 59–3. (*A*) Bowen's disease (squamous cell carcinoma in situ) Several adjacent lesions coalesced over the left eye. (*B*) Another lesion was found on the same cat located on the lateral thoracic wall. (*C*) Same cat 10 months following irradiation with strontium 90. (Courtesy of Dr. Jane Turrel, Pacifica, CA.)

cies,[17] usually in cats older than 8 years. Males appear to be at a higher risk.

Biologic Behavior

The majority of ceruminous gland tumors in cats are malignant (50 to 65%) and metastasize frequently.[18] The tumor metastasizes to local lymph nodes as well as to the lungs.

Clinical Signs

Clinical presentation of this tumor is usually as a unilateral mass in the external ear canal, although bilateral presentation is more common in the cat than in the dog. In most cases, otoscopic examination must be performed to visualize this tumor. On otoscopic examination, the mass is small, pink, well circumscribed, and often ulcerated; it is usually found near the tympanic membrane. A seropurulent discharge usually accompanies the mass and the ear canal must be cleaned before the lesion can be seen. Failure to clean the canal leads to an incorrect diagnosis of chronic otitis externa that is minimally responsive to topical medication. Occasionally, regional lymph node involvement may be seen, and rarely, the regional node involvement outgrows the primary tumor, resulting in a client's bringing in the cat because of a mass that is palpable in the parotid area.[18] Performing a biopsy is very important because these masses cannot be distinguished grossly from tissue hyperplasia or inflammatory granulation tissue.

Treatment

The treatment of choice is surgical excision. Because of the anatomic location of the tumor, resection of the lateral wall of the vertical canal or total ablation of the canal may need to be performed, depending on the invasive nature of the masses. Radiation therapy has been successful in treatment of localized adenocarcinomas. Because of the anatomic location and difficulty of complete surgical excision, the progno-

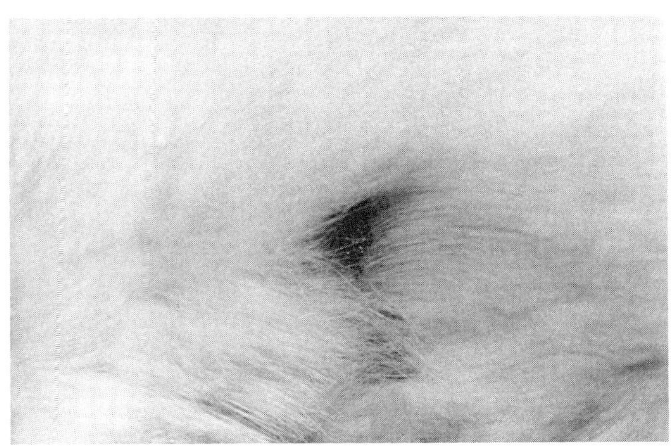

Figure 59–4. Basal cell tumor on the flank of a cat.

sis is fair to good with benign tumors and guarded with malignant tumors.

Mesenchymal Tumors

Fibrosarcomas

Fibrosarcomas are common malignant neoplasms of the cat arising from dermal or subcutaneous fibroblasts. Their benign counterpart, the fibroma, is less common.

Characteristics

Fibrosarcomas in cats may be either solitary or multiple. Some feline fibrosarcomas are viral-induced.[19] These tumors tend to be found in cats less than 5 years of age and are multicentric and significantly more invasive than the solitary fibrosarcomas found in older cats. A C-type oncornavirus, the feline sarcoma virus, has been implicated as the etiologic agent of the multicentric fibrosarcomas. The feline sarcoma virus is a mutant of the feline leukemia virus, and cats with feline sarcoma virus–induced fibrosarcomas test positive for feline leukemia virus antigen. Feline sarcoma virus is not associated with solitary fibrosarcomas in older cats.

Biologic Behavior

Most fibrosarcomas are poorly circumscribed and locally invasive and tend to infiltrate along tissue planes. They often recur after surgical removal. Metastasis occurs in 10 to 25% of cases, most commonly to the lungs.

Clinical Signs

Fibrosarcomas in older cats are usually solitary round to ovoid tumors that are subcutaneous to dermoepidermal in location and firmly attached to the overlying epidermis. They are firm to fleshy, variable in size, and poorly circumscribed. They often ulcerate, and they have a predilection for the limbs.[7] Multicentric fibrosarcomas are gray to white, firm, demarcated nodules that often become necrotic because rapid growth causes the mass to outgrow its blood supply (Fig. 59–5).

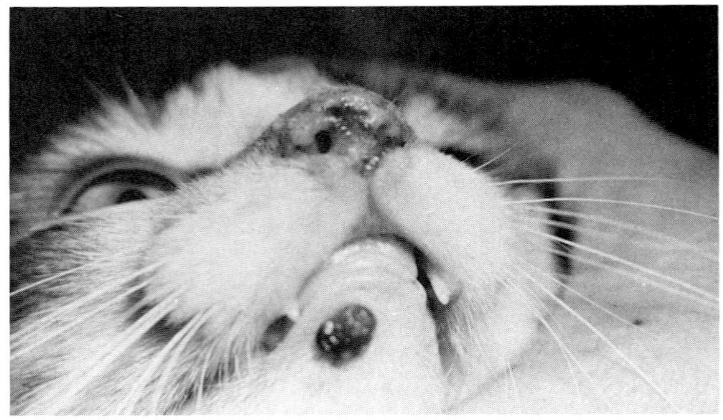

Figure 59–5. **Multifocal proliferative and ulcerative fibrosarcoma on the nose and chin of a cat. (Courtesy of Dr. Carol Foil, Louisiana State University, Baton Rouge, LA.)**

Treatment

The treatment of choice for fibrosarcomas is wide surgical excision. Unfortunately, many tumors recur after surgery. Cats with fibrosarcomas of the head, back, or limbs and with a high mitotic index on histopathologic examination have the poorest prognosis. When an extremity is involved, amputation should be considered. Fibrosarcomas respond poorly to chemotherapy. Radiation therapy may be helpful as an adjunct to surgery. No therapy is recommended for multicentric fibrosarcomas. On rare occasions, the multicentric form may spontaneously regress.[9]

Mast Cell Tumors

The mast cell tumor is a common lesion in the cat and is the only common skin tumor that is seen in cats younger than 1 year of age.

The "histiocytic" subtype of mast cell tumor is found most often in young cats and tends to be multiple.[7] This subtype has been observed most commonly in Siamese cats less than 4 years old, but it has also been seen in other breeds.[7,20-22] A second type, the "mast cell" type of mast cell tumor, occurs in cats older than 4 years of age and may be solitary or multiple.

Characteristics and Biologic Behavior

Controversy exists in the literature concerning the clinical characteristics and biologic behavior of mast cell tumors. Some investigators refer to the high malignancy rate and fatal nature of the disease, whereas others comment on the low rate of visceral metastasis despite recurrent cutaneous disease. Cutaneous mast cell tumors usually develop independently of the visceral form of the disease, but cases have been reported with concurrent cutaneous and visceral disease.[22] Most often, the skin is assumed to be the primary site, with visceral disease the result of metastasis. A case of diffuse cutaneous mastocytosis appearing as a generalized miliary papular and crusting disease with extension to the lymph nodes has been reported.[23]

Attempts have been made to correlate histologic grading with biologic behavior of these tumors, as has been done with canine cutaneous mast cell tumors. Although mast cell tumors can be categorized as well differentiated, intermediate, or poorly differentiated, all groups may exhibit benign behavior, thereby making this classification a less valuable prognostic indicator.[22] However, the feline tumors with an unusual degree of cellular atypia and high mitotic activity are the ones most likely to recur locally or metastasize.[19]

Clinical Signs

The typical "mast cell" type mast cell tumor is 2 to 3 cm in diameter, is found on the head or neck, and can occur in single or multiple form. Mast cell tumors can vary from this typical appearance and can appear as indolent, ulcerlike lesions on the lip, single or multiple papular and nodular lesions on a normal, alopecic, or ulcerated skin surface, or as plaques that frequently ulcerate and are pruritic.[21] Noncutaneous signs are rare and include gastric and duodenal ulcers and defective blood coagulation.[1]

The "histiocytic" type mast cell tumor is characterized

as a firm, 0.5 to 1.0-cm subcutaneous nodule. These tend to be multiple but can consist of one solitary subcutaneous nodule. They have a predilection for the head region.

Treatment

The treatment of choice is wide surgical excision with histologic or cytologic evaluation of the local lymph nodes for evidence of disease. Opinion reflected in the current literature is that there is a low metastatic potential for mast cell tumors in the cat. However, local recurrence rates vary from 25 to 50%. Most cats with cutaneous recurrences do not have evidence of metastasis or dissemination and remain lesion-free after subsequent excision.[24] Recurrent lesions can be surgically excised again or treated with benign neglect if they are small, static, and asymptomatic or no lymphadenopathy or evidence of paraneoplastic syndrome is present.[24] A more aggressive approach is surgical excision and systemic administration of prednisone (40 mg/m^2 by mouth every 24 hours for 1 week, then 20 mg/m^2 by mouth every other day).[25] Radiation therapy has also been recommended.[26] The majority of the histiocytic mast cell tumors spontaneously regress over a period of several months (see Chapter 51).

REFERENCES

1. Muller GH, Kirk RW, Scott DW. Small Animal Dermatology. 4th ed. Philadelphia: WB Saunders Co., 1989:844.
2. Wilcock BP, Yager JA, Zink MC. The morphology and behavior of feline cutaneous mastocytomas. Vet Pathol 1986;23:321.
3. Carpenter JL, Andrews LK, Holzworth J. Tumors and Tumor-like Lesions. In: Holzworth J, ed. Diseases of the Cat, Vol. 1. Philadelphia: WB Saunders Co., 1987:406.
4. Pulley LT, Stannard AA. Tumors of Skin and Soft Tissue. In: Moulton JE, ed. Tumors in Domestic Animals. 3rd ed. Berkeley: University of California Press. 1990:23.
5. Madewell BR, Theilen GH. Tumors of the Skin and Subcutaneous Tissues. In: Theilen GH, Madewell BR, eds. Veterinary Cancer Medicine, 2nd ed. Philadelphia: Lea & Febiger, 1987:233.
6. Susaneck SJ, Withrow SJ. Tumors of the Skin and Subcutaneous Tissues. In: Withrow SJ, MacEwen EG, eds. Clinical Veterinary Oncology. Philadelphia: JB Lippincott, 1989:139.
7. Miller MA, Nelson SL, Turk JR, et al. Cutaneous neoplasia in 340 cats. Vet Pathol 1991;28:389.
8. Pollack M, Martin RA, Diters RW. Metastatic squamous cell carcinoma in multiple digits of a cat: Case report. J Am Anim Hosp Assoc 1984;21:835.
9. Scott DW. Feline dermatology 1900–1978. A monograph. J Am Anim Hosp Assoc 1980;16:331.
10. Personal communication: Dr. Gary D. Norsworthy, San Antonio, TX, 1991.
11. Grier RL, Brewer WG, Theilen GH. Hyperthermic treatment of superficial tumors in cats and dogs. J Am Vet Med Assoc 1980;177:227.
12. Kabay MJ, Jones BR. Local current field radiofrequency hyperthermia for the treatment of superficial skin tumors in cats. N Z Vet J 1983;31:173.
13. Carlisle CH, Gould S. Response of squamous cell carcinoma of the nose of the cat to treatment with x-rays. Vet Radiol 1982; 23:186.
14. Turrel JM, Gross TL. Diagnosis and Treatment of Multicentric Squamous Cell Carcinoma in Situ (Bowen's Disease) of Cats. Proceedings, Veterinary Cancer Society, Minneapolis, MN, 1991:84.
15. Adams WM. Veterinary radiation therapy. Compend Contin Educ Pract Vet 1991;13:262.
16. Fehrer SL, Lin SH. Multicentric basal cell tumors in a cat. J Am Vet Med Assoc 1986;189:1469.
17. White SD, Ihrke PJ. Skin Tumors. In: Pratt PW, ed. Feline Medicine. Santa Barbara: American Veterinary Publications, 1983: 592.
18. Legendre AM, Krahwinkel DJ. Feline ear tumors. J Am Anim Hosp Assoc 1981;17:1035.
19. Harasen GLG. Multicentric fibrosarcoma in a cat and a review of the literature. Can Vet J 1984;25:217.
20. Wilcox BP, Yager JA, Zink MC. The morphology and behavior of feline cutaneous mastocytomas. Vet Pathol 1986;23:321.
21. Chastain CB, Turk MA, O'Brien D. Benign cutaneous mastocytomas in two litters of Siamese kittens. J Am Vet Med Assoc 1988;193:959.
22. Buerger RG, Scott DW. Cutaneous mast cell neoplasia in cats: 14 cases (1975–1985). J Am Vet Med Assoc 1987;190:1440.
23. Brown CA, Chalmers SA. Diffuse cutaneous mastocytosis in a cat. Vet Pathol 1990;27:366.
24. Buerger RG. Cutaneous Mast Cell Tumors. In: August JR, ed. Consultations in Feline Internal Medicine. Philadelphia: WB Saunders Co., 1991:95.
25. Couto CG. Oncology. In: Sherding RG, ed. The Cat: Diseases and Clinical Management. New York: Churchill Livingstone, 1989:589.
26. Nesbitt GH. Canine and Feline Dermatology; A Systematic Approach. Philadelphia: Lea & Febiger, 1983:125.

CHAPTER 60

◇ ◇ ◇

The Skin: Diseases of Unknown or Multiple Etiology

Sandra R. Merchant

The most common cutaneous diseases of unknown or multiple etiology are discussed in this chapter. Many of the conditions discussed here are cutaneous reaction patterns and not true disease entities.

Miliary Dermatitis

Miliary dermatitis has been described under several names in recent literature, including scabby cat disease and miliary eczema. Miliary dermatitis is not a disease but the clinical description of a cutaneous reaction pattern in the cat that is one of the most common feline skin disorders.[1,2]

Etiology

Multiple etiologies have been reported for miliary dermatitis (Table 60–1). By all accounts, flea allergic dermatitis is the most common cause of miliary dermatitis in the cat.[1,3] The percentage of miliary dermatitis cases secondary to flea allergy probably varies geographically.

Clinical Signs

Clinical signs are characterized by an eruption of papules, each of which is surmounted by a crust (Fig. 60–1). The lesions may be localized or generalized. If the papular eruption is localized, it is seen most often on the dorsum, especially on the neck, shoulder, or tail region. The presence of pruritus and alopecia is variable, although most cats with miliary dermatitis experience some amount of pruritis. Self-inflicted alopecia is usually seen in severe or chronic cases.

Diagnosis

Diagnosis of the underlying etiology is based on a thorough history, dermatologic examination, and the completion of several diagnostic tests. A skin scraping, culture for fungi, fecal examination, flea allergy test, and/or response to flea control measures (in areas with a flea problem) should constitute the minimum data base. If these procedures do not point to a diagnosis or flea control measures do not resolve the underlying disease, a 2-week trial of antibiotics, a food allergy elimination diet, intradermal skin testing, response to administration of ivermectin (to rule out several parasitic diseases), intestinal deworming, and discontinuation of any previously prescribed drug are indicated. The order in which these are performed depends on clinical suspicion, availability of the test, and cooperation and financial constraints of the owner. Tissue biopsy is frequently unrewarding but may indicate a fungal infection that was not obtained from culture samples, a skin parasite that was not seen on the skin scraping, bacterial folliculitis, or increased numbers of eosinophils (making the possibility of allergic/parasitic disease more likely).[4]

Therapy

Treatment is based on the definitive diagnosis. In the case of idiopathic miliary dermatitis (which should be the diagnosis in 10% or fewer of the cases), glucocorticoids are the initial treatment of choice. Many cats require 2 to 4 mg/kg/day of oral short-acting glucocorticoids for the initial dose. This should be reduced as soon as possible to as low a dose as possible to maintain the disease in remission. If long-term therapy is required, oral glucocorticoids should be given on an alternate-day treatment regimen or less often. A number of cats do not respond to oral glucocorticoids or become resistant to them with time. In these instances, 10 to 20 mg of methylprednisolone acetate (Depo-Medrol) may improve the disease. This should not be given any more often than every other month, preferably every 3 months. Side effects of steroid therapy should be monitored when long-term treatment is needed.

Progestational compounds (megestrol acetate, repositol progesterone, medroxyprogesterone acetate) have also been used in the treatment of miliary dermatitis, in the following dosages: megestrol acetate, 2.5 to 5.0 mg s.i.d. to every other day until lesions are resolved, followed by a maintenance dose of 2.5 to 5.0 mg weekly or biweekly when indicated; repositol progesterone, 2.2 to 22 mg/kg subcutaneously or intramuscularly, as needed; and medroxyprogesterone acetate, 50 to 175 mg subcutaneously or intramuscularly, as needed. The author does not use the progestational compounds to treat this disease and does

Table 60–1. Differential Diagnosis of Miliary Dermatitis

Flea allergy
Food allergy
Atopy
Otodectic mange (*Otodectes cynotis*)
Cheyletiellosis (*Cheyletiella blakei*)
Trombiculidiasis
Notoedric mange (*Notoedes cati*)
Ticks
Demodectic mange (*Demodex cati, Demodex* spp.)
Cat fur mite (*Lynxacarus radovsky*)—rare
Pediculosis (*Felicola subrostratus*)
Staphylococcal folliculitis
Dermatophytosis
Drug eruption—rare
Internal parasitism—rare
Feline hypereosinophilic syndrome—rare
Biotin deficiency—rare
Fatty acid deficiency—rare
Hormone hypersensitivity—rare
Idiopathic

not recommend their use. Side effects seen with megestrol acetate include polyphagia, weight gain, polydipsia, polyuria, personality changes, mammary gland changes, pyometra, stump pyometra, diabetes mellitus, and adrenocortical suppression[5] (see Chapter 7).

Eosinophilic Granuloma Complex

The eosinophilic granuloma complex is composed of four clinical-histologic syndromes—the indolent ulcer, the eosinophilic plaque, the linear granuloma, and the atypical form. The name is inaccurate because very few of these syndromes cause a peripheral or tissue eosinophilia and only one is actually a granuloma. More than one form may occur in a patient simultaneously or at separate times. All syndromes do respond to the same treatment, namely, glucocorticoids. These syndromes are probably best viewed as cutaneous reaction patterns rather than as true disease entities.[6]

Etiology

A plethora of diseases have been implicated in causing lesions of the eosinophilic granuloma complex. A clustering of cases from in-contact or related cats has suggested that infectious or genetic factors may be important in transmission.[1,7] In one study, feline leukemia virus was seen in 90% of cats with indolent ulcers,[7] but this association has not been reported since. Controversy exists as to whether lesions can be transmitted from one area to another area on the same cat with autologous tissue.[8,9] Viral particles resembling calicivirus have been seen on electron microscopy in reexamination of these lesions, but viral isolation procedures were not performed.[10] In another study, filamentous bacteria presumed to be anaerobic were seen on histopathologic examination of an oral eosinophilic granuloma. An anaerobic organism was not cultured, but this lesion responded partially to administration of metronidazole.[11] Antiepithelial antibodies have been seen in cats with eosinophilic ulcers.[12] However, these antibodies could be the result and not the cause of the disease.

Recently, parasitic and allergic diseases related to the eosinophilic granuloma complex have received the most attention. An atypical form of the complex that affects the bridge of the nose, the pinnae, and sometimes the footpads has proved to be secondary to mosquito bite hypersensitivity.[13] The complex has also been associated with atopy, food hypersensitivity, and flea bite hypersensitivity.[14]

Clinical Signs and Diagnosis

Indolent Ulcer (Rodent Ulcer, Eosinophilic Ulcer, Lip Ulcer)

This lesion is characterized by a well-circumscribed, reddish brown ulcerated area with raised borders and a central depression (Fig. 60–2). It is found more frequently in females and has a mean age of 6 years and a range of 9 months to 9 years. The lesions are seen most often on the upper lip but can occur in the oral cavity, on the lower lip, and on other body surfaces. Malignant transformation into squamous cell carcinoma or fibrosarcoma is rare.[1,7]

Differential diagnoses include bacterial or fungal infec-

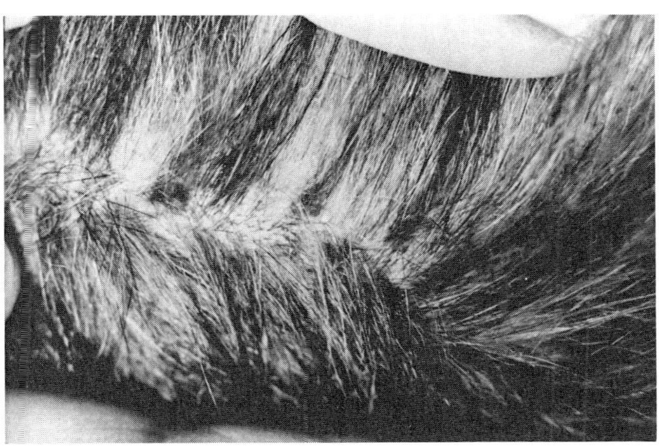

Figure 60–1. Lesions of miliary dermatitis.

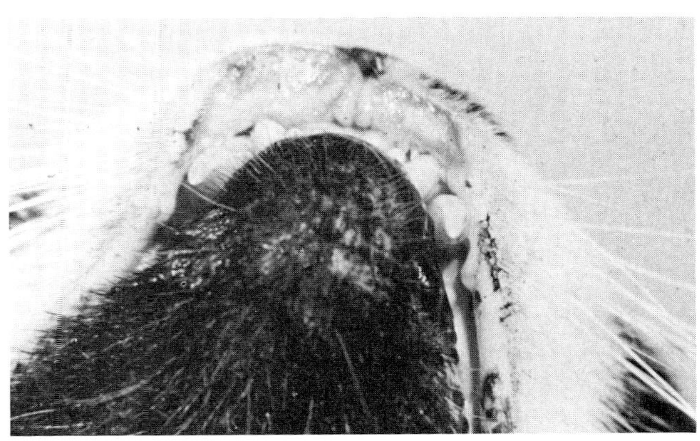

Figure 60–2. Indolent ulcer on the upper lip of a cat.

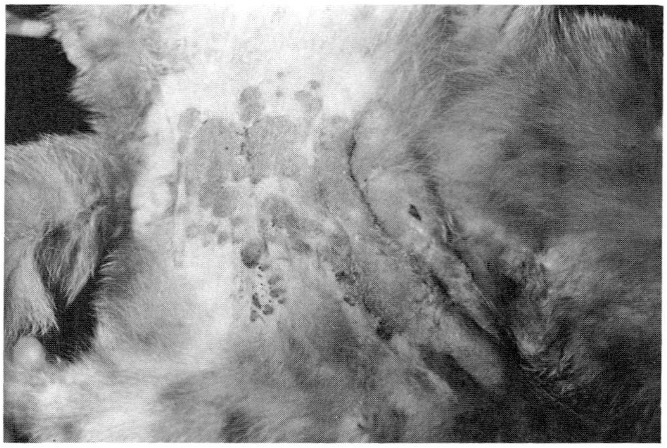

Figure 60–3. Atopic cat with eosinophilic plaques on the ventral abdomen. (Courtesy of Dr. Joy Barbet, Gainesville, FL.)

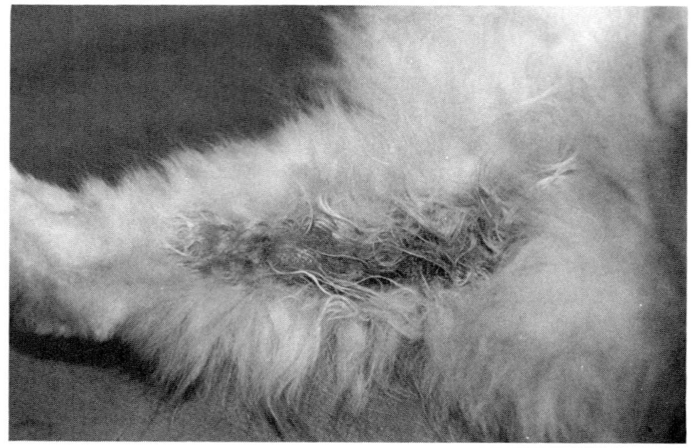

Figure 60–4. Raised linear (collagenolytic) granuloma on the caudal aspect of the rear leg. (Courtesy of Dr. Karin Beale, University of Florida, Gainesville, FL.)

tion, feline leukemia virus-associated ulcers, trauma, and neoplasia. The most common biopsy findings suggest a chronic ulcerative dermatitis with neutrophils, plasma cells, and mononuclear cells. However, in some cases there are increased eosinophils and collagenolysis with granulomatous inflammation. (This is more typical of the linear or collagenolytic form of the eosinophilic granuloma complex.)

Eosinophilic Plaque

These lesions are well circumscribed, raised, ulcerated, exudative, erythemic, and alopecic (Fig. 60–3). Lesions may be single or multiple. They most often occur on the abdomen and medial thighs but can be seen in the oral cavity and on other areas of the skin.

Pruritus is usually marked. Cats affected with this lesion range in age from 2 to 4 years with a mean age of 3 years.

Differential diagnoses include bacterial and fungal granulomas and neoplasia. Histopathologic examination reveals a spongiotic epidermitis with massive numbers of dermal eosinophils. This entity is usually accompanied by blood eosinophilia. This form is most closely associated with hypersensitivity disorders.

Linear Granuloma (Collagenolytic Granuloma)

Linear granulomas occur in young cats (usually 1 year of age) with a range of 6 months to 5 years, with a predisposition for females. Lesions are well circumscribed, raised, firm, yellowish to pink plaques. Lesions occurring on the caudal thighs are linear in configuration (Fig. 60–4); lesions on the face and in the oral cavity have a papular to nodular configuration (Fig. 60–5). Variations of the caudal thigh lesion, such as symmetric truncal bands or irregular linear bands anywhere on the body, have been seen.[6] The disease entity can also take the form of a swollen chin (Fig. 60–6). Tissue and blood eosinophilia is variable in the linear granuloma entity.

Differential diagnoses include bacterial and fungal granulomas and neoplasia. Histopathologic study reveals collagenolysis and palisading granulomatous inflammation, often associated with giant cell infiltration. Because of the consistent collagenolysis, this disease entity would be better termed collagenolytic granuloma.

Atypical Eosinophilic Granuloma Complex

A fourth, atypical cutaneous pattern of eosinophilic granuloma complex has been recently described. These cats have a papular eruption, erosions, crusting, and depigmentation of the skin over the bridge of the nose (Fig. 60–7), a papular eruption on the pinnae, erosive and granulomatous lesions, hyperkeratosis, and sometimes hyperpigmentation of the pads of the paws that is occasionally accompanied by swelling, tenderness, fissuring, and depigmentation. Most cats with this pattern have marked peripheral lymphadenopathy.[15]

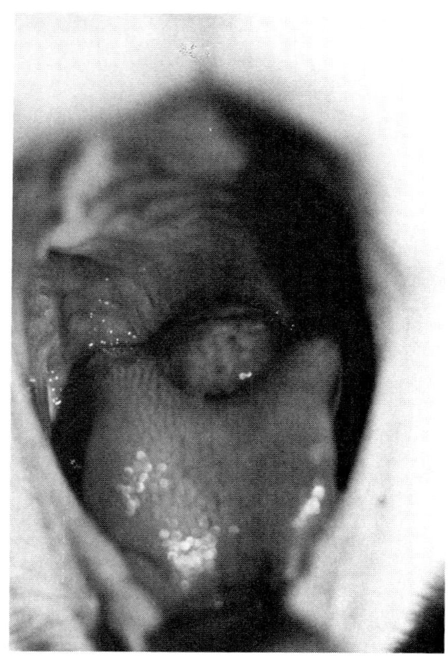

Figure 60–5. Nodular, pharyngeal (collagenolytic) granuloma in the oral cavity.

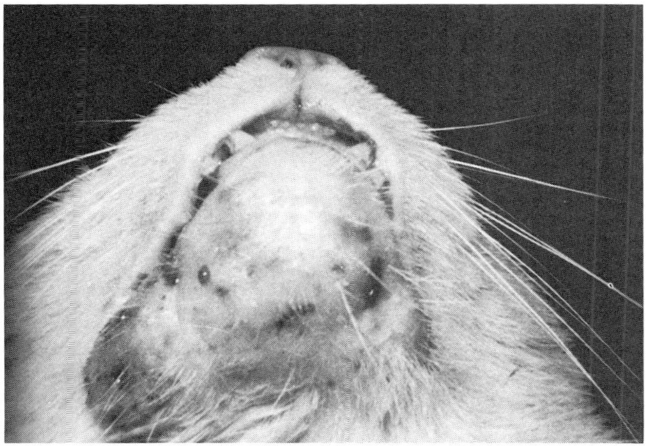

Figure 60–6. "Fat chin" (collagenolytic) granuloma.

Since all these disease entities include a differential diagnosis of neoplasia and infectious disease, performing a biopsy with or without a culture is in the best interest of the cat. Because mast cells accompany eosinophils in these lesions, careful histologic evaluation is needed to differentiate mast cell tumor from the eosinophilic granuloma complex. In cases of severe financial limitations on the part of the owner, diagnosis by medical therapy may be an alternative to biopsy.

Therapy

Glucocorticoids are the traditional therapy in this disease complex. However, some cases of eosinophilic granuloma complex have responded to the use of antibiotics. Trimethoprim potentiated sulfonamides, 120 mg b.i.d., cefadroxil, 100 mg b.i.d., or amoxicillin trihydrate plus clavulanate potassium, 62.5 mg b.i.d., have produced reduction or complete remission of disease.[6] This is a more benign therapy than glucocorticoids and may be utilized as the first line of therapy. If glucocorticoids are employed, prednisone or

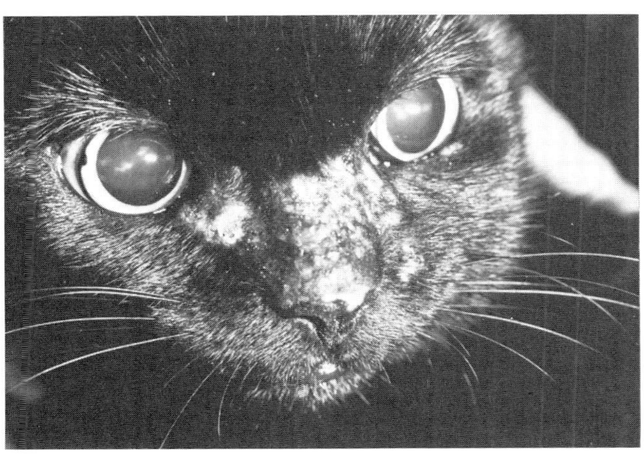

Figure 60–7. Atypical (mosquito bite hypersensitivity?) eosinophilic granuloma complex.

prednisolone is given at 2 to 4 mg/kg once daily until the lesions are healed. Alternatively, methylprednisolone acetate (Depo-Medrol) may be given subcutaneously or intramuscularly at 10 to 20 mg every 2 weeks, usually for three treatments. Although this interval is shorter than administration times generally recommended for other diseases, this regimen seems to produce much longer lasting remission than monthly injections. If the lesions recur, retreatment with glucocorticoids is in order, and maintenance therapy may need to be instituted consisting of alternate-day prednisone or prednisolone therapy or injection of methylprednisolone acetate every few months. Progestational compounds also have been used to treat this disease, but the author has not used and does not recommend these compounds.

If lesions become refractory to therapy, or if further diagnostic work is desired before medical therapy is instituted, a food trial with lamb babyfood or cooked lamb, intradermal skin testing, or testing for flea allergy followed by flea control in the environment can be instituted. This is especially relevant in the case of pruritic eosinophilic plaque. Because pruritis is more typical of the diseases for which tests are being performed. If atypical eosinophilic granuloma complex is seen on the ears, nose, and toes, changing the animal to a mosquito-free inside environment is warranted. Other methods that have occasionally been successful in refractory cases include surgical excision of localized disease, radiotherapy, cryosurgery, laser therapy, mixed bacteria vaccines, and immunomodulating drugs.[1,16-18]

Symmetric Alopecia

Hair loss is common in cats with skin disease, and it is usually patchy in distribution. Symmetric hair loss without skin disease is less commonly found.[1] Many different diseases can cause symmetric alopecia, either self-induced alopecia or non–self-induced (endocrine?) alopecia. The former category can be further divided into self-induced alopecia secondary to pruritus or secondary to psychogenic causes. The most common type by far is self-induced alopecia secondary to pruritus. Psychogenic alopecia runs a distant second, and non–self-induced symmetric (endocrine?) alopecia is considered rare in the cat.

Clinical Signs

Cats have symmetric hair loss of varying degrees of severity. It may be bilateral in distribution (Fig. 60–8). The most common areas of hair loss are the ventral abdomen (Fig. 60–9) and proximal thighs.[19] The next most common site of hair loss is over the lower back and rump. In some cases, multiple areas of alopecia become confluent and involve the whole trunk. A dermatitis may be associated with the hair loss, or the skin may be completely normal.

Clinical Evaluation

When evaluating the cat with symmetric alopecia, it must first be ascertained if the hair loss is self-induced. Information from the history may be helpful if the owner has noticed excessive licking, chewing, biting, or scratching. How-

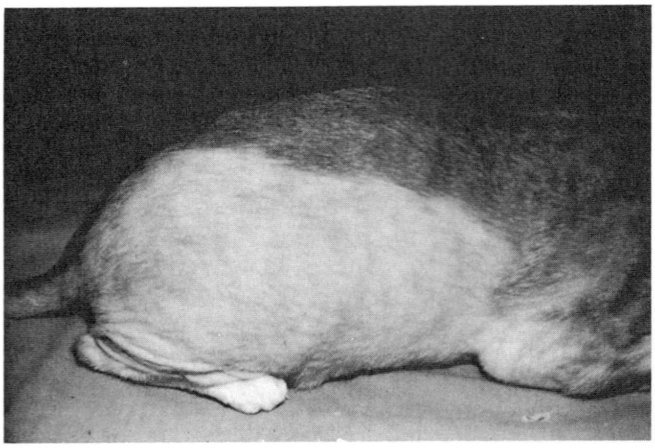

Figure 60–8. Bilateral symmetric alopecia secondary to flea allergic dermatitis. (Courtesy of Dr. Michele Brignac, Baton Rouge, LA.)

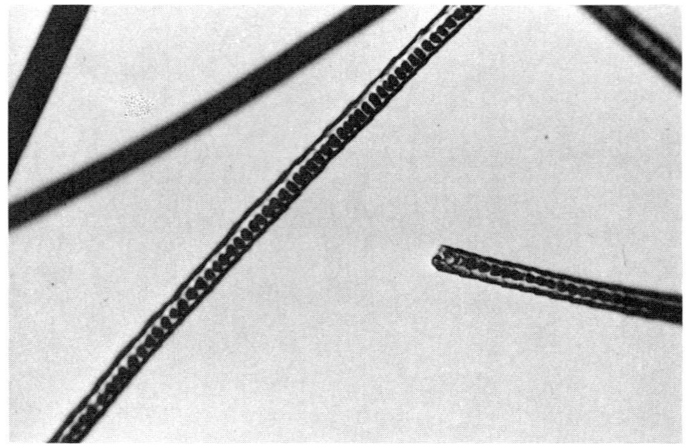

Figure 60–10. Note jagged broken end of hair, suggesting self-trauma. (Courtesy of Dr. Carol Foil, Louisiana State University, Baton Rouge, LA.)

ever, in many cases the cat is secretive about inflicting the self-trauma or the question to the owner is not phrased correctly. A very specific question should be formulated, such as, "Does your cat scratch, chew, lick, or groom excessively or repeatedly in one area?" In addition, hairballs or constipation may be signs of excessive grooming.

On dermatologic examination, ease of hair epilation, amount of broken hairs, and any involvement of the skin can be determined. In self-induced alopecia the hair does not epilate easily. Most of these cats have a certain amount of stubby, broken hair, but some cats can lick themselves bald with no evidence of stubby hair. Dermatitis of the skin may be seen with self-induced disease but is not present with non–self-induced alopecia.

Hair can be plucked and the distal ends examined microscopically. Jagged blunt ends suggest self-trauma (Fig. 60–10), whereas smooth tapered ends suggest hair loss that is not self-inflicted (Fig. 60–11) (see Chapter 12). If a question still remains concerning the nature of the alopecia, an Elizabethan collar can be placed on the cat for a few weeks. If the alopecia is self-induced, a small amount of new hair growth will be seen in that period of time. However, most of the time the nature of the hair loss can be ascertained without the use of an Elizabethan collar.

Diagnosis

If the disease is self-induced, as is the case in the vast majority of such patients, pruritic versus psychogenic origin needs to be determined. Since underlying pruritic diseases are

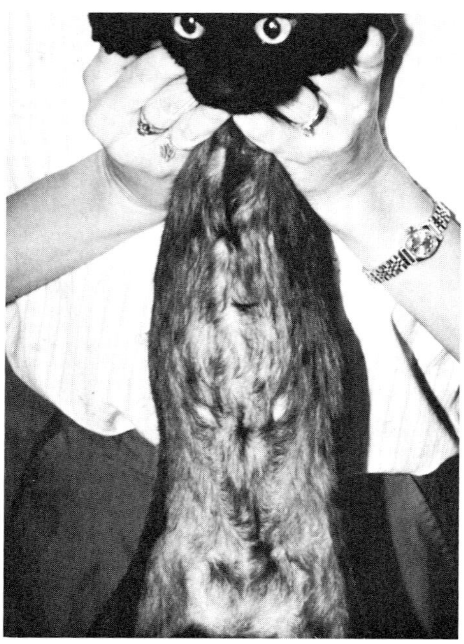

Figure 60–9. Alopecia on the abdomen of a cat with flea allergic dermatitis. (Courtesy of Dr. Gary Norsworthy, San Antonio, TX.)

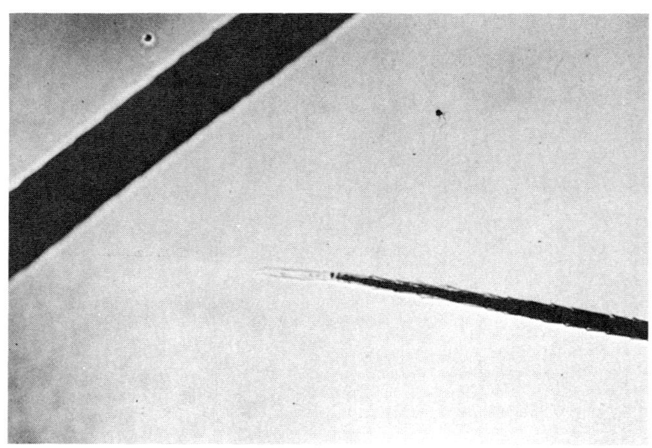

Figure 60–11. Note tapered end of hair, suggesting that the hair loss was not self-induced. (Courtesy of Dr. Carol Foil, Louisiana State University, Baton Rouge, LA.)

much more common than psychogenic alopecia, this possibility is explored first.

Self-Induced and Pruritic Alopecia

A skin scraping, fungal culture, fecal examination, and flea allergy test and/or flea control measures (in areas with fleas) should constitute the minimum data base. If these procedures do not point to a diagnosis or resolve the disease, a food allergy elimination diet or allergy testing or administration of ivermectin or intestinal deworming are in order. Successful treatment of the underlying pruritic disease will stop the excessive self-trauma and the hair will regrow.

If an exhaustive search for an underlying pruritic disease has not produced results, a trial therapeutic run with Depo-Medrol may help to differentiate between pruritic and psychogenic alopecia. In some cases, because of owner-imposed financial constraints, this test may be performed earlier in the diagnostic work-up. The clinician must be sure that the cat is not suffering from demodicosis or dermatophytosis. Most cases of pruritic alopecia respond to treatment with this glucocorticoid. However, a disease such as food allergy may not be fully responsive to glucocorticoids.

A cat with psychogenic alopecia does not respond to administration of glucocorticoids. However, personalities of some cats are altered by glucocorticoids, and psychogenic alopecia may potentially respond to these agents due to psychological effects instead of relief of pruritus.

Self-Induced and Psychogenic Alopecia

Cats most typically affected by psychogenic alopecia are the "high-strung" breeds: Siamese, Burmese, Abyssinian, and Himalayan. The history may be helpful in diagnosis and may include a recent major or minor change in the household, such as a new family member or pet, the loss of a family member or pet, a new house, a change of furniture, new restrictions in the areas accessible to the cat, altered work schedule of the owner, or a new animal in the outside environment seen from the window.

If the history and findings of the physical examination are supportive of psychogenic alopecia, altering the stressor is most helpful. If this is not possible, mood-modifying drugs may be tried. Phenobarbital at 2.2 to 6.6 mg/kg b.i.d. or diazepam at 1.25 to 2.5 mg b.i.d.[20] may be given until the excessive grooming behavior abates. The medication should then be gradually tapered. It can be completely discontinued in some cats, but the disease may recur when another stressor appears. Other cats require long-term or lifetime maintenance therapy with these agents at the lowest effective dose.

If a small amount of hair regrowth is not seen after the cat has worn an Elizabethan collar for 1 month, then the alopecia is definitely non–self-induced. Diseases that can cause this type of alopecia are very rare in the cat.

Non–Self-Induced Alopecia

Temporary stresses (e.g., antimitotic drugs, surgery, high fever) can interrupt hair growth. When the stress is removed, the hair continues to grow but is weakened at that point. This damaged hair breaks more easily, and as a result clinical alopecia is seen. This condition is called anagen defluxion.[20] Hair loss is seen within days of the insult.

In telogen defluxion, a stressful circumstance (such as high fever, surgery, queening) causes premature cessation of growth in anagen hair follicles. This is followed by a synchronization of the hair cycle of hairs in the resting or telogen phase. A few months later, a large number of these resting hairs are shed at the same time as new anagen hairs replace them. Again, clinical alopecia is seen.

Diffuse or symmetric alopecia is seen in association with hyperadrenocorticism, advanced diabetes mellitus, hyperthyroidism, advanced kidney disease, and chronic hepatic conditions.[19,21] Systemic signs should be obvious in these cats.

Sex hormone–associated alopecia is very rare in cats. Sex hormones can have anti-inflammatory and psychotropic effects on cats, and thus hair regrowth with sex hormone replacement therapy does not necessarily document a sex hormone–influenced hair loss.

In the case of anagen or telogen defluxion, no therapy is needed. The hairs are replaced and a normal hair cycle resumes. Treatment of the underlying endocrine disease resolves the endocrine alopecia. In one study of cats diagnosed with feline endocrine alopecia (but not proven hypothyroidism), treatment with liothyronine sodium at an initial dose of 20 μg b.i.d., and increasing this dose by 10 μg b.i.d. every third day to a maximum of 50 μg b.i.d., showed total hair regrowth in 73% of the cases within 12 weeks.[21]

Combined repositol diethylstilbestrol (0.625 mg) or estradiol (0.5 mg) and testosterone (12.5 mg) have been used to treat suspected sex hormone imbalance. Overdose of any of these sex hormones can cause severe liver disease in cats. Progestogens have also been utilized for suspected sex hormone imbalance. Megestrol acetate at 2.5 to 5.0 mg daily to every other day at induction, decreasing to 2.5 to 5.0 mg every 7 to 14 days, and medroxyprogesterone at 50 to 100 mg repeated in 3 to 6 months if needed, have been used in the cat.[20] The author does not use or recommend any of the preceding sex hormone replacement therapy because of its potential side effects compared with the relatively benign course of the clinical disease (cosmetic hair loss only).

Keratinization/Seborrheic Disorders

Disorders of keratinization are secondary to abnormal keratinocyte maturation, differentiation, and exfoliation. Feline acne, stud tail, and seborrheic syndrome are associated with keratinization abnormalities.

Feline Acne

Feline acne is a common disorder of unknown etiology. The severity of the disease is variable. Most affected cats have comedones on the chin and ventral to the lower lips that are usually asymptomatic. Occasionally, lesions can become secondarily infected and inflamed, resulting in papules, pustules, and edema (Fig. 60–12). Accompanying pruritus is variable with these lesions. The presence of *Malassezia canis* has been reported in acute cases of feline acne.[22] A biopsy reveals the organism in the hair follicles.

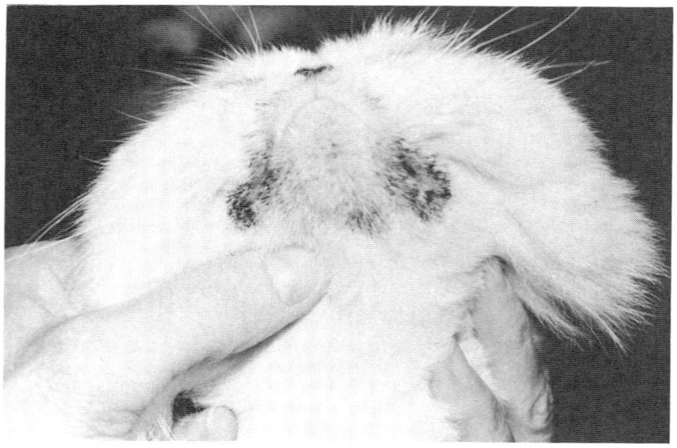

Figure 60–12. **Chin acne with a secondary bacterial infection showing a papular eruption with oozing. (Courtesy of Dr. Carol Foil, Louisiana State University, Baton Rouge, LA.)**

Differential diagnoses include abscesses, dermatophytosis, demodicosis, and the collagenolytic form of the eosinophilic granuloma complex. A skin scraping and fungal culture of the lesion should be performed in all cases. If the lesions do not respond to appropriate therapy, a bacterial culture, culture for *Malassezia canis,* and biopsy may be indicated.

Treatment of the mild "comedo" cases is unnecessary. If lesions are more severe, clipping the area and gentle daily washing with soap or detergent are effective. Benzoyl peroxide shampoo may be helpful because of its follicular flushing action. Benzoyl peroxide gel (5%) can be irritating to cats and is not usually used. If a bacterial infection is present, appropriate antibiotics given for a minimum of 2 to 3 weeks are indicated. Ketoconazole has been successfully used to treat yeast chin infections. Isotretinoin at 5 mg once a day is reported to be effective in the treatment of chin acne.[14] This disease can recur, and maintenance cleaning may be needed.

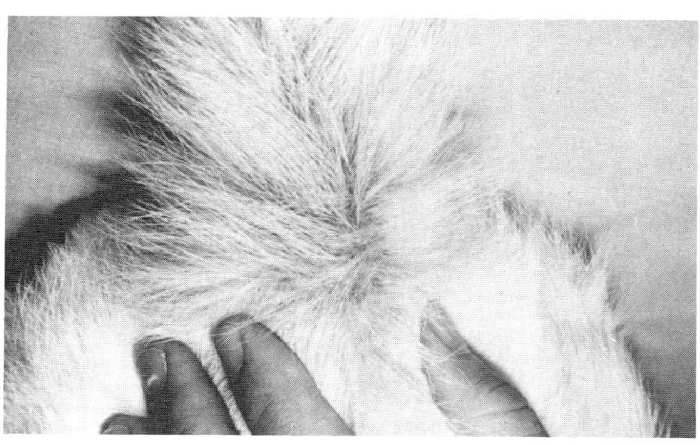

Figure 60–13. **Erythema and waxy yellow debris on the dorsum of a male cat with stud tail. (Courtesy of Dr. Nita Gulbas, Phoenix, AZ.)**

Stud Tail

The dorsum of the cat tail is rich in sebaceous and apocrine glands. Abnormal amounts of waxy exudate can accumulate in this region (Fig. 60–13). This is most commonly seen in intact males but can also be seen in females or castrated males.

In addition to the yellow wax accumulation, comedones, alopecia, and hyperpigmentation of the skin may be seen (stud tail). Occasionally, a secondary bacterial folliculitis and furunculosis may complicate the condition. The author has seen a case of stud tail in which a pure culture of *Malassezia canis* was obtained from the area.

Treatment of mild lesions is usually not necessary. In more severe cases, clipping the area and washing it with soap and water or using a degreasing benzoyl peroxide shampoo can be useful. Cleaning the area every few days may be required as maintenance therapy. Appropriate antibiotic therapy for a minimum of 2 to 3 weeks should be instituted if a secondary bacterial infection is present. If *Malassezia canis* is suspected, topical ketoconazole shampoo and administration of oral ketoconazole (at 10 mg/kg s.i.d. to b.i.d.) may be helpful. If the patient is an intact male, neutering often will be curative.

Seborrhea

Generalized seborrhea is an uncommon clinical condition in the cat; when it exists, it is usually secondary to other diseases, including cheyletiellosis, pediculosis, endoparasitism, dermatophytosis, environmental factors (low humidity and high temperature), overly frequent shampooing or powdering, nutritional disorders, systemic disease (diabetes mellitus, chronic liver disease, hyperthyroidism, systemic lupus erythematosus, feline leukemia virus infection), or drug eruption. An idiopathic generalized seborrhea, also called "the sticky cat," has been reported.[23] These cats are healthy in all respects except for the generalized seborrhea, and the condition can wax and wane despite therapy.

Work-up for the seborrheic cat should include a skin scraping and close examination for ectoparasites, a fungal culture, a fecal examination, and information on environmental living conditions, diet, and current topical or systemic medications. If these procedures do not lead to a diagnosis, blood studies consisting of a feline leukemia virus test, feline immunodeficiency virus (FIV) test, complete blood count, and chemistry panel should be performed.

Treatment should be aimed at the underlying disease. While the underlying disease is being addressed or if a diagnosis of idiopathic seborrhea is made, symptomatic therapy with antiseborrheic shampoos is indicated. Shampoos containing sulfur and salicylic acid combinations are best. Tar-based shampoos are potentially toxic in cats. For dry seborrhea, emollient shampoos and rinses may also be helpful.

REFERENCES

1. Scott DW. Feline dermatology 1900–1978: A monograph. J Am Anim Hosp Assoc 1980;16:331.

2. Ihrke PJ. The Miliary Eczema Complex. In: Pratt PW, ed. Feline Medicine. Santa Barbara: American Veterinary Publications, Inc., 1983:599.
3. Nesbitt GH. Feline Dermatoses. In: Nesbitt GH, ed. Dermatology. New York: Churchill Livingstone, 1987:209.
4. Gross TL, Kwochka KW, Kunkle GA. Corrrelation of histologic and immunologic findings in cats with military dermatitis. J Am Vet Med Assoc 1986;189:1322.
5. Kunkle GA. Feline dermatology. Vet Clin North Am (Small Anim Pract) 1984;14:1065.
6. Rosenkrantz WS. Eosinophilic Granuloma "Confusion." In: August JR, ed. Consultations in Feline Internal Medicine. Philadelphia: WB Saunders, 1991:121.
7. Scott DW. Observations on the eosinophilic granuloma complex in cats. J Am Anim Hosp Assoc 1975;11:261.
8. Hess PW, MacEwen EG. Feline Eosinophilic Granuloma. In: Kirk RW, ed. Current Veterinary Therapy VI. Philadelphia: WB Saunders, 1977:534.
9. Moriello KA, Kunkle G, Miller LM, et al. Lack of autologous tissue transmission of eosinophilic plaques in cats. Am J Vet Res 1990;51:995.
10. Neufield JL, Bertun L, Jeffrey KR. Eosinophilic granuloma in a cat. Recovery of virus particles. Vet Pathol 1980;17:97.
11. Russell RG, Slattum MM, Abkowitz J. Filamentous bacteria in oral eosinophilic granulomas of a cat. Vet Pathol 1988;25:249.
12. Gelberg HB, Lewis RM, Felsburg PJ, et al. Antiepithelial autoantibodies associated with the feline eosinophilic granuloma complex. Am J Vet Res 1985;46:263.
13. Mason KV, Evans AG. Mosquito bite-caused eosinophilic dermatitis in cats. J Am Vet Med Assoc 1991;198:2086.
14. Scott DW. Feline dermatology 1986 to 1988: Looking to the 1990s through the eyes of many counsellors. J Am Anim Hosp Assoc 1990;26:515.
15. Wilkinson GT, Bate MJ. A possible further clinical manifestation of the feline eosinophilic granuloma complex. J Am Anim Hosp Assoc 1984;20:325.
16. Manning TO, Crane SW, Scheidt VJ. Three cases of feline eosinophilic granuloma complex (eosinophilic ulcer) and observations on laser therapy. Semin Vet Med Surg Small Anim 1987;2:206.
17. Willsemse TA. Cryotherapy in Small Animal Dermatology. In: Kirk RW, ed. Current Veterinary Therapy VII. Philadelphia: WB Saunders, 1980:495.
18. MacEwen EG, Hess PW. Evaluation of the effect of immunomodulation on the feline eosinophilic granuloma complex. J Am Anim Hosp Assoc 1987;23:519.
19. Miller WH. Symmetrical truncal hair loss in cats. Compend Contin Educ Pract Vet 1990;12:461.
20. Muller GH, Kirk RW, Scott DW. Small Animal Dermatology, 4th ed. Philadelphia: WB Saunders 1989:699.
21. Thoday KL. Differential Diagnosis of Symmetric Alopecia in the Cat. In: Kirk RW, ed. Current Veterinary Therapy IX. Philadelphia: WB Saunders, 1986:545.
22. Moriella KA. The cutaneous mycoses of dogs and cats. Vet Reports 1988;1:9.
23. Longbottom GM. "Sticky cats." Vet Rec 1977;100:392.

CHAPTER 61

◇ ◇ ◇

Systemic Fungal Diseases

Sharon K. Fooshee and Benny J. Woody

Systemic fungal infections are relatively rare in the cat when compared to the frequency with which they occur in the dog. The reported incidence of feline mycotic disease should increase, however, as clinicians adopt a higher index of suspicion. Deep mycotic infections are most often associated with the feline respiratory tract, but they may be included in the differential diagnosis for many presenting complaints because of the myriad of potential clinical manifestations.

The major systemic mycotic diseases of cats are cryptococcosis, histoplasmosis, blastomycosis, and coccidioidomycosis. The etiology, epidemiology, pathogenesis, and clinical manifestations of each disease are presented; a summary of diagnostic and therapeutic protocols concludes each section. A summary of comments related to general aspects of antifungal therapy and the significance of public health concerns can be found at the end of the chapter.

Cryptococcosis

Etiology and Epidemiology

Cryptococcosis was first reported[1] in cats in 1951, and the first recognized case in a dog, shortly thereafter.[2] It is observed regularly, albeit infrequently, and represents the most common deep mycotic infection of cats.[3] Cryptococcosis is the only systemic fungal disease that is more prevalent in cats than in dogs.[4] There is no apparent breed or sex predisposition.[3,5] (In humans, males are more likely to be infected.[6]) Cryptococcosis has been reported in exotic felidae.[7]

The etiologic agent of this disease is *Cryptococcus neoformans,* a small, budding, yeastlike organism that has a characteristic thick mucopolysaccharide capsule, or "halo." While the presence of the capsule is variable in vitro, it is always present during the tissue, or yeast, phase.[8]

Once thought to exist solely in the yeast (asexual) form, a mycelial (sexual or perfect) form has been identified, but it is demonstrated only under specific laboratory conditions.[9] Identification of specific capsular antigens has resulted in recognition of four serotypes—A, B, C, and D—serotype A being most commonly associated with human infection.[10] Serotypes B and C are focused in southern California.[3] Feline serotypes have not been published as of this writing.

Unlike the other systemic fungal organisms, *C. neoformans* is not geographically isolated and is recognized worldwide.[11] The presence of pigeon droppings is known to favor growth of *C. neoformans,* because the organism is able to utilize for growth many of the nitrogen compounds in pigeon excreta.[3] Survival is enhanced by increased humidity.[12] The pigeon may serve as a fomite, but it does not become infected, as pathogenic species of *C. neoformans* do not grow at temperatures of 39°C or above.[3]

Inhalation of aerosolized particles is generally regarded as the primary route of infection for cats; the upper respiratory tract is the most common site of involvement. Although cryptococcal pneumonia does occur in cats, the mechanism by which pulmonary infection is established has not been clearly defined. When encapsulated, *C. neoformans* may measure 5 to 20 μm and would reasonably appear too large to penetrate into the alveolar spaces (1 to 2 μm).[13] However, the organism may not develop a capsule when grown on media or as it occurs in the environment. Hyperosmolarity is considered one factor that may inhibit capsule formation.[14] Pigeon feces are hyperosmolar and thus may promote development of unencapsulated organisms small enough to penetrate into terminal airways.[15] A potential role has been postulated for the more recently discovered mycelial phase and its smaller structural element, the basidiospore.[3,8,16]

Experimental attempts to infect cats by oral, subcutaneous, and intraperitoneal inoculation of organisms were unsuccessful; infection was established by intranasal, intratracheal, and intrathecal routes.[17] Primary cutaneous disease with no evidence of hematogenous or lymphatic dissemination was documented in three cats.[18] Another report describes the recovery of *C. neoformans* from a chronic ulcerated skin wound over the tibiotarsal joint of a cat; systemic involvement could not be demonstrated.[19]

Pathogenesis

Cell-mediated immunity provides the primary defense against establishment of deep mycotic infections.[20] The limited role of humoral immunity in controlling *C. neoformans* was demonstrated by comparing the course of fungal disease in normal and B-cell deficient mice: no difference was noted between groups.[21] Immunocompromised persons, particularly those who have a disease that suppresses the cellular immune system or who are being treated with immunosuppressive drugs, are known to be predisposed to cryptococcal infection.[22] Human immunodeficiency virus, the etiologic agent of acquired immunodeficiency syndrome (AIDS), and the feline leukemia virus (FeLV) and feline immunodeficiency virus (FIV) of cats are retroviruses well known for preferential suppression of cellular immunity. The opportunistic infection of AIDS patients with cryptococcosis is well documented.[23] Interestingly, a clear association between viral immunosuppression and cryptococcosis has not been identified in cats,[3] but many of the early cases described in the literature were not tested for FeLV. It would appear reasonable to expect immunosuppression to predispose cats to cryptococcal infection.

Immunosuppressed humans, already predisposed to cryptococcal infection, may undergo specific alterations of the immune system in response to the organism. Although this is speculative, it seems possible that these same changes might occur in infected cats. *C. neoformans* appears able to induce some degree of immunosuppression in the host. The polysaccharide capsule is believed to be responsible for inhibition of phagocytosis; the capacity of phagocytic cells to engulf the organism is increasingly diminished as greater amounts of capsular material are presented to the immune system.[24] The pathogenicity of the organism appears to be essentially lost when the capsule is removed.[8] Capsular polysaccharide also decomplements serum by activating the classical and alternate complement pathways, and it may block chemotaxis of neutrophils and monocytes.[25] Plasma cell function is inhibited[3]; antibody that is generated may later be adsorbed to the capsule surface.[8]

Histopathologic tissue sections may not always reflect a significant inflammatory response to the presence of the organism.[11] This may be related to antigens "hidden" beneath the mucopolysaccharide capsule that effectively avoid recognition by and provocation of the immune system. The capsule itself is considered immunologically inert because the polysaccharide does not evoke a significant response from the immune system.[26]

Clinical Signs

The organism appears to have the greatest affinity for the respiratory system; the skin and central nervous system rank second and third, respectively, in frequency of involvement.[27] Lesions tend to appear granulomatous or gelatinous.[28]

In general, respiratory infections tend to localize in the sinuses and upper airways of cats more often than in the lower respiratory tree,[3,4] though in a review of mycotic disease it was reported that pulmonary lesions were found in one fourth to half of cited infections in cats.[28,29] Clinical signs of lower airway involvement, such as coughing, are infrequently noted; sneezing, snuffling, and a variety of types of nasal discharges are more common (see Chapter 30). These may be temporarily responsive to antibiotic therapy. Cryptococcosis should be part of the differential diagnosis for any cat with chronic sinusitis.[4] Some cats present with the classic swelling across the bridge of the nose; others exhibit a fleshy, granulomatous-looking mass protruding from one or both nostrils. Submandibular lymphadenopathy may be present.

The skin and subcutaneous tissues are involved in approximately 40% of affected cats; lesions usually are on the face and head (Fig. 61–1).[3] Initially, most lesions appear as firm nodules that grow somewhat rapidly and eventually ulcerate, suggesting a neoplasm. Facial lesions frequently occur in concert with upper respiratory tract involvement

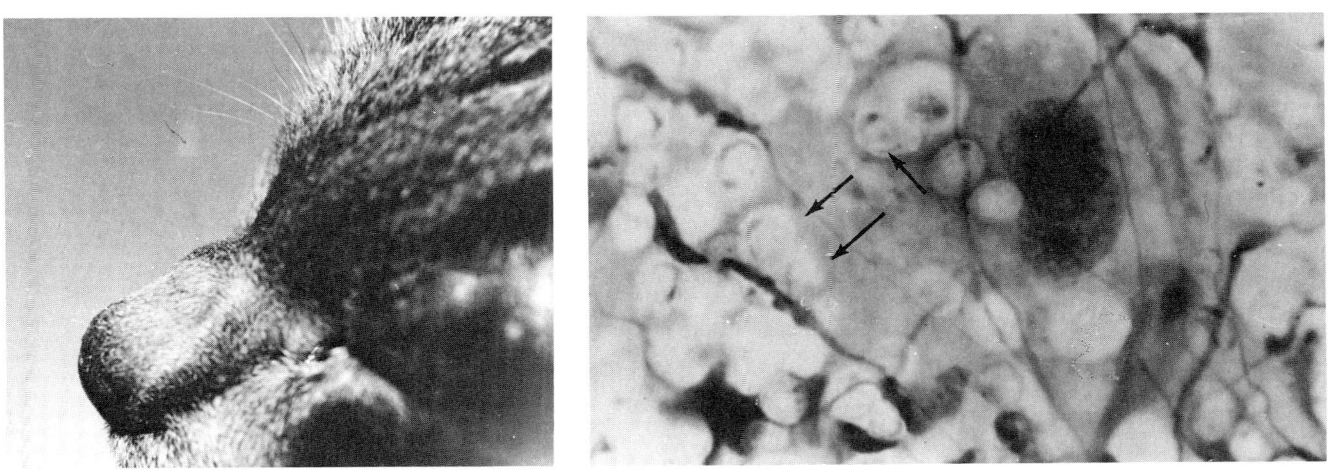

A B

Figure 61–1. (*A*) The swelling on the nose was the only external lesion on this cat. (*B*) The lesion was aspirated and the aspirate stained with Diff-Quik. The poorly staining organisms (*arrows*) are *Cryptococcus neoformans*. The organism, 5 to 20 μm diameter, is surrounded by a thick capsule. Budding from a narrow base is typical. (Courtesy of Dr. Gary D. Norsworthy, San Antonio, TX.)

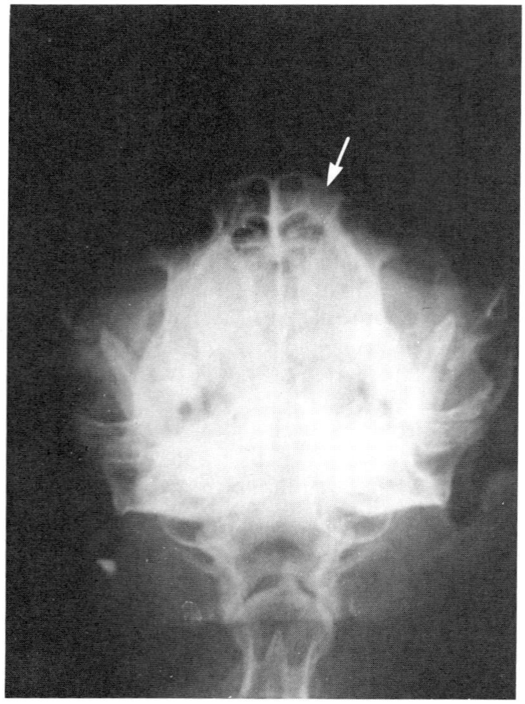

A

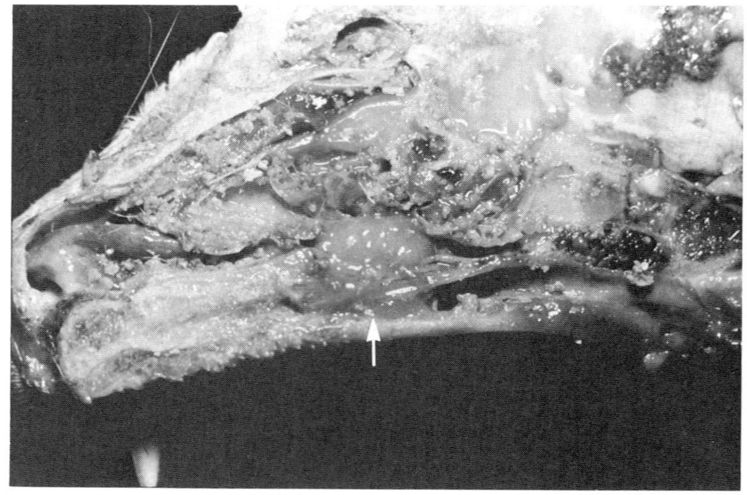

B

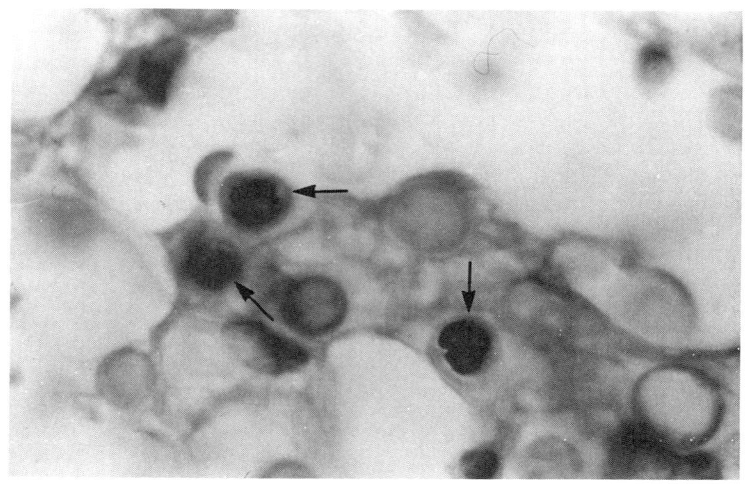

C

Figure 61–2. (*A*) This cat has a chronic, purulent nasal discharge of several months duration. There is radiographic evidence of frontal sinusitis, as evidenced by increased density of the left sinus (*arrow*). (*B*) Necropsy revealed copious purulent material in the nasal cavity (*arrow*) and frontal sinuses. (*C*) Hematoxylin-eosin stain of the tissues revealed *Cryptococcus neoformans* (*arrows*). (Courtesy of Dr. Gary D. Norsworthy, San Antonio, TX.)

(Fig. 61–2) or generalized cryptococcal skin disease.[27] Although primary cutaneous cryptococcosis has been reported, the vast majority of cases reflect multisystem involvement.[18,19] Cutaneous lesions are usually a manifestation of disseminated disease.[13]

The organism has a definite propensity for tissue of the central nervous system (CNS), but the route taken to achieve neural infection and the cause for CNS affinity have not been determined. Invasion through the cribriform plate or by hematogenous routes is likely.[3] Clinical CNS involvement is seen in fewer than 20% of cases, though about a third have CNS lesions at necropsy.[29] A wide variety of presentations may be observed with CNS infection; these may mimic other infections of the nervous system such as feline infectious peritonitis (FIP), toxoplasmosis, bacterial meningitis, and tumors such as lymphosarcoma. There is no particular pattern with regard to acuteness of onset or progression of signs.

Ocular lesions are common with feline cryptococcosis.[30] A wide variety of lesions have been reported, many of which have been reproduced by experimental introduction of infection via intracarotid injection of the organism.[31] Some of the more commonly reported ocular lesions are optic neuritis, panophthalmitis, chorioretinitis, and dilated, unresponsive pupils.[3,4,27] One or both eyes may be affected.

Diagnosis

The hemogram, biochemical profile, and urinalysis do not offer specific indications of cryptococcal infection, but they are useful tools for assessment of general health and the ability of major organ systems to withstand chemotherapy. Adjunctive tests to rule out other mutisystem infectious diseases (toxoplasmosis, FIP, FeLV, FIV) should be performed, because cryptococcosis may occasionally present in an unusual fashion. Skull or thoracic radiographs may be helpful in determining repiratory tract involvement.

C. neoformans has classically been identified with cytologic inspection of wet mounts or smears of exudative material. New methylene blue stain offers a fairly reliable means for identifying the organism in cytologic specimens. Wright's stain and Gram stain are considered less reliable by some authors.[32] India ink preparations are another well-known technique for cytologic identification of the yeast, but if this method is employed it is important to recognize that artifacts or other cells may be mistaken for fungal organisms.[3] The organism is 5 to 20 μm in diameter and surrounded by the characteristic thick capsule. Budding from a narrow base is typical. Presence of an associated local inflammatory response is variable; however, pyogranulomatous inflammation typifies most fungal infections.

Although it is not routinely needed, tissue biopsy may be indicated in particular cases. Routine staining with hematoxylin and eosin may fail to demonstrate the capsule, although the organism itself stains. Gomori's methenamine silver and periodic acid–Schiff (PAS) stains are useful for histopathologic studies. Mayer's mucicarmine is often recommended because it produces intense pink staining of the capsule.[3,5]

Laboratory culture of the organism is occasionally required, particularly for cerebrospinal fluid, as culture is more likely to render a diagnosis than cytologic study.[3] Sabouraud's dextrose agar without cycloheximide, a saprophyte inhibitor, is an ideal medium, although *C. neoformans* grows well on blood agar.[8] Dermatophyte test medium (DTM) should not be used because of the cycloheximide.[32]

Serologic testing is becoming a more reliable means of determining infection in both humans and cats, but the reliability of the different tests varies. The indirect fluorescent antibody test for serum has limited diagnostic value because it detects circulating antibody directed against cryptococcal antigen. It is less desirable than the latex agglutination test, which is specific for capsular antigen.

Historically, cryptococcus-infected patients may have no measurable antibody, whereas healthy persons, those with an early infection, and those who are recovering from active infection demonstrate measurable levels of antibody. Clinical cases of cryptococcosis may fail to demonstrate antibodies owing to complexing of circulating antibodies with polysaccharide capsular antigen in the blood.[8] Also, as previously described, the immune system may receive varying amounts of stimulus because fungal antigens may be "hidden" beneath the capsule and the capsule itself offers only minimal antigenic stimulus.[11] These variables make interpretation of antibody levels somewhat confusing and a poor way to confirm active disease.

The latex agglutination test (LAT) is considered the most sensitive and specific test in current use; serum, urine, or cerebrospinal fluid samples may be tested. In this test latex particles coated with *C. neoformans*–specific antibody form complexes with cryptococcal capsular antigen in vitro, resulting in clumping or agglutination of particles. At the present time this test is considered the only clinically reliable serologic test for use in veterinary medicine.[3] Localized and transient infections may result in false negative titers, whereas immune-mediated diseases and *Klebsiella* infections may result in false positives.[3,8,26]

In humans the LAT is purported to correlate well with severity of infection and to serve as a useful indicator of response to therapy. Progress in therapy is suggested by a fall in antigen load.[26] Favorable correlation has been found between cats with known infection and the LAT.[3,33,34] The usefulness of the test for evaluation of response to therapy in the cat is being investigated.[35] Results of the LAT should be evaluated in conjunction with other clinical indices to best assess response and appropriate duration of therapy.

Treatment

Potential therapeutic agents include ketoconazole (KCZ), amphotericin B, and flucytosine (known chemically as 5-fluorocytosine [5-FC]). Medleau and coinvestigators successfully treated cutaneous cryptococcosis with KCZ (10 mg/kg every 24 hours) for 5 months.[18] An extremely high dose—72 mg/kg/day—was used for a total of 10 months for another cat with cutaneous lesions; apparent cure was achieved without observed toxicity.[34] Noxon and coworkers achieved clinical remission in a cat with upper respiratory tract involvement at a dose of 1 mg/kg KCZ every 24 hours for 188 days.[36] Mikiciuk and associates reported clinical cure in a cat with nasal lesions using a combination of KCZ at 10 mg/kg every 12 hours and 5-FC at 125 mg every 24 hours for 81 days.[37] Because the blood-brain barrier results in poor distribution into the CNS, some do not recommend KCZ as single-agent therapy when there is nervous system involvement. Others recommend it but in higher doses (20 to 30 mg/kg/day divided into two doses).[4] Prolonged treatment for at least 3 to 6 months is recommended for all cases of cryptococcosis. Although the literature indicates that *C. neoformans* is less sensitive to KCZ than to amphotericin B, we have had success with KCZ in treating nasal cryptococcosis and find it an attractive alternative to amphotericin B because most cats tolerate it well. For many veterinarians, it has become the treatment of choice for this disease.[13] Itraconazole (ITZ), a pharmacologically related compound, is currently being investigated for use in cats. It holds promise because it appears to have fewer side effects and to achieve greater CNS penetration than KCZ.[13]

Amphotericin B is the single-agent therapy preferred by some for CNS cryptococcosis.[38] Localized cutaneous cryptococcosis has been successfully treated with amphotericin B alone[39] and by amphotericin B combined with 5-FC.[40] Wilkinson suggests a protocol of amphotericin B, 0.3 mg/kg intravenously (IV) three times per week.[11] Blood urea nitrogen (BUN) levels should be monitored frequently so that the drug may be discontinued temporarily if azotemia develops (i.e., BUN greater than 40 mg/dL).

Barrett and coworkers suggest 5-FC at a minimum dose of 100 mg/kg/day divided into four equal dosages.[40] Legendre recommends 200 mg/kg/day divided into six doses and suggests that it not be used as single-agent therapy because *C. neoformans* organisms rapidly develop resistance.[4] Combination therapy with amphotericin B and 5-FC has been shown to be additive, and possibly synergistic.[40] KCZ, alone or in combination with 5-FC, was less effective in experimental mice than amphotericin B alone.[41] In combination with KCZ, 5-FC has shown toxicity for the cat.[42]

All antifungals should be administered for several weeks after clinical remission. Ideally, treatment for cryptococcosis should be continued until a negative LAT is achieved. As previously mentioned, use of the LAT to assess response to therapy in cats is currently being investigated.[3]

Histoplasmosis

Etiology and Epidemiology

Human histoplasmosis was first reported from the Panama Canal Zone in 1906.[43] It was not until 1939 that the first natural infection in a dog was described,[44] and the first feline case followed in 1949.[45] While it is clear that natural infections do occur in cats, histoplasmosis is not frequently noted as a cause of clinical disease, although it probably is more common than blastomycosis or coccidioidomycosis.[46] Subjective evidence suggests that cats are fairly susceptible to this disease, although most infected cats probably develop only a transient, clinically inapparent infection.[47]

A predilection for a specific sex or cat breed is not apparent, although cats younger than 1 year appear to be preferentially infected.[48,49] Like the other deep mycotic agents, *Histoplasma capsulatum* is a dimorphic organism and shares a similar life cycle with the other dimorphic fungi.[49] The mycelial form produces two types of spores: macroconidia of 8 to 14 μm diameter, and the smaller microconidia, which measure 2 to 4 μm.

Like *C. neoformans,* this organism has worldwide distribution. In North America known endemic areas of infection include the St. Lawrence River Valley and the Mississippi River Valley and areas surrounding its tributary rivers, the Ohio, Tennessee, and lower Missouri.[28] The organism has been identified in nearly all states. A preponderance of cases have been reported from Texas and Oklahoma.[48,50–54]

Exposure to the common environment, as opposed to animal-to-human transmission, is thought to be responsible for concurrent infection in humans and animals. The organism is most frequently associated with topsoil enriched with feces of birds and bats.[49] Because of their higher body temperature, birds remain uninfected, although bats may develop disease.[55]

Establishment of infection is thought to be related to environmental exposure. Two routes of entry are postulated—respiratory and gastrointestinal—and most evidence clearly supports the respiratory route.[49] A case of primary gastrointestinal histoplasmosis in a cat has been reported.[50] Experimental attempts to reproduce infection by this route in dogs have been unsuccessful.[56]

Pathogenesis

Like other fungal diseases, containment of histoplasmosis depends on competency of the cell-mediated immune response. Humoral immunity is not protective.[55] Following inhalation of microconidia, organisms are engulfed by pulmonary phagocytes. Infection may then be eliminated or contained in the respiratory mononuclear phagocytic system. Dissemination from the respiratory tree most likely occurs via lymphatic or hematogenous routes.[57] Dissemination and exacerbation of clinical signs are reported in immunosuppressed humans and in those receiving prolonged glucocorticoid therapy[58]; the same phenomenon appears to be observable in dogs.[59] In cats, neither immunosuppression nor FeLV infection appears to be a predisposing factor for development of histoplasmosis.[47]

Clinical Signs

Signs of specific organ dysfunction are infrequently noted, and the most common presenting complaints are vague[47]: fever, weight loss, anorexia, and lethargy.[47,48,52] In contrast, disseminated disease in dogs is commonly manifested as chronic diarrhea.[60]

Usually, fewer than half of infected cats demonstrate overt evidence of organ-specific disturbance.[47] Since this is essentially, a disease of the mononuclear phagocyte system, hepatomegaly and splenomegaly may be observed.[61,62] Dyspnea and tachypnea are expected findings with diffuse pulmonary disease, although radiographic evidence of mycotic pneumonia may be present without apparent respiratory distress.[52] A miliary interstitial pattern in the lungs is the most commonly reported radiographic finding (Fig. 61–3*A*).[63] Fungal osteomyelitis has been reported in several cats.[53,54] Inflammatory ocular changes are a nonspecific but common finding.[52,64] Subcutaneous nodules may also be seen (Fig. 61–3*B*).

Laboratory profiles are normally nondiagnostic, although nonregenerative anemia and hypoalbuminemia are consistent findings.[47]

Diagnosis

To date, serologic and intradermal skin testing have not proven to be reliable indicators of infection or useful for staging confirmed infection. Serologic testing with a variety of fungal antigens has been described.[55] Cross-reaction with other fungal agents and lack of standardization in testing procedures render serologic evaluation a peripheral, adjunctive diagnostic tool.[60] Clinkenbeard and coworkers reported seronegativity for *Histoplasma* antibodies in two of four cats with confirmed infection.[48]

It is possible to identify the organism in peripheral blood smears, but this may not be a high-yield procedure. Nevertheless, the blood smear should be carefully examined before more invasive procedures are undertaken. The phagocytic white cells (monocytes, neutrophils) should be closely examined in large numbers. Because *Histoplasma* organisms are relatively small, they may be engulfed by the circulating phagocytes. In one study, the number of cats diagnosed with peripheral smears was increased by evaluating 1000 leukocytes or buffy coat smears, as opposed to the standard 100 cells (see Chapter 12).[48] Wolf reported four of 20 cats were diagnosed by blood smear examination.[52] Bone marrow aspiration appears to be a high-yield diagnostic procedure. In one retrospective study, organisms were found in the bone marrow of 11 of 12 cats that had marrow examinations.[48]

Because the organism does not stain well with hematoxylin and eosin, cytologic examination may actually be superior to biopsy and histopathologic inspection. In many cases a diagnosis may be easily achieved by cytologic inspection of fine-needle aspirates of organs or cutaneous lesions. The liver, spleen, and lymph nodes, accessible components of the mononuclear phagocyte system, frequently harbor the organism. Lung aspirates may also be helpful, although aspiration carries potentially significant risks for the patient.

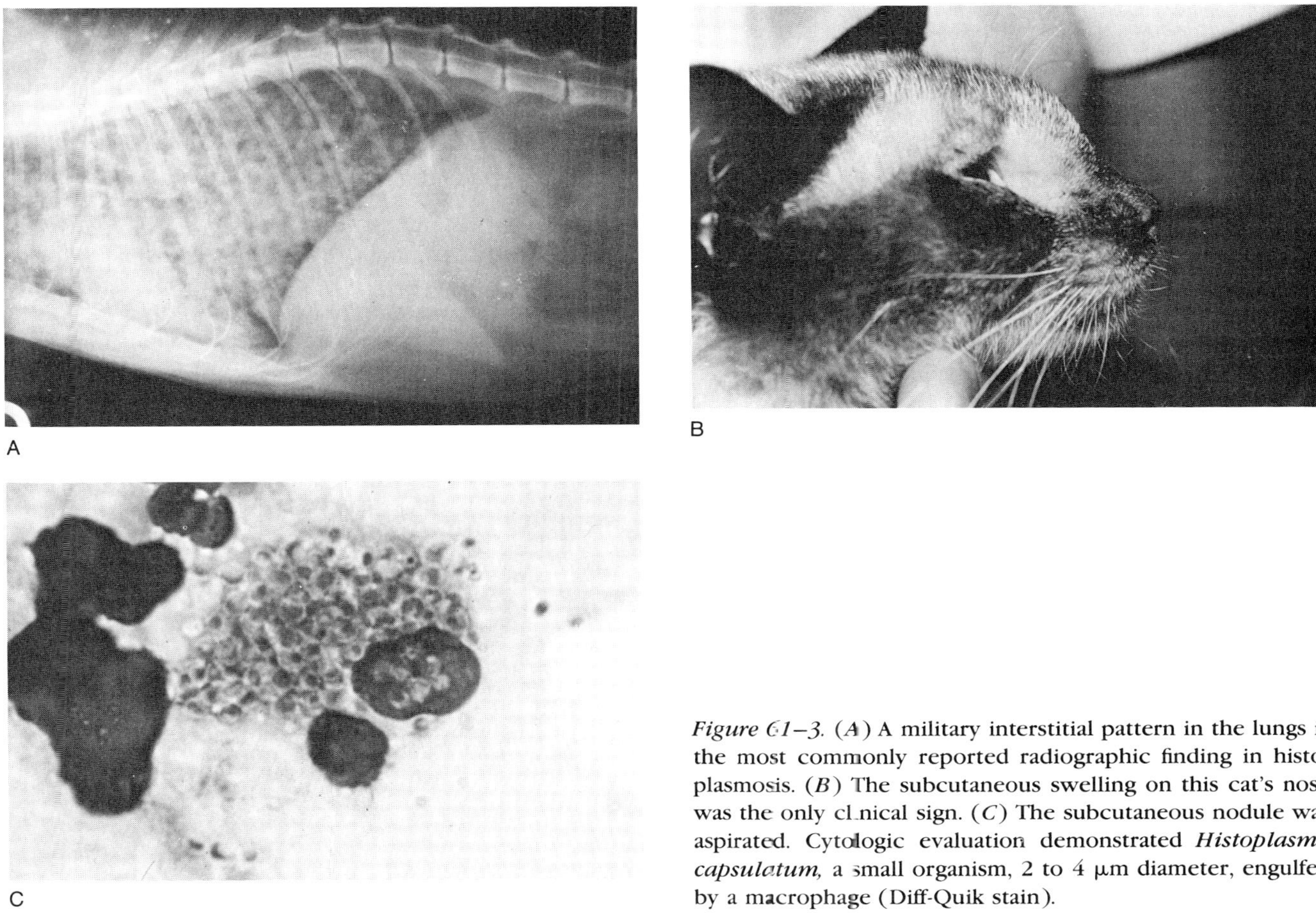

Figure 61–3. (*A*) A military interstitial pattern in the lungs is the most commonly reported radiographic finding in histoplasmosis. (*B*) The subcutaneous swelling on this cat's nose was the only clinical sign. (*C*) The subcutaneous nodule was aspirated. Cytologic evaluation demonstrated *Histoplasma capsulatum,* a small organism, 2 to 4 μm diameter, engulfed by a macrophage (Diff-Quik stain).

Cytologic evaluation of the yeast phase demonstrates a small organism, 2 to 4 μm in diameter (Fig. 61–3*C*). It is frequently found intracellularly engulfed by monocytes and macrophages. *Histoplasma capsulatum* organisms are banded by a characteristic halo which develops as the organism shrinks during fixing and staining.

Treatment

Amphotericin B and KCZ are the antifungal agents most commonly used to treat cats with histoplasmosis.

Breitschwerdt and coworkers described an unsuccessful course of therapy with amphotericin B in one cat with disseminated histoplasmosis.[61] Wolf and colleagues reported unsatisfactory results with amphotericin B in three of four cats in which it was used.[52] A satisfactory protocol could be 0.15 to 0.50 mg/kg IV every other day, to a cumulative dose of 4 mg/kg. Treatment should be discontinued if signs of renal toxicity appear.

Clinkenbeard and coworkers described three cats that were treated with KCZ at doses ranging from 10 to 30 mg/kg every 24 hours for as long as 10 weeks; two of the cats died and the third was euthanized.[48] One cat treated with 15 mg/kg every 24 hours for 5 months was still in remission at 37 months. Noxon and associates reported apparent success in treating one cat with KCZ at 20 mg/kg every 12 hours on alternate days for 78 days.[64] Reinstitution of therapy was necessary 8 months later, and the same dosage was administered for 129 additional days. A general recommendation of 10 to 20 mg/kg, daily or every other day as tolerated, can be made.[47]

Combination therapy with amphotericin B and KCZ is the preferred protocol of some clinicians. Some cats may not tolerate amphotericin B; in such cases KCZ becomes the treatment of choice. When possible, prolonged treatment with KCZ—for at least 6 months—is ideal.

Blastomycosis

Etiology and Epidemiology

Documented cases of human blastomycosis date to 1894, when the disease was first identified in skin lesions.[65] The first natural case of canine blastomycosis[66] was reported in 1912; feline blastomycosis[67] was not reported until 1961. Like the other deep mycoses, blastomycosis is only occasionally reported in cats. A clear predisposition for breed, age, or sex has not been demonstrated in cats.[68] Among both humans and dogs, males are preferentially infected.[68] While some cases may remain undiagnosed owing to a low index of suspicion, it appears that cats are less susceptible to *Blastomyces* infection than dogs. Blastomycosis has been reported in exotic felidae.[69]

Blastomyces dermatitidis, the etiologic agent of blastomycosis, is a dimorphic, saprophytic organism. It converts from the mycelial phase to the yeast phase in tissue. The yeast phase has a characteristic thick-walled appearance.

B. dermatitidis is principally a disease of North America.[68] Areas of endemic infection include the Mississippi, Missouri, Tennessee, and Ohio River basins and the central Atlantic states.[28,68]

As recently as 1985, the ecological niche for *B. dermatitidis* had not been conclusively determined. Although soil was thought to harbor the organism, the majority of attempts to culture it from soil were unsuccessful. In 1986, it was reported that the fungus has been readily isolated from soil samples taken at an environmental camp in Wisconsin.[70] This study was prompted by a large outbreak of infection in a group of visitors to the campsite. Of 95 persons evaluated, 48 were found to be infected. In dogs there is an association between exposure to wooded areas and infection.[71] This variable has not been investigated for cats.

The mode of establishment of infection in dogs is inhalation of airborne mycelial spores into the lower airways; the mechanism is likely the same for cats.

Pathogenesis

The lung is the primary focus of infection. If infection is not controlled or eliminated at this stage, dissemination by blood and lymphatics may occur. Following experimental infection of dogs, clinical signs and radiographic changes are not observed until 12 weeks postinoculation.[72] The incubation period for cats is unknown at present.

Dogs with natural disseminated blastomycosis had demonstrable deficiencies of the cell-mediated immune response; absolute lymphopenia, as well as decreased lymphocyte responsiveness, was observed.[73] Neither immunocompetence nor FeLV status of blastomycotic cats has been surveyed as of this writing. Of interest is the fact that *B. dermatitidis* is not generally regarded as an opportunistic pathogen of immunosuppressed humans.[74]

Clinical Signs

In feline cases reported to date, disseminated infection is frequently described. The related clinical signs are dyspnea, intermittent cough, ocular and CNS problems, fever, depression, anorexia, and weight loss.[28,75,76] Pulmonary signs are most common and usually suggest a progressive, ultimately fatal course of disease.[28] Pleural effusion has been reported in several cases.[75,77,78]

Ocular changes are consistent with inflammatory disease.[76,77] A variety of neurologic disturbances have been reported with feline blastomycotic meningitis.[75–77] Campbell and colleagues reported primary cutaneous blastomycosis in a cat presented for evaluation of a puncture wound to the leg.[79] No apparent response was noted after two antibiotic regimens: the leg continued to swell and developed draining tracts. *B. dermatitidis* organisms were found on histologic examination following limb amputation; systemic disease was not demonstrable in this animal.

Diagnosis

In most cases, blastomycosis may be diagnosed in cytologic preparations of tissue exudate, body fluids, impression smears, or aspirates. Recommended techniques include lung aspiration, bronchial brushing, lymph node aspirate, and examination of any draining tracts. *B. dermatitidis* organisms are usually plentiful and easily identified. The organism is 6 to 20 μm in diameter with a characteristic thick, double wall (Fig. 61–4). The associated inflammatory response is typically pyogranulomatous. A broad-based attachment observed during reproduction is helpful in distinguishing it from *C. neoformans.*

The organism may be identified in histopathologic sections but may not reliably stain with routine hematoxylin and eosin stain. Fungal stains, such as Gridley's, PAS, or Gomori's methenamine silver, are recommended. A minimum data base may not provide the diagnosis, but it should nevertheless be established to assess the overall health of the cat. Serologic testing for FeLV and FIV should be included in the health screen. Radiography may provide suggestive evidence, particularly with pulmonary involvement, and it is a recommended adjunct to the data base. A miliary interstitial pattern in the lung is the most commonly reported radiographic finding.[4]

For the canine patient, agar gel immunodiffusion (AGID) appears to have a high degree of sensitivity and specificity.[68] Reliability of the AGID in feline disease is unknown, but presumably a positive result would support the diagnosis. A positive result of AGID in an infected cat has been reported.[76] A negative result does not rule out blastomycosis. Promising new diagnostic tests, such as the immunoassay for detection of antigen-specific antibodies, are being developed in human medicine and await investigation in veterinary medicine.

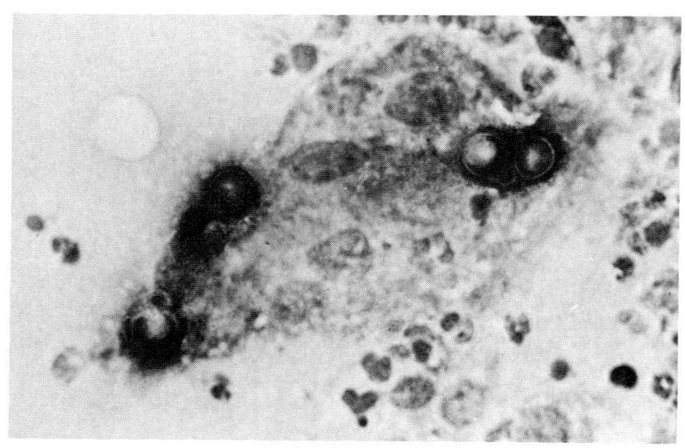

Figure 61–4. Cytologic preparations of tissue exudate, body fluids, impression smears, or aspirates may be used to identify *Blastomyces dermatitidis.* The organisms are usually plentiful and easily identified, being 6 to 20 μm diameter with a characteristic thick double wall. (Courtesy of Dr. R. L. Cowell, Oklahoma State University.)

Treatment

Combination chemotherapy with amphotericin B and KCZ offers the best chance for a successful therapeutic outcome. Renal function withstanding, a cumulative dose of at least 4 mg/kg amphotericin B should be given. Several protocols are available.[4,75] Initially, a small dose (0.1 to 0.25 mg/kg) may be administered IV over 30 minutes; the dose may be increased to 0.5 mg/kg if the BUN does not exceed 40 mg/dL. Treatments are given every other day or three times per week. If azotemia develops, amphotericin B therapy should be abandoned and KCZ initiated promptly. KCZ is recommended at 10 mg/kg every 12 hours for a minimum of 60 days. If cost and toxicity are not limiting factors, treatment with KCZ should extend to 4 to 6 months.

Coccidioidomycosis

Etiology and Epidemiology

The first case of human coccidioidomycosis was described in 1892.[80] Naturally occurring coccidioidomycosis was reported in dogs by Farness in 1940.[81] It is only in the last 25 years that this disease has been described in cats, and only a few such cases are reported to date.[82–85] Some speculate that cats may be inherently more resistant to infection than dogs.[86] Too few cases have been described to establish a predilection for breed, age, or sex in cats.

Coccidioidomycosis is caused by *Coccidioides immitis,* a saprophytic, dimorphic organism that is unique among the pathogenic fungi because it does not reproduce by budding.[87] The mycelium is filamentous with septate hyphae that divide the rectangular-shaped arthrospores into compartments. The arthrospores are easily detached and may be carried long distances by wind or as fomites.

Of all the deep mycotic agents, *C. immitis* has the most limited geographic distribution. It has been described in Central and South America as well as Mexico, but the arid southwestern United States is best known as an endemic area of infection. This area, geographically described as the lower Sonoran life zone, provides an ideal climate for persistence of the organism: high environmental temperatures during summer months, moderately wet winters, and sandy, alkaline soils.[28]

Pathogenesis

Inhalation of airborne arthrospores establishes an initial focus of infection in the lungs. Although this has not been described specifically for cats, it is well documented for humans and canines. The arthrospores penetrate into deeper pulmonary tissue and develop into gradually enlarging spherules. The nuclei in the spherules divide, forming endospores, which may then be released into the lymphatics. These endospores develop into new spherules, and the process is repeated.[86] Dissemination likely occurs through hematogenous and lymphatic routes.[86]

The life cycle of the fungus facilitates the process of respiratory infection. During periods of scant rainfall, the organism survives easily in dry soil. When a significant amount of rain does occur, the fungus multiplies in the mycelial form, releasing arthrospores to be carried by wind and on wild animals as fomites.[28] As noted for the other fungal infections, competence of the cell-mediated immune response dictates the course of infection. The animal may remain relatively asymptomatic or develop fulminant, ultimately fatal, disease. There is no evidence to date that associates FeLV or FIV infection with feline coccidioidomycosis.[88]

Clinical Signs

Both primary (localized) and disseminated coccidioidomycosis have been described in cats. Nonspecific clinical signs of anorexia and attendant weight loss are common in reported cases. Observed clinical and radiographic signs in the cases reported to date include chronic draining tracts, uveitis, dyspnea with pyogranulomatous pneumonia, and hilar lymphadenopathy and lameness.[82–85]

Diagnosis

Potentially valuable diagnostic techniques for identifying *C. immitis* include cytologic and histopathologic examination and fungal culture. Cytologic specimens may be obtained by fine-needle aspiration of lung parenchyma and lymph nodes, impression smears from draining tracts, transtracheal wash, and bronchial brushing. The organism may be seen in unstained preparations with reduced lighting. Ten percent potassium hydroxide may be used to clear these unstained slides.[83] *C. immitis* typically does not exfoliate in large numbers, so a diligent search may be required to locate the organism. It is large (approximately 50 to 100 μm diameter) and associated with a granulomatous inflammatory response (Fig. 61–5). Papanicolaou and PAS stains are recommended for cytologic preparations.[89] Best staining effects for tissue specimens are achieved with Grocott-Gomori's methenamine silver and PAS.

Serologic testing has not proven to be a reliable adjunct to the diagnostic plan. Complement fixation has been routinely negative, but one cat had a positive precipitin test.[83]

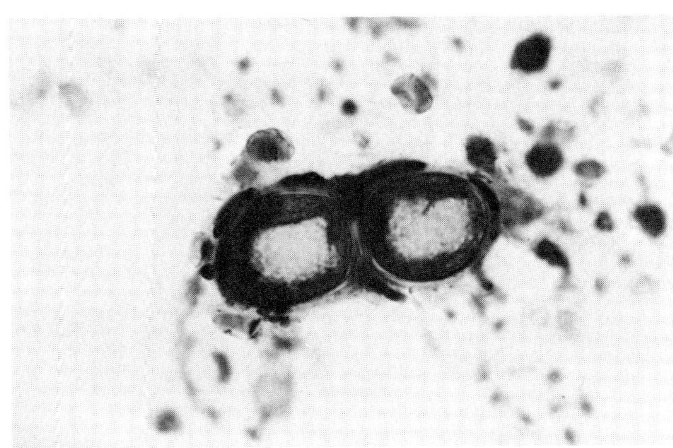

Figure 61–5. ***Coccidioides immitis*** **does not typically exfoliate in large numbers; therefore, a diligent search may be required to locate the organism. It is large, approximately 50 to 100 μm in diameter, and associated with a granulomatous inflammatory response. (Courtesy of Dr. R. L. Cowell, Oklahoma State University.)**

Treatment

Treatment of coccidioidomycosis in cats has not been specifically addressed in the literature. Amphotericin B is not particularly efficacious against *C. immitis.*[80] KCZ has demonstrated better activity against *C. immitis* in vitro and is probably the preferred drug for treatment.[86,89] It has been curative in a few cases.[89] A dose of 10 mg/kg once or twice daily is recommended.[4] Long-term therapy—at least 6 months—is desirable. Enucleation was curative in one case of disease localized to the eye.[85]

Antifungal Therapy

Amphotericin B

Amphotericin B is a polyene antibiotic that binds to ergosterol, the principal sterol compound in fungal cell membranes. This process results in altered membrane permeability and, ultimately, cell death. It has a wide spectrum of antifungal activity and, in decreasing order of susceptibility, demonstrates activity against *Blastomyces, Histoplasma, Cryptococcus,* and *Coccidioides* organisms.[90]

The necessity for intravenous administration and the toxicity of the drug are the major disadvantages. The nephrotoxicity of amphotericin B is the factor that most frequently limits duration of use. Arteriolar vasoconstriction leads to a decrease in glomerular filtration rate and altered tubule function.[91] The BUN should be monitored closely and therapy discontinued if azotemia develops. If extravasated, amphotericin B may cause severe perivascular irritation. The most common local side effect is thrombophlebitis.[92] In humans, it has been shown that rapid infusion and removal of the catheter after infusion reduce thrombophlebitis.

The 50-mg vial of amphotericin B may be reconstituted with sterile water and then divided into aliquots, which may be frozen for later use. Five percent dextrose in water is the only fluid recommended for use when administering the drug; lactated Ringer's solution and isotonic saline may cause precipitation of amphotericin B in solution. A general protocol for amphotericin B therapy in cats is 0.1 to 0.5 mg/kg every other day to a cumulative dose of 4 mg/kg. We prefer to begin with 0.1 mg/kg. If the BUN does not exceed 40 mg/dL, this dose is increased by 0.1 mg/kg at each dosing up to the maximum of 0.5 mg/kg per treatment. The drug is diluted in 50 mL of 5% dextrose and administered as a slow drip over 30 to 60 minutes. The BUN is evaluated prior to each treatment. Amphotericin B therapy is discontinued when the BUN exceeds 40 mg/dL, and fluid diuresis is then initiated. Amphotericin B therapy is reinstituted when the BUN falls below 30 mg/dL.

5-Fluorocytosine

We do not recommend 5-FC for treating fungal infections in cats, but some have used it successfully and may advocate its incorporation into the treatment protocol. An oral antifungal agent, 5-FC is converted to 5-fluorouracil (5-FU) within fungal cells; this antimetabolite interrupts DNA synthesis.[36] It has several advantages over amphotericin B: oral administration and rapid uptake from the gastrointestinal tract, CSF level comparable to 60% to 75% of serum level, and no nephrotoxicity.[11] It is more costly, however, and is frequently associated with rapid development of resistance by fungal organisms. Also, while some consider it less toxic than amphotericin B, it has its own spectrum of potential side effects, each of which must be considered with regard to the individual patient when considering a potential therapeutic protocol. Some of the side effects include bone marrow suppression leading to thrombocytopenia and leukopenia, vomiting and diarrhea, enterocolitis, and cutaneous lesions. Rapid, inexpensive, and simple enzymatic methods are available to determine serum levels of 5-FC.[93] Therapy should be discontinued or the dose decreased with impaired or diminishing renal function.

Clinical trials in humans have shown a synergistic effect between amphotericin B and 5-FC.[94] In combination with KCZ, 5-FC has significant toxicity for cats.[42]

Imidazole Derivatives

KCZ, the better-known imidazole compound, produces changes in fungal membrane permeability by interfering with synthesis of ergosterol, a component of the fungal cell membrane. It is considered fungistatic in therapeutic doses but in larger doses may be fungicidal.[95] KCZ demonstrates activity against *Histoplasma, Coccidioides,* and *Blastomyces* organisms but less activity against *Cryptococcus.* However, most cats tolerate KCZ so well that we utilize it to treat cryptococcosis. KCZ is administered orally and is well absorbed from the gastrointestinal tract, particularly when taken with food. Distribution to peripheral tissues achieves therapeutic levels in all but the CNS, eyes, and testes. The minimal side effects reported include anorexia, vomiting, diarrhea, elevated liver enzyme values, and icterus.[3] The increase in liver enzymes may have no clinical significance, but the chemistry profile should always be interpreted in conjunction with each individual patient's status. A study by Willard and coworkers detected no significant clinicopathologic changes in cats given 30 mg/kg daily for 30 days, a higher dose than is routinely used for antifungal therapy.[96] An extremely high dose of 72 mg/kg/day was tolerated longer than 6 months by one cat with cutaneous cryptococcosis.[34]

Because it is a fungistatic drug, a prolonged course of treatment is generally needed and, when used in concert with amphotericin B, it should be sequential to rather than concurrent with the fungicidal drug. Most cats tolerate a dose of 5 to 10 mg/kg every 12 hours. Relapses are not uncommon following discontinuation of KCZ, and, in most cases, it should be given a minimum of 4 to 6 months.

Itraconazole, a newer imidazole derivative, likely will gain wider clinical use in the future. It may be given orally or parenterally and may have less impact than KCZ on host steroid hormone production.[97] It is more potent than KCZ against *Blastomyces* and *Cryptococcus* organisms.[97] Its toxicity appears to be minimal compared to KCZ and amphotericin B.

Public Health Implications

Cryptococcosis is not considered contagious because the organism does not aerosolize from culture media or tissue infection.[3,4] However, direct inoculation of the yeast from nasal exudate or skin lesions into an open wound is a potential means of transmission. Consequently, care should be taken to avoid contact with exudative material.[11]

Histoplasmosis, blastomycosis, and coccidioidomycosis are also considered noncontagious infections, except perhaps by direct inoculation of the yeast phase into an open wound. Inoculation infection with blastomycosis was reported in a veterinarian who sustained a cut while performing a necropsy on an infected dog and in a veterinary technician who was bitten.[98,99] None of these three organisms should be cultured except by laboratories equipped with a biohazard safety hood, since the mycelial phase of each may aerosolize infectious particles. When a systemic fungal infection is identified in a cat, a concern for human health exists because of the shared potential source of environmental exposure. Immunosuppressed humans should be considered at risk.

REFERENCES

1. Curtis AJ. A case of torulosis in a domestic cat. Aust J Med Tech 1951;1:71.
2. Seibold HR, Roberts CS, Jordan EM. Cryptococcosis in a dog. J Am Vet Med Assoc 1953;122:213.
3. Medleau L, Barsanti JA. Cryptococcosis. In: Greene CE, ed. Infectious Diseases of the Dog and Cat. 2nd ed. Philadelphia: WB Saunders Co, 1990:687.
4. Legendre AM. Systemic Mycotic Infections. In: Sherding RG, ed. The Cat: Diseases and Clinical Management. New York: Churchill Livingstone, 1989:427.
5. Wolf AM, Troy GC. Deep Mycotic Diseases. In: Ettinger SJ, ed. Textbook of Veterinary Internal Medicine. 3rd ed. Philadelphia: WB Saunders Co, 1989:341.
6. Medoff G. Pulmonary Cryptococcosis. In: Braude AI, Davis CE, Fierer J, eds. Medical Microbiology and Infectious Diseases. Philadelphia: WB Saunders Co, 1986:855.
7. Beehler BA. Oral therapy for nasal cryptococcosis in a cheetah. J Am Vet Med Assoc 1982;181:1400.
8. Davis CE. Cryptococcus. In: Braude AI, Davis CE, Fierer J, eds. Medical Microbiology and Infectious Diseases. Philadelphia: WB Saunders Co, 1986:564.
9. Kwon-Chung KJ. A new genus, *Filobasidiella,* the perfect state of *C. neoformans.* Mycologia 1975;67:1197.
10. Drutz DJ. The Mycoses. In: Wyngaarden JB, Smith LH, eds. Cecil Textbook of Medicine. 18th ed. Philadelphia: WB Saunders Co, 1988:1837.
11. Wilkinson GT. Feline cryptococcosis: A review and seven case reports. J Small Anim Pract 1979;20:749.
12. Ishaq CM, Bulmer GS, Felton FG. An evaluation of various environmental factors affecting the propagation of *Cryptococcus neoformans.* Mycopathol Mycol Appl Toxicol 1968;35:81.
13. Medleau L. Feline Cryptococcosis. In: Kirk RW, ed. Current Veterinary Therapy X. Philadelphia: WB Saunders Co, 1989:1109.
14. Dykstra MA, Friedman L, Murphy JW. Capsule size of *Cryptococcus neoformans:* Control and relationship to virulence. Infect Immun 1977;16:129.
15. Powell KE, Bernhoff A, Dahl A, Weeks RJ, Tosh FE. Airborne *Cryptococcus neoformans:* Particles from pigeon excreta compatible with alveolar deposition. J Infect Dis 1972;125:412.
16. Cohen J. The pathogenesis of cryptococcosis. J Infection 1982;5:109.
17. Tumquest RU. Experimental Feline Cryptococcosis. Master's thesis. Ithaca, NY: Cornell University, 1968.
18. Medleau L, Hall EJ, Goldschmidt MH, Irby N. Cutaneous cryptococcosis in three cats. J Am Vet Med Assoc 1985;187:169.
19. Pal M, Mehrotra BS. Occurrence and etiologic significance of *Cryptococcus neoformans* in a cutaneous lesion of a cat. Mykosen 1983;26:608.
20. Graybill JR, Drutz DJ. Host defense in cryptococcosis. II. Cryptococcosis in the nude mouse. Cell Immunol 1978;40:263.
21. Monga DP, Kumar R, Mohapatra LN, Malaviya AN. Experimental cryptococcosis in normal and B cell–deficient mice. Infect Immun 1979;26:1.
22. Schimpf SC, Bennett JE. Abnormalities in cell-mediated immunity in patients with *Cryptococcus neoformans* infection. J Allerg Clin Immunol 1975;55:430.
23. Chuck SL, Sande MA. Infections with *Cryptococcus neoformans* in the acquired immunodeficiency syndrome. N Engl J Med 1989;321:794.
24. Bulmer GS, Sans MD. *Cryptococcus neoformans.* III. Inhibition of phagocytosis. J Bacteriol 1968;95:5.
25. Diamond RD, Erickson NF III: Chemotaxis of human neutrophils and monocytes induced by *Cryptococcus neoformans.* Infect Immun 1982;38:380.
26. Rippon JW. Cryptococcosis. In: Medical Mycology. 3rd ed. Philadelphia: WB Saunders Co, 1988:582.
27. Holzworth J, Blouin P, Conner MW. Mycotic Diseases. In: Holdzworth J, ed. Diseases of the Cat. Philadelphia: WB Saunders Co, 1987:320.
28. Roudebush P. Mycotic pneumonias. Vet Clin North Am, Small Anim Pract 1985:15:949.
29. Pedersen NC. Cryptococcosis. In: Feline Infectious Diseases. Goleta, CA: American Veterinary Publications, 1988:255.
30. Rosenthal JJ, Heidgerd J, Peiffer RL. Ocular and systemic cryptococcosis in a cat. J Am Anim Hosp Assoc 1981;17:307.
31. Blouin P. Experimental Feline Cryptococcosis: Characteristics and Pathogenesis of Ocular Lesions. PhD thesis. Davis, CA: University of California, 1979.
32. Ackerman L. Feline cryptococcosis. Compend Contin Educ 1988;10:1049.
33. Pentlarge VW, Martin RA. Treatment of cryptococcosis in three cats using ketoconazole. J Am Vet Med Assoc 1986;188:536.
34. Hansen BL. Successful treatment of severe feline cryptococcosis with long-term high doses of ketoconazole. J Am Anim Hosp Assoc 1987;23:193.
35. Medleau L, Marks MA, Brown J, Borges WL. Clinical evaluation of a cryptococcoal antigen latex agglutination test for diagnosis of cryptococcosis in cats. J Am Vet Med Assoc 1990;196:1470.
36. Noxon JO, Monroe WE, Chinn DR. Ketoconazole therapy in canine and feline cryptococcosis. J Am Anim Hosp Assoc 1986;22:179.
37. Mikiciuk MG, Fales WH, Schmidt DA. Successful treatment of feline cryptococcosis with ketoconazole and flucytosine. J Am Anim Hosp Assoc 1990;26:199.
38. Ribas JL, Braund KG. Fungal infections of the CNS in dogs and cats. Am Coll Vet Int Med Proceedings 1987;5.19–5.25.
39. Palumbo NE, Perri S. Amphotericin therapy in two cases of feline cryptococcosis. Vet Med/Small Anim Clin 1975;70:553.
40. Barrett R, Scott D. Treatment of feline cryptococcosis: Literature review and case report. J Am Anim Hosp Assoc 1975;11:511.
41. Graybill JR, Williams DM, VanCutsem E, et al. Combination therapy of experimental histoplasmosis and cryptococcosis with amphotericin B and ketoconazole. Rev Infect Dis 1980;2:551.
42. Fukay BP, Dion WM. Feline phaeohyphomycosis: Treatment with ketoconazole and 5-fluorocytosine. Can Vet J 1984;24:130.
43. Darling ST. A protozoon general infection producing pseudotubercles in the lungs and focal necrosis in the liver, spleen, and lymph nodes. J Am Med Assoc 1906;46:1283.
44. De Monbreun WA. The dog as a natural host for *Histoplasma capsulatum.* Am J Trop Med 1939;19:565.

45. Emmons CW. Histoplasmosis in animals. Trans NY Acad Sci, Ser. II, 1949;2:248.
46. Legendre AL. Systemic mycotic infections of dogs and cats. In: Scott FW, ed. Infectious Diseases. New York: Churchill Livingstone, 1986:29.
47. Clinkenbeard KD, Wolf AM, Cowell RL, Tyler RD. Feline disseminated histoplasmosis. Compend Contin Educ 1989;11:1223.
48. Clinkenbeard KD, Cowell RL, Tyler RD. Disseminated histoplasmosis in cats: 12 cases (1981–1986). J Am Vet Med Assoc 1987;190:1445.
49. Wolf AM. Histoplasmosis. In: Greene CE, ed. Infectious Diseases of the Dog and Cat. 2nd ed. Philadelphia: WB Saunders Co, 1990:679.
50. Stark DR. Primary gastrointestinal histoplasmosis in a cat. J Am Anim Hosp Assoc 1982;18:154.
51. Blass CE. Histoplasmosis in a cat. J Am Anim Hosp Assoc 1982; 18:468.
52. Wolf AM, Belden MN. Feline histoplasmosis: A literature review and retrospective study of 20 new cases. J Am Anim Hosp Assoc 1984;20:995.
53. Wolf AM. *Histoplasma capsulatum* osteomyelitis in the cat. J Vet Intern Med 1987;1:158.
54. Wolf AM. Successful treatment of disseminated histoplasmosis with osseous involvement in two cats. J Am Anim Hosp Assoc 1988;24:511.
55. Larsh HW, Hall K. *Histoplasma capsulatum*. In: Braude AI, ed. Microbiology and Infectious Diseases. Philadelphia: WB Saunders Co, 1981:654.
56. Farrell RL, Cole CR. Experimental canine histoplasmosis with acute fatal and chronic recovered courses. Am J Pathol 1968; 53:425.
57. Sherding RG. Systemic mycoses. Proceedings Am Anim Hosp Assoc, San Francisco, CA, 1989;363.
58. Kauffman CA, Israel KS, Smith JW et al. Histoplasmosis in immunosuppressed patients. Am J Med 1978;64:923.
59. Cole CR. Experimentally induced histoplasmosis in a dog. J Am Vet Med Assoc 1955;127:526.
60. Barsanti JA. Histoplasmosis. In: Greene CE, ed. Clinical Microbiology and Infectious Diseases of the Dog and Cat. Philadelphia: WB Saunders Co, 1984;687.
61. Breitschwerdt EB, Halliwell WH, Burk RL, Schmidt DA. Feline histoplasmosis. J Am Anim Hosp Assoc 1977;13:216.
62. Mahaffey E, Gabbert N, Johnson D, Guffy M. Disseminated histoplasmosis in three cats. J Am Anim Hosp Assoc 1977;13:46.
63. Wolf AM, Green RW. The radiographic appearance of pulmonary histoplasmosis in the cat. Vet Radiol 1987;28:34.
64. Noxon JO, Digilio K, Schmidt DA. Disseminated histoplasmosis in a cat: Successful treatment with ketoconazole. J Am Vet Med Assoc 1982;181:817.
65. Gilchrist TC, Stokes WR. A case of pseudo–lupus vulgaris caused by a *Blastomyces*. J Exp Med 1988;3:53.
66. Saunders LZ. Systemic fungus infections in animals: A review. Cornell Vet 1948;38:213.
67. Easton KL. Cutaneous North American blastomycosis in a Siamese cat. Can Vet J 1961;2:350.
68. Legendre AM. Blastomycosis. In: Greene CE, ed. Infectious Diseases of the Dog and Cat. 2nd ed. Philadelphia: WB Saunders Co, 1990:669.
69. Stroud RK, Coles BM. Blastomycosis in an African lion. J Am Vet Med Assoc 1980;177:842.
70. Klein BS, Vergeront JM, Weeks RJ, et al. Isolation of *Blastomyces dermatitidis* in soil associated with a large outbreak of blastomycosis in Wisconsin. N Engl J Med 1986;314:529.
71. Sarosi GA, Davies SF. Blastomycosis. Am Rev Respir Dis 1979;120:911.
72. Smith CD, Furcolow ML, Hulker PW. Effect of immunosuppressants on dogs exposed two and one-half years previously to *Blastomyces dermatitidis*. Am J Epidemiol 1976;104:299.
73. Legendre AM, Becker RU. Immunologic changes in acute canine blastomycosis. Am J Vet Res 1982;43:2050.
74. Dismukes WE. Blastomycosis: Leave it to beaver. N Engl J Med 1986;314:575.
75. Breider MA, Walker TL, Legendre AM, VanEe RT. Blastomycosis in cats: Five cases. J Am Vet Med Assoc 1988;193:570.
76. Miller PE, Miller LM, Schoster JV. Feline blastomycosis: A report of three cases and literature review (1961 to 1988). J Am Anim Hosp Assoc 1990;26:417.
77. Hatkin JM, Phillips WE, Utroska WR. Two cases of feline blastomycosis. J Am Anim Hosp Assoc 1979;15:217.
78. Nasisse MP, VanEe RT, Wright B. Ocular changes in a cat with disseminated blastomycosis. J Am Vet Med Assoc 1985;187: 629.
79. Campbell KL, Humphrey JA, Ramsey GH. Cutaneous blastomycosis. Feline Pract 1980;10:28.
80. Barsanti JA, Jeffery JL. Coccidioidomycosis. In: Greene CE, ed. Clinical Microbiology and Infectious Diseases of the Dog and Cat. Philadelphia: WB Saunders Co, 1984:710.
81. Famess OJ. Coccidioidal infection in a dog. J Am Vet Med Assoc 1940;97:263.
82. Reed RE, Hoge RS, Trautman RJ. Coccidioidomycosis in two cats. J Am Vet Med Assoc 1963;143:953.
83. Wolf AM. Primary cutaneous coccidioidomycosis in a dog and a cat. J Am Vet Med Assoc 1979;174:504.
84. Schwavz W. *Coccidioides immitis* infection in a cat. Southwest Vet 1981;24:94.
85. Angell JA, Shively JN, Merideth RE, et al. Ocular coccidioidomycosis in a cat. J Am Vet Med Assoc 1985;187:167.
86. Macy DW. Coccidioidomycosis. In: Kirk RW, ed. Current Veterinary Therapy IX. Philadelphia: WB Saunders Co, 1986:1076.
87. Kaplan W. Epidemiology of the principal systemic mycoses of man and lower animals and the ecology of their etiologic agents. J Am Vet Med Assoc 1973;163:1043.
88. Pedersen NC. Coccidioidomycosis. In: Feline Infectious Diseases. Goleta, CA: American Veterinary Publications, 1988:243.
89. Barsanti JA, Jeffery JL. Coccidioidomycosis. In: Greene CE, ed. Clinical Microbiology and Infectious Diseases of the Dog and Cat. 2nd ed. Philadelphia: WB Saunders Co, 1990:696.
90. Greene CE, O'Neal KG, Barsanti JA. Antimicrobial Therapy. In: Greene CE. Clinical Microbiology and Infectious Diseases of the Dog and Cat. Philadelphia: WB Saunders Co, 1984:172.
91. Rubin SI. Nephrotoxicity of Amphotericin B. In: Kirk RW, ed. Current Veterinary Therapy IX. Philadelphia: WB Saunders Co, 1986:1142.
92. Sarosi GA. Amphotericin B: Still the "gold standard" for antifungal therapy. Postgrad Med 1990;88:151.
93. Washbum RG, Klym DM, Kroll MH, Bennett JE. Rapid enzymatic method for measurement of serum flucytosine levels. J Antimicrob Chemother 1986;17:673.
94. Bennett JE. Flucytosine. Ann Intern Med 1977;86:319.
95. Dismukes WE, Stamm AM, Graybill JR, et al. Treatment of systemic mycoses with ketoconazole: Emphasis on toxicity and clinical responses in 52 patients. Ann Intern Med 1983;98:13.
96. Willard MD, Nachrciner RF, Howard VC, Fooshee SK. Effect of long-term administration of ketoconazole in cats. Am J Vet Res 1986;47:2510.
97. Willard MD. Treatment of Fungal and Endocrine Disorders with Imidazole Derivatives. In: Kirk RW, ed. Current Veterinary Therapy X. Philadelphia: WB Saunders Co, 1989:82.
98. Graham WR, Callaway JL. Primary inoculation of blastomycosis in a veterinarian. Am Acad Dermatol 1982;7:785.
99. Gnann JW, Bressler GS, Bodet A, Avent CK. Human blastomycosis after a dog bite. Ann Intern Med 1983;98:48.

CHAPTER 62

◇ ◇ ◇

Toxicoses and Toxins

Richard M. Groff, Joan M. Miller, Eric L. Stair, Jeffery O. Hall, Michael W. Knight, and William B. Buck

Initial Treatment

In most feline practices poisonings account for only a small percentage of the case load. Because of the critical nature of these cases, however, practitioners must have a basic understanding of how to treat poisoning emergencies.

Client Communication

Most toxicoses are first brought to the veterinarian's attention when a client who believes that the cat has been poisoned calls for professional advice. Frequently, the client's diagnosis is erroneous. If the client does seem to be describing a poisoning, a brief history should be obtained over the phone. The cat's age and weight are important, as is its physical condition prior to the suspected poisoning. Medications the cat takes are also relevant. The practitioner should identify the type of suspected toxin and the amount and concentration; the route and duration of exposure are vital. If reasonable potential for toxicosis exists the client should be instructed to bring the cat to the hospital immediately. The client should be encouraged to bring along packaging or product information on the suspected toxic substance if possible. Samples of the toxicant and vomitus also are helpful if the substance is not known for certain.

In most cases home treatment should not be recommended, as handling the patient could expose the owner to the toxin. Most important, in a true emergency valuable time may be lost while the client attempts a home remedy that will likely be ineffective. There are a few notable exceptions: If a topically exposed cat is asymptomatic, first-aid decontamination may prevent significant dermal absorption and ingestion by licking. If a cat has been exposed to a *powder* and is asymptomatic, the owner should be advised to wear gloves and to thoroughly vacuum the cat. (If the cat will not tolerate vacuuming, brushing is advised.) Once the powder has been removed by vacuuming or brushing, the cat should be rinsed with a mild detergent and warm water. If a *liquid* toxicant has been applied topically, the client should wear rubber gloves while rinsing the cat thoroughly.

If the cat has convulsions a large box, cat carrier, or blanket can be used as a makeshift stretcher. The client should be warned about the possibility of being bitten. Patients in status epilepticus should be lightly rinsed with warm water to prevent or ameliorate secondary hyperthermia and then should be transported to the hospital without further delay.

Professional Consultation

While the client is transporting the cat to the hospital, a member of the hospital staff should contact a veterinary poison control center that offers the services of a board-certified veterinary toxicologist. (Consultation with human poison control centers is discouraged because of species differences.) The National Animal Poison Control Center (NAPCC) is an excellent source of reliable information,* and many veterinary diagnostic laboratories also have competent professional personnel for consultation. The ubiquity of toxins in our world today and the extreme diversity of the chemicals in these poisons make consultation with a veterinary toxicologist very desirable. According to a leading veterinary attorney,[1] although the precedent has not yet been set, neglecting to consult with a toxicology specialist could be grounds for a malpractice suit in the event of therapeutic failure.

Determining Exposure Potential

Because many cats are exposed to toxic materials at subtoxic levels, determining this is an essential preliminary step before decontamination and antidote therapy. Some guidelines are relevant to the use of median lethal dose (LD_{50}) values: ten percent of an LD_{50} is considered a dose that could potentially cause actual clinical signs. Although references are made in this chapter to LD_{50}s, the clinician needs to be cautious in using this guide because LD_{50}s often are determined in laboratory animals, and there are species differences.

*National Animal Poison Control Center, College of Veterinary Medicine, University of Illinois: 1–800–548–2423 ($30 per case) or 1–900–680–0000 ($2.95 per minute).

Table 62–1. Calculation of Potential Toxic Exposure

Given situation:
1.5-ounce box of 0.005% brodifacoum and 10-lb, 3-year-old, neutered male cat. Owner thinks cat ingested 1 tablespoon.

Given factors:
1 tablespoon of toxin = 15 g*
LD_{50} of brodifacoum is 12 mg/lb

$$\text{Exposure (in mg)} = \text{Amount of toxin in grams} \times \text{Concentration of toxin}$$
$$= 15\text{ g} \times 0.00005$$
$$= 0.00075\text{ g}$$
$$= 0.75\text{ mg}$$

$$\text{Exposure (in mg/lb body weight)} = \frac{\text{exposure in mg}}{\text{weight of cat in lb}}$$
$$= 0.75\text{ mg/10 lb}$$
$$= 0.075\text{ mg/lb}$$

$$\text{Comparison to } LD_{50} = \frac{\text{exposure in mg/lb}}{LD_{50}}$$
$$= \frac{0.075\text{ mg/lb}}{12\text{ mg/lb}}$$
$$= 0.6\%$$

Since this amount is less than 10% of the LD_{50}, exposure would be considered minimal and treatment would not be required. If, however, the cat had a preexisting disease or was taking medication that might potentiate the toxin, decontamination should be considered.

*This factor is accepted by convention for all toxins.

Calculating exposure potential requires that the clinician determine the exposure in milligrams per pound; however, most clients express a pet's intake in tablespoons. By convention, 1 tablespoon of toxin equals 15 gm. (Table 62–1).

Emergency Stabilization

Treatment of intoxicated patients is prioritized once they have arrived at the hospital and it is determined that toxicosis exists. As in any emergency, the first consideration is treatment of life-threatening problems (Table 62–2).

The patient's *ventilation* should be assessed, and both tidal volume and respiratory rate closely monitored. Anesthesia or heavy sedation may be necessary if the patient exhibits seizures, tetany, or hypopnea. Respiration can often be normalized more quickly and effectively with intubation and manual or mechanical assistance. Blood gas analysis should be considered.

Oxygen supplementation should be implemented for cats that are hypotensive, hypoxemic, cyanotic, or hemoconcentrated. To patients that do not require intubation oxygen can be administered by cage, mask, or, most easily and effectively, by nasal catheter.[2]

Oxygen should be considered for any case of pulmonary exposure to dust, powder, liquid, or gas, but most importantly when the potential for carbon monoxide toxicosis exists, as oxygen is the specific antidote for this toxicant.

Cardiovascular support frequently is required, as many intoxicated cats become "shocky" because of either hypotension or hemoconcentration. Intravenous (IV) infusion of a balanced crystalloid solution is instituted, lactated Ringer's solution (LRS) being the fluid of choice until serum electrolytes, acid-base status, and chemistries have been evaluated.

If the heart rate or rhythm is abnormal an electrocardiogram (ECG) should be obtained and appropriate antiarrhythmic therapy instituted. If the practitioner has the capability to measure the patient's blood pressure, either directly or indirectly, this parameter should be closely monitored.

Cats may exhibit various symptoms related to *overstimulation of the central nervous system* (CNS), including seizures, muscle fasciculations, aggression, and increased response to external stimuli. Controlling these symptoms is essential. In all but the most severe cases, diazepam (Valium) should be administered. Diazepam is given intravenously in 0.5- to 1.25-mg increments to effect; occasionally a total dose of 20 mg is required.[3] If this dose of diazepam is ineffectual, heavy sedation or complete anesthesia can be introduced with a barbiturate. Phenobarbital, given IV up to 3 mg/lb, slowly to effect, provides sedation of extended duration and should be utilized for patients that do not respond to diazepam or when frequent administration of diazepam is required. Short-acting barbiturates such as thiamylal sodium are effective if prolonged anesthesia is not anticipated or if the patient is to be maintained on a gas anesthetic. If prolonged heavy sedation or anesthesia is necessary, pentobarbital (2 to 7 mg/lb IV slowly to effect) is the drug of choice.

For muscle fasciculations or tetany methocarbamol (Robaxin) can be an effective myasthenic agent when given IV, 20 to 100 mg/lb.

Table 62–2. Emergency Stabilization

Respiratory Support

Intubation and mechanical assistance
Oxygen supplementation
  Intubation
  Cage, mask, or nasal catheter

Cardiovascular Support

Shock
  LRS IV initially
  Secondary fluid choice based on serum electrolytes, acid-base status, and chemistries
ECG status
Blood pressure monitoring

CNS Support

Overstimulation (seizures, muscle fasciculations, aggressiveness, etc.)
  Diazepam: 0.5 to 1.25-mg increments IV to effect *or*
  Phenobarbital: up to 3 mg/lb IV, slowly to effect *or*
  Pentobarbital: 2–7 mg/lb IV, slowly to effect
    and
  Methocarbamol: 20–100 mg/lb IV

Hyperthermia

Control seizures or other forms of CNS stimulation
IV fluids plus tepid-water bath
Gastric lavage and enema with lukewarm water

The potential for phenothiazine tranquilizers to lower the seizure threshold in some patients is well-established. In certain instances of CNS overstimulation, however, particularly overdosing with amphetamines or exposure to a hallucinogen, phenothiazines can be very efficacious sedatives.

Convulsing cats often have some degree of hyperthermia. Caution should be used in controlling the temperature of these patients. Initial alleviation of the primary neurologic symptoms may be enough to reverse moderate hyperthermia. Cats with profound hyperthermia should have the initial symptoms treated and fluid therapy instituted while they are rinsed with tepid water. Gastric lavage and enema also can be performed using lukewarm water. This conservative approach is usually effective in controlling the temperature without inducing rebound hypothermia. Immersion in an ice bath or very cold water is contraindicated because it may cause cutaneous vasoconstriction. Because heat dissipation is a major function of the skin, decreasing circulation may prolong core hyperthermia, which is especially important as many of these patients are intubated and, therefore, unable to pant.

For severe CNS depression due to ingestion of sedatives, narcotics, anticonvulsants, or other toxins, CNS stimulants such as amphetamine, caffeine, or nikethimide are contraindicated. Evidence has shown that these drugs do not increase the survival rate, and many have a tendency to induce arrhythmias and seizures.[4] These cats should be detoxified and treated with respiratory and cardiovascular support and appropriate antidotes.

Diagnostic Evaluation

Once the cat is stabilized the history should be reviewed thoroughly. The poison, its strength, the duration of exposure, and the symptoms noted prior to admission should be noted, as well as the cat's health immediately prior to exposure. This point is well-illustrated by acetaminophen or ibuprofen toxicosis. The obvious abnormality in these patients at the time of examination is their toxicosis, but in most instances the medications were *administered* because the patient was ill. An extensive physical examination is in order once the cat is stable. Blood and urine should be obtained for a complete blood count (CBC), serum chemistry evaluation, and urinalysis. While waiting for these tests to be completed, a data base of blood urea nitrogen (BUN), blood glucose, hematocrit value, and total serum solids should be assembled. If the poison is an anticoagulant rodenticide or if there is evidence of coagulopathy or disseminated intravascular coagulation, a clotting profile and fibrin degradation product quantitation should be obtained.

Pulmonary exposure necessitates radiographic evaluation of the thorax. When the history indicates possible heavy metal exposure, abdominal radiographs should be included, although absence of radiopaque foreign material does not rule out this diagnosis.

If ethylene glycol ingestion is suspected, a serum ethylene glycol test should be performed (see below). If serum ethylene glycol testing is unavailable, the serum osmolality should be evaluated. A significant osmolal gap is very suggestive, if not diagnostic, of this poisoning.[5]

Decontamination Procedures

As the patient is being stabilized and completely evaluated, ongoing efforts are made to limit further absorption of the poison. This process, *decontamination,* includes gastric evacuation to remove toxin from the gastrointestinal tract and cathartics to expel toxin (Table 62–3).

Cats suspected of having ingested a poison are subjected to gastric evacuation if exposure occurred within 4 hours of admission for treatment. If the toxin is one that delays gastric emptying (e.g., anticholinergic agents) or

Table 62–3. Decontamination Procedures

Gastrointestinal Emptying

Emesis: NOTE: A cat that has not eaten in the last 2 hours should be fed a small meal before emesis is induced.
- Xylazine: 0.5 mg/lb IM or SC. Causes CNS and respiratory depression in some cats. May be reversed with yohimbine (0.02 mg/lb IV)
- Hydrogen peroxide (3%): 1.0 ml/lb; if emesis does not occur repeat once after 10 to 20 minutes.
- Syrup of ipecac: 1.5 mL/lb PO: dilute 1:1 with water and give by orogastric or nasogastric tube. *Do not use* Extract *of Ipecac.*

Gastric lavage
- Place large bore stomach tube (40 Fr OD) under sedation
- Flush with water several times
- Begin at 2 mL/lb; increase to 5 mL/lb

Absorbent therapy (follows gastrointestinal emptying)

Activated charcoal: 1–2 g/lb in a slurry of water (must be accompanied by cathartic unless included)
Repeat in 6 to 8 hours for toxins that return to the intestinal tract via enterohepatic recirculation.
Do not use if cat is constipated.
Products available:
- Toxiban suspension, 104 mg/mL; must add cathartic
- Actidose with Sorbitol, 208 mg/mL; cathartic included

Cathartics

To decrease bowel transit time. Cat must be well-hydrated and not have diarrhea. Cathartic should be used following activated charcoal that does not contain a cathartic.
- Magnesium sulfate (Epsom salts): ¼ level teaspoon/9 lb body weight
- Sodium sulfate (Glauber's salts): ¼ level teaspoon/9 lb body weight
- Sorbitol 70% (3 mL/kg)—an osmotic cathartic. This is most appropriate to use when repeated activated charcoal and a cathartic are needed. It has the least effect on overall electrolyte status.
- *Mineral oil is contraindicated.*

Dermal toxins

Powder, solid or liquid: vacuuming, brushing, shaving, or bathing
Oily toxicants: butter, peanut butter, mayonnaise, waterless hand cleaner

Pulmonary toxins

Remove from exposure
Support respiratory function

causes decreased gastrointestinal motility by inducing severe shock or convulsions, or if the toxin forms a gastric concretion or mass (e.g., aspirin), gastric evacuation may be effective as long as 12 to 18 hours after ingestion.[6]

The first method of gastric evacuation is the induction of emesis. It is considered if the patient is asymptomatic and the airway does not need to be protected. If the cat has not eaten in the last 2 hours it should be fed a small moist meal before vomiting is induced. A few precautions are important: Vomiting should not be induced if the cat is already vomiting or if the suspected poison is a corrosive or a hydrocarbon. If the cat is showing clinical signs of toxicity, vomiting may induce aspiration pneumonia. Inducing emesis of a toxin that causes seizures can precipitate seizures.

It should be noted that the results of emesis vary. One reference states that 40 to 60% of chyme in the stomach is emptied after vomiting.[7] Studies in humans have shown the stomach to empty from 7 to 70%.[8]

Vomiting can be induced in cats with several medications. Xylazine (Rompun) is an effective emetic when given intramuscularly (IM) or subcutaneously (SC) at 0.5 mg/lb, but it also results in slight sedation and respiratory depression.[5] These side effects outweigh its usefulness in many instances, although they may be reversed with yohimbine (Yobine). Three-percent hydrogen peroxide can be used because of its action as a gastric irritant. It is given in doses of approximately 1 mL/lb (up to 15 mL total dose), and this dose is repeated in 10 minutes if vomiting does not occur.[9]

Syrup of ipecac is efficacious in cats in doses of 1.5 mL/lb PO, although like other emetics it is not 100% effective. It should be diluted 1:1 with water and administered by orogastric or nasogastric tube. Onset of action of ipecac can be delayed; sometimes it takes 15 to 60 minutes to exert its effect. Obviously, during such a delay additional toxin can be absorbed. Emetine, the active ingredient in ipecac, also induces lacrimation and bronchial secretions, and it can be neurotoxic and cardiotoxic at high levels, occasionally resulting in fatal reactions.[9] *Syrup* of ipecac, *not extract* of ipecac, should be used. The extract is 14 times more potent, and extremely toxic. A major drawback to the use of ipecac is that it can significantly reduce the effectiveness of activated charcoal.[5] Neither apomorphine nor salt should be given as an emetic to cats.

The second method of gastric evacuation, lavage, is considered when (1) emetics fail, (2) the airway needs to be guarded, (3) massive ingestion has occurred, (4) a highly toxic substance has been ingested, or (5) the patient is symptomatic. It should not be used when the toxin is a corrosive that can weaken the esophagus or stomach. The patient is anesthetized or heavily sedated, and a cuffed endotracheal tube is placed. The cat is positioned in left lateral recumbency with its posterior elevated approximately 15 degrees. This position places the pylorus dorsally, to delay gastric emptying as the stomach is filled with irrigant, and places the end of the stomach tube ventrally in the cardia. A large-bore stomach tube is passed; the diameter should be as large as possible without damaging the esophagus. A multifenestrated soft rubber tube approximately three times the diameter of the endotracheal tube passes easily through the esophagus of most cats (e.g., a 40-Fr external diameter catheter for a 9-lb cat). The length of the tube is premeasured from the nose to the xiphoid area, then the tube is passed carefully into the stomach.

The stomach is emptied using gentle abdominal pressure. After initial evacuation, the stomach is lavaged with warm water, starting with a volume of approximately 2 mL/lb and increasing to 5 mL/lb as the stomach is emptied of ingesta. Initial wash material can be saved and frozen if analysis is desired. Activated charcoal in a dilute slurry can be utilized until clear fluid returns from the stomach. When this is accomplished, activated charcoal, 0.5 to 1.0 g/lb, can be instilled to absorb any remaining toxin. As with emesis, lavage is contraindicated if a corrosive substance was ingested. Lavage following ingestion of volatile liquid is very controversial, since occasionally aspiration can occur even when the airway is protected.

If the dose of poison ingested or the interval since ingestion suggests to the clinician that toxicant may be present in the intestine, intestinal decontamination with a through-and-through enema is warranted. A reservoir of warm water is elevated 3 to 4 feet above the cat, and a 15- to 25-Fr soft rubber catheter is placed in the colon to the level of the anterior portion of the descending colon. The bowel is irrigated until the lavage fluid is produced orally or until stomach contents (e.g., charcoal) are noted in the stool. The enema dilutes the toxin and facilitates catharsis.

Activated charcoal is the preferred absorbent after gastroenteric decontamination. This compound, which binds to most commonly ingested toxins, should be used routinely.

After gastric evacuation, activated charcoal is administered orally in a slurry of water at a dose of 1 to 4 g/lb.[10] The charcoal is easily dosed through the stomach tube if the patient has been anesthetized for lavage. If emesis has been induced with xylazine the patient should be sedate enough to allow passage of a stomach tube with the aid of a mouth gag. Activated charcoal can be administered with a stomach tube or PO in small amounts to unsedated patients. Activated charcoal is contraindicated with corrosives, since it does not bind to alkalis or mineral acids,[6] or if constipation is present; constipation may occur if a cathartic is not administered following activated charcoal. Administration of this drug should be repeated in 6 to 8 hours for toxins that return to the intestinal tract following enterohepatic recirculation.

A cathartic is used to decrease bowel transit time and so limit contact of the toxin with the bowel mucosa in order to decrease the dose absorbed. A cathartic should *not* be administered if the cat is dehydrated or has diarrhea; one *should* be administered after activated charcoal. Otherwise, the toxin-containing activated charcoal remains in the intestinal tract long enough for the toxin to be absorbed through the mucosa.

The cathartics of choice are magnesium sulfate (Epsom salts), sodium sulfate (Glauber's salts), and Sorbitol 70%. The first two are administered PO in a dose of ¼ level teaspoon per pound of body weight, and Sorbitol 70% is given at a dose of 1.36 mL/lb. Sodium sulfate may be more effective, but magnesium sulfate is easier to obtain since it is available at most retail pharmacies. Magnesium sulfate has the disadvantage of elevating the serum magnesium level in patients whose renal function is compromised. It should be used with caution in these patients. Magnesium sulfate is contraindicated for catharsis of toxins that cause bowel stasis, since an excessive amount of magnesium may be absorbed. It should not be given in repeated doses nor to cats with compromised renal function. Sorbitol is an osmotic cathartic that is gentler in its effect on the electrolyte status of the animal and should be the cathartic of choice when repeated charcoal is indicated.

Bulk cathartics may be indicated when a nontoxic, bulky product or a physical agent is ingested and its elimination needs to be aided. Activated charcoal is not given in this situation. Bran cereal, vegetable fiber (i.e., pumpkin, sweet potato) and psyllium (Vetasyl) 1 to 2 capsules per day or Metamucil (0.5 to 1.0 teaspoons every 12 to 24 hours) are the commonly used bulk cathartics.

Mineral oil has been touted as a cathartic, but it has been shown to bind with some fat-soluble toxins and coat the intestinal mucosa. Mineral oil may actually increase bowel transit time of certain poisons, thus enhancing absorption. Should the patient aspirate mineral oil, lipid pneumonitis will result. The use of mineral oil is generally discouraged.[4]

In case of cutaneous exposure the toxin should be removed with a combination of brushing, vacuuming (if tolerated), shaving, and bathing. In all instances gloves should be worn by the hospital workers treating the patient. If the toxin is a solid or powder the cat should be brushed thoroughly and vacuumed. Any remaining toxin should be removed by rinsing with copious volumes of warm water. A mild dishwashing detergent can be used to thoroughly clean the coat. Anecdotally, some practitioners have recommended emulsifying oily toxicants with butter, peanut butter, or mayonnaise prior to bathing. Mechanics' waterless hand cleaners such as Hand Cleaner are also effective when used to remove particularly stubborn oil-based toxins, but these products should be used with caution and washed off immediately after application since they can be toxic to the cat if absorbed dermally or ingested.

If pulmonary exposure occurs, detoxification is accomplished by removing the patient from the contaminated environment. Indications of exposure, especially from smoke inhalation, include singed guard hairs, the smell of smoke on the hair coat, carbonaceous sputum, respiratory abnormalities, and cyanotic or bright red mucous membranes. Continued detoxification usually depends on maintaining respiratory function.

Enhancing Elimination

Many compounds are secreted by the renal tubules or filtered by the glomeruli. If they are not reabsorbed, these are rapidly excreted in the urine. The rationale for forced diuresis relies on the ability of mannitol or furosemide to promote diuresis by elevating the osmotic pressure of the glomerular and tubular filtrates, thus hindering reabsorption of water and solutes (e.g., toxins).[10]

Forced diuresis is utilized only if a specific toxin is identified whose excretion is enhanced by this procedure. Once the poisoned cat is adequately hydrated, forced diuresis is instituted. Mannitol is administered IV, slowly in a dose of 1 g/lb every 6 hours, or furosemide is utilized IV at 2 mg/lb every 6 to 8 hours. Urine output and the cat's weight should be closely monitored and the rate of fluid administration adjusted accordingly to prevent dehydration.

Renal elimination of toxins can be further assisted when the poison is a weak acid or a weak base. To be effectively reabsorbed from the renal tubules a toxicant must be relatively nonpolar or un-ionized. Increasing the ionization of the chemical renders it less absorbable and increases its rate of elimination. This method of enhancing excretion is termed "ion trapping." Acid drugs are ionized in slightly alkaline urine and alkaline drugs in slightly acidic urine. Doses of sodium bicarbonate to alkalinize and ammonium chloride to acidify the urine vary, depending on the source. If ion trapping is being considered, a toxicologist should be consulted for the appropriate protocol.

The other factor to be considered in patient decontamination is prevention of reabsorption. Regardless of the route of absorption, if a toxin or its metabolites are excreted from the liver into bile there is a potential for intestinal absorption. If a toxin is recycled enterohepatically, steps taken to prevent its reintroduction to the splanchnic and systemic circulation increase the rate of elimination. Intestinal resorption is prevented by repeated doses of absorbent-activated charcoal with Sorbitol. It is for this reason that oral activated charcoal can be therapeutic in certain cases of dermal exposure. If the absorbent is repeated more than twice after initial decontamination the patient's electrolytes and hydration should be closely monitored. As with ion trapping, a toxicologist should be consulted to determine which toxins respond to this therapy.

Some renally excreted toxins respond to forced diuresis only to be resorbed through the bladder mucosa. Decontamination of these toxins can be hastened simply by placing an indwelling urinary catheter.

Specific Toxins

Rodenticides

In general, owing to their selective eating habits, cats are not as likely as dogs to ingest bait-type rodenticides. The clinician must decide if a significant exposure has occurred and what must be done to either prevent or treat clinical signs.

Anticoagulants

Anticoagulants are the most common household rodenticides. They act by interfering wtih epoxide reductase, an enzyme required to reactivate vitamin K in the liver. Synthesis of clotting factors II, VII, IX, and X requires vitamin K. In general, animals that are exposed to toxic doses of an anticoagulant show no signs until the preexisting clotting factors and active vitamin K are depleted. The prothrombin time (PT) is a valuable diagnostic tool, as early after exposure it indicates that factor VII (half-life 6.2 hours[11]) and the extrinsic pathway are ceasing to function. A PT longer than 15 seconds at a point 24 to 48 hours after exposure indicates the need to begin vitamin K_1 therapy.[12]

Predisposing factors that increase toxicity to anticoagulant rodenticides include certain drugs, disease states, and the age of the animal. Concurrent use of highly protein-bound drugs actually releases anticoagulant, since it is

Table 62–4. LD_{50} of Anticoagulant Rodenticides[14]

Rodenticide	LD_{50} (mg/kg)
Warfarin	5–50
Diphacinone	15
Brodifacoum	25*
Bromadiolone	25*

*When calculating exposure potential the practitioner should take into consideration that LD_{50} values for newer-generation anticoagulants are based on limited data.

bound to serum albumin. This increases its active form and increases clotting inhibition.[13]

Drugs such as corticosteroids, sulfonamides, and promazine-derivative tranquilizers are contraindicated. Very young animals with immature liver function have decreased amounts of circulating clotting factors. They show signs sooner even after exposure to smaller amounts. In general, LD_{50} values in cats can be used to estimate exposure potential. As a general rule, one tenth of the LD_{50} can be considered a minimum toxic dose. Much of the LD_{50} data on the newer generation of anticoagulants is based on very limited information. The LD_{50}s for several common anticoagulant rodenticides are listed in Table 62–4.

Generally, clinical signs of anticoagulants become evident some 2 to 5 days after exposure to a significant amount.[15] Very young, very old, and clinically ill animals can show signs within 24 hours. Preexisting liver or kidney disease or malabsorption syndrome can also shorten the interval until signs occur. Early signs include depression, anemia, anorexia, weakness, muscle soreness and stiffness, and intermittent cough. Petechiae, ecchymoses, epistaxis, hemoptysis, and joint swelling are later signs. Abdominal pain that is difficult to localize may be present. Sudden death without early signs can occur when hemorrhage occurs in the thoracic or abdominal cavity, pericardial sac, or cerebral vessels.

The most important part of dealing with such an exposure is determining if a significant amount of rodenticide has been ingested. This is done by comparing the amount of toxin ingested with its LD_{50} (see Tables 62–1 and 62–4). Early after exposure decontamination measures, including emesis and doses of activated charcoal and a cathartic, are very important. PT should be measured at 24, 48, and 72 hours after exposure, to determine if vitamin K therapy is indicated. Occasionally when the clinician knows a large amount has been ingested and the animal is in one of the more susceptible groups, it can be appropriate to begin vitamin K_1 therapy without performing a PT. If clinical signs are already obvious, treatment begins by stabilizing the animal.

Treatment involves basic life support, including oxygen and blood transfusions, if the cat is severely affected. Vitamin K_1 (phytonadione) is the treatment of choice in a dose of 1.5 to 2.5 mg/lb s.i.d. or divided b.i.d.[14,16] It can be given SC, IM, or PO. IV injection has caused anaphylaxis, but human products labeled for IV use are safe for cats. Optimally, after the animal is stabilized the oral route is preferred. Absorption is much enhanced when it is given with a fatty meal (e.g., canned food). If the animal is showing signs of bleeding, deep IM injection can cause hematoma formation. The animal also needs to be kept in a stress-free environment during treatment. Duration of treatment varies with the type of rodenticide ingested. Generally, for warfarin it is 10 to 14 days, for bromodiolone 21 days, for diphacinone 30 days, and for brodifacoum 30 days.

With any of these, prothrombin time should be checked 2 or 3 days after vitamin K_1 treatment is discontinued, to ensure that the course was long enough.

Differential diagnosis is very important, since rodenticide intoxication in cats can mimic other syndromes, including FeLV, FIV, liver disease, immune-mediated or inherited bleeding disorders, and disseminated intravascular coagulation.[17]

Relay toxicosis, also known as secondary toxicity, is toxicosis produced by ingestion of another animal that was poisoned by a rodenticide. In general this is not considered a problem unless the cat regularly eats exposed rodents. One report describes a cat that died after eating six warfarin-poisoned rats over an 8-day period.[18] Symptoms of food poisoning also can result from consuming dead rodents.

Cholecalciferol

Cholecalciferol (vitamin D_3) rodenticides increase circulating vitamin D metabolites, thus increasing circulating calcium. Calcium may increase to the extent that it causes dystrophic calcification and subsequent death.[16] Once the serum calcium value exceeds 12 mg/dL calcification of the tissues is likely.

Several cholecalciferol products are marketed that contain 0.075% of the active ingredient.[19] Cats are unlikely to ingest these products owing to their cereal bait composition, though this does occasionally occur.

The incidence of exposure is greatest for young cats, generally less than 1 year of age, probably owing to kittens' more indiscriminate eating habits. The minimum lethal dose is reported to be 1.9 to 2.4 mg of cholecalciferol per pound of body weight.[16] The clinical signs are divided into four syndromes: neurologic, cardiovascular, gastrointestinal, and renal.

Clinical signs usually occur within 12 to 36 hours after exposure. Generally seen are anorexia, depression, vomiting, polyuria, polydipsia, diarrhea, and renal pain. Occasionally, gastrointestinal and pulmonary bleeding, which may be confused with anticoagulant rodenticides, can result from the dystrophic calcification. Less common signs include cardiac arrhythmias and bradycardia. Death results from acute renal failure.

In the event of a significant exposure decontamination should be performed first (see Table 62–3). Repeated doses of activated charcoal should be given at 6- to 8-hour intervals, as vitamin D metabolites are recirculated in bile. The baseline serum profile, or at least a serum calcium level, should be determined at the time of presentation. The calcium level should be monitored daily for 3 days. Total chemistry panels make it possible to monitor for azotemia and hyperphosphatemia. The phosphorus level often rises 12 hours before the calcium level does, giving an early indication of toxicosis.[16]

Treatment consists of fluid therapy (0.9% saline continuous infusion) and furosemide (2.5 mg/lb IV followed by 1 to 2.5 mg/lb every 8 to 12 hours PO). Normal saline is the fluid of choice because it enhances calcium elimination. Supplementation of potassium chloride is usually necessary, since 0.9% saline is deficient in potassium. Use of IV fluids is preferred. One author states that SC administration may be sufficient if the serum calcium value does not exceed 15 mg/dL.[20] Fluid administration should be aimed at correcting dehydration, expanding plasma volume, and providing daily fluid needs. The amount should be two or three times the amount needed for maintenance (60 to 90 mL/lb/day).[21]

Prednisolone should be given in doses of 1 mg/lb every 12 hours, to inhibit osteoclast-activating factors, exert hypercalciuric effects, and decrease intestinal absorption of calcium. Salmon calcitonin (Calcimar) may be needed—2 to 3 IU/lb SC every 2 or 3 hours—until serum calcium stabilizes. Calcitonin is principally for use when the serum calcium level does not stabilize in response to administration of saline and prednisolone and when prolonged therapy (up to 4 weeks) is indicated. Calcitonin occasionally causes anaphylaxis, and it must be discontinued if untoward effects are observed. Adjuncts to treatment include low-calcium diet (Hill's Prescription Diet Feline s/d or Feline k/d) and protection from exposure to sunlight. Phosphate binders can also be useful to counteract hyperphosphatemia. Aluminum hydroxide (15 to 45 mg/lb/day in divided doses for up to 2 weeks) has been recommended.[21] Milk and other dairy products are contraindicated.

Treatment with diuretics and corticosteroids often needs to be continued as long as 2 weeks, since it may take that long for the serum calcium value to stay below 12 mg/dL. The serum calcium and BUN values need to be rechecked 24, 48, and 72 hours after treatment is discontinued. Prognosis depends on the clinical severity and the ability of the clinician to treat appropriately for the necessary period.

Bromethalin

A rodenticide containing 0.01% bromethalin is available as tan and as green pellets. The minimum toxic dose for cats is 1.5 g of bait per pound of body weight; the minimum lethal toxic dose is 2 g/lb.[16,22,23] In theory, a 10-lb cat would have to ingest almost 1 tablespoon of bait to get a minimal toxic dose. Bromethalin causes cerebral edema resulting from spongy degeneration of white matter, caused by uncoupling of oxidative phosphorylation. Vacuole formation also occurs between myelin sheaths, causing increased damage to nerve axons.[16,22-24] With doses at or near the LD_{50} clinical signs develop within 24 hours: weakness, severe muscle tremors, hyperthermia, extreme hyperexcitability, and seizures. Smaller doses produce slower onset of signs, generally between 24 and 96 hours after ingestion. These signs include hindlimb ataxia, paresis, and central nervous system (CNS) depression. Other signs include vomiting, coma, and mydriasis. Manifestations of both syndromes are severe, and death is very common once signs occur.[24]

Treatment is very unrewarding once clinical signs occur, so decontamination is very important. It should be given to any animal that has ingested more than 20% of the minimum toxic dose. Repeated doses of activated charcoal and cathartic should be given (see Table 62–3). Excretion of bromethalin is slow, and it has a plasma half-life of 5.6 days.[16] Some authors have advocated mannitol and dexamethasone to reduce the cerebral edema, but they have produced disappointing results.[22] Mannitol has risks in itself, so its use must be judiciously monitored. The balance of treatment is symptomatic and supportive.

Anthelminthics

Ivermectin

Owing to widespread availability of over-the-counter anthelminthics, toxicosis in small animals is not uncommon. Owners who administer products purchased in feed or grocery stores often overdose or misuse them. The most common agents of anthelminthic toxicosis in cats are ivermectin and piperazine.[32]

Ivermectin is an effective antiparasitic agent developed in the 1980s, originally for large animals. Structurally similar to milbemycin, it has been found to be effective against many nematodes and arthropods. Ivermectin is an agonist of the inhibitory neurotransmitter gamma-aminobutyric acid (GABA), in contrast to acetylcholine which is stimulatory. GABA is found only in the CNS of mammals. Ivermectin is a relatively safe anthelminthic, since it rarely crosses the blood-brain barrier.[26,27] It is not indicated for use in very young animals, as their blood-brain barrier is thought not to be fully developed. Originally a prescription preparation, it is now readily available in several over-the-counter preparations. It is approved for use in cattle, horses, and swine in doses of 90 μg/lb and in dogs for heartworm prevention at a dose of 3 μg/lb. It is not approved for use in cats.

Ivermectin has been shown to be effective in treating many external parasites of cats, such as *Otodectes, Cheyletiella,* and *Notoedres* species. The doses used have been between 90 and 180 μg/lb, PO or SC (see Chapter 57).[28-30] (One author [MM] knows of many practitioners who use it in the ear canal for *Otodectes* species, but no studies are available to prove its effectiveness.)

Toxicosis generally results when large-animal preparations are given without consideration for the cat's size. It is not unusual for an owner to give "a dab" of the paste formulation. Overdosing by a factor of ten (i.e., 1.0 mL instead of 0.1 mL) is not uncommon.

The interval from administration until onset of the first clinical signs is generally less than 24 hours. The most common clinical signs are ataxia (dragging hindlimbs), vocalizing, abnormal behavior (including biting and scratching), mydriasis, whole body tremors, lethargy, weakness or recumbency, transitory blindness (evidenced by walking into walls circling, loss of bilateral menace, head pressing, and slow, incomplete pupillary light reflex), bradycardia, hypothermia, slow respiratory rate, and coma. Less typical signs are seizures and death.[25,30,31]

A tentative diagnosis of ivermectin toxicosis should be considered when clinical signs, onset interval, and dose seem compatible. Most references indicate the minimum toxic dose for cats to be 230 μg/lb, but caution is advised because several cases have been reported to the NAPCC after a cat received the "recommended dose." Three cases in which ivermectin toxicity was apparent were in cats given 0.1 mL subcutaneously. The doses were 82, 100, and 143 μg/lb, respectively. The cats showed common signs of ataxia and varying degrees of depression. Two became comatose and then improved very slowly. They were euthanized, one at 8 days after injection and the other at 12 days. Since ivermectin is not approved for use in cats, the practitioner should consider the responsibility incumbent on extralabel usage.

Treatment requires persistent symptomatic care and fluid support. Treatment often requires days to weeks before animals fully respond. As evidenced by the cases described above, these cats may be severely affected for long periods, but if owners are willing the effort can prove rewarding. (One author [JMM] has spoken to one practitioner who reportedly treated a comatose cat for 18 days before it responded.)

These cats generally are not presented until signs appear. In the absence of CNS signs an overdose of oral ivermectin should be treated by inducing vomiting, if this can be done wtihin 1 hour (see Table 62–3). Activated charcoal and a cathartic should follow. Repeated doses of activated charcoal with an osmotic cathartic (every 8 to 12 hours) can be highly effective, because approximately 90% of ivermectin is excreted unchanged in the feces.[32] In dogs, the half-life is 1.8 days.[32] When the drug has been given by the SC route and the amount is considered life threatening, surgical débridement should be considered. It is thought that this could possibly lessen the amount absorbed. Good supportive care then becomes the principal form of therapy. Adequate nutritional and fluid support should be maintained. If the cat is comatose, frequent turning and maintaining normal body temperature are very important.

Picrotoxin, a GABA antagonist, has been shown to reverse severe depression from ivermectin in some dogs,[25,33] but it has not shown this effect after overdose in mice.[25] Physostigmine is a reversible cholinesterase inhibitor (the "original" carbamate) that has been used in severely affected dogs to increase responsiveness, muscle activity, respiratory rate, and eating and drinking, but it also has serious side effects, including cardiac arrhythmias and asystole. There are no studies or reports of use in cats, and at this time neither can be recommended for use in ivermectin toxicosis.[25]

Piperazine

Piperazine is one of the most common over-the-counter anthelminthics. It is available in numerous small-animal preparations labeled for both kittens and adult cats, and a large-animal preparation to be put in drinking water. For swine, cattle, and horses the dose is 50 mg/lb, and for dogs and cats 20 to 30 mg/lb. There are various salts of the drug, but the most common is piperazine adipate. Piperazine is also a GABA agonist.[25,33]

Clinical signs of toxicosis include ataxia, muscle weakness, intention tremors of the head and neck, diarrhea, vomiting, seizures, and behavior changes.[25,33,34] Doses between 10 and 50 mg/lb have been reported in cases of toxicosis.[25] Signs occur within 24 hours after exposure. Preexisting renal or CNS disease may predispose to toxicity.

Diagnosis of toxicosis relies on a history of exposure, appropriate clinical signs, and compatible time of onset of signs. Piperazine can be isolated from blood and urine, but this only confirms that exposure has occurred, not that the dose was toxic. In the rare event that death occurs, a complete necropsy is likely to discover other causes or concurrent organ dysfunction. Piperazine itself does not cause significant lesions.

Treatment consists of decontamination and supportive care (see Table 64–3). If ingestion occurred recently and no CNS signs are present, induction of vomiting is indicated. If more than 1 hour has elapsed, activated charcoal and a cathartic are appropriate. Sedatives should be used to control CNS stimulation (see Table 62–2). Good supportive care emphasizes nutritional and fluid support. Recovery is generally uneventful within a few days, and death is rare.

Pain Relievers

Cats ingest human medications, though not as frequently as dogs. Generally, a dog chews a bottle of medication that a cat will not. Cats are exposed when an owner drops a tablet that the cat proceeds to eat or when owners medicate with human products. Since cats do not metabolize drugs as efficiently as humans and dogs do through liver glucuronidation, they are predisposed to toxicity from what appears to be small amounts of medicine. People who perceive that an animal is in pain sometimes give it their own pain relievers, most often ibuprofen, acetaminophin, or aspirin.

Ibuprofen

Nonsteroidal antiinflammatory drugs (NSAIDs) have come into widespread use in the last 10 years. There are many drugs in this category, and they have a wide range of pharmacologic activity. The most common, ibuprofen, is now available over-the-counter in 200-mg tablets. The NSAIDs are antiprostaglandins that reduce pain, inflammation, and fever.[19]

In humans 80% of ibuprofen is absorbed from the gastrointestinal tract, and the plasma concentration peaks 1 or 2 hours after ingestion. It is excreted mainly through the kidneys; 50 to 60% of an oral dose is excreted within 24 hours.[35] Some biliary elimination of conjugates also occurs. Specific pharmacokinetics and pharmacodynamics of ibuprofen have not been determined in cats, and only limited information is available about dogs. The elimination half-life in dogs is reported to be 3.7 to 5.8 hours.[36] Dogs are considered at greater risk than humans for the toxic effects of NSAIDs because the half-life is longer in dogs and the gastrointestinal absorption rate is higher. Therefore, the drug persists longer in plasma.[37] Though these specifics have not been studied for cats, they are considered more sensitive than dogs to the toxic effects of NSAIDs.

Cats are at risk from any dose greater than 23 mg/lb, an amount that causes gastrointestinal irritation and hemorrhage. Signs include vomiting, anorexia, mild depression, hematemesis, and melena. Gastrointestinal upset can be seen as early as 4 to 6 hours after ingestion, but hemorrhage and ulceration may occur 12 hours to 4 days later. Ingestion of amounts greater than 140 mg/lb have caused acute renal failure. This can occur as early as 12 hours after exposure to a large amount, but it generally is delayed as long as 3 to 5 days. Renal failure usually is characterized by oliguria and azotemia, but, rarely, anuria occurs. Doses greater than

280 mg/lb have caused severe depression, coma, seizures, metabolic acidosis, respiratory depression, and death.[38,39]

Treatment should begin with decontamination (see Table 62–3). Repeating doses of activated charcoal without the cathartic is indicated, since bile metabolites are reabsorbed. Occasionally, ibuprofen tablets or capsules coalesce in the stomach and absorption is prolonged. Therefore, gastric emptying procedures can be useful even when a longer interval has elapsed (i.e., 6 to 8 hours).

Symptomatic care for anticipated clinical signs is very important. At doses greater than 23 mg/lb, gastrointestinal support is needed to protect against the expected effects of irritation, hemorrhage, and ulceration. H_2 antagonists such as cimetidine (Tagamet) and famotidine (Pepcid) are recommended. Cimetidine should be administered in doses of 2.3 mg/lb IV or PO two to four times daily. Famotidine is administered in doses of 1–2 mg/cat IV b.i.d. Sucralfate (Carafate) binds to ulcer sites, allowing them to heal.[35] The dose for cats is a quarter to a half tablet two to four times daily.[4]

The H_2 antagonist should not be given within 2 hours of sucralfate, lest the latter coat it and limit its bioavailability. The two drugs should be given for a period of 7 days. Mild gastrointestinal irritation can be treated symptomatically for several days with either a kaolin-pectin preparation (Kaopectate, 0.5 to 1.0 mL/lb every 2 to 12 hours) or nonabsorbable antacids such as magnesium or aluminum hydroxide (milk of magnesia, 5 to 15 mL once or twice daily; Maalox, 2 to 10 mL q.i.d.).[40] These can cause side effects and should not be used long or given to debilitated cats. Formulations with bismuth subsalicylate (Pepto Bismol) must be avoided as they may aggravate gastritis.

Fluid therapy is very important to replace fluid loss through vomiting or diarrhea and to protect the kidneys. Ensuring that urine output is adequate is very important, and a diuretic such as furosemide may be necessary. Renal function needs to be closely monitored when exposure approaches the 140 mg/lb range. The preferred fluid is 0.45% saline in 2.5% dextrose, or 0.9% saline given IV. Fluids should be given IV at least 48 to 72 hours. After ingestion of large amounts, the fluids are necessary to prevent damage to the kidneys, even if the cat appears clinically normal. Smaller doses may not cause renal failure, but renal *damage* can still occur; thus, the importance of fluid therapy. Electrolyte monitoring is very important as is observation for metabolic acidosis.

Occasionally seizures follow ingestion of a large amount of ibuprofen, and they should be treated as indicated in Table 62–2.

Acetaminophen

Acetaminophen is available in more than 200 formulations. The most familiar are Tylenol, Tempera, Panadol, and Datril. No dose of these is safe to give to cats.

In all species acetaminophen is metabolized principally to glucuronide and sulfate conjugates. Because cats are deficient in the enzyme glucuronyl transferase, more of the drug in the liver is metabolized by sulfation. When sulfate stores are depleted, metabolism proceeds via cytochrome P_{450} oxidation, and toxic metabolites are formed. Clinical signs occur when glutathione, which is present in both liver and red blood cells (RBCs), is depleted. Glutathione normally conjugates with these metabolites and makes possible their excretion as nontoxic conjugates. Once glutathione is depleted, the reactive metabolite covalently binds to other cell macromolecules, and tissue necrosis occurs.[41-44] In cats the depletion of glutathione in the RBCs leaves the cells unprotected from the oxidizing effects of the reactive metabolite, thus methemoglobinemia occurs. The larger the dose of acetaminophen the more toxic metabolites are formed.[45]

In studies to determine minimum toxic dose in cats clinical signs of salivation developed 30 minutes after dosing at 9 mg/lb. Generally, doses greater than 18 mg/lb cause serious clinical signs.[41] One study recorded death at 65 mg/lb, while a case report describes death in one cat that was given 250-mg tablets at an interval of 12 hours (35 mg/lb).[46,47] Because a diet containing propylene glycol (i.e., semimoist foods) predisposes cats to methemoglobinemia, the toxic dose of acetaminophen may be smaller for cats fed such food.[48]

Clinical signs include hypersalivation, vomiting, depression, weakness, cyanosis, facial edema, anemia, methemoglobinemia, hemoglobinuria, hematuria, and tachypnea.[49] Without treatment coma and death are common. Diagnosis is based on a history of exposure and on clinical signs and laboratory evidence. A dose of 28 mg/lb produced 21.7% methemoglobinemia 4 hours later.[45] With 55 mg/lb methemoglobinemia was 45.5%, and these cats had facial edema associated with squinting and pawing at the face.[45] Generally, hematological studies reveal a decreased hematocrit, methemoglobinemia, Heinz body formation, reticulocytosis, hemolysis, leukocytosis, and prolonged PT. Liver enzyme values in cats may be marginally elevated. Elevated BUN value and evidence of hemoglobinuria may also be seen.[45]

Successful treatment requires decontamination, basic life support, and administration of sulfhydryl groups to which the toxic metabolites react, permitting excretion.[43,50] In the rare event that a cat is presented before onset of clinical signs, induction of vomiting should be attempted although tablet expulsion is not common. Activated charcoal and a cathartic are usually more efficacious. The use of *N*-acetylcysteine (Mucomyst) in 5% solution would be indicated if the dose is greater than 18 mg/lb or if clinical signs are present.[41]

Mucomyst is available in 10 and 20% solutions and should be diluted to 5%. If signs are severe, a dose of 130 mg/lb IV has been advocated by the NAPCC. In general, the initial dose is 65 mg/lb IV or PO.[47,50,51] If activated charcoal was given, acetylcysteine should not be given PO for at least 2 hours. When acetylcystine is given intravenously a bacteriostatic filter is recommended, though the preparation comes in a sterile ampules and no adverse effects have been reported when the 5% solution is used without filtration if it is mixed in an aseptic manner. Acetylcysteine is actually thought to be best utilized when given PO. The initial dose is followed by 32 mg/lb q.i.d. for 3 days. Monitoring is recommended as the drug is discontinued, since some cats need a longer course of therapy.

Vitamin C is also recommended, since it is a reducing agent. The effects are delayed as long as 3 to 5 days in humans, so it is much less effective in the management of acute methemoglobinemia.[52] Its usefulness has not been proven in acetaminophen toxicosis. The currently recommended dose is 14 mg/lb q.i.d., SC, IM, or PO.

Cimetidine has also been suggested for acetaminophen toxicosis. It inhibits the cytochrome P_{450} system in the liver, and, so, prevents formation of toxic metabolites through this system without inhibiting the glucuronide or sulfate pathway. This may protect against hepatotoxicity by inhibiting covalent binding of the toxic metabolites to hepatocytes,[44] and it may be more useful in dogs, which more often exhibit hepatotoxicity.

The remainder of therapy is supportive. Fluid therapy is important in preventing dehydration and renal damage from hemoglobinuria. Monitoring for metabolic acidosis is also important. Oxygen therapy is often indicated for severely cyanotic cats. Rarely, blood transfusions may be indicated if an animal develops profound anemia. Corticosteroids and antihistamines are contraindicated, as their metabolism may enhance the toxicity of acetaminophen. If affected cats are treated early and aggressively the prognosis is good. Once recovered, they suffer no long-term deleterious effects on their organ systems.[42,45]

Ruling out other toxicoses may be necessary when an animal presents with clinical signs that are similar to those of acetaminophen toxicosis. Other drugs that produce similar clinical findings include pyridium, napthalene, saponins, thiazide dyes, sulfonamides, aniline compounds, diaminodiphenylsulfate (Dapsone) Dipyrone, benzocaine, and methionine.[30,53] Manifestations of lead, copper, or zinc toxicosis may also be similar, but these are rare in cats.

Aspirin

Worldwide, aspirin is the most purchased over-the-counter drug. Because of its availability it is frequently administered to cats for relief of pain or fever. Although it is considerably safer than acetaminophen,[54] its prolonged half-life (37.6 hours)[55] makes repeated administration dangerous.

Aspirin has therapeutic indications for felines. It is commonly used to prevent thrombus formation in cats with cardiomyopathy. It may also be used for management of inflammatory and degenerative diseases. Owing to its prolonged half-life, the recommended dosage is 5 to 10 mg/lb every 48 hours. This is equivalent to a half to a whole baby aspirin tablet or an eighth to a quarter regular-strength adult tablet (82 mg) every 48 hours. For very old or very young cats and for cats with renal or hepatic disease, even this dose may be excessive.[56]

Sulfasalazine, a salicylate-containing drug used to treat ulcerative colitis, is formulated so that it is carried to the colon before it is cleaved into its active components. Although it can be safely used in cats they must be monitored for signs of toxicosis.

Aspirin toxicosis manifests as depression, anorexia, vomiting, gastric hemorrhage, toxic hepatitis, anemia, bone marrow hypoplasia, hyperpnea, and fever.[57] Treatment should consist of decontamination (see Table 62–3) and supportive care. IV fluid therapy is often required when gastrointestinal signs are severe. Blood transfusion may be necessary if gastrointestinal bleeding is severe or if anemia or bone marrow hypoplasia occurs.

Insecticides

Most feline insecticide poisonings are related to flea control products. Other products used as insecticides (roach control, ant bait, fly bait) can be dangerous, but problems are reported less frequently. These other household insecticides, which usually contain the same classes of compounds as flea control products, are mentioned under the appropriate headings.

Veterinarians and staff members who sell insecticides need to make their clients aware that these products should be used only on healthy animals. Owners of long-haired cats should also be informed that larger amounts of dermally applied insecticides may be absorbed owing to prolonged contact with the wet product. Cat owners may be unaware or may disregard health problems that might make a product more toxic. Clinic staff should have a good understanding of product contents and potential problems. It bears stressing that any insecticides can produce toxicosis given the "right" circumstances.

Organophosphorus and Carbamates

Organophosphorus (OP) and carbamate insecticides are used frequently as premise sprays, for home or yard treatment. Some are also directly applied to animals as dust, shampoo, spray, dip, or in a flea collar. There are many formulations for each of these products. When toxicosis is suspected, it is a good idea to have owners bring the product to the veterinarian so the active ingredients can be determined.

Some of the common organophosphorus compounds are chlorpyrifos, diazinon, dichlorovos (DDVP), fenthion, malathion, phosmet, and propetamphos. The more commonly recognized carbamate insecticides are bendiocarb, carbaryl (Sevin), carbofuran, fenoxycarb, methomyl, and propoxur (Baygon).

Adverse effects can occasionally be seen with any of the products listed, even if they are used per instructions. The age of the animal, its genetic makeup, preexisting medical problems, and other concurrent insecticide exposure can all be factors in whether or not an animal will exhibit clinical signs. Certain drugs may lower the threshold for toxicosis if given prior to exposure to OP or carbamates. Phenothiazines, inhalation anesthetics, and other drugs that either compete for esterases utilized by OP and carbamate compounds or have a neuromuscular-blocking activity should not be used if the animal was recently exposed to an OP or carbamate.[58] Usually, problems observed in cats involve misuse of the product. "Extralabel" use of insecticides on cats, whether in higher concentration than specified or by using a preparation not labeled for use on or around cats, is strongly contraindicated.

Since both OP and carbamate insecticides act by binding to acetylcholinesterase they both exhibit similar clinical effects. Onset of clinical signs is usually rapid (within several hours) but occasionally, it can be delayed as long as several days, and with some of the more lipophilic compounds signs may persist several weeks. Cats are particularly susceptible to delayed onset after chlorpyrifos poisoning.[58] These animals may appear somewhat normal for several days and then become depressed and anorectic; they may even die if proper treatment measures are not instituted. In most cats toxic effects are typical muscarinic signs (hypersalivation, bradycardia, lacrimation, urinary incontinence, increased bronchial secretions, gastrointestinal hypermotility, and miosis). These signs may be masked, however, by sympathetic stimulation, which can reverse muscarinic effects. For example, a number of cats have very dilated pupils. Nicotinic signs generally follow and include muscle stiffness, fasciculations weakness, paralysis, seizures, and tremors.[58] When death occurs, it can usually be attributed to respiratory complications.

Preliminary diagnosis may be based on a history of recent environmental or animal application or exposure and clinical signs compatible with OP or carbamate intoxication. LD_{50}s of common insecticides are listed in Table 62–5. Bradycardia or miosis that does not respond to a preanesthetic dose of atropine (0.01 to 0.03 mg/lb IV) is suggestive of OP or carbamate toxicosis. In cats, marked depression of cholinesterase activity accompanies exposure to OP and carbamate compounds. In live animals, whole blood cholinesterase is the only means of determining depressed cholinesterase enzyme activity. Enzyme depression may be noted even in asymptomatic animals. Post mortem, samples may be analyzed at some laboratories for cholinesterase depression or for the presence of OP or carbamate compounds. Since tissue concentrations decrease quickly, tissues must be taken rapidly and frozen. Contact should be made with the laboratory prior to submission to confirm its analytic capability and to learn its requirements for tissue types and amounts. Tissues for submission should include brain (sagittal half to include cerebrum, cerebellum, and brain stem), body fat, liver (half), stomach and intestinal contents, and, if dermal exposure is suspected, skin with subcutaneous tissue.[58,59]

The first response to toxicosis involving OP or carbamate insecticide is measures to sustain life. Maintenance of a patent airway and oxygen should be supplied if needed. Control of seizures is the first priority (see Table 62–2). Cats that exhibit severe life-threatening muscarinic signs should be administered atropine sulfate at the therapeutic dose of 0.1 mg/lb (10 times the preanesthetic dose); a quarter of this dose is given IV and the rest SC or IM. Atropine acts by blocking muscarinic receptors, thus mitigating the parasympathomimetic effects of the OP or carbamate insecticide.[60] Once initial atropinization is accomplished (miosis, drying of respiratory and oral secretions), as clinical signs (increased bronchial secretions, bradycardia) return more atropine should be administered in smaller doses to effect. Pralidoxime chloride (2-PAM; Protopam) should also be used in conjunction with atropine sulfate for OP toxicosis.† 2-PAM is not beneficial for carbamate toxicosis because it does not interact with the carbamylated acetylcholinesterase in the same manner as with phosphorylated acetylcholinesterase.[61] 2-PAM should be dosed 5 to 10 mg/lb IM, SC, or IV slowly over 30 minutes, two or three times daily to control nicotinic signs. If the second or third treatment produces no response, discontinuation of 2-PAM should be considered. From NAPCC experience, 2-PAM may be needed as long as several weeks, especially with chlorpyrifos toxicosis. Cats that suffer with dermal exposure should be bathed in a mild detergent soap to remove remaining insecticide. Repeated dosing with activated charcoal and a cathartic (given with the initial dose of charcoal) should be considered after ingestion or dermal exposure, to promote enhanced elimination and quicker recovery. Grooming habits of cats can turn dermal exposure into oral exposure.

Table 62–5. LD_{50}s of Common Organophosphorus and Carbamate Insecticides

Organophosphorus	LD_{50}* (mg/kg)	Carbamate	LD_{50}* (mg/kg)
Malathion	1375	Carbaryl (Sevin)	500
Diazinon	300	Propoxur (Baygon)	90
Fenthion	250	Bendiocarb	40
Chlorpyrifos	135	Methomyl	17
Phosmet	113	Carbofuran	8
Propetamphos	83		
Dichlorovos (DDVP)	56		

*LD_{50}s are for albino rats and are given as a general guide for relative toxicity. They are not useful for anticipating general clinical effects.[59]

Chlorpyrifos toxicosis in cats bears special mention. Affected cats often show signs for several days after initial exposure. Typically, they become anorexic and ataxic, even to the extent of dragging their hindlimbs. Tremors and fasciculations may also be seen. Ventroflexion of the neck is a prominent sign and should be differentiated from that due to hypokalemia. 2-PAM should be given in doses ranging from 5 to 10 mg/lb, not to exceed 20 mg/lb in 24 hours. Some authors believe action of 2-PAM is enhanced by concurrent use of atropine, but in the absence of muscarinic signs this would not be indicated. These cats need good nursing care and special attention to nutrition. A nasogastric tube, or even an esophagostomy tube, may be necessary to ensure adequate alimentation (see Chapter 5). Treatment of these cats often continues several days to weeks before nicotinic signs resolve. Occasionally, cats have been known to relapse, in which case they need to be treated again with 2-PAM.

Pyrethrins

Natural pyrethrins and the synthetic pyrethrins (pyrethroids), while generally regarded as relatively safe for use in cats, are the toxicants in a large percentage of feline cases handled by the NAPCC. A list of the common products appears in Table 62–6. These compounds are applied directly to cats or to the environment and are usually combined with various synergists. The synergists increase the duration of action of the pyrethrins by inhibiting oxidative metabolism of the insecticide. Some of the more common synergists include piperonyl butoxide and *N*-octyl-bicycloheptene dicarboximide (MGK 264). Pyrethrins and pyrethroids are susceptible to degradation in the environment by ultraviolet light, acids, or alkalis. The pyrethroids were developed to increase availability, light stability, and insecti-

† 2-PAM comes in increments of 1 g sterile powder to be reconstituted with 20 mL sterile water for injection (included). Once reconstituted, the solution equals 50 mg/mL and must be refrigerated in the dark to maintain a 2-week shelf life, according to the manufacturer.

Table 62–6. Some Commonly Used Pyrethrin and Pyrethroid Insecticides

Allethrin	Permethrin
Cyfluthrin	Phenothrin
Cypermethrin	Pyrethrin I
Deltamethrin	Resmethrin
Fenvalerate	Tetramethrin

cide activity. They are generally considered more toxic than the pyrethrins.

N,N-diethyl-*m*-toluamide (Deet), an insect repellent, has been used with fenvalerate, a pyrethroid, sometimes resulting in disturbances of the CNS.[62] Insect growth regulators such as methoprene and fenoxycarb mimic and interfere with hormones of the insect. They pose minimal hazard to cats and are often combined with the pyrethrins.

Problems that occur with these compounds are generally mild and usually involve product misuse, but occult preexisting medical problems account for some.

Onset of clinical signs is generally abrupt (30 minutes to several hours) and is rarely delayed beyond 24 hours. After dermal application the most commonly reported clinical sign in cats is foaming or drooling from the mouth, which often follows the cat's grooming itself. Shivering is frequently recognized and may be due to hypothermia. It is very important to distinguish between shivering, muscle tremors, and seizures, since owners often have difficulty doing so. Vomiting and diarrhea can also follow acute exposure. Depression and lethargy, along with anorexia of several days' duration after a toxic exposure, are less common sequelae. Cats may exhibit hyperesthesia, restlessness, and hiding for several days after an exposure.

Appropriate clinical signs following recent exposure are the predominant criteria used to gain a diagnosis. Ante- or post mortem, laboratory sudmission is relatively ineffective at confirming more than exposure to the product.

The most common treatment for cats presented for hypersalivation and shivering is a lukewarm mild detergent bath followed by thorough drying with a towel. A cat presented having seizures or tremors may be treated according to guidelines in Table 62–2. Maintenance of a patent airway is also a priority. After the cat has been stabilized, a bath with a mild detergent soap should remove a majority of the insecticide and carriers. Repeated doses of activated charcoal and a cathartic with first dose of charcoal are indicated for animals that exhibit moderate to severe CNS signs. Atropine is not antidotal and is not indicated unless severe bradycardia or significant respiratory distress results from increased secretions. Further treatment includes symptomatic and supportive care (maintaining proper body temperature, hydration, and parenteral nutrition if necessary).

Cats appear to be especially sensitive to permethrin, and possibly to other pyrethroids. Neurologic signs frequently seen with permethrin toxicosis include tremor, depression, seizure, and ataxia and incoordination.[63] Several products on the market to which cats are commonly exposed are labeled solely for dogs. A cat can be adversely affected by playing with and biting a dog in an area where permethrin has been applied. Most problems, however, result from extralabel use of the products. Therefore, the clinician and staff should be vigilant in urging owners against extralabel use of canine products on cats. Treatment is the same for the pyrethrins but it may have to be continued longer.

Rotenone

Rotenone, an insecticide used on crops and animals, is more toxic than the pyrethrins. For animal use it is found in flea dips, sprays, and powders. Flea dips containing rotenone should be diluted with more water for cats than for dogs and should not be used on kittens. Rotenone is metabolized in the liver and should not be used on animals whose liver function is compromised. Rotenone dips used in higher concentrations than specified on the label are believed to cause many of the problems seen in cats. Clinical signs of toxicosis can include hypersalivation, vomiting, depression, hypothermia, ataxia and incoordination, muscle tremors or fasciculations, seizures, and dypsnea. Diagnosis is based on appearance of appropriate clinical signs following exposure.

After the animal is stabilized, removal of the insecticide with a lukewarm bath with a mild detergent soap is the required treatment. Maintenance of a patent airway and oxygen therapy may be necessary for dyspneic patients. Cats with muscle tremors or fasciculations should be treated with diazepam IV, starting at doses of 2.5 mg and given to effect. Symptomatic and supportive care should follow initial lifesaving measures (maintaining proper body temperature, hydration, and parenteral nutrition if necessary).

Boric Acid

Boric acid is used alone or in combination as an insecticide for control of roaches, ants, and flies. It has also been recommended for use in feline litter boxes and elsewhere because of its weak fungistatic and bacteriostatic effects.[64] Cats are often exposed by walking through dust put down for insects. Subsequent grooming to remove the dust from their paws results in ingestion. How much boric acid must be ingested to initiate toxicosis is not well-documented for cats, but no deaths or serious systemic effects were observed in dogs given 0.5 to 1.4 g/lb boric acid PO. Most of the dogs vomited; however, repeated small doses of boric acid tend to be more toxic than a single large dose.[64] Boric acid is also concentrated in the kidneys before excretion. The kidneys are the organs most damaged by ingestion of very large amounts. Renal excretion is comparatively slow.[65]

The most common clinical sign of acute exposure is vomiting. Other common signs include hypersalivation, diarrhea, depression, and anorexia. Less common signs are weakness, ataxia, tremors, seizures, and bloody stool. Signs rarely progress beyond those listed, but additional clinical signs may be seen with chronic ingestion.

Diagnosis is based on known exposure and on clinical signs compatible with toxicosis. Laboratory analysis for boric acid is possible but it confirms only exposure. Tissue levels associated with toxicosis have not been well-established in cats.

If the animal is not already vomiting emesis is recommended. Activated charcoal is not as effective for boric acid ingestion, and it must be administered in five to ten times the usual recommended dose, according to studies in vitro.[64] Diazepam should be administered IV to effect for seizure or tremor control (see Table 62–3). Symptomatic and supportive care should include fluid diuresis and gastrointestinal protectants.

d-Limonene

d-Limonene is a natural oil extract of citrus fruits. It is insecticidal and is an ingredient in shampoos, sprays, and dips for animal use. *d*-Limonene may be found alone or combined with other insecticides or insecticide synergists. Cats are very tolerant of *d*-limonene alone but may be more susceptible to products containing *d*-limonene plus other insecticides or synergists. Cats treated with *d*-limonene at 15 times the recommended concentration in the final dip solution survived with no supportive or detoxification treatment, though they did display temporary signs of toxicosis.[66] Combination products containing *d*-limonene may be much more toxic, producing serious clinical signs or death at similar concentrations or slightly above that of *d*-limonene by itself. These formulations, however, are usually diluted to the right concentration for spraying, which reduces the chance of overdosing the animal.[66]

The most frequently recognized clinical sign when *d*-limonene is used alone is hypersalivation, which lasts 15 minutes to 1 hour and may be independent of other symptoms. Cats with more severe signs may exhibit mild to moderate muscle tremors that resemble shivering, beginning approximately 30 minutes after treatment and lasting as long as 4 hours. These cats may also develop mild to extremely severe ataxia. Hypothermia may also be seen in animals treated with concentrations that elicit tremors or severe ataxia. Male cats dipped with a concentrated solution of *d*-limonene may have areas of erythema or excoriation on the scrotal skin, as a result of licking to relieve dermal irritation.[57] Diagnosis is based primarily on known exposure to products containing *d*-limonene and on clinical signs consistent with toxicosis from *d*-limonene, with or without other insecticides or synergists.

Decontamination is the primary therapy for cats that show clinical signs of *d*-limonene poisoning. A lukewarm bath with a mild detergent soap should be used to remove any remaining dermal insecticide, along with symptomatic and supportive care. Special mention needs to be made of hypothermia and its treatment. Diligent monitoring and maintenance of the cat's body temperature near normal are necessary, as studies have shown animals to become hypothermic when they are exposed to higher than recommended concentrations of *d*-limonene.[67]

Pennyroyal Oil

Pennyroyal oil is related to turpentine and is sometimes marketed as an insect repellent or herbal fragrance.[68] Owners have been known to apply the oil directly to the animal's coat or to place on it a collar impregnated with pennyroyal and other essential oils (citrus, citronella, eucalyptus, and bay—all also potentially toxic). Pennyroyal oil exerts its primary toxic effects on the central nervous system, kidneys, and liver.[69] Typical clinical signs include hypersalivation, vomiting, diarrhea, depression, anorexia, ataxia and incoordination, weakness, and hypothermia.

The potential for aspiration of oil should discourage use of emesis for decontamination. Activated charcoal and a cathartic are indicated with this toxicosis also. Removing pennyroyal oil from the skin with a lukewarm bath in a mild detergent soap is essential. *N*-acetyl cysteine has been used experimentally to try to prevent liver damage from pennyroyal oil and its metabolites. Acetylcysteine appears to have a wide margin of safety, so administration presents little toxic hazard relative to the potential benefits.[69] Symptomatic and supportive care should occur in conjunction with the above-mentioned treatments.

Plants

Plant toxicoses are less common in cats than in other species. Being carnivores, more finicky eaters, and often being restricted to life indoors, cats generally are not exposed to as many toxic plants. Nevertheless, their habit of chewing on grasses and other plants can predispose them to ingest such plants, especially indoor cats that are exposed to plants only periodically. The playful nature of cats also increases plant exposure, as they like to play with dangling leaves and often bite or eat them. The most common feline plant exposure inquiries received at the NAPCC are listed in Table 62–7. The following review of poisonous plants that may be of concern in feline practice is not comprehensive, so plants not specifically mentioned should *not* be considered nontoxic.

Nontoxic Plants

Many indoor and outdoor plants are considered nontoxic to cats, but the fact is that many of them have never actually been tested on cats (see Easter lily and tiger lily below). A great number of indoor plants currently are considered nontoxic to cats, but even "nontoxic" plants have the potential to cause them gastrointestinal upset since green plant material is foreign material to a carnivore's digestive tract. Physical irritation by ingested plant material is generally thought to account for the digestive upset caused by nontoxic plants. In some cases of digestive upset associated with nontoxic plant ingestion, no treatment is necessary, but demulcents such as kaolin-pectin preparations (0.5 to 1.0 mL/lb every 2 to 12 hours) may decrease the duration of clinical signs.

Table 62–7. Plants Most Commonly Involved in Exposure Inquiries at NAPCC, 1990–1991

Common Name	Scientific Name
Althea*	*Hibiscus* spp.
Azalea	*Rhododendron* spp.
Chinese evergreen	*Aglaonema modestum*
Cyclamen	*Cyclamen* spp.
Dumbcane	*Diefenbachia* spp.
Easter lily	*Lilium longiflorum*
English ivy	*Hedera helix*
Catnip	*Nepeta cataria*
Peace lily	*Spathiphyllum* spp.
Philodendron	*Philodendron* spp.
Poinsettia	*Euphorbia pulcherrima*

*Nontoxic

Catnip

Catnip (*Nepeta cataria*) is a plant of the mint family that is frequently used in cat toys. Cats appear to be attracted to the plant or plant material, and some display altered neurologic activity after exposure. Neurologic effects are generally seen with inhalation exposure to the aromatics of the plant, but ingestion of the plant produces only the mild gastric upset typical of "nontoxic" plants. The active principle for catnip does not appear to be neuroactive when ingested. The absence of neurologic effects when ingested could be explained by poor gastrointestinal absorption or extensive first-pass liver metabolism. The active principle of catnip is thought to be a constituent of the plant's volatile oil, neptalactone, and to be chemically similar to that of a sedative compound in *Valerion* species.[70]

The clinical presentation of inhalation exposure to catnip varies from sedative to excitatory. Some cats exposed to catnip, actually become aggressive,[71] but the most common effects include mild depression, rolling, mild ataxia, and an almost euphoric appearance. Clinical signs associated with catnip exposure generally require no specific therapy, owing to their short duration. Removing the source of exposure and keeping the cat undisturbed usually result in a return to normal within 1 to 2 hours.

Easter Lily and Tiger Lily

Both Easter lily (*Lilium longiflorum*) and tiger lily (*Lilium tigrinum*) have been considered nontoxic plants, but findings at the NAPCC and subsequent research indicate they are nephrotoxic to cats.[72,73] During 1990 the NAPCC handled five cases of Easter lily ingestion in cats. All experienced renal failure and died or were euthanized. In the five 1990 cases ingestion of leaves or flowers was incriminated; the number of leaf ingested ranged from three to ten per cat. Analysis of the prior year's data also indicated a high incidence of clinical signs that were associated with renal failure, but follow-up information was not available for most of those cases. Subsequent evaluation of tiger lily cases revealed an identical syndrome.

Common clinical signs associated with ingestion of Easter- or tiger lily are associated with renal failure and gastritis. Cats begin vomiting within a few minutes to hours after ingestion, but this subsides after 6 to 12 hours. Anorexia, also a prominent finding, persists for the duration of the syndrome. By 24 to 72 hours after exposure the cats again began vomiting and develop severe dehydration, anuria, and increased creatinine, potassium, phosphorus, and BUN values. Experimentally, evidence of renal damage is seen as early as 12 hours after exposure with the onset of polyuria and dehydration. Urine is generally found to be isothenuric containing numerous tubular epithelial casts, protein, and glucose. Death due to renal failure or euthanasia generally occurs by 3 to 6 days after exposure. Histopathologic evaluation reveals congestion in the liver and lung, but the predominant finding is extensive renal tubule necrosis. It has been observed that a few tubular epithelial cells contained mitotic figures, and the basement membrane appeared still to be intact.

To date, successful treatment protocols necessitate early intervention. When decontamination was accomplished by 6 hours after exposure and fluid diuresis was maintained at least 24 hours, the survival rate was 100%. On the other hand, cases that had progressed past 18 to 24 hours before the animal was presented for treatment were not successfully treated. In a single case of survival after the onset of renal failure it was found that daily peritoneal dialysis of two weeks' duration resulted in return to normal of all urinary parameters and clinical condition. At autopsy histologic evidence of beginning regeneration of the renal tubule epithelium supported peritoneal dialysis as a treatment after the onset of renal failure.

Oxalate Plants

Plant oxalate can occur as soluble oxalic acid or insoluble calcium oxalate crystals. The insoluble calcium oxalate crystals are found in many common houseplants (see Table 62–8). Plant-derived insoluble calcium oxalate crystals are different from those seen microscopically in urine sediment. Plant oxalate crystals are sharp and needlelike. Although oxalate plants generally contain *either* the soluble or insoluble form, there is evidence that some plants contain both.[6]

Clinical manifestations of calcium oxalate crystal toxicosis are generally limited to the oral cavity and digestive tract. The crystals, being sharp, tend to penetrate mucosal surfaces, resulting in irritation, pain, and swelling. There have also been indications of a histamine component to the swelling.[74] This toxicosis can present as oropharyngeal irritation and swelling with salivation or gastrointestinal irritation and swelling with accompanying vomiting and diarrhea, or both. Rarely, oral swelling can result in airway obstruction and dyspnea.

Oxalic acid toxicosis presents as renal failure. Oxalic acid is absorbed and binds to circulating calcium, which is filtered and precipitated in the renal tubules. The resulting calcium oxalate crystals are the same as those seen in ethylene glycol toxicosis. Clinical signs result from renal failure, and possibly hypocalcemia.

Treatment of calcium oxalate crystal toxicosis is aimed at decreasing the irritation and swelling. The oral cavity should be washed thoroughly to remove any remaining plant material and free crystals. Steroids and antihistamines should be given to decrease the swelling, but antihistamines have shown beneficial results in only a minority of the studies. Gastrointestinal demulcents, such as kaolin-pectin prep-

Table 62–8. Common Plants That Contain Calcium Oxalate Crystals

Common Name	Scientific Name
Caladium	*Caladium* spp.
Calla or arum lily	*Zantedeschia aethiopica*
Cuckoo pint	*Arum maculatum*
Dumbcane	*Dieffenbachia* spp.
Elephant's ear	*Alocasia* or *Colocasia*
Jack-in-the-pulpit	*Arisaema triphyllum*
Malanga	*Xanthosoma* spp.
Mother-in-law plant	*Monstera* spp.
Peace lily	*Spathiphyllum* spp.
Philodendron	*Philodendron* spp.
Pothos or devil's ivy	*Epiprenum* spp.

arations (0.5 to 1.0 mL/lb every 2 to 12 hours) may help decrease the irritation to the gastric mucosa. The clinical course usually lasts 2 to 6 hours, but it can persist several days. Since there is at least some evidence that these plants may also contain oxalic acid, feeding milk provides a calcium source that can bind the free oxalic acid to produce insoluble complexes that cannot be absorbed.

Gastrointestinal Irritants

The poinsettia plant (*Euphorbia pulcherrima*) was long considered a very toxic plant, but this is no longer accepted. Review of the literature finds that its reputation originated with a single case of a child who ingested poinsettia leaves and died.[74] Studies in rats, mice, and rabbits have not shown the plant to be particularly lethal. In cats it is common to see a syndrome of gastric upset following ingestion of poinsettia, but some cats show no effect. Clinical signs of vomiting, abdominal pain, and diarrhea can occur. A gastric demulcent such as a kaolin-pectin preparation (0.5 to 1.0 mL/lb every 2 to 12 hours) is generally all that is required to treat more severely affected cats, but they should be watched for possible secondary dehydration.

Both English ivy (*Hedera helix*) and cyclamen (*Cyclamen* species) can cause severe gastrointestinal effects in cats. Both plants contain complex saponins that produce a very profound gastrointestinal effect as well as systemic ones. Although the entire plant can be toxic, the most toxic portion of cyclamen is the tuber; for English ivy it is the fruits and seeds. The primary effects can include profuse vomiting, salivation, hematemasis, diarrhea with or without blood, anorexia, and abdominal pain.[74-77] Death from ingestion of large amounts is reportedly due to secondary complications of the gastroenteritis or respiratory collapse. Depression and coma may also follow ingestion of significant amounts.

For cyclamen or English ivy ingestion early decontamination is performed when possible. Once clinical signs appear demulcents, such as kaolin-pectin mixtures at 0.5 to 1.0 mL/lb every 2 to 12 hours, are indicated, as well as fluid and electrolyte replacement. Death is not common, but prolonged support may be required.

Cardiotoxic Plants

The azaleas (*Rhododendron* species) are very toxic and ingestion of only a small amount produces a profound effect. The azaleas contain a cardiac glycoside, grananotoxins, and the signs much resemble those of an overdose of digoxin.[74-76,78] The leaves, flowers, stems, roots, and nectar from the flowers are toxic. Even honey produced from the nectar has been reported to be toxic. With marginal exposure the primary clinical effects are vomiting and diarrhea, but salivation is also common. When larger amounts are ingested bradycardia, hypotension, arrhythmias, shock, dyspnea, tremors, seizures, and cardiac failure can result. The cause of death, cardiac failure, is due to sustained depolarization of myocardial cells.

Treatment of cardiac glycoside toxicosis includes decontamination (see Table 62–3) and reversal of the cardiac effects. Because of the potency of grananotoxin, azalea ingestion warrants gastric lavage even if spontaneous emesis has occurred. Activated charcoal should be instilled into the stomach after the lavage (1 gm/lb). Monitoring cardiac function is imperative. Bradycardia, and to some degree hypotension, are responsive to atropine, but it should be utilized only when clinical signs indicate the need. The clinical syndrome generally persists 24 to 36 hours.

Preliminary findings at the NAPCC indicate that the digoxin antibody used to treat human digoxin overdose may have some cross-reactivity with other cardiac glycosides. In ingestions that should have been lethal to both dogs and goats, they were saved by the use of this monoclonal antibody. The dose, however, has not been determined for domestic animals (nor for nondigoxin cardiac glycosides), and the drug is very expensive. For animals that do not respond to general treatment it may be of value.

Ethylene Glycol

Ethylene glycol (1,2-ethylene diol) is odorless, colorless, and viscous with a sweet to bittersweet taste. Most commercial antifreeze preparations contain 95 to 97% ethylene glycol. Ethylene glycol undergoes no significant degradation over time in an automotive coolant system,[79] and most automobile manufacturers recommend a 50% solution. Poisonings are more frequent during the colder months, although problems are encountered year-round. Cats are thought to be less likely than dogs (by 25 to 50%) to become intoxicated, although variables such as environment and ownership may influence exposure potential.[80]

Following ingestion, ethylene glycol is assumed to be rapidly absorbed, since clinical CNS depression occurs within 30 minutes. Peak blood levels occur at 3 hours in cats.[80] It is metabolized principally in the liver, and toxic metabolites are formed. Alcohol dehydrogenase converts ethylene glycol to glycoaldehyde, which is very potent but very unstable. Glycoaldehyde is metabolized to glycolic acid, which constitutes 30 to 45% of the approximately dozen or so metabolites (such as oxalic acid, formic acid, benzoic acid, hippuric acid).[81] Glycolic acid is more toxic than ethylene glycol, is fairly stable and slowly excreted, and is primarily responsible for the very high anion gap.[80,82] Cats produce more oxalic acid than some other species and are very prone to form urinary oxalate crystals. Ethylene glycol is filtered by the glomeruli and passively reabsorbed by the distal convoluted tubules and collecting ducts.[82] For untreated cats, the serum half-life of ethylene glycol is 2 to 5 hours; for cats treated with ethanol 3 hours after being given lethal oral doses of ethylene glycol it is 29 hours. Thus, early treatment of ethanol ingestion in cats significantly increases the amount of unchanged ethylene glycol excreted in the urine and the time frame (up to 72 hours or longer) in which elimination is accomplished.[80] The minimum lethal dose for cats is reported to be 0.6 mL/lb of concentrated (commercial) ethylene glycol.[80-82] Thus, the average 8- to 10-lb cat could receive a potentially lethal dose by ingesting approximately 1 teaspoon of a concentrated commercial antifreeze preparation. This lethal dose compares to 0.7 mL/lb for humans and 2.0 to 3.0 mL/lb for dogs.[80-82]

Common findings in untreated cats are listed in Table 62–9. Other than causing CNS depression, vomiting, and osmotic diuresis, prior to catabolism ethylene glycol does not have major acute toxic effects. It is the parent metabo-

Table 62–9. Common Findings in Untreated Cats with Ethylene Glycol Poisoning[80,83-85]

Clinical Signs

Vomiting within 30–60 minutes
Depresssion, ataxia, disorientation, anorexia, panting within 3 hours
Hypothermia within 9 hours

Hematologic Findings

CBC: Mature neutrophilia, lymphopenia, increased total PCV, but may be unremarkable over 72 hours
Total protein: Increased
Hyperglycemia: Within 3 to 9 hours; may be marked
Hypocalcemia: Within 6 to 9 hours; may be marked
BUN and creatinine: Increased above normal range by 12 hours; may continue slow rise with treatment over 72 hours
Serum potassium: Increased above normal by 9 hours
Serum phosphorus: Steady to marked increase by 12 hours
Anion gap: Increases above normal by 6 hours; remains elevated without treatment but decreases with early treatment
Osmolal gap: Increases above normal by 1 hour; remains elevated through 72-hour treatment period
Metabolic acidosis: By 6 to 9 hours
Blood pH: Decreased by 1–2 hours
Serum HCO_3: Decreased by 1–2 hours
Serum ethylene glycol concentration: Peaks at 3 hours, then declines sharply to steadily over 48–72 hours; concentration is dose and treatment dependent

Urine Findings

Specific gravity: Less than 1.020 within 3 hours; approaches isosthenuria (1.008 to 1.012) by 6–12 hours
Calcium oxalate crystals: May be seen within 6 hours; may be none or many, with several forms present
Granular casts, renal epithelial cells: May be few to none
Glucose: May detect trace (with elevated serum glucose)
Hematuria: May see at 3–4 hours

lites that are responsible for the various associated pathophysiologic changes. Initially, vomiting is due to direct gastric irritation and activation of the chemoreceptor trigger zone by the parent compound. Late in the course of toxicity it is due to metabolite-induced uremia. Early vomition is often absent from the clinical history. Early CNS effects resemble those of alcohol intoxication in humans and include dose-related degrees of staggering, stupor, delerium, depression, and weakness. With clinical progression, tachypnea, tachycardia, miosis, vocalization, tremors, seizures, or coma may occur. Stages and signs can overlap or wax and wane throughout the course. Dogs typically exhibit early diuretic-induced polyuria and polydipsia, but cats may not. Dehydration may be fairly marked, and the patient may present with an empty bladder. Hypothermia is the norm, but hyperthermia may be associated with muscle or seizure activity. In essentially all cases blood values reveal increased BUN and creatinine; most reveal elevated phosphorus and glucose levels and decreased calcium levels; and fewer cats have a low level of chloride and elevated potassium. Oxalate crystalluria may be noted early, but multiple samples may be needed before crystals are found. The crystals are not limited to one shape or type, and mixed forms are often noted. In untreated cases, vomition, anuria, abdominal pain, seizure, coma, or death ensue by 18 to 24 hours. The renal dysfunction during this time is probably due to the direct cytotoxic effects of the ethylene glycol metabolites on the renal tubule epithelium.[80] Many patients are admitted in acute renal failure. Postmortem lesions may reveal gastric hyperemia, petechiation, and renal edema. Renal histopathology is fairly diagnostic of oxalate nephrosis. Also, renal tissue calcium concentrations in poisoned animals are generally well above the norm for cats and dogs. Elevated renal calcium concentrations (above 4000 ppm) generally is noted with ethylene glycol and cholecalciferol intoxication.[86]

The osmolal gap and the anion gap are being used more frequently as diagnostic aids, because ethylene glycol toxicosis is one of the few clinical conditions (including diabetic ketoacidosis and methanol intoxication) that causes both a high osmolal gap and high anion gap metabolic acidosis.[80] The osmolal gap is a reflection of the presence in serum of an osmotically active substance not normally found there. It is expressed thus:

$$\text{Osmolal gap} = (\text{measured osmolality}) - (\text{calculated osmolality})^*$$

The osmolal gap increases by 1 hour after ingestion, owing to the influence of osmotically active ethylene glycol and its metabolites, and it remains significantly increased through 72 hours. The magnitude of the increase in serum osmolality is directly proportional to the dose of ethylene glycol ingested.[80] Normal serum osmolality is 280 to 310 mOsm/kg water, and the normal gap is 5 to 10 mOsm/kg water in dogs and cats. An osmolal gap value greater than 10 mOsm should arouse suspicion of ethylene glycol intoxication. Gap values as high as 60 to 100 mOsm are noted. Other disorders that contribute to elevated serum osmolality are ketoacidotic diabetes mellitus, severe lactic acidosis, and other toxicoses: alcohol (ethanol, methanol, isopropanol), mannitol, sorbitol (e.g., in various commercial liquid activated charcoal preparations), iodinated intravenous contrast media, ethyl ether, and trichloroethane.

The anion gap is the difference between the measured cations and the measured anions in the serum:

$$\text{Anion gap} = (Na^+ + K^+) - (HCO_3 + Cl^-)$$

The gap value represents the unmeasured anions normally present in serum (proteins, organic adds, sulfates, phosphates). In ethylene glycol intoxication the anion gap rises above the normal value, owing to accumulation in blood of acid metabolites of ethylene glycol, principally glycolic acid. The normal anion gap is 10 to 25 mEq/L, but it can be as

*A local laboratory will need a serum sample to determine measured osmolality. Calculated osmolality is derived using the equation:

$$\frac{1.86\,(Na^+ + K^+) + \text{glucose}}{18} + \frac{\text{BUN}}{2.9} + 9.0$$

great as 40 mEq with ethylene glycol toxicosis. Other causes to be considered when the anion gap is elevated are methanol, salicylate, or paraldehyde intoxication, diabetic ketoacidosis, and lactic acidosis.

Commercial ethylene glycol test kits are available for use in veterinary practice, and though they have their limitations, they can be a valuable aid in establishing a diagnosis. These kits, available through most major veterinary drug distributors, are cost effective and easy to use. One such test kit, Ethylene Glycol Test Kit, has a shelf life of 2 years, requires a minimum of 0.5 mL of blood, and costs about $9 per test. The test is strictly qualitative, but it is set to detect ethylene glycol in concentration of 50 mg/dL, the level that is used to establish a diagnosis of ethylene glycol intoxication in humans and dogs. Because this test was developed for use in dogs its sensitivity to lower levels of ethylene glycol that could be toxic to cats might be limited. Also, compounds such as formaldehyde and other *cis* 1,2-diols (such as propylene glycol) yield a false-positive result. Propylene glycol is contained in such medications as injectable diazepam and pentobarbital, in semimoist cat foods, and in some liquid activated charcoal preparations. Ethanol does not interfere with the test. Clinicians who have access to a local hospital or other laboratory with mechanized analytic capabilities for ethylene glycol may want to arrange to have standing access to such capabilities. Otherwise, the ethylene glycol test kit can augment the workup.

Successful treatment is directed at early interruption of the initial step in metabolism (considering early peak time), which would allow ethylene glycol to be excreted unchanged through the kidneys. When early detection of ingestion occurs, activated charcoal with a saline cathartic should be administered PO. In dogs, 4-methylpyrazole has been used with greater success (over ethanol) as a blocking agent. However, controlled studies in cats show 4-methylpyrazole to be significantly less effective than ethanol. Therefore, it cannot be recommended as an alternative to ethanol in cats, even though ethanol treatment of intoxicated cats has proven less than satisfactory.[80] The recommended dose for cats is 2.3 mL/lb of 20% ethanol in saline, IV or IP, every 6 hours for five treatments then every 8 hours for four treatments.[85] It is important to remember that, like ethylene glycol, ethanol causes direct CNS depression, increased hyperosmolality, and osmotic diuresis. The established dose for ethanol should be regarded only as a guide; it may need to be adjusted for the individual case. Sodium bicarbonate is used to treat the metabolic acidosis that accompanies the intoxication. If at all possible, the clinician should obtain blood gas values, or at the least a serum bicarbonate level. (Total CO_2 can approximate.) The amount of bicarbonate (in milliequivalents) to be given the patient is calculated from the base deficit:

$$0.5 \times \text{body weight (kg)} \times (24 - \text{plasma } HCO_3 \text{ [mEq/L]})$$

If possible, the base excess should be determined again prior to any additional bicarbonate administration. If laboratory assistance is not available, the published dose of 5% sodium bicarbonate in saline may be administered IV or intraperitoneally (IP).[83] The interval and duration are the same as for ethanol, but again it is important that these doses serve only as guides; they likely will need to be adjusted as the case evolves. Fluid therapy should be aggressive and strict attention should be paid to maintaining urine output and preventing overhydration. Furosemide can be used to enhance excretion of ethylene glycol. Mannitol, if used, interferes with osmolal data, as does the ethanol treatment. Peritoneal dialysis has been used successfully to enhance removal of ethylene glycol, and it should be considered in any situation. Hemoperfusion is used routinely in human medicine but currently is less practical than peritoneal dialysis in veterinary medicine. Pyridoxine and thiamine are cofactors in the metabolic pathway and, hypothetically, could enhance the outcome to an unknown degree.

The window of opportunity for successful treatment of ethylene glycol toxicity occurs early and is rather narrow. This necessitates rapid diagnosis and early aggressive intervention to ensure optimal case management and outcome. The ingested dose of ethylene glycol and the time lapse before beginning treatment are significant determinants of recovery success. The difference between beginning treatment at 4 hours versus 8 hours post-ingestion may make a significant difference in the patient's final outcome.[83] A poor to grave prognosis is indicated when the patient is presented more than 12 hours after ingestion, when BUN and creatinine values are elevated, or when the patient does not show improvement after 24 hours of aggressive treatment. Late-stage ethylene glycol poisoning can be treated, but results are usually disappointing. Cats that recover following early intervention and treatment should be monitored for a minimum of 1 to 2 weeks for evidence of renal insufficiency. A portion of the patients experience complete recovery, and another portion develop some degree of compensated renal failure. Ingested dose, time of clinical presentation, follow-up clinical data, age, and previous health status must all be factored in to arrive at a reasonable prognosis. Patients with variable chronic renal damage are often manageable and should be considered for salvage.

REFERENCES

1. Wilson J. Personal communication. 1991.
2. Fitzpatrick FK, Crowe DT. Nasal oxygen administration in dogs and cats: Experimental and clinical investigations. J Am Anim Hosp Assoc 1986;22:293.
3. Atkins CE, Johnson RK. Clinical toxicities of cats. Vet Clin North Am 1975;5:623.
4. Gelman CJE, Connor CS. Rational Use of Antidotes. In: Bayer MJ, Rumack BH, Wanke LA, eds. Toxicological Emergencies. Bowie, MD Brady Co, 1989:69.
5. Mount ME. Toxicology. In: Ettinger SJ, ed. Textbook of Veterinary Internal Medicine. 3rd ed. Philadelphia: WB Saunders Co, 1989:456.
6. Wanke LA. Prevention of Absorption. In: Bayer Rumack BH, Wanke, LA, eds. Toxicological Emergencies. Bowie, MD: Brady Co, 1984:37.
7. Beasley VR, Dorman DC. Management of toxicoses. Vet Clin North Am, Small Anim Pract 1990;20:307.
8. Haddad LM, Roberts JR. A General Approach to the Emergency Management of Poisoning. In: Clinical Management of Poison-

ing and Drug Overdose. 2nd ed. Philadelphia: WB Saunders Co, 1990:14.

9. Jenkins WL. Drugs Acting on the Digestive System. In: Booth NH, McDonald LE, eds. Veterinary Pharmacology and Therapeutics. 6th ed. Ames, IA: Iowa State University Press, 1988:657.
10. Buck WB, Osweiler GD, Van Gelder GA. Management and Treatment of Toxicoses. In: Buck WB, Osweilor GD, Van Gelder GA, eds. Clinical and Diagnostic Veterinary Toxicology. 3rd ed. Dubuque, IA: Kendall/Hunt, 1985:23.
11. Mount ME, Woody BJ, Murphy MJ. The Anticoagulant Rodenticides. In: Kirk RW, ed. Current Veterinary Therapy IX, Small Animal Practice. Philadelphia: WB Saunders Co, 1986:156.
12. Mount ME. Diagnosis and Therapy of Anticoagulant Rodenticides. Vet Clin North Am (Small Anim Pract) 1988;18:115.
13. Beasley VR, Buck WB. Warfarin and Other Anticoagulant Poisonings. In: Kirk RW, ed. Current Veterinary Therapy VIII, Small Animal Practice. Philadelphia: WB Saunders Co, 1983:101.
14. Murphy M, Gerkin D. The Anticoagulant Rodenticides. In: Kirk RW, ed. Current Veterinary Therapy X. Philadelphia: WB Saunders Co, 1989:1430.
15. Osweiler GD, Carson TL, Buck WB, Van Gelder GA. Rodenticides. In: Osweiler GD, Carson TL, Buck WB, Van Gelder GA, eds. Clinical and Diagnostic Veterinary Toxicology. 3rd ed. Dubuque, IA: Kendall/Hunt, 1985:327.
16. Dorman DC. Anticoagulant, cholecalciferol, and bromethalin-based rodenticides. Vet Clin North Am (Small Anim Pract) 1990;20:339.
17. Dodd WJ. Bleeding Disorders. In August JR, ed. Consultations in Feline Internal Medicine. 1st ed. Philadelphia: WB Saunders Co, 1991:383.
18. Prier RF. Evaluation of the hazard of secondary poisoning by warfarin-poisoned rodents. J Am Vet Med Assoc 1961;140:351.
19. Rubin SI, Papich MG. Nonsteroidal Anti-inflammatory Drugs. In: Kirk RW, ed. Current Veterinary Therapy X. Philadelphia: WB Saunders Co, 1989:47.
20. Carothers M, Chew DJ. Management of cholecalciferol rodenticide toxicity. Compend Contin Educ 1991;13:1058.
21. Chew DJ, Carothers M. Hypercalcemia. Vet Clin North Am (Small Anim Pract) 1989;19:265.
22. Dorman DC, Parker AJ, Dye JA, Buck WA. Bromethalin neurotoxicosis in the cat. Prog Vet Neurol 1990;1:1898.
23. Dorman DC, Parker AJ, Buck WB. Bromethalin toxicosis in the dog. Part II: Selected treatments for the toxic syndrome. J Am Vet Med Assoc 1990;26:595.
24. Martin T, Johnson B. A suspected case of bromethalin toxicity in a domestic cat. Vet Human Toxicol 1989;3:2395.
25. Lovell RA. Ivermectin and Piperazine Toxicosis in Dogs and Cats. Vet Clin North Am (Small Anim Pract) 1990;20:453.
26. Barragry TB. A review of the pharmacology and clinical uses of ivermectin. Can Vet J 1987;28:512.
27. Bennett DG. Clinical pharmacology of ivermectin. J Am Vet Med Assoc 1986;189:100.
28. Song MD. Using ivermectin to treat feline dermatoses caused by external parasites. Vet Med 1991;86:498.
29. Bevier DE. Parasitic dermatoses in the dog and cat. I and II. In: Proceedings of the American Animal Hospital Association 57th Annual Meeting, Denver, CO, 1990:549.
30. Franc M, Dorchies PH, Soubeyroux H. Studies on the treatment of otocariasis in cats with ivermectin. Rev Med Vet 1985; 136: 683.
31. Houston D. Extralabel use of drugs. J Am Vet Med Assoc 1985;187:671.
32. Ray DE. Pesticides Derived from Plants and Other Organisms. In: Hayes WJ, ed. Handbook of Pesticide Toxicology. New York: Academic Press, 1991;2:622.
33. Hartigan PJ, Woolsicroft GJ. Piperazine toxicity. Vet Rec 1989;120:70.
34. Stoffman AE, Braithwaite A. Piperazine overdose in a kitten. Can Vet J 1976;17:140.
35. McEvoy GK. American Hospital Formulary Service Drug Information. 32nd ed. 1991:1185.
36. Scherkl R. Pharmokinetics of ibuprofen in the dog. J Vet Pharmacol Ther 1987;10:261.
37. Spyridakis LK, Bacia JJ, Barsanti JA. Ibuprofen toxicosis in a dog. J Am Vet Med Assoc 1986;188:918.
38. Kore AM. Ibuprofen. In: Kirk RW, ed. Current Veterinary Therapy XI. Philadelphia: WB Saunders Co, 1992:191.
39. Kore AM. Toxicology of nonsteroidal antiinflammatory drugs. Vet Clin North Am (Small Anim Pract) 1990;20:419.
40. Plumb DC. Veterinary Drug Handbook. 1st ed. White Bear Lake. Pharma Vet, 1991:152.
41. Cullison RF. Acetaminophen toxicosis in small animals: Clinical signs, mode of action and treatment. Compend Contin Educ 1984;6:315.
42. Hjelle JJ, Grauer GF. Acetaminophen toxicosis in dogs and cats. J Am Vet Med Assoc 1986;188:742.
43. Nash SL, Oehme FW. A review of acetaminophens effect on methemoglobin, glutathione and some related enzymes. Vet Human Toxicol 1984;26:123.
44. Savides MC, Oehme FW. Acetaminophen and its toxicity. J Appl Toxicol 1983;3:96.
45. Savides MC, Oehme FW, Nash SL, Leipold HW. The toxicity and biotransformation of single doses of acetaminophen in dogs and cats. Toxicol Appl Pharmacol 1984;74:26.
46. Anvik JO. Acetaminophen toxicosis in a cat. Can Vet J 1984; 25:445.
47. Gaunt SD, Baker DC, Green RA. Clinicopathologic evaluation of *N*-acetylcysteine therapy in acetaminophen toxicosis in the cat. Am J Vet Res 1981;42:1982.
48. Weiss DJ, McClay CB, Christopher MM, et al. Effects of propylene glycol–containing diets on acetaminophen-induced methemoglobinemia in cats. J Am Vet Med Assoc 1990;196:1816.
49. Finco DR, Duncan JR, Schall WD, Prasse KW. Acetaminophen toxicosis in the cat. J Am Vet Med Assoc 1975;166:469.
50. Savides MC, Oehme FW, Leipold HW. Effects of various antidotal treatments on acetaminophen toxicosis and biotransformation in cats. Am J Vet Res 1985;46:1485.
51. St. Omer VV, McKnight ED. Acetylcysteine for treatment of acetaminophen toxicosis in the cat. J Am Vet Med Assoc 1980; 176:911.
52. Bolyai J, Smith RP, Gray CT. Ascorbic acid and chemically induced methemoglobinemias. Toxicol Appl Pharmacol 1972; 21:176.
53. Tvedten H. Erythrocyte Disorders. In: Willard MD, Tvedten H, Turnwald GH, eds. Diagnosis by Laboratory Methods. Philadelphia: WB Saunders Co, 1989:47.
54. Cotter S, Holzworth J. Disorders of the Hematopoietic System. In: Holzworth J, ed. Diseases of the Cat: Medicine and Surgery. Vol. 1 Philadelphia: WB Saunders Co, 1987:758.
55. Davis LE, Westfall BA. Species differences in biotransformation and excretion of salicylate. Am J Vet Res 1972;33:1253.
56. Conlon PD. Nonsteroidal drugs used in the treatment of inflammation. Vet Clin North Am (Small Anim Pract) 1988;18: 1115.
57. Booth NM. Veterinary Pharmacology and Therapeutics. 6th ed. Ames, IA: Iowa State University Press, 1988:329.
58. Fikes JD. Organophosphorus and carbamate insecticides. Vet Clin North Am (Small Anim Pract) 1990;20:356.
59. Thomson WT. Agricultural Chemicals. Book 1. Fresno, CA: Thomson Publications, 1989:21.
60. Adams HR. Cholinergic Pharmacology: Autonomic Drugs. In: Booth NH, McDonald LE, eds. Veterinary Pharmacology and Therapeutics. 6th ed. Ames, IA: Iowa State University Press, 1988:128.

61. Ecobichon DJ. Toxic Effects of Pesticides. In: Amdur MO, Doull J, Klaassen CD, eds. Casarett and Doull's Toxicology: The Basic Science of Poisons. 4th ed. New York: Pergamon Press, 1991: 592.
62. Dryden MW, Neal JJ. Concepts of flea control. Companion Anim Pract, Parasitol/Dermatol 1989;19:20.
63. Trammel HL, Buck WB. Tenth Annual Report of the Illinois Animal Poison Information Center. Vol. 2, Dubuque, IA: Kendall/Hunt Publishing, 1990:452.
64. Kiesche-Nesselrodt A, Hooser SB. Boric acid. Vet Clin North Am (Small Anim Pract) 1990;20 369.
65. Beasley VR, Dorman DC, Fikes JD. Boric Acid. In: Beasley VR, Dorman DC, Fikes JD. Boric Acid, eds. A Systems Affected Approach to Veterinary Toxicology. Urbana, IL: University of Illinois College of Veterinary Medicine, 1990:346.
66. Beasley VR, Dorman DC, Fikes JD. Citrus Oil Extracts. In: Beasley VR, Dorman DC, Fikes JD, eds. A Systems Affected Approach to Veterinary Toxicology. Urbana, IL: University of Illinois College of Veterinary Medicine, 1990:188.
67. Hooser SB. Effects of an insecticidal dip containing *d*-limonene in the cat. J Am Vet Med Assoc 1986;189:905.
68. Gunby P. Plants known for centuries still causes problems today. J Am Med Assoc 1979;241:2246.
69. Poisindex CD-ROM. Pennyroyal oil. Denver: Micromedex, 1991.
70. Poisindex CD-ROM. Catnip. Denver: Micromedex, 1991.
71. Diamond BL. The catnip mystique. Cat Fancy 1989;7:16.
72. Hall JO. Are Easter lilies toxic to cats? In: NAPI Net Report 1990;3(2):1.
73. Gathings AM. Acute renal failure in a cat: Was it the tiger lily? In: NAPI Net Report 1991;3(2):2.
74. Spoerke DG, Smolinske SC. Toxicity of Houseplants. 1st ed. Boca Raton, FL CRC Press, 1990.
75. Kingsbury JM. Poisonous Plants of the United States and Canada. Englewood Cliffs, NJ: Prentice-Hall, 1964.
76. Poisindex CD-ROM. English ivy. Denver: Micromedex, 1991.
77. Poisindex CD-ROM. Cyclamen. Denver: Micromedex, 1991.
78. Poisindex CD-ROM. Rhododendron. Denver: Micromedex, 1991.
79. McKenzie DA (Union Carbide, Inc.). Personal communication. 1986.
80. Dial SM. 4-Methylpyrazole as an antidote for ethylene glycol intoxication in dogs and cats. PhD dissertation, Colorado State University, 1988.
81. Poisindex CD-ROM. Glycols. Denver: Micromedex, 1991.
82. Beasley VR, Buck WB. Acute ethylene glycol toxicosis: A review. Vet Human Toxicol 1980;22:255.
83. Penumarthy L, Oehme FW. Treatment of ethylene glycol toxicosis in cats. Am J Vet Res 1975;36:209.
84. Thrall MA, Grauer GP, Kendall NM, et al. Clinicopathologic findings in dogs and cats with ethylene glycol intoxication. JAVMA 1984;184:37.
85. Grauer GF, Thrall MAH. Ethylene Glycol (Antifreeze) Poisoning. In: Kirk RW, ed. Current Veterinary Therapy X. Philadelphia: WB Saunders Co, 1986:206.
86. Poppenga RH, Braselton WE. Effective use of analytical laboratories. Vet Clin North Am (Small Anim Pract) 1990;20:304.

CHAPTER 63

◇ ◇ ◇

Upper Respiratory Infections

Gary D. Norsworthy

The sneezing cat has always been a common patient in veterinary practices. Several diseases may cause sneezing, including viral rhinitis, bacterial rhinitis, irritant and allergic rhinitis, nasopharyngeal polyps, nasal foreign bodies (Fig. 63–1, *A* and *B*), and nasal tumors. However, most sneezing cats have viral respiratory infections. At one time, sneezing cats were seen almost daily. However, since the introduction of vaccines against the major viral respiratory agents, the incidence of sneezing cats has dropped markedly.

Sneezing is the most common clinical sign seen in cats with viral upper respiratory diseases (URDs). Because most viral respiratory agents cause pathologic conditions involving the upper respiratory tract, the diseases they cause are commonly referred to as upper respiratory diseases (URDs) or upper respiratory infections (URIs). In this discussion, the terms URD and URI imply a viral etiology.

There are two distinct forms of URI in the cat. The acute form is associated with sneezing, conjunctivitis, fever, and frequently, anorexia. Acute URIs generally last about 1 week. The chronic form is a sequela of the acute form. It occurs because most recovered cats become viral carriers and have either chronic signs of URI or asymptomatic periods followed by periods of URI.

Etiologic Agents

More than 90% of feline URIs are caused by two viruses: feline herpesvirus I (FHV-I) (also known as the feline rhinotracheitis virus) and the feline calicivirus (FCV).[1] The feline reovirus and possibly some feline coronaviruses also cause URIs. Nonviral agents that may affect the upper respiratory tract include *Chlamydia psittaci* and *Cryptococcus neoformans.*

Rates of Infection

The infection rate for URIs varies greatly because of the numerous factors involved when any infectious agent challenges the cat's immune system. The most critical factor for URI in cats is their age. When maternal antibodies decline, a kitten becomes susceptible to challenges from viruses transmitted from cats with acute infections or from cats that are virus-shedding carriers. Kittens that are infected with viral respiratory agents at a very young age have high mortality rates. Most fatal infections occur in kittens that are 8 to 10 weeks of age.[2]

The second most important factor influencing the development of URIs in cats is population density. When several litters of kittens are housed with several adults, and the latter are viral carriers and chronic viral shedders, the infection rate will be very high. If URIs are a problem in multicat households or catteries, the kittens must be separated from the adult carriers until the kittens have completed an adequate vaccination program.

Other factors that affect the infection rate include the virulence of the viral strains present, the amount of the inoculum (degree of exposure), the level of sanitation (including proper ventilation), concomitant diseases (especially the feline leukemia virus [FeLV] and the feline immunodeficiency virus [FIV]), the cat's nutritional status, and the competence of the cat's immune system.[3] It should be noted that these factors are important determinants of infection rates for all infectious diseases.

Transmission

The two major viruses causing URIs in cats—FHV-I and FCV—may be transmitted in several ways. The most common mode of transmission is direct contact between cats. When an affected cat sneezes, the viral particles become aerosolized and may provide a source of infection for other cats in the immediate area. Macrodroplets deposited by sneezing may account for the spread of viral particles up to 4 feet away.[4] The viral particles may persist on fomites for short periods of time; therefore, proper cleaning and disinfecting are worthwhile efforts in preventing the spread of disease. In utero infections may occur as well.

In multicat households and catteries, the importance of carrier cats cannot be overemphasized. These cats provide a constant source of virus for kittens and newly acquired or visiting adults.[5]

Feline Viral Rhinotracheitis

Feline viral rhinotracheitis (FVR) is the disease caused by FHV-I. FHV-I replicates in the nasal turbinates, conjunctiva,

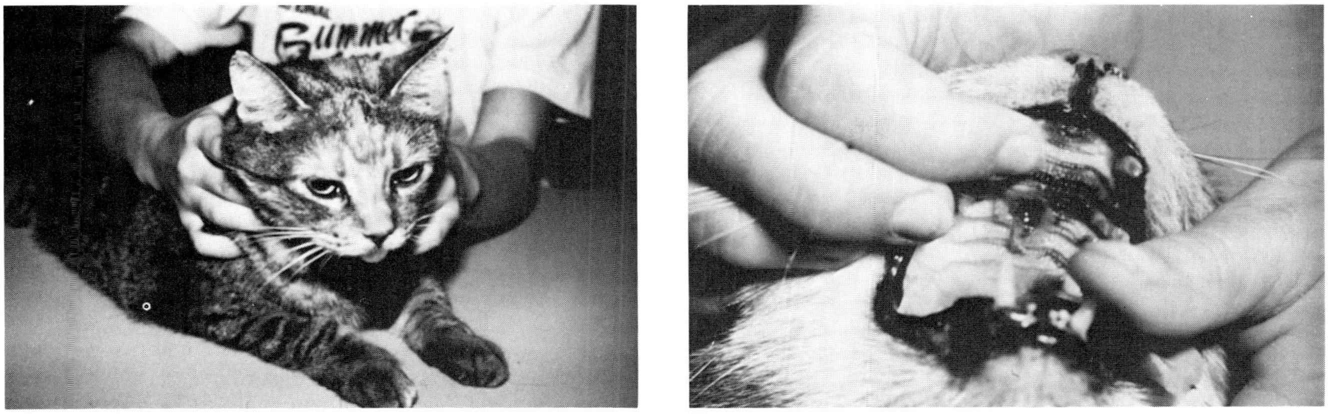

A B

Figure 63–1. (*A*) This cat was presented for an acute onset of sneezing. Although a URI is the most common cause of acute-onset sneezing, a thorough inspection of the mouth should be part of the physical examination. (*B*) A pellet was found in the hard palate of this cat. It had penetrated the nasal cavity and was causing sneezing. Its removal proved curative

cornea, soft palate, tonsils, and occasionally, in the trachea.[6] It may cause pathologic changes in all of these sites, as well as clinical signs relating to the affected tissues.

Clinical Signs

The clinical signs of FVR begin with sneezing and may include rhinitis, conjunctivitis (including corneal ulceration) (Figs. 63–2 and 63–3), and occasionally, tracheitis and bronchitis. Affected cats exhibit one or more of the following: fever, anorexia, thick ocular and/or nasal exudates, open-mouthed breathing, coughing, and rales. When kittens are affected in utero, they may exhibit these signs at birth or a few days thereafter. They generally die within 1 to 3 weeks.[6]

Sequelae

FHV-I affects the turbinate mucosa and the turbinate bones themselves. The damage done by the virus allows opportunistic bacteria, such as *Pseudomonas aeruginosa,* and opportunistic fungi, such as *C. neoformans,* to institute chronic infections in the maxillary and ethmoid turbinates. If these organisms ascend into the frontal sinuses, a chronic sinusitis may result. A chronic infection in either or both locations will result in the cat having a chronic, purulent nasal discharge and recurrent bouts of sneezing.[7] Chronic rhinitis and frontal sinusitis respond poorly to medical treatment, so surgical therapy is usually required (see Chapters 30 and 55).

Cats with corneal ulcers should be treated aggressively; otherwise, corneal penetration and panophthalmitis is likely (Fig. 63–4).

Carrier State

One of the characteristics of most herpes viruses is the development of a carrier state following an acute infection. This is also true of FHV-I. In one experimental study, 82% of affected unvaccinated cats became chronic carriers.[8] Al-

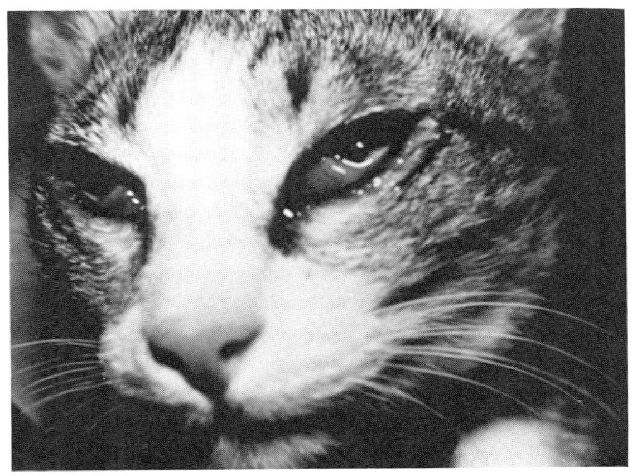

Figure 63–2. Conjunctivitis is a common finding in cats with URI secondary to FHV, FRV, feline respiratory coronavirus, or *Chlamydia psittaci* infection. It is not a typical finding in FCV infections.

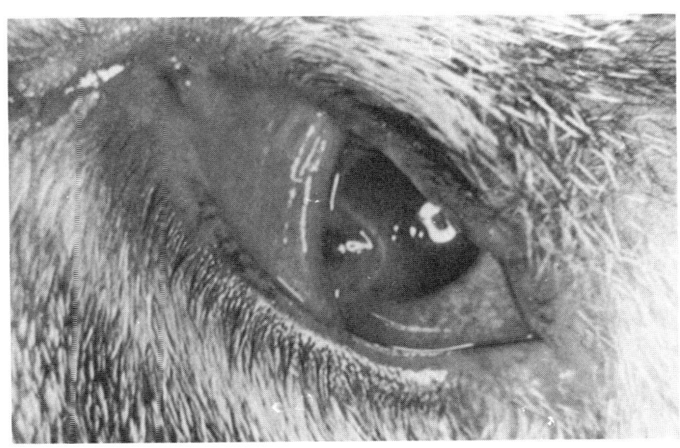

Figure 63–3. Corneal ulceration may result from FHV infections.

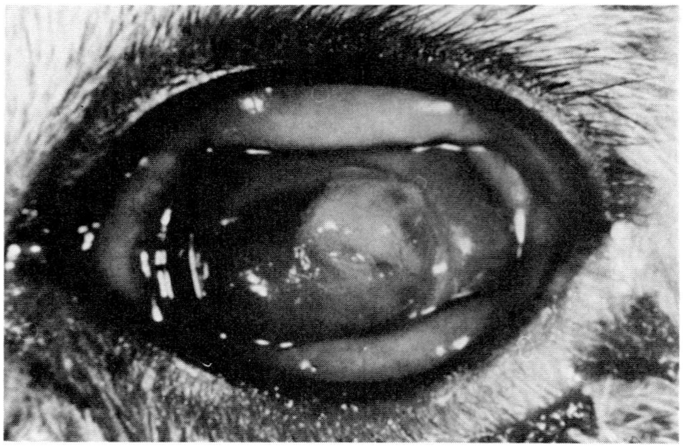

Figure 63–4. **Panophthalmitis is a possible sequela of FHV-induced corneal ulcers. It is important, therefore, to treat these ulcers aggressively.**

though the exact incidence is unavailable for multicat households and catteries, it is likely to be similarly high. Fortunately, only about 50% of chronic carriers are actually able to shed virus; however, the implications in those situations involving many cats housed together is staggering.

The carrier state has two phases. There is a *latent phase* in which the cat is asymptomatic and does not shed virus. During this phase, the virus cannot be cultured by routine oropharyngeal or nasal collection because it is not replicating. In the active phase, there is proliferation and shedding of the virus, which may or may not be accompanied by clinical signs of URI.[9] Cats remain carriers for years despite vaccinations.[3]

A recurrence of viral shedding occurs approximately 7 days following any of several types of stressful situations.[8] Moving a cat from one environment to another or the onset of another disease can provide adequate stress for this to occur. Parturition and lactation frequently cause a queen to become an active viral shedder, resulting in exposure of her kittens in utero or at a very early age. If these kittens develop clinical disease, they may subsequently become carriers themselves, perpetuating the disease within the household or cattery.[10]

Carrier cats shed about the same amount of virus as do cats with acute infections. If the carrier cat has an exacerbation of clinical signs, including sneezing accompanied by nasal and oropharyngeal discharges, the likelihood of transmission is as great as if that cat had an initial infection. However, if the carrier cat is shedding virus but does not have clinical signs, more direct contact is needed for transmission, and the likelihood of transmission is significantly lessened.[10]

Disinfection of Premises

FHV-I has a lipoprotein envelope, making it quite susceptible to chemical destruction and drying. At room temperature, FHV-I is generally inactivated within 18 to 24 hours. Therefore, if this virus is the only viral agent causing disease, prolonged environmental contamination is not likely to occur, and extensive disinfection is not necessary.[11]

Feline Calicivirus Infection

FCV represents a single major antigenic type with multiple subtypes. These subtypes have varying degrees of antigenic cross-reactivity[6] and varying degrees of pathogenicity. Some are nearly nonpathogenic and cause very mild clinical signs, whereas others cause severe disease.

FCV replicates on the epithelium of the oral cavity, the tongue, the tonsils, the nasal cavity, and the pulmonary interstitium. It causes clinical signs involving those tissues.[12]

Clinical Signs

The clinical signs of FCV infections are more variable than those of FHV-I infections because of the variety of subtypes. Some cats have a few, minimal clinical signs; others are severely ill with multiple clinical signs. The typical manifestations include: sneezing, fever, anorexia, drooling (Fig. 63–5) secondary to ulcers of the hard palate and tongue (Fig. 63–6), ulcers of the nasal philtrum, lips, and footpads, and ocular and nasal exudates. More unusual manifestations include interstitial pneumonia, tracheobronchitis, diarrhea, myalgia, a stiff gait, and hyperesthesia.[6] The 2280 and LLK strains have been associated with a transient limping syndrome accompanied by fever in kittens. The polyarthritis is related to intra-articular cartilage damage.[13]

Carrier State

FCV may be isolated from the oropharynx of some healthy cats that have no history of overt respiratory disease.[14] In one study it was isolated from the oropharynx of 80% of a group of cats with chronic stomatitis;[15] it has also been found in cats with persistent conjunctivitis, gingivitis, and periodontal disease. However, the significance of FCV in either of these situations remains unclear.[3]

These findings make it difficult to interpret the significance of the behavior of FCV following a primary infection. Following such an infection, the cat may continuously shed virus for weeks, months, or even for the remainder of the cat's life. The viral shedding state is not influenced by the presence or absence of stress, but is continuous.[3] In one

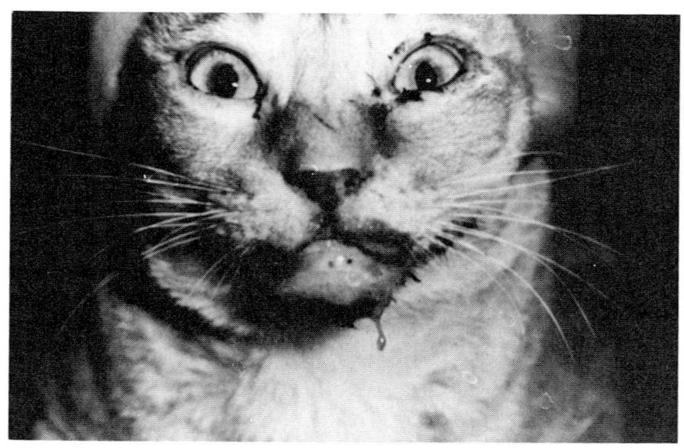

Figure 63–5. **Drooling may be profuse in FCV-induced oral ulceration.**

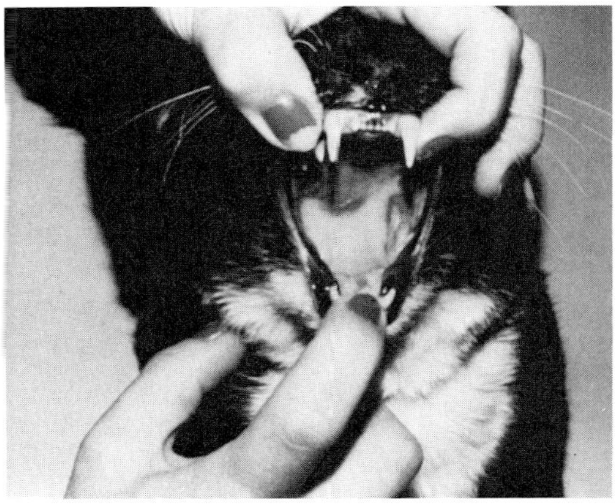

Figure 63–6. Ulceration of the tongue and hard palate is a common finding in FCV infections.

study, the virus was shed for up to 186 days, with viral shedding terminating abruptly. Following elimination of the virus, the recovered cat appears to be rather resistant to new infections with FCV.[16]

Disinfection of Premises

The FCV does not have an envelope, making it resistant to lipotrophic solvents and disinfectants. It is somewhat resistant to environmental conditions; most strains survive about 8 days in dry conditions and 10 days in damp conditions.[11]

If this virus is involved in a URI outbreak in a multicat setting, infection of other cats in the environment may occur. Aggressive use of virucidal disinfectants and elimination of damp conditions are recommended.

Minor Respiratory Pathogens

There are four pathogens that account for less than 10% of primary feline URIs: *C. psittaci,* feline mycoplasma, feline reovirus, and a feline coronavirus.[1] Most often, they occur as secondary pathogens to FVR or FCV.

C. psittaci causes a disease known as pneumonitis. Its incidence in feline respiratory infections is about 5%.[1] Its major clinical sign is a mucopurulent conjunctivitis. Sneezing and fever are also usually present. This organism is sensitive to chloramphenicol and tetracycline, administered parenterally or as ophthalmic preparations. A vaccine is available against *C. psittaci,* and is frequently part of a combination feline respiratory vaccine.

Feline mycoplasma is another minor respiratory pathogen. It causes a pseudomembranous conjunctivitis. It, too, is sensitive to chloramphenicol and tetracycline administered parenterally or as an ophthalmic preparation. There is no vaccine for this organism.

The feline reovirus and a feline respiratory coronavirus have been identified as causes of sneezing and conjunctivitis. These are mild infections against which there are no vaccines.

C. neoformans is another potential pathogen of the upper respiratory tract. It is generally associated with a purulent nasal discharge and will cause chronic signs of systemic illness. Aggressive chemotherapy using ketoconazole and/or amphotericin B is necessary (see Chapter 30).

Diagnosis of Upper Respiratory Infections

A presumptive diagnosis of a URI can be made from a history of frequent sneezing and fever. If one wishes to differentiate FVR from FCV infection, the following are "exclusive" characteristics:[3]

FVR conjunctivitis, ulcerative keratitis, rhinitis

FCV: ulcerative glossitis, acute pneumonia, limping

However, one should remember that a cat is not limited to one disease at a time; these diseases may occur simultaneously. In addition, both of these conditions are quickly complicated by the presence of opportunistic viruses and bacteria Therefore, in the course of routine veterinary practice, an attempt to differentiate between FVR and FCV is likely to lead one to erroneous results. Viral isolation can be performed when differentiation is necessary.

Treatment

Acute Infections

Outpatient versus Inpatient Setting

The first decision concerning treatment is whether the cat should be treated as an outpatient or whether it should be hospitalized. Several factors must be considered in this decision:

- Hospitalize an affected cat only if adequate isolation facilities are available. These cats are very contagious and may spread disease to any cat nearby.
- If the owner has several unaffected cats at home, hospitalization can serve to eliminate exposure of the healthy cats.
- The most important reason for hospitalization is based on the cat's appetite and availability of proper home care. If the cat is eating and appropriate antibiotic therapy and supportive care can be given at home, outpatient care is appropriate. However, if the cat is not eating, or will not get appropriate care at home, hospitalization is preferred.

Medical Treatment

There are no systemic antiviral agents that are efficacious for cats with URI. Fortunately, these viral organisms produce acute infections for only 5 to 10 days. However, during the acute phase, opportunistic bacteria frequently complicate the disease, compromising the cat's ability to recover. Therefore, the objective of treatment is to eliminate secondary bacterial infections with antibiotics and provide supportive care for the cat.

Antibiotics. Antibiotic selection should be based on the understanding that a number of bacterial organisms are likely to be present. Some antibiotics may have adverse side effects in some cats, including appetite suppression and aggravation of fever. Because these cats may have nasal obstruction and oral ulcers, an antibiotic that can be administered with a minimal amount of stress to the cat is preferred. Small tablets or oral liquids should be chosen.

When the cat is treated as an outpatient, this author's preference is to prescribe small amoxicillin tablets (Amoxi-Tabs), amoxicillin liquid (Amoxi-Drop), clavulanic acid-amoxicillin in tablet or liquid form (Clavamox), or enrofloxacin (Baytril). When the cat is hospitalized as a result of severe disease, injectable enrofloxacin (Baytril), gentamicin (Gentocin), or amikacin (Amiglyde-V) in combination with injectable amoxicillin (Amoxi-Inject) or ampicillin (Polyflex) are reliable therapeutic choices. The parenteral route of administration is preferred because it minimizes the likelihood of absorption problems.

Although two of the minor respiratory pathogens are sensitive to chloramphenicol and tetracycline, the parenteral form of these drugs should not be considered first-choice forms of therapy for two reasons. The incidence of *C. psittaci* and mycoplasma as primary pathogens is 10% or less; therefore, their presence is unlikely. Additionally, these drugs often cause appetite depression and fever.

Ophthalmic antibiotics can be an effective adjunct to therapy for conjunctivitis or ulcerative keratitis. Steroids should not be a component of the drug selected owing to the attendant risk of inducing or aggravating corneal ulcers. Oxytetracycline (Terramycin) or chloramphenicol (Chloromycetin ophthalmic) are good choices because of their efficacy against *C. psittaci* and feline mycoplasma.

Two ophthalmic antiviral agents are available for treating corneal ulcerations secondary to FHV-I. The recommended dosages for these agents are as follows:

Idoxuridine, 0.1% (Stoxil or Herplex): 1 drop to the affected eye(s) q1h during waking hours[17]

Trifluridine, 1% (Viroptic): 1 drop to the affected eye(s) q2h during waking hours[18]

Both: Treat until reepithelialization has occurred, then administer q4h for another 2 weeks.

Supportive Care. Supportive care begins with cleaning any discharge from the eyes and nostrils to make the cat more comfortable and to minimize appetite suppression. This should be done for both outpatients and hospitalized patients. Some practitioners have found intranasal decongestants to be helpful.[19] Afrin nasal spray is often preferred, but can cause a nasal secretory rebound if used frequently. The appropriate dosage is 1 drop instilled once daily in alternating nostrils. However, some cats resist intranasal medications so strongly that the benefits of therapy may not outweigh the stress induced. Cats with URIs should be kept in a warm environment to retard viral replication. The administration of oral, subcutaneous (SC), or intravenous (IV) fluids will help to reduce the tenacity of discharges from the eyes and nose. Warm humidification of inspired air will also facilitate this.

It is essential that proper nutrition be maintained; if it is not, a curable disease can become fatal. There are three reasons why a cat with a URI may stop eating; these possibilities should be explored during the physical examination.

1. If the cat's nose is severely congested, the cat will be unable to smell and thus will stop eating.
2. If the cat's temperature exceeds 104°F, eating will stop in most cases.
3. If the cat develops painful oral or lingual ulcers, the cat will stop eating even if its appetite is normal.

Oral feeding by syringe, as described in Chapter 5, can be done by some clients on some cats. Orogastric tube feeding, also described in Chapter 5, is the most practical method for the hospitalized cat. This may also be performed twice daily in outpatients if the owner's schedule will permit frequent trips to the hospital. Extreme care should be taken in passing the orogastric tube in an affected cat because a cat with heavy nasal discharges may be very resistant to tube passage, which may result in the tube being passed into the trachea. The tube and mouth speculum should be disinfected following use owing to the contagious nature of respiratory pathogens.

Chronic Infections

Viral Carriers

Treatment of cats that are viral carriers can be frustrating, as there is no treatment available for eliminating the carrier state. FHV-I infections may persist for the duration of a cat's life. FCV infections are usually not life-long disease states, but they may persist for several weeks or months.

Recurrences of viral shedding and of clinical signs are stress-induced in FHV-I infections. Therefore, minimizing stress and maximizing healthy living conditions are important factors in treatment. These cats should be maintained on a well-balanced diet and kept in an environment with good ventilation and sanitation. Overcrowding, the major cause of multicat household and cattery problems, should be prevented or solved. Current vaccinations should be maintained. FeLV- and FIV-infected cats should be removed from the household or cattery. Spaying queens to prevent pregnancy and lactation is also advisable. Unfortunately, many of these suggestions are not well received by owners of multicat households or catteries.

Chronic Sneezing

The chronically sneezing cat typically has a chronic, purulent nasal discharge. Medical treatment of this cat is generally not rewarding. When antibiotics are administered, the sneezing nasal discharge often will subside. However, when the antibiotics are discontinued, the problems generally return. Similar results often occur with the use of antihistamines.

The most practical medical treatment for this cat, in the author's experience, is the use of an injectable penicillin G procaine/penicillin G benzathine combination (Ambi-Pen). The appropriate dose for a 9-lb cat is 2 mL administered SC. Many cats will have a good response for 30 to 45 days from one injection, at which time dosing can be repeated. Most cats respond better to this treatment regimen than to oral antibiotics, and many can be maintained reasonably well for several months or even years.

Surgical treatment for chronic rhinitis and sinusitis is discussed in Chapter 55.

Prevention

The ideal vaccine is safe, causes no undesirable side effects, imparts complete immunity, and prevents the development of a carrier state.[20] Unfortunately, the ideal vaccine does not exist for feline URI. In reality, we are vaccinating cats against serious disease and not against infection.[21]

A number of parenteral vaccines proven to be effective in field use are currently available to protect the cat against FHV-I, FCV, and *C. psittaci.* Because maternal antibodies for these viruses do not wane until about 7 to 8 weeks, they should be administered at about 8 to 9 weeks of age and again at 12 to 14 weeks of age. Many practitioners administer a third vaccination at 16 weeks of age. It is important that the final vaccination not be given before 12 weeks of age. Annual revaccination is recommended.

The parenteral vaccines provide good protection against the development of clinical signs of URI without causing viral shedding. However, the carrier state may still develop if the vaccinated cat receives a natural challenge with FHV-I.[21] There is no evidence that vaccination terminates the carrier state of FHV-I or FCV.

Care should be taken in the administration of parenteral vaccine. If it is inadvertently placed on ocular or respiratory mucous membranes, signs of infection may occur.[22] Additionally, ulcerative stomatitis may occur if vaccine remains on the skin owing to a faulty injection technique and the cat licks the injection site

Intranasal vaccines are composed of modified viruses that cannot replicate except in the feline conjunctiva and turbinate mucosa. They are not blocked by maternal antibodies and produce solid immunity within 5 to 6 days.[23] Based on those facts, these vaccines would appear to be ideal for use in cats. Unfortunately, however, they result in sneezing and oculonasal discharges that may become chronic in a significant number of cats. They also cause shedding of virulent virus for up to 3 months. Therefore, most practitioners do not use them for routine vaccinations. Their use is generally reserved for special situations.

One of the special situations for which the use of intranasal vaccine is indicated is to protect exposed cats in an outbreak of URI. If an intranasal vaccine is given 4 days before a natural challenge, the cat will probably be protected against URI. If they are given 24 hours before a natural challenge, the clinical signs will be much less severe than normal.[23]

Prevention of URI in multicat households and catteries can be very difficult unless adequate isolation facilities exist. If litters of kittens are born and reared in the same room with adults that are carriers, the kittens will be exposed within a few days of birth. They will invariably develop disease as soon as their maternal antibodies wane. They then become carriers and the cycle continues. Prevention requires that this cycle be broken. Chronically infected cats and carriers should be identified and removed from the premises or housed separately from noninfected cats. Pregnant queens should be isolated and should remain isolated with their litters until their kittens have completed an adequate course of vaccinations.

The following vaccination program was developed by the Cornell Feline Health Center to protect kittens in multicat settings from becoming infected:

- Administer intranasal vaccine at 2 weeks of age.
- Administer injectable vaccine at 4 weeks of age.
- Wean kittens by 6 weeks of age.
- Separate kittens from adult cats until 4 months of age.
- Administer injectable vaccine at 8 and 14 weeks of age.
- When the kittens are 16 weeks old, return them to the normal population.

Public Health Considerations

Clients frequently question whether upper respiratory pathogens can be transmitted from cats to humans. Apparent incidences of transmission are believed to be coincidental because there is no evidence that FHV-1 or FCV can infect humans.[1] However, on rare occasions, *C. psittaci* in cats has been reported to be a source of transient, mild conjunctivitis in humans.[24] However, these conjunctival infections are effectively treated with ophthalmic tetracycline or chloramphenicol.

Conclusions

Viral URIs in cats are common, but their incidence has decreased since the advent of protective vaccines. Affected cats may sneeze for a few days and recover, or they may become seriously ill. Few will die if proper antibiotic and supportive therapy is instituted.

REFERENCES

1. Ford RB. Viral upper respiratory infection in cats. Compend Contin Educ Pract Vet 1991;13:593.
2. August JR. Feline viral respiratory disease. Vet Tech 1986;7:88.
3. August JR. Feline Viral Diseases. In: Ettinger SJ, ed. Textbook of Veterinary Internal Medicine, 3rd ed. Philadelphia: WB Saunders, 1989 312.
4. Povey RC, Johnson RH. Observations on the epidemiology and control of viral respiratory disease in cats. J Small Anim Pract 1970;11:485.
5. Gaskell RM. An Update on Feline Upper Respiratory Disease (URD). In Grunsell CSG, Hill FWG, Raw R-E, eds. The Veterinary Annual, 26th Issue. Bristol: Scientechnica, 1986:318.
6. Scott, FW: Feline Viral Respiratory Infections. In: Scott FW, ed. Contemporary Issues in Small Animal Practice, Vol. 3. New York: Churchill Livingstone, 1986:155.
7. Ford RB. The Respiratory System. In: Pratt PW, ed. Feline Medicine. Santa Barbara: American Veterinary Publications, 1983: 316.
8. Gaskell RM, Povey RC. Experimental induction of feline viral rhinotracheitis virus reexcretion in FVR-recovered cats. Vet Rec 1977;100:128.

9. Povey RC. A review of feline viral rhinotracheitis (feline herpesvirus 1 infection). Comp Immunol Microbiol Infect Dis 1979;21:373.
10. Gaskell RM, Povey RC. Transmission of feline viral rhinotracheitis. Vet Rec 1982;11:359.
11. Povey RC, Johnson RH. Observations on the epidemiology and control of viral respiratory disease in cats. J Small Anim Pract 1971;12:233.
12. Wardley RC, Povey RC. The pathology and sites of persistence associated with three different strains of feline calicivirus. Res Vet Sci 1977;23:15.
13. Pedersen NC, Meric SM, Johnson L, Plucker S, Theilen GH. A transient febrile "limping" syndrome of kittens caused by two different strains of feline calicivirus. Feline Pract 1984;14:32.
14. Wardley, RC. Feline respiratory viruses—Their prevalence in clinically healthy cats. J Small Anim Pract 1974;15:579.
15. Thompson RR. Association of calicivirus infection with chronic gingivitis and pharyngitis in cats. J Am Anim Pract 1984;25:207.
16. Wardley RC, Povey RC. The clinical disease and patterns of excretion associated with three different strains of feline calicivirus. Res Vet Sci 1976;23:7.
17. Gustafson DP. Antiviral therapy. Vet Clin North Am (Small Anim Pract) 1986;16:1181.
18. Nasisse MP. Manifestations, diagnosis and treatment of ocular herpesvirus infection in the cat. Compend Contin Educ Pract Vet 1982;4:962.
19. Hawkins EC. Chronic viral upper respiratory disease in cats: Differential diagnoses and management. Compend Contin Educ Pract Vet 1988;10:1003.
20. August JR. Feline Preventive Health Care and Infectious Disease Control. In: Sherding RG, ed. Diseases of the Cat: Diagnosis and Management. New York: Churchill Livingstone, 1990;197.
21. Goddard LE. Feline viral rhinotracheitis—Host versus herpes. Feline Pract 1986;16:36.
22. Povey RC, Wilson MR. A comparison of inactivated feline viral rhinotracheitis and feline caliciviral disease vaccines with live-modified viral vaccines. Feline Pract 1978;8:35.
23. Cocker FM. Responses of cats to nasal vaccination with a live, modified feline herpesvirus type 1. Res Vet Sci 1986;41:323.
24. Greene CE. Chlamydial Infections. In: Greene CE, ed. Infectious Diseases of the Dog and Cat. Philadelphia: WB Saunders, 1990:443.

CHAPTER 64

◇ ◇ ◇

Zoonotic Diseases

Gary D. Norsworthy

A number of diseases of humans may be transmitted by, or are associated with, the cat. A comprehensive list of these is given in Table 64–1. This list contains several diseases that are rare in the United States. However, other diseases on this list are of significance to the veterinary practitioner. This chapter discusses the public health significance of four of these.

Cat Bites to Humans

Despite the domestic nature of the cat, cats inflict bites of varying degrees of severity on humans. An estimated 100,000 to 200,000 Americans are bitten annually by cats.[1-3] Women are twice as likely to be bitten as men, and one half to two thirds of the victims are younger than 20 years of age.[3]

The cat's method of biting differs from that of the dog. Typically, a dog will bite the victim, clench its teeth, and shake its head, creating an open laceration. However, cats typically produce only puncture wounds with their four canine teeth. This difference in the nature of dog and cat bites accounts for the significant variations in infection rates. Only 3% to 5% of dog bites will become infected.[4,5] However, up to 50% of cat bites are associated with infection.[3,6] The most commonly isolated organisms from bite wounds that become infected are *Pasteurella multocida, Staphylococcus* species, *Streptococcus* species, *Klebsiella,* and *Enterobacter* species.[7] It is not surprising that these are the same organisms typically found in cat fight abscesses.

Although not all cat bites become infected, those that do may cause local and systemic consequences severe enough to require hospitalization and surgical debridement (Fig. 64–1). Several risk factors have been identified that increase the chances for infection. These include the presence of punctures instead of lacerations, a bite location on the hand or foot, a treatment delay of more than 12 hours, a victim younger than 2 years of age or older than 50 years of age, corticosteroid therapy or immune disorders, diabetes mellitus, asplenism, and alcoholism.[8]

Initial Treatment

It is not the author's purpose to encourage self-treatment of one's bite wounds or that of one's employees or clients. However, appropriate treatment during the initial few minutes after a bite may greatly reduce the likelihood of infection. Scrubbing of the wound should be avoided, but pressure irrigation is very beneficial.[2,9,10] High pressure (50 to 70 lb per square inch) is required, as low pressure is ineffective. The simplest acceptable method is to use a 19-gauge needle and a 35-mL syringe. Another acceptable method involves the use of a 20-gauge needle attached to a 500-mL plastic normal saline bag. An average of 150 to 250 mL of irrigation solution should be used.[11] The use of detergents and antiseptics is generally discouraged because they may harm tissue and increase healing time.[12] Following irrigation of the wound the victim should be referred to a physician for further treatment. In the case of a cat bite, a reluctant victim should be strongly encouraged to seek professional treatment owing to the high incidence of infection and the possible severe (and expensive) consequences.

Cat Scratch Disease

Cat scratch disease (CSD) has also been termed cat scratch fever, but the latter name has fallen into disuse because less than 50% of affected patients actually develop a fever. It is a relatively common disease that is associated with the cat.

Etiology

Although CSD was considered to be an infectious disease for more than 50 years, the etiologic agent eluded detection until 1983. At that time, Wear and colleagues isolated a gram-negative pleomorphic bacterium from lymph nodes, primary inoculation sites, and ocular lesions of patients with this disease.[13] This bacterium was observed within the walls of capillaries and within microabscesses when stained with Warthin-Starry silver impregnation stain.[14,15] It may appear to be delicate and slightly curved, or it may be rodlike with bulbous ends; it is thought to be an inhabitant of the cat's mouth. It has been named *Afipia felis.*[16]

Transmission

The primary inoculation site is on the extremities, although it has also been reported to occur on the head or neck.[15] A cat scratch is the most commonly implicated means of

Table 64–1. Zoonotic Diseases of Cats

Disease	Mode of Transmission
Parasitic Diseases	
Visceral larva migrans *Toxocara canis*	Soil contamination (feces)
Cutaneous larva migrans (feces) *Ancylostoma caninum* *A. braziliense*	Soil contamination
Dipylidiasis	Intermediate host (flea)
Dirofilariasis (mosquito) *Dirofilaria immitus*	Intermediate host
Toxoplasmosis *Toxoplasma gondii*	Direct (feces)
Giardiasis *Giardia lamblia*	Direct transmission not proven
Cryptosporidiosis *Cryptosporidium* species	Direct
Diseases Transmitted by Ectoparasites	
Plague *Yersinia pestis*	Intermediate host (flea); direct (bite, scratch)
Tularemia *Francisella tularensis*	Intermediate host (tick); direct (bite, scratch)
Bacterial Infections	
Campylobacteriosis *Campylobacter jejuni*	Direct (feces)
Salmonellosis *Salmonella* species	Direct (feces)
Cat scratch disease Gram-negative bacillus	Direct (scratch, bite)
Mycotic Infections	
Dermatomycosis *Microsporum canis*	Direct (hair)
Sporotrichosis *Sporothrix schenckii*	Direct (skin lesion)
Miscellaneous	
Bites	Direct
Rabies	Direct (bite)
Flea and mite dermatitis	Direct

Adapted from Miller JB. Small Animal Zoonoses. In: Ettinger SJ, ed. Textbook of Veterinary Internal Medicine, 3rd ed. Philadelphia: WB Saunders, 1989:188.

transmission, although some cases are related to a cat licking a skin abrasion.[17] One study of 595 patients revealed that 84% were younger than 21 years of age, and 52% were younger than 12 years of age. In less than 5% of the families studied was a second family member affected. When this occurred, the second patient was rarely a parent. Multiple cases within a family typically would occur within a 3-week period, suggesting that the period of cat transmission is quite short.[18] Human-to-human transmission has not been reported, so patients do not require isolation or quarantine.[18]

Diagnosis

A reliable CSD antigen skin test with a high degree of specificity has been used extensively at Walter Reed Army Medical Center.[18] However, there is currently no test antigen commercially available. Any skin test that is performed is generally done with antigen prepared from previous cases at the same hospital. Presently, diagnosis is generally based upon typical clinical signs and a history of a cat scratch (or bite). Confirmation is based on the presence of a swollen lymph node and histopathologic study of the bacterium using the Warthin-Starry stain. Identification of the organism is most accurate during the first 3 to 4 weeks after the onset of illness.[13]

Clinical Signs

Typically, CSD is characterized by a lesion at the primary inoculation site consisting of a papule or skin pustule that appears 3 to 10 days after exposure. Lymphadenopathy develops about 2 weeks after the exposure and is generally painful. Fever of 1 to 7 days' duration occurs only about 30%

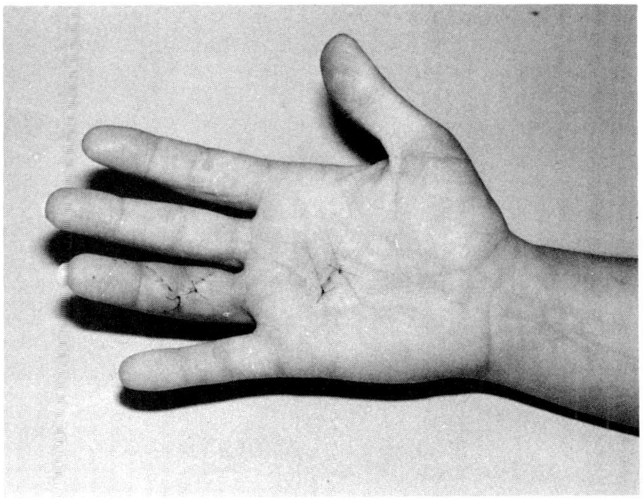

Figure 64–1. The surgical incisions on this veterinary technician's hand were made for drainage of an infection induced by a cat bite. She was hospitalized for 4 days and missed 10 days of work.

of the time. The disease is generally self-limiting.[18] However, patients that are immunocompromised, such as those with human immunodeficiency virus (HIV) infection, may become bacteremic and develop endocarditis, liver abscesses, and unusual histiocytoid or epithelial hemangiomas.[16]

Treatment and Prognosis

Because this is a self-limiting disease, it has been managed with symptomatic therapy, including surgical drainage of affected lymph nodes.[16] However, a recent study reported a dramatic response to oral ciprofloxacin (Cipro) (500 mg b.i.d.) in five patients with CSD.[19] Two of the five had failed to improve with treatment with other antibiotics. Prior to this report, no antimicrobial drug has been found that would produce consistently good clinical response.

Disposition of the Infecting Cat

There are three factors to consider when deciding about the disposition of the cat:

1. The cat, which is generally a kitten, is generally contagious for only 2 to 3 weeks.
2. Less than 5% of other family members that have been scratched by the same cat will develop the disease.
3. Relapses or second infections following recovery from CSD have not been reported.[20]

Prevention

The following recommendations have been offered to cat owners who are concerned about CSD[18]:

1. Declaw your cat.
2. Wash cuts and scratches promptly, and do not allow a cat to lick an open wound.
3. Wash your hands after playing with or petting a cat.
4. Avoid cat and dog scratches by handling pets gently.

Dermatophytosis

Dermatophytosis is commonly called ringworm. Feline cases may be caused by several species of fungal organisms but are most commonly attributable to *Microsporum canis, Trichophyton mentagrophytes,* and *M. gypseum.* All three organisms are transmissible to humans. Affected cats typically have circular, alopecic lesions (ringworm lesions) on any portion of the body that is covered by hair. However, they may also have a more diffuse, generalized form without the classical ringworm lesions. In addition, they may be asymptomatically infected. Both asymptomatic and symptomatic infections serve as a source of infection for other cats, dogs, and humans. Conversely, humans may be a source of dermatophytoses for cats.[21]

Predisposing Factors

There are several predisposing factors that increase the incidence of dermatophytoses in humans or cats.[22-24] Immune status is a major factor. Humans and cats without prior exposure, or with immunosuppression, have increased susceptibility to the disease. Several environmental factors also may predispose one to infection, including contamination, crowding, high humidity, poor ventilation, and darkness. General physical condition becomes a factor if the nutritional level is poor or if other debilitating diseases are present. Age also appears to be a factor, as children have a higher incidence of dermatophytoses than adults. However, several studies suggest that a lack of previous exposure may be the main reason that children are more easily affected.[21]

Transmission and Outcome of Exposure

Transmission occurs by both direct and indirect contact. Fomites, such as bedding and grooming equipment, are frequently involved in transmission. Cats with symptomatic and asymptomatic infections may transmit the infection by direct contact or by serving as a source of fungal spores. Spores can remain viable for years under normal, indoor conditions.[24,25] Infected bedding is one of the most common sources of cat-to-cat transmission. Beds and furniture used by cats may be a source of spores that may infect other pets or family members.

Exposure to a dermatophyte does not ensure an infection. Rather, such exposure will result in one or more of several possibilities:[24,25]

1. The fungus may be removed mechanically from the host before infection occurs.
2. Normal skin flora may successfully compete with the fungus, preventing fungal growth.
3. The fungus may establish residence without producing gross lesions (i.e., an asymptomatic infection).
4. The fungus may establish residence and produce active lesions (i.e., a symptomatic infection).

The average incubation period is about 1 to 2 weeks. However, under some circumstances, the incubation period may be as long as 6 weeks.[21]

Cats are frequently presented to practitioners for examination because a family member has dermatophytosis. The cat should be examined thoroughly; however, the owner should be informed that dermatophyte transmission is also possible from dogs and other humans. It should also be noted that infected cats and dogs may be the recipients, and not the sources, of infection from humans. If children are involved, schoolmates or playmates should also be considered as possible sources.

Diagnosis

The diagnosis of dermatophytosis is based on the history, physical examination (to detect characteristic lesions), Wood's light examination, potassium hydroxide preparations, fungal culture, and (rarely) skin biopsy.[21,25] Scott and Horn have made two classic observations about feline and canine dermatophytosis:[21]

1. Most skin lesions that look like ringworm are not ringworm.
2. Many skin lesions that look like other types of lesion are actually ringworm.

Their observations underscore the importance of laboratory evaluations when considering this disease. However, several of the previously mentioned methods are not totally reliable. Although *M. canis* accounts for 98% of feline infections, the Wood's light examination will only produce positive results in the presence of *M. canis, M. audouinii,* and *M. distortum,* and then only 30% of the time.[26] In addition, the light must be turned on for 5 to 10 minutes before its use to prevent an even greater false-negative rate. Experienced dermatologists or mycologists have a 40% false-negative rate when using potassium hydroxide preparations.[24,25] Therefore, the most reliable diagnostic method is fungal culture.

As previously mentioned, cats are frequently presented for examination when a family member is infected. Because many cats are asymptomatic carriers, a proper examination should include a fungal culture using the sterile toothbrush method (the MacKenzie brush technique). A sterile toothbrush is brushed through the cat's haircoat to accumulate spores that may be entrapped in hair and keratin debris. The toothbrush is then shaken to remove excess debris and gently pressed into the culture medium.[21]

Treatment

There are two goals for treatment of the cat with dermatophytosis:

1. To rid the cat of symptomatic and asymptomatic infection
2. To prevent contagion by direct contact and environmental contamination

Although dermatophytosis is frequently self-limiting in cats,[24,25] proper treatment will eliminate environmental contamination, prevent reinfection, and prevent transmission to other pets and humans. With proper topical treatment, the period of contagion is only about 1 week. Without topical treatment, contagion may continue for 30 to 45 days. Treatment must also be aimed at eliminating transmission via fomites. The bedding of all affected cats and humans should be washed in hot, bleach-containing water. For more details on all aspects of dermatophytosis, including treatment, see Chapter 56.

Toxoplasmosis

Toxoplasmosis is the feline zoonotic disease that generates the most inquiry from pregnant women and women contemplating pregnancy. It has been called the "*Ladies Home Journal* disease" because its association with the cat was widely publicized in that popular women's magazine in the 1970s. Although the disease is quite rare in domestic cats, its potential for causing significant disease in fetuses and young children justifies some measure of concern.

Role of the Cat

Although up to 80% of cats in the United States have serologic evidence of exposure to *Toxoplasma gondii,* they rarely develop clinical toxoplasmosis. However, because domestic (and wild) cats are the only known definitive host, they may serve as a source of infection for humans. Infections are acquired by ingesting any of the three stages of *T. gondii.* Because *T. gondii* can infect any warm-blooded animal or bird, cats that are prone to hunting (especially those that hunt mice and birds) and cats that are fed uncooked or unfrozen meats are at greatest risk. The highest incidence of *T. gondii* in meats prepared for human consumption is found in pork. Therefore, cats ingesting uncooked pork are at greatest risk of ingesting bradyzoite-containing tissue cysts.[27,28] After the cysts are ingested, the cyst wall is dissolved in the stomach and small intestines. The bradyzoites penetrate the epithelial cells of the small intestine and initiate their reproductive cycle, resulting in the production of oocysts. Oocysts are then passed in the cat's feces and become the source of infection to other species, including humans. However, the oocysts must sporulate before they become infective. This process takes 1 to 5 days after excretion. Oocyte shedding normally lasts up to 2 weeks and occurs only once in a cat's lifetime.[29] Handling and petting a cat are very unlikely means of transmission.[25] Although most bradyzoites enter the cat's epithelial cells, some penetrate the lamina propria of the small intestine and multiply as tachyzoites. Within a few hours, the organisms may spread to extraintestinal tissues via the lymph and blood. Ultimately, tissue cysts develop. These are dormant and persist for months, years, or even for the remainder of the cat's life. Under normal conditions, even if these cysts rupture, the cat's immune system will be able to kill the bradyzoites. However, in immunosuppressed cats, it is possible for multiplication to occur, leading to another period of oocyst shedding or clinical disease. However, the number of oocysts shed this second time is far less than the number shed during a primary infection.[27]

Human Infections

Approximately one third of the United States population has serologic evidence of a past infection with *T. gondii.*[30] Humans may become infected by the ingestion of sporulated oocyts passed in cat feces 1 to 5 days prior to ingestion. Humans may also become infected by the ingestion of bradyzoite-containing tissue cysts in uncooked meats, especially pork. Studies have shown that meat-borne transmission is the most common mode of transmission in the U.S. population.[31] Two uncommon modes of transmission to humans are transfusions of platelets and blood cells, and organ transplants.[27]

Human Disease

Normal adults who are infected with *T. gondii* may have subclinical infections or they may experience adenopathy, fever, malaise, or headache.[32] Most infections go undiagnosed; without laboratory testing, these infections may be diagnosed as influenza, since they are characterized by flu-like symptoms. It has been estimated that 15% of the cases of unexplained lymphadenopathy are attributable to toxoplasmosis.[33] Severe systemic disease is common in persons concomitantly infected with HIV or in those receiving immunosuppressive therapy.[34]

Approximately 30% of women of childbearing age in the United States have protective antibodies against *T. gondii*. If a previously uninfected woman acquires a *T. gondii* infection while pregnant, there is a 20% to 50% probability that her fetus will also be infected.[35] In the United States, it is estimated that such infections occur in 1 of 1,000 live births, resulting in a rate of 0.1%.[36,37] Most of the infected babies will be normal at birth, but will develop disease later in life.

Factors to Consider

Veterinarians are frequently asked to make recommendations concerning cats and pregnant women. They may also be asked to confirm advice given by physicians. Unfortunately, some physicians are either uninformed or prejudiced against cat ownership, and some clients will be given recommendations that are neither valid nor reasonable. A number of factors should be considered when assisting a pregnant client in deciding what should be done with a cat during her pregnancy.

A positive *T. gondii* serum antibody titer in a woman or a cat does not indicate active infection unless a rising titer is demonstrated 2 to 4 weeks later. It is more likely to mean that the woman or the cat has immunity. However, serologic testing of women during pregnancy will often not allow one to make a definitive distinction between an active infection and a previous infection. If at all possible, serologic testing should be done prior to a pregnancy.[38]

A negative *T. gondii* serum antibody titer in cats or women means that there has been no prior exposure, and future infection is possible. Therefore, healthy seropositive cats are safer pets than seronegative cats because secondary shedding of oocysts is unlikely in the former.[38]

There is a 33% chance of fetal infection in women having a primary infection during pregnancy.[39] A subsequent pregnancy will produce normal, unaffected offspring, even if reexposure has occurred.[33] In the United States, the incidence of *T. gondii* infection in infants is about 0.1%.

Recommendations

Current studies have shown that having a pet cat, having direct contact with cats around the house, or working with cats in a veterinary hospital do not increase the likelihood of contracting toxoplasmosis.[40] One study even showed that persons with cats were *less* likely to be seropositive than those without cats.[41] However, because toxoplasmosis can be a serious disease, especially in pregnant women, several recommendations are appropriate in minimizing exposure to *T. gondii*.[27]

Cats should only be fed cat commercial food or cooked meat. Freezing of meats reduces infectivity but does not consistently prevent it.[42] For best protection from toxoplasmosis, cats should be kept indoors to prevent them from hunting or foraging for food. Raw garbage and dead animals can be a source of *T. gondii*.

Because oocysts must be present in a cat's feces before transmission occurs, a weekly fecal examination is an effective way to ensure safety to the pregnant woman. However, this is rarely feasible. A more practical suggestion is for pregnant women to have their husbands change the cat's litter box. Feces should be removed daily to prevent sporulation from occurring in the litter box.

Hands should be washed thoroughly with soap and water after touching any meat. Cutting boards, sink tops, knives, and other materials coming in contact with uncooked meat should be washed with soap and water. Meat of any animal, but especially pork, should be cooked to an internal temperature of 70°C (160°F) before human or animal consumption, and tasting of meat during the cooking process should be avoided.

As the cat's major role in *T. gondii* transmission is its ability to contaminate the soil with massive numbers of oocysts, gloves should be worn while gardening to avoid coming in contact with those oocysts.[38] Vegetables should be washed thoroughly before eating because of possible contact with cat feces.

When farm cats are involved, dead animals, especially pigs, should be removed promptly to prevent scavenging by cats Cats should not be allowed near pregnant sheep or goats. Aborted ovine fetal membranes should not be handled with bare hands, and should be buried or incinerated, as *T. gondii* is a cause of ovine abortions. Grain bins should be kept covered to prevent fetal contamination by cats.

An experimental vaccine that has been shown to protect 84% of cats challenged with *T. gondii* has been developed.[43] If this vaccine becomes commercially available, it will be indicated for use in farm cats, free-roaming cats, and cats in households with pregnant women or women anticipating pregnancy.

Summary

Because *T. gondii* can be acquired from sources other than cats, disposal of cats will not ensure protection from toxoplasmosis. Special attention should be paid to the handling and cooking of foodstuffs, including meats and vegetables. Keeping a cat indoors and feeding it only commercial food will virtually eliminate the cat as a threat for transmitting *T. gondii*. If pregnant women honor these recommendations, the chances of a cat being a source of toxoplasmosis to her unborn child is virtually nil.

REFERENCES

1. Pinckney LE, Kennedy LA. Traumatic deaths from dog attacks in the United States. Pediatrics 1982;69:193.
2. Veitch JM, Omer GE. Case report: Treatment of cat bite injuries to the hand. J Trauma 1979;19:201.
3. Kizer KW. Epidemiologic and clinical aspects of animal bite injuries. J Am Coll Emerg Physicians 1979;8:134.
4. Goldstein EJC, Citron DM, Finegold SM. Dog bite wounds and infection: A prospective clinical study. Ann Emerg Med 1980; 9:508.
5. Saphir DA, Carter GR. Gingival flora of the dog with special reference to bacteria associated with bites. J Clin Microbiol 1976;3:334.
6. Douglas LG. Bite wounds. Am Fam Physician 1975;11:93.
7. Marcy SM. Infections due to dog and cat bites. Pediatr Infect Dis 1982;1:351.
8. Callaham ML. Treatment of common dog bites: Infection risk factors. J Am Coll Emerg Physicians 1978;7:83.
9. Rodeheaver GT, Pettry D, Thacker JG. Wound cleansing by high pressure irrigation. Surg Gynecol Obstet 1975;141:357.
10. Stevenson TR, Thacker JG, Rodeheaver GT. Cleansing the traumatic wound by high pressure syringe irrigation. J Am Coll Emerg Physicians 1976;5:17.
11. Underman AE. Bite wounds inflicted by dogs and cats. Vet Clin North Am (Small Anim Pract) 1987;17(1):195.
12. Hawkins J, Paris PM, Stewart RD. Mammalian bites: Rational approach to management. Postgrad Med 1983;73:52.
13. Wear DJ, Margileth AM, Hadfield TL. Cat scratch disease: A bacterial infection. Science 1983;221:1403.
14. Carithers HA. Cat-scratch disease: Notes on its history. Am J Dis Child 1970;139:1124.
15. Margileth AM, Wear DJ, Hadfield TL. Cat scratch disease: Bacteria in skin at the primary inoculation site. J Am Med Assoc 1984;252:928.
16. Goldstein EJC. Household pets and human illness. Infect Dis Clin North Am 1991;93:117.
17. Margileth AM. Cervical adenitis. Pediatr Rev 1985;7:13.
18. Margileth AM. Cat scratch disease: A therapeutic dilemma. Vet Clin North Am (Small Anim Pract) 1987;17(1):91.
19. Holley HP. Successful treatment of cat-scratch disease with ciprofloxacin. J Am Med Assoc 1991;265:1563.
20. Margileth AM. Cat Scratch Disease. In: Wyngaarden JB, Smith LH, eds. Cecil Textbook of Medicine, 17th ed. Philadelphia: WB Saunders, 1985:1618.
21. Scott DW, Horn HT Jr. Zoonotic dermatoses of dogs and cats. Vet Clin North Am (Small Anim Pract) 1987;17(1):133.
22. Fitzpatrick TB, Eisen AZ, Wolff K. Dermatology in General Medicine, 2nd ed. New York: McGraw-Hill, 1979.
23. Hernandez AD. An approach to the diagnosis and therapy of dermatophytosis. Int J Dermatol 1980;19:540.
24. Scott DW. Feline dermatology 1900–1978: A monograph. J Am Anim Hosp Assoc 1980;16:331.
25. Muller GH, Kirk RW, Scott DW. Fungal Diseases. In: Muller GH, Kirk RW, Scott DW, eds. Small Animal Dermatology, 3rd ed. Philadelphia: WB Saunders, 1983:243.
26. Thomas MLE, Scheidt VJ, Walker RL. Inapparent carriage of *Microsporum canis* in cats. Compend Contin Educ Pract Vet 1989;11:563.
27. Dubey JP. Toxoplasmosis. J Am Vet Med Assoc 1986;189:166.
28. Dubey JP. Toxoplasmosis in cats. Feline Pract 1986;16(4):12.
29. Dreesen DW, Lubroth JS. The life cycle of *Toxoplasma gondii:* An illustrative view. Compend Contin Educ Pract Vet 1983;5: 456.
30. Remington JS. Toxoplasmosis in the adult. Bull NY Acad Med 1974;50:21.
31. Jones TC. Toxoplasmosis. In: Kaye D, Rose LF, eds. Fundamentals of Internal Medicine. St. Louis: CV Mosby, 1983:498.
32. Elliott DL, Tolle SW, Goldberg L, Miller JB. Pet-associated illness. J Am Anim Hosp Assoc 1986;22:387.
33. Krick JA, Remington JS. Toxoplasmosis in the adult—An overview. N Engl J Med 1978;298:550.
34. Frenkel JK, Nelson BM, Arias-Stella J. Immunosuppression and toxoplasmic encephalitis. Clinical and experimental findings. Hum Pathol 1975;6:97.
35. Remington JS, Desmonts G. Toxoplasmosis. In: Remington JS, Klein JO, eds. Infectious Diseases of the Fetus and Newborn Infant. Philadelphia: WB Saunders, 1976:191.
36. Frenkel JK. Toxoplasma in and around us. Biol Sci 1973;23:343.
37. Wilson CB, Remington JS. What can be done to prevent congenital toxoplasmosis? Am J Obstet Gynecol 1980;138:357.
38. August JR, Chase TM. Toxoplasmosis. Vet Clin North Am (Small Anim Pract) 1987;117(1):55.
39. Desmonts G, Couvreur J. Congenital toxoplasmosis: A prospective study of 378 pregnancies. N Engl J Med 1974;290:1110.
40. Reif JS. Toxoplasmosis: Assessment of the role of cats in human infection. Compend Contin Educ Pract Vet 1980;2:810.
41. Ganley JP, Comstock GW. Association of cats and toxoplasmosis. Am J Epidemiol 1980;111:238.
42. Dubey JP, Frenkel JK. Experimental Toxoplasma infection in mice with strains producing oocysts. J Parasitol 1973;59:505.
43. Frenkel JK, Pfefferkorn ER, Smith DD, et al. Prospective vaccine prepared from a new mutant of *Toxoplasma gondii* for use in cats. Am J Vet Res 1991;52:759.

APPENDIXES

◇ ◇ ◇

A. Drug Formulary: Alphabetical by Generic Name
B. Drug Formulary: Alphabetical by Trade Name
C. Drug Formulary: Alphabetical by Indication
D. Conversion Table: Weight to Body-Surface Area
E. Medication Dosage Charts
F. Differential Overview

INTRODUCTION TO THE DRUG FORMULARY (APPENDIXES A, B, AND C)

The information concerning drugs used for feline diseases is beyond the memory of any practitioner. Therefore, this drug formulary (Appendixes A, B, and C) is assembled as a reference source.

In her recent extensive list of drugs used in cats, Dr. Dawn Boothe noted that less than 20% of them are approved by the Food and Drug Administration (FDA) for use in the cat.[1] The use of drugs in animals in a manner not specifically approved by the FDA is termed *extralabel use.* This includes the use of a drug in a species, for an indication, or at a dosage not stated in the labeling. The Food, Drug, and Cosmetic Act completely prohibits the extralabel use of animal drugs. However, the FDA realizes that for some diseases in animals there is no approved drug. It also recognizes that the label dosages of some drugs have been found to be clinically ineffective and that it is not economically feasible for the drug manufacturer to conduct the research necessary to change the labeling. Therefore, the FDA has adopted a position of regulatory discretion and developed an extralabel policy. This policy is designed to protect the public and to provide the veterinarian rational options for therapy.

According to the extralabel policy, the FDA will not ordinarily recommend regulatory action in the case of a veterinarian using extralabel indications and dosages in nonfood animals unless there is a clear threat to the public health, the health and welfare of the animal treated, or other serious consequences. This policy is based on the assumption that a bona fide veterinarian-client-patient relationship exists.[2] Most of the drugs in this formulary are used in the cat in an extralabel manner. If the practitioner is not familiar with the use of any particular drug, consultation with others who are knowledgeable in this area is recommended. Dosages should be regarded as averages; individualization may be necessary for any given patient. Since recommendations for extralabel drug dosages are constantly subject to review and change, one should strive to keep abreast of the current veterinary literature.

How to Use This Drug Formulary

This formulary is intended to be extremely user friendly; it is designed with the busy practitioner in mind. The following features should be understood before beginning to use it.

1. Appendix A is alphabetical by generic name. Appendix B is alphabetical by trade name. Appendix C is alphabetical by indication. This triple listing maximizes one's likelihood of finding the drug desired.
2. The dosages are listed and calculated in apothecary units instead of metric units. In spite of our government's best efforts a few years ago, most practitioners think in apothecary units in order to communicate with our clients.
3. The dosages are calculated on the basis of specific tablet or capsule size or of the concentrations available for each specific drug. The tablet or capsule size and/or the concentrations are specified with each listing to avoid confusion.
4. The dosages are calculated for the "textbook 10-pound cat." Most adult cats are very near this weight so the calculated dosages can often be used without conversion. Since 10 is a round number, needed adjustments can generally be performed rapidly in one's head.
5. A separate listing is made for each indication since dosages generally vary from one indication to the next for the same drug.
6. References in the literature vary for recommended dosages for many of these drugs. A concerted effort was made to use the most current and reliable sources for information. However, one should expect to find other recommendations in other formularies.

The following format is used for listing each generic drug:

Generic name Trade name
Disease or indication Reference/Chapter number

Dosage
How supplied
Administration dosage
Administration dosage continued (if needed)/Comments

Disease or Indication is used to designate a particular use for this drug. If this drug is specific for a particular disease, the disease is listed. However, some drugs are used for clinical signs common to many diseases, such as vomiting or diarrhea. In these instances, the clinical sign is designated.

Dosage is expressed in milligram per pound of body weight with a designation of time intervals and route of administration, i.e., 4.5 mg/lb b.i.d. PO.

How Supplied lists the available sizes or concentrations of the drug that have significance to the cat. If a larger size or higher concentration is available but its dosage is much less convenient than others available, it is omitted.

For *tablets or capsules, Administration Dosage* begins with the size of tablet or capsule designated and expresses the dosage as the number of tablets or capsules per 10 pounds of body weight. The listing "100 mg: 0.5/10 lb b.i.d. PO" means that one half of a 100-mg tablet or capsule is given twice daily by mouth to a 10-pound cat.

For *oral liquids or injectable drugs, Administration Dosage* is expressed in the number of milliliters per 10 pounds of body weight. The listing "100 mg/mL: 1 mL/10 lb b.i.d. PO" means 1 mL of a 100 mg/mL liquid is given twice daily by mouth to a 10-pound cat. Oral liquids or injectable drugs can be differentiated according to route of administration (PO versus IV, IM, or SQ).

Since many of the drugs listed are intended for human use, the calculated portion of the tablet or capsule may not be convenient for accurate dosing in a 10-pound patient. When this occurs, one is encouraged to crush the tablet or open the capsule into a small bottle of palatable liquid and figure the dose based on the concentration of the mixture. Vitamino 4X (TechAmerica Veterinary Products, Kansas City, MO) is palatable and available in a 1-ounce bottle. It is but one of several liquids suitable for this purpose.

Every effort has been made to provide accurate dosages. However, a few mistakes are inevitable. If a listed dose does not seem reasonable, please make an effort to verify what is listed. A reference is given for each dosage.

Abbreviations used are:

mg	milligrams
mL	milliliter
tbsp	tablespoon
tsp	teaspoon
lb	pounds
e.o.d.	every other day or q48h
s.i.d.	once daily or q24h
b.i.d.	twice daily or q12h
t.i.d.	three times daily or q8h
q.i.d.	four times daily or q6h
p.r.n.	as needed
qxh	every x hours
qxd	every x days
qxw	every x weeks
qxm	every x months
PO	per os or orally
SQ	subcutaneously
IM	intramuscularly
IV	intravenously
tab	tablet
cap	capsule
inj	injectable
susp	suspension
soln	solution
liq	liquid
OTC	over the counter
BW	body weight
CM	cardiomyopathy
NSAI	nonsteroidal antiinflammatory

REFERENCES

1. Booth DM. Drug therapy in cats: Recommended dosing regimens. J Am Vet Med Assoc 1990;196:1845.
2. Talbot RB. Pharmaceutical Product Regulation by the Federal Government. In: Talbot RB, ed. Veterinary Pharmaceuticals and Biologicals. Lenexa, KS: Veterinary Medicine Publishing Co, 1990:917.

APPENDIX A
DRUG FORMULARY: ALPHABETICAL BY GENERIC NAME

Acebutolol Sectral
Cardiac disease: beta-blocker 44
100 mg/cat s.i.d. PO
Cap: 200 & 400 mg
200 mg: 0.5/cat s.i.d. PO

Acetaminophen Tylenol
Contraindicated 4

Acetazolamide Diamox
Glaucoma 44
2.5–5 mg/lb IV single dose, then 1–5 mg/lb t.i.d. PO
Tab: 125 & 250 mg; inj: 100 mg/mL when reconstituted with 5 mL
100 mg/mL: 0.25–0.5 mL/10 lb IV single dose; then 125 mg: 0.1–0.4/10 lb t.i.d. PO

Acetohydroxamic acid (AHA) Lithostat
Urine crystal dissolution 44
5 mg/lb s.i.d.–b.i.d. PO
Tab: 250 mg
250 mg: 0.2/10 lb s.i.d.–b.i.d. PO
May cause oral ulcers

Acetylcysteine Mucomyst
Toxicity (moderate): acetaminophen Chapter 62
64 mg/lb PO IV; then 32 mg/lb q6h for 3+ doses
Soln: 100 & 200 mg/mL (10% & 20%)
100 mg/mL: 6 mL/10 lb, 200 mg/mL: 3 mL/10 lb PO IV. Give IV in 5% dextrose over 20 min; then 100 mg/mL: 3 mL/10 lb PO q6h for 3+ doses

Acetylcysteine Mucomyst
Toxicity (severe): acetaminophen Chapter 62
128 mg/lb PO IV; then 32 mg/lb q6h for 3+ doses
Soln: 100 & 200 mg/mL (10% & 20%)
100 mg/mL: 12 mL/10 lb, 200 mg/mL: 6 mL/10 lb PO IV. Give IV in 5% dextrose over 20 minutes; then 100 mg/mL: 3 mL/10 lb PO q6h for 3+ doses

Acetylpromazine PromAce
Thromboembolism 2
0.11–0.22 mg/lb t.i.d. PO SC
Tab: 10 & 25 mg; inj: 10 mg/mL
10 mg/mL: 0.1–0.2 mL/10 lb t.i.d. SC; 10 mg: 0.1–0.2 tab t.i.d.

Note: The references for this appendix appear on pages 626–627.

Acetylpromazine PromAce
Tranquilization 3
0.45–0.9 mg/lb PO p.r.n.
Tab: 10 & 25 mg
10 mg: 0.5–1.0/10 lb PO p.r.n.

Acetylpromazine PromAce
Vomiting/nausea due to renal failure Chapter 31
0.05 mg/lb PO IM b.i.d.
Tab: 10 & 25 mg; inj: 10 mg/mL
10 mg: 0.05/10 lb PO b.i.d.; 10 mg/mL: 0.05 mL/10 lb IM b.i.d.

Activated charcoal Actidose-Aqua
Toxicity general 8
0.3–0.6 g/lb as slurry p.r.n. (q8–12h) PO
208 mg/mL in 25-g and 50-g susp (aqueous)
208 mg/mL: 15–30 mL as slurry PO q8–12h PO
Contains a cathartic

Activated charcoal ToxiBan Granules or Suspension
Toxicity: general 43
0.5–1.0 g/lb PO; may be repeated in 12 hr
Susp: 1 g/4.5 mL; granules: mix 1 part to 5–7 parts cold water
22–45 mL/10 lb PO; may be repeated in 12 hr
2 g ToxiBan granules = activity of 9 mL ToxiBan Suspension

Acyclovir Zovirax
Viral infections, especially herpes 44
50 mg/cat t.i.d. PO
Cap: 200 mg
200 mg: 0.25/cat t.i.d. PO

Albendazole Valbazen
Paragonimus infection 43
11 mg/lb b.i.d. PO × 10 days
Susp: 113.6 mg/mL
113.6 mg/mL: 1 mL/10 lb b.i.d. PO × 10 days

Albutrol Proventil, Ventolin
Bronchoconstriction 44
1.25 mg/cat b.i.d.–t.i.d. PO
Tab: 5 mg
5 mg: 0.25/cat b.i.d.–t.i.d. PO

Aloe vera cream Dermaide Aloe Cream
Burns 43
Apply to thickness of ⅛″–¼″ q.i.d. for several days, then s.i.d.–b.i.d.
4-oz jars
⅛″–¼″ q.i.d. for several days, then s.i.d.–b.i.d.

Alprazolam Xanax
Urine spraying 44
0.25 mg/cat b.i.d. PO
Tab: 0.25 & 0.5 mg
0.25 mg: 1/cat b.i.d. PO

Aluminum acetate, Burow's solution Domeboro solution
Wounds, open 5
1–2 tab/pint water; apply topically q8h
2.2 g tab and powder packets
1–2 tabs or packets/pint water; apply topically q8h
Store solution less than 7 days

Aluminum carbonate gel Basaljel
Hyperphosphatemia Chapter 31
15–45 mg/lb s.i.d. in food
Cap: 500 mg
500 mg: 0.3–0.9/10 lb s.i.d. in food
Open capsule and mix powder in food

Aluminum hydroxide gel Amphojel
Hyperphosphatemia 6
5–15 mg/lb t.i.d.
Tab: 300 & 600 mg; susp: 64 mg/mL
64 mg/mL: 0.8–2.3 mL/10 lb t.i.d.; 300 mg: 0.2–0.6 tab/10 lb t.i.d.

Amikacin Amiglyde
Bacterial infections 7
2.3 mg/lb t.i.d. SC (3.5 mg/lb b.i.d. SC)
Inj: 50 & 250 mg/mL
50 mg/mL: 0.5 mL/10 lb t.i.d. SC or 0.7 mL/10 lb b.i.d. SC

Aminopentamide Centrine
Vomiting 8
0.1–0.4 mg/cat b.i.d.–t.i.d. SC IM PO
Tab: 0.2 mg; inj: 0.5 mg/mL
0.2 mg: 0.5 tab: up to 10 lb, 1 tab: 11–20 lb b.i.d.–t.i.d.
0.5 mg/mL: 0.2 mL: up to 10 lb, 0.4 mL: 11–20 lb b.i.d.–t.i.d. SC

Aminophylline Aminophylline USP
Bronchoconstriction 8
2–4 mg/lb b.i.d. PO, 1–3 mg/lb b.i.d. IV
Tab: 100 & 200 mg
100 mg: 0.2–0.4/10 lb b.i.d. PO

Amitraz Mitaban
Demodicosis Chapter 57
0.125% topically (½ recommended strength)
Soln to dilute: 19.9%
0.125% soln: apply topically q7d until skin scraping is negative
Dilute 1 bottle (10.6 mL) with 4 gal water

Amitriptyline Elavil
Hair pulling 3
5–10 mg/cat s.i.d. PO
Tab: 10 mg
10 mg: 0.5–1.0/cat s.i.d. PO

Amitriptyline Elavil
Self-mutilation 3
5–10 mg/cat s.i.d. PO
Tab: 10 mg
10 mg: 0.5–1.0/cat s.i.d. PO

Ammonium chloride Uroeze
Alkaline urine 9
0.8–1.0 g/day PO or 140 mg/lb/day PO
Tab: 500 mg (chewable): powder: 650 mg/¼ tsp
500 mg: 1/10 lb b.i.d.–t.i.d. PO; powder: ¼ tsp/10 lb b.i.d. PO

Amoxicillin Amoxi-Tab, Amoxil
Bacterial infections 47
5 mg/lb b.i.d. PO IM SC
Tab: 50 & 100 mg; susp: 25 & 50 mg/mL; Inj: 100 & 250 mg/mL
50 mg: 1/10 lb b.i.d. PO; 50 mg/mL: 1 mL/10 lb b.i.d. PO; 100 mg/mL: 0.5/10 lb b.i.d. IM SC

Amoxicillin/clavulanic acid Clavamox
Bacterial infections 5
6.25 mg/lb b.i.d. PO
Tab: 62.5 & 125 mg; susp: 62.5 mg/mL
62.5 mg: 1/10 lb b.i.d. PO; 62.5 mg/mL: 1 mL/10 lb b.i.d. PO

Amphotericin B Fungizone
Fungal infections: systemic Chapter 61
0.05–0.25 mg/lb IV e.o.d. for total dose of 2 mg/lb
5 mg/mL when diluted in 50-mg vial
5 mg/mL: 0.1–0.5 mL/10 lb IV e.o.d.; max total dose: 2 mg/lb
Dilute with 5% dextrose in water (only); may be frozen

Ampicillin sodium Polyflex
Bacterial infections 47
3 mg/lb b.i.d. IM SC
100 mg/mL when diluted
100 mg/mL: 0.3 mL/10 lb b.i.d. IM SC

Ampicillin trihydrate Principen
Bacterial infections 47
5–25 mg/lb t.i.d. PO
Cap: 250 & 500 mg; susp: 25 & 50 mg/mL
250 mg: 0.2–1/10 lb t.i.d. PO; 50 mg/mL: 1–5 mL/10 lb t.i.d.

Amprolium Corid
Coccidiosis 51
50–100 mg/lb s.i.d. PO for 7–12 days
Oral soln: 96 mg/mL (9.6%)
96 mg/mL: 5–10 mL/10 lb s.i.d. PO for 7–12 days

Amrinone Inocor
Cardiac: dilated CM 12
0.23–0.46 mg/lb IV
5 mg/mL
5 mg/mL: 0.45–0.9 mL/10 lb IV

Apomorphine HCl Apomorphine USP
Toxicity (to induce emesis) 11
0.018 mg/lb IV; 0.036 mg/lb SC IM
Tab: 6 mg to make 1 mg/mL soln (dissolve in 6 mL PSS)
1 mg/mL: 0.2 mL/10 lb IV; 0.4 mL/10 lb SC IM
Because of potential CNS excitation, another emetic should be used instead

Ascorbic acid Vitamin C
Toxicity: acetaminophen Chapter 62
15 mg/lb q.i.d. PO IM
Tab: 250 & 500 mg
250 mg: 2/10 lb b.i.d. PO; 500 mg: 1/10 lb b.i.d. PO

Asparaginase Elspar
See L-Asparaginase

Aspirin Ecotrin, Ascriptin
Pain 8
75–80 mg/cat q48–72h PO
Tab: Baby aspirin: 83 mg; regular strength: 325 mg
83 mg: 1/10 lb q72h PO; 325 mg: 0.25/10 lb q72h PO

Aspirin Ecotrin, Ascriptin
Thromboembolism 8
14 mg/lb q72h PO
Tab: Baby aspirin: 83 mg; regular strength: 325 mg
83 mg: 1/10 lb q72h PO; 325 mg: 0.25/10 lb q72h PO

Aspirin Ecotrin, Ascriptin
Uveitis Chapter 36
75–80 mg/cat q48–72h PO
Tab: Baby aspirin: 83 mg; regular strength: 325 mg
83 mg: 1/10 lb q72h PO; 325 mg: 0.25/10 lb q72h PO

Atenolol Tenormin
Cardiac: hypertrophic CM 11
6.25–12.5 mg/cat s.i.d. PO
Tab: 50 & 100 mg
50 mg: 0.12–0.25/cat s.i.d. PO

Atropine Atropine USP
Cardiac: bradycardia 8
0.02 mg/lb IV IM SC
Inj: 0.5 mg/mL (small animal); 15 mg/mL (large animal)
0.5 mg/mL: 0.5 mL/10 lb q6h IV IM SC

Atropine Atropine USP
Salivation: excessive 8
0.02 mg/lb IV IM SC
Inj: 0.5 mg/mL (small animal); 15 mg/mL (large animal)
0.5 mg/mL: 0.5 mL/10 lb q6h IV IM SC

Atropine Atropine USP
Toxicity: carbamate 14
0.1–0.25 mg/lb; give ¼ dose IV, remainder SC IM p.r.n.
Inj: 0.5 mg/mL (small animal); 15 mg/mL (large animal)
0.5 mg/mL: 2.0–20.0 mL/10 lb: ¼ dose IV, remainder SC IM p.r.n.
Repeat every 3–6 hr p.r.n.

Atropine Atropine USP
Toxicity: organophosphate 14
0.1–0.25 mg/lb; give ¼ dose IV, remainder SC IM p.r.n.
Inj: 0.5 mg/mL (small animal); 15 mg/mL (large animal)
0.5 mg/mL: 2.0–20.0 mL/10 lb: ¼ dose IV, remainder SC IM p.r.n.
Repeat every 3–6 hr p.r.n.

Auranofin Ridaura
Autoimmune skin diseases 44
0.8 mg/lb b.i.d. PO
Cap: 3 mg
3 mg: 2.6/10 lb b.i.d. PO

Auranofin Ridaura
Rheumatoid arthritis 44
0.8 mg/lb b.i.d. PO
Cap: 3 mg
3 mg: 2.6/10 lb b.i.d. PO

Aurothioglucose Solganol
Pemphigus 15
Treat q7d 1st: 1 mg IM; 2nd: 2 mg IM; 3rd–7th: 0.45 mg/lb IM
Inj: 50 mg/mL
Treat q7d, 50 mg/mL: 1st: 0.02 mL IM; 2nd–12th: 0.2 mL IM
May increase to 0.3 mL; when in remission treat q30d

Azathioprine Imuran
Autoimmune hemolytic anemia 11
0.9 mg/lb s.i.d. PO
Tab: 50 mg
50 mg: 0.2/10 lb s.i.d. PO

Azathioprine Imuran
Inflammatory bowel disease Chapter 48
0.14 mg/lb e.o.d. PO
Tab: 50 mg
50 mg: 0.03/10 lb e.o.d. PO (may safely use up to ¼ tab in many 10 lb cats)
Crush and mix with palatable liquid

Azathioprine Imuran
Pemphigus 11
0.9 mg/lb s.i.d. PO
Tab: 50 mg
50 mg: 0.2/10 lb s.i.d. PO

Benzocaine Cetacaine
Contraindicated 8

Benzyl alcohol Benzyl Alcohol USP
Contraindicated 16

Benzyl peroxide shampoo Oxydex Shampoo
Acne Chapter 60
Shampoo chin s.i.d. until healed
Do not use cream form of 5% benzyl peroxide

Betamethasone Betasone
Atopy 44
0.1–0.2 mg/lb SC IM once
Inj: 7 mg/mL
7 mg/mL: 0.14–0.28 mL/10 lb SC IM once

Betamethasone Betasone
Uveitis Chapter 36
3.5 mg/cat subconjunctivally
Inj: 7 mg/mL
7 mg/mL: 0.5 mL subconjunctivally

Bethanechol Urecholine
Bladder atony 8
1.25–5 mg/cat t.i.d. PO
Tab: 5, 10, 25, & 50 mg
5 mg: 0.25–1.0/cat t.i.d. PO

Bisacodyl Dulcolax
Constipation 8
2–5 mg/cat s.i.d.–b.i.d. PO
Tab: 5 mg; suppositories: 10 mg
5-mg tabs: 0.2–1.0/cat s.i.d.–b.i.d. PO; 10 mg suppositories: 0.1–0.5/cat s.i.d.–b.i.d.
Takes 6–12 hr to take effect; do not give if dehydrated or obstructed

Bismuth subsalicylate Pepto-Bismol
Diarrhea 8
0.5–1 mL/lb q4–6h PO
Tab: 262 mg; susp: 17.5 mg/mL
Tab: 0.25–0.5/10 lb q4–6h PO; susp: 5–10 mL/10 lb q4–6h PO
Max: 15 mL or 1 tab/day because of salicylate toxicity

Bran Bran
Constipation 8
1 to 2 tbsp/400 g food
Cereals
1–2 tbsp/400 g food

Brewer's yeast Brewer's Yeast
Folic acid deficiency 5
0.1 g/lb once daily PO
Tab: 390 mg
390 mg: 2.5/10 lb s.i.d. PO

Bunamidine Scolaban
Tapeworm infestation 5
11–23 mg/lb PO
Tab: 100, 200, and 400 mg
100 mg: 0.5–1.0/10 lb PO; fast 3 hr before and after administration

Buprenorphine Buprenex
Pain 43
Cat: 0.0045 mg/lb IM IV b.i.d.
Soln: 3 mg/mL
3 mg/mL: 0.015 mL IM IV b.i.d.

Busulfan Myleran
Neoplasia 44
2 mg/m^2 s.i.d. PO
Tab: 2 mg
2 mg: 0.5/10 lb s.i.d. PO

Butorphanol Torbutrol/Torbugesic
Pain 11, 36
0.05–0.1 mg/lb IV t.i.d.; 0.1–0.2 mg/lb t.i.d. IM SC; 0.25 mg/lb t.i.d. PO
Tab: 1, 5, & 10 mg; Inj: 0.5 mg/mL (Torbutrol) & 10 mg/mL (Torbugesic)
5 mg: 0.5/10 lb t.i.d. PO; 0.5 mg/mL: 1–2 mL/10 lb IV t.i.d.
0.5 mg/mL: 2–4 mL/10 lb t.i.d. IM SC; 10 mg/mL: 0.1–0.2 mL/10 lb t.i.d. IM SC

Calcitonin Calcimar
Toxicity: calciferol Chapter 62
2–3 IU/lb q2–3h SC
Inj: 200 IU/mL
200 IU/mL: 0.1–0.15 mL/10 lb q2–3h SC until serum calcium goes down to normal and stabilizes

Calcitonin Calcimar
Toxicity: vitamin D Chapter 62
2–3 IU/lb q2–3h SC
Inj: 200 IU/mL
200 IU/mL: 0.1–0.15 mL/10 lb q2–3h SC until serum calcium stabilizes

Calcium Calcium USP
Hypocalcemia 8
Inj: 100 mg/mL (10%) Calcium gluconate
Calcium gluconate (10%): 5–10 mL/cat slow IV to effect; monitor serum calcium
Goal is to maintain serum calcium at 8.5–9.5 mg/dL

Calcium carbonate Calcet
Hypocalcemia 43
22 mg/lb b.i.d.–t.i.d. PO
Tab: 240 mg
240 mg: 1/10 lb b.i.d.–t.i.d. PO

Calcium chloride Calcium Chloride, USP
Cardic arrest 43
4.5 mg/lb IV
Soln: 100 mg/mL (10%)
100 mg/mL (10% soln): 0.45 mL/10 lb

Calcium disodium EDTA Calcium Disodium Versenate
Toxicity: chelating agent Chapter 62
12 mg/lb q.i.d. SC
Inj: 200 mg/mL (dilute to 10 mg/mL in 5% dextrose)
10 mg./mL: 12 mL/10 lb q.i.d. SC

Calcium gluconate, 10% Calcium gluconate 10% USP
Hyperkalemia: severe Chapter 40
0.25 mg/lb IV
Inj: 10% soln (100 mg/mL)
100 mg/mL: 0.02 mL/10 lb IV

Calcium gluconate, 10% Calcium gluconate 10% USP
Uterine inertia Chapter 54
1–2 mL/cat IV with oxytocin
Inj: 10% soln (100 mg/mL)
10%: 1–2 mL/cat IV with oxytocin

Captan-50 WP Orthocide
Dermatophytosis 17
2 tbsp/gal water; 2×/wk for 2 wk, then 1×/wk for 4–6 wk
50% wettable powder (nurseries)
1.5 tbsp/L water: 2×/wk × 2, then q7d × 4–6 wk
Make fresh each time; use gloves and sponge on; shake well

Captopril Capoten
Cardiac: dilated CM 8
2–3 mg/cat t.i.d. PO, 3–6.25 mg/cat b.i.d. PO
Tab: 25, 50, 75, & 100 mg
25 mg: 0.12/cat t.i.d. or 0.12–0.25/cat b.i.d.; if anorexia occurs, reduce dose by 50%; do not use with furosemide

Carbenicillin Geopen/Geocillin
Bacterial infections 5
6.8 mg/lb t.i.d. PO IV
Tab: 382 mg; inj: 250 mg/mL when diluted
382 mg: 0.2/10 lb t.i.d. PO; 250 mg/mL: 0.3 mL t.i.d. IV

Cefaclor Ceclor
Bacterial infections 43
2–9 mg/lb t.i.d. PO
Cap: 250 & 500 mg
250 mg: 1/10–1/3/10 lb t.i.d. PO

Cefadroxil Cefa-Tabs, Cefa-Drops
Bacterial infections 11
10 mg/lb b.i.d. PO
Tab: 50, 100, & 200 mg; susp: 50 mg/mL
100 mg: 1/10 lb b.i.d. PO; susp: 2 mL/10 lb b.i.d. PO

Cefamandole nafate Mandol
Bacterial infections 11
2.7–18 mg/lb t.i.d.–q.i.d. IM IV
10 mg/mL, 20 mg/mL, and 100 mg/mL
20 mg/mL: 1.3–9.0 mL/10 lb t.i.d.–q.i.d. IM IV

Cefazolin Kefzol, Ancef
Bacterial infections 5
5–10 mg/lb t.i.d.–q.i.d. IM IV
Inj: 100 mg/mL
100 mg/mL: 0.5–1.0 mL/10 lb t.i.d.–q.i.d. IM IV

Cefotaxime sodium Claforan
Bacterial infections 8
9–36 mg/lb q.i.d. IM IV
Inj: 100 mg/mL
100 mg/mL: 0.9–3.6 mL/10 lb q.i.d. IM IV

Cefoxitin Mefoxin
Bacterial infections 8
10–15 mg/lb t.i.d. IM IV
Inj: 100 mg/mL
100 mg/mL: 1–1.5 mL/10 lb t.i.d. IM IV

Cephalexin Keflex
Bacterial infections 8
10–15 mg/lb t.i.d.–q.i.d. PO
Tab: 250 & 500 mg; susp: 125 & 250 mg/mL
250 mg: 0.4–0.6/10 lb t.i.d.–q.i.d. PO; 125 mg/mL: 0.8 mL/10 lb t.i.d.–q.i.d. PO

Cephalothin Keflin
Bacterial infections 50
4.5–9 mg/lb q6h IV
Inj: 100 mg/mL when reconstituted
100 mg/mL: 0.45–0.9 mL/10 lb q6h IV

Cephapirin Cefadyl
Bacterial infections 43
4.5 mg/lb IM, IV t.i.d.–q.i.d.
Inj: 33 mg/mL (500 mg/15 mL) & 66 mg/mL (1,000 mg/15 mL)
33 mg/mL: 1.4 mL/10 lb IM, IV t.i.d.–q.i.d.; 66 mg/mL: 0.7 mL/10 lb IM, IV t.i.d.–q.i.d.

Cephradine Anspor, Velosef
Bacterial infections 10
9 mg/lb q.i.d. PO, 4.5 mg/lb q.i.d. IM IV
Cap: 250 & 500 mg; susp: 25 & 50 mg/mL; inj: 50 mg/mL
250 mg: 0.4/10 lb q.i.d. PO; 25 mg/mL: 3.6 mL/10 lb q.i.d. PO
50 mg/mL: 1.8 mL/10 lb q.i.d. IM IV

Charcoal, activated Actidose-Aqua
See Activated charcoal

Chlorambucil Leukeran
Immune-mediated diseases 5
2 mg/cat e.o.d. PO
Tab: 2 mg
2 mg: 1/cat e.o.d. PO

Chlorambucil Leukeran
Neoplasia Chapter 51
2 mg/m^2 e.o.d. PO
Tab: 2 mg
2 mg: 0.3/10 lb e.o.d. PO

Chloramphenicol Medicol, Chloromycetin
Bacterial infections 8
7–9 mg/lb b.i.d.–t.i.d. PO SC IV
Tab/cap: 50, 100, 200, & 500 mg; inj: 100 mg/mL
100 mg: 0.7–0.9/10 lb b.i.d. PO; 100 mg/mL: 0.7–0.9 mL/10 lb SC IV

Chloramphenicol ophthalmic Chloromycetin
Conjunctivitis: *Chlamydia* 10
Ophthalmic ointment
Apply to eye(s) q3h

Chlordiazepoxide Librium
Anorexia 19
1.25–2.5 mg/cat s.i.d.–t.i.d. PO
Cap: 5, 10, & 25 mg
5 mg: 0.25–0.5/cat s.i.d.–t.i.d. PO

Chlorhexidine diacetate Nolvasan Solution
Dermatophytosis 17
25 mL soln/L water (2%) applied topically
2% soln: applied topically

Chlorhexidine diacetate Nolvasan/Chlorhexiderm
Dermatophytosis Chapter 56
Shampoo every 5–7 days

Chlorinated hydrocarbons Chlorinated Hydrocarbons
Contraindicated 8

Chlorpheniramine maleate Teldrin, Chlor-Trimeton Maleate
Pruritus 20 & 21
2 mg/cat b.i.d. PO
Tab: 4 mg; cap: 8 & 12 mg
4 mg: 0.5/cat b.i.d.–t.i.d. PO; 8 mg: 0.25/cat b.i.d.–t.i.d. PO

Chlorpromazine hydrochloride Thorazine
Toxicity: amphetamine Chapter 62
5–6 mg/lb IV
Inj: 25 mg/mL
25 mg/mL: 2.0–2.4 mL/10 lb IV
For lethal doses only

Chlorpromazine hydrochloride Thorazine
Tranquilization 8
1–2 mg/lb b.i.d.–t.i.d. PO; 0.2 mg/lb t.i.d.–q.i.d. IM IV
Tab: 10, 25, 50, & 100 mg; inj: 25 mg/mL
10 mg: 1–2/10 lb b.i.d.–t.i.d. PO; 25 mg/mL: 0.1 mL/10 lb t.i.d.–q.i.d. IM IV

Chlorpropamide Diabinese
Diabetes insipidus Chapter 22
5–20 mg/lb/day s.i.d. PO
Tab: 100 & 250 mg
100 mg: 0.5–2/10 lb s.i.d. PO

Chlorthiazide Diuril
Cardiac: diuretic 8
9–18 mg/lb b.i.d. PO
Tab: 250 & 500 mg; susp: 50 mg/mL
250 mg: 0.4–0.7/10 lb b.i.d. PO; 50 mg/mL: 1.8–3.6 mL/10 lb b.i.d. PO

Chlorthiazide Diuril
Pulmonary edema 8
9–18 mg/lb b.i.d. PO
Tab: 250 & 500 mg; susp: 50 mg/mL
250 mg: 0.4–0.7/10 lb b.i.d. PO; 50 mg/mL: 1.8–3.6 mL/10 lb b.i.d. PO

Cimetidine Tagamet
Gastritis due to renal failure Chapter 31
2 mg/lb b.i.d.–t.i.d. PO SC
Tab: 200 & 300 mg; inj: 150 mg/mL
200 mg: 0.1/10 lb b.i.d.–t.i.d. PO; 150 mg/mL: 0.02 mL/10 lb b.i.d.–t.i.d. SC

Cimetidine Tagamet
Mast cell tumor Chapter 51
2.3 mg/lb t.i.d. PO
Tab: 200 & 300 mg
200 mg: 0.1/10 lb t.i.d. PO

Cimetidine Tagamet
Toxicity: acetaminophen 22
2.5–5 mg/lb b.i.d.–t.i.d. PO IV IM
Tab: 200 & 300 mg; inj: 150 mg/mL
200 mg: 0.1–0.2/10 lb b.i.d.–t.i.d. PO; 150 mg/mL: 0.2–0.3 mL/10 lb b.i.d.–t.i.d. IV IM

Cimetidine Tagamet
Toxicity: NSAI (gastric ulcers) Chapter 62
2–5 mg/lb q6–8h PO; 5 mg/lb q6h IV (slow infusion over 30 min)
Tab: 200 & 300 mg; inj: 150 mg/mL
200 mg: 0.1–0.25/10 lb q6–8h PO; 150 mg/mL: 0.33 mL/10 lb IV as slow infusion over 30 min

Ciprofloxacin Cipro
Bacterial infections: soft tissue, bone 8
5–7 mg/lb b.i.d. PO
Tab: 250, 500, & 750 mg
250 mg: 0.2–0.3/10 lb b.i.d. PO

Ciprofloxacin Cipro
Bacterial infections: urinary 8
2–4 mg/lb b.i.d. PO
Tab: 250, 500, & 750 mg
250 mg: 0.1–0.2/10 lb b.i.d. PO

Clindamycin Antirobe
Bacterial infections 8
2.5 mg/lb b.i.d. PO
Cap: 25, 75, & 150 mg; susp: 25 mg/mL
25 mg: 1/10 lb b.i.d. PO; 25 mg/mL: 1 mL/10 lb b.i.d. PO

Clindamycin Antirobe
Bacterial osteomyelitis 8
5 mg/lb s.i.d.–b.i.d. PO
Cap: 25, 75, & 150 mg; susp: 25 mg/mL
25 mg: 2/10 lb s.i.d.–b.i.d. PO; 25 mg/mL: 2 mL/10 lb s.i.d.–b.i.d. PO

Clindamycin Antirobe
Toxoplasmosis 23
6 mg/lb b.i.d. PO × 2–6 wk
Cap: 25, 75, & 150 mg
25 mg: 2.5/10 lb b.i.d. PO; 75 mg: 1/10 lb b.i.d. PO for 2–6 wk

Clotrimazole Veltrim/Lotrimin
Dermatophytosis Chapter 56
Cream
Apply to lesions topically b.i.d.

Colistimethate sodium Coly-Mycin
Bacterial infections 5
0.5 mg/lb q.i.d. IM
Inj: 15 mg/mL when diluted
15 mg/mL: 0.3 mL/10 lb q.i.d. IM

Cortisone acetate Cortone Acetate
Hypoadrenocorticism 43
0.45 mg/lb s.i.d. PO, IM
Tab: 25 mg; inj: 25 mg/mL
25 mg: 0.2/10 lb s.i.d. PO; 25 mg/mL: 0.2 mL/10 lb s.i.d. IM

Cyclizine lactate Marezine
Vomiting 8
2 mg/lb t.i.d. PO IM
Tab: 50 mg; inj: 50 mg/mL
50 mg: 0.4/10 lb t.i.d. PO; inj: 0.4 mL/10 lb t.i.d. IM

Cyclophosphamide Cytoxan
Immune-mediated anemia 11
3 mg/lb s.i.d. PO for 3 days; then 1 mg/lb s.i.d. PO
Tab: 25 & 50 mg
25 mg: 1.2/10 lb s.i.d. PO for 3 days; then 0.4/10 lb s.i.d. PO
See reference for long-term use

Cyclophosphamide Cytoxan
Neoplasia Chapter 51
50 mg/m^2 e.o.d. PO; 100–200 mg/m^2 q7d then 250 mg/m^2 q3wk
Tab: 25 & 50 mg; inj: 20 mg/mL
25 mg: 0.5/10 lb e.o.d. PO; 20 mg/mL: 1.4–2.8 mL/10 lb q7d then 3.3 mL/10 lb q3wk
See Table 51–2 for combination therapy

Cyproheptadine Periactin, Vimicon
Anorexia 44
0.25 mg/lb t.i.d. PO
Tab: 4 mg
4 mg: 0.6/10 lb t.i.d. PO
Note: Has caused aggression in some cats

Cythioate Proban
Flea infestation 8
0.7–1.4 mg/lb PO q72–96h
Tab: 30 mg
30 mg: 0.5/10 lb q72–96h

Cythioate Proban
Flea infestation 11
0.1 mg/lb PO 2×/wk
Tab: 30 mg; liq: 16 mg/mL (1.6%)
30 mg: 0.5/10 lb q3–4d PO; 16 mg/mL: 0.6 mL/10 lb q3–4d PO

Cytosine arabinoside (cytarabine) Cytosar
Neoplasia Chapter 51
100 mg/m^2 q24h for 2–4 days IV SC; 10 mg–m^2 q24h for 14 days IV SC
20 mg/mL when diluted
20 mg/mL: 1.35 mL/10 lb q24h for 2–4 days IV SC; 0.14 mL/10 lb q24h for 14 days IV SC; see Table 51–2 for combination therapy

Dacarbazine DTIC-Dome
Neoplasia: lymphoreticular 11
200–250 mg/m^2 s.i.d. IV for 5 days, repeat q3wk; or 300 mg/m^2 q3w IV
10 mg/mL when diluted
10 mg/mL: 5–6.25 mL/10 lb s.i.d. IV for 5 days, repeat q3w or 7.5 mL/10 lb q3w IV

Delmadione Unavailable in United States
Estrus prevention Chapter 54
Unavailable: PO q7d or SC q6m

Demecarium bromide Humorsol
Glaucoma Chapter 36
2 drops in affected eye s.i.d.–b.i.d.
Ophthalmic drops: 0.125% & 0.25%
Both: 2 drops in affected eye s.i.d–b.i.d.
Titrate dosage interval based on effects

Desferoxamine Desferal
Toxicity: iron (in vitamins) Chapter 62
20 mg/lb q6–8h IM IV (slow drip)
Inj: 250 mg/mL
250 mg/mL: 0.8 mL/10 lb IM or slow IV infusion (less than 0.3 mL/10 lb/hr)

Desmopressin acetate DDAVP
Diabetes insipidus Chapter 22
1–2 drops in alternating eyes s.i.d.–b.i.d.
Nasal spray: 100 μg/mL
1–2 drops in alternating eyes s.i.d.–b.i.d.
1 drop contains 1.5–4.0 μg; *very expensive*

Desmopressin acetate DDAVP
Diabetes insipidus 5
2–4 drops s.i.d.–b.i.d. intranasally or in conjunctival sac
Inj: 4 μg/mL DDAVP; nasal spray 2.5 mL/vial
2–4 drops s.i.d.–b.i.d. intranasally or in conjunctival sac

Desoxycorticosterone acetate DOCA Injection
Hypoadrenocorticism 8
0.5–1 mg/cat s.i.d. IM
Inj: 5 mg/mL
0.1–0.2 mL/cat s.i.d. IM

Desoxycorticosterone pivalate Percortin IM Repository
Hypoadrenocorticism 8
5–50 mg/cat q30d IM
6.25 mg/mL
6.25 mg/mL: 1–8 mL/cat q30d IM

Dexamethasone Azium
Autoimmune diseases 8
0.45 mg/lb s.i.d. IV IM
Inj: 2 & 4 mg/mL
2 mg/mL: 2 mL/10 lb s.i.d. IV IM; 4 mg/mL: 1 mL/10 lb s.i.d. IV IM

Dexamethasone Azium
Neoplasia 8
0.45 mg/lb s.i.d. IV IM
Inj: 2 & 4 mg/mL
2 mg/mL: 2 mL/10 lb s.i.d. IV IM; 4 mg/mL: 1 mL/10 lb s.i.d. IV IM

Dexamethasone Azium
Pruritus 8
0.06–0.2 mg/lb s.i.d. PO IV IM
Tab: 0.25, 0.5, 1 & 1.5 mg; inj: 2 & 4 mg/mL
2 mg/mL: 0.3–1 mL/10 lb s.i.d. IV IM; 4 mg/mL: 0.2–0.5 mL/10 lb s.i.d. IV IM
1 mg: 0.6–2.0/10 lb s.i.d. PO

Dexamethasone Azium
Shock 8
2.3 mg/lb p.r.n. IV
Inj: 2 & 4 mg/mL
2 mg/mL: 12 mL/10 lb; 4 mg/mL: 6 mL/10 lb p.r.n. IV

Dexamethasone Azium
Spinal cord trauma Chapter 45
0.5–1.0 mg/lb IV initially, then 0.025 mg/lb IM q8h × 3 days, then tapered
Inj: 2 & 4 mg/mL
2 mg/mL: 2.5–5 mL/10 lb IV initially then 1.5 mL/10 lb q8h IM × 3 days, then tapered over the next 10–14 days

Dexamethasone Azium
Uveitis Chapter 36
0.1–0.2 mg/lb s.i.d. PO SC IV
Tab: 0.25, 0.5, 1 & 1.5 mg; inj: 2 & 4 mg/mL
0.25 mg: 4–8 s.i.d. PO; 1.0: 1–2/10 lb s.i.d. PO; 2 mg/mL: 0.5–1.0/10 lb s.i.d. SC IV

Dextran 75, in saline Dextran 6%
Frostbite 43
5–10 mL/lb/day IV in saline in first 24 hr
6% dextran 40, in saline
50–100 mL/10 lb IV in saline in first 24 hr

Dextran 75, in saline Dextran 6%
Shock 43
5–10 mL/lb/day IV in saline in first 24 hr
6% dextran 40, in saline
50–100 mL/10 lb IV in saline in first 24 hr

Dextromethorphan Tussar DM (+ chlorpheniramine & pseudoephedrine)
Cough 24
0.9 mg/lb q.i.d PO
3 mg/mL
3 mg/mL: 3 mL/10 lb q.i.d. PO

Dextrose 20% Dextrose USP 20%
Renal failure: intense diuresis Chapter 31
2 mL/min for 10–15 min, then 1 mL/min to a total dose of 10–30 mL/lb
Inj: 200 mg/mL (20%)
2 mL/min for 10–15 min, then 1 mL/min to a total dose of 10–30 mL/lb

Diazepam Valium
Aggression 3
1–2 mg/cat b.i.d.
Tab: 2, 5, & 10 mg
2 mg: 0.5–1.0 b.i.d. for 1–2 mo, then gradually reduce; may need p.r.n.

Diazepam Valium
Anorexia 8
0.1 mg/lb s.i.d.–b.i.d. IV PO
Tab: 2, 5, & 10 mg; inj: 5 mg/mL
2 mg: 0.5/10 lb s.i.d.–b.i.d. PO; 5 mg/mL: 0.2 mL s.i.d.–b.i.d. IV

Diazepam Valium
Dysuria 9
1 mg t.i.d. PO
Tab: 2, 5, & 10 mg
2 mg: 0.5/cat t.i.d. PO

Diazepam Valium
Fear 3
1–2 mg/cat b.i.d.
Tab: 2, 5, & 10 mg
2 mg: 0.5–1.0 b.i.d. for 1–2 mo, then gradually reduce; may need p.r.n.

Diazepam Valium
Seizures (maintenance) 8
0.1–0.3 mg/lb t.i.d. PO
Tab: 2, 5, & 10 mg
2 mg: 0.5–1.5/10 lb t.i.d. PO
t.i.d. essential; therefore, many problems with client compliance

Diazepam Valium
Status epilepticus Chapters 23 & 62
0.5–1.25 mg increments (up to 20 mg/cat) IV to effect
Inj: 5 mg/mL
5 mg/mL: 0.1–0.25 mL increments (up to 4 mL/cat) IV
Must be given IV; IM does not achieve adequate blood levels

Diazepam Valium
Tranquilization 8
0.1–0.2 mg/lb IV IM
Inj: 5 mg/mL
5 mg/mL: 0.2–0.4 mL/10 lb IV
Less than 5 mg total dose

Diazepam Valium
Urine spraying 3
1–2 mg/cat b.i.d.
Tab: 2, 5, & 10 mg
2 mg: 0.5–1.0 b.i.d. for 1–2 mo, then gradually reduce; may need p.r.n.

Diazepam Valium
Vertigo (vestibular disease) Chapter 17
2–3 mg t.i.d.–q.i.d. PO
Tab: 2, 5, & 10 mg
2 mg: 1.0–1.5 t.i.d.–q.i.d. PO
Reduce dose if sedation occurs

Diazoxide Proglycem
Insulinoma: hypoglycemia 25
Initially: 5 mg/lb s.i.d.; gradually increase to 20 mg/lb s.i.d. according to glucose
Cap: 50 mg; susp: 50 mg/mL
50 mg: 1/10 lb s.i.d. PO; 50 mg/mL: 1 mL/10 lb s.i.d. PO; gradually increase to 2 cap or 2 mL/10 lb PO according to glucose level

Dichlorphenamide Daranide
Glaucoma Chapter 36
1–2 mg/lb b.i.d.–t.i.d. PO
Tab: 50 mg
50 mg: 0.2–0.4/10 lb b.i.d.–t.i.d. PO

Dichlorvos Task
Helminths 43
5–10 mg/lb PO; repeat in 3 wk
Tab: 10, & 25 mg
25 mg: 2–4/10 lb PO; repeat in 3 wk

Dicloxacillin Dynapen, Dicloxin
Bacterial infections 5
5–25 mg/lb t.i.d. PO
Cap: 250 & 500 mg
250 mg: 0.2–1.0/10 lb t.i.d. PO

Diethylcarbamazine Difil, Carbam, Nemacide
Helminths 47
25–50 mg/lb once PO; repeat in 3 wk
Tab: 200 & 300 mg; syrup: 60 mg/mL
200 mg: 1.25–2.5/10lb once PO; 60 mg/mL: 4.2–8.3 mL/10 lb once PO
Repeat in 3 wk

Diethylcarbamazine Dirocide
Heartworm (prevention) 47
3 mg/lb s.i.d. PO
Tab: 50 & 100 mg; syrup: 60 mg/mL
50 mg: 0.6/10 lb s.i.d. PO; 60 mg/mL: 0.5 mL/10 lb s.i.d. PO

Digestive enzymes Prozyme
Diarrhea 10
¼ tsp with each meal, not to exceed 1 tsp/day
Powder
¼ tsp/cat with meal, not to exceed 1 tsp/day

Digoxin Cardoxin, Lanoxin
Cardiac: dilated CM 8
0.0023–0.0045 mg/lb PO q48–72h
Tab: 0.125, 0.25, 0.5 mg
0.125 mg: 0.25/10 lb q48–72h

Dihydrotachysterol DHT, Intensol Liquid
Hypocalcemia 11
0.014 mg/lb/day for 3–4 days, then 0.005–0.009 mg/lb/day or 1–2 drops s.i.d.–b.i.d. PO
Tab: 0.125, 0.2, & 0.4 mg; liq: 0.2 mg/mL
0.2 mg/mL: 1–2 drops s.i.d.–b.i.d. PO, or 0.7 mL/10 lb/s.i.d. for 3–4 days, then 0.25–0.45 mL/10 lb/s.i.d.

Diltiazem HCl Cardizem
Cardiac: hypertrophic CM 8
0.7–0.9 mg/lb t.i.d. PO
Tab: 30, 60, 90, & 120 mg
30 mg: 0.25–0.33/cat b.i.d.–t.i.d. PO
Adjust to heart rate (<180)

Dimenhydrinate Dramamine
Motion sickness 5
4 mg/lb t.i.d. PO
Tab: 50 mg
50 mg: 0.8/10 lb t.i.d. PO

Dimercaprol BAL in Oil
Toxicity: heavy metal Chapter 62
1.1–2.3 mg/lb IM q4h 1st 2 days; q8h, 3rd day; b.i.d. × 10
Inj: 100 mg/mL
100 mg/mL: 0.1–0.2 mL/10 lb IM
Give q4h for 2 days, q8h on 3rd day, then b.i.d. × 10 until recovery

Dioctyl sulfosuccinate Colace, Surfak
Constipation 26
50 mg/cat s.i.d.–b.i.d. PO
Cap: 50 mg
50 mg: 1/cat s.i.d.–b.i.d. PO
Oral liquid not recommended because of very bad taste

Diphenhydramine HCl Benadryl
Mast cell tumor 8
1–2 mg/lb t.i.d. PO
Cap: 25 & 50 mg; elixir: 2.5 mg/mL
25 mg: 0.4–0.8/10 lb t.i.d. PO; 2.5 mg/mL: 4–8 mL/10 lb PO t.i.d.

Diphenoxylate Lomotil
Diarrhea 8
0.125 mg/lb b.i.d. PO
Tab: 2.5 mg; liq: 0.5 mg/mL
2.5 mg: 0.5/10 lb b.i.d. PO; 0.5 mg/mL: 2.5 mL/10 lb b.i.d. PO

Dipyrone Novin
Fever 8
0.25 mL/cat t.i.d. SC IM IV × 2, then s.i.d.–b.i.d. SC IM IV
Inj: 500 mg/mL (50% soln)
500 mg/mL: 0.25 mL/cat t.i.d. SC IM IV × 2, then s.i.d.–b.i.d.

Dl-methionine Methio-Form
Urine acidifier 9
1.0–1.5 g/cat/day
Tab: 500 mg
500 mg: 1–1.5 b.i.d.–t.i.d. according to urine pH

DMSO Rismo-50
Dysuria 9
10–20 mL of 1:10 (10%) soln
99% DMSO; dilute 1:10 to make 10% soln
10% soln: 10–20 mL in bladder for 10 min; repeat once in 2 wk

Dobutamine Dobutrex
Cardiac: dilated CM 12
0.45–2.3 µg/lb/min IV infusion
Inj: 1,250 µg/mL when diluted with 200 mL lactated Ringer's
1,250 µg/mL: 0.004–0.02 mL/10 lb IV infusion

Docusate calcium/sodium Surfak/Colace
Constipation 5
50 mg/cat s.i.d.–b.i.d. PO
Cap: 50 mg
50 mg: 1/cat s.i.d.–b.i.d. PO
Oral liquid not recommended because of bad taste

Dopamine Intropin
Renal shutdown Chapter 31
0.9–2.3 µg/lb/min IV with diuretics
Inj: 40 mg/mL (dilute to 0.04 mg/mL with lactated Ringer's)
0.04 mg/mL: 0.22–0.58 mL/10 lb IV
See Chapter 31 before administering

Dopamine Intropin
Shock: cardiogenic 12
0.45–2.3 µg/lb/min IV infusion
Inj: 40 mg/mL (dilute to 0.04 mg/mL with lactated Ringer's)
0.04 mg/mL: 0.11–0.6 mL/10 lb IV infusion

Doxapram Dopram
Apnea 5
2.3–4.5 mg/lb IV; neonates: 1–5 mg SC, sublingual, or umbilical vein
Inj: 20 mg/mL
20 mg/mL: 1.1–2.2 mL/10 lb, IV
Neonates: 20 mg/mL: 0.05–0.25 mL SC, sublingual, or umbilical vein

Doxorubicin Adriamycin
Neoplasia Chapter 51
20–30 mg/m^2 q3w IV
Inj: 2 mg/mL when diluted
2 mg/mL: 2.5–3.8 mL/10 lb q3w IV
See Table 51-2 for combination therapy

Doxycycline Vibramycin, Doxytabs
Bacterial infections 5
Loading: 2.3 mg/lb; then 1.1 mg/lb 12 hr later, then 1.1 mg/lb s.i.d. PO
Tab: 100 mg; cap: 50 & 100 mg
50 mg: loading: 0.5/10 lb PO followed in 12 hr by 0.25/10 lb PO, then 0.25/10 lb s.i.d. PO
Susp: 5 mg/mL

Doxycycline Vibramycin, Doxytabs
Rickettsial infections 5
Loading: 2.3 mg/lb; then 1.1 mg/lb 12 hr later, then 1.1 mg/lb s.i.d. PO
Susp: 5 mg/mL
Tab: 100 mg; cap: 50 & 100 mg
50 mg: loading: 0.5/10 lb PO followed in 12 hr by 0.25/10 lb PO, then 0.25/10 lb s.i.d. PO

Echothiophate Phospholine Iodide
Glaucoma Chapter 36
2 drops on affected eye s.i.d.–b.i.d.
Ophthalmic drops: 0.06%, 0.12%, and 0.25%
All concentrations: 2 drops in affected eye s.i.d.–b.i.d.
Begin with 0.06%; increase strength if needed to produce results

Edrophonium chloride Tensilon
Myasthenia gravis 27
0.1–1.0 mg IV slowly
Inj: 10 mg/mL
10 mg/mL: 0.01–0.1 mL/10 lb IV slowly
May cause bradycardia; have atropine ready if needed

EDTA EDTA USP
See Calcium EDTA

Enalapril Vasotec
Hypertension 11
0.11–0.23 mg/lb e.o.d. PO
Tab: 2.5, 5, & 10 mg
2.5 mg: 0.5–1.0/10 lb e.o.d. PO; 5 mg: 0.2–0.4/10 lb e.o.d. PO

Enflurane Ethrane
Anesthesia 43
Induction: 2–3%; maintenance: 1.5–3%

Enrofloxacin Baytril
Bacterial infections 47
1 mg/lb b.i.d. PO IM
Tab: 5, 20, & 60 mg; inj: 22.7 mg/mL
5 mg: 2/10 lb b.i.d. PO; 20 mg: 0.5/10 lb b.i.d. PO; 22.7 mg/mL: 0.5 mL/10 lb b.i.d. IM

Ephedrine Marax
Bronchoconstriction 8
0.45 mg/lb PO t.i.d.
Tab: 25 mg; syrup: 1.25 mg/mL
25 mg: 0.2/10 lb t.i.d. PO; 1.25 mg/mL: 4 mL t.i.d. PO

Epinephrine Adrenalin
Cardiac arrest 8
0.05 mL/lb of 1:1,000 soln IV IM SC intrapulmonary
1:1,000 soln: dilute to 1:10,000 to use
1:10,000: 0.5 mL/10 lb IV IM SC intrapulmonary

Epinephrine Epifrin
Horner's syndrome Chapter 35
2 drops in affected eye t.i.d.–q.i.d.
Ophthalmic: 1–2%
1 or 2%: 2 drops in affected eye t.i.d.–q.i.d.

Epsiprantel Cestex
Tapeworm infestation 43
1.14 mg/lb PO
Tab: 12.5, 25, 50, & 100 mg
12.5 mg: 1/10 lb PO
Not for kittens less than 7 wk of age

Erythromycin Erythrocin
Bacterial infections 8
5.0 mg/lb t.i.d. PO
Tab: 250 & 500 mg; oral susp: 40 mg/mL and 80 mg/mL
Tab: 0.2/10 lb t.i.d. PO
40 mg/mL: 1.2 mL/10 lb t.i.d. PO; 80 mg/mL: 0.6 mL/10 lb t.i.d. PO

Erythropoietin, human recombin Epogen, Procrit
Anemia secondary to renal failure 53
Initially: 50–240 U/lb IV, SC 3 ×/wk
Inj: 1,000 & 2,000 U/mL
1,000 U/mL: 0.5–2.4 mL/10 lb 3 ×/wk initially, then reduce
2,000 U/mL: 0.25–1.2 mL/10 lb 3 ×/wk initially, then reduce

Estradiol cypionate ECP
Mismating Chapter 54
250 μg/cat IM 36–48 hr postcoitus
Inj: 2 mg/mL
2 mg/mL: 0.12 mL/cat IM 36–48 hr postcoitus
Retards embryo transport in oviduct

Estradiol cypionate ECP
Mismating Chapter 54
125–250 μg/cat IM once, up to 6 days after end of estrus
Inj: 2 mg/mL
2 mg/mL: 0.06–0.12 mL/cat IM 36–48 hr postcoitus
Blocks implantation or is embryotoxic

Ethacrynate sodium Edecrin
Cardiac: diuretic 43
0.1–0.2 mg/lb q4–12h IV IM
Tab: 25 & 50 mg
25 mg: 0.1/10 lb

Ethanol Everclear
Toxicity: ethylene glycol 1
2.5 mg/lb IV q4h × 5, then q.i.d. × 4
Inj: 200 mg/mL (20% soln)
20% soln: 8 mL/10 lb IV q4h × 5, then q.i.d. × 4 + $NaHCO_3$ & lactate Ringer's IV
$NaHCO_3$ & IV lactated Ringer's needs to be given during treatment period

Famotidine Pepcid
Gastric Ulcer 54
1–2 mg s.i.d. PO; 1–2 mg b.i.d. IV
Oral susp.: 8 mg/mL; Inj: 10 mg/mL
Susp: 8 mg/mL: 0.12–0.25 mL/10 lb s.i.d. PO; 10 mg/mL: 0.1–0.2 mL/10 lb b.i.d. IV

Fenbendazole Panacur
Helminths 8
23 mg/lb PO once
Powder: 222 mg/g; paste & susp: 100 mg/mL
0.4 tsp/10 lb PO once

Fenthion Pro-Spot
Flea infestation 8
0.035 mg/lb topically q7d
Topical soln: 56 mg/mL (5.6%) & 138 mg/mL (13.8%)
56 mg/mL: 1 drop/10 lb topically q7d

Ferrous sulfate Lixotinic, Feosol
Anemia: iron deficiency 8
23–136 mg/lb s.i.d. PO
Lixotinic: 16.6 mg/mL; Feosol: cap: 250 mg & elixir: 44 mg/mL
Lixotinic: 16.6 mg/mL: 14–88 mL/10 lb s.i.d. PO
Feosol: 44 mg/mL: 5.4–34 mL/10 lb s.i.d. PO; 250 mg: 1–6/10 lb s.i.d. PO

Flubiprofen, 0.03% Ocufen
Uveitis Chapter 36
Apply topically q6h
Topical susp: 0.03%
0.03%: apply topically q6h

Flucytosine (5-FC) Ancobon
Systemic fungal diseases 43
15–20 mg/lb t.i.d.–q.i.d. PO
Cap: 250 & 500 mg
250 mg: 0.6–0.8/10 lb t.i.d.–q.i.d. PO

Fludrocortisone acetate Florinef
Hypoadrenocorticism 8
0.1–0.2 mg/cat s.i.d. PO
Tab: 0.1 mg
0.1 mg: 1–2/10 lb s.i.d. PO
Dose usually needs to be adjusted (up) during first 6–18 mo into therapy

Flumethasone Flucort
Pruritus 8
0.03–0.125 mg/cat s.i.d. IV IM SC PO
Tab: 0.0625 mg; soln: 0.5 mg/mL
0.0625 mg: 0.5–2.0/cat s.i.d. PO; 0.5 mg/mL: 0.06–0.25 mL/cat s.i.d. IV IM SC

Flunixin meglumine Benamine
Inflammation 4
0.5 mg/lb IV q7d for 3 injections
Inj: 50 mg/mL
50 mg/mL: 0.1 mL/10 lb IV q7d for 3 injections

Flurazepam HCl Dalmane
Anorexia 28
0.05–0.1 mg/lb s.i.d.–b.i.d. PO
Cap: 15 & 30 mg
15 mg: 0.05–0.1/10 lb s.i.d.–b.i.d. PO

Folic acid Folic Acid Tabs (Danbury)
Folic acid deficiency due to pyrimethamine 43
1 mg/cat s.i.d. PO
Tab: 1 mg
1 mg: 1/cat s.i.d. PO

Follicle-stimulating hormone FSH-P
Estrus induction Chapter 54
2 mg/cat IM s.i.d. until estrus (max: 5 days)
Inj: 5 mg/mL
5 mg/mL: 0.4 mL/cat IM s.i.d. until estrus (max: 5 days)
House with cycling queen & provide 14+ hr of light

Furosemide Lasix
Cardiac: diuretic 8
0.11–2.3 mg/lb b.i.d.–q.i.d. PO
Tab: 12.5 & 50 mg; syrup: 10 mg/mL (1%)
12.5 mg: 0.25–2/10 lb b.i.d.–q.i.d. PO; 10 mg/mL: 0.1–2.0 mL/10 lb b.i.d.–q.i.d. PO

Furosemide Lasix
Diuresis: forced Chapter 62
2 mg/lb IV q6–8h
Inj: 50 mg/mL
50 mg/mL: 0.4 mL/10 lb IV q6–8h

Furosemide Lasix
Pulmonary edema 8
0.11–2.3 mg/lb b.i.d.–q.i.d. PO
Tab: 12.5 & 50 mg; syrup: 10 mg/mL (1%)
12.5 mg: 0.25–2/10 lb b.i.d.–q.i.d. PO; 10 mg/mL: 0.1–2.0 mL/10 lb b.i.d.–q.i.d. PO

Gentamicin sulfate Gentocin
Baterial infections 8
1.1 mg/lb b.i.d. IM SC
Inj: 40, 50, & 100 mg/mL
40 mg/mL: 0.3 mL/10 lb b.i.d. IM SC; 50 mg/mL: 0.2 mL/10 lb b.i.d. IM SC

Gentamicin sulfate Gentocin Ophthalmic
Conjunctivitis: bacterial 10
Apply to affected eye b.i.d.–q.i.d.
Ophthalmic soln & ointment
Apply to affected eye b.i.d.–q.i.d.

Gentamicin sulfate + betamethasone Gentocin Durafilm
Conjunctivitis: bacterial 10
Apply to affected eye b.i.d.–q.i.d.
Ophthalmic soln
Apply to affected eye b.i.d.–q.i.d.

Gentamicin sulfate + betamethasone Gentocin Otic
Otitis: bacterial 10
Apply to affected ear canal b.i.d.
Otic soln
Apply to affected ear canal b.i.d.

Glucagon Glucagon
Hypoglycemia: short-term 43
0.01 mg/lb IV
Inj: 0.02 mg/mL
0.02 mg/mL: 5 mL/10 lb IV

Glipizide Glucotrol
Diabetes mellitus (Type II) Chapter 34
2.5–10 mg/cat b.i.d. PO
Tab: 5 mg
5 mg: ¼–2 b.i.d. PO adjusted to fasting blood glucose

Glycerin Glycerin USP
Glaucoma Chapter 36
0.25–0.5 g/lb b.i.d. PO
Liq: 99.5%
99.5% liq: 2.5–5 mL/10 lb b.i.d. PO
Mix in palatable liq or milk; may cause nausea or diarrhea

Glycopyrrolate Robinul
Cardiac: bradycardia 5
0.005 mg/lb IM IV SC; divide dose ½ IV and ½ SC
Inj: 0.2 mg/mL
0.2 mg/mL: 0.5 mL/10 lb: ½ IV and ½ SC

Glycopyrrolate Robinul
Salivation: excessive 5
0.005 mg/lb IM IV SC; divide dose ½ IV and ½ SC
Inj: 0.2 mg/mL
0.2 mg/mL: 0.5 mL/10 lb: ½ IV and ½ SC

Gonadotropin-releasing hormone Cystorellin
Ovulation induction Chapter 54
25 μg/cat IM on Day 2 of estrus
Inj: 50 μg/mL
50 μg/mL: 0.5 mL/cat IM on Day 2 of estrus

Griseofulvin microsize Fulvicin U/F
Dermatophytosis Chapter 56
5–25 mg/lb PO b.i.d.
Tab: 125, 250, & 500 mg; susp: 25 mg/mL
125 mg: 0.4–2.0/10 lb; 250 mg: 0.2–1/10 lb; 25 mg/mL: 1–2 mL/10 lb b.i.d. PO
Give with fatty meal; treat for 4–6 wk

Griseofulvin ultramicrosize Fulvicin P/G, Gris-PEG
Dermatophytosis Chapter 56
2.3–4.6 mg/lb b.i.d. PO
Tab: 125 & 250 mg
125 mg: 0.2–0.4/10 lb b.i.d. PO
Treat for 4–6 wk; fatty meal not necessary

Halothane Fluothane
Anesthesia 43
Induction: 3%; maintenance: 0.5–1.5%
Induction: 3%; maintenance: 0.5–1.5%

Heparin Heparin USP
Disseminated intravascular coagulation 8
45–114 U/lb t.i.d. IV SC
Inj: 1,000 U/mL
1,000 IU/mL: 0.5–1.0 mL/10 lb t.i.d. IV SC

Heparin Heparin USP
Thromboembolism 30
1,000 U/cat IV then 25 U/lb q6–8h
Inj: 1,000 U/mL
1,000 U/mL: 1 mL/cat, then 0.25 mL/10 lb q6–8h to maintain clotting time at 2–2.5 times pretreatment value

Hetacillin Hetacin K
Bacterial infections 10
10 mg/lb b.i.d. PO
Tab: 50, 100, & 200 mg
50 mg: 2/10 lb b.i.d. PO; 100 mg: 1/10 lb b.i.d. PO

Hexachlorophene PHisoHex
Contraindicated 31

Human chorionic gonadotropin Follutein
Cystic ovarian follicles Chapter 54
250 IU/cat IM s.i.d. × 2
Inj: 1,000 IU/mL
1,000 IU: 0.25 mL/cat IM s.i.d. × 2
Controversial efficacy

Human chorionic gonadotropin Follutein
Ovulation induction 43
100–500 IU IM following follicle-stimulating hormone (FSH) or mating
Inj: 1,000 IU/mL
1,000 IU/mL: 0.1–0.5 mL/10 lb IM following FSH or mating

Human chorionic gonadotropin Follutein
Ovulation induction Chapter 54
500 IU/cat IM on Day 1 or Days 1 & 2 of estrus
Inj: 1,000 IU/mL
1,000 IU/mL: 0.5 mL/cat IM on Day 1 or Days 1 & 2 of estrus

Human chorionic gonadotropin Follutein, Chortropin
Anestrus: induce ovulation 29
250 IU IM on Day 1 & 2 of estrus, and after FSH inj have been discontinued
1,000 IU/mL when reconstituted
1,000 IU/mL: 0.25 mL/10 lb IM on Day 1 & 2 of estrus and after FSH inj have been discontinued

Hydralazine Apresoline
Cardiac: afterload reducer 8
2.5 mg/cat b.i.d. PO
Tab: 10, 25, 50, & 100 mg
25 mg: 1/cat b.i.d. PO

Hydrochlorothiazide HydroDiuril
Diabetes insipidus Chapter 22
12.5 mg/cat b.i.d. PO
Tab: 25 mg
25 mg: 0.5/10 lb b.i.d. PO

Hydrochlorothiazide HydroDiuril
Hypertension Chapter 36
12.5 mg/cat b.i.d. PO
Tab: 25 mg
25 mg: 0.5/cat b.i.d. PO

Hydrochlorothiazide HydroDiuril
Retinal detachment (hypertension) Chapter 36
12.5 mg/cat b.i.d. PO
Tab: 25 mg
25 mg: 0.5/cat b.i.d. PO

Hydrochlorothiazide Hydrochlorothiazide USP
Cardiac: diuretic 8
1–2 mg/lb b.i.d. PO
Tab: 25 & 50 mg
25 mg: 0.4–0.8/10 lb b.i.d. PO

Hydrocodone Hycodan, Tussigon
Coughing 8
2.5–5 mg/cat b.i.d.–t.i.d. PO
Tab: 5 mg; syrup: 5 mg/mL
5 mg: 0.5–1.0/cat b.i.d. PO; 5 mg/mL: 0.5–1.0 mL/cat b.i.d.–t.i.d. PO

Hydrocortisone sodium succinate Solu-Cortef
Asthma 43
0.5–1.5 mg/lb IV
Inj: 50 mg/mL & 125 mg/mL
50 mg/mL: 0.1–0.3 mL/10 lb IV; 125 mg/mL: 0.04–0.12 mL/10 lb IV

Hydrocortisone sodium succinate Solu-Cortef
Shock 43
4–10 mg/lb IV
Inj: 50 mg/mL & 125 mg/mL
50 mg/mL: 0.8–1 mL/10 lb IV; 125 mg/mL: 0.3–0.8 mL/10 lb IV

Hydrogen peroxide 3% Hydrogen Peroxide USP
Emesis induction Chapter 62
5–10 mL/cat q10m PO until emesis occurs
Soln: 3%
5–10 mL/cat q10m PO until emesis occurs

Hydrogen peroxide 3% Hydrogen Peroxide USP
Toxicosis Chapter 62
5–10 mL/cat q10m PO until emesis occurs
Soln: 3%
5–10 mL/cat q10m PO until emesis occurs

Idoxuridine Stoxil, Herplex
Corneal ulcer: herpes virus 32
1 drop of 0.1% soln topically q1h or 0.5% ointment topically q2h
0.1% soln, 0.5% ointment
0.1% soln: 1 drop topically q1h; 0.5% ointment: topically q2h

Insulin, intermediate NPH, Lente
Diabetes mellitus 33
0.25–2.0 U/lb SC s.i.d.–b.i.d.
Inj: 100 U/mL
100 U/mL: 0.05–0.2 mL/10 lb SC s.i.d.–b.i.d.; begin at low end of dose range and adjust according to glucose curve

Insulin, long-acting Ultralente
Diabetes mellitus 33
0.25–2.0 U/lb SC s.i.d.–b.i.d.
Inj: 100 U/mL
100 U/mL: 0.05–0.2 mL/10 lb SC s.i.d.–b.i.d.; begin at low end of dose range and adjust according to glucose curve

Insulin, short-acting Regular Purified Pork Insulin
Diabetes mellitus 33
2–5 U/cat IM SC p.r.n., based on blood glucose
Inj: 100 U/mL
100 U/mL: 0.02–0.05 mL/cat IM SC according to blood glucose

Insulin/glucose Regular Insulin + Glucose
Hyperkalemia, severe Chapter 31
4 U/cat total dose (in glucose)
Regular insulin inj: 100 U/mL
Insulin/glucose mixture: 16 mL/cat IV slowly as total dose
Mix 1 U (0.01 mL) of regular insulin in 4 mL of 50% glucose

Iodine Organidin
Asthma 8
50–100 mg/cat s.i.d. PO
Tab: 30 mg; oral liq: 50 mg/mL (5%); elixir 12 mg/mL (1.2%)
30 mg: 1.5–3.0/cat PO, 50 mg/mL: 1–2 mL/cat PO; 12 mg/mL: 4–8 mL/cat s.i.d. PO

Iodine (polyhydroxydine) Xenodine
Dermatophytosis Chapter 56
Apply to lesions topically b.i.d.
Topical soln
Apply to lesions topically b.i.d.

Iodine aqueous organic Iodine USP, aqueous
Corneal ulcers, herpesvirus Chapter 35
Apply diluted (1:20 with saline) topically q4–6h
Topical soln: aqueous
1:20 dilution: apply topically to cornea q4–6h

Iohexol Omnipaque
Myelography 43
0.12–0.18 mL/lb in subarachnoid space
Inj: 240 mg iodine/mL
240 mg iodine/mL: 1.2–1.8 mL/10 lb in subarachnoid space

Ipecac syrup Ipecac Syrup USP
Toxicity 11
1.5 mL/lb PO
15 mL and 30 mL bottles
15 mL/10 lb PO; do *not* use extract of ipecac
May take 1 hr to work; can reduce effectiveness of activated charcoal

Iron dextran Armidexan, Ferrextran 100
Anemia: iron deficiency 11
2.2–4.5 mg/lb b.i.d. IM
Inj: 100 & 200 mg/mL
100 mg/mL: 0.25 mL/10 lb b.i.d. IM

Isoflurane Aerrane
Anesthesia 43
Induction: 5%; maintenance: 1.5–2.5%
Induction: 5%; maintenance: 1.5–2.5%

Isopropamide iodide Darbid
Cardiac: bradycardia 43
0.1–0.2 mg/lb b.i.d.–t.i.d. PO
Tab: 5 mg
5 mg: 0.2–0.4/10 lb b.i.d.–t.i.d. PO

Isopropamide iodide Darbid
Cardiac: heart blocks 43
0.1–0.2 mg/lb b.i.d.–t.i.d. PO
Tab: 5 mg
5 mg: 0.2–0.4/10 lb b.i.d.–t.i.d. PO

Isoproterenol Isuprel
Cardiac: bradycardia 11
0.1–0.2 mg q.i.d. IV SC; 15–30 mg q4–6h PO
Tab: 10 & 15 mg; inj: 0.2 mg/mL
0.2 mg/mL: 0.5–1.0 mL q.i.d. IV SC; 10 mg: 1.5–3.0 q4–6h PO
0.2 mg/mL: slow IV drip with dextrose (5 mL in 250 mL)

Isoproterenol Isuprel
Cardiac: heart blocks 11
0.1–0.2 mg q.i.d. IV SC; 15–30 mg q4–6h PO
Tab: 10 & 15 mg; inj: 0.2 mg/mL
0.2 mg/mL: 0.5–1.0 mL q.i.d. IV SC; 10 mg: 1.5–3.0 q4–6h PO
0.2 mg/mL: slow IV drip with dextrose (5 mL in 250 mL)

Isotretinoin Accutane
Acne 34
0.9 mg/lb s.i.d. PO
Cap: 10, 20, 40 mg
10 mg: 1/10 lb s.i.d. PO

Intraconazole Not currently available
Systemic fungal diseases 35
2.3 mg/lb b.i.d. PO

Ivermectin Ivomec
Cheyletiellosis Chapter 57
100–200 μg/lb q14d for 2 treatments SC
Inj: 10 mg/mL (1%)
10 mg/mL: 0.1 mL/10 lb q14d for 2 treatments SC

Ivermectin Ivomec
Ear mites Chapter 57
100–200 μg/lb q14d for 5 treatments SC
Inj: 10 mg/mL (1%)
10 mg/mL: 0.1 mL/10 lb q14d for 5 treatments SC
Can be used on kittens 8 wk and older

Ivermectin Ivomec
Notoedric mange (scabies) Chapter 57
100–200 μg/lb q14d for 2 treatments SC
Inj: 10 mg/mL (1%)
10 mg/mL: 0.1 mL/10 lb q14d for 2 treatments SC

Kaolin-pectin Kaopectate
Diarrhea 11
0.5–1 mL/lb q2–6h PO
OTC liq
Liq: 5–10 mL/10 lb q2–6h PO

Ketamine Ketaset, Vetalar
Anesthesia 5
10–15 mg/lb IM; 1–2 mg/lb IV
Inj: 100 mg/mL
100 mg/mL: 1.0–1.5 mL/10 lb IM or 0.1–0.2 mL/10 lb IV

Ketamine Ketaset, Vetalar
Restraint 5
1–5 mg/lb IM
Inj: 100 mg/mL
100 mg/mL: 0.1–0.5 mL/10 lb IM

Ketoconazole Nizoral
Dermatophytosis Chapter 56
4.6 mg/lb s.i.d. PO
Tab: 200 mg
200 mg: 0.25/10 lb s.i.d. PO

Ketoconazole Nizoral
Systemic fungal diseases Chapter 61
2.5–5 mg/lb b.i.d. PO
Tab: 200 mg
200 mg: 0.12–0.25/10 lb b.i.d. PO for 1 mo past clinical signs
May be used concurrent with or after amphotericin B

L-Asparaginase Elspar
Neoplasia Chapter 51
182 IU/lb q1–3w SC; 10,000 IU/m^2 q1–3w IM
1,000 IU/mL
1,000 IU/mL: 1.8 mL/10 lb q1–3w SC; 2.7 mL/10 lb q1–3w IM
See Table 51-2 for combination therapy

L-Thyroxine Synthroid, Thyro-Tabs
Hypothyroidism/postthyroidectomy 38
0.1 mg/cat b.i.d.
Tab: 0.1 & 0.2 mg
0.1 mg: 1 tab/cat b.i.d.; give for 1 mo post bilateral thyroidectomy

Lactated Ringer's solution Lactated Ringer's solution
Fluid maintenance Chapter 34
30 mL/lb/24 hr
IV, SC soln
IV, SC soln: 300 mL/10 lb/24 hr

Lactated Ringer's solution Lactated Ringer's solution
Shock Chapter 44
6.8 mL/lb IV in 1st hour, then slowed
IV soln: 68 mL/10 lb IV in 1st hr, then slowed

Lactulose Cephulac, Chronulac
Hepatic encephalopathy 39
0.05 mL/lb b.i.d.–t.i.d. PO to start, then adjust to maintain soft stool
Syrup: 667 mg/mL
667 mg/mL: 0.5 mL/10 lb t.i.d. PO, then adjust to maintain soft stool

Levamisole Tramisol, Levasole
Immunostimulation 11
1 mg/lb 3 ×/wk PO
36 mg/mL when reconstituted (pig wormer)
36 mg/mL: 0.3 mL/10 lb 3 ×/wk PO

Levamisole Tramisol, Levasole
Lungworms 11
10–20 mg/lb PO e.o.d. for 5–6 treatments
Oblet: 184 mg; soln: 36 mg/mL when reconstituted (pig wormer)
184 mg: 0.5–1.0/10 lb; 36 mg/mL: 3–6 mL/10 lb PO e.o.d. for 5–6 treatments

Levamisole Tramisol, Levasole
Microfilaria of heartworms 40
5 mg/lb s.i.d. PO for 7–12 days
Oblet: 184 mg; soln: 36 mg/mL when reconstituted (pig wormer)
184 mg: 0.25 s.i.d. PO for 7–12 days
36 mg/mL: 1.5 mL/10 lb s.i.d. PO for 7–12 days

Lidocaine HCl (without epinephrine) Xylocaine
Cardiac: vent premature complexes 8
0.11–0.23 mg/lb IV over 5-min period, p.r.n.
Inj: 20 mg/mL
20 mg/mL: 0.1–0.2 mL/10 lb IV over 5-min period, p.r.n.

Lidocaine HCl (without epinephrine) Xylocaine
Cardiac: vent tachycardia 8
0.11–0.23 mg/lb IV over 5-min period, p.r.n.
Inj: 20 mg/mL
20 mg/mL: 0.1–0.2 mL/10 lb IV over 5-min period, p.r.n.

Lime sulfur solution Lym-Dyp
Dermatophytosis Chapter 56
2 oz/gal water applied topically
Concentrate: 50 mg/mL (5%)
Concentration: 2 oz/gal water applied topically q7d until skin scraping is negative

Lime sulfur solution Lym-Dyp
Notoedric mange Chapter 57
2 oz/gal water applied topically
Concentrate: 50 mg/mL (5%)
50 mg/mL: 2 oz/gal water applied q5d for 6–8 treatments

Lime sulfur solution Lym-Dyp
Pediculosis (lice) Chapter 57
2 oz/gal water applied topically
Concentrate: 50 mg/mL (5%)
50 mg/mL: 2 oz/gal water topically twice at 10–14 day interval

Lincomycin Lincocin
Bacterial infections 11
PO: 10 mg/lb b.i.d. PO; 7 mg/lb t.i.d. PO; 5 mg/lb b.i.d. IM IV
Tab: 100, 200, & 500 mg; liq: 50 mg/mL; inj: 100 mg/mL
100 mg: 1/10 lb b.i.d. PO; 100 mg: 0.7/10 lb t.i.d. PO; 50 mg/mL: 2 mL/10 lb b.i.d. PO
100 mg/mL: 0.5 mL/10 lb b.i.d. IM IV

Liothyronine sodium Cytobin
Endocrine-deficiency alopecia Chapter 60
20 μg/cat b.i.d. PO × 3, then increase by 10 μg q3d to 60 μg/cat
Tab: 60 & 120 μg
60 μg: 0.33/cat b.i.d. PO × 3, then increase by ⅙ tab up to 1 tab/cat

Liothyronine sodium Cytobin
Hypothyroidism 42
1 μg/lb b.i.d. PO
Tab: 60 & 120 μg
60 μg: 0.17/10 lb b.i.d. PO; 120 μg: 0.3/10 lb b.i.d. PO

Liothyronine sodium Cytobin, Cytomel
T_3 suppression test 41
25–30 μg q8h for 7 doses
Tab: 60 μg (Cytobin), 25 μg (Cytomel)
60 μg: 0.5/10 lb q8h × 7; 25 μg: 1.0/10 lb q8h × 7 doses
Run T_3 & T_4 before 1st dose & 2–4 hr after last dose

Loperamide Imodium (A–D)
Diarrhea 8
0.05–0.14 mg/lb s.i.d.–b.i.d. PO
Cap: 2 mg; liq: 0.2 mg/mL
2 mg: 0.25–0.75/10 lb s.i.d.–b.i.d. PO; 0.2 mg/mL: 2.5–7 mL/10 lb s.i.d.–b.i.d. PO

Lysine-8-vasopressin Diapid
Central diabetes insipidus 43
1–2 sprays in each nostril s.i.d.–t.i.d.
0.185 mg [50 USP posterior pituitary (pressor) U]/mL
1–2 sprays in each nostril s.i.d.–t.i.d.

Mafenide 10% Sulfamylon Cream
Burns 43
Apply to thickness of 0.25–0.50″ b.i.d.; wash off once daily

Magnesium hydroxide Milk of Magnesia
Constipation 43
5–15 mL/cat s.i.d.–b.i.d. PO
5–15 mg/cat s.i.d.–b.i.d. PO

Magnesium sulfate Epsom's Salts
Cathartic Chapter 62
115 mg/lb PO (¼ level tsp/10 lb)
Epsom's salts powder
¼ level tsp/10 lb in water PO
May be mixed with activated charcoal slurry

Mannitol Manniject
Edema of CNS 5
0.5–1.0 g/lb q.i.d. IV
Inj: 200 mg/mL
200 mg/mL: 20–40 mL/10 lb q.i.d. IV
Administer slowly; repeat dose cautiously

Mannitol Manniject
Glaucoma Chapter 36
0.5–1 g/lb IV
Inj: 200 mg/mL
200 mg/mL: 2.5–5 mL/10 lb IV
Effects in 30 min; duration: 6–10 hr

Mannitol Manniject
Oliguric renal failure Chapter 31
0.25–0.5 g/lb IV over 15–20 min
Inj: 200 mg/mL
200 mg/mL: 12.5–25.0 mL/10 lb IV over 15–20 min

Meclizine Antivert
Vomiting 35
1.8 mg/lb s.i.d. PO
Tab: 25 & 50 mg
25 mg: 0.5–1.0/10 lb s.i.d. PO

Medium chain triglyceride oil MCT Oil
Hepatic encephalopathy 11
0.5–1 mL/lb/day PO in food
Quarts: no concentration given
5–10 mL/10 lb/day PO in food

Medroxyprogesterone acetate Depo-Provera
Urine spraying 3
4.5–9 mg/lb SC IM
Inj: 100 & 400 mg/mL
100 mg/mL: 0.5–1.0 mL/10 lb SC IM

Megestrol acetate Ovaban
Acne Chapter 7
5 mg/cat s.i.d. PO × 7, then 5 mg/cat q7d
Tab: 5 & 20 mg
5 mg: 1/cat s.i.d. PO × 7, then 1/cat q7d

Megestrol acetate Ovaban
Asthma 8
5 mg/cat s.i.d. PO × 4, then q7d × 4
Tab: 5 & 20 mg
5 mg: 1/cat s.i.d. PO × 4, then 1/cat q7d × 4

Megestrol acetate Ovaban
Dysuria Chapter 40
5 mg/cat s.i.d. PO × 5–7
Tab: 5 & 20 mg
5 mg: 1/cat s.i.d. PO × 5–7

Megestrol acetate Ovaban
Eosinophilic granuloma complex Chapter 60
5 mg/cat s.i.d. PO × 7, then 5 mg/cat q7d
Tab: 5 & 20 mg
5 mg: 1/cat s.i.d. PO × 7, then 1/cat q7d

Megestrol acetate Ovaban
Eosinophilic keratitis Chapter 35
5 mg/cat s.i.d. PO × 7, then 5 mg/cat e.o.d., then 5 mg/cat q7d
Tab: 5 & 20 mg
5 mg: 1/cat s.i.d. PO × 7, then 1/cat e.o.d., then 1/cat q7d

Megestrol acetate Ovaban
Estrus prevention Chapter 54
2.5 mg/cat q7d PO up to 18 mo
Tab: 5 & 20 mg
5 mg: 0.5/cat q7d PO up to 18 mo
Begin during anestrus

Megestrol acetate Ovaban
Estrus prevention Chapter 54
2.5 mg/cat s.i.d. PO up to 60 days
Tab: 5 & 20 mg
5 mg: 0.5/cat s.i.d. PO up to 60 days
Begin during interestrus

Megestrol acetate Ovaban
Estrus suppression Chapter 54
5 mg/cat s.i.d. PO × 3, then 2.5–5 mg/cat q7d
Tab: 5 & 20 mg
5 mg: 1/cat s.i.d. PO × 3, then 0.5–1 mg/cat q7d
Begin during estrus

Megestrol acetate Ovaban
Gingivitis Chapter 52
5 mg/cat s.i.d. PO × 7, then 5 mg/cat q7d
Tab: 5 & 20 mg
5 mg: 1/cat s.i.d. PO × 7, then 1/cat q7d

Megestrol acetate Ovaban
Miliary dermatitis: idiopathic Chapter 60
Initially: 2.5–5.0 mg/cat s.i.d.–e.o.d. PO; maintenance: 2.5–5.0 mg/cat q7–14d PO
Tab: 5 & 20 mg
5 mg: 0.5–1.0/cat s.i.d.–e.o.d. PO initially, then 0.5–1.0/cat q7–14d PO

Megestrol acetate Ovaban
Pruritus Chapter 60
5 mg/cat s.i.d. PO × 7, then 5 mg/cat q7d
Tab: 5 & 20 mg
5 mg: 1/cat s.i.d. PO × 7, then 1/cat q7d

Megestrol acetate Ovaban
Vomiting: idiopathic Chapter 24
5 mg/cat s.i.d. PO × 7, then 5 mg/cat q7d
Tab: 5 & 20 mg
5 mg: 1/cat s.i.d. PO × 7, then 1/cat q7d

Meperidine Demerol
Pain 8
1–2 mg/lb p.r.n. IM
Inj: 50 mg/mL
50 mg/mL: 0.2–0.5 mL/10 lb p.r.n. IM

Metaproterenol Metaprel
Bronchoconstriction 11
0.22 mg/lb q.i.d. PO
Tab: 10 & 20 mg; syrup: 2 mg/mL
10 mg: 0.25/10 lb q.i.d. PO; 2 mg/mL: 1 mL/10 lb q.i.d. PO

Metaraminol Aramine
Shock 43
0.005–0.05 mg/lb IV slowly
Inj: 10 mg/mL
10 mg/mL: 0.005–0.05 mL/10 lb IV slowly to effect

Methazolamide Neptazane
Glaucoma Chapter 36
1–2 mg/lb b.i.d.–t.i.d. PO
Tab: 50 mg
50 mg: 0.2–0.4/10 lb b.i.d.–t.i.d. PO

Methimazole Tapazole
Hyperthyroidism: medical (only) treatment 8
2.5–10 mg/cat s.i.d.–b.i.d. PO
Tab: 5 mg
5 mg: 0.5–2.0/cat s.i.d.–b.i.d. PO
Monitor T_4 q2–4m
Susp: 10 mg/mL*

Methimazole Tapazole
Hyperthyroidism: prethyroidectomy Chapter 46
5–10 mg/cat s.i.d. × 7–14
Tab: 5 mg
5 mg: 1–2/cat s.i.d. × 7–14, then recheck T_4
Susp: 10 mg/mL*

Methionine (D-L) Methio-Form
Urinary acidifier 8
100 mg/lb t.i.d. PO
Tab: 500 mg; granules: 242 mg/g
500 mg: 2/10 lb t.i.d. PO; granules: 2 tsp/10 lb t.i.d. PO

Methocarbamol Robaxin
Muscle spasm, pain 8
20 mg/lb loading t.i.d. PO IV IM; 10–20 mg/lb (maintenance) t.i.d. PO
Tab: 500 & 750 mg; inj: 100 mg/mL (do not refrigerate)
Loading: 500 mg: 0.5/10 lb; 100 mg/mL: 2 mL/10 lb t.i.d. PO IV IM
Maintenance: 500 mg: 0.2–0.5/10 lb t.i.d. PO

Methocarbamol Robaxin
Tetany, muscle fasciculation Chapter 62
20–100 mg/lb IV
Inj: 100 mg/mL
100 mg/mL: 2–10 mL/10 lb IV

Methohexital Brevital
Anesthesia 43
2.5% soln: 5 mg/lb IV to effect
Soln: 25 mg/mL
2.5%: 2 mL/10 lb IV (give ½ as bolus, then to effect)

Methotrexate Rheumatrex
Neoplasia Chapter 51
2.5–5.0 mg/m^2 g2–3w PO; 10–15 mg/m^2 q1–3w IV
Tab: 2.5 mg; inj: 12.5 mg/mL when diluted (with 5% dextrose)
2.5 mg: 0.27–0.54/10 lb q2–3w PO; 12.5 mg/mL: 0.22–0.33 mL/10 lb q1–3w IV
See Table 51-2 for combination therapy

Methoxyflurane Metofane
Anesthesia 43
Induction: 3%; maintenance: 0.5–1.5%
Induction: 3%; maintenance: 0.5–1.5%

Methoxyprogesterone acetate Depo-Provera
Miliary dermatitis: idiopathic Chapter 60
50–175 mg/cat SC IM p.r.n.
Inj: 100 & 400 mg/mL
100 mg/mL: 0.5–1.75 mL/cat SC IM p.r.n.

Methylene blue Methylene Blue USP
Contraindicated

Methylprednisolone (Depo) Depo-Medrol
Eosinophilic granuloma complex Chapter 60
10–20 mg/cat SC IM q14d for 1–3 treatments
Inj: 20 & 40 mg/mL
20 mg/mL: 0.5–1.0 mL/cat SC IM q14d for 1–3 treatments

Methylprednisolone (Depo) Depo-Medrol
Miliary dermatitis: idiopathic Chapter 60
10–20 mg/cat SC IM q60–90d
Inj: 20 & 40 mg/mL
20 mg/mL: 0.5–1.0 mL/cat SC IM q60–90d

Methylprednisolone (Depo) Depo-Medrol
Pruritus 8
0.45 mg/lb q7–14d IM or 20 mg/cat IM once
Inj: 20 & 40 mg/mL
20 mg/mL: 0.25 mL/10 lb IM q7–14 days or 1 mL/cat IM once

Methylprednisolone (Depo) Depo-Medrol
Uveitis Chapter 36
10 mg subconjunctivally once
Inj: 20 & 40 mg/mL
40 mg/mL: 0.25 mL subconjunctivally once

Methylprednisolone sodium succinate Solu-Medrol
Spinal cord injury 37
13.5 mg/lb; 15 min later give 1 mg/lb/hr over next 24 hr IV
Inj: 40 mg/mL
40 mg/mL: 3.4 mL initially; 15 min later give 0.25 mL/hr/10 lb IV
Give 2nd and subsequent doses as continuous IV drip

Methyltestosterone Metandren
Muscle wasting 43
0.45–0.9 mg/lb s.i.d. PO
Tab: 10 & 25 mg
10 mg: 0.5–1/10 lb s.i.d. PO; 25 mg: 0.02–0.4/10 lb s.i.d. PO

Metoclopramide Reglan
Vomiting 22
0.05–0.15 mg/lb b.i.d. IM PO
Tab: 5 & 10 mg; syrup: 1 mg/mL; inj: 5 mg/mL
5 mg: 0.2–0.4/10 lb b.i.d. PO; 10 mg: 0.1–0.2/10 lb b.i.d. PO
1 mg/mL: 0.5–1.5/10 lb b.i.d. PO; 5 mg/mL: 0.1–0.2 mL/10 lb b.i.d. IM

Metoprolol Lopressor
Hypertension 11
2–15 mg t.i.d. PO
Tab: 50 & 100 mg
50 mg: 0.04–0.3/10 lb t.i.d. PO

Metronidazole Flagyl
Bacterial infections 8
4.5–6.8 mg/lb t.i.d.–q.i.d. PO
Tab: 250 & 500 mg
250 mg: 0.1/10 lb t.i.d.–q.i.d. PO
Susp: 65 mg/mL*

Metronidazole Flagyl
Fungal infections 8
4.5–6.8 mg/lb t.i.d.–q.i.d. PO
Tab: 250 & 500 mg
250 mg: 0.1/10 lb t.i.d.–q.i.d. PO
Susp: 65 mg/mL*

Metronidazole Flagyl
Giardiasis 8
4.5 mg/lb b.i.d. PO × 5
Tab: 250 & 500 mg
250 mg: 0.1/10 lb b.i.d. PO × 5
Susp: 65 mg/mL*

Metronidazole Flagyl
Gingivitis 8
23 mg/lb PO s.i.d.
Tab: 250 & 500 mg
250 mg: 0.9/10 lb s.i.d. PO
Susp: 65 mg/mL*

Metronidazole Flagyl
Inflammatory bowel disease Chapter 48
5–10 mg/lb b.i.d.–t.i.d. PO
Tab: 250 & 500 mg
250 mg: 0.2–0.4/10 lb b.i.d.–t.i.d. PO
Susp: 65 mg/mL*

Mibolerone Cheque-Drops
Contraindicated Chapter 54

Miconazole Conofite
Dermatophytosis Chapter 56
Cream or lotion
Apply to lesions topically b.i.d.

Milk of Magnesia Phillip's Milk of Magnesia
Constipation 35
2–6 mL/cat PO
Tab: 311 mg; susp: 81 mg/mL
311 mg: 0.5–1.5/cat PO; susp: 2–6 mL/cat PO

Milrinone Not available yet
Cardiac: hypertrophic CM 12
0.23–0.45 mg/lb b.i.d. PO

Mineral oil Mineral oil
Constipation 45
5–20 mL b.i.d. orally or rectally
Liq
5–20 mL/cat b.i.d. PO (orogastric tube) or rectally

Minocycline HCl Minocin
Bacterial infections 11
11.4 mg/lb b.i.d. PO
Tab & Cap: 50 & 100 mg; susp: 10 mg/mL
50 mg: 2/10 lb; 100 mg: 1/10 lb; 10 mg/mL: 10 mL/10 lb b.i.d. PO

Mitotane Lysodren
See O,p'DDD

Mitoxantrone HCl Novantrone
Neoplasia 11
6.25 mg/M^2 every 3 wk IV
Inj: 2 mg/mL
2 mg/mL: 0.8 mL/10 lb q21d IV

Morphine Morphine
Pain 8
0.05 mg/lb IM SC
Inj: 15 mg/mL
15 mg/mL: 0.03 mL/10 lb IM SC

Nafcillin sodium Nafcil, Unipen
Bacterial infections 11
4.5 mg/lb q.i.d. PO IM
Tab: 500 mg; cap: 250 mg; soln: 50 mg/mL; inj: 50 mg/mL (diluted)
250 mg: 0.1/10 lb; 50 mg/mL: 1 mL/10 lb q.i.d. PO
50 mg/mL: 1 mL/10 lb q.i.d. IM (more dilute than manufacturer recommends)

Nalbuphine Nubain
Pain 8
0.34–0.68 mg/lb IV
Inj: 10 & 20 mg/mL
10 mg/mL: 0.3–0.7 mL/10 lb IV

Nalorphine HCl Nalline
Narcotic reversal 43
0.05 mg/lb IV; max 1 mg
Inj: 5 mg/mL
5 mg/mL: 0.1 mL/10 lb IV; may be repeated once

Naloxone HCl Narcan
Narcotic reversal 5
0.02 mg/lb IV IM SC
Inj: 0.02, 0.4, & 1.0 mg/mL
0.02 mg/mL: 10 mL/10 lb IV IM SC; 0.4 mg/mL: 0.5 mL/10 lb IV IM SC

Nandrolone decanoate Deca-Durabolin
Anemia secondary to renal failure Chapter 31
0.45 mg/lb q7d IM
Inj: 25 & 50 mg/mL
25 mg/mL: 0.2 mL/10 lb q7d IM

Nandrolone decanoate Deca-Durabolin
Anorexia 5
0.45 mg/lb q7d IM
Inj: 25 & 50 mg/mL
25 mg/mL: 0.2 mL/10 lb q7d IM

Neomycin Bio-Sol
Hepatic encephalopathy 39
10 mg/lb b.i.d.–t.i.d. PO
Tab: 70 mg; liq: 50 & 200 mg/mL
70 mg: 1.5/10 lb b.i.d.–t.i.d. PO; 50 mg/mL: 2 mL/10 lb b.i.d.–t.i.d. PO
200 mg/mL: 0.5 mL/10 lb b.i.d.–t.i.d. PO

Neostigmine Stiglyn, Prostigmin
Myasthenia gravis 11
0.2 mg p.r.n. IV
Inj: 2.0 mg/mL
2 mg/mL: 0.1 mL p.r.n. IV

Niclosamide Yomesan
Tapeworm infestation 43
70 mg/lb PO after 12 hr fast; repeat in 2–3 wk
Tab: 500 mg
500 mg: 1.4/10 lb PO after 12 hr fast; repeat in 2–3 wk

Nikethamide Coramine
CNS depression: drug-induced 43
3.5–14 mg/lb IV, IM, SC
Inj: 250 mg/mL (25%)
250 mg/mL: 0.2–0.5 mL/10 lb IV, IM, SC

Nitroglycerin Nitrostat Ointment, 2%
Cardiac: vasodilator 8
⅛–¼ inch topically q.i.d.
15 mg/inch topical paste (2%)
⅛–¼ inch topically *on skin* q.i.d.
Do not allow to contact human skin

Norfloxacin Noroxin
Bacterial infections 8
10 mg/lb b.i.d. PO
Tab: 400 mg
400 mg: 0.25/10 lb b.i.d. PO

Norfloxacin Noroxin
Bacterial infections: urinary 8
2.3 mg/lb b.i.d. PO
Tab: 400 mg
400 mg: 0.06/10 lb b.i.d. PO

Nystatin Mycostatin
Candida infections 11
100,000 IU q.i.d. PO
Tab: 500,000 IU; liq: 100,000 IU/mL
500,000: 0.2/cat q.i.d. PO; 100,000 IU/mL: 1 mL/cat q.i.d. PO

O,p′-DDD (Mitotane) Lysodren
Hyperadrenocorticism 8
11.4 mg/lb PO s.i.d.
Tab: 500 mg
500 mg: 0.2/10 ib s.i.d. PO until in remission, then p.r.n.
Given to effect based on results of ACTH stimulation test

Omeprazole Prilosec (formerly Losec)
Esophagitis 46
0.32 mg/lb s.i.d. PO
Cap: 20 mg
20 mg: 0.2/10 lb s.i.d. PO
Must repackage granules in gelatin capsule or give via orogastric tube

Omeprazole Prilosec (formerly Losec)
Gastric ulcers 46
0.32 mg/lb s.i.d. PO
Cap: 20 mg
20 mg: 0.2/10 lb s.i.d. PO
Must repackage granules in gelatin capsule or give via orogastric tube

Oxacillin, sodium Oxacillin
Bacterial infections 8
5–10 mg/lb q.i.d. PO
Cap: 250 & 500 mg; liq: 50 mg/mL
250 mg: 0.2–0.4/10 lb q.i.d. PO; 50 mg/mL: 1–2 mL/10 lb q.i.d. PO

Oxazepam Serax
Anorexia 28
0.14–0.18 mg/lb s.i.d.–t.i.d.
Tab: 15 mg 5-sided; cap: 10, 15, & 30 mg
10 mg: 0.2/10 lb; 15 mg: 0.1/10 lb s.i.d.–t.i.d.

Oxtriphylline Choledyl
Bronchoconstriction 11
4.5–6.8 mg/lb t.i.d.–q.i.d. PO
Tab: 100 & 200 mg; elixir: 20 mg/mL
100 mg: 0.5–0.7/10 lb t.i.d.–q.i.d. PO; 20 mg/mL: 3.5 mL/10 lb

Oxybutynin HCl Ditropan
Detrussor hyperreflexia 11
0.5 mg/cat b.i.d. PO
Tab: 5 mg; oral syrup: 1 mg/mL
5 mg: 0.1/cat b.i.d. PO; 1 mg/mL: 0.5 mL/cat b.i.d. PO
May take up to 3 wk to be effective

Oxymetazoline HCl Afrin Pediatric Drops
Nasal congestion 52
Nose drops: 0.025%
1 drop s.i.d. in alternating nostrils

Oxymetholone Anadrol-50
Anorexia 8
0.05–0.5 mg/lb s.i.d. PO
Tab: 50 mg
50 mg: 0.01–0.1/10 lb s.i.d. PO

Oxymorphone Numorphan
Anesthesia 8
0.2–0.7 mg/lb p.r.n. IV IM SC
Inj: 1 & 1.5 mg/mL
1 mg/mL: 2.0–3.5 mL/10 lb; 1.5 mg/mL: 1.3–4.7 mL/10 lb p.r.n. IV IM SC

Oxytetracycline Terramycin; Liquamycin
Bacterial infections 8
7 mg/lb t.i.d. PO; 3.2 mg/lb b.i.d. IM IV
Cap: 250 mg; inj: 50 mg/mL
250 mg: 0.3/10 lb t.i.d. PO; 50 mg/mL: 0.6 mL/10 lb b.i.d. IM IV
May cause significant pyrexia in some cats

Oxytetracycline Terramycin; Liquamycin
Rickettsial infections 8
7 mg/lb t.i.d. PO; 3.2 mg/lb b.i.d. IM IV
Cap: 250 mg; inj: 50 mg/mL
250 mg: 0.3/10 lb t.i.d. PO; 50 mg/mL: 0.6 mL/10 lb b.i.d. IM IV
May cause significant pyrexia in some cats

Oxytetracycline ophthalmic Terramycin
Conjunctivitis: *Chlamydia* 10
Ophthalmic ointment
Apply to eye(s) 2–4 × /day

Oxytocin Oxytocin USP
Uterine inertia Chapter 54
2–4 IU/cat IM q20m
Inj: 10 & 20 IU/mL
10 IU/mL: 0.2–0.4 mL/cat IM q20m

Oxytocin Pitocin
Dystocia 8
0.5–3.0 U/cat p.r.n. IV IM; 2.0–4.0 U/cat IV q20m × 2
Inj: 20 IU/mL
20 IU/mL: 0.03–0.2 mL/10 lb p.r.n. IV IM; 0.1–0.2 mL/cat IV q20m × 2
Precede 2nd treatment with calcium gluconate infusion

Pancreatin Viokase
Pancreatic insufficiency 8
0.5–1 tsp PO with food
Tab: 425 mg; powder: 2.8 g/tsp
Tab: 3–6/day PO with food; powder: 0.5–1 tsp/day PO with food

Pancuronium bromide Pavulon
Ophthalmic surgery 8
0.03–0.5 mg/lb p.r.n. IV
Inj: 1 & 2 mg/mL
1 mg/mL: 0.3–5.0 mL/10 lb p.r.n. IV

Paregoric Donnagel-PG
Diarrhea 8
0.023–0.027 mg/lb b.i.d.–t.i.d. PO
Liq 0.8 mg/mL (with 24 mg opium/oz)
0.8 mg/mL: 0.3–0.4 mL/10 lb b.i.d.–t.i.d. PO

Penicillin G potassium Pentids, Pfizerpen
Bacterial infections 5
20,000 IU/lb q.i.d. PO; 10,000 IU/lb q4h IV IM SC
Tab: 125, 250, & 500 mg; inj: 100,000 U/mL when reconstituted
125 mg: 1/10 lb q.i.d. PO; 100,000 U/mL: 1 mL/10 lb q4h IV IM SC

Penicillin G procaine Penicillin G Procaine
Bacterial infections 5
10,000 IU/lb s.i.d.–b.i.d. IM SC
Inj: 300,000 IU/mL
300,000 IU/mL: 0.3 mL/10 lb s.i.d.–b.i.d. IM SC

Penicillin G, benzathine Flo-cillin, Pen-BP-48, Dual-Pen
Bacterial infections 5
20,000 IU/lb q5d IM
Inj: 150,000 IU Penicillin G procaine and 150,000 IU Penicillin G benzathine/mL
150,000 + 150,000 IU/mL: 1.2/10 lb q5d IM

Penicillin V Veetids
Bacterial infections 43
5 mg/lb t.i.d. PO
Tab: 250 & 500 mg; susp: 25 & 50 mg/mL
250 mg: 0.2/10 lb t.i.d. PO
25 mg/mL: 2 mL/10 lb t.i.d. PO; 50 mg/mL: 1 mL/10 lb t.i.d. PO

Penicillin, procaine Crysticillin 300 AS
Actinomycosis 43
10,000–20,000 U/lb b.i.d. IM, SC
Inj: 300,000 U/mL
300,000 U/mL: 0.33–0.67 mL/10 lb b.i.d. IM, SC

Penicillin, procaine Crysticillin 300 AS
Leptospirosis 43
10,000–20,000 U/lb b.i.d. IM, SC
Inj: 300,000 U/mL
300,000 U/mL: 0.33–0.67 mL/10 lb b.i.d. IM, SC

Pentazocine Talwin
Analgesia 8
0.45–1.4 mg/lb p.r.n. SC IM
Inj: 30 mg/mL
30 mg/mL: 0.15–0.46 mL/10 lb p.r.n. SC IM

Pentazocine Talwin
Sedation 8
0.45–1.4 mg/lb p.r.n. SC IM
Inj: 30 mg/mL
30 mg/mL: 0.15–0.46 mL/10 lb p.r.n. SC IM

Pentobarbital sodium Pentobarbital USP
Anesthesia 8
10–15 mg/lb p.r.n. IV
Inj: 64.8 mg/mL
64.8 mg/mL: 1.5–2.3 mL/10 lb p.r.n. IV

Pentobarbital sodium Pentobarbital USP
Status epilepticus Chapter 23
Slowly IV to effect (up to 12 mg/lb)
Inj: 64.8 mg/mL
64.8 mg/mL: Up to 2 mL slowly IV to effect
If other depressants given prior, *dose very carefully*

Petrolatum, white & liquid Laxatone
Hair balls 10
Oral paste
Initially: 0.5–1.0 tsp × s.i.d. 2–3 days, then 0.25–0.5 tsp s.i.d. 2–3×/wk

Phenazopyridine AzoGantrasin, Pyridium
Containdicated

Phenobarbital Phenobarbital USP
Seizures (maintenance) Chapter 23
1.0 mg/lb b.i.d. PO
Tab: 16.2 mg (¼ grain)
16.2 mg (¼ grain): 0.6/10 lb b.i.d. PO
Adjust to serum level of 15–40 μg/mL or to effect

Phenobarbital Phenobarbital USP
Status epilepticus 8
3 mg/lb s.i.d.–q.i.d. IV IM
Inj: 65 mg/mL (1 grain)
65 mg/mL: 0.5 mL/10 lb s.i.d.–q.i.d. IV IM

Phenobarbital Phenobarbital USP
Vertigo (vestibular disease) Chapter 17
⅛–¼ grain/cat b.i.d. PO
Tab: 16.2 mg (¼ grain)
16.2 mg (¼ grain): 0.5–1.0/cat b.i.d. PO
Reduce dosage if sedation occurs

Phenoxybenzamine Dibenzyline
Dysuria 9
0.23 mg/lb b.i.d.–t.i.d. PO
Cap: 10 mg
10 mg: 0.25/10 lb b.i.d.–t.i.d. PO

Phenylbutazone Butazolin
Pain 8
5.5–7.3 mg/lb PO b.i.d. on alternating weeks
Tab: 100 & 200 mg
100 mg: 0.5/10 lb b.i.d. PO alternating weeks
Use cautiously: potentially serious side effects

Phenylephrine Neo-Synephrine
Horner's syndrome Chapter 35
2 drops in affected eye t.i.d.–q.i.d.
Ophthalmic drops: 2.5%
2.5%: 2 drops in affected eye t.i.d.–q.i.d.

Phenylephrine Neo-Synephrine
Nasal congestion 44
1–2 drops in alternating nostrils e.o.d.
Nasal spray: 0.25–1% soln
1–2 drops in alternating nostrils e.o.d.

Phenylephrine Neo-Synephrine
Prolapsed third eyelids Chapter 35
2 drops in affected eye t.i.d.–q.i.d.
Ophthalmic drops: 2.5%
2.5%: 2 drops in affected eye t.i.d.–q.i.d.

Phenylpropanolamine Ornade, Comtrex, Triaminic
Urinary incontinence 8
6.25–12.5 mg/cat b.i.d.–t.i.d. PO
Cap: 75 mg (Ornade); 12.5 mg (Comtrex & Triaminic)
12.5 mg: 0.5–1.0/cat b.i.d.–t.i.d. PO; 75 mg: 0.1–0.2/cat b.i.d.–t.i.d. PO

Phenytoin Dilantin
Seizures 8
9 mg/lb q7d PO
Cap: 30, 50, & 100 mg
30 mg: 3/10 lb q7d PO
Use only if other anticonvulsants do not work

Phosphate enemas Fleet
Contraindicated 8

Phytonadione (Vitamin K_1) AquaMEPHYTON, Mephyton
Toxicity: anticoagulants Chapter 62
0.7–1.2 mg/lb b.i.d. PO SC
Tab: 5 mg; inj: 2 & 10 mg/mL
5 mg: 1.4–2.4/10 lb PO b.i.d.; 10 mg/mL: 0.7–1.2 mL/10 lb SC b.i.d.

Pilocarpine Pilocarpine Ophthalmic USP 2%
Glaucoma Chapter 36
2 drops in affected eye b.i.d.–q.i.d.
Ophthalmic drops: 0.5–10%
2%: 2 drops in affected eye b.i.d.–q.i.d.
Concentrations over 4% usually produce vomiting

Piperazine Sargeants Worm Away for Cats
Roundworm infestation 47
20–30 mg/lb once PO
Cap: 140 mg
140 mg: 1.4–2.1/10 lb once PO
Repeat in 3 wk

Potassium chloride Potassium Chloride USP
Hypokalemia 8
IV according to serum K+
Inj: 2 mEq/mL
2 mEq/mL: add to IV fluids dependent upon serum K+ level
See Chapter 34 for complete instructions

Potassium gluconate Tumil-K, Kaochlor, Kaon
Hypokalemia 10
5–10 mEq/day; when stable reduce to 2–6 mEq/day
Powder: 8 mEq/tsp; tab: 6.7 & 10 mEq; elixir: 1.3 mEq/mL
8 mEq/tsp: 0.25–0.75 tsp/day PO; 6.7 mEq: 0.75–1.5/day PO
10 mEq: 0.5–1.0/day PO; 1.3 mEq/mL: 1.5/4.5 mL/day PO

Potassium permanganate (1:2,000) Potassium Permanganate
Strychnine toxicosis 43
2.5 mL/lb in gastric lavage
Soln: 1:2,000
1:2,000: 25 mL/10 lb in gastric lavage

Povidone iodine solution Betadine Solution
Dermatophytosis 17
42 mL soln/L water applied topically
Soln: 100 mg/mL (10%)
100 mg/mL: 42 mL of soln/L water applied topically

Pralidoxime (2-PAM) Protopam
Toxicity: heavy metal Chapter 62
5–10 mg/lb b.i.d.–t.i.d. PO SC IM (slowly IV over 30 min) for days/weeks
Inj: 50 mg/mL when reconstituted
50 mg/mL: 1–2 mL/10 lb PO SC IM (slowly IV over 30 min)
Administer for days or weeks until nicotinic signs resolve

Pralidoxime (2-PAM) Protopam
Toxicity: organophosphates Chapter 62
5–10 mg/lb b.i.d.–t.i.d. PO SC IM (slowly IV over 30 min) for days/weeks
Inj: 50 mg/mL when reconstituted
50 mg/mL: 1–2 mL/10 lb PO SC IM (slowly IV over 30 min)
Administer for days or weeks until nicotinic signs resolve

Praziquantel Droncit
Tapeworm infestation 11
115–250 mg/lb once PO
Tab: 23 mg; inj: 57 mg/mL
23 mg: 0–4 lb: 0.5 tab; 5–11 lb: 1 tab; >11 lb: 1½ tab

Prednisolone acetate Meticorten
Hypoadrenocorticism 43
0.05–0.1 mg/lb b.i.d. IM
Inj: 10 & 40 mg/mL
10 mg/mL: 0.05–0.1 mL/10 lb b.i.d. IM

Prednisolone acetate, 1% Pred-Forte, Econopred
Uveitis Chapter 36
Topical: 1%
1%: Apply topically q4–6h

Prednisolone sodium phosphate Prednis-A-Vet
Shock 43
5 mg/lb IV
Inj: 20 mg/mL
20 mg/mL: 2.5 mL/10 lb IV

Prednisolone sodium succinate Solu-Delta-Cortef
Asthma 43
0.5–1.4 mg/lb IV, IM
Inj: 10 & 50 mg/mL
10 mg: 0.5–1.4 mL/10 lb IV, IM

Prednisolone sodium succinate Solu-Delta-Cortef
Shock 43
5–11.4 mg/lb IV
Inj: 10 & 50 mg/mL
10 mg/mL: 5–11.4 mL/10 lb IV; 50 mg/mL: 1–2.3 mL/10 lb IV

Prednisolone, prednisone Prednisolone USP
Asthma 8
0.9–1.8 mg/lb q4–6h IV; 5 mg/cat s.i.d.–e.o.d. PO
Tab 5 & 20 mg; inj: 20 mg/mL
20 mg/mL: 0.5–1 mL/10 lb q4–6h IV; 5 mg: 1/cat s.i.d.–e.o.d. PO

Prednisolone, prednisone Prednisolone USP
Autoimmune hemolytic anemia 43
0.25–1 mg/lb b.i.d. PO
Tab: 5 & 20 mg
5 mg: 0.5–2.0/10 lb b.i.d. PO

Prednisolone, prednisone Prednisolone USP
Autoimmune thrombocytopenia 43
0.25–0.8 mg/lb b.i.d. PO; taper to 0.2–0.5 mg/lb q2–3d PO
Tab: 5 & 20 mg
5 mg: 0.5–1.6/10 lb b.i.d. PO; taper to 0.4–1.0/10 lb q2–3d PO

Prednisolone, prednisone Prednisolone USP
Cerebral edema from brain tumor 43
0.2–0.45 mg/lb s.i.d.–e.o.d. PO
Tab: 5 & 20 mg
5 mg: 0.4–0.9/10 lb s.i.d.–e.o.d. PO

Prednisolone, prednisone Prednisolone USP
Cholangitis: lymphocytic 43
0.1–1.0 mg/lb b.i.d. PO
Tab: 5 & 20 mg
5 mg: 0.2–2.0/10 lb b.i.d. PO

Prednisolone, prednisone Prednisolone USP
Colitis: eosinophilic Chapter 48
0.5–2.0 mg/lb s.i.d. PO; taper slowly to e.o.d.
Tab: 5 & 20 mg
5 mg: 1–4/10 lb s.i.d. PO; taper slowly to e.o.d.

Prednisolone, prednisone Prednisolone USP
Colitis: plasmacytic/lymphocytic Chapter 48
0.5–2.0 mg/lb s.i.d. PO; taper slowly to e.o.d.
Tab: 5 & 20 mg
5 mg: 1–4/10 lb s.i.d. PO; taper slowly to e.o.d.

Prednisolone, prednisone Prednisolone USP
Enteritis: eosinophilic Chapter 48
0.5–2.0 mg/lb s.i.d. PO; taper slowly to e.o.d.
Tab: 5 & 20 mg
5 mg: 1–4/10 lb s.i.d. PO; taper slowly to e.o.d.

Prednisolone, prednisone Prednisolone USP
Enteritis: plasmacytic/lymphocytic Chapter 48
0.5–2.0 mg/lb s.i.d. PO; taper slowly to e.o.d.
Tab: 5 & 20 mg
5 mg: 1–4/10 lb s.i.d. PO; taper slowly to e.o.d.

Prednisolone, prednisone Prednisolone USP
Eosinophilic granuloma complex Chapter 60
1–2 mg/lb s.i.d. PO until healed
Tab: 5 & 20 mg
5 mg: 2–4/10 lb s.i.d. PO until healed

Prednisolone, prednisone Prednisolone USP
Food allergy 43
0.2 mg/lb s.i.d. PO; taper weekly
Tab: 5 & 20 mg
5 mg: 0.4/10 lb s.i.d. PO

Prednisolone, prednisone Prednisolone USP
Gastritis: eosinophilic Chapter 48
0.1–0.4 mg/lb b.i.d. PO; taper over 3 mo
Tab: 5 & 20 mg
5 mg: 0.2–0.8/10 lb b.i.d. PO; taper over 3 mo

Prednisolone, prednisone Prednisolone USP
Gastritis: plasmacytic/lymphocytic Chapter 48
0.1–0.4 mg/lb b.i.d. PO; taper over 3 mo
Tab: 5 & 20 mg
5 mg: 0.2–0.8/10 lb b.i.d. PO; taper over 3 mo

Prednisolone, prednisone Prednisolone USP
Gingivitis: plasma cell 43
1–2 mg/lb s.i.d. PO
Tab: 5 & 20 mg
5 mg: 2–4/10 lb s.i.d. PO; 20 mg: 0.5–1/10 lb s.i.d. PO

Prednisolone, prednisone Prednisolone USP
Hypoadrenocorticism 43
0.1–0.2 mg/lb s.i.d.–e.o.d. PO
Tab: 5 & 20 mg
5 mg: 0.2–0.4/10 lb s.i.d.–e.o.d. PO

Prednisolone, prednisone Cortisate-20
Immune-mediated diseases 8
0.9–2.3 mg/lb s.i.d.–b.i.d. IM SC PO
Tab: 5 & 20 mg; inj: 20 mg/mL
5 mg: 2–5/10 lb s.i.d.–b.i.d. PO; 20 mg: 0.5–1/10 lb s.i.d.–b.i.d. PO
20 mg/mL: 0.5–1 mL/10 lb s.i.d.–b.i.d. IM SC

Prednisolone, prednisone Prednisolone USP
Inflammatory bowel disease Chapter 48
0.1–0.4 mg/lb b.i.d. PO; taper over 3 mo
Tab: 5 & 20 mg
5 mg: 0.2–0.8/10 lb b.i.d. PO; taper over 3 mo

Prednisolone, prednisone Prednisolone USP
Lupus 43
1 mg/lb s.i.d. PO; taper to 0.5 mg/lb e.o.d. PO (or less)
Tab: 5 & 20 mg
5 mg: 2/10 lb s.i.d. PO; taper to 1/10 lb e.o.d. PO (or less)

Prednisolone, prednisone Prednisolone USP
Mast cell tumor Chapter 59
40 mg/m^2 s.i.d. × 7 PO, then 20 mg/m^2 e.o.d. PO
Tab: 5 & 20 mg
5 mg: 2/10 lb (0.27 m^2) s.i.d. × 7 PO, then 1/10 lb e.o.d. PO

Prednisolone, prednisone Prednisolone USP
Miliary dermatitis: idiopathic Chapter 60
1–2 mg/lb s.i.d. until response, then reduce to lowest dose e.o.d.
Tab: 5 & 20 mg; inj: 20 mg/mL
5 mg: 2–4/10 lb s.i.d. until response, then reduce to lowest dose e.o.d.

Prednisolone, prednisone Prednisolone USP
Neoplasia 18
20–40 mg/m^2 s.i.d. or e.o.d. PO
Tab: 5 & 20 mg
5 mg: 1–2/10 lb (0.27 m^2) s.i.d. or e.o.d. PO
See Table 51-2 for combination therapy

Prednisolone, prednisone Prednisolone USP
Polymyositis 43
1 mg/lb s.i.d. PO, IM
Tab: 5 & 20 mg; inj: 20 mg/mL
5 mg: 2/10 lb s.i.d. PO; 20 mg/mL: 0.5 mL/10 lb s.i.d. IM

Prednisolone, prednisone Prednisolone USP
Pruritus 8
0.23–0.45 mg/lb b.i.d.–t.i.d. IM PO
Tab: 5 & 20 mg; inj: 20 mg/mL
5 mg: 0.5–1/10 lb b.i.d.–t.i.d. PO; 20 mg/mL: 0.1–0.2 mL/10 lb b.i.d.–t.i.d. IM

Prednisolone, prednisone Prednisolone USP
Pulmonary eosinophilic infiltrates 43
0.2–0.45 mg/lb s.i.d. PO
Tab: 5 & 20 mg
5 mg: 0.4–0.9/10 lb s.i.d. PO

Prednisolone, prednisone Prednisolone USP
Rheumatoid arthritis 43
1 mg/lb s.i.d. PO; taper to 0.5 mg/lb e.o.d. PO (or less)
Tab: 5 & 20 mg
5 mg: 2/10 lb s.i.d. PO; taper to 1/10 lb e.o.d. PO (or less)

Prednisolone, prednisone Cortisate-20
Shock 8
2.5–5 mg/lb q1–10h IV
Inj: 20 mg/mL
20 mg/mL: 1.25–2.5 mL/10 lb q1–10h IV

Prednisolone, prednisone Prednisolone USP
Systemic lupus erythematosus 43
1 mg/lb b.i.d. PO until remission, then taper
Tab: 5 & 20 mg
5 mg: 2 b.i.d. PO until remission, then taper

Prednisolone, prednisone Prednisolone USP
Toxicity: cholecalciferol Chapter 62
1 mg/lb q12h
Tab: 5 & 20 mg
5 mg: 2/10 lb q12h

Prednisolone, prednisone Prednisolone USP
Ulcers, eosinophilic 43
1–2 mg/lb s.i.d. PO
Tab: 5 & 20 mg; inj: 20 mg/mL
5 mg: 2–4 s.i.d. PO; 20 mg: 0.5–1.0/10 lb s.i.d. PO

Prednisolone, prednisone Prednisolone USP
Urethritis, persistent hematuria 43
2.5–5.0 mg/cat s.i.d–e.o.d. PO
Tab: 5 & 20 mg
5 mg: 0.5–1/10 lb s.i.d.–e.o.d. PO

Prednisolone, prednisone Prednisolone USP
Uveitis Chapter 36
0.5 mg/lb b.i.d. PO
Tab: 5 & 20 mg
5 mg: 1 b.i.d. PO

Procainamide Pronestyl-SR
Arrhythmias 8
2.3–4.5 mg/lb t.i.d.–q.i.d. PO
Tab & cap: 250 mg
250 mg: 0.1–0.2/10 lb t.i.d.–q.i.d. PO

Prochlorperazine Compazine
Vomiting 35; 11
0.23 mg/lb t.i.d.–q.i.d. PO; 0.06 mg/lb b.i.d. IM
Tab: 5, 10, & 25 mg; inj: 5 mg/mL
5 mg: 0.5/10 lb t.i.d.–q.i.d. PO; 5 mg/mL: 0.12 mL/10 lb b.i.d. IM

Progesterone, reposital Progesterone, USP
Miliary dermatitis: idiopathic Chapter 60
1–10 mg/lb SC IM p.r.n.
Inj: 50 mg/mL
50 mg/mL: 0.2–2.0 mL/10 lb SC IM p.r.n.
Other drugs are generally more efficacious

Promazine Sparine
Sedation 43
1–2 mg/lb IM
Inj: 50 mg/mL
50 mg/mL: 0.2–0.4 mL/10 lb IM

Propantheline Pro-Banthine
Diarrhea 8
0.11 mg/lb t.i.d. PO
Tab: 7.5 & 15 mg
7.5 mg: 0.15/10 lb t.i.d. PO

Propantheline Pro-Banthine
Dysuria 8
0.11 mg/lb t.i.d. PO
Tab: 7.5 & 15 mg
7.5 mg: 0.15/10 lb t.i.d. PO

Propranolol HCl Inderal
Cardiac: tachycardia 8
<10 lb: 5 mg/cat b.i.d.–t.i.d. PO; >10 lb: 5 mg/cat b.i.d.–t.i.d. PO
Tab: 10 & 20 mg
10 mg: 0.25/cat <10 lb BW; 0.5/cat >10 lb BW b.i.d.–t.i.d. PO

Proprionobacterium acnes ImmunoRegulin
Gingivitis: plasmacytic/lymphocytic Chapter 52
0.5 mL/cat 2 ×/wk IV for 3 wk, then tapered
Inj: 0.4 mg/mL
0.4 mg/mL: 0.5 mL/cat 2×/wk IV for 3 wk, then tapered
Maintenance dose every 2–4 wk

Proprionobacterium acnes ImmunoRegulin
Immune suppression 8
7 μg/lb IV q3–4d
Inj: 0.4 mg/mL
0.4 mg/mL: 0.5 mL/10 lb q3–4d

Propylthiouracil PTU USP
Hyperthyroidism: prethyroidectomy 8
50 mg/cat b.i.d.–t.i.d. PO
Tab: 50 mg
50 mg: 1/cat b.i.d.–t.i.d. PO
Use only if cat has reactions to methimazole

Prostg F2a (dinoprost tromethamine) Lutalyse
Abortion induction Chapter 54
250 μg/lb s.i.d. IM × 2 after Day 40
5 mg/mL
5 mg/mL: 0.5 mL/10 lb s.i.d. IM × 2 after Day 40 of pregnancy

Prostig F2a (dinoprost tromethamine) Lutalyse
Pyometra Chapter 54
100 μg/lb s.i.d. IM × 2, then 250 μg/lb s.i.d. IM × 3
Inj: 5 mg/mL
5 mg/mL: 0.2 mL/10 lb s.i.d. IM × 2, then 0.5 mL/10 lb s.i.d. IM ×3

Psyllium Vetasyl
Constipation Chapter 62
1–2 cap/cat s.i.d. in food
Cap
1–2 cap/cat s.i.d. in food

Psyllium + coarse bran Metamucil
Constipation 45
1–3 tsp/cat s.i.d.–b.i.d.
Powder (OTC)
Powder: 1–3 tsp/cat s.i.d.–b.i.d. in food
Takes 12–24 hr to take effect

Pumpkin pie filling Pumpkin pie filling
Constipation 45
1–4 tbsp/cat/day in food
Grocery store
1–4 tbsp/cat/day in food

Pyrantel pamoate Strongid-T, Nemex
Helminths 11
4.5 mg/lb PO, repeat in 3 wk
Tab: 22.7 mg; liq: 50 mg/mL (Strongid-T), 2.27 mg/mL (Nemex)
22.7 mg: 2/10 lb; 50 mg/mL: 1 mL/10 lb PO; 2.27 mg/mL: 20 mL/10 lb PO
Repeat in 3 wk

Pyridostigmine Mestinon
Myasthenia gravis 8
1–5 mg/cat IV
Inj: 5 mg/mL; syrup: 12 mg/mL
5 mg/mL: 0.2–1 mL/cat IV; administer anticholinergic first

Pyrilamine Histavet-P
Histamine release 47
0.5–1.0 mg/lb b.i.d.–t.i.d. SC IM IV
Inj: 20 mg/mL
20 mg/mL: 0.25–0.5 mL/10 lb SC IM IV

Pyrimethamine Daraprim
Toxoplasmosis 11
0.45 mg/lb s.i.d. PO × 3, then 0.23 mg/lb s.i.d.
Tab: 25 mg
25 mg: 0.2/10 lb s.i.d. PO × 3, then 0.1/10 lb s.i.d.
Used in conjunction with sulfas

Quinacrine Atabrine
Coccidiosis 51
4.5 mg/lb s.i.d. PO for 5 days
Tab: 100 mg
100 mg: 0.45/10 lb s.i.d. PO for 5 days

Quinidine Quinaglute, Cardioquin
Cardiac: atrial fibrillation 8
9–18 mg/lb t.i.d.–q.i.d. PO
Tab: 324 mg
324 mg: 0.25–0.5/10 lb t.i.d.–q.i.d. PO

Quinidine Quinaglute, Cardioquin
Cardiac: ventricular premature complexes 8
9–18 mg/lb t.i.d.–q.i.d. PO
Tab: 324 mg
324 mg: 0.25–0.5/10 lb t.i.d.–q.i.d. PO

Ranitidine Zantac
Gastritis due to renal failure Chapter 31
1–2 mg/lb b.i.d. PO SC
Syrup: 16.8 mg/mL; inj: 25 mg/mL
16.8 mg/mL: 0.6–1.2 mL/10 lb b.i.d. PO; 25 mg/mL: 0.4–0.8 mL/10 lb b.i.d. SC

Ranitidine Zantac
Mast cell tumor Chapter 51
1 mg/lb t.i.d. PO
Syrup: 16.8 mg/mL
16.8 mg/mL: 0.6 mL/10 lb t.i.d. PO

Ranitidine Zantac
Ulcers: gastrointestinal 8
0.23 mg/lb b.i.d. PO IV
Syrup: 16.8 mg/mL; inj: 25 mg/mL
16.8 mg/mL: 0.15 mL/10 lb b.i.d. PO; 25 mg/mL: 0.1 mL/10 lb b.i.d. IV

Rifampin Rifamate, Rimactane
Aspergillosis 43
5–9 mg/lb PO t.i.d. with amphotericin and flucytosine

Rifampin Rifamate, Rimactane
Histoplasmosis of CNS 43
5–9 mg/lb PO t.i.d. with amphotericin and flucytosine
Cap: 300 mg
300 mg: 0.2–0.3/10 lb t.i.d. with amphotericin and flucytosine

Silver nitrate solution Silver Nitrate Solution USP
Burns 43
Saturate wet topical dressings s.i.d.–b.i.d.
Soln: 5 mg/mL (0.5%)
Saturate wet topical dressings s.i.d.–b.i.d.

Silver sulfadiazine Silvadene Cream
Burns 43
Apply light coating b.i.d. × several days, then s.i.d.
Cream: 1%
Apply light coating b.i.d. × several days, then s.i.d.

Sodium bicarbonate Sodium bicarbonate USP
Acidemia secondary to renal failure Chapter 31
4–6 mEq/lb b.i.d. PO
Baking soda: ⅓ teaspoon = 1 g = 12 mEq
Baking soda: ¾ teaspoon/10 lb b.i.d. PO in food

Sodium bicarbonate Sodium bicarbonate USP
Hyperkalemia: severe Chapter 31
0.23–0.45 mEq/lb IV
Inj: 50 mEq/mL (5%); 84 mEq/mL (8.4%)
50 mEq/mL: 0.5–0.9 mL/10 lb IV; 84 mEq/mL: 0.03–0.05 mL/10 lb IV

Sodium chloride Salt
Toxicity 11
1–3 tsp with warm water PO
OTC
1–3 tsp with warm water PO to induce vomiting

Sodium hypochlorite Clorox
Dermatophytosis 17
100 mL/L water
OTC (bleach)
100 mL/L of water applied topically
Caution: may change color of hair

Sodium iodide Sodium Iodide USP
Sporotrichosis Chapter 56
10 mg/lb b.i.d. PO
Inj: 20% aqueous soln
20% soln: 0.5 mL/10 lb b.i.d. PO
Give IV solution orally; mix with cream or milk to increase palatability

Sodium phosphate Sodium phosphate oral solution USP
Hypercalcemia 43
Dilute 1–3 g with water (1:1); give 10–20 mL PO s.i.d.–t.i.d. until stool soft
Soln: 30 mL
Dilute 1–3 g with water (1:1); give 10–20 mL PO s.i.d.–t.i.d. until stool is soft

Sodium sulfate Glauber's Salts
Cathartic Chapter 62
115 mg/lb PO
Powder
¼ level tsp/10 lb in water PO
May be mixed with activated charcoal slurry

Sodium sulfate GoLYTELY
Toxicity: acetaminophen 11
23 mg/lb q4h using 1.6% soln
16 mg/mL (GoLYTELY)
GoLYTELY: 14.4 mL/10 lb PO

Sodium thiopental Pentothal
Anesthetic 43
1.4–6.8 mg/lb IV to effect
Inj: 25 mg/mL (2.5%) & 50 mg/mL (5%)
2.5%: 0.6–2.7 mL/10 lb IV to effect

Spironolactone Aldactone
Cardiac: diuretic 11
0.9–1.8 mg/lb s.i.d. PO
Tab: 25 mg
25 mg: 0.3–1.0/10 lb s.i.d. PO

Spironolactone/hydrochlorothiazide Aldactazide
Cardiac: diuretic 43
1 mg/lb b.i.d. PO
Tab: 50 mg (25 + 25 mg)
Tab: 0.2/10 lb b.i.d. PO

Spironolactone/hydrochlorothiazide Aldactazide
Hypertension 43
0.5–1 mg/lb b.i.d. PO
Tab: 50 mg (25 + 25 mg)
50 mg: 0.1–0.2/10 lb b.i.d. PO

Stanozolol Winstrol
Anemia secondary to renal failure Chapter 31
0.5–2 mg/cat s.i.d. PO; 4.5–11.4 mg/lb PO, IM q7d
Tab: 2 mg; inj: 50 mg/mL
2 mg: 0.5–2/cat s.i.d. PO or 2.5–10 q7d PO; 50 mg/mL: 1–2 mL/10 lb q7d IM

Stanozolol Winstrol
Anorexia 8
0.5–2 mg/cat s.i.d. PO; 4.5–11.4 mg/lb PO, IM q7d
Tab: 2 mg; inj: 50 mg/mL
2 mg: 0.5–2/cat s.i.d. PO or 2.5–10 q7d PO; 50 mg/mL: 1–2 mL/10 lb q7d IM

Succinylcholine Anectine, Sucostrin
Muscle paralysis induction 43
0.027 mg/lb IV
Inj: 20 mg/mL
20 mg/mL: 0.01 mL/10 lb IV

Sucralfate Carafate
Ulceration: gastrointestinal 8
18 mg/lb PO t.i.d.
Tab: 1 g
1 g: 0.2/10 lb t.i.d. PO

Sucralfate Carafate
Toxicity: NSAI Chapter 62
250–500 mg/cat b.i.d.–t.i.d. PO
Tab: 1 g
1 g: 0.25–0.5/cat b.i.d.–t.i.d. PO

Sulfadiazine Tribrissen, Di-Trim
Coccidiosis 43
14 mg/lb t.i.d. PO × 5–7 days
Tab: 100 mg (of 120 mg tab) & 400 mg (of 480 mg tab)
100 mg: 1.4/10 lb t.i.d. PO × 5–7 days

Sulfadiazine Tribrissen, Di-Trim
Nocardiosis 43
Tab: 100 mg (of 120 mg tab) & 400 mg (of 480 mg tab)
480 mg: 2.1 PO × 1 dose, then 1 b.i.d. PO/10 lb

Sulfadiazine Tribrissen, Di-Trim
Toxoplasmosis 43
20 mg/lb b.i.d.–t.i.d. PO × 14 days
Tab: 100 mg (of 120 mg tab) & 400 mg (of 480 mg tab)
100 mg: 2/10 lb b.i.d.–t.i.d. PO × 14 days; 400 mg: 0.5/10 lb b.i.d.–t.i.d. PO × 14 days

Sulfadimethoxine Albon
Coccidiosis 11
Initial: 25 mg/lb; subsequent daily dose 12.5 mg/lb for 9 days
Tab: 125 & 250 mg; oral soln: 50 mg/mL
125 mg: 2/10 lb s.i.d. PO initially, then 1/10 lb s.i.d. PO × 9
50 mg/mL: 5 mL/10 lb s.i.d. PO initially, then 2.5 mL/10 lb s.i.d. PO × 5

Sulfadimethoxine + ormetroprim Primor
Coccidiosis 51
25 mg/lb + 5 mg/lb s.i.d. PO up to 23 days
Tab: 240 mg (200 + 40); 600 mg (500 + 100)
240 mg: 1.25/10 lb s.i.d. PO up to 23 days

Sulfasalazine Azulfidine
Inflammatory bowel disease Chapter 48
7–10 mg/lb b.i.d.–t.i.d. PO
Tab: 500 mg; susp: 50 mg/mL
500 mg: 0.14–0.2/10 lb b.i.d.–t.i.d. PO; 50 mg/mL: 1.4–2.0 mL/10 lb b.i.d.–t.i.d. PO
Watch for anemia and anorexia

Taurine Taurine
Cardiac: dilated CM 12
250–500 mg/cat b.i.d. PO
Tab: 250 mg
250 mg: 1–2/cat b.i.d. PO

Taurine Taurine
Seizures (maintenance) Chapter 23
500 mg/cat b.i.d. PO
Tab: 250 mg
250 mg: 2/cat b.i.d. PO
Only effective in selected cases

Terbutaline Brethine
Bronchoconstriction 8
1.25–2.5 mg/cat b.i.d.–t.i.d. PO
Tab: 2.5 & 5 mg
2.5 mg: 0.5–1/cat b.i.d.–t.i.d. PO; 5 mg: 0.25–0.5/cat b.i.d.–t.i.d. PO

Testosterone, methyl Metandren
Anabolic effects 43
0.5–1.0 mg/lb s.i.d. PO
Tab: 10 & 25 mg; cap: 5 & 10 mg
10 mg: 0.5–1.0/10 lb s.i.d. PO

Testosterone, methyl Metandren
Galactorrhea 43
0.5–1 mg/lb IM once or s.i.d. PO × 5–7 days
Tab: 10 & 25 mg; cap: 5 & 10 mg
10 mg: 0.5–1.0/10 lb s.i.d. PO × 5–7 days

Tetracycline HCl Achromycin
Bacterial infections 8
4.5–11.4 mg/lb b.i.d.–t.i.d. PO
Tab: 250 & 500 mg; susp: 25 mg/mL
250 mg: 0.25–0.5/10 lb b.i.d.–t.i.d. PO; 25 mg/mL: 1.8–4.6 mL/10 lb b.i.d.–t.i.d. PO

Tetracycline HCl Achromycin
Epiphora Chapter 35
5–10 mg s.i.d. PO
Susp: 25 mg/mL; tab: 250 & 500 mg
25 mg/mL: 0.2–0.4 mL/10 lb s.i.d. PO

Tetracycline/Novobiocin/Prednisolone Delta Albaplex
Bacterial infections 10
5–8 lb: 1 tab b.i.d. PO; 9–15 lb: 2 tab b.i.d. PO
Tab: 60 mg tetracycline, 60 mg novobiocin, and 1.5 mg prednisolone
5–8 lb: 1 tab b.i.d. PO; 9–15 lb: 2 tab b.i.d. PO

Theophylline Theo-Dur
Bronchoconstriction 8
1.8 mg/lb b.i.d. PO
Tab: 100 mg
100 mg: 0.2/10 lb b.i.d. PO

Thiabendazole Equizole
Aspergillosis 43
5 mg/lb in 10–20 mL water; flush b.i.d. × 10 days or 5 mg/lb b.i.d. PO × 6 wk
Susp: 4 g/oz (133 mg/mL)
133 mg/mL: 0.4 mL in 10–20 mL water/10 lb; flush b.i.d. × 10 days
133 mg/mL: 0.4 mL/10 lb b.i.d. PO × 6 wk

Thiabendazole Tresaderm
Dermatophytosis Chapter 56
Apply to lesions topically b.i.d.
Topical soln
Apply to lesions topically b.i.d.

Thiacetarsemide Caparsolate
Heartworms 8
1 mg/lb IV b.i.d. × 2
Inj: 10 mg/mL
10 mg/mL: 1 mL/10 lb b.i.d. × 2 days
See Chapter 7 for conflicting recommendations

Thiacetarsemide Caparsolate
Hemobartonellosis 8
0.45 mg/lb s.i.d. q48h IV
Inj: 10 mg/mL
10 mg/mL: 0.5 mL q48h for 2 doses IV

Thiamine hydrochloride Thymine Hydrochloride USP
Thiamine deficiency 8
50 mg/cat s.i.d.–b.i.d. PO IM
Tab: 50 & 100 mg: inj: 100 mg/mL
50 mg: 1/cat s.i.d.–b.i.d. PO; 100 mg: 0.5/cat s.i.d.–b.i.d. PO
100 mg/mL: 0.5 mL/cat s.i.d.–b.i.d. IM

Thiamylal Bio-Tal
Anesthesia 5
8 mg/lb IV
Inj: 20 mg/mL (2%) (other dilutions possible)
20 mg/mL: 4 mL/10 lb IV (give ⅓ as bolus, then to effect)

Thiethylperazine Torecan
Vomiting 44
5 mg/cat b.i.d. or p.r.n. PO; 0.1–0.2 mg/lb SC b.i.d.
Tab: 10 mg; inj: 5 mg/mL
10 mg: 0.5/cat b.i.d. or p.r.n. PO; 5 mg/mL: 0.2–0.4 mL/10 lb SC b.i.d.

Thyroxine Synthroid
See L-Thyroxine

Ticarcillin Ticar
Bacterial infections 11
6.8–11.4 mg/lb t.i.d. IM IV
Inj: 100 mg/mL when reconstituted
100 mg/mL: 0.7–1.14 mL/10 lb t.i.d. IM IV

Ticarcillin/clavulanate Timentin
Bacterial infections 50
18 mg/lb q6h IV, IM
Inj: 200 mg/mL when reconstituted
200 mg/mL: 0.9 mL/10 lb q6h IV, IM

Tiletamine/zolazepam Telazol
Anesthesia 45
4–6 mg/lb IM
Inj: 100 mg/mL
100 mg/mL: 0.4–0.6 mL/10 lb IM

Timilol Timoptic
Glaucoma 44
1–2 drops b.i.d. in eyes
Ophthalmic drops
1–2 drops b.i.d. in eyes

Tobramycin Nebcin
Bacterial infections 8
0.9 mg/lb t.i.d. SC
Inj: 40 mg/mL when reconstituted
40 mg/mL: 0.2 mL/10 lb t.i.d. SC

Tolazoline Priscoline HCl
Cardiac: vasodilator 8
0.9 mg/lb IV
Inj: 25 mg/mL
25 mg/mL: 0.4 mL/10 lb IV

Tolazoline Priscoline HCl
Toxicity: xylazine Chapter 62
2.3–4.5 mg/lb IV
Inj: 25 mg/mL
25 mg/mL: 1.0–1.8 mL/10 lb IV

Triamcinolone Vetalog
Pruritus 8
0.05–0.1 mg/lb IM SC
Inj: 2 & 6 mg/mL
2 mg/mL: 0.25–0.5 mL/10 lb IM SC

Triethylene thiophosphoramide Thiotepa
Neoplasia: bladder 43
30 mg/m^2 q3–4w intravesicularly
Inj: 10 mg/mL when reconstituted with 1.5 mL sterile injection water
10 mg/mL: 0.8 mL/10 lb (0.27 m^2) q3–4w intravesicularly

Trifluridine Viroptic
Keratitis: herpes virus 48
1 drop in affected eye topically q2h during waking hours
1% soln
1 drop in affected eye topically q2h during waking hours

Triiodothyronine (T_3) Cytobin
Hypothyroidism 43
2 μg/lb b.i.d.–t.i.d. PO
Tab: 60 & 120 μg
60 μg: 0.33/10 lb b.i.d.–t.i.d. PO

Trimethobenzamide Tigan
Contraindicated

Trimethoprim + sulfadiazine Tribrissen, Di-Trim
Bacterial infections 11
13.6 mg/lb PO SC s.i.d. or 7 mg/lb PO SC b.i.d.
Tab: 120 & 480 mg; inj: 240 mg/mL (24%) & 480 mg/mL (48%)
120 mg: 1/10 lb s.i.d. or 0.5/10 lb PO b.i.d.
240 mg/mL: 0.5 mL/10 lb s.i.d. SC or 0.25 mL/10 lb b.i.d. SC

Trimethoprim + sulfamethoxazole Bactrim
Bacterial infections 8
7 mg/lb b.i.d. PO
Tab: 480 mg; susp: 48 mg/mL
480 mg: 0.1/10 lb b.i.d. PO; 48 mg/mL: 1.5 mL/10 lb b.i.d. PO

Tripelennamine HCl PBZ
Pruritus 8
0.45 mg/lb b.i.d. PO IM
Tab: 25, 50, & 100 mg; elixir: 5 mg/mL
25 mg: 0.25/10 lb b.i.d. PO; 5 mg/mL: 1 mL/10 lb b.i.d. PO

Tylosin Tylan
Bacterial infections 8
3 mg/lb b.i.d. IM IV
Inj: 50 & 200 mg/mL
50 mg/mL: 0.6 mL/10 lb b.i.d. IM IV

Tylosin Tylan
Bacterial overgrowth 11
20–40 mg/lb t.i.d. PO
Soluble powder
Soluble powder: 0.25–0.5 tsp t.i.d. in food

Tylosin Tylan
Colitis 11
5 mg/lb b.i.d. PO
Soluble powder
Soluble powder: 1/16 tsp b.i.d. in food (a pinch)

Vancomycin Vancocin
Bacterial infections 11
2.3–4.5 mg/lb q.i.d. PO; 9 mg/lb b.i.d. IV
Cap: 125 & 250 mg; soln: 100 mg/mL; inj: 50 mg/mL
125: 0.2–0.5/10 lb q.i.d. PO; 100 mg/mL: 0.5 mL/10 lb q.i.d. PO
125 mg/mL: 0.2–0.4 mL/10 lb b.i.d. IV

Vasopressin in Oil Pitressin tannate in oil
Diabetes insipidus Chapter 22
1–2 U q24–72h SC IM
Inj: 5 U/mL
5 U/mL: 0.2–0.4 mL/10 lb q24–72h SC IM
Give p.r.n. based on polyuria

Vasopressin, aqueous Pitressin
Diabetes insipidus: central 43
10 mU p.r.n. IV, IM
Inj: 20 U/mL
20 U/mL diluted 100:1 with PSS to 0.2 U/mL (20 mU/mL): 0.5 mL/cat p.r.n. IV, IM

Vinblastine Velban
Neoplasia 11
2 mg/m^2 q7d IV or 0.023–0.045 mg/lb q7d IV
Inj: 1 mg/mL
1 mg/mL: 0.5 mL/10 lb q7d IV or 0.2–0.4 mL/10 lb q7d IV

Vincristine Oncovin
Neoplasia Chapter 51
0.5–0.75 mg/m^2 q1–3w IV
1 mg/mL
1 mg/mL: 0.13–0.19 mL/10 lb q1–3w IV
See Table 51-2 for combination therapy

Vitamin C Vitamin C, USP
Toxicity: acetaminophen Chapter 62
14 mg/lb q.i.d. SC, IM, PO
Cap: 250 mg; inj: 250 mg/mL
250 mg: 0.6/10 lb q.i.d. PO; 250 mg/mL: 0.6 mL/10 lb q.i.d. PO

Vitamin D DHT Tabs, Dihydrotachysterol
Hypocalcemia 8
Initial: 0.01–0.02 mg/lb s.i.d. PO × 3; maintenance: 0.005–0.01 mg/lb s.i.d.–e.o.d. PO
Tab: 0.125, 0.2, & 0.4 mg
Initial: 0.125 mg: 0.5–1/10 lb s.i.d. PO × 3
Maintenance: 0.125 mg: 0.25–0.5/10 lb s.i.d.–e.o.d. PO

Vitamin E Aquasol E
Steatitis 43
Cap: 100 & 400 IU; drops: 50 IU/mL
100 mg: 0.5–1/10 lb b.i.d. PO; 50 IU/mL: 1–2 mL/10 lb b.i.d. PO

Vitamin K$_1$ AquaMEPHYTON
Toxicity Chapter 62
2.3 mg/lb s.i.d.–b.i.d. SC, then 0.5–1.0 mg/lb b.i.d. PO
Tab: 5 mg; inj: 2 & 10 mg/mL
10 mg/mL: 2.1 mL/10 lb s.i.d.–b.i.d. SC, then 0.5–1.0 mg/lb b.i.d. PO
Oral therapy may be needed up to 24 days for 2nd-generation products

Warfarin sodium Coumadin, Panwarfin, Sofarin
Thromboembolism 49 & 8
0.045 mg/lb s.i.d. PO
Tab: 2 & 5 mg
2 mg: 1.4/10 lb s.i.d. PO
Check prothrombin time at 8–10 hr; postpill should be 15–20 sec

Water Water
Gastric lavage Chapter 62
Initial: 2 mL/lb; repeat increasing to 5 mL/lb
Repeat until 3 clean rinses occur

Xylazine Rompun, Anased
Emetic Chapter 62
0.5 mg/lb SC IM
Inj: 20 & 100 mg/mL
20 mg/mL: 0.25 mL/10 lb SC IM

Xylazine Rompun, Anased
Sedation and analgesia 8
0.45–1 mg/lb IM SC
Inj: 20 & 100 mg/mL
20 mg/mL: 0.2–0.5 mL/10 lb IM SC

Yohimbine Yobine
Toxicity: xylazine Chapter 62
0.02 mg/lb IV (IM SC)
Inj: 2 mg/mL
2 mg/mL: 0.1 mL/10 lb IV (IM SC)

*Island Pharmacy Services, 1-800-328-7060. This pharmacy will compound custom drugs in a liquid form in a taste that is accepted by cats.

APPENDIX B
DRUG FORMULARY: ALPHABETICAL BY TRADE NAME

Trade Name	Generic Name
Accutane	Isotretinoin
Achromycin	Tetracycline HCl
Actidose-Aqua	Activated charcoal
Adrenalin	Epinephrine
Adriamycin	Doxorubicin
Aerrane	Isoflurane
Afrin Pediatric Drops	Oxymetazoline HCl
Albon	Sulfadimethoxine
Aldactazide	Spironolactone, hydrochlorothiazide
Aldactone	Spironolactone
Amiglyde	Amikacin
Aminophylline USP	Aminophylline
Amoxi-Tab, Amoxil	Amoxicillin
Amphojel	Aluminum hydroxide gel
Anadrol-50	Oxymetholone
Ancobon	Flucytosine (5-FC)
Anectine, Sucostrin	Succinylcholine
Anspor, Velosef	Cephradine
Antirobe	Clindamycin
Antivert	Meclizine
Apomorphine USP	Apomorphine HCl
Apresoline	Hydralazine
AquaMEPHYTON	Vitamin K_1
AquaMEPHYTON, Mephyton	Phytonadione (vitamin K_1)
Aquasol E	Vitamin E
Aramine	Metaraminol
Armidexan, Ferrextran 100	Iron-dextran
Atabrine HCl	Quinacrine
Atropine USP	Atropine
Azium	Dexamethasone
Azo Gantrisin, Pyridium	Phenazopyridine
Azulfidine	Sulfasalazine
Bactrim	Trimethoprim + sulfamethoxazole
BAL in Oil	Dimercaprol
Banamine	Flunixin meglumine
Basaljel	Aluminum carbonate gel
Baytril	Enrofloxacin
Benadryl	Diphenhydramine HCl
Benzyl Alcohol USP	Benzyl alcohol
Betadine Solution	Povidone iodine solution
Betasone	Betamethasone
Bio-Sol	Neomycin
Bio-Tal	Thiamylal
Bran	Bran
Brethine	Terbutaline sulfate
Brevital	Methohexital
Brewer's Yeast	Brewer's Yeast
Buprenex	Buprenorphine
Butazolidin	Phenylbutazone
Calcet	Calcium carbonate
Calcimar	Calcitonin
Calcium Chloride USP	Calcium chloride
Calcium Disodium Versenate	Calcium disodium EDTA
Calcium Gluconate 10% USP	Calcium gluconate 10%
Calcium USP	Calcium
Caparsolate	Thiacetarsemide
Capoten	Captopril
Carafate	Sucralfate
Cardizem	Diltiazem HCl
Cardoxin, Lanoxin	Digoxin
Ceclor	Cefaclor
Cefa-Tabs, Cefa-Drops	Cefadroxil
Cefadyl	Cephapirin
Centrine	Aminopentamide
Cephulac, Chronulac	Lactulose
Cestex	Epsiprantel
Cetacaine	Benzocaine

Note: The references for this appendix appear on pages 626–627.

Trade Name	Generic Name
Cheque-Drops	Mibolerone
Chlorinated Hydrocarbons	Chlorinated hydrocarbons
Chloromycetin	Chloramphenicol ophthalmic
Choledyl	Oxtriphylline
Cipro	Ciprofloxacin
Claforan	Cefotaxime sodium
Clavamox	Amoxicillin, clavulanic acid
Clorox	Sodium hypochlorite
Colace, Surfak	Docusate calcium
Coly-Mycin	Colistimethate sodium
Compazine	Prochlorperazine
Conofite	Miconazole
Coramine	Nikethamide
Corid	Amprolium
Cortisate-20	Prednisolone, prednisone
Cortone Acetate	Cortisone acetate
Coumadin, Panwarfin, Sofarin	Warfarin sodium
Crysticillin 300 AS	Penicillin, procaine
Cystorellin	Gonadotropin-releasing hormone
Cytobin, Cytomel	Triiodothyronine (T_3), Liothyronine sodium
Cytosar	Cytosine arabinoside (cytarabine)
Cytoxan	Cyclophosphamide
Dalmane	Flurazepam HCl
Daranide	Dichlorphenamide
Daraprim	Pyrimethamine
Darbid	Isopropamide iodide
DDAVP	Desmopressin Acetate
Deca-Durabolin	Nandrolone decanoate
Delta Albaplex	Tetracycline, novobiocin/prednisolone
Demerol	Meperidine
Depo-Medrol	Methylprednisolone (depo)
Depo-Provera	Methoxyprogesterone acetate
Dermaide Aloe Cream	Aloe vera cream
Desferal	Desferoxamine
Dextran 6%	Dextran 75, in saline
Dextrose USP 20%	Dextrose, 20%
DHT Tabs, Dihydrotachysterol	Vitamin D
DHT, Intensol Liquid	Dihydrotachysterol
Diabinese	Chlorpropamide
Diamox	Acetazolamide
Diapid	Lysine-8-vasopressin
Dibenzyline	Phenoxybenzamine
Difil, Carbam, Nemacide	Diethylcarbamazine
Dilantin	Phenytoin
Dirocide	Diethylcarbamazine
Ditropan	Oxybutynin HCl
Diuril	Chlorthiazide
Dobutrex	Dobutamine
DOCA Injection	Desoxycorticosterone acetate
Domeboro Solution	Aluminum acetate, Burow's solution
Donnagel-PG	Paregoric
Dopram	Doxapram HCl
Dramamine	Dimenhydrinate
Droncit	Praziquantel
DTIC-Dome	Dacarbazine
Dulcolax	Bisacodyl
Dynapen, Dicloxin	Dicloxacillin
Ecotrin/Ascriptin	Aspirin
ECP	Estradiol cypionate
Edecrin	Ethacrynate sodium
EDTA USP	EDTA
Elavil	Amitriptyline
Elspar	Asparaginase, L-Asparaginase
Epifrin	Epinephrine
Epogen, Procrit	Erythropoietin, human recombinent
Epsom's Salts	Magnesium sulfate
Equizole	Thiabendazole
Erythrocin	Erythromycin
Ethrane	Enflurane
Everclear	Ethanol
Flagyl	Metronidazole
Fleet	Phosphate enemas
Flo-cillin, Pen-BP-48, Dual-Pen	Penicillin G, benzathine
Florinef	Fludrocortisone acetate
Flucort	Flumethasone
Fluothane	Halothane
Folic Acid Tabs	Folic acid
Follutein, Chortropin	Human chorionic gonadotropin
FSH-P	Follicle-stimulating hormone
Fulvicin P/G, Gris-PEG	Griseofulvin ultramicrosize
Fulvicin U/F	Griseofulvin microsize
Fungizone	Amphotericin B
Gentocin	Gentamicin sulfate
Gentocin Durafilm	Gentamicin sulfate + betamethasone
Gentocin Ophthalmic	Gentamicin sulfate
Gentocin Otic	Gentamicin sulfate + betamethasone

Trade Name	Generic Name
Geopen, Geocillin	Carbenicillin
Glauber's Salts	Sodium sulfate
Glucagon	Glucagon
Glucotrol	Glipizide
Glycerin USP	Glycerin
GoLYTELY	Sodium sulfate
Heparin USP	Heparin
Hetacin K	Hetacillin
Histavet-P	Pyrilamine
Humorsol	Demecarium bromide
Hycodan, Tussigon	Hydrocodone
Hydrochlorthiazide USP	Hydrochlorthiazide
HydroDiuril	Hydrochlorothiazide
Hydrogen Peroxide USP	Hydrogen peroxide 3%
ImmunoRegulin	*Proprionibacterium acnes*
Imodium (A-D)	Loperamide
Imuran	Azathioprine
Inderal	Propranolol HCl
Inocor	Amrinone
Intropin	Dopamine
Iodine USP, aqueous	Iodine, aqueous organic
Ipecac Syrup USP	Ipecac syrup
Isuprel	Isoproterenol
Ivomec	Ivermectin
Kaopectate	Kaolin-pectin
Keflex	Cephalexin
Keflin	Cephalothin
Kefzol, Ancef	Cefazolin
Ketaset, Vetalar	Ketamine
Lactated Ringer's solution	Lactated Ringer's solution
Lasix	Furosemide
Laxatone	Petrolatum, white & liquid
Leukeran	Chlorambucil
Librium	Chlordiazepoxide
Lincocin	Lincomycin
Lithostat	Acetohydroxamic acid (AHA)
Lixotinic, Feosol	Ferrous sulfate
Lomotil	Diphenoxylate
Lopressor	Metoprolol
Lutalyse	Prostig F2a (dinoprost tromethamine)
Lym-Dyp	Lime sulfur solution
Lysodren	Mitotane, O,p′-DDD (Mitotane)
Mandol	Cefamandole nafate
Manniject	Mannitol
Marax	Ephedrine
Marezine	Cyclizine lactate
MCT Oil	Medium-chain triglyceride oil
Medicol, Chloromycetin	Chloramphenicol
Mefoxin	Cefoxitin
Mestinon	Pyridostigmine
Metamucil	Psyllium + coarse bran
Metandren	Methyltestosterone; testosterone, methyl
Metaprel	Metaproterenol
Methio-Form	Dl-methionine, methionine (D-L)
Methylene Blue USP	Methylene blue
Meticorten	Prednisolone acetate
Metofane	Methoxyflurane
Milk of Magnesia	Magnesium hydroxide
Mineral oil	Mineral oil
Minocin	Minocycline HCl
Mitaban	Amitraz
Morphine	Morphine
Mucomyst	Acetylcysteine
Mycostatin	Nystatin
Myleran	Busulfan
Nafcil, Unipen	Nafcillin sodium
Nalline	Nalorphine HCl
Narcan, P/M Naloxone HCl	Naloxone HCl
Nebcin	Tobramycin
Neo-Synephrine	Phenylephrine
Neptazane	Methazolamide
Nitrostat Ointment, 2%	Nitroglycerin
Nizoral	Ketoconazole
Nolvasan Solution	Chlorhexidine diacetate
Nolvasan/Chlorhexiderm	Chlorhexidine diacetate
Noroxin	Norfloxacin
Novantrone	Mitoxantrone HCl
Novin	Dipyrone
NPH, Lente	Insulin, intermediate
Nubain	Nalbuphine
Numorphan	Oxymorphone
Ocufen	Flubiprofen 0.03%
Omnipaque	Iohexol
Oncovin	Vincristine
Organidin	Iodine
Ornade, Comtrex, Triaminic	Phenylpropanolamine
Orthocide	Captan-50 WP
Ovaban	Megestrol acetate
Oxacillin	Oxacillin, sodium
Oxydex Shampoo	Benzyl peroxide shampoo

Trade Name	Generic Name
Oxytocin USP	Oxytocin
Panacur	Fenbendazole
Pavulon	Pancuronium bromide
PBZ	Tripelennamine HCl
Penicillin G Procaine	Penicillin G procaine
Pentids, Pfizerpen	Penicillin G potassium
Pentobarbital USP	Pentobarbital sodium
Pentothal	Sodium thiopental
Pepcid	Famotidine
Pepto-Bismol	Bismuth subsalicylate
Percorten IM Repository	Desoxycorticosterone pivalate
Periactin, Vimicon	Cyproheptadine
Phenobarbital USP	Phenobarbital
Phillips' Milk of Magnesia	Milk of magnesia
PHisoHex	Hexachlorophene
Phospholine Iodide	Echothiophate
Pilocarpine Ophthalmic USP, 2%	Pilocarpine
Pitocin	Oxytocin
Pitressin	Vasopressin, aqueous
Pitressin Tannate in Oil	Vasopressin in oil
Polyflex	Ampicillin sodium
Potassium Chloride USP	Potassium chloride
Potassium permanganate	Potassium permanganate (1:2,000)
Pred-Forte, Econopred	Prednisolone acetate 1%
Prednis-A-Vet	Prednisolone sodium phosphate
Prednisolone USP	Prednisolone, prednisone
Prilosec (formerly Losec)	Omeprazole
Primor	Sulfadimethoxine + ormetroprim
Principen	Ampicillin trihydrate
Priscoline	Tolazoline HCl
Pro-Banthine	Propantheline bromide
Pro-Spot	Fenthion
Proban	Cythioate
Progesterone USP	Progesterone, reposital
Proglycem	Diazoxide
PromAce	Acetylpromazine
Pronestyl-SR	Procainamide
Protopam chloride	Pralidoxime (2-PAM)
Proventil, Ventolin	Albuterol sulfate
Prozyme	Digestive enzymes
PTU USP	Propylthiouracil
Quinaglute, Cardioquin	Quinidine
Reglan	Metoclopramide

Trade Name	Generic Name
Regular Insulin + Glucose	Insulin/glucose
Regular Purified Pork Insulin	Insulin, short-acting
Rheumatrex	Methotrexate
Ridaura	Auranofin
Rifamate, Rimactane	Rifampin
Rismo-50	DMSO
Robaxin	Methocarbamol
Robinul	Glycopyrrolate
Rompun, Anased	Xylazine
Salt	Sodium chloride
Sargeants Worm Away for Cats	Piperazine
Scolaban	Bunamidine
Sectral	Acebutolol HCl
Serax	Oxazepam
Silvadene Cream	Silver sulfadiazine
Silver Nitrate Solution USP	Silver nitrate solution
Sodium Bicarbonate USP	Sodium bicarbonate
Sodium Iodide USP	Sodium iodide
Sodium Phosphate Oral Solution USP	Sodium phosphate
Solganal	Aurothioglucose
Solu-Cortef	Hydrocortisone sodium succinate
Solu-Delta-Cortef	Prednisolone sodium succinate
Solu-Medrol	Methylprednisolone sodium succinate
Sparine	Promazine HCl
Stiglyn, Prostigmin	Neostigmine
Stoxil, Herplex	Idoxuridine
Strongid, Nemex	Pyrantel pamoate
Sulfamylon Cream	Mafenide 10%
Surfak	Docusate calcium
Synthroid	Thyroxine
Synthroid, Thyro-Tabs	L-Thyroxine
Tagamet	Cimetidine
Talwin	Pentazocine
Tapazole	Methimazole
Task	Dichlorvos
Taurine	Taurine
Telazol	Tiletamine/zolazepam
Teldrin, Chlor-Trimeton	Chlorpheniramine maleate
Tenormin	Atenolol
Tensilon	Edrophonium chloride
Terramycin, Liquamycin	Oxytetracycline
Theo-Dur	Theophylline
Thiotepa	Triethylene thiophosphoramide

Trade Name	Generic Name
Thorazine	Chlorpromazine HCl
Thymine Hydrochloride USP	Thiamine HCl
Ticar	Ticarcillin
Tigan	Trimethobenzamide
Timentin	Ticarcillin/clavulanate
Timoptic	Timilol
Torbutrol/Torbugesic	Butorphanol
Torecan	Thiethylperazine
ToxiBan, Granules or Suspension	Activated charcoal
Tramisol, Levasole	Levamisole
Tresaderm	Thiabendazole
Tribrissen, Di-Trim	Sulfadiazine, Trimethoprim + sulfadiazine
Tumil-K, Kaochlor, Kaon	Potassium gluconate
Tussar DM (+ chlorpheniramine & pseudoephedrine)	
Tylan	Tylosin
Tylenol	Acetaminophen
Ultralente	Insulin, long-acting
Urecholine	Bethanechol
Uroeze	Ammonium chloride

Trade Name	Generic Name
Valbazen	Albendazole
Valium	Diazepam
Vancocin	Vancomycin
Vasotec	Enalapril
Veetids	Penicillin V
Velban	Vinblastine
Veltrim/Lotrimin	Clotrimazole
Vetalog	Triamcinolone
Vetasyl	Psyllium
Vibramycin, Doxytabs	Doxycycline
Viokase	Pancreatin
Viroptic	Trifluridine
Vitamin C	Ascorbic acid
Winstrol	Stanozolol
Xanax	Alprazolam
Xenodine	Iodine (polyhydroxydine)
Xylocaine	Lidocaine HCl (without epinephrine)
Yobine	Yohimbine
Yomesan	Niclosamide
Zantac	Ranitidine
Zovirax	Acyclovir

APPENDIX C
DRUG FORMULARY: ALPHABETICAL BY INDICATION

Indication	Drug
Abortion induction	Prostig F2a (dinoprost tromethamine)
Acidemia secondary to renal failure	Sodium bicarbonate
Acne	Benzyl peroxide shampoo Isotretinoin Megestrol acetate
Actinomycosis	Penicillin, procaine
Aggression	Diazepam
Anabolic effects	Testosterone, methyl
Analgesia	Pentazocine
Anemia secondary to renal failure	Erythropoietin, human recombinant Nandrolone decanoate Stanozolol
Anemia: iron deficiency	Ferrous sulfate Iron dextran
Anesthesia	Enflurane Halothane Isoflurane Ketamine Methohexital Methoxyflurane Oxymorphone Pentobarbital sodium Sodium thiopental Thiamylal Tiletamine, zolazepam
Anestrus: induce ovulation	Human chorionic gonadotropin
Anorexia	Chlordiazepoxide Cyproheptadine Diazepam Flurazepam HCl Nandrolone decanoate Oxazepam Oxymetholone Stanozolol
Apnea	Doxapram
Arrhythmias	Procainamide

Indication	Drug
Aspergillosis	Rifampin Thiabendazole
Asthma	Hydrocortisone sodium succinate Iodine Megestrol acetate Prednisolone sodium succinate Prednisolone, prednisone
Atopy	Betamethasone
Autoimmune diseases	Dexamethasone
Autoimmune hemolytic anemia	Azathioprine Prednisolone, prednisone
Autoimmune skin diseases	Auranofin
Autoimmune thrombocytopenia	Prednisolone, prednisone
Bacterial infections	Amikacin Amoxicillin Amoxicillin, clavulanic acid Ampicillin sodium Ampicillin trihydrate Carbenicillin Cefaclor Cefadroxil Cefamandole nafate Cefazolin Cefotaxime sodium Cefoxitin Cephalexin Cephalothin Cephapirin Cephradine Chloramphenicol Clindamycin Colistimethate sodium Dicloxacillin Doxycycline Enrofloxacin Erythromycin Gentamicin sulfate Hetacillin Lincomycin

Indication	Drug
Bacterial infections (*cont.*)	Metronidazole Minocycline HCl Nafcillin, sodium Norfloxacin Oxacillin, sodium Oxytetracycline Penicillin G, potassium Penicillin G, procaine Penicillin G, benzathine Penicillin V Tetracycline HCl Tetracycline, novobiocin, prednisolone Ticarcillin Ticarcillin, clavulanate Tobramycin Trimethoprim + sulfadiazine Trimethoprim + sulfamethoxazole Tylosin Vancomycin
Bacterial infections, soft tissue/bone	Ciprofloxacin
Bacterial infections, urinary	Ciprofloxacin Norfloxacin
Bacterial osteomyelitis	Clindamycin
Bacterial overgrowth	Tylosin
Bladder atony	Bethanechol
Bronchoconstriction	Albutrol Aminophylline Ephedrine Metaproterenol Oxtriphylline Terbutaline Theophylline
Burns	Aloe vera cream Mafenide 10% Silver nitrate solution Silver sulfadiazine
Candida infections	Nystatin
Cardiac arrest	Calcium chloride Epinephrine
Cardiac: afterload reducer	Hydralazine
Cardiac: atrial fibrillation	Quinidine
Cardiac: beta-blocker	Acebutolol
Cardiac: bradycardia	Atropine Glycopyrrolate Isopropamide iodide Isoproterenol
Cardiac: dilated CM	Amrinone Captopril Digoxin Dobutamine Taurine
Cardiac: diuretic	Chlorthiazide Ethacrynate sodium Furosemide Hydrochlorthiazide Spironolactone Spironolactone/hydrochlorothiazide
Cardiac: heart blocks	Isopropamide iodide Isoproterenol
Cardiac: hypertrophic CM	Atenolol Diltiazem HCl Milrinone
Cardiac: tachycardia	Propranolol HCl
Cardiac: vasodilator	Nitroglycerin Tolazoline
Cardiac: vent premature complexes	Lidocaine HCl (without epinephrine)
Cardiac: vent tachycardia	Lidocaine HCl (without epinephrine)
Cardiac: ventricular premature complexes	Quinidine
Cathartic	Magnesium sulfate Sodium sulfate
Central diabetes insipidus	Lysine-8-vasopressin
Cerebral edema from brain tumors	Prednisolone, prednisone
Cheyletiellosis	Ivermectin
Cholangitis, lymphocytic	Prednisolone, prednisone
CNS depression (drug-induced)	Nikethamide
Coccidiosis	Amprolium Quinacrine Sulfadiazine Sulfadimethoxine Sulfadimethoxine + ormentoprim
Colitis	Tylosin
Colitis, eosinophilic	Prednisolone, prednisone
Colitis, plasmacytic/lymphocytic	Prednisolone, prednisone
Conjunctivitis, bacterial	Gentamicin sulfate Gentamicin sulfate + betamethasone
Conjunctivitis: *Chlamydia*	Chloramphenicol ophthalmic Oxytetracycline ophthalmic
Constipation	Bisacodyl Bran Dioctyl sulfosuccinate Docusate sodium Magnesium hydroxide Milk of Magnesia Mineral oil Psyllium + coarse bran Pumpkin pie filling
Corneal ulcer: herpes virus	Idoxuridine Iodine, aqueous organic

Indication	Drug
Cough	Dextromethorphan
Coughing	Hydrocodone
Cystic ovarian follicles	Human chorionic gonadotropin
Demodicosis	Amitraz
Dermatophytosis	Captan-50 WP Chlorhexidine diacetate Clotrimazole Griseofulvin microsize Griseofulvin ultramicrosize Iodine (polyhydroxydine) Ketoconazole Lime sulfur solution Miconazole Povidone iodine solution Sodium hypochlorite Thiabendazole
Detrussor hyperreflexia	Oxybutynin HCl
Diabetes insipidus	Chlorpropamide Desmopressin acetate Hydrochlorothiazide Vasopressin in oil
Diabetes insipidus, central	Vasopressin, aqueous
Diabetes mellitus	Glipizide Insulin, intermediate Insulin, long-acting Insulin, short-acting
Diarrhea	Bismuth subsalicylate Digestive enzymes Diphenoxylate Kaolin-pectin Loperamide Paregoric Propantheline
Disseminated intravascular coagulation	Heparin
Diuresis	Furosemide
Dystocia	Oxytocin
Dysuria	Diazepam DMSO Megestrol acetate Phenoxybenzamine Propantheline
Ear mites	Ivermectin
Edema of CNS	Mannitol
Emesis induction	Hydrogen peroxide 3%
Emetic	Xylazine
Endocrine deficiency alopecia	Liothyronine sodium
Enteritis, eosinophilic	Prednisolone, prednisone
Enteritis, plasmacytic/ lymphocytic	Prednisolone, prednisone
Eosinophilic granuloma complex	Megestrol acetate Methylprednisolone (Depo) Prednisolone, prednisone

Indication	Drug
Eosinophilic keratitis	Megestrol acetate
Epiphora	Tetracycline HCl
Esophagitis	Omeprazole
Estrus induction	Follicle-stimulating hormone
Estrus prevention	Delmadione Megestrol acetate
Estrus suppression	Megestrol acetate
Fear	Diazepam
Fever	Dipyrone
Flea infestation	Cythioate Fenthion
Fluid maintenance	Lactated Ringer's solution
Folic acid deficiency due to pyrimethamine	Folic acid
Folic acid deficiency	Brewer's Yeast
Food allergy	Prednisolone, prednisone
Frostbite	Dextran 75, in saline
Fungal infections	Metronidazole
Fungal infections, systemic	Amphotericin B
Galactorrhea	Testosterone, methyl
Gastric lavage	Water
Gastric ulcers	Famotidine
Gastritis due to renal failure	Cimetidine Ranitidine
Gastritis, eosinophilic	Prednisolone, prednisone
Gastritis, plasmacytic/ lymphocytic	Prednisolone, prednisone
Gastrointestinal ulceration	Sucralfate
Giardiasis	Metronidazole
Gingivitis	Megestrol acetate Metronidazole
Gingivitis, plasma cell	Prednisolone, prednisone
Glaucoma	Acetazolamide Demecarium bromide Dichlorphenamide Echothiophate Glycerin Mannitol Methazolamide Pilocarpine Timilol
Hair balls	Petrolatum, white & liquid
Hair pulling	Amitriptyline
Heartworm prevention	Diethylcarbamazine
Heartworms	Thiacetarsemide
Helminths	Dichlorvos Diethylcarbamazine Fenbendazole Pyrantel pamoate
Hemobartonellosis	Thiacetarsemide

Indication	Drug
Hepatic encephalopathy	Lactulose Medium-chain triglyceride oil Neomycin
Histamine release	Pyrilamine
Histoplasmosis of CNS	Rifampin
Horner's syndrome	Epinephrine Phenylephrine
Hyperadrenocorticism	O,p′-DDD (mitotane)
Hypercalcemia	Sodium phosphate
Hyperkalemia, severe	Calcium gluconate 10% Insulin/glucose Sodium bicarbonate
Hyperphosphatemia	Aluminum carbonate gel Aluminum hydroxide gel
Hypertension	Enalapril Hydrochlorothiazide Metoprolol Spironolactone/ hydrochlorothiazide
Hyperthyroidism: medical (only) treatment	Methimazole
Hyperthyroidism: Pre-thyroidectomy	Methimazole Propylthiouracil
Hypoadrenocorticism	Cortisone acetate Desoxycorticosterone acetate Desoxycorticosterone pivalate Fludrocortisone acetate Prednisolone acetate Prednisolone, prednisone
Hypocalcemia	Calcium Calcium carbonate Dihydrotachysterol Vitamin D
Hypoglycemia (short-term)	Glucagon
Hypokalemia	Potassium chloride Potassium gluconate
Hypothyroidism	Liothyronine sodium Triiodothyronine (T_3)
Hypothyroidism, post-thyroidectomy	L-Thyroxine
Immune-mediated anemia	Cyclophosphamide
Immune-mediated diseases	Chlorambucil Prednisolone, prednisone
Immune suppression	Levamisole *Proprionibacterium acnes*
Inflammation	Flunixin meglumine
Inflammatory Bowel Disease	Azathioprine Metronidazole Prednisolone, prednisone Sulfasalazine
Insulinoma: hypoglycemia	Diazoxide
Keratitis: herpes virus	Trifluridine

Indication	Drug
Leptospirosis	Penicillin, procaine
Lungworms	Levamisole
Lupus	Prednisolone, prednisone
Mast cell tumor	Cimetidine Diphenhydramine HCl Prednisolone, prednisone Ranitidine
Microfilaria of heartworms	Levamisol
Miliary dermatitis, idiopathic	Megestrol acetate Methoxyprogesterone acetate Methylprednisolone (Depo) Prednisolone, prednisone Progesterone, reposital
Mismating	Estradiol cypionate
Motion sickness	Dimenhydrinate
Muscle paralysis induction	Succinylcholine
Muscle spasm, pain	Methocarbamol
Muscle wasting	Methyltestosterone
Myasthenia gravis	Edrophonium chloride Neostigmine Pyridostigmine
Myelography	Iohexol
Narcotic reversal	Nalorphine HCl Naloxone HCl
Nasal congestion	Oxymetazoline HCl Phenylephrine
Neoplasia	Busulfan Chlorambucil Cyclophosphamide Cytosine arabinoside (cytarabine) Dexamethasone Doxorubicin L-Asparaginase Methotrexate Mitoxantrone HCl Prednisolone, prednisone Vinblastine Vincristine
Neoplasia, bladder	Triethylene thiophosphoramide
Neoplasia, lymphoreticular	Dacarbazine
Nocardiosis	Sulfadiazine
Notoedric mange	Lime sulfur solution
Notoedric mange (scabies)	Ivermectin
Oliguric renal failure	Mannitol
Ophthalmic surgery	Pancuronium bromide
Otitis, bacterial	Gentamicin sulfate + betamethasone
Ovulation induction	Gonadotropin-releasing hormone Human chorionic gonadotropin

Indication	Drug
Pain	Aspirin Buprenorphine Butorphanol Meperidine Morphine Nalbuphine Phenylbutazone
Pancreatic insufficiency	Pancreatin
Paragonimus	Albendazole
Pediculosis (lice)	Lime sulfur solution
Pemphigus	Aurothioglucose Azathioprine
Plasmacytic/lymphocytic gingivitis	*Proprionibacterium acnes*
Polymyositis	Prednisolone, prednisone
Prolapsed third eyelids	Phenylephrine
Pruritus	Flumethasone Methylprednisolone (Depo) Chlorpheniramine maleate Dexamethasone Megestrol acetate Prednisolone, prednisone Triamcinolone Tripelennamide HCl
Pulmonary edema	Chlorthiazide Furosemide
Pulmonary eosinophilic infiltrates	Prednisolone, prednisone
Pyometra	Prostig F2a (dinoprost tromethamine)
Renal failure: intense diuresis	Dextrose 20%
Renal shutdown	Dopamine
Restraint	Ketamine
Retinal detachment (hypertension)	Hydrochlorothiazide
Rheumatoid arthritis	Prednisolone, prednisone Auranofin
Rickettsial infections	Doxycycline Oxytetracycline
Roundworm infestation	Piperazine
Salivation	Atropine Glycopyrrolate
Sedation	Pentazocine Promazine
Sedation and analgesia	Xylazine
Seizures	Phenytoin
Seizures (maintenance)	Diazepam Phenobarbital Taurine
Self-mutilation	Amitriptyline
Shock	Dexamethasone Dextran 75, in saline Hydrocortisone sodium succinate Lactated Ringer's solution Metaraminol Prednisolone sodium phosphate Prednisolone, prednisone
Shock: cardiogenic	Dopamine
Spinal cord trauma	Dexamethasone Methylprednisolone sodium succinate
Sporotrichosis	Sodium iodide
Status epilepticus	Diazepam Pentobarbital sodium Phenobarbital
Steatitis	Vitamin E
Strychnine toxicosis	Potassium permanganate (1:2,000)
Systemic fungal diseases	Flucytosine (5-FC) Itraconazole Ketoconazole
Systemic lupus erythematosus	Prednisolone, prednisone
T_3 suppression test	Liothyronine sodium
Tapeworm infestation	Bunamidine Epsiprantel Niclosamide Praziquantel
Tetany, muscle fasciculation	Methocarbamol
Thiamine deficiency	Thiamine hydrochloride
Thromboembolism	Acetylpromazine Aspirin Heparin Warfarin sodium
Toxicity (to induce emesis)	Apomorphine HCl Acetylcysteine
Toxicity: acetaminophen	Ascorbic acid Cimetidine Sodium sulfate
Toxicity: amphetamines	Chlorpromazine hydrochloride
Toxicity: anticoagulants	Phytonadione (Vitamin K_1)
Toxicity: calciferol	Calcitonin
Toxicity: carbamate	Atropine
Toxicity: chelating agent	Calcium disodium EDTA
Toxicity: cholecalciferol	Prednisolone, prednisone
Toxicity: ethylene glycol	Ethanol
Toxicity: general	Activated charcoal Ipecac syrup Sodium chloride Vitamin K_1

Indication	Drug
Toxicity: heavy metal	Dimercaprol Pralidoxime (2-PAM)
Toxicity: iron (in vitamins)	Desferoxamine
Toxicity: NSAI	Sucralfate
Toxicity: NSAI (gastric ulcers)	Cimetidine
Toxicity: organophosphate	Atropine Pralidoxime (2-PAM)
Toxicity: vitamin D	Calcitonin
Toxicity: xylazine	Tolazoline Yohimbine
Toxicosis	Hydrogen peroxide 3%
Toxoplasmosis	Clindamycin Pyrimethamine Sulfadiazine
Tranquilization	Acetylpromazine Chlorpromazine hydrochloride Diazepam
Ulcers, eosinophilic	Prednisolone, prednisone
Ulcers, gastrointestinal	Ranitidine
Urethritis, persistent hematuria	Prednisolone, prednisone
Urinary acidifier	Ammonium chloride Methionine (D-L)
Urinary incontinence	Phenylpropanolamine
Urine acidifier	Dl-methionine
Urine crystal dissolution	Acetohydroxamic acid (AHA)
Urine spraying	Alprazolam Diazepam Medroxyprogesterone acetate
Uterine inertia	Calcium gluconate 10% Oxytocin
Uveitis	Aspirin Betamethasone Dexamethasone Flubiprofen 0.03% Methylprednisolone (Depo) Prednisolone acetate 1% Prednisolone, prednisone
Vertigo (vestibular disease)	Diazepam Phenobarbital
Viral infections, especially herpes	Acyclovir
Vomiting	Aminopentamide Cyclizine lactate Meclizine Metoclopramide Prochlorperazine Thiethylperazine
Vomiting, idiopathic	Megestrol acetate
Vomiting/nausea due to renal failure	Acetylpromazine
Wounds, open	Aluminum acetate, Burow's solution

REFERENCES FOR APPENDIXES A, B, C

1. Dial SM, Thrall MA, Hamar DW. 4-Methylpyrazole as treatment for naturally acquired ethylene glycol intoxication in dogs. J Am Vet Med Assoc 1989;195:73.
2. Pion PD, Kittleson MD. Therapy for Feline Aortic Thromboembolism. In: Kirk RW, ed. Current Veterinary Therapy X. Philadelphia: WB Saunders, 1989:295.
3. Marder AR. Psychotropic drugs and behavior therapy. Vet Clin N Am, Sm Anim Pract 1991;21:329.
4. Potthoff A, Carithers RW. Pain and analgesia in dogs and cats. Compend Cont Ed Pract Vet 1989;11:887.
5. Kirk RW, Bonagura JD. Table of Common Drugs: Approximate Doses. In: Kirk RW, ed. Current Veterinary Therapy X, Philadelphia: WB Saunders, 1989:1370.
6. Mikiciuk MG, Thornhill JA. Control of parathyroid hormone in chronic renal failure. Compend Cont Ed Pract Vet 1989;11:831.
7. Jernigan AD, Wilson RC, Hatch RC. Pharmacokinetics of amikacin in cats. Am J Vet Res 1988;49:355.
8. Boothe DM. Drug therapy in cats: Recommended dosing regimens. J Am Vet Med Assn 1990;196:1845.
9. Ross LA. Treating FUS in unobstructed cats and preventing its recurrence. Vet Med 1990;85:1218.
10. Product Information. In: Talbot RB, ed. Veterinary Pharmaceuticals and Biologicals, 7th ed. Lenexa, KS: Veterinary Medicine Publishing Co, 1991/1992:1.
11. Allen DG. Drugs: Approximate Dose and Routes of Administration. In: Allen DG, ed. Small Animal Medicine. Philadelphia: JB Lippincott, 1991:1099.
12. Bonagura JD.Cardiovascular Diseases. In: Sherding RG, ed. The Cat: Diseases and Clinical Management. New York: Churchill Livingstone, 1989:649.
13. Rentko VT, Cotter SM. The procedures for treating anemic cats. Vet Med 1990;85:605.
14. Stamathis G, ed. Veterinary Drug Formulary: Cornell Research Foundation Inc. Baltimore: Williams & Wilkins, 1985:1.
15. Griffin CE. Recognizing and treating pemphigus foliaceus in cats. Vet Med 1991;86:513.
16. Cullison RF. Toxicosis in cats from use of benzyl alcohol in lactated Ringer's solution. J Am Vet Med Assoc 1983;182:61.
17. Medleau L, White-Weithers NE. Dermatophytosis in cats. Compend Cont Ed Pract Vet 1991;13:557.
18. Kitchell BE. Feline Geriatric Oncology. Compend Cont Ed Pract Vet 1990;12:51.
19. Norsworthy GD. Providing nutritional support for anorectic cats. Vet Med 1991;86:589.
20. Miller WH. Symmetrical truncal hair loss in cats. Compend Cont Ed Pract Vet 1990;12:461.
21. Miller WH, Scott DW. Efficacy of chlorpheniramine maleate for management of pruritus in cats. J Am Vet Med Assoc 1990;197:67.
22. Rubin SI. Diagnosis and management of chronic renal failure in geriatric cats. Compend Cont Ed Pract Vet 1989;11:1065.
23. Lappin MR, Greene CE, Winston S, et al. Clinical feline toxoplasmosis. J Vet Int Med 1989;3:139.
24. Product Information. In: Barnhart ER, pub. Physicians Desk Reference, 44th ed. Oradell, NJ: Medical Economics Co Inc, 1990:1.
25. Leifer CE. Hypoglycemia. In: Kirk RW, ed. Current Veterinary Therapy IX. Philadelphia: WB Saunders, 1986:982.
26. Burrows CF. Constipation, Obstipation, and Megacolon. In: August JR, ed. Consultations in Feline Internal Medicine. Philadelphia: WB Saunders Co, 1991:445.
27. Braund KG. Myopathies in dogs and cats: Reviewing the conditions of unknown and exogenous origin. Vet Med 1986;81:918.
28. Crowe DT. Nutrition in critical patients: administering the support therapies. Vet Med 1989;84:152.

29. Feldman EC, Nelson RW. Feline Reproduction. In: Canine and Feline Endocrinology and Reproduction. Philadelphia: WB Saunders, 1987:525.
30. Fox PR. Myocardial Diseases. In: Ettinger SJ. Textbook of Veterinary Internal Medicine, 3rd ed. Philadelphia: WB Saunders, 1989:1097.
31. Thompson JP, Senior DF, Pinson DM, Moriello KA. Neurotoxicosis associated with the use of hexachlorophene in a cat. JAVMA 1987;190:1311.
32. August JR. Feline Viral Diseases. In: Ettinger SJ, ed. Textbook of Veterinary Internal Medicine, 3rd ed. Philadelphia: WB Saunders, 1989:312.
33. Nelson RW. Therapeutic Complications of Diabetes Mellitus. In: August JR, ed. Consultations in Feline Internal Medicine. Philadelphia: WB Saunders, 1991:257.
34. Rosenkrantz WS. The pathogenesis, diagnosis, and management of feline acne. Vet Med 1991;86:504.
35. Boothe DM. Feline Pharmacology. In: Feline Medicine Seminar, Texas A&M University. College Station, Texas, January, 1991.
36. Sawyer DC, Rech RH. Analgesia and behavioral effects of butorphanol, nalbuphine, and pentazocine in the cat. J Am Anim Hosp Assoc 1987;23:438.
37. Siemering GB. Drug improves results in dogs with herniated disk, paralysis. DVM Mag 1991;3:6.
38. Feldman EC, Nelson RW. Hyperthyroidism and Thyroid Tumors. In: Pedersen D, ed. Canine and Feline Endocrinology and Reproduction. Philadelphia: WB Saunders, 1987:91.
39. Center SA. Hepatic Lipidosis. In: August JR, ed. Consultations in Feline Internal Medicine. Philadelphia: WB Saunders, 1991:349.
40. Center SA, Randolph JF. Eosinophilia. In: August JR, ed. Consultations in Feline Internal Medicine. Philadelphia: WB Saunders, 1991:349.
41. Peterson ME, Graves TK, Gamble DA. Triiodothyronine(T_3) Suppression Test. J Vet Int Med 1990;4:233.
42. Dodds J. Feline Endocrine Diseases. DVM Mag 1990;21:48.
43. Morgan RV. American Animal Hospital Association Formulary, 2nd ed. Denver, CO: American Animal Hospital Association, 1988.
44. Mandelker L. Burns Veterinary Supply Pharmaceutical Index. New York: Burns Veterinary Supply, 1991.
45. Hoskins JD. Management of fecal impaction. Compend Cont Ed Pract Vet 1990;12:1579.
46. Jenkins CC, DeNovo RC. Omeprazole: A potent antiulcer drug. Compend Cont Ed Pract Vet 1991;13:1578.
47. Wilcke JR. List of Useful Drugs and Their Approximate Doses. In: Talbot RB, ed. Veterinary Pharmaceuticals and Biologicals, 7th ed. Lenexa, KS: Veterinary Medicine Publishing Co, 1991/1992:928.
48. Szymanski CM, Latimer CA. Diseases of the Eye. In: Sherding RG, ed The Cat: Diseases and Clinical Management. New York: Churchill Livingstone, 1989:1639.
49. Bernstein M. Feline Hyperthyroidism. Western Veterinary Conference, Las Vegas, NV, 1990.
50. Brown SA. Appropriate Use of Antimicrobial Agents. In: August JR, ed. Consultations in Feline Internal Medicine. Philadelphia: WB Saunders, 1991:583.
51. Lindsay DS, Blagburn BL. Coccidial Parasites of Dogs and Cats. Compend Cont Ed Pract Vet 1991;13:759.
52. Hawkins EC. Chronic viral upper respiratory disease in cats: differential diagnosis and management. Compend Cont Ed Pract Vet 1988;10:1003.
53. Densford LE. Synthetic hormone reverses anemia in dogs and cats with renal failure. Vet Prod News 1991;3:1.
54. Center S. Feline Liver Diseases. Proceedings: American Association of Feline Practitioners, Fall Meeting, Scottsdale, AZ, 1992.

APPENDIX D
CONVERSION TABLE: WEIGHT TO BODY-SURFACE AREA

Kilograms	Pounds	Meter^2
0.5	1.1	0.06
1.0	2.2	0.10
2.0	4.4	0.15
3.0	6.6	0.20
4.0	8.8	0.25
5.0	11.0	0.29
6.0	13.2	0.33
7.0	15.4	0.36
8.0	17.6	0.40
9.0	19.8	0.43
10.0	22.0	0.46
11.0	24.2	0.49

Note: This table is calculated for dogs; however, it can be used for cats. For more precise values for cats, use the following formula:

$$\text{BSA in m}^2 = \frac{10 \times W^{2/3}}{10^4}$$

BSA = body surface area; m^2 = square meters; W = weight in grams.

Adapted from Theilen GH. Veterinary Medical Oncology. In: Ettinger SJ, ed. Textbook of Veterinary Internal Medicine, 1st ed. Philadelphia: WB Saunders, 1975:127.

APPENDIX E
MEDICATION DOSAGE CHARTS

The following tables are designed to allow rapid calculation of medication dosages. The tables are designed for administration to a 10-lb cat. This amount was chosen because many adult cats have a body weight of approximately 10 lb and because this number can be transposed more easily than any other for other body weights.

On each table the dosages in mg/kg and in mg/lb are listed in the first two columns. The pill size or liquid concentration is listed in the other columns. By reading across, one can quickly determine the number of pills or the number of milliliters for most commonly used medications.

Dosage Chart: Number of Milliliters for 10-lb Cat

Dose, mg/kg	Dose, mg/lb	Concentration, mg/mL													
		.5	1	5	10	20	25	50	75	100	200	250	300	400	500
.02	.01	.2	.1												
.04	.02	.4	.2												
.07	.03	.6	.3	.1											
.09	.04	.8	.4	.1											
.11	.05	1.0	.5	.1	.1										
.13	.06	1.2	.6	.1	.1										
.15	.07	1.4	.7	.1	.1										
.18	.08	1.6	.8	.2	.1										
.20	.09	1.8	.9	.2	.1										
.22	.10	2.0	1.0	.2	.1	.1									
.44	.20	4.0	2.0	.4	.2	.1	.1								
.66	.30	6.0	3.0	.6	.3	.1	.1	.1							
.88	.40	8.0	4.0	.8	.4	.2	.2	.1	.1						
1.10	.50	10.0	5.0	1.0	.5	.2	.2	.1	.1	.1					
1.32	.60	12.0	6.0	1.2	.6	.3	.2	.1	.1	.1					
1.54	.70	14.0	7.0	1.4	.7	.3	.3	.1	.1	.1					
1.76	.80	16.0	8.0	1.6	.8	.4	.3	.2	.1	.1					
1.98	.90	18.0	9.0	1.8	.9	.5	.4	.2	.1	.1					
2.20	1.00	20.0	10.0	2.0	1.0	.5	.4	.2	.1	.1	.1				
2.42	1.10		11.0	2.2	1.1	.6	.4	.2	.1	.1	.1				
2.64	1.20		12.0	2.4	1.2	.6	.5	.2	.2	.1	.1				
2.86	1.30		13.0	2.6	1.3	.7	.5	.3	.2	.1	.1	.1			
3.08	1.40		14.0	2.8	1.4	.7	.6	.3	.2	.1	.1	.1			
3.30	1.50		15.0	3.0	1.5	.8	.6	.3	.2	.2	.1	.1	.1		
3.52	1.60		16.0	3.2	1.6	.8	.6	.3	.2	.2	.1	.1	.1		
3.74	1.70		17.0	3.4	1.7	.8	.7	.3	.2	.2	.1	.1	.1		
3.96	1.80		18.0	3.6	1.8	.9	.7	.4	.2	.2	.1	.1	.1		
4.18	1.90		19.0	3.8	1.9	.9	.8	.4	.3	.2	.1	.1	.1		
4.40	2.00		20.0	4.0	2.0	1.0	.8	.4	.3	.2	.1	.1	.1	.1	
4.84	2.20			4.4	2.2	1.1	.9	.4	.3	.2	.1	.1	.1	.1	
5.28	2.40			4.8	2.4	1.2	1.0	.5	.3	.2	.1	.1	.1	.1	
5.72	2.60			5.2	2.6	1.3	1.0	.5	.3	.3	.1	.1	.1	.1	.1
6.16	2.80			5.6	2.8	1.4	1.1	.6	.4	.3	.1	.1	.1	.1	.1
6.60	3.00			6.0	3.0	1.5	1.2	.6	.4	.3	.1	.1	.1	.1	.1
7.70	3.50			7.0	3.5	1.8	1.4	.7	.5	.3	.2	.1	.1	.1	.1
8.80	4.00			8.0	4.0	2.0	1.6	.8	.5	.4	.2	.2	.1	.1	.1
9.90	4.50			9.0	4.5	2.2	1.8	.9	.6	.5	.2	.2	.1	.1	.1
11.00	5.00			10.0	5.0	2.5	2.0	1.0	.7	.5	.2	.2	.2	.1	.1
13.20	6.00			12.0	6.0	3.0	2.4	1.2	.8	.6	.3	.2	.2	.1	.1
15.40	7.00			14.0	7.0	3.5	2.8	1.4	.9	.7	.3	.3	.2	.2	.1
17.60	8.00			16.0	8.0	4.0	3.2	1.6	1.1	.8	.4	.3	.3	.2	.2
19.80	9.00			18.0	9.0	4.5	3.6	1.8	1.2	.9	.5	.4	.3	.2	.2
22.00	10.00			20.0	10.0	5.0	4.0	2.0	1.3	1.0	.5	.4	.3	.2	.2
26.40	12.00				12.0	6.0	4.8	2.4	1.6	1.2	.6	.5	.4	.3	.2
30.80	14.00				14.0	7.0	5.6	2.8	1.9	1.4	.7	.6	.5	.3	.3
35.20	16.00				16.0	8.0	6.4	3.2	2.1	1.6	.8	.6	.5	.4	.3
39.60	18.00				18.0	9.0	7.2	3.6	2.4	1.8	.9	.7	.6	.5	.4
44.00	20.00				20.0	10.0	8.0	4.0	2.7	2.0	1.0	.8	.7	.5	.4
46.20	21.00					10.5	8.4	4.2	2.8	2.1	1.1	.8	.7	.5	.4
48.40	22.00					11.0	8.8	4.4	2.9	2.2	1.1	.9	.7	.6	.4
50.60	23.00					11.5	9.2	4.6	3.1	2.3	1.1	.9	.8	.6	.5
52.80	24.00					12.0	9.6	4.8	3.2	2.4	1.2	1.0	.8	.6	.5
55.00	25.00					12.5	10.0	5.0	3.3	2.5	1.2	1.0	.8	.6	.5
66.00	30.00					15.0	12.0	6.0	4.0	3.0	1.5	1.2	1.0	.8	.6
77.00	35.00					17.5	14.0	7.0	4.7	3.5	1.8	1.4	1.2	.9	.7
88.00	40.00					20.0	16.0	8.0	5.3	4.0	2.0	1.6	1.3	1.0	.8
99.00	45.00						18.0	9.0	6.0	4.5	2.2	1.8	1.5	1.1	.9
110.00	50.00						20.0	10.0	6.7	5.0	2.5	2.0	1.7	1.2	1.0
121.00	55.00							11.0	7.3	5.5	2.8	2.2	1.8	1.4	1.1
132.00	60.00							12.0	8.0	6.0	3.0	2.4	2.0	1.5	1.2
143.00	65.00							13.0	8.7	6.5	3.2	2.6	2.2	1.6	1.3
154.00	70.00							14.0	9.3	7.0	3.5	2.8	2.3	1.8	1.4
165.00	75.00							15.0	10.0	7.5	3.8	3.0	2.5	1.9	1.5
176.00	80.00							16.0	10.7	8.0	4.0	3.2	2.7	2.0	1.6
187.00	85.00							17.0	11.3	8.5	4.2	3.4	2.8	2.1	1.7
198.00	90.00							18.0	12.0	9.0	4.5	3.6	3.0	2.2	1.8
209.00	95.00							19.0	12.7	9.5	4.8	3.8	3.2	2.4	1.9
220.00	100.00							20.0	13.3	10.0	5.0	4.0	3.3	2.5	2.0

Dosage Chart: Number of Pills for 10-lb Cat

Dose, mg/kg	Dose, mg/lb	Size, mg .1	.2	.3	.4	.5	1.0	2.0	3.0	4.0	5.0	10.0	25.0	50.0	62.5	100	200	250	500	1000
.02	.0	1.0	.5	.3	.2	.2	.1	.1												
.04	.0	2.0	1.0	.7	.5	.4	.2	.1	.1	.1										
.07	.0	3.0	1.5	1.0	.7	.6	.3	.1	.1	.1	.1									
.09	.0	4.0	2.0	1.3	1.0	.8	.4	.2	.1	.1	.1									
.11	.1	5.0	2.5	1.7	1.2	1.0	.5	.2	.2	.1	.1	.1								
.13	.1		3.0	2.0	1.5	1.2	.6	.3	.2	.1	.1	.1								
.15	.1		3.5	2.3	1.8	1.4	.7	.4	.2	.2	.1	.1								
.18	.1		4.0	2.7	2.0	1.6	.8	.4	.3	.2	.2	.1								
.20	.1		4.5	3.0	2.2	1.8	.9	.4	.3	.2	.2	.1								
.22	.1		5.0	3.3	2.5	2.0	1.0	.5	.3	.2	.2	.1								
.44	.2				5.0	4.0	2.0	1.0	.7	.5	.4	.2	.1							
.66	.3						3.0	1.5	1.0	.8	.6	.3	.1	.1						
.88	.4						4.0	2.0	1.3	1.0	.8	.4	.2	.1	.1					
1.10	.5						5.0	2.5	1.7	1.2	1.0	.5	.2	.1	.1	.1				
1.32	.6							3.0	2.0	1.5	1.2	.6	.2	.1	.1	.1				
1.54	.7							3.5	2.3	1.8	1.4	.7	.3	.1	.1	.1				
1.76	.8							4.0	2.7	2.0	1.6	.8	.3	.2	.1	.1				
1.98	.9							4.5	3.0	2.2	1.8	.9	.4	.2	.1	.1				
2.20	1.0							5.0	3.3	2.5	2.0	1.0	.4	.2	.2	.1	.1			
2.42	1.1								3.7	2.8	2.2	1.1	.4	.2	.2	.1	.1			
2.64	1.2								4.0	3.0	2.4	1.2	.5	.2	.2	.1	.1			
2.86	1.3								4.3	3.2	2.6	1.3	.5	.3	.2	.1	.1	.1		
3.08	1.4								4.7	3.5	2.8	1.4	.6	.3	.2	.1	.1	.1		
3.30	1.5									3.8	3.0	1.5	.6	.3	.3	.2	.1	.1		
3.52	1.6									4.0	3.2	1.6	.6	.3	.3	.2	.1	.1		
3.74	1.7									4.2	3.4	1.7	.7	.3	.3	.2	.1	.1		
3.96	1.8									4.5	3.6	1.8	.7	.4	.3	.2	.1	.1		
4.18	1.9									4.8	3.8	1.9	.8	.4	.3	.2	.1	.1		
4.40	2.0									5.0	4.0	2.0	.8	.4	.3	.2	.1	.1		
4.84	2.2										4.4	2.2	.9	.4	.4	.2	.1	.1		
5.28	2.4										4.8	2.4	1.0	.5	.4	.2	.1	.1		
5.72	2.6											2.6	1.0	.5	.4	.3	.1	.1	.1	
6.16	2.8											2.8	1.1	.6	.4	.3	.1	.1	.1	
6.60	3.0											3.0	1.2	.6	.5	.3	.1	.1	.1	
7.70	3.5											3.5	1.4	.7	.6	.3	.2	.1	.1	
8.80	4.0											4.0	1.6	.8	.6	.4	.2	.2	.1	
9.90	4.5											4.5	1.8	.9	.7	.5	.2	.2	.1	
11.00	5.0											5.0	2.0	1.0	.8	.5	.2	.2	.1	.1
13.20	6.0												2.4	1.2	1.0	.6	.3	.2	.1	.1
15.40	7.0												2.8	1.4	1.1	.7	.3	.3	.1	.1
17.60	8.0												3.2	1.6	1.3	.8	.4	.3	.2	.1
19.80	9.0												3.6	1.8	1.4	.9	.5	.4	.2	.1
22.00	10.0												4.0	2.0	1.6	1.0	.5	.4	.2	.1
26.40	12.0												4.8	2.4	1.9	1.2	.6	.5	.2	.1
30.80	14.0													2.8	2.2	1.4	.7	.6	.3	.1
35.20	16.0													3.2	2.6	1.6	.8	.6	.3	.2
39.60	18.0													3.6	2.9	1.8	.9	.7	.4	.2
44.00	20.0													4.0	3.2	2.0	1.0	.8	.4	.2
46.20	21.0													4.2	3.4	2.1	1.1	.8	.4	.2
48.40	22.0													4.4	3.5	2.2	1.1	.9	.4	.2
50.60	23.0													4.6	3.7	2.3	1.1	.9	.5	.2
52.80	24.0													4.8	3.8	2.4	1.2	1.0	.5	.2
55.00	25.0													5.0	4.0	2.5	1.2	1.0	.5	.2
66.00	30.0														4.8	3.0	1.5	1.2	.6	.3
77.00	35.0															3.5	1.8	1.4	.7	.3
88.00	40.0															4.0	2.0	1.6	.8	.4
99.00	45.0															4.5	2.2	1.8	.9	.5
110.00	50.0															5.0	2.5	2.0	1.0	.5
121.00	55.0																2.8	2.2	1.1	.6
132.00	60.0																3.0	2.4	1.2	.6
143.00	65.0																3.2	2.6	1.3	.7
154.00	70.0																3.5	2.8	1.4	.7
165.00	75.0																3.8	3.0	1.5	.8
176.00	80.0																4.0	3.2	1.6	.8
187.00	85.0																4.2	3.4	1.7	.8
198.00	90.0																4.5	3.6	1.8	.9
209.00	95.0																4.8	3.8	1.9	.9
220.00	100.0																5.0	4.0	2.0	1.0

APPENDIX F DIFFERENTIAL OVERVIEW

Gerard J. Rubin

These lists of differential diagnoses based on clinical signs are separated into diseases that are common, uncommon, and rare. An attempt is also made to separate the diseases systematically. They are intended to be both comprehensive lists of diseases that should be considered and a means for the practitioner to locate diseases quickly.

Abdominal Pain

Common

Food allergy, Food intolerance, Food hypersensitivity
Gastritis, Hemorrhagic gastroenteritis, Enteritis
Gastrointestinal foreign body
Peritonitis
Intraabdominal neoplasia
Abdominal trauma
Pancreatitis, Pancreatic neoplasia
Hepatitis, Hepatic neoplasia
Nephritis, Pyelonephritis
Urolithiasis, Nephrolithiasis
Cystitis
Cystic endometrial hyperplasia, Metritis, Pyometra
Organophosphate/carbamate toxicity
Panleukopenia, Feline distemper, Feline enteritis

Uncommon

Chemical toxicosis
  Arsenic toxicity
  Lead toxicity
  Phosphorus poisoning
  Zinc phosphide poisoning
Hypoadrenocorticism, Addison's disease
Mast cell tumor, Mastocytoma, Mast cell sarcoma, Mastocytosis
Splenitis
Salmonellosis
Gnathostomiasis, Stomach worms
Platynosomiasis, Liver fluke, Lizard poisoning
Pseudotuberculosis, Yersiniosis

Rare

Vacor (Pyriminil) poisoning

Abnormal Behavior

Common

Deficient socialization
Stress
Psychogenic alopecia/dermatitis
Nymphomania
Pseudopregnancy, Pseudocyesis
Intracranial neoplasia
Ischemic encephalopathy
Epilepsy Convulsion, Seizure
Hydrocephalus
Vestibular disease
Otitis media/interna
Hearing loss
Blindness
Glaucoma
Cataracts
Hyperthyroidism
Feline immunodeficiency virus
Toxoplasmosis
Cuterebriasis, Grubs
Systemic diseases
Hepatic cirrhosis, Liver cirrhosis
Hepatic lipidosis, Fatty liver disease

Uncommon

Rabies
Feline polioencephalomyelitis
Encephalitozoonosis
Ceroid lipofuscinosis, Familial amaurotic idiocy
GM_2 gangliosidosis
Portal systemic shunt, Portal vascular anomalies
Hyperinsulinism
Hyperadrenocorticism, Cushing's syndrone
Hypothyroidism
Diabetes mellitus
Pituitary neoplasia
Chemical toxins
  Lead toxicity
  Sodium fluoroacetate poisoning

Abortion, Stillbirth (see Chapter 54)

Common

Feline chlamydiosis, Feline pneumonitis
Feline leukemia virus
Panleukopenia, Feline distemper, Feline enteritis
Feline herpesvirus infection, Feline rhinotracheitis
Feline infectious peritonitis/serositis
Cystic endometrial hyperplasia, Metritis, Pyometra
Trauma

Malnutrition
Severe systemic diseases
Stress
Chemical toxins
Drugs during pregnancy
  Griseofulvin
  Organophosphate/carbamate toxicity

Uncommon
Feline immunodeficiency virus
Campylobacteriosis
Salmonellosis
Mycoplasma
Other bacterial infections
Toxoplasmosis
Lethal genes

Abscessation, Fistulae

Common
Foreign-body puncture wounds
Bite wounds
Flea-allergy dermatitis, Flea-bite hypersensitivity
Surgical stitch abscesses and fistulae
Periodontitis, Periodontal disease
Bacterial conjunctivitis
Mastitis, Mammary gland neoplasia

Uncommon
Nodular panniculitis, Steatitis
Folliculitis, Furunculosis
Orbital cellulitis, Retrobulbar abscess
Dacryocystitis
Actinomycosis
Nocardiosis
Mycoplasma
Pseudotuberculosis, Yersiniosis
Bubonic plague, Sylvatic plague
Mycetoma
Phaeohyphomycosis, Chromomycosis
Dermatophilosis, Cutaneous streptothricosis
Orchitis
Melanoma, Melanosarcoma
Intestinal obstruction, Pseudoobstruction
Anal sacculitis, Anal sac abscess
Perianal fistula

Alopecia (see Chapters 56–60)

Common
Bacterial dermatitis, Pyoderma
Dermatophytosis, Ringworm
Scabies, Notoedric mange, Sarcoptic mange
Fleas, Flea-allergy dermatitis, Flea-bite hypersensitivity
Myiasis, Fly blown
Cuterebriasis, Grubs
Indolent ulcer, Rodent ulcer, Eosinophilic ulcer
Eosinophilic plaque, Lick granuloma
Feline miliary dermatitis
Food allergy, Food intolerance, Food hypersensitivity
Atopy, Allergic inhalant dermatitis, Allergic dermatitis
Allergic contact dermatitis, Contact hypersensitivity
Irritant contact dermatitis
Seborrhea, Keratinization disorders
Feline endocrine alopecia
Telogen defluxion
Psychogenic alopecia/dermatitis, Neurodermatitis
Burns
Hyperthyroidism

Uncommon
Congenital
Hypotrichosis
Alopecia areata
Folliculitis, Furunculosis
Anal sacculitis
Zygomycosis, Pythiosis, Phycomycosis
Pelodera dermatitis, Rhabditic dermatitis
Trombiculidiasis, Chiggers, Harvest mites
Demodectic mange, Follicular mange, Demodicosis
Lynxacariasis, Cat fur mite
Hypothyroidism
Hyperadrenocorticism, Cushing's syndrome
Systemic lupus erythematosus
Pemphigus complex
Toxic epidermal necrolysis, Lyell disease
Nodular panniculitis, Steatitis
Basal cell tumor, Basal cell carcinoma
Fibroma, Fibrosarcoma
Ovarian neoplasia

Rare
Leishmaniasis
Thallium poisoning
Cutaneous asthenia, Ehlers-Danlos syndrome, Dermatospraxis

Anemia (see Chapter 16)

Common
Nutritional deficiency
Chronic infection
Trauma
Burns
Abscesses
Neoplasia
Hemobartonellosis, Feline infectious anemia
Feline immunodeficiency virus
Feline leukemia virus
Lymphosarcoma
Myeloproliferative diseases
Feline infectious peritonitis/serositis
Histoplasmosis
Hookworm disease, Ancylostomiasis
Scabies, Notoedric mange, Sarcoptic mange
Pneumonia
Pyothorax, Empyema
Pleural effusion, Thoracic effusion
Mediastinal neoplasia
Gastrointestinal neoplasia
Colonic neoplasia, Cecal neoplasia, Rectal neoplasia
Peritonitis
Hepatic lipidosis, Fatty liver disease

Hepatitis, Hepatic neoplasia
Urinary tract trauma
Renal glomerular disease
Renal insufficiency, Renal failure, Uremia
Renal neoplasia
Cystic endometrial hyperplasia, Metritis, Pyometra
Hyperthyroidism, Thyrotoxicosis
Diabetes mellitus
Chemical toxins
  Acetaminophen toxicity
  Aspirin toxicity
  Cancer chemotherapy
  Anticoagulant poisoning

Uncommon

Iron deficiency anemia of kittens
Immune-mediated disease
  Systemic lupus erythematosus
Chemical toxins
  Chloramphenicol toxicity
  Phenol toxicity
  Excessive estrogens
  Lead toxicity
  Arsenic toxicity
  Urinary antiseptics with methylene blue
  Phenazopyridine
  Benzocaine
  Phenacetin
  Propylene glycol
  Methionine
  Onions
Stomatitis, Glossitis, Gingivitis
Gastritis
Gastric ulceration
Protein-losing enteropathy
Granulomatous enteritis, Regional enteritis, Crohn's disease
Lymphocytic/plasmacytic enteritis
Eosinophilic gastroenteritis, Hypereosinophilic syndrome
Intestinal obstruction
Portal systemic shunt, Portal vascular anomalies
Hepatic cirrhosis
Cholangiohepatitis, Cholangitis
Cardiovascular neoplasia
Pericardial effusion, Cardiac tamponade
Endocarditis/myocarditis
Hydronephrosis
Nephrotic syndrome
Pyelonephritis
Renal amyloidosis
Renal congenital disease
Renal secondary hyperparathyroidism
Urinary bladder neoplasia
Ovarian neoplasia
Hypoadrenocorticism, Addison's disease
Hypothyroidism
Pituitary neoplasia
Hypersomatotropism, Acromegaly
Hemangioma, Hemangiosarcoma
Mast cell tumor, Mastocytoma, Mast cell sarcoma, Mastocytosis
Plasma cell myeloma
Pseudotuberculosis, Yersiniosis
Tuberculosis
Zygomycosis, Pythiosis, Phycomycosis
Coccidioidomycosis, San Joaquim Valley fever
Blastomycosis, North American blastomycosis
Babesiosis
Coccidiosis
Dirofilariasis, Heartworm disease
Strongyloidiasis
Pediculosis, Lice
Snakebite, Snake venom poisoning
Feline myeloproliferative disease
Feline progressive polyarthritis

Rare

Neonatal isoerythrolysis
Coagulation defects; Factor VIII, IX, or XII deficiency
Gastrinoma, Zollinger-Ellison syndrome

Anisocoria, Pupils Unequal (see Chapter 36)

Common

Head trauma
Feline leukemia virus

Uncommon

Feline infectious peritonitis/serositis
Hypoplasia/aplasia optic nerve
Snakebite, Snake venom poisoning
Brachial plexus nerve root avulsion
Oculomotor nerve damage, Third cranial nerve damage
Pseudorabies, Aujeszky's disease, Mad itch

Arrhythmia, Cardiac Irregularity

Common

Mitral valve dysplasia
Tricuspid valve dysplasia
Ventricular septal defect
Patent ductus arteriosus
Aortic stenosis
Hypertrophic cardiomyopathy
Dilated cardiomyopathy
Endocarditis/myocarditis
Pericardial effusion, Cardiac tamponade
Acute renal failure, Acute nephrosis
Renal insufficiency, Renal failure
Pancreatitis, Pancreatic neoplasia
Mediastinal neoplasia
Epilepsy, Convulsions, Seizures
Head injuries
Brain neoplasia
Burns
Hypoadrenocorticism, Addison's disease
Hyperthyroidism, Thyrotoxicosis
Chemical toxins
  Cardioglycosides
  Antiarrhythmic drugs
  Heavy metal poisons

Uncommon
Hypopituitarism
Toxoplasmosis
Cardiac neoplasia
Endocardial fibroelastosis
Common atrioventricular canal, Endocardial cushion defect
Restrictive cardiomyopathy, Intermediate cardiomyopathy
Pseudorabies, Aujeszky's disease, Mad itch

Rare
Sodium fluoroacetate poisoning
American trypanosomiasis, Chagas' disease

Arthritis

Common
Feline infectious peritonitis/serositis
Feline chlamydiosis, Feline pneumonitis
Degenerative joint disease, Osteoarthritis, Osteoarthrosis
Feline progressive polyarthritis
Infectious arthritis, Infectious inflammatory joint disease

Uncommon
Immune-mediated arthritis
  Systemic lupus erythematosus
  Rheumatoid arthritis
Hypersomatotropism, Acromegaly
Pituitary neoplasia

Ascites, Abdominal Distension, Bloat

Fluid, solid masses, or gas in the peritoneal cavity may appear the same and sometimes cannot be distinguished without centesis, radiographs, ultrasound, palpation, or other diagnostic procedures.

Common
Ventricular septal defect
Hypertrophic cardiomyopathy
Dilated cardiomyopathy
Hepatitis, Hepatic neoplasia
Pancreatitis
Splenic neoplasia
Renal neoplasia
Hydronephrosis
Urinary obstruction, Feline urologic syndrome, Urine retention
Urinary tract trauma
Ureteral obstruction
Leukemia virus infection
Feline infectious peritonitis/serositis
Peritonitis
Intestinal obstruction, Pseudoobstruction
Intestinal neoplasia
Megacolon
Hepatic cirrhosis, Liver cirrhosis
Cystic endometrial hyperplasia, Metritis, Pyometra

Uncommon
Patent ductus arteriosus
Pulmonic stenosis
Atrial septal defect
Tricuspid valve dysplasia
Restrictive cardiomyopathy, Intermediate cardiomyopathy
Pericardial effusion, Cardiac tamponade
Cardiac neoplasia, Cardiovascular neoplasia
Gastric retention
Lymphocytic/plasmacytic enteritis
Granulomatous enteritis, Regional enteritis, Crohn's disease
Protein-losing enteropathy
Atresia ani, Imperforate anus, Rectal aplasia
Portal systemic shunt, Portal vascular anomalies
Pancreatic neoplasia
Nephrotic syndrome
Renal amyloidosis
Renal glomerular disease, Glomerulonephritis
Uterine neoplasia
Ovarian neoplasia
Hemangioma, Hemangiosarcoma
Mast cell tumor, Mastocytoma, Mast cell sarcoma, Mastocytosis
Hyperadrenocorticism, Cushing's syndrome
Pituitary neoplasia
Actinomycosis
Nocardiosis
Tuberculosis
Dirofilariasis, Heartworm disease
Ascariasis, Ascaridiasis, Roundworms
Platynosomiasis, Liver fluke, Lizard poisoning
Opisthorchis infection; Bile, pancreatic duct, intestinal fluke

Rare
American trypanosomiasis, Chagas' disease

Ataxia, Incoordination (see Chapter 17)

Common
Smoke inhalation
Intracranial neoplasia, Brain tumor
Vestibular disease
Epilepsy, Convulsion, Seizure
Otitis media/interna
Spinal cord neoplasia intramedullary
Spinal cord neoplasia extramedullary
Intervertebral disk disease
Chemical toxins
  Nonsteroidal antiinflammatory drug toxicity
  Acetaminophen toxicity
  Aspirin toxicity
  Organophosphate/carbamate toxicity
Feline infectious peritonitis, Infectious serositis
Panleukopenia, Feline distemper, Feline enteritis
Hepatic cirrhosis
Hepatic lipidosis, Fatty liver disease
Aortic, arterial thromboembolism
Hypoglycemia
Hypokalemia
Hypocalcemia

Uncommon
Globoid cell leukodystrophy, Krabbe's disease
Mucopolysaccharidosis; Hurler's, Maroteaux-Lamy syndrome
Glycogenosis, Glycogen storage disease

Mannosidosis
Neuroaxonal dystrophy
Spongiform degeneration
Ceroid lipofuscinosis, Familial amaurotic idiocy
Sphingomyelinosis, Niemann-Pick disease
GM_2 gangliosidosis, Sandhoff's disease
GM_1 gangliosidosis
Feline polioencephalomyelitis
Cerebellar hypoplasia, Cerebellar malformation
Hydrocephalus
Nutritional secondary hyperparathyroidism
Hyperinsulinism
Hypoparathyroidism
Pituitary neoplasia
Hypopituitarism
Chemical toxins
- Chloramphenicol toxicity
- Aminoglycoside toxicity
- Phenol toxicity
- Ethylene glycol toxicity
- Lead toxicity
- Arsenic toxicity
- Zinc phosphide poisoning
- Phosphorus poisoning
- Metaldehyde poisoning

Rabies
Pseudorabies, Aujeszky's disease, Mad itch
Cryptococcosis
Encephalitozoonosis
Babesiosis
Toxoplasmosis
Dirofilariasis, Heartworm disease
Cuterebriasis, Grubs
Portal systemic shunt, Portal vascular anomalies
Puerperal tetany, Eclampsia

Rare
Pyriminil (Vacor) poisoning

Blindness (see Chapters 35, 36)

Common
Intracranial neoplasia, Brain tumor
Ischemic encephalopathy
Epilepsy, Convulsion, Seizure
Cataract, Lens opacity, Lens capsule opacity
Hypoplasia/aplasia optic nerve
Optic neuritis
Retinal detachment
Retinal hemorrhage
Retinal degeneration, Retinal atrophy
Chorioretinitis
Uveitis
Panophthalmitis
Glaucoma
Hypertension
Feline herpesvirus infection, Feline rhinotracheitis
Feline leukemia virus
Feline infectious peritonitis/serositis
Lymphosarcoma
Ocular trauma

Uncommon
Congenital
Congenital nystagmus
Microphthalmia
Retrobulbar abscess
Retrobulbar mass
Inherited progressive retinal atrophy
Portal systemic shunt, Portal vascular anomalies
Ceroid lipofuscinosis, Familial amaurotic idiocy
Sphingomyelinosis, Niemann-Pick disease
GM_1 gangliosidosis
GM_2 gangliosidosis, Sandhoff's disease
Hydrocephalus
Granulomatous meningoencephalomyelitis
Reticulosis
Pituitary neoplasia
Hyperinsulinism
Panleukopenia, Feline distemper, Feline enteritis
Toxoplasmosis
Cryptococcosis
Coccidioidomycosis, San Joaquim Valley fever
Blastomycosis, North American blastomycosis
Dirofilariasis, Heartworm disease
Lead toxicity
Taurine deficiency

Rare
Vacor (Pyriminil) poisoning

Blisters, Vesicles

Common
Chemical, actinic, thermal burns
Irritant contact dermatitis

Uncommon
Pemphigus complex
Toxic epidermal necrolysis, Lyell disease
Erythema multiforme

Bradycardia, Heart Rate <100 bpm

Common
Dilated cardiomyopathy, Congestive cardiomyopathy
Heart block
Shock
Renal insufficiency, Renal failure, Uremia, Azotemia
Chemical toxins
- Digitalis toxicity
- Organophosphate/carbamate toxicity
- Narcotics
- Acetylpromazine

Uncommon
Glycogenosis, Glycogen storage disease
Restrictive cardiomyopathy, Intermediate cardiomyopathy
Sick sinus syndrome
Hypothyroidism
Primary hyperparathyroidism
Pseudohyperparathyroidism, Hypercalcemia of malignancy
Hypoadrenocorticism, Addison's disease

Hypoglycemia
Hyperkalemia

Rare
Key-Gaskell syndrome, Dysautonomia, Autonomic polyganglionopathy

Breath Odor Abnormal, Halitosis (see Chapter 52)

Common
Renal insufficiency, Renal failure, Uremia, Azotemia
Stomatitis, Glossitis, Gingivitis
Periodontitis, Periodontal disease
Buccal, Pharyngeal, Esophageal foreign body

Uncommon
Renal secondary hyperparathyroidism
Diabetic ketoacidosis
Esophageal ulceration
Bronchiectasis
Metaldehyde poisoning

Capillary Refill Time Prolonged >2 Sec

Common
Dilated cardiomyopathy, Congestive cardiomyopathy
Heart failure
Shock
Hypovolemia

Uncommon
Hypoadrenocorticism, Addison's disease
Nonketotic hyperosmolar diabetes

Capillary Refill Time Decreased <1 Sec

Hypertropic cardiomyopathy
Vasodilation
Vasodilating drugs
- Angiotensin converting enzyme inhibitors
  - Captopril
  - Enalopril
- Isosorbide dinitrate
- Nitroglycerin
- Hydralazine

Hyperthyroidism, Thyrotoxicosis
Cardiac stimulants
B_2 adrenergic drugs

Cerebellar Signs

Cerebellar signs are related to disease of the cerebellum or the cerebellar tracts. They include hypermetria (over-action), spasticity, broad-based stance, swaying of the body, intention tremors, oscillatory nystagmus, absent menace response, and ataxia.

Common
Panleukopenia virus
Aortic, arterial thromboembolism
Cranial trauma
Chemical toxins

Uncommon
Cerebellar malformation, Cerebellar hypoplasia
Caudal intracranial neoplasia
Mannosidosis
Neuroaxonal dystrophy
Spongiform degeneration
Ceroid lipofuscinosis, Familial amaurotic idiocy

Chemosis, Scleral Edema (see Chapter 35)

Common
Keratoconjunctivitis sicca
Viral conjunctivitis
Feline chlamydiosis, Feline pneumonitis
Bacterial conjunctivitis
Allergic conjunctivitis
Uveitis

Uncommon
Exophthalmia
Orbital cellulitis, Retrobulbar abscess
Orbital neoplasia, Orbital tumor
Parasitic conjunctivitis

Circling

Circling is usually toward the affected side, but not always.

Common
Vestibular disease
Meningitis
Ischemic encephalopathy
Hepatic encephalopathy
Epilepsy, Convulsion, Seizure
Cryptococcosis
Head trauma
Otitis media/interna
Feline infectious peritonitis/serositis

Uncommon
Intracranial neoplasia
Meningioma
Pituitary neoplasia
Hydrocephalus
Hypersomatotropism, Acromegaly
Dirofilariasis, Heartworm disease
Encephalitozoonosis
Toxoplasmosis
Hypoglycemia

Coagulation Defects, Abnormal Bleeding

Common
Feline leukemia virus
Chemical toxins
- Anticoagulant poisoning
- Aspirin toxicity

Nonsteroidal antiinflammatory drug toxicity
Excessive estrogen
Liver disease
Uremia
Inflammatory disorders
Immune disorders
Autoimmune thrombocytopenia

Uncommon
Snakebite, Snake venom poisoning
Systemic lupus erythematosus
Immune-mediated thrombocytopenia
Myeloproliferative diseases
Disseminated intravascular coagulation
Chemical toxins
High doses of penicillin
Trimethoprim/sulfadiazine
High-molecular-weight dextrans
Modified live virus vaccines

Rare
Factor VIII, IX, or XII deficiency

Coma, Unconscious

Common
Smoke inhalation
Head trauma
Epilepsy, Convulsion, Seizure
Cerebrovascular disease
Toxoplasmosis
Cryptococcosis
Feline infectious peritonitis/serositis
Hypoxia
Chemical toxins
Anesthetic/sedative overdose
Ethylene glycol poisoning
Uremia
Liver disease
Heart failure
Shock

Uncommon
Intracranial neoplasia
Intracranial hemorrhage
Snakebite, Snake venom poisoning
Encephalomyelitis
Granulomatous meningoencephalitis
Hypoglycemia
Hyperinsulinism
Hypoadrenocorticism, Addison's disease
Electric cord shock
Cerebral parasites
Diabetic ketoacidosis
Cerebral mycotic infections
Cerebral parasitic migration

Constipation/Obstipation

Constipation must be distinguished from dyschezia (painful defecation). Constipation is the presence of hard feces in the rectum and may cause dyschezia. Pain when attempting to defecate may result in constipation.

Common
Electrolyte disturbance
Hypokalemia
Rectal foreign body
Neuromuscular disease
Manx cat syndrome
Constipating drugs
Diuretics
Barium sulfate
Idiopathic megacolon

Uncommon
Colonic neoplasia, Cecal neoplasia, Rectal neoplasia
Rectal deviation, Diverticulum, Sacculation
Proctitis
Rectal prolapse
Rectal stricture
Anal neoplasia
Anal sac impaction, Anal sac disease
Perianal fistula
Perineal hernia
Chemical toxins
Lead toxicity
Hypothyroidism
Hyperparathyroidism
Pseudohyperparathyroidism, Hypercalcemia of malignancy
Renal secondary hyperparathyroidism
Nutritional secondary hyperparathyroidism
Vaginal/vulval neoplasia

Rare
Key-Gaskell syndrome, Dysautonomia, Autonomic polyganglionopathy

Convulsion, Fit, Seizure

Seizure must be distinguished from syncope. Seizure is excessive neuronal activity that may be evidenced by excessive motor or autonomic activity. Syncope is depressed neuronal activity, especially of the cerebrum expressed as a depression of motor activity and/or consciousness.

Common
Feline leukemia virus infection
Feline infectious peritonitis, Infectious serositis
Mycotic infections
Cryptococcosis
Chemical toxins
Ethylene glycol toxicity
Organophosphate toxicity
Carbamate toxicity
Hypokalemia
Cranial trauma
Intracranial neoplasia, Brain tumor
Idiopathic epilepsy
Hydrocephalus
Heat stroke
Myocarditis
Vegetative valvular endocarditis
Arterial thromboembolism
Ischemic encephalopathy, Cerebral vascular accident, Stroke
Hepatic cirrhosis, Liver cirrhosis

Renal insufficiency, Renal failure, Uremia, Azotemia
Kidney anomalies, Renal congenital disease
Hormonal
  Hyperinsulinism
  Hypoparathyroidism
  Pituitary neoplasia, Tumor
  Hypersomatotropism, Acromegaly

Uncommon
Rabies
Aujeszky's disease
Feline immunodeficiency virus infection
Nocardiosis
Intracranial abscess
Aspergillosis
Encephalitozoonosis
Toxoplasmosis
Portal systemic shunt, Portal vascular anomalies
Snakebite, Snake venom poisoning
Dirofilariasis, Heartworm disease
Chemical toxins
  Chlorinated hydrocarbon toxicity
  Zinc phosphide poisoning
  Phosphorus poisoning
  Metaldehyde poisoning
  Strychnine poisoning
  Lead toxicity
Feline polioencephalomyelitis
Thiamine deficiency
Mucopolysaccharidosis, Hurler's, Maroteaux-Lamy syndrome
Glycogenosis, Glycogen storage disease
Hypoglycemia
Hyperosmolality
Hypoxia
Cerebral hemorrhage, Cerebral vascular accident, Stroke
Ceroid lipofuscinosis, Familial amaurotic idiocy
GM_2 gangliosidosis, Sandhoff's disease
GM_1 gangliosidosis
Puerperal tetany, Eclampsia
Smoke inhalation

Rare
Thallium poisoning
Sodium fluoroacetate poisoning

Corneal Ulcer (see Chapter 35)

Common
Dacryocystitis
Uveitis
Viral conjunctivitis
Feline herpesvirus infection, Feline rhinotracheitis
Bacterial infection
Foreign body
Keratoconjunctivitis sicca
Trauma
Chemical irritant
  Soaps
  Caustics
Dust

Uncommon
Blink response absent
Trigeminal nerve paralysis
Facial nerve paralysis
Eyelid defect
Entropion
Ectropion
Ectopic cilia
Distichiasis
Trichiasis
Palpebral neoplasia

Coughing

Common
Tracheitis
Bronchitis
Allergic bronchitis, Bronchial asthma, Feline asthma
Bronchiectasis, Chronic dilation of bronchi
Pneumonia
Inhalant irritants
Respiratory foreign body
Aspiration pneumonia
Feline asthma, Allergic pneumonitis
Eosinophilic pneumonitis
Feline herpesvirus infection, Feline rhinotracheitis
Histoplasmosis
Toxoplasmosis
Pulmonary neoplasia
Pulmonary edema
Pulmonary infarction
Smoke inhalation
Mediastinal neoplasia
Pyothorax, Empyema
Pleural effusion, Thoracic effusion
Heart failure
Endocarditis/myocarditis, Vegetative valvular endocarditis
Esophagitis
Esophageal obstruction, stricture; Periesophageal obstruction
Megaesophagus, Esophageal hypomotility
Obesity

Uncommon
Sinusitis
Pharyngitis
Nasal pharyngeal polyps
Laryngeal neoplasia
Tracheal collapse
Tracheal hypoplasia
Tracheal neoplasia
Pneumothorax
Diaphragmatic hernia
Hiatal hernia, Gastroesophageal intussusception
Pectus excavatum, Funnel chest
Actinomycosis
Nocardiosis
Bubonic plague, Sylvatic plague
Tuberculosis
Aspergillosis
Cryptococcosis
Coccidioidomycosis, San Joaquim Valley fever

Blastomycosis, North American blastomycosis
Dirofilariasis, Heartworm disease
Aelurostrongylosis
Capillariasis
Paragonimiasis
Esophageal neoplasia
Cardiac neoplasia
Pericardial effusion, Cardiac tamponade
Vascular ring anomalies, Persistent right aortic arch
Mitral valve dysplasia
Ventricular septal defect
Aortic stenosis
Patent ductus arteriosus
Abdominal masses

Rare
ANTU poisoning
Thallium poisoning

Crying, Vocalization

Common
Epilepsy, Convulsion, Seizure
Mastitis
Agalactia, Lactation deficiency
Nymphomania
Siamese cats
Estrus
Blindness
Hearing loss
Cerebral arterial embolism

Uncommon
Encephalitozoonosis
Trichinellosis, Trichinosis
Glycogenosis, Glycogen storage disease, Hypoglycemia
Pseudorabies, Aujeszky's disease, Mad itch
Pseudotuberculosis, Yersiniosis
Intracranial neoplasia, Brain tumor

Rare
Sodium fluoroacetate poisoning

Cyanosis, Mucous Membranes Bluish Coloration

Common
Bronchitis
Bronchiectasis
Allergic bronchitis, Bronchial asthma, Feline asthma
Pulmonary neoplasia
Airway obstruction
Endotracheal tube obstruction
Pneumonia
Pulmonary edema
Pulmonary atelectasis
Pulmonary emphysema
Pulmonary infarction
Hypoxia
Mediastinal neoplasia
Pneumothorax
Diaphragmatic hernia
Pyothorax, Empyema
Pleural effusion, Thoracic effusion
Chemical toxins
  Acetaminophen toxicity
  Organophosphate/carbamate toxicity

Uncommon
Laryngeal neoplasia, Tracheal neoplasia
Laryngeal paralysis
Pectus excavatum, Funnel chest
Paragonimiasis
Hiatal hernia, Gastroesophageal intussusception
Tricuspid valve dysplasia
Endocardial fibroelastosis
Tetralogy of Fallot
Common atrioventricular canal
Pulmonic stenosis
Chemical toxins
  Chlorinated hydrocarbon toxicity
  Strychnine poisoning
  Metaldehyde poisoning

Rare
ANTU poisoning
Sodium fluoroacetate poisoning

Deafness

Common
Congenital (may occur with blue iris color)
Otitis media/interna
Trauma
Senility

Uncommon
Hydrocephalus
Chemical toxins
  Lead toxicity
  Aminoglycoside medication
Neoplasia

Rare
Ceroid lipofuscinosis, Familial amaurotic idiocy

Dermatitis (see Chapters 56–60)

Common
Bacterial dermatitis, Pyoderma
Ear mites, Otodectic mange
Psychogenic alopecia/dermatitis, Neurodermatitis
Seborrhea, Keratinization disorders
Irritant contact dermatitis
Allergic contact dermatitis, Contact hypersensitivity
Atopy, Allergic inhalant dermatitis, Allergic dermatitis
Acne, Atypical pyoderma
Folliculitis, Furunculosis
Fistula
Feline miliary dermatitis
Eosinophilic plaque, Lick granuloma
Indolent ulcer, Rodent ulcer, Eosinophilic ulcer

Pediculosis, Lice
Fleas, Flea-allergy dermatitis, Flea-bite hypersensitivity
Demodectic mange, Follicular mange, Demodicosis
Cheyletiellosis, Walking dandruff
Scabies, Notoedric mange, Sarcoptic mange
Dermatophytosis, Ringworm
Feline immunodeficiency
Eosinophilic gastroenteritis, Hypereosinophilic syndrome

Uncommon

Systemic lupus erythematosus
Plasma cell pododermatitis
Calcinosis circumscripta
Nodular panniculitis, Steatitis
Toxic epidermal necrolysis, Lyell disease
Linear granuloma
Mycetoma
Phaeohyphomycosis, Chromomycosis
Zygomycosis, Pythiosis, Phycomycosis
Candidiasis
Dermatophilosis, Cutaneous streptothricosis
Lynxacariasis, Cat fur mite
Trombiculidiasis, Chiggers, Harvest mites
Hookworm dermatitis, Ancylostomiasis, Uncinariasis
Pelodera dermatitis, Rhabditic dermatitis
Myiasis, Fly blown

Rare

Ectopic ureter
Leishmaniasis

Diarrhea (see Chapter 24)

Diarrhea must be distinguished from fluid leakage during constipation and fecal incontinence due to the inability to retain feces in the rectum.

Common

Food allergy, Food intolerance, Food hypersensitivity
Overfeeding
Abrupt dietary change
Ingestion of irritating material
Stress
Gastritis
Eosinophilic gastroenteritis
Intestinal obstruction
Pseudoobstruction
Inflammatory bowel disease
Malabsorption
Protein-losing enteropathy
Lymphocytic/plasmacytic enteritis
Colitis
Intestinal neoplasia
  Lymphosarcoma
  Adenocarcinoma
  Mast cell tumor, Mastocytoma, Mast cell sarcoma, Mastocytosis
Hypereosinophilic syndrome
Colonic neoplasia
Peritonitis
Exocrine pancreatic insufficiency
Pancreatitis
Hepatic lipidosis, Fatty liver syndrome
Liver neoplasia
Liver cirrhosis
Cholangiohepatitis
Cholangitis
Viral diarrhea
  Feline immunodeficiency virus
  Feline leukemia virus
  Panleukopenia, Feline distemper, Feline enteritis
  Feline calicivirus infection
Campylobacteriosis
Salmonellosis
Histoplasmosis
Coccidiosis
Tapeworm infestation
Hookworm disease, Ancylostomiasis
Ascariasis, Ascaridiasis, Roundworms
Chemical toxins
  Antibiotics
  Chloramphenicol toxicity
  Parasiticides
  Nonsteroidal anti-inflammatory drug toxicity
  Acetaminophen toxicity
  Salicylate
  Organophosphate/carbamate toxicity
Diabetes mellitus
Hypoadrenocorticism, Addison's disease
Hyperthyroidism, Thyrotoxicosis
Mediastinal neoplasia, tumor
Hydronephrosis
Pyelonephritis
Renal insufficiency, Renal failure, Uremia, Azotemia
Kidney anomalies, Renal congenital disease
Cystic calculi
Urethral obstruction
Cystic endometrial hyperplasia, Metritis, Pyometra
Epilepsy, Convulsions, Seizures, Fits
Idiopathic epilepsy

Uncommon

Pancreatic neoplasia
Portal systemic shunt, portal vascular anomalities
Bile duct rupture
Gallbladder rupture
Cholelithiasis
Choledocolithiasis
Granulomatous enteritis, Regional enteritis, Crohn's disease
Short bowel syndrome
Cecal neoplasia
Rectal prolapse
Rectal neoplasia
Anal neoplasia, Tumor
Perianal fistula
Rotavirus
Astrovirus
Escherichia coli
Clostridium difficile
Clostridium perfringens
Tyzzer's disease
Tuberculosis, Mycobacteria

Pseudotuberculosis, Yersiniosis
Actinomycosis
Nocardiosis
Zygomycosis, Pythiosis, Phycomycosis
Aspergillosis
Sporotrichosis
Candidiasis
Toxoplasmosis
American trypanosomiasis, Chagas' disease
Amebiasis
Pentatrichomoniasis, Trichomoniasis
Platynosomiasis, Liver fluke, Lizard poisoning
Opisthorchis infection; Bile, pancreatic duct, intestinal fluke
Ollulanus, Stomach worms
Whipworms, Trichuriasis
Strongyloidiasis
Chemical toxins
  Digitalis
  Lactulose
  Anticancer drugs
  o,p'-DDD-(Lysodren, mitotane)
  Lead toxicity
  Arsenic toxicity
  Metaldehyde poisoning
  Herbicides
  Fungicides
Certain house plants
Nonketotic hyperosmolar diabetes
Diabetic ketoacidosis
Hypothyroidism
Nodular panniculitis
Vitamin E deficiency, Steatitis
Pancreatitis
Ureteral obstruction
Vesicoureteral reflux
Nephrotic syndrome
Renal calculi
Uterine neoplasia

Rare
Thallium poisoning
Mucopolysaccharidosis; Hurler's, Maroteaux-Lamy syndrome
Mannosidosis
Gastrinoma, Zollinger-Ellison syndrome

Dyschezia, Painful Defecation

Dyschezia must be distinguished from constipation. Constipation may or may not be present. The hallmark of dyschezia is the frequent attempts at painful defecation.

Common
Constipation
Obstipation
Bite wound
Vicious trauma
Spinal trauma
Pelvic trauma
Foreign body
Colonic neoplasia, Cecal neoplasia, Rectal neoplasia
Colonic obstruction
Colonic atony
Megacolon
Proctitis
Rectal stricture
Rectal-colonic prolapse
Neuromuscular disease

Uncommon
Intussusception
Anal sac impaction, Anal sac disease
Anal sacculitis, Anal sac abscess
Anal neoplasia
Perianal fistula
Perineal hernia
Amebiasis
Myiasis
Pregnancy
Cachexia
Hyperkalemia
Hypercalcemia
Hyperparathyroidism
Hypothyroidism
Hyperthyroidism
Chemical-induced
Anticholinergics
Anticonvulsants
Barium sulfate
Diuretics
Heavy metal toxicity
Cessation of laxatives

Dysphagia

Dysphagia is a difficulty of swallowing and should not be confused with anorexia, the lack of desire to eat, or emesis/regurgitation, the return of food after it has been swallowed. These conditions may overlap. With dysphagia the cat usually appears hungry.

Common
Periodontitis, Periodontal disease
Stomatitis, Glossitis, Gingivitis
Megaesophagus, Esophageal hypomotility
Esophageal obstruction, Periesophageal obstruction
Esophagitis
Nasalpharyngeal polyp
Mediastinal neoplasia

Uncommon
Salivary mucocele, Sialocele, Ranula
Salivary gland neoplasia
Esophageal diverticulum
Esophageal neoplasia
Hiatal hernia, Gastroesophageal intussusception
Rabies
Coccidioidomycosis, San Joaquim Valley fever
Snakebite, Snake venom poisoning

Rare
Key-Gaskell syndrome, Dysautonomia, Autonomic polyganglionopathy

Dyspnea (see Chapter 18)

Common

Rhinitis
Nasal-pharyngeal polyp
Nasal-passage neoplasia
Sinusitis
Laryngospasm, Laryngeal spasm
Bronchitis
Allergic bronchitis, Bronchial asthma, Feline asthma
Bronchiectasis
Emphysema
Pulmonary atelectasis
Pulmonary neoplasia
Pneumonia
  Viral
  Bacterial
  Mycotic
Parasitic tracheobronchitis/pneumonia
  Aelurostrongylosis
  Paragonimiasis
Inhalation pneumonia
Pulmonary edema
Mediastinal neoplasia
Pneumothorax
Diaphragmatic hernia, Peritoneal pericardial diaphragmatic hernia
Pleural effusion, Thoracic effusion
Pyothorax, Empyema
Burns, Smoke inhalation
Irritant contact dermatitis
Hyperthyroidism, Thyrotoxicosis
Chemical toxins
  Organophosphate/carbamate toxicity
  Anticoagulant poisoning
Feline chlamydiosis, Feline pneumonitis
Feline leukemia virus
Feline infectious peritonitis/serositis
Feline calicivirus infection
Feline herpesvirus infection
Histoplasmosis
Toxoplasmosis
Pericardial effusion, Cardiac tamponade
Endocarditis/myocarditis, Vegetative valvular endocarditis
Hypertrophic cardiomyopathy
Dilated cardiomyopathy
Electric shock
Esophagitis
Esophageal obstruction
Megaesophagus, Esophageal hypomotility

Uncommon

Nephrotic syndrome
Laryngeal neoplasia, Tracheal neoplasia
Laryngeal paralysis
Pectus excavatum, Funnel chest
Myasthenia gravis
Multiple cartilaginous exostoses, Osteochondromatosis
Myositis ossificans, Fibrodysplasia ossificans
Pituitary neoplasia
Hypersomatotropism, Acromegaly
Chemical toxins
  Chlorinated hydrocarbon toxicity
  Zinc phosphide poisoning
Actinomycosis
Nocardiosis
Pseudotuberculosis, Yersiniosis
Bubonic plague, Sylvatic plague
Tuberculosis
Pox virus infection
Pseudorabies, Aujeszky's disease, Mad itch
Cryptococcosis
Coccidioidomycosis, San Joaquim Valley fever
Blastomycosis, North American blastomycosis
Dirofilariasis, Heartworm disease
Snakebite, Snake venom poisoning
Cleft palate
Salivary mucocele, Sialocele, Ranula
Esophageal neoplasia
Hiatal hernia, Gastroesophageal intussusception
Protein-losing enteropathy
Vascular ring anomalies, Persistent right aortic arch
Cardiovascular neoplasia
Restrictive cardiomyopathy, Intermediate cardiomyopathy
Tricuspid valve dysplasia
Mitral valve dysplasia
Tetralogy of Fallot
Endocardial fibroelastosis
Common atrioventricular canal, Endocardial cushion defect
Ventricular septal defect
Atrial septal defect
Pulmonic stenosis
Aortic stenosis
Patent ductus arteriosus

Rare

ANTU poisoning
Thallium poisoning
Sodium fluoroacetate poisoning

Dystocia (see Chapter 54)

Common

Emaciation
Obesity
Trauma
Cystic endometrial hyperplasia, metritis, Pyometra
Ectopic pregnancy
Death of feti
Fetus abnormal size
Abnormal fetal presentation
Loss of amniotic fluid
Uterine contractions insufficient, Oxytocin deficiency
Malformation of pelvic canal

Uncommon

Rectal prolapse
Uterine prolapse
Uterine torsion
Hypocalcemia
Hypoglycemia
Neoplasia

Dysuria, Painful Urination (see Chapter 40)

Dysuria and strangiuria, difficult urination, may frequently be mistaken for dyschezia and vice versa. It is necessary to determine which function is painful or difficult. Usually a full bladder is present during dysuria, but not necessarily.

Common

Urinary obstruction, Feline urologic syndrome, Urine retention
Urethritis, Urethral inflammation
Urethral stricture due to previous catheterization
Urinary bladder neoplasia
Urolithiasis
Cystitis
Ureteral obstruction

Uncommon

Ectopic ureter
Nephrolithiasis
Hydronephrosis
Perineal hernia

Edema

Edema (fluid in the tissue) should be distinguished from cellulitis (subcutaneous inflammation) and subcutaneous emphysema (air in the tissues). Cellulitis is frequently accompanied by pain and emphysema by crepitation.

Common

Right heart failure
Pulmonic stenosis
Dilated cardiomyopathy
Lymphocytic/plasmacytic enteritis
Granulomatous enteritis, Regional enteritis, Crohn's disease
Protein-losing enteropathy
Hepatic cirrhosis
Hypoproteinemia
Burns
Mammary gland neoplasia
Mediastinal neoplasia
Lymphosarcoma
Renal insufficiency
Renal glomerular disease, Glomerulonephritis

Uncommon

Tricuspid valve dysplasia
Tetralogy of Fallot
Nephrotic syndrome
Hookworm dermatitis, Ancylostomiasis, Uncinariasis
Chemical toxins
  Acetaminophen toxicity
Hypersomatotropism, Acromegaly
Pituitary neoplasia
Hypothyroidism
Food allergy, Food intolerance, Food hypersensitivity
Erythema multiforme
Hypertrophic osteopathy, Hypertrophic pulmonary osteoarthropathy
Galactostasis
Renal amyloidosis
Poxvirus infection

Emesis, Vomiting (see Chapter 24)

Emesis should be distinguished from regurgitation whenever possible. It is the forceful ejection of food and/or fluid from the stomach and proximal duodenum after stimulation of the vomiting center in the medulla oblongata. The afferent impulses that stimulate the vomiting center come from the pharynx, stomach, duodenum, heart, uterus, kidney, urinary bladder, liver, brain, chemoreceptor trigger zone on the floor of the fourth ventricle, and semicircular canals of the ear. The efferent impulses of vomition are carried by the vagus nerve. The animal senses the start of vomition, hypersalivation begins, followed by repeated swallowing movements, and then retching movements. These movements consist of forceful contraction of the abdominal muscles and the diaphragm against a closed glottis, the gastroesophageal sphincter relaxes and food and fluid pass retrograde through the esophagus and pharynx and out the mouth and nose.

Common

Acute renal failure
Renal glomerular disease, Glomerulonephritis
Renal insufficiency, Renal failure, Uremia, Azotemia
Pyelonephritis
Ureteral obstruction
Urinary obstruction, Feline urologic syndrome, Urine retention
Urinary tract trauma
Urolithiasis
Cystitis
Cystic endometrial hyperplasia, Metritis, Pyometra
Bronchitis
Bronchiectasis, Chronic dilation of bronchi
Pneumonia
Mediastinal neoplasia
Vestibular disease
Epilepsy, Convulsion, Seizure
Otitis media/interna, Otitis interna
Periodontitis, Periodontal disease
Stomatitis, Glossitis, Gingivitis
Eosinophilic gastroenteritis, Hypereosinophilic syndrome
Gastric retention
Gastric ulceration
Gastritis
Intestinal obstruction, Pseudoobstruction
Lymphocytic/plasmacytic enteritis
Megacolon
Gastrointestinal neoplasia
Viral diarrhea
Peritonitis
Pancreatitis
Hepatitis, Hepatic neoplasia
Cholangitis, Cholangiohepatitis
Hepatic cirrhosis
Hepatic lipidosis, Fatty liver disease
Mast cell tumor, Mastocytoma, Mast cell sarcoma, Mastocytosis
Food allergy, Food intolerance, Food hypersensitivity

Hyperthyroidism, Thyrotoxicosis
Hypertrophic cardiomyopathy
Chemical toxins
  Insecticide toxicity
  Organophosphate/carbamate toxicity
  Chlorinated hydrocarbon toxicity
  Medications
  Cardioglycosides
  Antibiotics
  Nonsteroidal antiinflammatory drug toxicity
  Acetaminophen toxicity
  Aspirin toxicity
  Apomorphine
  Morphine
  Xylazine
  Ammonium chloride
  Mebendazole
  Cancer chemotherapy drugs
Ascariasis, Ascaridiasis, Roundworms
Panleukopenia, Feline distemper, Feline enteritis
Feline calicivirus infection

Uncommon

Pancreatic neoplasia
Bile duct rupture, Gallbladder rupture
Cholelithiasis, Choledocolithiasis
Portal systemic shunt, Portal vascular anomalies
Perineal hernia
Anal sacculitis, Anal sac abscess
Anal sac impaction, Anal sac disease
Rectal stricture
Rectal deviation, Diverticulum, Sacculation
Granulomatous enteritis, Regional enteritis, Crohn's disease
Aortic, Arterial thromboembolism, Saddle clot thrombus
Restrictive cardiomyopathy, Intermediate cardiomyopathy
Dilated cardiomyopathy, Congestive cardiomyopathy
Vesicoureteral reflux
Nephrolithiasis
Hydronephrosis
Nephrotic syndrome
Renal amyloidosis, Amyloidosis
Renal congenital disease
Renal secondary hyperparathyroidism
Ovarian neoplasia
Uterine neoplasia
Smoke inhalation
Diaphragmatic hernia
Peritoneal/pericardial diaphragmatic hernia
Pectus excavatum, Funnel chest
Systemic lupus erythematosus
Nodular panniculitis, Steatitis
Nonketotic hyperosmolar diabetes
Diabetic ketoacidosis
Hypoadrenocorticism, Addison's disease
Pseudohyperparathyroidism, Hypercalcemia of malignancy
Hyperparathyroidism
Hypoparathyroidism
Chemical toxicity
  Chloramphenicol toxicity
  Ethylene glycol toxicity
  Lead toxicity
  Arsenic toxicity
  Rodenticide
  Vitamin D_3 rodenticide toxicity
  Cholecalciferol toxicity
  Zinc phosphide poisoning
  Phosphorus poisoning
  Metaldehyde poisoning
Campylobacteriosis
Salmonellosis
Pseudotuberculosis, Yersiniosis
Pseudorabies, Aujeszky's disease, Mad itch
Toxoplasmosis
Babesiosis
Zygomycosis, Pythiosis, Phycomycosis
Candidiasis
Eurytrema infection, Pancreatic fluke infection
Platynosomiasis, Liver fluke, Lizard poisoning
Opisthorchis infection; Bile, pancreatic duct, intestinal fluke
Stomach worms
  Ollulanus
  Physaloptera
  Gnathostomiasis
Dirofilariasis, Heartworm disease
Strongyloidiasis

Rare

ANTU poisoning
Thallium poisoning
Sodium fluoroacetate poisoning
Vacor (Pyriminil) poisoning
Gastrinoma, Zollinger-Ellison syndrome

Epiphora, Hyperlacrimation (see Chapter 35)

Common

Dust
Irritating vapors
Uveitis
Ulcerative keratitis, Corneal sequestrum
Allergic conjunctivitis
Viral conjunctivitis
  Feline herpesvirus infection, Feline rhinotracheitis
  Feline calicivirus infection
  Reovirus
Bacterial conjunctivitis
Glaucoma
Ocular neoplasia
Feline leukemia virus
Dacryocystitis
Obstructed nasolacrimal duct
Blepharitis
Conjunctival dermoid, Sebaceous cyst, Epidermoid cyst
Symblepharon
Ectropion
Entropion
Trichiasis
Distichiasis

Uncommon

Organophosphate/carbamate toxicity
Blastomycosis, North American blastomycosis

Parasitic conjunctivitis
Thelazia
Eyelid agenesis, Eyelid coloboma
Imperforate puncta

Episodic, Intermittent Weakness

Common

Anemia
Hypoglycemia
Hypokalemia
Heart failure
Hypertrophic cardiomyopathy
Dilated cardiomyopathy, Congestive cardiomyopathy
Aortic, arterial thromboembolism, Saddle clot thrombus
Endocarditis/myocarditis, Vegetative valvular endocarditis
Cardiac arrhythmia
Pericardial effusion
Hypoxia
Respiratory disease
Respiratory tract obstruction
Pleural effusion, Thoracic effusion
Osteomyelitis
Arthritis/polyarthritis
Myositis/polymyositis
Neuritis/polyneuritis
Neural tumors
Feline infectious peritonitis/serositis
Feline leukemia virus
Chemical toxins
Sedative/tranquilizers

Uncommon

Myasthenia gravis
Glycogenosis, Glycogen storage disease
Episodic weakness of young Burmese cats
Hyperkalemia
Hyponatremia
Hypernatremia
Hypocalcemia
Hypercalcemia
Hypophosphatemia
Hypomagnesemia
Hyperosmolality
Hypothyroidism
Hypoadrenocorticism, Addison's disease
Hyperadrenocorticism, Cushing's disease
Hyperinsulinism
Pancreatic tumor
Nephrotic syndrome
Hypertrophic osteodystrophy
Bone neoplasia
Systemic lupus erythematosus
Rheumatoid arthritis
Feline immunodeficiency virus
Cryptococcosis
Blastomycosis, North American blastomycosis
Coccidioidomycosis, San Joaquim Valley fever
Phaeohyphomycosis, Chromomycosis
Histoplasmosis
Toxoplasmosis
Granulomatous meningoencephalitis, Reticulosis

Epistaxis, Nosebleed

Common

Anticoagulant poisoning
Hemangioma, Hemangiosarcoma
Rhinitis, Rhinosinusitis
Nasal passage neoplasia
Nasal passage foreign body
Trauma

Uncommon

Aspergillosis
Babesiosis
Dirofilariasis, Heartworm disease
Immune-mediated coagulation defects
Disseminated intravascular coagulation

Rare

Coagulation defects; Factor VIII, IX, or XII deficiency

Erythema, Skin Reddened (see Chapters 56–60)

Common

Thermal, chemical, actinic burns
Mammary hyperplasia, Mammary fibroepithelial hyperplasia
Hemangioma, Hemangiosarcoma
Psychogenic alopecia/dermatitis, Neurodermatitis
Irritant contact dermatitis
Allergic contact dermatitis, Contact hypersensitivity
Atopy, Allergic inhalant dermatitis, Allergic dermatitis
Acne, Atypical pyoderma
Feline miliary dermatitis
Eosinophilic plaque, Lick granuloma
Bacterial dermatitis, Pyoderma
Scabies, Notoedric mange, Sarcoptic mange
Blepharitis
Hypereosinophilic syndrome

Uncommon

Keratoses
Systemic lupus erythematosus
Xanthomatosis
Erythema multiforme
Linear granuloma
Trombiculidiasis, Chiggers, Harvest mites
Pelodera dermatitis, Rhabditic dermatitis
Hookworm dermatitis, Ancylostomiasis, Uncinariasis

Rare

Leishmaniasis
Thallium poisoning

Excoriation, Self-Mutilation

Common

Eosinophilic gastroenteritis, Hypereosinophilic syndrome
Allergies
Allergic conjunctivitis
Bacterial dermatitis, Pyoderma
Scabies, Notoedric mange, Sarcoptic mange
Fleas, Flea-allergy dermatitis, Flea-bite hypersensitivity

Pediculosis, Lice
Seborrhea, Keratinization disorders
Otitis, Ear mites, Otodectic mange
Cheyletiella, Walking dandruff

Uncommon
Trombiculidiasis, Chiggers
Harvest mites
Lynxacariasis, Cat fur mite
Chemical reactions
Methimazole reaction

Exostoses Palpable

Common
Bone neoplasia
Chronic progressive polyarthritis

Uncommon
Multiple cartilaginous exostoses, Osteochondromatosis

Fecal Incontinence

Fecal incontinence should be distinguished from diarrhea. It is the uncontrolled loss of normal fecal matter from the rectum.

Common
Sacrocaudal dysgenesis, Sacrococcygeal dysgenesis, Spina bifida
Spinal cord tumors (extramedullary), Spinal neoplasia (extramedullary)
Intervertebral disk disease
Proctitis
Surgical procedures on rectum, anus, or perineum

Uncommon
Cerebral disease
Brain stem disease
Spinal dysraphism, Syringomyelia
Aortic, arterial thromboembolism, Saddle clot thrombus
Manx cat syndrome

Rare
Key-Gaskell syndrome, Dysautonomia, Autonomic polyganglionopathy

Femoral Pulse Deficit

During examination of the cardiovascular system, the femoral pulses should be palpated while the heart is auscultated with a stethoscope. Every cardiac beat should be accompanied by a peripheral pulse; its absence is called *pulse deficit* and indicates a nonproductive cardiac impulse.

Common
Atrial fibrillation
Atrial premature complexes
Ventricular premature complexes
Mitral valve dysplasia
Tricuspid valve dysplasia
Ventricular septal defect
Patent ductus arteriosus
Aortic stenosis
Hypertrophic cardiomyopathy
Dilated cardiomyopathy
Endocarditis/myocarditis
Pericardial effusion, Cardiac tamponade
Acute renal failure, Acute nephrosis
Renal insufficiency, Renal failure
Pancreatitis, Pancreatic neoplasia
Mediastinal neoplasia
Epilepsy, Convulsions, Seizure
Head injuries
Brain neoplasia
Burns
Hypoadrenocorticism, Addison's disease
Hyperthyroidism, Thyrotoxicosis
Chemical toxins
  Cardioglycosides
  Antiarrhythmic drugs
  Heavy metal poisons

Uncommon
Ventricular fibrillation
Hypopituitarism
Toxoplasmosis
Cardiac neoplasia
Endocardial fibroelastosis
Common atrioventricular canal, Endocardial cushion defect
Restrictive cardiomyopathy, Intermediate cardiomyopathy
Pseudorabies, Aujeszky's disease, Mad itch

Rare
Sodium fluoroacetate poisoning
American trypanosomiasis, Chagas' disease

Femoral Pulse Weak or Thready

Common
Burns
Severe debilitating systemic diseases
Shock
Hypovolemia
Peritonitis
Pericardial effusion
Bacterial endocarditis/myocarditis
Aortic, arterial thromboembolism, Saddle clot thrombus
Hypertrophic cardiomyopathy
Patent ductus arteriosus
Aortic stenosis

Uncommon
Cardiovascular neoplasia
Restrictive cardiomyopathy, Intermediate cardiomyopathy
Dilated cardiomyopathy, Congestive cardiomyopathy
Aortic insufficiency
Hypoadrenocorticism, Addison's disease

Rare
Sodium fluoroacetate poisoning
American trypanosomiasis, Chagas' disease

Gait Abnormal

When an animal exhibits an abnormal gait it should be determined whether a musculoskeletal, vascular, neurologic, or combined abnormality is present.

Common

Hypokalemia
Spondylitis, Discospondylitis, Vertebral osteomyelitis
Degenerative joint disease, Osteoarthritis, Osteoarthrosis
Cruciate ligament rupture
Patella luxation/subluxation, Patella instability
Infectious arthritis, Infectious inflammatory joint disease
Chronic progressive polyarthritis
Bone neoplasia
Spinal cord tumors
Peripheral nerve disease
Trauma
Nail bed disease
Foreign body

Uncommon

Hookworm dermatitis, Ancylostomiasis, Uncinariasis
Myositis ossificans, Fibrodysplasia ossificans
Neuroaxonal dystrophy
Cerebellar hypoplasia, Cerebellar malformation
Mannosidosis
Spinal dysraphism, Syringomyelia
Sacrocaudal dysgenesis, Sacrococcygeal dysgenesis, Spina bifida
Aortic arterial thromboembolism, Saddle clot thrombus

Rare

Mucopolysaccharidosis, Hurler's, Maroteaux-Lamy syndrome

Head Tilt

Head tilt is usually toward the affected side (ear down toward the affected side, nose up and away from the affected side).

Common

Otitis media/interna
Ear mites, Otodectic mange
Otic tumors
Vestibular disease
Heat prostration

Uncommon

Aortic arterial thromboembolism
Cerebral vascular hemorrhage
Dirofilariasis, Heartworm disease
Migrating parasites
Mycotic infections
Toxoplasmosis
Intracranial neoplasia, Brain tumor

Heinz Body Anemia (see Chapter 16)

Common

Abscesses
Peritonitis
Chronic renal failure
Peritonitis
Upper respiratory tract diseases
Diabetes mellitus
Hyperthyroidism
Lymphosarcoma
Acetaminophen toxicity
Aspirin toxicity
Cancer chemotherapy

Uncommon

Urinary antiseptics with methylene blue
Phenazopyridine
Benzocaine
Phenacetin
Propylene glycol
Methionine
Onions
Stomatitis, Glossitis, Gingivitis
Intestinal obstruction

Hematemesis, Vomitus Hemorrhagic (see Chapter 24)

After severe vomiting most cats produce a small amount of blood in the vomitus. Hematemesis is the presence of large amounts of blood, or "coffee ground" vomitus.

Common

Renal insufficiency, Renal failure
Gastric ulceration
Duodenal ulceration
Gastritis

Uncommon

Renal congenital disease
Mast cell tumor, Mastocytoma, Mast cell sarcoma, Mastocytosis
Arsenic toxicity
Zinc phosphide poisoning
Rodenticide, Vitamin D_3 toxicity, Cholecalciferol toxicity
Anticoagulant poisoning
Esophageal neoplasia
Gastric neoplasia
Hepatic cirrhosis

Rare

Thallium poisoning
Gastrinoma, Zollinger-Ellison syndrome

Hematochezia, Feces Hemorrhagic (see Chapter 24)

Dark digested blood mixed well into the feces indicates a lesion in the upper digestive tract. Red blood streaks on the surface of the stool indicates a lesion in the colon, rectum, or anus.

Common

Eosinophilic gastroenteritis, Hypereosinophilic syndrome
Lymphocytic/plasmacytic enteritis
Granulomatous enteritis, Regional enteritis, Crohn's disease

Inflammatory bowel disease, Colitis
Intestinal neoplasia
Intestinal foreign body
Megacolon
Colonic neoplasia, Cecal neoplasia, Rectal neoplasia
Rectal stricture
Proctitis
Anal neoplasia
Hookworm disease, Ancylostomiasis
Whipworms, Trichuriasis
Nonsteroidal antiinflammatory drug toxicity
Food allergy, Food intolerance, Food hypersensitivity
Renal insufficiency, Renal failure

Uncommon
Chemical toxins
  Anticoagulant poisoning
  Rodenticide, Vitamin D_3 toxicity, Cholecalciferol toxicity
  Arsenic toxicity
Renal congenital disease
Pancreatitis
Pancreatic neoplasia
Salmonellosis
Tyzzer's disease
Campylobacteriosis
Histoplasmosis
Coccidiosis
Amebiasis
Strongyloidiasis
Trichinellosis, Trichinosis

Rare
Thallium poisoning

Hematuria (see Chapter 40)

Common
Urinary obstruction, Feline urologic syndrome, Urine retention
Urethritis, Urethral inflammation
Urinary tract trauma
Urinary bladder neoplasia
Urolithiasis
Cystitis
Ureteral obstruction
Acute renal failure, Acute nephrosis
Cystic endometrial hyperplasia, Metritis, Pyometra
Renal glomerular disease, Glomerulonephritis

Uncommon
Vesicoureteral reflux
Renal neoplasia
Nephrolithiasis
Hydronephrosis
Nephrotic syndrome
Pyelonephritis
Renal amyloidosis, Amyloidosis
Diabetes mellitus
Chemical toxins
  Arsenic toxicity
  Phosphorus poisoning
  Anticoagulant poisoning

Hepatomegaly

Common
Right heart congestive failure
Dilated cardiomyopathy
Eosinophilic gastroenteritis, Hypereosinophilic syndrome
Intestinal neoplasia
Hepatic lipidosis, Fatty liver disease
Hepatic neoplasia
Pancreatitis
Leukemia virus infection
Hemobartonellosis, Feline infectious anemia

Uncommon
Systemic lupus erythematosus
Pulmonic stenosis
Ventricular septal defect
Common atrioventricular canal, Endocardial cushion defect
Endocardial fibroelastosis
Tricuspid valve dysplasia
Restrictive cardiomyopathy, Intermediate cardiomyopathy
Pancreatic neoplasia
Tuberculosis
Pseudotuberculosis, Yersiniosis
Histoplasmosis
Babesiosis
Dirofilariasis, Heartworm disease
Opisthorchis infection; Bile, pancreatic duct, intestinal fluke
Platynosomiasis, Liver fluke, Lizard poisoning
Hypersomatotropism, Acromegaly
Pituitary neoplasia
Hyperadrenocorticism, Cushing's syndrome
Diabetes mellitus
Mast cell tumor, Mastocytoma, Mast cell sarcoma, Mastocytosis
Hemangioma, Hemangiosarcoma
Cutaneous lymphosarcoma, Malignant lymphoma, Mycosis fungoides
Hypervitaminosis A
Sphingomyelinosis, Niemann-Pick disease
Mannosidosis
Glycogenosis, Glycogen storage disease
Mucopolysaccharidosis, Hurler's, Maroteaux-Lamy syndrome

Rare
American trypanosomiasis, Chagas' disease

Horner's Syndrome

Horner's syndrome is a complex of signs due to disruption somewhere along the sympathetic pathway from the hypothalamus, through the cervical spinal cord region, to the second thoracic cord segment, then through the vagosympathetic trunk to segments of the optic globe. Lesions along this pathway may cause miotic pupil, drooped upper lid, sunken eyeball, and prolapsed nictitating membrane.

Common
Otitis media/interna
Injury to brachial plexus
Feline leukemia virus
Mediastinal neoplasia

Uncommon
Neoplasia of sympathetic pathway
Cervical/thoracic spinal cord injury
Cervical/thoracic spinal cord neoplasia
Cavernous sinus infection or neoplasia
Ischemic, necrotizing, fibrocartilaginous embolic myelopathy
Forelimb amputation

Rare
Hypothalamic disease

Hyperesthesia (see Chapter 45)

Common
Nodular panniculitis, Feline steatitis
Spinal cord neoplasia
Spondylitis, Discospondylitis, Vertebral osteomyelitis

Uncommon
Feline polioencephalomyelitis
Hypervitaminosis A
Chemical toxins
  Lead toxicity
  Chlorinated hydrocarbon toxicity
  Zinc phosphide poisoning
  Metaldehyde poisoning
Rabies
Pseudorabies, Aujeszky's disease, Mad itch

Hypersalivation, Ptyalism

Common
Epilepsy, Convulsion, Seizure
Irritant contact dermatitis
Chemical toxins
  Phenol toxicity
  Acetaminophen toxicity
  Aspirin toxicity
  Organophosphate/carbamate toxicity
  Glucocorticoids
Feline calicivirus infection
Periodontitis, Periodontal disease
Stomatitis, Glossitis, Gingivitis
Lymphocytic/plasmacytic stomatitis
Oral foreign body
Esophagitis
Esophageal obstruction/stricture, Periesophageal obstruction

Uncommon
Chemical toxins
  Lead toxicity
  Arsenic toxicity
  Chlorinated hydrocarbon toxicity
  Metaldehyde poisoning
Chemicals with a bitter taste
  Oral ketamine
  Oral Gastrografin-76
  Oral liquid chloramphenicol
  Oral liquid dioctyl sodium sulfosuccinate (DSS)
Snakebite, Snake venom poisoning
Ingestion of frogs
Dirofilariasis, Heartworm disease
Rabies
Pseudorabies, Aujeszky's disease, Mad itch
Salivary neoplasia
Esophageal neoplasia
Hiatal hernia, Gastroesophageal intussusception
Cholangiohepatitis Cholangitis
Portal systemic shunt, Portal vascular anomalies

Rare
ANTU poisoning

Icterus, Jaundice (see Chapter 20)

The three major causes of icterus are intravascular hemolysis, biliary stasis, and hepatic parenchymal disease.

Common
Feline leukemia virus
Feline infectious peritonitis/serositis
Panleukopenia, Feline distemper, Feline enteritis
Hemobartonellosis, Feline infectious anemia
Intravascular hemolysis
Peritonitis
Pancreatitis
Hepatotoxins
Chemical toxins
  Aspirin toxicity
  Acetaminophen toxicity
Hepatitis
Hepatic neoplasia
Hepatic cirrhosis
Hepatic lipidosis, Fatty liver disease
Cholangiostasis
Cholangiohepatitis, Cholangitis

Uncommon
Immune-mediated disease
Systemic lupus erythematosus
Diabetes mellitus
Chemical toxins
  Phenol toxicity
  Phosphorus poisoning
Babesiosis
Toxoplasmosis
Tyzzer's disease
Pseudotuberculosis, Yersiniosis
Histoplasmosis
Platynosomiasis, Liver fluke, Lizard poisoning
Opisthorchis infection; Bile, pancreatic duct, intestinal fluke
Pancreatic neoplasia
Bile duct rupture, Gallbladder rupture
Cholelithiasis, Choledocolithiasis

Infertility (see Chapter 54)

When infertility exists, it must be determined whether the tom or the queen is at fault.

Common
Overbreeding
Psychogenic

Feline leukemia virus
Feline immunodeficiency virus
Feline infectious peritonitis/serositis
Toxoplasmosis
Hemobartonellosis
Cystic endometrial hyperplasia, Metritis, Pyometra
Vaginitis
Cachexia
Renal failure
Hepatic failure
Orchitis
Bilateral cryptorchidism

Uncommon

Hyperadrenocorticism
Hypoadrenocorticism
Pancreatic insufficiency

Jaw Pain, Mouth Opening Painful

Common

Rhinitis
Sinusitis
Periodontitis, Periodontal disease
Stomatitis, Glossitis, Gingivitis
Lymphocytic/plasmacytic stomatitis
Feline immunodeficiency virus
Foreign body in mouth
Tonsilitis
Fractured jaw

Uncommon

Myositis
Retrobulbar abscess
Pharyngitis

Lymphadenopathy, Lymph Node Enlarged (see Chapter 21)

Common

Hypereosinophilic syndrome
Lymphocytic/plasmacytic stomatitis
Lymphocytic/plasmacytic enteritis
Intestinal neoplasia
Feline leukemia virus
Feline immunodeficiency virus
Hemobartonellosis, Feline infectious anemia
Scabies, Notoedric mange, Sarcoptic mange
Demodectic mange, Follicular mange, Demodicosis
Fleas, Flea-allergy dermatitis, Flea-bite hypersensitivity
Feline miliary dermatitis
Bacterial dermatitis, Pyoderma
Acne, Atypical pyoderma
Food allergy, Food intolerance, Food hypersensitivity
Squamous cell carcinoma
Cat bite wounds
Superficial foreign body

Uncommon

Systemic lupus erythematosus
Feline leprosy
Bubonic plague, Sylvatic plague
Botryomycosis, Bacterial granuloma
Nocardiosis
Actinomycosis
Blastomycosis, North American blastomycosis
Coccidioidomycosis, San Joaquim Valley fever
Cryptococcosis
Histoplasmosis
Sporotrichosis
Phaeohyphomycosis, Chromomycosis
Toxoplasmosis
Mast cell tumor, Mastocytoma, Mast cell sarcoma, Mastocytosis
Hemangiosarcoma
Fibrosarcoma
Malignant melanoma, Melanosarcoma
Cutaneous lymphosarcoma, Malignant lymphoma, Mycosis fungoides
Chronic progressive polyarthritis

Rare

American trypanosomiasis, Chagas' disease

Mammary Gland Enlarged, Swollen (see Chapter 54)

Common

Mammary gland neoplasia
Galactostasis
Mastitis
Mammary hyperplasia, Mammary fibroepithelial hyperplasia

Miosis, Pupil Constricted

Pupillary constriction can be caused by depression of sympathetic control or overstimulation of parasympathetic activity.

Common

Mediastinal neoplasia
Brachial plexus nerve root avulsion
Ischemic, necrotizing, fibrocartilaginous embolic myelopathy
Intracranial neoplasia
Otitis media/interna
Organophosphate/carbamate toxicity
Uveitis
Head injuries
Horner's syndrome
Acetylcholinergic medications, especially ophthalmic
Pain

Uncommon

Rabies

Rare

Vacor (Pyriminil) poisoning

Mydriasis, Pupil Dilated

Pupillary dilation can be caused by depression of parasympathetic control or overstimulation of sympathetic activity.

Common
Excitement, Fear, Stress
Ischemic encephalopathy
Retinal detachment
Hypoplasia/aplasia optic nerve
Blindness
Oculomotor nerve damage, Third cranial nerve damage
Retinal degeneration, Retinal atrophy
Glaucoma
Leukemia virus infection

Uncommon
Chemical toxins
  Lead toxicity
  Strychnine poisoning
Blastomycosis
Rabies

Rare
Key-Gaskell syndrome, Dysautonomia, Autonomic polyganglionopathy
Vacor (Pyriminil) poisoning

Murmur

Common
Innocent murmur
Valvular stenosis
Valvular insufficiency
Endocarditis/myocarditis, Vegetative valvular endocarditis
Hypertrophic cardiomyopathy
Hyperthyroidism
Dilated cardiomyopathy, Congestive cardiomyopathy
Ventricular septal defect
Hyperthyroidism

Uncommon
Mediastinal neoplasia
Diaphragmatic hernia
Peritoneal/pericardial diaphragmatic hernia
Pectus excavatum, Funnel chest
Pituitary neoplasia
Hypersomatotropism
Dirofilariasis, Heartworm disease
Restrictive cardiomyopathy, Intermediate cardiomyopathy
Tricuspid valve dysplasia
Mitral valve dysplasia
Endocardial fibroelastosis
Tetralogy of Fallot
Common atrioventricular canal, Endocardial cushion defect
Atrial septal defect
Pulmonic stenosis
Aortic stenosis
Patent ductus arteriosus

Rare
Mucopolysaccharidosis, Hurler's, Maroteaux-Lamy syndrome

Muscle Atrophy, Wasting

Common
Infectious arthritis, Infectious inflammatory joint disease
Degenerative joint disease, Osteoarthritis, Osteoarthrosis
Aortic, arterial thromboembolism, Saddle clot thrombus
Peripheral nerve damage
Cachexia

Uncommon
Chronic progressive polyarthritis
Muscular dystrophy
Hyperadrenocorticism, Cushing's syndrome

Nasal Discharge (see Chapter 30)

Common
Nasal foreign body
Nasal trauma
Rhinitis
  Allergic
  Viral
  Bacterial
  Mycotic
Sinusitis
Periodontitis, Periodontal disease
Stomatitis, Gingivitis, Glossitis
Nasal-pharyngeal polyp
Pneumonia
Irritant contact dermatitis
Food allergy, Food intolerance, Food hypersensitivity
Feline chlamydiosis, Feline pneumonitis
Feline calicivirus infection
Feline herpesvirus infection, Feline rhinotracheitis

Uncommon
Cleft palate
Nasal passage neoplasia
Parasitic tracheobronchitis/pneumonia
Protothecosis
Aspergillosis
Cryptococcosis
Actinomycosis
Nocardiosis
Bubonic plague, Sylvatic plague
Coagulation defects, Abnormal bleeding

Rare
Thallium poisoning

Neck Ventroflexion (see Chapter 28)

Common
Hypokalemia
Taurine deficiency

Uncommon
Thiamine deficiency
Polymyopathy
Cervical myelopathy

Nystagmus, Rapid Eye Movement

Common
Vestibular disease
Cerebellar hypoplasia, Cerebellar malformation

Brain stem lesion
Cranial trauma
Otitis media/interna
Intracranial neoplasia, Brain tumor
Aortic, arterial thromboembolism
Rapid head movement (doll's eye movement), Normal heat stroke
Chemical toxins

Uncommon

Hydrocephalus
Mannosidosis
Neuroaxonal dystrophy
Ceroid lipofuscinosis, Familial amaurotic idiocy
Metaldehyde poisoning
Cryptococcosis
Panleukopenia, Feline distemper, Feline enteritis
Feline infectious peritonitis/serositis
Granulomatous meningoencephalitis, Reticulosis
Rabies
Pseudorabies, Aujeszky's disease, Mad itch
Congenital nystagmus
Chediak-Higashi syndrome

Ocular Discharge (see Chapter 35)

Common

Rhinitis
Sinusitis
Food allergy, Food intolerance, Food hypersensitivity
Atopy
Feline chlamydiosis, Feline pneumonitis
Feline reovirus infection
Feline calicivirus infection
Feline herpesvirus infection, Feline rhinotracheitis
Bacterial conjunctivitis
Mycoplasma
Uveitis
Ulcerative keratitis, corneal sequestrum
Allergic conjunctivitis
Keratoconjunctivitis sicca
Dusty environment
Irritating vapors

Uncommon

Nasal passage neoplasia
Parasitic tracheobronchitis/pneumonia
  Paragonimiasis
  Aelurostrongylus
Actinomycosis
Nocardiosis
Bubonic plague, Sylvatic plague
Feline ocular melanoma, Uveal malignant melanoma
Conjunctival squamous cell carcinoma
Parasitic conjunctivitis, Thelazia

Rare

Mucopolysaccharidosis, Hurler's, Maroteaux-Lamy syndrome

Paralysis (see Chapter 17)

During the examination of a paralytic animal attempt should be made by reflex examination to distinguish between lower and upper motor neuron disease.

Common

Ischemic encephalopathy
Intracranial neoplasia, Brain tumor
Spinal injury
Spinal cord neoplasia
Spondylitis; Discospondylitis; Vertebral osteomyelitis
Intervertebral disc disease
Peripheral nerve injury
Peripheral nerve neoplasia
Leukemia virus infection
Feline infectious peritonitis/serositis
Aortic, arterial thromboembolism
Hypertrophic cardiomyopathy
Dilated cardiomyopathy

Uncommon

Sacrolcaudal dysgenesis, Sacrococcygeal dysgenesis, Spina bifida
Spinal dysraphism, Syringomyelia
Ischemic, necrotizing, fibrocartilaginous embolic myelopathy
Globoid cell leukodystrophy, Krabbe's disease
Feline polioencephalomyelitis
Mucopolysaccharidosis, Hurler's syndrome, Maroteaux-Lamy syndrome
Ceroid lipofuscinosis, Familial amaurotic idiocy
Sphingomyelinosis, Niemann-Pick disease
GM_2 gangliosidosis, Sandhoff's disease
GM_1 gangliosidosis
Multiple cartilaginous exostoses, Osteochondromatosis
Bone neoplasia
Myositis ossificans, Fibrodysplasia ossificans
Otitis media/interna
Xanthomatosis
Hyperinsulinism
Diabetes mellitus
Hyperadrenocorticism, Cushing's syndrome
Chemical toxins
  Ethylene glycol toxicity
  Arsenic toxicity
  Organophosphate/carbamate toxicity
Rabies
Cryptococcosis
Toxoplasmosis
Encephalitozoonosis
Cuterebriasis, Grubs
Snakebite, Snake venom poisoning
Salivary neoplasia
Restrictive cardiomyopathy, Intermediate cardiomyopathy

Rare

Thallium poisoning
Vacor (Pyriminil) poisoning

Pollakiuria, Frequent Urination (see Chapter 40)

Pollakiuria, frequent urination, should be distinguished from polyuria (increased amount of urine) if possible. Irritation to the urinogenital tract may result in frequent attempts at urination, which can be interpreted as increased urination, but is seldom accompanied by polydipsia. Polyuria is usually accompanied by increased thirst. A polyuric cat may also show pollakiuria.

Common
Urinary obstruction, Feline urologic syndrome, Urine retention
Urethritis, Urethral inflammation
Cystitis
Cystic calculi
Urinary bladder neoplasia
Vaginitis

Uncommon
Ureteral obstruction
Vesicoureteral reflux
Renal neoplasia
Hydronephrosis
Nephrotic syndrome
Pyelonephritis
Renal congenital disease
Renal secondary hyperparathyroidism
Uterine neoplasia
Diabetes mellitus
Pseudohyperparathyroidism, Hypercalcemia of malignancy
Hyperparathyroidism
Hypoparathyroidism
Hyperthyroidism, Thyrotoxicosis
Pituitary neoplasia
Central diabetes insipidus
Hypersomatotropism, Acromegaly
Hepatic neoplasia
Portal systemic shunt, Portal vascular anomalies
Hepatic cirrhosis
Cholangiohepatitis, Cholangitis
Hepatic lipidosis, Fatty liver disease

Polydipsia (see Chapter 22)

Polydipsia should be distinguished from unproductive attempts at water consumption due to dysphagia or the inability to lap water. This may be the result of a buccal or glossal foreign body or disease. Many cats, when very ill, will hang over a waterbowl without imbibing.

Common
Renal glomerular disease
Renal insufficiency, Renal failure, Uremia, Azotemia
Renal congenital disease
Pyelonephritis
Cystitis
Cystic endometrial hyperplasia, Metritis, Pyometra
Epilepsy, Convulsion, Seizure
Burns
Diabetes mellitus
Hyperthyroidism, Thyrotoxicosis
Rodenticide, Vitamin D_3 toxicity, Cholecalciferol toxicity
Pancreatitis
Heart failure

Uncommon
Renal neoplasia
Hydronephrosis
Nephrotic syndrome
Renal amyloidosis
Renal secondary hyperparathyroidism
Nephrogenic diabetes insipidus
Ureteral obstruction
Vesicoureteral reflux
Urinary bladder neoplasia
Uterine neoplasia
Mediastinal neoplasia
Nonketotic hyperosmolar diabetes
Diabetic ketoacidosis
Hyperadrenocorticism, Cushing's syndrome
Hypoadrenocorticism, Addison's disease
Pseudohyperparathyroidism, Hypercalcemia of malignancy
Hyperparathyroidism
Hypoparathyroidism
Pituitary neoplasia
Central diabetes insipidus
Hypersomatotropism, Acromegaly
Intracranial neoplasia
Chemical toxins
  Ethylene glycol toxicity
  Nonsteroidal antiinflammatory drug toxicity
  Arsenic toxicity
Leukemia virus infection
Gastric neoplasia
Gastric ulceration
Gastritis
Intestinal obstruction, Pseudoobstruction
Pancreatic neoplasia
Hepatic neoplasia
Portal systemic shunt, Portal vascular anomalies
Hepatic cirrhosis
Cholangiohepatitis, Cholangitis
Hepatic lipidosis, Fatty liver disease

Rare
Gastrinoma, Zollinger-Ellison syndrome

Polymyositis

Common
Immune-mediated disease
  Systemic lupus erythematosus
  Rheumatoid arthritis
  Eosinophilic myositis
Trauma

Uncommon
Toxoplasmosis
Trichinosis
Viral diseases
Ischemic neuromyopathy
Idiopathic feline polymyopathy
Hypothyroidism

Polyneuritis

Common
Immune-mediated disease
  Systemic lupus erythematosus
Chemical toxins
  Lead toxicity
  Organophosphate/carbamate toxicity
Diabetes mellitus

Hyperadrenocorticism, Cushing's disease, Uremia
Neoplasia
Nutritional deficiencies
  Taurine deficiency
  Thiamine deficiency

Uncommon
Lysosomal storage diseases

Polyphagia, Increased Appetite

Common
Hyperthyroidism, Thyrotoxicosis
Hyperadrenocorticism, Cushing's syndrome
Diabetes mellitus
Epilepsy, Convulsion, Seizure
Infiltrative bowel disease
  Lymphocytic/plasmacytic enteritis
  Eosinophilic gastroenteritis
  Lymphosarcoma
Protein-losing enteropathy
Exocrine pancreatic insufficiency
Parasitism

Uncommon
Hypersomatotropism, Acromegaly
Pituitary neoplasia
Hyperinsulinism
Hypothalamic dysfunction
Mediastinal neoplasia
Lymphangiectasia

Polyuria, Increased Urination (see Chapter 22)

Polyuria, increased amount of urine, should be distinguished from pollakiuria (frequent urination) if possible. Irritation to the urinogenital tract may result in frequent attempts at urination, which can be interpreted as increased urination, but is seldom accompanied by polydipsia. Polyuria is usually accompanied by increased thirst. A polyuric cat may also exhibit pollakiuria.

Common
Renal glomerular disease
Renal insufficiency, Renal failure, uremia, azotemia
Renal congenital disease
Pyelonephritis
Ureteral obstruction
Cystitis
Cystic endometrial hyperplasia, Metritis, Pyometra
Pancreatitis
Hepatic cirrhosis
Cholangiohepatitis, Cholangitis
Diabetes mellitus
Rodenticide, Vitamin D_3 toxicity, Cholecalciferol toxicity

Uncommon
Renal neoplasia
Hydronephrosis
Nephrotic syndrome
Renal amyloidosis
Renal secondary hyperparathyroidism
Nephrogenic diabetes insipidus
Vesicoureteral reflux
Urinary bladder neoplasia
Uterine neoplasia
Mediastinal neoplasia
Intracranial neoplasia
Nonketotic hyperosmolar diabetes
Diabetic ketoacidosis
Hyperadrenocorticism, Cushing's syndrome
Hypoadrenocorticism, Addison's disease
Pseudohyperparathyroidism, Hypercalcemia of malignancy
Hyperparathyroidism
Hypoparathyroidism
Hyperthyroidism, Thyrotoxicosis
Pituitary neoplasia
Central diabetes insipidus
Hypersomatotropism, Acromegaly
Leukemia virus infection
Pancreatic neoplasia
Hepatic neoplasia
Portal systemic shunt, Portal vascular anomalies
Hepatic lipidosis, Fatty liver disease

Proprioception Deficit

Common
Spondylitis, Discospondylitis, Vertebral osteomyelitis
Ischemic encephalopathy
Cerebellar hypoplasia, Cerebellar malformation
Cerebral disease
Cerebral neoplasia
Cerebral trauma
Brain stem disease
Spinal cord disease
Spinal cord neoplasia
Spinal cord trauma
Peripheral nerve disease

Uncommon
Sphingomyelinosis, Niemann-Pick disease
Neuroaxonal dystrophy
Mannosidosis

Pruritus (see Chapters 56–60)

Common
Hypereosinophilic syndrome
Eosinophilic plaque, Lick granuloma
Blepharitis
Allergic conjunctivitis
Feline miliary dermatitis
Acne, atypical pyoderma
Food allergy, Food intolerance, Food hypersensitivity
Atopy, Allergic inhalant dermatitis, Allergic dermatitis
Allergic contact dermatitis, Contact hypersensitivity
Irritant contact dermatitis
Seborrhea, Keratinization disorders
Bacterial dermatitis, Pyoderma

Mycotic infection
Scabies, Notoedric mange, Sarcoptic mange
Trombiculidiasis, Chiggers, Harvest mites
Cheyletiellosis, Walking dandruff
Fleas, Flea-allergy dermatitis, Flea-bite hypersensitivity
Pediculosis, Lice
Ear mites, Otodectic mange, Otitis
Tapeworm infestation

Uncommon
Poxvirus infection
Feline leprosy
Botryomycosis, Bacterial granuloma
Hookworm dermatitis, Ancylostomiasis, Uncinariasis
Pelodera dermatitis, Rhabditis, Rhabditic dermatitis
Lynxacariasis, Cat fur mite
Demodectic mange, Follicular mange, Demodicosis
Pemphigus complex
Squamous cell carcinoma
Cutaneous lymphosarcoma, Malignant lymphoma, Mycosis fungoides
Burns

Pupillary Light Reflex Decreased

Common
Metabolic disorders
Drugs
- Atropine
- Neosynephrine
- Organophosphate/carbamate

Excessive sympathetic tone
- Fright, Fear, Pain

Horner's syndrome

Uncommon
Diencephalon dysfunction
- Thalamus, Hypothalamus

Midbrain lesions
Oculomotor nerve lesion
Lesions of the pons

Pyoderma, Skin Purulent
(see Chapters 56–60)

Common
Bacterial dermatitis
Allergic contact dermatitis, Contact hypersensitivity
Irritant contact dermatitis
Food allergy, Food intolerance, Food hypersensitivity
Atopy, Allergic inhalant dermatitis, Allergic dermatitis
Acne, Atypical pyoderma
Eosinophilic plaque, Lick granuloma
Feline miliary dermatitis
Seborrhea, Keratinization disorders
Psychogenic alopecia/dermatitis, Neurodermatitis
Burns
Skin-fold dermatitis, Intertriginous dermatitis
Fleas, Flea-allergy dermatitis, Flea-bite hypersensitivity
Scabies, Notoedric mange, Sarcoptic mange
Pediculosis, Lice

Uncommon
Pemphigus complex
Erythema multiforme
Toxic epidermal necrolysis, Lyell disease
Nodular panniculitis, Steatitis
Xanthomatosis
Cutaneous lymphosarcoma, Malignant lymphoma, Mycosis fungoides
Botryomycosis, Bacterial granuloma
Pelodera dermatitis, Rhabditis, Rhabditic dermatitis
Demodectic mange, Follicular mange, Demodicosis
Hookworm dermatitis, Ancylostomiasis, Uncinariasis
Feline impetigo

Pyuria, Urine Purulent

Common
Acute renal failure, Acute nephrosis
Pyelonephritis
Urinary obstruction, Feline urologic syndrome, Urine retention
Urethritis, Urethral inflammation
Urinary bladder neoplasia
Urolithiasis
Cystitis
Cystic endometrial hyperplasia, Metritis, Pyometra
Diabetes mellitus

Uncommon
Vesicoureteral reflux
Nephrolithiasis

Rales, Wheezes

Common
Bronchitis
Bronchiectasis, Chronic dilation of bronchi
Allergic bronchitis, Bronchial asthma, Feline asthma
Parasitic tracheobronchitis/pneumonia
- Aelurostrongylosis
- Paragonimiasis

Pneumonia
Emphysema
Atelectasis
Pulmonary neoplasia
Mediastinal neoplasia
Pectus excavatum, Funnel chest

Uncommon
Renal insufficiency, Renal failure, Uremia
Renal congenital disease, Renal familial disease
Diaphragmatic hernia
Peritoneal/pericardial diaphragmatic hernia
Anticoagulant poisoning
Esophageal diverticulum
Megaesophagus, Esophageal hypomotility
Gastroesophageal reflux
Restrictive cardiomyopathy, Intermediate cardiomyopathy
Dilated cardiomyopathy, Congestive cardiomyopathy
Hypertrophic cardiomyopathy

Rare
ANTU poisoning

Rectal Bleeding

Dark digested blood mixed well into the feces indicates a lesion in the upper digestive tract. Red blood streaks on the surface of the stool indicate a lesion in the colon, rectum, or anus.

Common
Colonic neoplasia, Cecal neoplasia, Rectal neoplasia
Rectal stricture
Proctitis
Inflammatory bowel disease, Colitis
Rectal foreign body
Malicious trauma

Uncommon
Anal neoplasia
Anal gland abscess
Perianal fistula
Amebiasis

Regurgitation

Regurgitation should not be confused with vomiting. It is the discharging through the mouth or nose of undigested food or fluid from the pharynx, esophagus, or stomach without any overt retching activity. It is locally mediated in contrast to vomiting, which is centrally mediated.

Common
Mediastinal neoplasia
Esophagitis
Esophageal obstruction, stricture; Periesophageal obstruction
Megaesophagus, Esophageal hypomotility
Esophageal diverticulum
Esophageal trauma
Gastric retention

Uncommon
Myasthenia gravis
Polymyositis
Esophageal neoplasia
Vascular ring anomalies, Persistent right aortic arch
Hiatal hernia, Gastroesophageal intussusception
Lead toxicity
Systemic lupus erythematosus
Hypoadrenocorticism

Rare
Key-Gaskell syndrome, Dysautonomia, Autonomic polyganglionopathy
Gastrinoma, Zollinger-Ellison syndrome

Seborrhea, Keratinization Disorders

Common
Hypereosinophilic syndrome
Food allergy, Food intolerance, Food hypersensitivity
Atopy, Allergic inhalant dermatitis, Allergic dermatitis
Miliary dermatitis
Bacterial dermatitis, Pyoderma
Mycotic infection
Scabies, *Notoedres cati, Sarcoptes scabiei*
Cheyletiella spp
Pediculosis, Lice
Internal parasites
Nutritional deficiency

Uncommon
Congenital
Lynxacariasis, Cat fur mite
Cutaneous lymphoma
Growth-hormone–responsive dermatitis
Hyperadrenocorticism
Hypothyroidism
Immune-mediated
Feline leukemia virus
Hepatic disease
Kidney disease

Sneezing

Common
Sinusitis
Rhinitis
- Viral
- Feline calicivirus infection
- Feline herpesvirus infection, Feline rhinotracheitis
- Feline infectious peritonitis/serositis
- Bacterial
- Mycoplasmal
- *Chlamydia psittaci*
- Fungal
- Aspergillosis
- Cryptococcosis

Bacterial conjunctivitis
Foreign body
Bite wounds
Dental disease
- Tooth root abscess

Allergic
- Food allergy, Food intolerance, Food hypersensitivity

Uncommon
Cleft palate
Nasalpharyngeal polyp
Nasal passage neoplasia
Parasitic tracheobronchitis/pneumonia
- Aelurostrongylus abstrusus

Nasal hemorrhage

Splenomegaly

Common
Anesthesia/sedation
Congestive right heart failure
Neoplasia
Hemangioma, Hemangiosarcoma
Mastocytoma, Mast cell sarcoma, Mastocytosis

Histoplasmosis
Hemobartonellosis, Feline infectious anemia
Leukemia virus infection
Intestinal neoplasia
Eosinophilic gastroenteritis, Hypereosinophilic syndrome

Uncommon
Cutaneous lymphosarcoma, Malignant lymphoma, Mycosis fungoides
Xanthomatosis
Pseudotuberculosis, Yersiniosis
Tuberculosis
Sporotrichosis
Babesiosis
Dirofilariasis, Heartworm disease
Systemic lupus erythematosus

Rare
Mucopolysaccharidosis, Hurler's, Maroteaux-Lamy syndrome
Sphingomyelinosis, Niemann-Pick disease
American trypanosomiasis, Chagas' disease

Spraying, Inappropriate Urination (see Chapter 26)

Common
Normal territorial marking
Antagonistic encounters
Stress
Estrous females

Uncommon
Abnormal behavior
Anabolic steroids
Incomplete ovariectomy

Steatorrhea, Fecal Fat Increased

Common
Excessive fat ingestion
Giardiasis
Histoplasmosis
Exocrine pancreatic insufficiency
Intestinal neoplasia
Eosinophilic gastroenteritis, Hypereosinophilic syndrome
Lymphocytic/plasmacytic enteritis

Uncommon
Protein-losing enteropathy

Stomatitis, Gingivitis, Glossitis (see Chapter 52)

Common
Immune-mediated disease
- Plasma cell gingivitis/pharyngitis
- Lymphocytic/plasmacytic stomatitis

Viral
- Feline immunodeficiency virus
- Feline calicivirus
- Feline herpesvirus, Feline rhinotracheitis
- Feline leukemia virus

Bacteria
- Hemolytic streptococci
- *Staphylococcus* spp
- *Pseudomonas* spp
- *Proteus* spp
- *Escherichia coli*
- *Nocardia*

Ulcerative necrotizing stomatitis
- *Spirochaeta*
- Fusiform bacteria

Fungi
- Candidiasis

Periodontitis, Periodontal disease
Dental plaque
Awns, burrs, splinters
Rubber bands, strings
Systemic disease
Respiratory disease
Hepatic, liver disease
Thermal, electrical, chemical burns
Renal disease
Uremia
Nutritional deficiency

Uncommon
Immune-mediated diseases
- Systemic lupus erythematosus
- Pemphigus complex
- Eosinophilic granuloma complex

Hypothyroidism
Diabetes mellitus
Neoplasia
Chemical toxins, caustics

Rare
Thallium toxicity

Strangiuria, Urination Difficult (see Chapter 40)

Strangiuria, pollakiuria, dysuria, dyschesia, and tenesmus are sometimes difficult to identify. Attempt should be made, by questioning the owner or by direct observation, to identify the clinical sign.

Common
Vaginal/vulval neoplasia
Ureteral obstruction
Cystitis
Urolithiasis
Urinary bladder neoplasia
Urinary tract trauma
Urethritis
Urinary obstruction, Feline urologic syndrome, Urine retention
Arthritis

Uncommon
Hydronephrosis
Nephrolithiasis
Ectopic ureter

Syncope, Fainting

Syncope must be distinguished from seizure, narcolepsy, or cataplexy. Seizures are due to excessive neuronal activity, whereas syncope is caused by depressed neuronal activity. This is usually a result of decreased circulation, hypopoxia, or metabolic disturbance. Narcolepsy and cataplexy are forms of syncope related to inappropriate sleep tendencies.

Common

Congestive heart failure
Cardiac neoplasia, Cardiovascular neoplasia
Pericardial effusion, Cardiac tamponade
Myocarditis
Vegetative valvular endocarditis
Hypertrophic cardiomyopathy
Chronic obstructive lung disease
Mediastinal neoplasia, Tumor
Heatstroke
Hyperthyroidism
Hypokalemia
Hypoxemia
Anemia
Acute generalized hemorrhage
Chemical toxins
- Diuretics
- Tranquilizers
- Vasodilators
- Alpha-adrenergic blockers
- Chloramphenicol toxicity

Uncommon

Congenital cardiac malformations
Aortic stenosis
Restrictive cardiomyopathy, Intermediate cardiomyopathy
Dilated cardiomyopathy, Congestive cardiomyopathy
Atrioventricular block
Atrial standstill
Severe ventricular arrhythmias
Cerebral arterial infarction
Cerebral hemorrhage
Cerebral trauma
Cerebral neoplasia
Hypoadrenocorticism
Hyperinsulinism
Pancreatic tumor
Polycythemia, hemoconcentration

Tachycardia, Heart Rate Rapid >240 bpm

Common

Fright, Fear, Stress
Congenital
- Patent ductus arteriosus
- Aortic stenosis
- Ventricular septal defect

Hypertrophic cardiomyopathy
Gastritis
Pancreatitis
Peritonitis
Hyperthyroidism, Thyrotoxicosis
Uremia
Pyometra, Endometritis
Pneumonia
Pulmonary edema
Anemia
Fever, Hyperthermia
Bacterial infections
Viral
- Feline immunodeficiency virus
- Feline calicivirus
- Feline herpesvirus, Feline rhinotracheitis
- Feline leukemia virus

Hemobartonellosis
Chemical toxins
- Aspirin toxicity
- Acetaminophen toxicity

Uncommon

Immune-mediated diseases
- Systemic lupus erythematosus
- Autoimmune hemolytic anemia
- Autoimmune thrombocytopenia

Congenital
- Pulmonic stenosis
- Common atrioventricular canal, Endocardial cushion defect
- Tetralogy of Fallot
- Endocardial fibroelastosis
- Mitral valve dysplasia
- Tricuspid valve dysplasia
- Restrictive cardiomyopathy, Intermediate cardiomyopathy

Dilated cardiomyopathy, Congestive cardiomyopathy
Aortic, arterial thromboembolism, Saddle clot thrombus
Endocarditis/myocarditis, Vegetative valvular endocarditis
Dirofilariasis, Heartworm disease
Pericardial effusion, Cardiac tamponade
Cardiac neoplasia, Cardiovascular neoplasia
Peritoneal pericardial diaphragmatic hernia
Chemical toxins
- Anticoagulant poisoning
- Ethylene glycol toxicity
- Chloramphenicol toxicity
- Catecholamines
- Anticholinergics

Hemangioma, Hemangiosarcoma
Puerperal tetany, Eclampsia
Mediastinal neoplasia
Heat prostration

Rare

American trypanosomiasis, Chagas' disease
Sodium fluoroacetate poisoning
ANTU poisoning

Tenesmus, Straining

It is sometimes difficult to determine whether straining is due to an attempt to defecate or urinate. The positions assumed over the litter pan may be similar.

Common

Urinary obstruction, Feline urologic syndrome, Urine retention

Urinary incontinence
Urethritis, Urethral inflammation
Urinary tract trauma
Urinary bladder neoplasia
Urolithiasis
Cystitis
Ureteral obstruction
Vaginal/vulval neoplasia
Anal neoplasia
Perineal hernia
Perianal fistula
Anal sacculitis, Anal sac abscess
Anal sac impaction, Anal sac disease
Proctitis
Rectal prolapse
Rectal stricture
Rectal foreign body
Rectal deviation, diverticulum, sacculation
Colonic neoplasia, Cecal neoplasia, Rectal neoplasia
Megacolon
Inflammatory bowel disease, Colitis

Uncommon
Hydronephrosis
Amebiasis
Campylobacteriosis
Salmonellosis
Atresia ani, Imperforate anus, Rectal aplasia
Granulomatous enteritis, Regional enteritis, Crohn's disease

Tires Easily

Common
Bronchitis
Bronchiectasis
Pneumonia
Pulmonary edema
Emphysema
Atelectasis
Pleural effusion
Pericardial effusion
Heart failure

Uncommon
Pectus excavatum, Funnel chest
Aelurostrongylosis
Paragonimiasis
Dirofilariasis
Myopathy
Myasthenia gravis
Hypoadrenocorticism
Feline infectious peritonitis/serositis
Feline leukemia virus
Feline immunodeficiency virus

Urinary Bladder Distension

Common
Urinary bladder neoplasia
Urethral calculi
Urethral neoplasia
Spinal injury
Spinal neoplasia
Intervertebral disk disease

Uncommon
Urethritis
Brain stem disease

Urinary Incontinence

Common
Urinary obstruction, Feline urologic syndrome, Urine retention
Stress
Cystitis
Urolithiasis
Nephrolithiasis
Neurogenic
Spinal shock
Spinal cord lesions
Spinal neoplasia
Vertebral trauma
Intervertebral disk disease
Urinary bladder lesion
Prolonged urine retention
Urinary bladder neoplasia
Drugs
- Corticosteroids
- Diuretics

Senility
Estrogen-responsive urinary incontinence

Uncommon
Congenital
Ectopic ureters
Iatrogenic
Ureterovaginal fistula
Sacrocaudal dysgenesis, Sacrococcygeal dysgenesis, Spina bifida
Spinal dysraphism, Syringomyelia
Upper motor neuron disease
Lower motor neuron disease
Myelitis
Bladder dyssynergia
Idiopathic, Unknown

Rare
Mucopolysaccharidosis, Hurler's, Maroteaux-Lamy syndrome
Key-Gaskell syndrome, Dysautonomia, Autonomic polyganglionopathy

Urticaria

Common
Food allergy, Food intolerance, Food hypersensitivity
Atopy, Allergic inhalant dermatitis, Allergic dermatitis
Allergic contact dermatitis, Contact hypersensitivity

Vaginal Discharge (see Chapter 54)

Common

Trauma
Vaginal/vulval neoplasia
Cervicitis/vaginitis
Uterine neoplasia
Cystic endometrial hyperplasia, Metritis, Pyometra

Uncommon

Vaginal herpesvirus infection
Rectal vaginal fistula

Rare

Tuberculosis

Visual Deficit (see Chapters 35, 36)

Common

Epilepsy, Convulsion, Seizure
Retinal dysplasia
Glaucoma
Cataract
Nuclear sclerosis
Uveitis
Keratitis
Corneal edema
Uremia
Senility
Panleukopenia, Feline distemper, Feline enteritis
Feline infectious peritonitis/serositis
Feline leukemia virus
Chemical toxins

Uncommon

Glycogenosis, Glycogen storage disease, Hypoglycemia

Acknowledgment: The editor would like to express thanks to Carter-Melloy Corporation for the use of this material, which is the basis of their diagnostic computer program "Feline Associate." Information concerning this program can be obtained by contacting Carter-Melloy Corporation, PO Box 9219, College Station, TX 77841.

REFERENCES

1. August JR, ed. Consultations in Feline Internal Medicine. Philadelphia: WB Saunders, 1991.
2. Braund KG, ed. Clinical Syndromes in Veterinary Neurology. Baltimore: William & Wilkins, 1986.
3. Ettinger SJ, ed. Textbook of Veterinary Internal Medicine: Diseases of the Dog and Cat, 3rd ed. Philadelphia: WB Saunders, 1989.
4. Feldman EC, Nelson RW, eds. Canine and Feline Endocrinology and Reproduction. Philadelphia: WB Saunders, 1987.
5. Fenner WR, ed. Quick Reference to Veterinary Medicine, 2nd ed. Philadelphia: JB Lippincott, 1991.
6. Gelatt KN, ed. Textbook of Veterinary Ophthalmology. Philadelphia: Lea & Febriger, 1981.
7. Georgi JR, Georgi ME, eds. Parasitology for Veterinarians, 5th ed. Philadelphia: WB Saunders, 1990.
8. Greene CE, ed. Clinical Microbiology and Infectious Diseases in Dog and Cat, 2nd ed. Philadelphia: WB Saunders, 1990.
9. Kirk RW, Bistner SI, Ford RB, eds. Handbook of Veterinary Procedures and Emergency Treatment, 5th ed. Philadelphia: WB Saunders, 1990.
10. Morgan RV, ed. Handbook of Small Animal Practice. New York: Churchill Livingstone, 1988.
11. Muller GH, Kirk RW, Scott DW, eds. Small Animal Dermatology, 4th ed. Philadelphia: WB Saunders, 1989.
12. Sherding RG, ed. The Cat: Diseases and Clinical Management. New York: Churchill Livingstone, 1989.

INDEX

Page numbers followed by *t* and *f* denote tables and figures, respectively.

Abbocath short catheter, 477
Abdomen
  fluid-filled, palpation of, 110
  palpation of, 36, 106, 110, 425
    in abdominal trauma, 394
    diagnosis of pregnancy by, 462
  physical examination of, 36
Abdominal cavity, fluid in
  aspiration of, 110–111
  identification of, 110
Abdominal disease, differential diagnosis of, 355
Abdominal distention, differential diagnosis of, 638
Abdominal effusions, cytologic findings with, 111–113, 112*f*
Abdominal masses
  cytologic findings with, 106–107
  palpation of, 106
Abdominal pain, differential diagnosis of, 635
Abdominal pressure wraps, contraindications to, 394
Abdominal trauma, caused by high-rise fall, 394
Abdominal wall injuries, caused by high-rise fall, 394
Abdominocentesis, indications for, 394
Abnormal behavior. *See* Behavioral problems
Abnormal gait, differential diagnosis of, 651
Abortion(s), 470*f*, 470–473
  caused by infectious agents, 365, 470–472
  differential diagnosis of, 635–636
  induction of, 463
Abscess(es). *See also specific type*
  differential diagnosis of, 636
  nonhealing, associated with feline immunodeficiency virus, 349, 349*f*
  secondary to cat fights, cytologic findings with, 99*f*, 108
Abscess drainage, 479, 479*f*
  postoperative care for, 479
  surgical technique for, 479
Absence seizures, 220*t*
Abyssinian, 4, 4*f*
  diseases of eyelid in, 320*t*
  nervous system disorders in, 165*t*
  periodontitis in, 442
Abyssinian ticked tabby pattern, 3
Acaricide, for otodectic mange, 512
Accordion pleating, 118, 118*f*
Accu-Chek II meter, 311
ACD. *See* Acid-citrate-dextrose
Acepromazine. *See* Acetylpromazine
Acetaminophen, 559–560
  anemia caused by, 160
  contraindications to, 48
  toxicosis, 385–387
    treatment of, 385–387
N-Acetylcysteine, 385–387, 559, 563
β-D-*N*-Acetylhexosaminidase deficiency, 346
Acetylpromazine
  dosage and administration of, 114, 284
  for feline asthma, 235
  for hypertrophic cardiomyopathy, 247
  indications for, 71–72, 114, 119, 284, 498
  for thromboembolic disease, 253
Acetylpromazine-oxymorphone, indications for, 498
Acid-citrate-dextrose, for anticoagulation, 65
Acidemia, in chronic renal disease, 284
Acidifiers. *See* Urinary acidifiers
Acid orlein Giemsa staining (AOG), 506
Acidosis, 310
  treatment of, 310–311
Acid-to-base status, evaluation of, with diuresis, 282
Acne, 537–538, 538*f*
Acoustic impedance, in ultrasonography, 144
Acoustic shadowing artifact, in ultrasonography, 144, 147, 148*f*, 150*f*
Acromegaly
  in diabetic cats, 315
  diagnosis of, 211, 211*t*
  etiology of, 211
  PU/PD syndrome caused by, 210–211
ACTH. *See* Adrenocorticotropic hormone
Actinobacillus, 442
Actinomyces, 509
Activated clotting time, 88
  normal value for, 82
Activated partial thromboplastin time, normal value for, 82
Acute necrotizing ulcerative gingivitis, 444
Adenine arabinoside, indications for, 328
Adenitis, 327
Adenocarcinoma
  gastrointestinal, 226, 431
    caused by megestrol acetate, 50*f*
  mammary, cytologic findings with, 106*f*, 109
  nasal, 433–434
  pulmonary, 434–435
  renal, 435
Adenomas
  nasal, 434
  thyroid. *See* Hyperthyroidism; Thyroid adenomas
Adenomatous hyperplasia, of thyroid gland, 401
ADH. *See* Antidiuretic hormone
Adrenalin. *See* Epinephrine
Adrenocorticotropic hormone level, test for, 88
  normal value, 83
Adrenocorticotropic hormone stimulation test, 88
  in diagnosis of PU/PD syndrome, 210, 210*t*, 214
Adriamycin, indications for, 431
Aelurostrongylus abstrussus infestation, test for, 88
Aerophagia, 173, 175*f*
Aerosol transmission of infectious diseases, 420
AErrane. *See* Isoflurane
Afrin nasal spray, 574
Agar gel immunodiffusion, 546
Age, assessment of, by examination of teeth, 34, 34*f*
Aggregate reticulocytes, 158, 159*f*, 159–160
Aggression, 240–243
  fear-induced or defensive, 242–243
  idiopathic, 243
  interfeline, 240–242, 241*t*
  intermale, 240–241
  patient monitoring with, 243
  play, 242
  redirected, 242
  related to being petted, 243
  territorial, 240–241, 243
  toward people, 241*t*, 242–243
AGID. *See* Agar gel immunodiffusion
A/G ratio. *See* Albumin/globulin ratio
AHA. *See* Autoimmune hemolytic anemia
AI. *See* Artificial insemination
Air embolism, secondary to pneumocystography, 128
Airway diseases/disorders, dyspnea caused by, 177
Airway suctioning, for hypertrophic cardiomyopathy, 247
Alanine aminotransferase, test for
  diseases affecting, 86
  normal value, 82
Albumin, 461
  test for
    diseases affecting, 86
    normal value, 82–83
Albumin/globulin ratio, test for, normal value, 82
Alimentary lymphosarcoma, 428
Alkaline phosphatase, test for
  diseases affecting, 86
  normal value, 82
Alkalizing agents, drug interactions, 52*t*
Allergens, causing feline asthma, 231
  control of, 234
Allergic gastroenteritis, 223–224
Allergic inhalant dermatitis, 521–523
  clinical signs of, 521–522, 522*f*
  diagnosis of, 522
  immunotherapy for, 523, 523*t*
  pathogenesis of, 521
  therapy for, 522–523
Allescheria, 509
Alopecia
  differential diagnosis of, 636
    laboratory testing for, 93
  identification of, 32, 33*f*
  non–self-induced, 537
  pruritic, 537
  psychogenic, 537
  self-induced, 537
  symmetric, 535–537
    clinical evaluation of, 535–536, 536*f*
    clinical signs of, 535, 536*f*
    diagnosis of, 536–537
Alpha-fetoprotein, 461
ALT. *See* Alanine aminotransferase
Aluminum hydroxide, 559
  drug interactions, 52*t*
Alveolar bone, 291, 291*f*
Alveolar pulmonary pattern, 182
Ambi-Pen. *See* Penicillin G procaine/penicillin G benzathine combination
American Bobtail, 4
American Cat Show, 3
American Curl, 4–5
  longhair, 4*f*, 4–5
  shorthair, 4–5, 5*f*
American Shorthair, 5, 5*f*
  autonomic polyganglionopathy in, 321
American Wirehair, 5–6, 6*f*
Amiglyde. *See* Amikacin
Amiglyde-V. *See* Amikacin

Amikacin
for acute upper respiratory infections, 574
drug interactions, 52*t*
for feline asthma, 235
for pyrothorax, 456
Aminoglycosides
drug interactions, 52*t*
for neurologic disease, 168
for pyothorax, 456
Aminopentamide, 262
Aminophylline
dosage, 234*t*
for feline asthma, 235
for heartworm disease, 382
for hypertrophic cardiomyopathy, 247
Amitraz, 513–515
Amitriptyline, 238
Ammonium chloride, 50, 372
drug interactions, 52*t*
A-mode, 145
Amoxicillin, 44
for acute upper respiratory infections, 574
for cholangitis/cholangiohepatitis, 262
for feline asthma, 235
indications for, 374, 456, 479–480
for lymphocytic cholangitis/cholangiohepatitis, 263
prophylactic, for inflammatory bowel disease, 414
Amoxicillin/clavulanic acid, 44
for acute upper respiratory infections, 574
for eosinophilic granuloma complex, 535
indications for, 456, 479
Amoxi-Tabs. *See* Amoxicillin
Amphotericin B, 548
for blastomycosis, 547
for cryptococcosis, 543
drug interactions, 52*t*
for histoplasmosis, 545
for toxoplasmosis, 168
Ampicillin
for acute upper respiratory infections, 574
antimicrobial therapy with, 168
for cholangitis/cholangiohepatitis, 262
indications for, 456
Amplitude mode, 145
Amylase
test for
diseases affecting, 86
normal value, 82
urinary, normal value, 84
Anabolic steroids
contraindications to, 410*t*
indications for, 284
Anadrol-50. *See* Oxymethalone
Anaerobic infection, 455–456
common characteristics of, 456*t*
Anagen defluxion, 537
Anechoic images, 145
Anemia, 64, 157–163. *See also* Autoimmune hemolytic anemia; Heinz body hemolytic anemia; Hemobartonellosis; Nonregenerative anemia; Regenerative anemia
aplastic, caused by feline leukemia virus, 365
bone marrow response to, 159–162
caused by medications, 160, 384–385, 387
clinical signs of, 157
concurrent causes of, 162
definition of, 157
diagnosis of, 157–159, 158*f*, 159*t*
with blood smear, 64, 157, 158*f*, 384, 385*f*
with Coombs test, 160–162
flow chart for, 161*f*
differential diagnosis of, 64, 636–637
Heinz-body, 160
hemolytic, 159–160
hemorrhagic, 159–160
historical perspective on, 157
iron deficiency, 162
laboratory testing for, 157
mechanisms of, 159, 389
medication-induced, 162
muscle weakness caused by, 258
Anemic retinopathy, 343
Anesthesia, 56–61
adverse reactions to, 59
prevention of, 59–60
art of, 56
and fractious cat, 59–61
intubation for, 58
monitoring during, 56, 58–59
options for, 56–58
principles of, 56
Anesthesia circuit, non-rebreathing, 58
Anesthetic(s), 56–61
antagonist, 57*t*
concentrations, 57*t*
contraindications to, 472
dosages, 57*t*
inhalant, for restraint, 373
local, drug interactions, 53*t*
Anesthetic combinations
antagonists, 57*t*
concentrations, 57*t*
dosages, 57*t*
Anesthetic monitors, 58–59, 59*t*
Anestrus, 458, 461
lactational, 465
Angiocardiography
indications for, 177
nonselective, 138, 138*f*
of aorta, 137, 137*f*
of cardiomyopathy, 245, 247*f*, 248, 249*f*, 251
of saddle thrombus, 253, 253*f*
Angiocath short catheter, 477
Angular process, 291*f*
Animal Blood Bank, 65
Anion gap, 566–567
test for
diseases affecting, 86
normal value, 82
Anisocuria, differential diagnosis of, 637
Anisocytosis, of erythrocytes, 160
Ankyloblepharon, 321
Anodontia, 303
Anogenital reflex, definition of, 39
Anophthalmia, 317
Anorectic cat(s)
administration of fluid to, 41
force feeding of
complications of, 42
methods for, 41–43, 42*f*
schedule for, 41
with surgically implanted feeding tubes, 42–43, 411, 483–486
with idiopathic hepatic lipidosis, feeding methods for, 411
nutritional needs of, 40
selection of diet for, 40–41
stimulation of appetite in, 40, 42*t*, 285, 285*t*, 411
syringe feeding of, at home, 42
Anorexia, 40–43
after removal of urethral obstruction, 375
causes of, 41*t*
secondary disorders associated with, 40
treatment of
chemotherapeutic methods for, 40, 42*t*
physical methods for, 40–43
Antacids, drug interactions, 52*t*
Anterior uveitis, 332
associated with feline immunodeficiency virus, 333–334, 334*f*
associated with feline infectious peritonitis, 334, 334*f*
associated with feline leukemia virus, 333, 333*f*
associated with toxoplasmosis, 334, 334*f*
clinical signs of, 332–333
diagnosis of, 334–335
etiology of, 332–334
treatment of, 335
Anthelminthics, 557–558
Antibiotic(s). *See also* Aminoglycosides
for acute upper respiratory infections, 573–574
for chronic nasal discharge, 272
contraindications to, 472
for eosinophilic granuloma complex, 535
for feline asthma, 231, 235
indications for, 372, 374, 395, 479
for lymphocytic cholangitis/cholangiohepatitis, 262–263
for neonatal bacterial sepsis, 466
prophylactic, for inflammatory bowel disease, 414
for pyothorax, 456
for suppurative cholangitis/cholangiohepatitis, 262
topical, for corneal injury, 318
Antibody tests, versus antigen tests, 81
Anticancer drugs, 427*t*. *See also* Chemotherapy
contraindications to, 472
Anticholinergics, contraindications to, 498
Anticoagulant rodenticides, 555–556
median lethal doses of, 556*t*
Anticoagulants, for blood transfusion, 65
Anticonvulsants
contraindications to, 472
maintenance therapy with, 221
Antidiuretic hormone, 207
deficiency, 208
treatment of, 216
partial production of, 208
synthetic analogues of, 216
Antifungal therapy, 548
contraindications to, 472
for toxoplasmosis, 168
Antigen tests, versus antibody tests, 81
Antihistamines
for allergic inhalant dermatitis, 522
for chronic nasal discharge, 272
for flea allergic dermatitis, 519–521
indications for, 525
Anti-inflammatory agents, contraindications to, 472
Antimicrobial therapy, for neurologic disease, 168–169
Antiprostaglandin drugs, indications for, 252
Antirobe. *See* Clindamycin
Antispasmodic drugs
dosage and administration of, 49
indications for, 374
side effects of, 49
Antithyroid drugs
continuous management of hyperthyroidism with, 406–407
indications for, 404
side effects of, 407
Antivertigo therapy, 169
Antiviral agents, ophthalmic, 574
Aorta, nonselective angiogram of, 137, 137*f*
Aortic embolus, radiologic findings with, 137, 137*f*
apALERT. *See* Vet Alarm Respiratory Monitor
Appetite, increased. *See* Polyphagia
Appetite-stimulating drugs
dosage and administration of, 42*t*, 285*t*
indications for, 40, 285, 411
Apple core appearance, of intestinal lesions, 118
Apresoline. *See* Hydralazine
APTT. *See* Activated partial thromboplastin time
Aqueous, flow of, 338
Arginine, dietary, for hepatic lipidosis, 411*t*
Arrhythmia, differential diagnosis of, 637–638
Arterial pH, estimation of, based on serum total CO_2 and degree of hyperventilation, 310, 310*t*
Arthritis
differential diagnosis of, 638
treatment of, 49
Arthus-type vasculitis. *See* Disseminated pyogranulomatous vasculitis
Artificial insemination, 466–467
Artificial tears, indications for, 326–327
Ascites
diagnosis of, with abdominal fluid aspiration, 113
differential diagnosis of, 638
ultrasonographic evaluation of, 151, 152*f*
Ascorbic acid, 387
Asian Leopard cat, 6–7
Aspartate aminotransferase
elevated levels of, in thromboembolic disease, 252
test for, normal value, 82
Aspiration cytology. *See* Cytology; Tissue aspiration
Aspiration pneumonia, 182, 187*f*
Aspirin
contraindications to, 49
for dilated cardiomyopathy, 250
dosage and administration of, 49
drug interactions, 52*t*
for heartworm disease, 382
for hypertrophic cardiomyopathy, 247
indications for, 358
rate of excretion, 48
safe dosage interval for, 48
for thromboembolic disease, 252–253
for thrombus prevention, 251, 254
toxicity, 560
AST. *See* Aspartate aminotransferase
Asteroid hyalosis, 338
Asthma, 182, 185*f*, 231–235
clinical signs of, 231–232

Asthma (*continued*)
  diagnosis of, 232–234, 232*f*–234*f*
    with lung aspiration, 107
  pathophysiology of, 231
  pharmacological treatment of, 234*t*
  prognosis for, 235
  severe, 182, 187*f*
  staging of, 232, 232*t*
  treatment of, 234–235
    goals of, 234
Ataxia/paresis, 164–171. *See also* Paralysis
  breed predilections for, 165*t*
  classification of, DAMNIT scheme for, 165*t*
  clinical presentation of, 165–167
  diagnostic plan for, 167–168, 168*t*
  differential diagnosis of, 167, 167*t*, 638–639
  history with, 164
  neurologic examination of, 164–165
  physical examination of, 164
  signalment, 164
  therapy for, 168–169
  time/sign progression of, 165*t*
Atopy. *See* Allergic inhalant dermatitis
Atresia, lacrimal punctum, 327
Atropine. *See also* Diphenoxylate with atropine
  dosage, 56, 65, 234*t*
  for feline asthma, 234
  indications for, 169, 335
  ophthalmic ointment, indications for, 318
Atropine sulfate, for toxicosis, 561
Attenuation, in ultrasonography, 144
Aurothioglucose
  dosage and administration of, 444
  indications for, 444
Autoimmune disease, involving oral cavity, 444
Autoimmune hemolytic anemia, 160–162
Autonomic polyganglionopathy, 321–322
Avon Skin-So-Soft, 520
Awn hairs, 4
Ayres T Anesthesia Circuit, 58
Azaleas, 565
Azathioprine
  indications for, 358, 444
  for inflammatory bowel disease, 414
  for plasmacytic-lymphocytic stomatitis, 444
  side effects of, 414
Azo Gantrisin. *See* Phenazopyridine
Azotemia, 276
  definition of, 274
  etiology of, 276–277
  prerenal, 248
  types of, 276*t*, 276–277
Azulfidine. *See* Sulfasalazine

Bacillus piriformis, 261
Back pain, differential diagnosis of, 399
Bacterial contamination, of blood for transfusion, 67
Bacterial cystitis, 377
  after perineal urethrostomy, 496
Bacterial enteritis/colitis, 225
  diagnosis of, 225
Bacterial flora, of colon, normal, 225*f*
Bacterial infections
  abortions caused by, 472
  gastrointestinal, 225
Bacterial keratitis, 328
Bacterial pneumonia, 182, 186*f*
Bacterial sepsis, neonatal, 466
Bacteroides, 442
Baermann technique, 88
Baking soda, for bicarbonate therapy, 284
Balinese, 6, 6*f*
Banamine. *See* Flumixin meglumine
Barbiturates
  contraindications to, 221
  drug interactions, 52*t*
  indications for, 56, 373, 500, 552
Barium
  for esophagagram, 114
  for gastrointestinal series, 115, 118*f*, 177
  powdered, 119
Barium enema, 119–121
  clinical indications for, 119
  common lesions diagnosed with, 121, 121*f*
  goals of, 119
  materials for, 121
  normal findings with, 121, 121*f*
  technique for, 121
Baroreceptors, 207
Basal cell tumors, 528, 529*f*
  cytologic findings with, 110, 110*f*
Basal energy requirement, 40
Basaljel capsules, 283
Basophils, test for, diseases affecting, 85
Bauer Temno Biopsy Needle, 425
Bayer Children's Aspirin. *See* Aspirin
Baygon. *See* Propoxur
Baytril. *See* Enrofloxacin
B-complex vitamins, 410
BDC. *See* Bile duct carcinoma
Beckman Glucose Analyzer, 311
Beeper, 59, 59*t*
Beeper Plus, 59
Behavioral problems, 236–243. *See also* Clawing; Elimination behavior problems; Spraying
  differential diagnosis of, 399, 635
  prevention of, 243
Bendiocarb, 560–561
Bengal, 6*f*, 6–7
Benzocaine
  anemia caused by, 160, 387
  contraindications to, 48
Benzodiazepines
  contraindications to, 410*t*
  to stimulate appetite in anorectic cats, 40, 42*t*, 285, 285*t*, 411
Benzyl alcohol, contraindications to, 48
BER. *See* Basal energy requirement
Bereavement, definition of, 73
Bereavement reactions
  in adolescents, 75
  in children, 74–75
  definition of, 73
Betamethasone, dosage and administration of, 335
Betasone. *See* Betamethasone
Bethanechol, 375
Beuthanasia-D Solution, 72
BHV-4 (strain FCAHV), 369–370
Bicarbonate
  for oliguria, 280
  serum, estimation of arterial pH with, 310, 310*t*
  test for, diseases affecting, 86
Bicarbonate deficit
  associated with metabolic acidosis, 282
  calculation of, 282
Bicarbonate replacement, 282
Bi-color Persian, 20
Bile acid concentrations, test for, 88–89
  normal value, 82
Bile duct carcinoma, 432
Bile pigment deposition, 195
Bile sludging, 263, 264*f*
Bile stasis, ultrasonographic findings with, 146, 147*f*–148*f*
Biliary cirrhosis, 263, 263*f*
  definition of, 261
Biliary obstruction
  icterus caused by, 197*f*, 197–198
  treatment of, 263–264
Bilirubin
  direct, normal value for, 82
  test for, diseases affecting, 86
  total, normal value for, 82
  urinary, normal value for, 84
Biochemical profile
  in diagnosis of feline infectious peritonitis, 357
  in diagnosis of thromboembolic disease, 252–253
  diseases affecting, 86–88
  normal values for, 82
Biopsy(ies), 425–426. *See also specific type*
Biopsy specimen, versus cytologic specimen, 95
Bio-Tal. *See* Thiamylal sodium
Birman, 7, 7*f*
  diseases of eyelid in, 320*t*
Bisacodyl, 419*t*
Bismuth subsalicylate, 49, 559
Bite wounds. *See also* Cat bites
  abscesses/cellulitis secondary to, cytologic findings with, 99*f*, 108
  characteristics of, 479
  nonhealing, associated with feline immunodeficiency virus, 349, 349*f*
  transmission of feline immunodeficiency virus via, 348
  transmission of feline leukemia virus via, 361
Bladder
  filling defects of, radiologic findings with, 128, 131*f*, 133*f*
  ruptured, radiologic findings with, 127, 130*f*
  ultrasonographic evaluation of, 150, 150*f*
Bladder atony, after catheterization, 375
Bladder catheter(s)
  in closed urinary collecting system, 281, 281*t*
  indwelling, for removal of urethral obstruction, 374, 374*f*, 375
  for removal of urethral obstructions, 373, 373*f*, 492
Bladder catheterization
  fluid therapy after, 374–375
  with French catheter, 124, 126*f*
  restraint for, 372–373, 373*f*
Bladder distention, differential diagnosis of, 663
Bladder injuries, caused by high-rise fall, 394
Bladder marsupialization, 479–480
  indications for, 375
  results of, 480
  surgical technique for, 479–480, 480*f*
Bladder palpation, diagnosis of feline urologic syndrome with, 371
Bladder polyps, radiologic findings with, 128, 131*f*
Bladder tumors, 377, 435
  radiologic findings with, 128, 131*f*
Blastomyces dermatitides, 333, 344, 546, 546*f*
Blastomycosis, 182, 189*f*, 344, 545–547
  clinical signs of, 546
  diagnosis of, 546, 546*f*
  etiology and epidemiology of, 545–546
  pathogenesis of, 546
  public health implications of, 549
  treatment of, 547
Bleach
  household
    destruction of feline infectious peritonitis virus with, 352
    destruction of feline leukemia virus with, 361
    for disinfection of multicat facilities, 424
  as irrigant for root canal procedures, 299
Bleeding, abnormal, differential diagnosis of, 640–641
Bleeding time, normal value for, 82
Blepharitis, 322, 323*t*
Blindness, 33, 33*f*
  differential diagnosis of, 639
Blink reflex, 319
Blisters, differential diagnosis of, 639
Bloating, differential diagnosis of, 638
Blood
  enzyme-linked immunosorbent assay of, 81
  filtering of, for transfusion, 67
  storage of, 65
  warming of, for transfusion, 67
Blood collection, 62, 62*f*, 62–63, 63*f*
  equipment for, 62
  for transfusion, 65
Blood glucose level test, blood collection for, 62, 62*f*
Blood loss
  anemia caused by, 159
  chronic, 162
  regenerative anemias secondary to, 162
Blood profile
  amount of blood necessary for, 62
  for cardiac disease, 248
  for chronic renal disease, 275
Blood smear
  collection for, 62, 62*f*
  for diagnosis of anemia, 64, 157, 158*f*, 384, 385*f*
  white blood cell estimation from, 93
Blood transfusions, 64–68
  administration rate, 66
  adverse reactions to, 66–67
  bacterial contamination of blood used for, 67
  blood collection for, 65
  blood storage for, 65
  circulatory overload caused by, 67
  complications associated with, 67
  crossmatching for, 66
  donor for, 65
  filtering and warming of blood for, 67
  goal of, 67
  hemorrhage caused by, 67
  indications for, 64–66
  major determinants for, 65
  methods for, 65*f*, 65–66
  quantity of blood needed for, 67–68
    formulas for, 67, 67*t*
  for shock from abdominal hemorrhage, 394
  testing of packed cell volume with, 67–68

Blood typing, 66*t*, 66–67
Blood urea nitrogen
elevated levels of, 274
in chronic renal disease, 276–277
test for
diseases affecting, 87–88
normal value, 82
Blood values, at different ages, 83
Blunt trauma, diagnosis of, with liver aspirate, 104
B-mode, 145
Body, disposition of, after euthanasia, 72
Body fluid aspiration, 110–113
other tests used in conjunction with, 110
technique for, 110
Body or horizontal ramus, 291*f*
Body splint, 394–395
Body temperature. *See also* Fever
fluctuations in, 191
normal, 191
regulation of, 191
Body water regulation, normal, 207
Boldenone undecylenate
preparations, 42*t*
recommended dosage, 42*t*
Bombay, 7, 7*f*
Bond buttons, for tooth movement, 302
Bone marrow
chemotherapy-induced toxicity involving, 426–427
tests of, normal values for, 83
Bone marrow activity, indicators of, 64, 65*f*, 160
Bone marrow aspiration, 89–90, 89*f*–90*f*
for anemia, 162
Bone marrow biopsy, indications for, 194
Bone marrow response, to anemia, 159–162
Bone marrow suppression
anemia caused by, 159
diseases causing, 85
Bone tumors, 432–433
incidence of, 432
rare primary, 433
secondary, 433
Boric acid, 562–563
Bowel disease. *See* Gastrointestinal disorders; Gastrointestinal infections; Infiltrative bowel disease; Inflammatory bowel disease; Vomiting/diarrhea
Bowen's disease, 528, 529*f*
Bowman's membrane, 328
Brachicladium, 509
Brachycephalic breeds
congenital orbital disorders in, 317
prognathic malocclusion in, 301–302
Brachygnathic malocclusions, 301, 302*f*, 302–303
Bradycardia, differential diagnosis of, 639–640
Bran supplementation, 414, 555
Breath odor, abnormal
caused by cervical line lesions, 294
differential diagnosis of, 640
Breed(s), 3–27
CFA registration of, 3–4
definition of, 3
evolution of, 3
and human preferences, 3
Breeding. *See also* Reproduction
guidelines for, 37
normal, 466
repeated, and failure to ovulate, 468–469
Breeding soundness examination, 466
Breed registries, 3
Brethine. *See* Terbutaline
Brightness mode, 145
British Shorthair, 7–8, 8*f*
autonomic polyganglionopathy in, 321
British Ticks. *See* Abyssinian
Brodifacoum, 556
Bromadiolone, 556
Bromethalin rodenticides, 557
Bronchial asthma. *See* Asthma
Bronchial gland, adenocarcinoma of, 434–435
Bronchial obstruction, 177
Bronchial pattern, 182
in asthmatic cat, 233*f*
Bronchial thickening, in asthmatic cat, 232, 233*f*
Bronchoalveolar lavage, indications for, 176
Bronchodilation, for feline asthma, 234*t*, 234–235
Bronchospasm, in feline asthma, 231
alleviation of, 234
Buffy coat prep, 90
BUN. *See* Blood urea nitrogen
Bunny Cats. *See* Abyssinian
Buphthalmia, 339, 339*f*, 340
Burmese, 8*f*, 8–9
corneal sequestrum in, 330
CVF/MW complex in, 256, 258
diseases of eyelid in, 320*t*
predilection for nervous system disorders, 165*t*
predilection for periodontitis in, 443
predilection for seizure disorders among, 219*t*
Burmese shuffle, 9
Burmilla, 9
Burr
repair of chipped tooth with, 298
tooth extraction with, 298
for treatment of enamel hypoplasia, 304
Butorphanol, 253, 393
Butterfly catheters, 477
for blood transfusions, 65, 65*f*
placement of, procedure for, 477–478

Cage/carrier, 28
removal of cat from, 28–29
Cage confinement
for cardiomyopathy, 247, 249
indications for, 251
for thromboembolic disease, 253
CAHV. *See* Cell-associated herpesvirus
Calcimar. *See* Calcitonin
Calcitonin, 557
Calcium, test for
diseases affecting, 86–87
normal value, 82
Calcium carbonate
drug interactions, 52*t*
sources of, 285*t*
Calcium gluconate
for hypocalcemia, 406
indications for, 374
for oliguria, 280
Calcium hydroxide
for pulpotomy, 299
for root canal procedures, 295
Calcium lactate, for hypocalcemia, 406
Calcium oxalate crystals, 372
Calcium salts, drug interactions, 52*t*
Calcium supplementation, for hypocalcemia, 406
Calculi
cholecystic, ultrasonographic findings with, 146, 148*f*
cystic, ultrasonographic findings with, 150, 150*f*
ultrasonographic characteristics of, 145
Calculus removal, 441
California Spangled Cat, 9
Campylobacteriosis, 225
Campylobacter jejuni, 225
Cancer cells, metastatic, morphologic characteristics of, 202
Canine coronavirus, 352
Caparsolate. *See* Thiacetarsamide
Capillaria aerophila infestation, test for, 88
Capillary refill time
decreased (less than 1 sec), differential diagnosis of, 640
prolonged (more than 2 sec), differential diagnosis of, 640
Capoten. *See* Captopril
Capsules
administration of, 45*f*, 45–47, 46*f*
versus tablets, 44
dissolving in liquids, 47
masking taste/lubricating of, 45
Captan, for dermatophytosis, 507*t*
Captopril
contraindications to, 247
for dilated cardiomyopathy, 250
Car accidents, head injuries from, 447
Carafate. *See* Sucralfate
Carbamate insecticides, 560–561
lethal doses of, 561*t*
Carbaryl, toxicity, 560–561
Carbaryl shampoo, for demodectic mange, 515
Carbofuran, 560–561
Carbon dioxide, total, normal value for, 82
Carbonic anhydrase inhibitor diuretics, for glaucoma, 340
Cardiac disease, 244. *See also* Cardiomyopathy; Thromboembolic disease
Cardiac glycoside toxicosis, 565
Cardiac irregularity, differential diagnosis of, 637–638
Cardiomegaly, in heartworm-infected cat, 379, 381*f*
Cardiomyopathy, 244–252. *See also* Hypertrophic cardiomyopathy
congestive
radiologic findings with, 138, 138*f*
ultrasonographic findings with, 152, 152*f*
diagnosis of, 112*t*
with body fluid aspiration, 111
dilated, 248*f*–249*f*, 248–250
incidence of, 244
major forms of, 244, 245*t*
presumptive diagnosis of, 251–252
factors used to establish, 251
treatment based on, 251–252
restrictive, 250–251
taurine-related, 244, 248, 250
and thromboembolism, 252
ultrasonographic findings with, 152–153
Cardiotoxic plants, 565
Cardiovascular support, for toxicosis, 552, 552*t*
Cardiovascular system, radiologic evaluation of, 137–138
Cardizem Tablets. *See* Diltiazem
Carlin IV Feeding Splint, 478
Carnitine, dietary, for hepatic lipidosis, 410, 411*t*
Carpal injuries, caused by high-rise fall, management of, 395
Carriers. *See* Cage/carrier
Casec Powder, 41
Castration
and intermale aggression, 240
and reduction in marking behavior, 238
Cataracts, 336*f*, 336–338
diabetic, 336
formation of, 33, 33*f*
traumatic, 336, 337*f*
treatment of, 337–338
Cat bag, 29
Cat bites. *See also* Bite wounds
to humans, 577, 579*f*
Cat Book Poems, The, 14, 22
Cat Fanciers' Association, 3–4
registration of breeds with, 3
Cat Fancy Magazine, 72
Cat fur mite, 515–516, 517*f*
Cathartics, for toxicosis, 554–555
Catheter(s). *See* Bladder catheter(s); Intravenous catheter(s)
Catheterization. *See* Bladder catheterization; Intravenous catheterization
Catnip, 564
CatScan B, 376
CatScan G, 312
CatScan pH, 376
Cat scratch disease, 577–579
Cat scratch disease antigen skin test, 578
Cat shows, 3–4
Cattery(ies)
control of infectious diseases in, 422
definition of, 420
management of dermatophytosis in, 508
prevention of upper respiratory infections in, 575
Caudal lung lobes, interstitial infiltrates in, in heartworm-infected cat, 379, 381*f*
Caudal pulmonary arteries, blunting of, in heartworm-infected cat, 379, 382*f*
Cavity classification, Black's modified, 295
Cavity varnish, 298
CBC. *See* Complete blood count
CCHS. *See* Cholangitis/cholangiohepatitis syndrome
CCV. *See* Canine coronavirus
CDI. *See* Central diabetes insipidus
Cefadroxil, 44, 262, 535
Cefa-Tabs. *See* Cefadroxil
CEJ. *See* Cementoenamel junction
Celiogram, 141, 142*f*
Cell-associated herpesvirus, feline urologic syndrome caused by, 369
Cell collection techniques, for cytology, 96–98
Cell-mediated immune response, in feline infectious peritonitis, 353
Cells, normal, characteristics of, 100
Cellular patterns, basic, cytologic interpretation of, 98*t*, 98*f*–99*f*, 98–100
Cellulitis
oral, 290
orbital, 318–319
periorbital, 318–319
secondary to cat fights, cytologic findings with, 99*f*, 108

Cemento-enamel junction, lesions at, 293–294
Cementum, 291, 291*f*
Central diabetes insipidus, 208
  water deprivation testing in, 216, 216*t*
Central nervous system disorders. *See also* Ataxia/paresis; Paralysis
  caused by *Cryptococcus neoformans,* 542
  caused by noneffusive feline infectious peritonitis, 355
  differential diagnosis of, 428
Central nervous system support, for toxicosis, 552, 552*t,* 553
Central nervous system tumors, 169, 428
Centrine. *See* Aminopentamide
Cephalic vein
  blood collection from, 62, 62*f*
  catheterization, 477–478, 478*f*
  drug administration through, for euthanasia, 72
Cephalosporins
  drug interactions, 52*t*
  for neurologic disease, 168
Cephulac. *See* Lactulose
Cerebellar signs, differential diagnosis of, 640
Cerebrospinal fluid analysis
  in evaluation of neurologic disease, 168
  indications for, 194
  normal values for, 84
Cerumen gland tumors, 528–530
Ceruminolytic agent, indications for, 511–512
Cervical area, physical examination of, 35
Cervical line lesions, 293–297
  classification of, 295
  clinical signs of, 294
  diagnosis of, 294–296
  etiology of, 293–294
  history of, 293
  incidence of, 293–294
  restoration of, 295
  stage I (cementum or enamel only), 295, 295*f*
  stage II (through cementum/enamel into dentin), 295
  stage III (through dentin into pulp cavity), 295–296, 296*f*
  stage IV (extensive structural damage, fragile tooth), 296, 296*f*
  stage V (crown lost, roots still present), 296
  treatment of, 294–297
Cervical stimulation. *See* Coital stimulation
Cervical ventroflexion, 256–260
  definition of, 256, 257*f*
  differential diagnosis of, 655
Cervical ventroflexion/muscle weakness complex, 256
  clinical signs of, 256, 257*f*
  diagnosis of, 257–258
  differential diagnosis of, 258
  etiology of, 256–257
  incidence of, 256
  treatment of, 258–260
Cesarean section, indications for, 464
Cetacaine. *See* Benzocaine
CFA. *See* Cat Fanciers' Association
Chalazion, 322
Charcoal, activated, 554–555
  contraindications to, 555
Charges, for euthanasia, 72
Chartreux, 9, 9*f*
Chemosis, differential diagnosis of, 640
Chemotherapeutic drugs, 427*t*
Chemotherapy, 426–427
  contraindications to, 472
  toxicity, 426–427
Chemotherapy protocols, for lymphosarcoma, 429*t,* 429–430
Chemstrip bG reagent strips, 311
Cherry eye, 326
Chest, physical examination of, 35–36
Chest drainage, closed, indications for, 497
Cheyletiella, 513, 513*f*
Cheyletiellosis, 513–514
  clinical signs of, 513
  diagnosis of, 513–514
  etiology and pathogenesis of, 513, 513*f*
  therapy for, 514
Chiggers, 515
Children, bereavement reactions in, 74–75
Chlamydia psittaci, 421, 573, 575
  effects on reproduction, 472
Chlamydiosis
  in multicat facilities, 421, 423
  vaccination against, recommendations for, 423*t*
Chlorambucil
  dose, 427*t*
  route of administration, 427*t*
  toxicity, 427*t*
Chloramphenicol
  for cholangitis/cholangiohepatitis, 262
  complications of, 162
  contraindications to, 49, 168, 410*t,* 574
  dosage and administration of, 49
  drug interactions, 52*t*
  for hemobartonellosis, 390
  ophthalmic, indications for, 574
  side effects of, 390
Chlorazol, in fungal stains, 506, 506*t*
Chlordane, contraindications to, 48
Chlor-Ethamine, 372
Chlorhexiderm. *See* Chlorhexidine
Chlorhexidine, 442
  for dermatophytosis, 507*t*
Chloride, test for, normal value, 82
Chlorinated hydrocarbons, 48
Chlorpheniramine, 522
Chlorphenolac formulation
  for diagnosis of ringworm, 506, 507*f*
  recipe for, 506*t*
Chlorpropamide, 216
Chlorpyrifos, 560–561
Cholangiohepatitis. *See also* Cholangitis/cholangiohepatitis syndrome
  definition of, 261
  diagnosis of, with liver aspirate, 104
Cholangitis, definition of, 261
Cholangitis/cholangiohepatitis syndrome, 197, 197*f,* 261–265. *See also* Biliary cirrhosis; Lymphocytic cholangitis/cholangiohepatitis
  classification of, 261
  sequelae and complications of, 263–265, 264*f*
  suppurative, 261–262
Cholecalciferol rodenticides, 556–557
Cholecystic calculi, ultrasonographic findings with, 146, 148*f*
Cholelithiasis, 197, 197*f,* 264
  radiographic appearance of, 264, 264*f*
  treatment of, 264
Cholesterol, test for, normal value, 82
Cholesterol-to-triglyceride ratio, 287
Choline, dietary, for hepatic lipidosis, 411*t*
Cholinesterase, test for, 90–91
Chondromas, 433
Chondrosarcoma, 433
Choroid, 332
Chromosomal abnormalities, 473
Chronic interstitial nephritis, 274
Chronic renal disease, 274–286
  acidemia in, 284
  anemia caused by, 162
  diagnosis of, 274–275
    clinical history in, 274
    laboratory testing in, 275, 275*t*
    physical examination in, 274–275, 275*t*
    radiology and ultrasonography in, 277–278
    renal biopsy in, 278–279
  initial care for, 279–280
  long-term medical management of, 282–285
  minimizing stress for cat with, 285
  nausea/vomiting in cats with, 284
  nutritional support in, 282
  patient monitoring in, 282
  positive nutritional state in, maintenance of, 284–285
  slowing progression of, 282–283
  treatment of, 279–285
Chronic renal failure, 166, 274
  diuresis for, 280–282
  preazotemic, 214
Chylothorax, 287–289
  clinical signs of, 287
  cytologic findings with, 288, 289*f*
  definition of, 287
  diagnosis of, 287–288
    with body fluid aspiration, 111, 111*f*
    criteria for, 112*t*
  etiology of, 287, 288*t*
  laboratory testing with, 287
  physical examination of cats with, 287
  prognosis for, 289
  radiographic findings with, 287, 288*f*
  secondary to diaphragmatic hernia, 288
  surgical treatment of, 288–289
  treatment of, 288–289, 497
Chylous fluid
  characteristics of, 289*t*
  diagnosis of, 287–288, 289*t*
Ciliary body, 332
Cimetidine
  dosage and administration of, 284, 434
  indications for, 284, 434, 559–560
CIN. *See* Chronic interstitial nephritis
Ciproflaxin, for cat scratch disease, 579
Circling, differential diagnosis of, 640
Circulatory overload, caused by blood transfusion, 67
Cirrhosis. *See* Biliary cirrhosis
Cisterna magna, landmarks for, 134–135
CITE COMBO FeLV antigen/FIV antibody test kit, 350
CITE FIV antibody test kit, 350
CITE Semi-Quant T4 Test Kit, 402
Citrate-phosphate-dextrose-adenine, for anticoagulation, 65
Citrate toxicity, caused by blood transfusions, 67
Citrulline, dietary, for hepatic lipidosis, 411*t*
Cladosporium, 509
Clavamox. *See* Amoxicillin/clavulanic acid
Clawing, 239–240
  causes of, 239
  diagnosis of, 239
  treatment of, 240
Clearing agents, recipes for, 506*t*
Clindamycin
  indications for, 456
  for plasmacytic-lymphocytic stomatitis, 444
  for toxoplasmosis, 168, 345
CLL. *See* Cervical line lesions
Clotrimazole, for dermatophytosis, 507*t*
CMIR. *See* Cell-mediated immune response
Coagulation defects, differential diagnosis of, 640–641
COAP, 429*t*
Coccidioides immitis, 333, 344, 547, 547*f*
Coccidioidomycosis, 344, 547–548
  clinical signs of, 547
  diagnosis of, 547, 547*f*
  etiology and epidemiology of, 547
  pathogenesis of, 547
  public health implications of, 549
  treatment of, 548
Coccidiosis, 224–225
  diagnosis of, 224
Cochran IV Splint, 478
Coiled spring appearance, of small bowel, 118
Coital stimulation
  inadequate, 469
  induction of ovulation by, 458–459
Coitus, unsuccessful, 469
Cold agglutinins, 389
Colectomy, subtotal, 416, 417*f,* 480–481
  results of, 481
  surgical technique for, 480–481, 481*f*
Colibar-V, 114
Colitis. *See also* Enteritis/colitis
  idiopathic, 225
  treatment of, 414
Collagenolytic granuloma. *See* Linear granuloma
Coloboma, 320*f,* 321
  treatment of, 321, 321*f*
Colon, normal bacterial flora of, 225*f*
Colorpoint Shorthair, 9–10, 10*f*
Coma, differential diagnosis of, 641
Complete blood count
  diseases affecting, 84–86
  normal values for, 82
Conceptus, proteins produced by, 461
Condyloid process, 291*f*
Confinement, for urination/defecation problems, 239. *See also* Cage confinement
Conjunctival disease, 327–328
Conjunctival emphysema, 327
Conjunctivitis, 328
  chlamydial, 325, 325*f*
  diagnosis of, 329*t*
  etiology of, 329*t*
  neonatal, prior to lid separation, 321, 322*f*
  symptoms of, 329*t*
  treatment of, 329*t*
Conofite. *See* Miconazole

Constipation
differential diagnosis of, 641
drugs used to treat, categories of, 418*t*
Contact allergic dermatitis, 523–524
clinical signs of, 523, 523*f*
diagnosis of, 524
pathogenesis of, 523
therapy for, 524
Convulsions, differential diagnosis of, 641–642
Coombs test, 389–390
diagnosis of anemias with, 160–162
Copal varnish, 298
Copulation, failure of, 468
Cornea, anatomy of, 328
Corneal disease, 328–331
differential diagnosis of, 331
Corneal edema, 339, 339*f*
Corneal reflex, definition of, 39
Corneal sequestrum, 330
diagnosis of, 330, 330*f*
incidence of, 330
treatment of, 330
type I, 330*f*
Corneal ulcer, differential diagnosis of, 642
Cornification, 459, 459*f*
Cornish Rex, 10, 10*f*
Coronavirus, 224, 348, 352. *See also* Feline enteric coronavirus
respiratory infection caused by, 573
Coronavirus titers
for diagnosis of feline infectious peritonitis, 357
procedures for, 357
Coronoid process, 291*f*
Corticomedullary junction, hyperechoic ring at, 149
Corticosteroids
for allergic inhalant dermatitis, 522
contraindications to, 262, 472
drug interactions, 52*t*
for eosinophilic granuloma complex, 446
for feline asthma, 234*t*
for immunosuppressed cats, 364
indications for, 340, 444
for lymphocytic cholangitis/cholangiohepatitis, 263
ocular effects of, 335
precautions with, 335
for shock, 393–394
for spinal cord trauma, 395
for toxicosis, 557
for uveitis, 335
Cortisol, test for, normal value, 83
Cotter's COP Protocol, 429*t*
Coughing, 172
in asthmatic cat, 231, 232*f*
caused by chylothorax, 287
differential diagnosis of, 642–643
Coxofemoral joint, luxated, physical examination for, 35, 35*f*
CPDA-1. *See* Citrate-phosphate-dextrose-adenine
CPK. *See* Creatine phosphokinase
Crackles, definition of, 173*t*
Cranial embolism, 252
CrCl. *See* Creatinine clearance
CRD. *See* Chronic renal disease
Creatine phosphokinase
elevated levels of, in thromboembolic disease, 252–253
test for, normal value, 82
Creatinine
elevated levels of, 274
in chronic renal disease, 276–277
test for, normal value, 82
urinary, normal value for, 84
Creatinine clearance test, 91. *See also* Endogenous creatinine clearance
CRF. *See* Chronic renal failure
Crossmatching, for blood transfusions, 66
Crown, 300
indications for, 300
procedures for, 300
Crown amputation, indications for, 302–303
Crying, differential diagnosis of, 643
Cryoepilation, for distichia, 322
Cryptococcosis, 344, 540–543
clinical signs of, 541–542, 541*f*–542*f*
diagnosis of, 542–543
etiology and epidemiology of, 540
pathogenesis of, 540–541
public health implications of, 548–549
treatment of, 543
Cryptococcus neoformans, 266, 333, 344, 502, 540
identification of, 272, 273*f,* 541*f*–542*f,* 542–543
respiratory infection caused by, 571, 573
Cryptosporidiosis, 225
CSD. *See* Cat scratch disease
Ctenocephalides felis, 518
C:T ratio. *See* Cholesterol-to-triglyceride ratio
Cultures, indications for, 194. *See also specific type*
Curettes, for prophylactic dental care, 441
Curled ear. *See* American Curl
Curvularia, 509
Cutauxzoon felis, 160
Cuterebra, 516, 516*f*
CVF/MW complex. *See* Cervical ventroflexion/muscle weakness complex
Cyanosis, differential diagnosis of, 643
Cyclamen, 565
Cyclophosphamide
dose, 427*t*
indications for, 358, 444
route of administration, 427*t*
side effects of, 427
toxicity, 427*t*
Cycloplegics, indications for, 335
Cyclosporine, 327
Cycylophosphamide, indications for, 431
Cymric, 10–11, 11*f*
Cyst(s)
intrapulmonary, ruptured, 182, 183*f*
pulmonary, caused by *Paragonimus kellicolli,* 182, 183*f*
subcapsular renal, radiologic findings with, 122
ultrasonographic characteristics of, 145
Cystic calculi, ultrasonographic findings with, 150, 150*f*
Cystic ovarian follicles, 468, 468*f*
Cystitis
bacterial, 377, 496
chronic, radiologic findings with, 127, 129*f*
Cystocentesis
with large urethral plug, 375
prior to removal of urethral plug, 373
Cystogram. *See* Urinary cystogram
Cystoisospora, 224
Cystorellin. *See* Gonadotropin-releasing hormone
Cystotomy, for feline urologic syndrome, 372
Cytauxzoon felis, 157, 158*f,* 161
Cytauxzoonosis, 161
Cytobin. *See* Liothyronine
Cytologic interpretation, 98–100
Cytologic specimen, preparation of, 95–96
Cytology, 95–113
benefits of, 95
cell collection techniques for, 96–98
equipment for, 95–96
fluid, in diagnosis of chylothorax, 288, 289*f*
versus histopathology, 95
indications for, 193–194
Cytomel. *See* Liothyronine
Cytoxan. *See* Cyclophosphamide

Dacryocystitis, 327
DAMNIT [mnemonic], 165*t,* 218–219
Daranide. *See* Dichlorphenamide
Datril. *See* Acetaminophen
DDAVP Nasal Spray, 216
Deafness, differential diagnosis of, 643
Death. *See* Euthanasia; Grief management
Deca-Durabolin. *See* Nandrolone decanoate
Decholin. *See* Dehydrocholic acid
Deciduous teeth, retained, 301, 301*f,* 303
Declawing. *See* Onychectomy
Decontamination procedures, for toxicosis, 553*t,* 553–555
Deep digital flexor tendonectomy, 482–483, 483*f*–484*f*
Deet. *See N,N*-Diethyl-*m*-toluamide
Defecation, painful. *See* Dyschezia
Defecation problems, 239
treatment of, 239
Defensive aggression, 242–243
treatment of, 242–243
Degenerative disease, 165
Dehydration
clinical signs of, 279, 279*t*
degree of
based on clinical signs, 410*t*
estimation of, 308, 308*t*
Dehydrocholic acid, 262
contraindications to, 264
Delivery, difficult, 37
Delmadinone acetate, for estrus prevention/suppression, 461
Demecarium bromide, for glaucoma, 340
Demethylchlortetracycline, drug interactions, 53*t*
Demodectic mange, 514–515
clinical signs of, 514, 515*f*
diagnosis of, 514–515
etiology and pathogenesis of, 514, 514*f*
therapy for, 515
Demodex cati, 514, 514*f*
Dental anatomy, 291, 291*f*
Dental care
after treatment of cervical line lesions, by owner, 296
home, 442
in prevention of periodontal disease, 441, 441*t*
Dental charting, 292–293, 293*f*
Dental diseases/disorders, 290–304. *See also* Oral diseases
acquired, 303–304
congenital, 303
examination of cat with, 290
history of cat with, 290
Dental elevators, for tooth extraction, 298
Dental films, 297, 440, 448
Dental injuries
caused by high-rise fall, management of, 398
traumatic. *See* Tooth fracture(s)
Dental laminar epithelium, tumors of, 445
Dental nomenclature and formulae, 292*t*
Dental occlusion
correct, 301
incorrect. *See* Malocclusions
Dental sealer cements, for root canal procedures, 300
Dental terms, 292*t*
Dental work. *See* Crown; Orthodontics; Root canal(s); Tooth extraction
Dentin, 291, 291*f*
Dentinal sealer/conditioner, 298
Depo-Medrol. *See* Methylprednisolone acetate
Depo-Provera. *See* Medroxyprogesterone acetate
Dermal masses/ulceration, 95
cytologic findings with, 108*f,* 108–110, 109*f*
Derma Shield, 480
Dermatitis
allergic drug reaction, 524–525
allergic inhalant, 521–523
contact allergic, 523–524
differential diagnosis of, 643–644
flea allergic, 518–521
food allergic, 521
miliary, 532–533
Dermatophytes, 504
Dermatophyte test media, 505–506
Dermatophytosis, 504–508, 579–580
antifungal therapy for, 507–508
clinical signs of, 504–505, 505*f*
diagnosis of, 505–506, 580
with fungal culture, 505–506, 505*f*–506*f*
with microscopic examination of hair and scale, 506, 506*t,* 507*f*
with Wood's light examination, 506
etiology of, 504
pathophysiology of, 504, 505*f*
predisposing factors for, 579
transmission and outcome of exposure, 579–580
treatment of, 49, 580
in catteries, 508
with topical agents, 507, 507*t*
Derm Caps, 522–523
Dermoids, 322
Descemet's membrane, 328
Descemet's striae, 340
Desmopressin acetate, 216
Devon Rex, 11, 11*f*
Deworming, 38
Dexamethasone
contraindications to, 410*t*
dosage and administration of, 234*t,* 335
for feline asthma, 234
indications for, 173, 330
for shock, 394
test for
indications for, 214
normal value, 83

Dextrose
  in intense diuresis, 281–282
  for oliguric renal failure, 280
Diabetes insipidus, 207. *See also* Central diabetes insipidus; Nephrogenic diabetes insipidus
  incidence of, 214
  primary, 208
  treatment of, 216
Diabetes mellitus, 305–316
  caused by hyperadrenocorticism, 210
  classification of, 306
  clinical pathology of, 306
  clinical signs of, 305
    education of owner about, 312
  complicated (ketoacidotic), 305
    treatment of, 308–310
  diagnosis of, 306
  differential diagnosis of, 305
    by clinical trial, 307
  effects of concomitant disease on, 314
  etiology of, 305
  feline form, peculiarities of, 313
  history with, 305
  PU/PD syndrome caused by, 207–208, 208*t*, 211
  related to megestrol acetate, 313
  risk factors for, 305
  transient, 306, 313
  treatment of, 306
    with exogenous injected insulin, 306–307
  type I, 306
  type II, 306
  uncomplicated, 305
    treatment of, 307–308
Diabetic cat(s)
  acromegaly in, 315
  boarding, 315
    prolonged or frequent, 314
  consistent feeding of, 313
  drugs contraindicated for, 314
  estrus/pregnancy in, 313
  fluid therapy for, 308
  high-fiber diet for, 308
  home monitoring of, 312–313
  hyperadrenocorticism in, 314
  hyperosmolarity in, 310
  hypoglycemia in, 313
  improper diet for, 313–314
  interval feeding of, 313
  irregular activity level of, 314
  in multicat households, 314
  obesity in, 314
  regulation difficulties with, causes of, 313–315, 314*f*
  regulation of sodium concentration in, 308–309
  serum potassium levels in, 309–310
  veterinary monitoring of, 312
Diabetic cataracts, 336
Diabetic neuropathy, 305, 306*f*
Diabinese. *See* Chlorpropamide
Diaphragm
  fenestration of, for chylothorax, 289
  flattening of, in asthmatic cat, 232, 232*f*
Diaphragmatic hernia, 178, 180*f*, 190
  caused by high-rise fall, 394
  chylothorax secondary to, 288
  pericardial, 178, 181*f*
  radiologic findings with, 141, 142*f*
Diarrhea. *See* Vomiting/diarrhea
Diazepam. *See also* Ketamine, combined with diazepam
  for aggression, 242
  for central nervous system overstimulation, 552
  dosage, 42*t*, 169, 239
  for hyperesthesia syndrome, 400
  indications for, 42, 169, 285, 374–375
  as maintenance anticonvulsant, 221
  for marking behavior, 238–239
  preparations, 42*t*
  for psychogenic alopecia, 537
  for seizure control, 220
  side effects of, 239
  tolerance, 239
  for toxicosis, 562–563
  for urge incontinence, 372
Diazinon, 560–561
Dibenzyline. *See* Phenoxybenzamine
Dichlorovos (DDVP), 560–561
Dichlorphenamide, 340
Die Keen, 300
Diestrus, 458
Diet(s). *See also* Food; Nutrition
  bland, for vomiting/diarrhea, 223
  for cats with chronic renal disease, 284–285
  for cats with hepatic lipidosis, 410–411, 411*t*
  for diabetic cat, 313–314
  dry food, and feline urologic syndrome, 375
  effects on water consumption and urine production, 207
  and food allergic dermatitis, 521
  high-fiber
    commercially available, 308
    for diabetic cat, 308
  hypoallergenic, 414
  low-gluten, 414
  during pregnancy, 462
  and presumptive diagnosis of cardiomyopathy, 251
  restricted-protein, recipe for, 285*t*
  selection of, for anorectic cats, 40–41
  soft-moist, 384, 387
Dietary indiscretion, 223
Dietary palatability, increasing, 284–285
Diethylcarbamazine, 383
N,N-Diethyl-*m*-toluamide, 562
Diethylstilbestrol, 537
Differential overview, 624–664
Difficult cat. *See* Fractious cat
Diffuse hepatic disease, ultrasonographic findings with, 146, 146*f*
Diffuse renal parenchymal disease, ultrasonographic findings with, 149, 149*f*
Difil. *See* Diethylcarbamazine
Digestive system, radiologic evaluation of, 114–121
Digitalis glycosides, drug interactions, 52*t*
Digitalis toxicity, 250
Digoxin
  contraindications to, 247
  for dilated cardiomyopathy, 249–250
  maintenance dosage, 250
Digoxin elixir, contraindications to, 250
Dihydrostreptomycin, drug interactions, 52*t*
Dihydrotachysterol, 406
Dilantin. *See* Diphenylhydantoin
Dilated cardiomyopathy, 248*f*–249*f*, 248–250
Diltiazem
  for hypertrophic cardiomyopathy, 247
  for thromboembolic disease, 253
Dimethyl sulfoxide
  contraindications to, 472
  in fungal stains, 506, 506*t*
Diphacinone, 556
Diphenoxylate with atropine
  for diarrhea, 223
  dosage and administration of, 49
Diphenylhydantoin, contraindications to, 221
Dirofilaria immitis, 379
Dirofilaria immitis infection. *See* Heartworm disease
Dirofilariasis, 227
Diro-Form. *See* Diethylcarbamazine
Disease control
  in multicat facilities, 420–424
  principles of, 421–424
Disinfectants/detergents, household
  destruction of feline infectious peritonitis virus with, 352
  destruction of feline leukemia virus with, 361
  for disinfection of multicat facilities, 424
Disinfection
  of multicat facilities, 423–424
  of premises
    for feline calicivirus infection, 573
    for feline viral rhinotracheitis, 572
Disseminated pyogranulomatous vasculitis, associated with feline infectious peritonitis, 353
Distant enhancement artifact, in ultrasonography, 145, 147*f*–148*f*, 151*f*
Distemper. *See* Feline panleukopenia
Distichiasis, 322
Diuresis, 280–282
  fluid, 281
  forced, for toxicosis, 555
  indications for, 280–281
  intense, 281–282
  monitoring of, 281
  types of, 280–281
Diuretics. *See also* Thiazide diuretics
  carbonic anhydrase inhibitor, for glaucoma, 340
  for oliguric renal failure, 280
  side effects of, 207
  for toxicosis, 557
Diuril. *See* Thiazide diuretics
DM. *See* Diabetes mellitus
DMSO. *See* Dimethyl sulfoxide
Domestic breeds
  nervous system disorders among, 165*t*
  pyothorax among, 454
  seizure disorders among, 219*t*
Domestic Shorthair
  periodontitis in, 443
  pyothorax in, 454
Domoso Solution, nasal flushes with, for chronic nasal discharge, 273
Dosage charts, 631–633
Down hair, 10
Doxorubicin
  dose, 427*t*
  route of administration, 427*t*
  toxicity, 427*t*
Doxycycline
  drug interactions, 53*t*
  for hemobartonellosis, 390
Doxy-Tabs. *See* Doxycycline
Dragster posture, 458
Dreschlera, 509
Drug(s)
  anemia caused by, 162
  to be avoided, 48–49
  to be used with certain restrictions, 49–50
  nonliquid, administration of, 44–47, 45*f*–46*f*
  oral, 44–47
Drug eruption (allergy), 524–525, 525*f*
Drug formulary, 585–627
  alphabetical by generic name, 587–613
  alphabetical by indication, 621–626
  alphabetical by trade name, 615–619
  how to use, 585–586
Drug interactions, 52*t*–53*t*, 54
Drug metabolism, 48
Drug peculiarities, 48–55
Drug toxicity, 48
DTM. *See* Dermatophyte test media
Dulcolax. *See* Bisacodyl
Duodenal gas, acoustic shadowing caused by, 147–148
Dycal, 299
Dying-back neuropathy, 169
Dyschezia
  definition of, 416
  differential diagnosis of, 416, 645
Dysphagia, differential diagnosis of, 645
Dyspnea, 172–190
  acute onset of, 172
  in asthmatic cat, 231
  in cardiac disease, 244, 248, 250, 252
  caused by airway diseases/disorders, 177
  caused by extrapulmonary diseases and disorders, 177–178
  caused by multiple mechanisms, 190
  caused by pulmonary diseases/disorders, 182
  definition of, 172, 173*t*
  differential diagnosis of, 174*t*, 355, 646
  diseases causing, classification of, 177–190
  etiology of, 172
  terminology and clinical findings with, 172
Dyspneic cats
  physical examination of, 172–173
  sternal recumbency in, 172, 173*f*
Dystocia, 37, 464–465
  diagnosis of, 464
  differential diagnosis of, 646
  fetal, 464, 464*f*
  maternal, 464, 465*f*
Dysuria
  definition of, 370
  differential diagnosis of, 647
  nonresponsive to treatment, 377

Ear(s), physical examination of, 33
Ear infections, radiologic findings with, 139, 139*f*
Ear mites. *See* Otodectic mange
Ear trim, 483, 484*f*
Easter lily, 564
Echidnophaga gallinacea, 518
Echocardiography
  in diagnosis of cardiomyopathy, 251
  of dilated cardiomyopathy, 248, 249*f*
  of heartworm disease, 379–382, 382*f*–383*f*
  of hypertrophic cardiomyopathy, 245, 247*f*

Echocardiography (*continued*)
indications for, 177
of restrictive cardiomyopathy, 250–251
Echogenic images, 145
Echothiophate, for glaucoma, 340
ECP. *See* Estradiol cypionate
Ectoparasitism, 511, 518
Ectopia lentis, 336
Ectopic pregnancy, 464–465
Ectropion, 322, 323*f*
surgical correction of, 322, 324*f*
Edema
pulmonary, 182, 185*f*–186*f*
treatment of, 169
Effectors, 191
EGC. *See* Eosinophilic granuloma complex
Egyptian Mau, 11–12, 12*f*
predilection for nervous system disorders in, 165*t*
predilection for seizure disorders in, 219*t*
Electrical axis, normal value for, 84
Electrical cords, oral burns caused by chewing on, 448
Electric shock, bronchial pattern caused by, 233*f*
Electrocardiography
of dilated cardiomyopathy, 248
of hyperkalemia, 309, 309*t*, 310*f*
of hypertrophic cardiomyopathy, 245
of restrictive cardiomyopathy, 251
Electroejaculation, 466
Electrolyte(s), serum levels of, in chronic renal disease, 276
Electrolyte solution
for diabetic cat, 308
for hyperosmolarity, 310
for hypokalemic polymyopathic cat, 258–259
for idiopathic hepatic lipidosis, 410
for vomiting/diarrhea, 223
Electromyography, 194
Electrophoresis, serum, in diagnosis of feline infectious peritonitis, 357
Elimination behavior problems, 236–239
causes of, 236–238, 237*f*
diagnosis of, 238, 238*t*
treatment of, 238–239
ELISA. *See* Enzyme-linked immunosorbent assay
Elixophyllin. *See* Theophylline
Elizabethan collar, indications for, 536–537
Embryo transfer, 469
Emergency stabilization, for toxicosis, 552–553, 553*t*
Emesis. *See* Vomiting/diarrhea
Emetine, 554
Emollients, 418*t*–419*t*
Emphysema
conjunctival, 327
vesicular, 231
Empyema, definition of, 454
Enamel, 291, 291*f*
Enamel hypoplasia, 303
treatment of, 303–304
EnCC. *See* Endogenous creatinine clearance
Encephalopathy, hepatic, 265
Endocrine tests, normal values for, 83
Endodontia. *See* Crown amputation; Pulp capping
Endodontics. *See* Root canal(s)
Endogenous creatinine clearance, 276
indications for, 214
protocol for determining, 215*t*
Endogenous pyrogen, 191
Endometrial hyperplasia, 462, 469
Endometritis, 463, 469–470
Endoscopy
fiberoptic, indications for, 194
tracheal, indications for, 176
Endostops, 299
End-stage renal disease, radiologic findings with, 122
End-stage renal failure, definition of, 274
Enema(s), 418*t*. *See also* Barium enema
for intestinal decontamination, 554
phosphate, contraindications to, 49
English ivy, 565
Enrofloxacin
for acute upper respiratory infections, 574
for cholangitis/cholangiohepatitis, 262
for feline asthma, 235
indications for, 44, 456, 466, 487
Enteritis/colitis. *See also* Feline panleukopenia virus
bacterial, 225
diagnosis of, 225
Enterobacter, 577
Entropion, 322, 324*f*
Environmental adaptation, and evolution of cat breeds, 3
Environmental control, of fleas, 520–521
Environmental decontamination, for dermatophytosis, 507–508
Enzyme-linked immunosorbent assay, 81
for feline immunodeficiency virus, 350
for feline leukemia virus, 360–363, 365–367
for heartworm antigens, 379
Eosinophil(s)
morphologic characteristics of, 202
test for, diseases affecting, 85
Eosinophilic granuloma complex, 445–446, 533–535
atypical, 534–535, 535*f*
clinical signs of, 445–446, 533–535, 533*f*–535*f*
cytologic findings with, 108, 109*f*
diagnosis of, 533–535, 533*f*–535*f*
etiology of, 533
treatment of, 446, 535
Eosinophilic keratitis, 330, 331*f*
Eosinophilic lymphadenitis, 204, 205*f*
Eosinophilic plaque, 446, 534, 534*f*
Eosinophilic ulcers, 445
EP. *See* Endogenous pyrogen
Epidermal masses/ulceration, 95
cytologic findings with, 108*f*, 108–110, 109*f*
Epilepsy. *See also* Seizure disorder(s)
definition of, 218
incidence of, 218
primary generalized
clinical presentation of, 219
definition of, 218
secondary generalized, definition of, 218
Epinephrine
dosage, 234*t*
for feline asthma, 234
indications for, 322–323, 525
Epiphora, 33, 322, 327
differential diagnosis of, 648–649
Episcleral vessels, venous injection and congestion of, 339
Epistaxis, differential diagnosis of, 649
Epithelial tumors, 526–530
cytologic findings with, 205, 205*f*
malignant, cytologic findings with, 205, 205*f*
Epogen. *See* r-HuEPO
Epsom salts. *See* Magnesium sulfate
Equipoise. *See* Boldenone undecylenate
Eruption times, 292*t*
Erythema, differential diagnosis of, 649
Erythremic myelosis, 160
diagnosis of, with spleen aspiration, 105
Erythroblastopenia. *See* Nonregenerative anemia
Erythrocyte refractile bodies, 384
Erythrocytes. *See* Red blood cells
Erythromycin
for cholangitis/cholangiohepatitis, 262
drug interactions, 52*t*
Erythropoiesis, 159–160, 160*t*
Erythropoietin product, formulated. *See* r-HuEPO
Erythropoietin production, lack of, in chronic renal disease, 283
Escherichia coli, 462, 465, 479
polyuria caused by, 209
Esophageal tumors, 432
radiologic findings with, 114
Esophagitis, gastric, radiologic findings with, 114
Esophagogram, 114
clinical indications for, 114
common lesions diagnosed with, 114, 115*f*–116*f*
goals of, 114
materials for, 114
normal findings with, 114, 115*f*
technique for, 114
Esophagostomy tube
for force feeding, 42–43, 411
placement of, 483–486
results of, 486
surgical technique for, 483–486, 485*f*
removal of, 486
Esophagus
displacement or perforation of, radiologic findings with, 114
foreign bodies in, radiologic findings with, 114
inflammation of, radiologic findings with, 114
strictures of, radiologic findings with, 114
Estradiol
production, during pregnancy, 463
for sex hormone imbalance, 537
Estradiol cypionate, 460
side effects of, 460
Estrogen
drug interactions, 53*t*
multiple exposures to, 462
Estrogen analogs, contraindications to, 472
Estrus, 458
behavioral, promotion of, 467
in diabetic cats, 313
failure to exhibit, 467
induction of, 460–461
pharmacologic, 467
onset of, 36
persistent or prolonged, 468
possible outcomes of, 458–459, 459*f*
prediction of, 459, 459*f*, 467
prevention or suppression of, 461
permanent, 461
pubertal
absence of, 473
failure to exhibit, 467
signs of, 37, 467
Estrus cycle
control of, 460–461
stages of, 458–459
Ether clearance test, 91, 289*t*
Ethylenediaminetetra-acetic acid, 390
Ethylene glycol, 258, 565
toxicity, 166, 553, 565–567, 566*t*
ultrasonographic findings with, 149, 149*f*
Ethylene glycol test kits, 567
Eugenol liquid, in sealer cement for root canal procedures, 300
Euglycemic glucosuria, PU/PD syndrome caused by, 211
Euphorbia pulcherrima. *See* Poinsettia
Euthanasia, 69–72
charges for, 72
disposition of body after, 72
explaining what to expect during, 71
expression of sympathy after, 72, 73*f*
filling void left by, 70
grief management after, 72–76
grief of other pets after, 72
indications for, 69
owner's presence during, 71
supporting decision for, 70–71
technique for, 71–72
terms to use and terms to avoid with, 69
timing of, 70
who should make decision for, 69–70
Eutrombicula, 515
Excisional biopsy, 426
Excoriation, differential diagnosis of, 649–650
Excretory urography, 122
clinical indications for, 122
common lesions diagnosed with, 122, 123*f*–126*f*
complications of, 122
in diagnosis of chronic renal disease, 278
goal of, 122
indications for, 435
materials for, 122
normal findings with, 122, 123*f*
technique for, 122
Exodontia. *See* Tooth extraction
Exophiala, 509
Exostoses, palpable, differential diagnosis of, 650
Exotic Shorthair, 12, 12*f*
Expiration, forced, 231
Exploratory surgery, indications for, 194
Exposure keratopathy, caused by chronic glaucoma, 339, 339*f*
Extensor postural thrust, definition of, 39
Extraction, dental. *See* Tooth extraction
Eye(s). *See also under* Ocular
effects of noneffusive feline infectious peritonitis on, 355
extraocular diseases of, 317–331
intraocular diseases of, 332–347
opening of, in kittens, 38
physical examination of, 33
posterior segment of
clinical examination of, 341
diseases of, 341–343
Eyelid(s). *See also* Third eyelid
anatomy of, 319

Eyelid(s) (*continued*)
  diseases of, 319–326, 320*t*
    acquired, 319
  lacerations in, 325
  opening of, 38
  premature opening of, 326
  squamous cell carcinoma of, 325–326, 327*f*
Eyelid agenesis, 320*f*, 321
  treatment of, 321, 321*f*
Eyelid tumors, 325–326
Eyelid ulcers, geriatric-associated, 326
Eye movement, rapid, differential diagnosis of, 655–656

Face, asymmetry of, 290
Facial disfigurement, caused by wry mouth, 303
Facial paralysis, 323
Facial trauma, caused by high-rise fall, 397–398
Fading kitten syndrome, 66, 466
FAID. *See* Feline acquired immunodeficiency syndrome
Fainting, differential diagnosis of, 662
Falciform fat, in liver ultrasound, 146, 146*f*
Fall(s). *See also* High-rise syndrome
  common injuries caused by, 392
  vestibular mechanism during, 392
Farm cats, 420
  control of infectious diseases among, 423
Fat absorption test, 91
Fatigue, differential diagnosis of, 663
Fat supplementation, indications for, 288
Fatty acid preparations, for allergic inhalant dermatitis, 522–523
5-FC. *See* 5-Fluorocytosine
FCRD. *See* Feline central retinal degeneration
FCV. *See* Feline calicivirus infection
FD. *See* Fluid diuresis
Fear, aggression caused by, 242–243
Fecal Baermann technique, indications for, 177
Fecal examinations
  in diagnosis of intestinal parasites, 224
  indications for, 234
Fecal fat, increased, differential diagnosis of, 661
Fecal incontinence, differential diagnosis of, 650. *See also* Elimination behavior problems
Feces hemorrhagic, differential diagnosis of, 651–652
Fecundity, of queens, factors influencing, 461
FECV. *See* Feline enteric coronavirus
Feeding syringes, 42
Feeding Tube and Urethral Catheter, 41, 497
Feeding tubes, 41
  for kittens or small cats, 42
  sterilization of, 42
  surgically implanted, 42–43
Fees, for euthanasia, 72
Felicola subrostratus, 515, 515*f*
Feline acquired immunodeficiency syndrome, 364
Feline asthma. *See* Asthma
Feline calicivirus, 266
  and feline urologic syndrome, 369
  periodontitis associated with, 438
  transmission of, 570
  upper respiratory infection caused by, 570
  vaccination against, recommendations for, 423*t*
Feline calicivirus infection, 572–573
  carrier state, 572–573
  clinical signs of, 572, 572*f*–573*f*
  differential diagnosis of, 573
  disinfection of premises for, 573
  in multicat facilities, 421–423
Feline central retinal degeneration, 341, 342*f*–343*f*
Feline enteric coronavirus, 224, 352
  clinical presentation of, 224
  heat-labile properties of, 352
  transmission of, 352
  treatment of, 224
Feline enteric coronavirus infection, 352
Feline heartworm disease, 227
Feline herpesvirus, 266
  transmission of, 570
  upper respiratory infection caused by, 570
Feline herpesvirus infection
  effects on reproduction, 471–472
  in multicat facilities, 421–423
Feline herpesvirus keratitis, 328, 330*f*
  diagnosis of, 328
  treatment of, 328
Feline immunodeficiency virus
  anemia caused by, 162
  and bite wounds, 479
  1991 colloquium on, 350
  gastrointestinal infections caused by, 224
  interaction with griseofulvin, 349–350
  intraocular inflammation associated with, 333–334, 334*f*
  neoplasia associated with, 349
  periodontal disease associated with, 438
  transmission of, 348
Feline immunodeficiency virus antibody, detection of, 350
Feline immunodeficiency virus infection, 348–351
  acute stage (primary illness), clinical findings with, 348–349
  chronic/terminal stage
    clinical findings with, 349
    diseases and lesions associated with, 349*t*, 349*f*
  clinical findings with, 348–350
  diagnosis of, 350
  differential diagnosis of, 362
  incidence of, 348
  latent stage, clinical findings with, 349
  in multicat facilities, 421–423
  prevention of, 350
  risk factors for, 348
  treatment of, 49, 168, 350
Feline immunodeficiency virus test, 81, 160
Feline infectious anemia (FIA). *See* Hemobartonellosis
Feline infectious peritonitis, 81, 352–359
  anemia caused by, 162
  in cattery/multicat household situations, 358–359
  clinical signs of, 358
  counseling owners of cats with, 358
  diagnosis of, 112*t*, 345–346, 356–357
    with abdominal fluid aspiration, 111
    antemortem, 357
    with body fluid aspiration, 99*f*, 111
    future tests for, 357
    with liver aspiration, 104
    with lung aspiration, 107
    renal biopsy in, 279
    tests of greater reliability for, 356–357
    tests of lesser reliability for, 357
  differential diagnosis of, 355–356
  effects on reproduction, 471
  effusive, 353–354
    abdominal form of, 354, 355*f*
    pleural effusion caused by, 354 354*f*–355*f*
  lung sclerosis/consolidation caused by, 182, 184*f*
  in multicat facilities, 422–423, 471
  neonatal, 471
  noneffusive, 354–355
    central nervous system manifestations of, 355
    multiple pyogranulomas caused by, 355, 355*f*
    ocular manifestations of, 355
    radiographic findings with, 355, 356*f*
  ocular manifestations of, 345*f*, 345–346
  prevention of, 358
  prognosis for, 358
  radiologic findings with, 122, 124*f*
  treatment of, 168, 358
  uveitis associated with, 334, 334*f*
  vaccination against, 471
    recommendations for, 423*t*
Feline infectious peritonitis virus, 352
  antibodies, 353
  destruction of, by household disinfectants, detergents, 352
  gastrointestinal infections caused by, 224
  heat-labile properties of, 352
  pathophysiology of, 353
  strains, pathogenicity for, 352, 353*t*
  transmission of, 352–353
Feline leukemia virus, 360–368
  anemia caused by, 162
  and bite wounds, 479
  1991 colloquium on, 367
  control of, 365–367
  gastrointestinal infections caused by, 224
  historical perspective on, 157, 360
  immune carriers of, 363
  neoplastic disease associated with, 166, 333, 333*f*, 363, 427
  ocular manifestations of, 346, 346*f*
  pathway of, 361–362, 362*t*
  periodontal disease associated with, 438
  public health significance of, 368
  retinal dysplasia caused by, 341
  test and removal program for, 365, 365*t*
  tests/testing for, 361
    guidelines for, 367
    selection of, 363, 363*t*
  transmission of, 361
  vaccination against, 360, 365–367
    guidelines for, 367
    recommendations for, 423*t*
    testing of healthy cats prior to, 365–366, 366*f*
    vaccines available for, 366–367
  virology, 360
Feline leukemia virus infection, 363–365, 364*t*
  degenerative, 364–365
  differential diagnosis of, 362
  effects on reproduction, 470–471
  immune response to, 362
  incidence of, 360–361
  in multicat facilities, 421, 423, 471
  outcome of, 362–363, 363*t*
  persistent viremia in response to, 362–363
  proliferative, 363
  treatment of, 168
  viral latency in response to, 363
Feline leukemia virus test, 64, 81
Feline Mouth Speculum, 41
Feline oncornavirus cell membrane antigen test, detection of feline leukemia virus with, 360–363, 367
Feline panleukopenia
  clinical presentation of, 224
  diagnosis of, 224
  in multicat facilities, 421, 423
Feline panleukopenia virus, 224
  effects on reproduction, 471
  fetal infection by, 471
  retinal dysplasia caused by, 341, 342*f*
  vaccination against, 38
    recommendations for, 423*t*
Feline parvovirus (FPV). *See* Feline panleukopenia virus
Feline sarcoma virus, 360
Feline T-lymphocyte virus (FTLV). *See* Feline immunodeficiency virus
Feline urologic syndrome, 369–378
  clinical signs of, 370–371
  diagnosis of, 371
  etiology of, 369–370
  nonobstructed form
    clinical signs of, 370*f*, 370–371
    diagnosis of, 371
    treatment of, 371–372
  obstructed form
    clinical signs of, 371
    diagnosis of, 371
    reobstruction after treatment of, 375
    treatment of, 372–375, 479, 491–496, 493*f*–495*f*
    urethral plugs found in, 370, 370*f*
    in which urethral plug cannot be relieved, 375, 375*f*
  prevention and home monitoring of, 376
  terminology, 369
  treatment of, 371–375
Feline viral rhinotracheitis, 570–572
  carrier state, 571–572
  clinical signs of, 571, 571*f*
  differential diagnosis of, 573
  disinfection of premises with, 572
  in multicat facilities, 421
  sequelae, 571, 572*f*
  vaccination against, recommendations for, 423*t*
Felis libyca, 11
Fel-O-Vax, 366
FeLV. *See* Feline leukemia virus
Female cats
  catheterization of, 124, 126*f*
  characteristics of, 36
Female reproduction, 458–466
Femoral fracture
  comminuted, 481, 482*f*
    repair of, 481–482
    results of repair of, 482
    surgical technique for repair of, 481–482, 482*f*
  management of, 395–396
  physical examination for, 35, 35*f*
Femoral pulse, weak or thready, differential diagnosis of, 650
Femoral pulse deficit, differential diagnosis of, 650

Femur, proximal, medullary cavity of, blood transfusion into, 65–66
Fenchlorphos, for demodectic mange, 515
Fenoxycarb, 560–561
Fenthion, 560–561
Feral cats, 420
  control of infectious diseases among, 423
Ferrous sulfate, for iron deficiency anemia, 162
Fertilization, 461
  failure of, 469
  in vitro, 469
Fetal death, 470, 470*f*
Fetal infection, by panleukopenia virus, 471
Fetal injury, due to fetotoxic drugs, 472
Fetal resorptions, associated with feline leukemia virus, 365
Fetotoxic drugs, 472
Fever
  definition of, 191
  true, 193
    function of, 191
Fever of unknown origin, 191–194
  definition of, 191
  diagnosis of, 192–194
    ancillary tests for, 193–194
  etiology of, 191–192, 192*t*
    in human patients, 192*t*
  history of cat with, 193
  laboratory evaluation of, 193, 194*t*
  physical examination of cat with, 193
  physiology/pathophysiology of, 191
FHV. *See* Feline herpesvirus
Fiberoptic endoscopy, indications for, 194
Fibrinogen, test for
  in diagnosis of feline infectious peritonitis, 357
  normal value, 82
Fibroadenomatosis, caused by megestrol acetate, 51, 51*f*
Fibroadenomatous mammary hyperplasia, 463
Fibroma
  nasal, 434
  ossifying, 433
Fibropapilloma, nasal, 434
Fibrosarcoma
  of bone, 433
  nasal, 434
  oral, 431, 444–445
  of skin, 530, 530*f*
Fibular fracture, management of, 396, 396*f*
Fight(s). *See* Bite wounds
Fight or flight reflex, 305
  and anesthesia, 59
Fine-needle aspiration. *See* Tissue aspiration
FIP. *See* Feline infectious peritonitis
Fistulae, differential diagnosis of, 636
Fits, differential diagnosis of, 641–642
FIV. *See* Feline immunodeficiency virus
Flagyl. *See* Metronidazole
Flea(s)
  anemia caused by, 162
  life cycle of, 518
Flea allergic dermatitis, 518–521
  clinical signs of, 518–519, 519*f*
  diagnosis of, 519*f*, 519–520
  etiology and pathogenesis of, 518–519
  symmetric alopecia secondary to, 535, 536*f*
  therapy for, 520
Flea control
  on animal, 520
  in environment, 520–521
Flea preparations, allergic reactions to, 356*f*, 523, 523*f*, 536
Flea testing, 519, 519*f*
Fleet Enema. *See* Phosphate enemas
Fleshing, palpation to assess degree of, 32
Fluid aspiration, 97–98, 113. *See also* Body fluid aspiration
Fluid cytology, in diagnosis of chylothorax, 288, 289*f*
Fluid diuresis, 281
  for nausea, 284
Fluid-filled structures, ultrasonographic characteristics of, 145
Fluid therapy. *See also* Electrolyte solution
  after rehydration, for oliguric renal failure, 280
  after removal of urethral obstruction, 374–375
  for anorectic cat, 41
  for chronic renal failure, evaluation of, 279–280
  components of, 259*t*, 279*t*
  for dehydration, in chronic renal disease, 279–280
  for diabetic cat, 308
  for dilated cardiomyopathy, 250
  for hypokalemic polymyopathic cat, 258–259
  indications for, 262
  for neonatal bacterial sepsis, 466
  for pyothorax, 456
  for shock, 393–394
Flumixin meglumine, 49
Fluoride gels, in treatment of cervical line lesions, 296–297
Fluoride toxicity, 442
Fluoride varnish, 295
5-Fluorocytosine, 548
  for cryptococcosis, 543
  for toxoplasmosis, 168
5-Fluorouracil, 547
Fluothane. *See* Halothane
Focal hepatic disease
  classification of, 147*t*
  ultrasonographic findings with, 146, 147*f*
Focal lesions, types of, 147*t*
Focal renal parenchymal disease, ultrasonographic findings with, 149, 149*f*
FOCMA. *See* Feline oncornavirus cell membrane antigen
Follicle-stimulating hormone, estrus induction with, 460–461
Follicular conjunctivitis, due to chlamydia, 325, 325*f*
Follutein. *See* Human chorionic gonadotropin
Food. *See also* Diet(s); Nutrition
  hiding medications in, 44–45
  withholding of, for vomiting/diarrhea, 223
Food allergic dermatitis, 521
  cutaneous signs of, 521, 521*f*
  diagnosis of, 521
  pathogenesis of, 521
  therapy for, 521
Force feeding, 40–43
  of anorectic cats with hepatic lipidosis, 411
  complications of, 42
  esophagostomy tube for, 42–43, 411
    placement of, 483–486
  of kittens or small cats, 42
  methods for, 41–43, 42*f*
  objectives of, 40
  schedule for, 41
Foreign bodies
  in esophagus, radiologic findings with, 114
  in gastrointestinal tract, 224
  in intestine, radiologic findings with, 118, 118*f*, 118, 119*f*
  nasal, 266, 267*f*
Foreign body granulomas, cytologic findings with, 99*f*, 108
FP. *See* Feline panleukopenia
FPL. *See* Feline panleukopenia
FPV. *See* Feline panleukopenia virus
Fractional excretion, 274
Fractious cat
  administration of anesthesia to, 59–61
  management of, 29–30
  sedation of, for euthanasia, 71–72
Fracture(s). *See also specific type*
  caused by high-rise falls, management of, 395–397
  open, management of, 395–396
Fracture fixation, nylon bands for, 488–490
French catheter, 124, 374, 374*f*
French feeding tube, 41
Frontal sinuses, 266, 269*f*
  common lesions of, radiologic findings with, 140, 140*f*–141*f*
  infection of
    chronic, treatment of, 486
    radiologic findings with, 141*f*
  radiographic findings with, 139–140, 140*f*, 269*f*–270*f*
Frontal sinusitis, treatment of, 273
Frontal sinus obliteration, 486–488
  results of, 487–488
  surgical technique for, 486–487, 487*f*
FSA. *See* Fibrosarcoma
FSH. *See* Follicle-stimulating hormone
5-FU. *See* 5-Fluorouracil
Fulvicin. *See* Griseofulvin
Fungal culture, of hair, 505–506, 505*f*–506*f*
Fungal granulomas, cytologic findings with, 105*f*, 108, 108*f*
Fungal infections, 504–511
  deep (systemic). *See* Systemic fungal infections
  intermediate, 508–510
  superficial, 504–508
Fungassay. *See* Dermatophyte test media
Fungizone. *See* Amphotericin-B
FUO. *See* Fever of unknown origin
Fur. *See* Hair coat
Fur mite, 515–516, 517*f*
Furosemide
  contraindications to, 173
  for dilated cardiomyopathy, 249
  dosage and administration of, 173
  drug interactions, 53*t*
  for heartworm disease, 382
  for hypertrophic cardiomyopathy, 247
  indications for, 173, 251, 262, 448
  for oliguric renal failure, 280
  for toxicosis, 557
FUS. *See* Feline urologic syndrome
Fusiformis species, 479
Fusion teeth, 303
FVR. *See* Feline viral rhinotracheitis

Gait, abnormal, differential diagnosis of, 651
β-Galactosidase deficiency, 346
Gallbladder
  distention of, 263, 264*f*
  ultrasonographic evaluation of, 146–147, 147*f*–148*f*
Gamma-glutamyl transpeptidase, test for, normal value, 82
Gangliosidosis, ocular manifestations of, 346
Gastric adenocarcinoma, caused by megestrol acetate, 50*f*
Gastric esophagitis, radiologic findings with, 114
Gastric evacuation, for toxicosis, 553–554
Gastric lavage, for toxicosis, 554
Gastric masses, intraluminal, cytologic findings with, 106, 106*f*
Gastric ulcers
  perforated, radiologic findings with, 117, 117*f*
  radiologic findings with, 117, 117*f*–118*f*
Gastritis, uremic, treatment of, 284
Gastroenteritis
  allergic, 223–224
  radiologic findings with, 117
Gastroesophageal intussusception, radiologic findings with, 114, 116*f*
Gastrografin
  versus barium, for gastrointestinal series, 115, 118*f*
  complications of, 114
  contraindications to, 119
  for esophagogram, 114
  for gastrointestinal series, 115, 119
Gastrointestinal disorders. *See also* Vomiting/diarrhea
  dietary factors in, 223–224
  primary, 223–226
Gastrointestinal drugs, contraindications to, 472
Gastrointestinal infections, 224–225
  bacterial, 225
  protozoal, 225
  viral, 224
Gastrointestinal lymphosarcoma, 226, 431–432
  radiologic findings with, 118, 120*f*
Gastrointestinal series, 115–119, 177
  clinical indications for, 115
  common lesions diagnosed with, 117*f*, 117–118, 118*f*
  goals of, 115
  materials for, 115–116
  normal findings with, 116*f*, 116–117, 117*f*
  technique for, 116
Gastrointestinal tract
  chemotherapy-induced toxicity involving, 427
  foreign bodies in, 224
  ultrasonographic evaluation of, 150–151
Gastrointestinal tumors, 226, 431–432
  cytologic findings with, 106–107
Gastrostomy tube, 43
Gathering, 118, 118*f*
Gel Kam, 297
Gemination teeth, 303, 303*f*
Generalized retinal degeneration, 342
Genetic defects, 472–473
Gentamicin
  for acute upper respiratory infections, 574
  for cholangitis/cholangiohepatitis, 262
  in combination with penicillin derivative, for pyothorax, 456
  contraindications to, 340
  drug interactions, 52*t*–53*t*
  for feline asthma, 235

Gentamicin (*continued*)
for frontal sinus obliteration, 487
indications for, 466
GentiVac FeLV, 366
Gentocin. *See* Gentamicin
Geographic restrictions, and evolution of cat breeds, 3
Gestation. *See* Pregnancy
GFR. *See* Glomerular filtration rate
GGTP. *See* Gamma-glutamyl transpeptidase
GH. *See* Growth hormone
Giant cell tumor, 433
Giant inflammatory cells, morphologic characteristics of, 202
Giardia lamblia, 224
Giardiasis, 224–225
Gingiva 291, 291*f*
Gingiva bleeding, caused by periodontal disease, 439, 439*f*
Gingival health, nutrition and, 438–439
Gingival margin, 291, 291*f*
Gingival retraction cord
epinephrine-type, contraindications to, 295
indications for, 295
Gingival sulcus, 291, 291*f*
depth, measurement of, 291–292
Gingival tumors, 431
Gingivitis
acute necrotizing ulcerative, 444
associated with feline immunodeficiency virus, 349, 349*f*
differential diagnosis of, 661
Gingivitis index, 440*t*
Glass ionomer restoratives, 295
Glauber's salts. *See* Sodium sulfate
Glaucoma, 338–341
acute, treatment of, 340
chronic, treatment of, 340
classification of, 339
clinical signs of, 339*f,* 339–340
definition of, 338
diagnosis of, 340
medical treatment of, 340
pain caused by, 339
primary, 339
secondary, 339
secondary to anterior uveitis, treatment of, 340
surgical treatment of, 341
Glipizide, 307
Globulin, test for
diseases affecting, 87
normal value, 82–83
Glomerular filtration rate, 276
Glomerulonephritis, immune complex, caused by feline leukemia virus, 365
Glossitis, differential diagnosis of, 661
Glucocorticoids
contraindications to, 410*t*
for eosinophilic granuloma complex, 535
for flea allergic cat, 519–520
for miliary dermatitis, 532
Glucometers, 311
home use of, 312
Glucose
administration of, indications for, 374
test for
diseases affecting, 87
normal value, 82
urinary
normal value for, 84
testing of, 281
Glucose curve, 311
failure to perform, 313
Glucose monitoring
home, 312–313
veterinary, 312
Glucosuria, 281, 306
euglycemic, PU/PD syndrome caused by, 211
Glucotrol. *See* Glipizide
Glucuronide, 48
Glucuronyltransferase, deficient stores of, and drug metabolism, 48
Glutathione, 48
Glycerin, for glaucoma, 340
Glycopyrrolate
dosage, 56
indications for, 498
GM. *See* Gangliosidosis, ocular manifestations of
GnRH. *See* Gonadotropin-releasing hormone
Gold salts, for plasmacytic-lymphocytic stomatitis, 444
Gonadotropin-releasing hormone, 459
administration of, for ovulation induction, 460
Grand mal seizures. *See* Tonic-clonic seizures
Granulocytic cells, in bone marrow, test for, normal value, 83
Granulomas
foreign body, cytologic findings with, 99*f,* 108
fungal, cytologic findings with, 105*f,* 108, 108*f*
vaccine reaction, cytologic findings with, 99*f,* 108
Grief
definition of, 73
of other pets, after euthanasia, 72
Grief management, 72–76
children and, 74–75
recommendations for the veterinarian, 75–76
terminology for, 73
Grief manifestation, 74
Grief process, 73–74
Grief work, definition of, 73
Griseofulvin
contraindications to, 49, 472
for dermatophytosis, 507–508
drug interactions, 53*t*
indications for, 49
interaction of feline immunodeficiency virus and, 349–350
toxicity, 508
Growth hormone, excessive levels of, 210
Gutta-percha points, in feline dentistry, 295, 300, 300*f*

Hair
fungal culture of, 505–506, 505*f*–506*f*
microscopic examination of, for diagnosis of ringworm, 506, 506*t,* 507*f*
Hair balls, radiologic findings with, 118, 119*f*
Hair coat
physical examination of, 32–33
types of hair in, 10
Hair loss. *See* Alopecia
Halitosis
caused by cervical line lesions, 294
differential diagnosis of, 640
Halothane
dosage, 58
indications for, 58, 373, 486, 498
for seizure control, 221
Handling/addressing, of patient, guidelines for, 28–30
Hard palate, red line lesion across, 443, 443*f*
Hard palate defects, 449–451
Hard palate separations, 447, 447*f*
management of, 397, 397*f*
treatment of, 447
Hardy's Test and Removal Program, 360
Harelip, 450, 450*f*
treatment of, 450–451
Havana Brown, 12–13, 13*f*
Haws, 322
Hb. *See* Hemoglobin
HBHA. *See* Heinz body hemolytic anemia
HCG. *See* Human chorionic gonadotropin
HCM. *See* Hypertrophic cardiomyopathy
Hct. *See* Hematocrit
Head, asymmetry of, 290
Head tilt, differential diagnosis of, 651
Heart. *See also under* Cardiac
nonselective angiogram of, 138, 138*f*
ultrasonographic evaluation of, 152–153
Heart disease
and chronic renal failure, 278
ultrasonographic findings with, 152–153
Heartgard-30. *See* Ivermectin
Heart rate
normal, 84
over 100 bpm, differential diagnosis of, 639–640
rapid (more than 240 bpm), differential diagnosis of, 662
Heartworm disease, 227, 379–383
acute form, 379
chronic form, 379, 380*f*
clinical signs of, 379
diagnosis of, 379–382
echocardiographic findings with, 379–382, 382*f*–383*f*
feline and canine differences in 379
prevention of, 383
radiographic findings with, 379, 380*f*–382*f*
treatment of, 50, 382–383
ultrasonographic findings with, 153*f*
Heartworm test, 81
indications for, 232
Heat. *See* Estrus
Heat conservation, 191
Heat loss, 191
Heat production, 191
Hedera helix. *See* English ivy
Heinz bodies, 157, 158*f,* 384, 385*f*
staining of, 160, 162*f*
Heinz body hemolytic anemia, 160, 384–388
blood smear findings with, 384, 385*f*
clinical signs of, 384
differential diagnosis of, 651
specific oxidants causing, 384–387
treatment of, 387
Heinz body stain, 91–92
Helminths, 224
Hemangiosarcoma, 433
diagnosis of, with spleen aspiration, 105–106
Hematemesis, differential diagnosis of, 651
Hematochezia, differential diagnosis of, 651–652
Hematocrit
interpretation of, 279*t*
normal value, 82
Hematocrit tube, 63
Hematologic values
diseases affecting, 84–86
normal, 82
Hematology, in diagnosis of feline infectious peritonitis, 357
Hematoma, urinary system, radiologic appearance of, 128, 133*f*
Hematopoiesis, extramedullary, 160
Hematuria
caused by feline urologic syndrome, 371
differential diagnosis of, 652
Hemobartonella felis, 64, 65*f,* 157, 158*f,* 159, 161–162, 389
and nonregenerative anemias, 390–391
test for, 390
transmission of, 390
Hemobartonellosis, 157, 159–161, 389–391
clinical signs of, 390
diagnosis of, 390
hematologic signs of, 390, 390*f*
hemolysis-producing, 198
historical perspective on, 389
incidence of, 389
mechanisms of, 389
predisposing conditions for, 389
treatment of, 50, 390
Hemoglobin
test for
diseases affecting, 84–85
normal value, 82
values, at different ages, 83
Hemolymphatic neoplasms, 427–430
Hemolysis
anemia caused by, 159
caused by propylthiouracil, 162
diseases causing, 85
icterus secondary to, 195–196
regenerative anemias secondary to, 160–162
Hemolytic anemia, 159–160
Hemoperitoneum, caused by high-rise fall, 394
Hemorrhage
caused by blood transfusion, 67
caused by tissue aspiration, 104
diagnosis of, with abdominal fluid aspiration, 111
pulmonary, 182, 184*f*
retinal, 343, 343*f*–344*f*
subconjunctival, 328
Hemorrhagic anemia, 159–160
Hemostatic values, normal, 82
Heparin
for anticoagulation, 65
complications of, 254
dosage and administration, 254
indications for, 253–254
Hepatic disease
diffuse, ultrasonographic findings with, 146, 146*f*
focal
classification of, 147*t*
ultrasonographic findings with, 146, 147*f*
PU/PD syndrome caused by, 208*t,* 209–210
Hepatic encephalopathy, 265
Hepatic fibrosis, ultrasonographic findings with, 146, 146*f*
Hepatic lipidosis. *See* Idiopathic hepatic lipidosis
Hepatic parenchymal diseases, ultrasonographic findings with, 146

Hepatic shunts, 196, 197*f*
Hepatic tumors, 432
Hepatitis, bacterial, diagnosis of, with liver aspirate, 104
Hepatobiliary tumors, 432
Hepatocellular disease, icterus secondary to, 196–197, 197*f*
Hepatocytes
  evaluation of, in diagnosis of idiopathic hepatic lipidosis, 408–409
  normal, 409*f*
Hepatoencephalopathy, treatment of, 410
Hepatomegaly, differential diagnosis of, 652
Hernia
  diaphragmatic, 178, 180*f*, 190
    caused by high-rise fall, 394
    chylothorax secondary to, 288
    radiologic findings with, 141, 142*f*
  hiatal, radiologic findings with, 114
  pericardial diaphragmatic, 178, 181*f*
Herpesvirus. *See* Feline herpesvirus
Hexachlorophene, contraindications to, 48–49
Hiatal hernia, radiologic findings with, 114
High-fiber diet
  commercially available, 308
  for diabetic cat, 308
High-rise syndrome, 392–398
  abdominal trauma in, 394
  clinical findings with, 392
  facial trauma in, 397–398, 447
  management principles with, 395–398
  orthopedic trauma in, 395
  pathophysiology of, 392
  physical examination of cat with, 392–393
  shock in, 393–394
  spinal injuries in, 394–395
  thoracic trauma in, 393, 393*f*
  treatment principles for, 392–395
Himalayan, 20
  corneal sequestrum in, 330
  predilection for periodontitis in, 442
Hirschsprung's disease, 416
Histopathology
  versus cytology, 95
  indications for, 194
Histoplasma capsulatum, 272, 333, 344, 502, 544
Histoplasmosis, 344, 544–545
  clinical signs of, 544, 545*f*
  cytologic findings with, 108, 108*f*
  diagnosis of, 544–545
    with liver aspirate, 104, 105*f*
  etiology and epidemiology of, 544
  pathogenesis of, 544
  public health implications of, 549
  pulmonary, 182, 188*f*
  radiologic findings with, 118, 120*f*
  treatment of, 545
History of patient, 31–32
Homeostasis, renal contributions to, 274, 275*t*
Honeycomb appearance, with urinary cystogram, 128, 132*f*
Hookworms, 224
  anemia caused by, 162
Horizontal ramus, fractures of, 448–449
Hormone levels, associated with reproduction, 460, 460*t*
Hormone replacement therapy
  for eosinophilic granuloma complex, 446
  for PU/PD syndrome, 216
Horner's syndrome, 323, 324*f*
  differential diagnosis of, 652–653
  etiology of, 323
  treatment of, 323
Hospital cat, 28
Hot packs, for thromboembolic disease, 253
Houseplants. *See* Plant(s)
Housesoiling. *See* Elimination behavior problems
Howell-Jolly bodies, 64, 157, 158*f*, 160
HRS. *See* High-rise syndrome
Human(s). *See also* Children; Owner; Pregnant women
  aggression towards, 241*t*, 242–243
  cat bite wounds to, 577, 579*f*
  transmission of infectious diseases to cats by, 420–421
Human chorionic gonadotropin
  administration of, for ovulation induction, 460, 469
  in combination with pregnant mare serum gonadotropin, for estrus induction, 460
Humeral fracture, management of, 395–396
Humidification, of cat's atmospheric environment, for chronic nasal discharge, 272
Humorsol. *See* Demecarium bromide
Humulin L. *See* Insulin, intermediate-acting
Humulin N. *See* Insulin, intermediate-acting
Humulin R. *See* Insulin, regular
Humulin U Ultralente. *See* Insulin, long-acting
HWD. *See* Heartworm disease
Hydralazine
  contraindications to, 247
  for dilated cardiomyopathy, 250
Hydration deficit
  calculation of, 279, 279*t*
  replacement of, 279
Hydrochlorothiazide
  for hypertrophic cardiomyopathy, 247
  indications for, 216–217, 343
Hydrocortisone, indications for, 262
HydroDIURIL. *See* Hydrochlorothiazide
Hydrogen peroxide, for bleaching of teeth, 304
Hydrometra, 463, 463*f*
Hydronephrosis, radiologic findings with, 122, 124*f*
Hydroureter, radiologic findings with, 122
Hydrozide injection. *See* Hydrochlorothiazide
Hyperadrenocorticism
  in diabetic cats, 314
  diagnosis of, 210, 210*t*
  PU/PD syndrome caused by, 208*t*, 210, 214
Hyperbilirubinemia, 195
Hypercalcemia, 226–227
  PU/PD syndrome caused by, 209
Hyperechoic images, 145
Hyperesthesia, differential diagnosis of, 653
Hyperesthesia syndrome, 399–400
  clinical signs of, 399
  diagnosis of, 399–400
  differential diagnosis of, 399
  treatment of, 400
Hyperestrogenism, 468
Hyperglycemia
  nondiabetic causes of, 306
  persistent, 306
  rebound, 311–312, 312*f*
  transient, 305–306
Hyperkalemia, 309
  electrocardiographic findings in, 309, 309*t*, 310*f*
  treatment of, 280, 309
Hyperlacrimation. *See* Epiphora
Hypernatremia, treatment of, 309
Hypernatremic myopathy, CVF/MW complex caused by, 256
Hyperosmolarity
  in diabetic cats, 310
  treatment of, 310
Hyperplasia
  adenomatous, of thyroid gland, 401
  fibroadenomatous mammary, 463
  lymphoid, 203
    cytologic evaluation of, 203, 203*f*
  of third eyelid follicles, 325, 325*f*
Hyperproteinemia, in cats with feline infectious peritonitis, 356
Hypersalivation, differential diagnosis of, 653
Hypersensitivity diseases, of skin, 518–525
Hypersensitivity reaction
  classification of, 518
  in feline asthma, 231
    prevention of, 234
Hypertension
  associated with hyperthyroidism, 402
  in cats with chronic renal disease, 283
  clinical signs of, 244
Hypertensive retinopathy, 342–343, 343*f*
Hyperthermia. *See also* Fever
  definition of, 191
  emergency stabilization of, 552*t*, 553
  etiology of, 191
Hyperthyroidism, 227, 401–407
  apathetic, 401
  borderline cases of, tests for, 404
  cardiovascular findings in, 402
  clinical signs of, 401
  concurrent diseases, 404
  continuous medical management of, 406–407
  definitive treatment of, 405–407
    sequelae, 407
  diagnosis of, 209, 402–404
  differential diagnosis of, 404
  etiology of, 401
  hypertrophic cardiomyopathy caused by, 244
  initial treatment of, 404–405
  PU/PD syndrome caused by, 207–208, 208*t*, 209–211
  renal disease associated with, 403–404
  surgical treatment of, 405–406, 406*t*, 498–499, 499*f*–500*f*
Hypertrophic cardiomyopathy, 244–248, 245*f*
  clinical signs and findings with, 244
  diagnosis of, 245, 246*f*–247*f*
  prognosis for, 248
  pulmonary edema caused by, 182, 186*f*
  radiologic findings with, 138
  signalment, 244–248, 245*f*
  treatment of, 245–247
  ultrasonographic findings with, 152*f*, 153
Hyperventilation, degree of, estimation of arterial pH with, 310, 310*t*
Hypoadrenocorticism, 226
  diagnosis of, 210*t*
  PU/PD syndrome caused by, 210
Hypoallergenic diets, 414
Hypocalcemia, 406
Hypoechoic images, 145
Hypoglycemia, in diabetic cat, 313
Hypokalemia
  in diabetic cats, 309–310
    treatment of, 310
  and diuresis of anorectic cats, 282
  pathogenesis of, 257
  PU/PD syndrome caused by, 210
  treatment of, 259–260
Hypokalemic polymyopathy
  CVF/MW complex caused by, 256–257
  diagnosis of, 257–258
  treatment of, 258–259
Hypoluteoidism, 472
Hyponatremia, 309
Hyposensitization, for allergic inhalant dermatitis, 523, 523*t*
Hypothalamus
  release of antidiuretic hormone from, 207
  thermoregulatory functions of, 191

^{131}I. *See* Radioiodine
Iams Feline, 414
IBD. *See* Inflammatory bowel disease
Ibuprofen, 558–559
Icterus, 64, 195–198
  biochemical, 195
  caused by biliary obstruction, 197*f*, 197–198
  clinical, 195
  combined mechanisms causing, 198
  definition of, 195
  diagnosis of, 195, 196*t*
    basic biochemical tests for, 196*t*
  differential diagnosis of, 653
  on hard palate, 157
  historical perspective on, 195
  secondary to hemolysis, 195–196
  secondary to hepatocellular disease, 196–197, 197*f*
  underlying mechanisms of, 195–198, 196*t*
  variability in, 195
IDDM. *See* Insulin-dependent diabetes mellitus
Idiopathic aggressive behavior, 243
  treatment of, 243
Idiopathic colitis, 225
Idiopathic epilepsy. *See* Primary generalized epilepsy
Idiopathic hepatic lipidosis, 195, 408–412
  diagnosis of, 408–409
    with liver aspirate, 104, 105*f*
  diets for cats with, 410–411, 411*t*
  drugs to avoid in cats with, 410*t*
  etiology of, 408
  feeding methods for cats with, 411
  history and clinical signs of, 408
  initial treatment of, 410, 410*t*
  laboratory findings with, 408, 409*t*
  long-term therapy for, 410
  nosocomial, 411
  ultrasonographic findings with, 146, 146*f*
Idiopathic vomiting syndrome, 226
  diagnosis of, 226
  treatment of, 226
Idoxuridine, 574
  indications for, 328
α-1-Iduronidase deficiency. *See* Mucopolysaccharidosis
IFA test. *See* Indirect fluorescent antibody test
IHL. *See* Idiopathic hepatic lipidosis
Ilial wing, palpation of, 35, 35*f*

Image display modes, in ultrasonography, 145
Imidazole derivatives, 548
Immune complex glomerulonephritis, caused by feline leukemia virus, 365
Immune stimulation, cytologic evaluation of, from lymph node aspirates, 203
Immunoglobulin E antibodies, and atopy, 521
ImmunoRegulin, for plasmacytic-lymphocytic stomatitis, 444
Immunosuppression
  caused by feline leukemia virus, 364
  in cryptococcosis, 541
Imuran. *See* Azathioprine
Inbreeding, 472–473
Incisional biopsy, 426
Incisive bone, 290, 291*f*
Incoordination, differential diagnosis of, 638–639
Inderal. *See* Propranolol
Indirect fluorescent antibody test, 81, 157
  in detection of feline leukemia virus, 360–363, 365, 367
Indolent ulcers, 445, 533*f*, 533–534
Induction chambers, 60, 60*f*
Infarction, 166
Infection(s). *See specific type*
Infectious agents, abortion caused by, 470–472
Infectious diseases, 166
  common in multicat facilities, 421–422
  control of, general principles of, 420–421
  transmission of, 420
    barriers against, 420
    by humans, 420–421
Infertility. *See also* Reproductive failure
  differential diagnosis of, 653–654
  female, 467–473
  male, 467
Infiltrative bowel disease, radiologic findings with, 118, 120*f*, 121
Inflammatory bowel disease, 225, 413–415
  characterization of, 225
  diagnosis of, 225, 414
  etiology of, 413
  history and clinical signs of, 413–414
  pathophysiology and histopathology of, 413
  treatment of, 414
Inflammatory cellular subpatterns, 100
Inflammatory disease, 166
  anemia caused by, 162
  chronic, differential diagnosis of, 356
Inflammatory lesions, cytologic characterization of, 108
Inflammatory pattern
  acute, 100
  aseptic, 98, 99*f*, 100
  chronic, 100
  classification of, 98, 100
  cytologic interpretation of, 98, 99*f*
  eosinophilic, 98, 100
  granulomatous, 98, 100
  mixed with neoplastic pattern, 99*f*, 99–100
  purulent, 98, 100
  pyogranulomatous, 98, 100
  septic, 98, 99*f*, 100
  subacute, 100
Infraorbital foramen, 291*f*
Injections
  guidelines for, to minimize negative reactions, 29, 29*f*
  in presence of owner, 29
Insect growth regulator (IGR), 520
Insecticides, 560–563
Insulin
  dilution of, 306–307
  exogenous injected, 306–307
  human-derived, 307
  initial dose of, 308, 311
  intermediate-acting, 307
  long-acting, 307
  mixing of, 313
  regular, 307, 374
  types of
    comparison of, 307*t*
    by length of action, 307, 307*t*
    by source, 307, 307*t*
Insulin administration
  educating owner about, 307
  goal of, 307–308
  owner's failure with, 313
Insulin-dependent diabetes mellitus, 306
Insulin/dextrose, for oliguria, 280
Insulin incompatibility, 315
Insulin resistance, 315
Insulin syringes, 307
Insulin tolerance test, 311
Integrators, 191
Intense diuresis, 281–282
Interceptor. *See* Milbemycin oxime
Interestrus, 458
Interstitial lung diseases, 182
Interstitial pattern, 182
Intervertebral disks, ruptured, radiologic findings with, 136, 136*f*
Intestinal biopsy, diagnosis of inflammatory bowel disease with, 414
Intestinal decontamination, treatment of, 554
Intestinal mast cell tumors, 434
Intestinal obstruction, radiologic findings with, 118, 119*f*–120*f*
Intestinal parasites, 224
  in kittens, 38
Intestinal tumors, 431–432
  cytologic findings with, 106–107
Intestinal ulcers
  perforated, radiologic findings with, 117, 118*f*
  radiologic findings with, 117, 117*f*–118*f*
Intestine, foreign bodies in, radiologic findings with, 118, 118*f*, 119*f*
Intracath long catheter, 477
Intranasal vaccines, 575
Intraocular neoplasm, 346
Intraocular pressure
  elevation of, 338. *See also* Glaucoma
  measurement of, 339
Intraoral radiographic films, 297, 440 448
Intrapulmonary cysts, ruptured, 182, 183*f*
Intravenous catheter(s), types of, 477
Intravenous catheterization, 477–479
  procedures for, 477–479
  sites for, 477
Intravenous pyelogram. *See* Excretory urography
Intubation, 58
Intussusception
  gastroesophageal, radiologic findings with, 114, 116*f*
  of small bowel, radiologic findings with, 118, 120*f*
  ultrasonographic appearance of, 150, 151*f*
In vitro fertilization, 469
Iodine
  aqueous organic, indications for, 328
  for dermatophytosis, 507*t*
Iohexol, 134
Ipecac, 554
Irides, mottled appearance of, 33
Iris, 332
  melanoma of, 335
Iris color, change in, 33
Iron deficiency anemia, 162
Iron products, drug interactions, 53*t*
Ischemia, 166
Ischial tuberosity, palpation of, 35, 35*f*
Ischiocavernous myectomy, 488
  results of, 488
  surgical technique for, 488
Ischium, point of, palpation of, 35 35*f*
Isoflurane
  dosage, 58
  indications for, 58, 373, 486, 498
  for seizure control, 221
Isotretinoin, contraindications to, 472
Itraconazole, 548
Ivermectin, 557–558
  for cheyletiellosis, 514
  for microfilaria, 383
  for notoedric mange, 513
  for otodectic mange, 512
  prevention of heartworm disease with, 383
  toxicity, 557–558

Japanese Bobtail, 3, 13*f*, 13–14
Jaundice. *See* Icterus
Javanese, 14, 14*f*
Jaw fractures. *See* Mandibular trauma
Jaw pain, differential diagnosis of, 654
Jenotone, 372
Journal of the American Veterinary Medical Association, report on 1991 colloquium on feline leukemia virus, 367
Jugular vein
  blood collection from, 63, 63*f*
  catheterization, 477–478

Kanamycin, drug interactions, 52*t*
Kaolin-pectin preparations
  drug interactions, 53*t*
  for toxicosis, 559, 563–565
Kaon Elixir. *See* Potassium gluconate
Kaopectate. *See* Kaolin-pectin preparations
KCS. *See* Keratoconjunctivitis sicca
KCZ. *See* Ketoconazole
Keratinization/seborrheic disorders, 537–538
  differential diagnosis of, 660
Keratitis
  bacterial, 328
  eosinophilic, 330, 331*f*
  feline herpesvirus, 328, 330*f*
Keratoconjunctivitis sicca, 327
Keratopathy
  exposure, caused by chronic glaucoma, 339, 339*f*
  striate, 340
Ketamine
  antagonist, 57*t*
  combined with acepromazine
    advantages and indications for, 57–58
    concentrations, 57*t*
    contraindications to, 65
    disadvantages of, 58
    dosage, 57, 57*t*
  combined with Beuthanasia-D Solution, for euthanasia, 72
  combined with diazepam
    advantages and indications for, 57, 60
    for anesthesia induction, 500
    antagonist, 57*t*
    concentrations, 57*t*
    disadvantages of, 57
    dosage, 57*t*
    dosage, for 10-lb cat, 57, 57*t*, 60, 65
    for splinting of fractures, 395
  combined with xylazine, recommended dosage, 57*t*
  concentrations, 57*t*
  contraindications to, 498
  dosage, 57*t*
  duration of effects, 61
  for feline asthma, 235
  indications for, 373
  oral administration of, through open-end feline urinary catheter, 60*f*, 60–61
  side effects of, 60*f*, 61
Ketaset. *See* Ketamine
Ketoacidotic cat, treatment of, 308–310
Ketoconazole
  for blastomycosis, 547
  for coccidiomycosis, 548
  for cryptococcosis, 543
  for dermatophytosis, 508
  dosage and administration of, 548
  for histoplasmosis, 545
  indications for, 502, 509, 548
  side effects of, 548
  for stud tail, 538
  for toxoplasmosis, 168
Ketones, urinary, normal value for, 84
Ketonuria, 310
Key–Gaskell syndrome. *See* Autonomic polyganglionopathy
Kidney(s). *See also under* Renal
  effects of antidiuretic hormone of, 207
  hypoechoic, 149
  normal size of, 277
  palpation of, 275
  response to diuresis, 282
  subcapsular cyst of, radiologic findings with, 122
  ultrasonographic evaluation of, 148–149
    techniques for, 149
Kidney enlargement, cytologic findings with, 107
Kitten(s), 37–39
  in breeding cattery, and control of infectious diseases, 420, 422
  fading, 66, 466
  guidelines for raising, 37
  intestinal parasites in, 38
  in multicat facilities, prevention of upper respiratory infections among, 575
  neonatal, 38
    conjunctivitis in, 321, 322*f*
    death of, 466
  as new pet, instructions for owner of, 37
  normal development in, 38–39
  opening of eyes in, 38
  orphaned, raising, 38
  vaccinations of, 38

Klebsiella, 577
Klinefelter's syndrome, 473
KOH. *See* Potassium hydroxide
Korat, 14*f*, 14–15
  nervous system disorders in, 165*t*
  seizure disorders in, 219*t*

Laboratory tests/testing, 81–94
  antigen versus antibody, 81
  diseases affecting, 84–88
  important concepts about, 81
  normal values for, 81–84
  sensitivity of, 81
  specificity of, 81
Lacrimal apparatus, diseases of, 326–327
Lacrimal gland
  abscess of, 326
  inflammation of, 327
Lacrimal punctum atresia, 327
Lactate dehydrogenase
  elevated levels of, in thromboembolic disease, 252–253
  test for, normal value, 82
Lactated Ringer's solution, 308
  indications for, 374, 387, 552
  potassium content of, 259
  for shock, 393
Lactational anestrus, 465
Lactulose
  dosage and administration of, 410
  indications for, 265, 410
Lagophthalmos, 325
  treatment of, 325, 326*f*
Lameness, physical examination for, 35
Lanacaine. *See* Benzocaine
Landau reflex, definition of, 39
Lanoxin. *See* Digoxin
Laparotomy, 469
  liver biopsy taken via, 262
Lasix. *See* Furosemide
Latex agglutination test (LAT), 543
Laxatives
  bulk-forming, 418*t*–419*t*
  stimulant, 418*t*–419*t*
Laxatone-Evsco. *See* White petrolatum
LD_{50}. *See* Median lethal dose
LDH. *See* Lactate dehydrogenase
Lead poisoning, treatment of, 169
Leiomyoma, gastrointestinal, 226
Leiomyosarcoma, gastrointestinal, 226
Lens
  anatomy of, 335–336
  cloudiness of, 33, 33*f*
  diseases of, 335–338
  metabolism in, 336
  subluxation of, 336, 337*f*
Lens displacement, 337
Lens luxation, 336–337, 337*f*
Lens position, changes in, 336–337
Lens transparency, changes in, 336
Lente. *See* Insulin, intermediate-acting
Lentivirus, 348. *See also* Feline immunodeficiency virus
Lentivirus infection
  detection of, 350
  treatment of, 350
Lesion(s)
  malignant, cytologic findings with, 100
  solid and cystic, ultrasonographic characteristics of, 145
Lesion localization
  with nervous system disease, 164–165
  with seizure disorders, 218–219
Lethal dose, median, 551
Leukemias, 430. *See also* Feline leukemia virus infection
Leukocell, 366
Leukocytes, 157
Levamisole
  for microfilaria, 383
  for plasmacytic-lymphocytic stomatitis, 444
Levasole. *See* Levamisole
Levator palpebrae superioris muscle, 319
LH. *See* Luteinizing hormone
Lice, 515, 515*f*
Lid margins, black pigment depositions on, 33, 34*f*
Lidocaine
  indications for, 49, 58
  preparations, 49
Ligation, nylon bands for, 488–490
  indications for, 490
Liking for cats, demonstration of, 28
Lilium longiflorum. *See* Easter lily
Lilium tigrinum. *See* Tiger lily
Limb fractures/luxations, caused by high-rise fall, management of, 395–397
Lime sulfur
  for demodectic mange, 515
  for dermatophytosis, 507*t*
  for notoedric mange, 513
d-Limonene, 563
Lincomycin, drug interactions, 53*t*
Lindane, contraindications to, 48
Linear array scanner, 145
Linear granuloma, 445, 534, 534*f*–535*f*
Lingual tumors, 431
Liothyronine, in diagnosis of hyperthyroidism, 404
Lipase, test for
  diseases affecting, 86
  normal value, 82
Lip avulsion, 447
  treatment of, 447
Lipidosis. *See* Idiopathic hepatic lipidosis
Lipocytes, morphologic characteristics of, 206, 206*f*
Lipoma, cytologic findings with, 108–109, 109*f*
Lips, black pigment depositions on, 34, 34*f*
Lip ulcers, 455, 533*f*, 533–535
Liquid(s), dissolving medications in, 47
Liquid medications, administration of, 44
Litter, nonabsorbable, for home urine monitoring, 312, 376
Litter box
  cat's aversion to, 238–239
  maintenance of, 239
Litter size, average, 461
Liver. *See also under* Hepatic; Raw liver
  cirrhosis of, 263, 263*f*
  hyperechoic, 146*f*
  percutaneous fine-needle aspiration of
    in diagnosis of idiopathic hepatic lipidosis, 408
    procedures for, 409–410
  ultrasonographic evaluation of, 146, 146*f*
    technique for, 146
Liver aspirates, normal, 98*f*, 408, 409*f*
Liver aspiration, 104
  common feline diseases diagnosed by, 104, 105*f*
  in diagnosis of idiopathic hepatic lipidosis, 408
  for idiopathic hepatic lipidosis, 408, 409*f*
  for lymphocytic cholangitis/cholangiohepatitis, 262, 263*f*
  procedures for, 409–410
  technique for, 104, 104*f*
Liver biopsy, indications for, 262
Liver disease. *See also* Cholangitis/cholangiohepatitis syndrome
  classification of, 146
  ultrasonographic findings with, 146, 146*f*–147*f*
Lochia, 465
Lomotil. *See* Diphenoxylate with atropine
Long catheters, 477
  placement of, procedure for, 478–479
Longhair. *See* American Curl, longhair; Oriental Longhair
Longhair Scottish Fold, 15, 15*f*
Lower gastrointestinal series. *See* Gastrointestinal series
Lower urinary tract diseases, 376–377. *See also* Feline urologic syndrome
Low-gluten diets, 414
LRS. *See* Lactated Ringer's solution
Lumbar spine
  L-5/L-6 vertebra, landmarks for, 136
  L-6/L-7 vertebra, landmarks for, 134*f*, 136
Lumbar spondylosis, treatment of, 49
Lung. *See also under* Pulmonary
Lung abscess, diagnosis of, with lung aspiration, 107
Lung aspiration, 107
  common feline diseases diagnosed by, 107
  complications of, 107
  indications for, 176
  technique for, 107
Lung lacerations, 182
Lung parenchyma, tearing of, 182, 183*f*
Lung sclerosis/consolidation, 182, 184*f*
Lungworm infestation, test for, 88
Lutalyse. *See* Prostaglandin $F_{2\alpha}$
Luteal period
  abnormal events of, 462–463
  normal events of, 461–462
Luteinizing hormone, 459–460
Luxations. *See also specific type*
  caused by high-rise falls, management of, 395–397
LymDyp. *See* Lime sulfur
Lymphadenitis, 203–204
  cytologic evaluation of, 202–203, 203*f*–205*f*
  eosinophilic, 204, 205*f*
  granulomatous/pyogranulomatous, 203, 203*f*–204*f*
  neutrophilic, 203–204, 204*f*
  primary, 203
  purulent, 203, 203*f*
  secondary, 203
Lymphadenopathy, 199–206
  differential diagnosis of, 654
  etiology of, 199
  evaluation of, 199, 200*f*, 206
Lymph node(s), enlarged, 193
Lymph node aspirates
  cell types observed in, 201–202
  cytologic evaluation of, 202–205
    flow chart for, 200*f*
  excessive cell rupturing in, 202, 202*f*, 204–205
  interpretations of, 203–205
    basis for, 202–203
  normal, 202
  staining used with, 201
Lymph node aspiration
  accidental aspiration of nonlymphoid tissue during, 206, 206*f*
  combination cytology preparation with, 199–201, 201*f*
  indications for, 193–194
  sample collection and preparation, 199–201
  techniques for, 199–201
Lymph node excisional biopsy, indications for, 206
Lymphoblasts, morphologic characteristics of, 201, 205
Lymphocytes
  large. *See* Lymphoblasts
  mature (small), morphologic characteristics of, 201
  medium-sized, morphologic characteristics of, 201
  test for
    diseases affecting, 85
    normal value, 82
  traumatized or ruptured, differentiation of, 204–205
  values, at different ages, 83
Lymphocytic cholangitis/cholangiohepatitis, 262–263
  clinical and laboratory findings with, 262
  diagnosis of, 262, 263*f*
  incidence of, 262
  prognosis for, 263
  treatment of, 262–263
Lymphoglandular bodies, 202
Lymphoid hyperplasia, 203
  cytologic evaluation of, 203, 203*f*
Lymphoid leukemia, 428
Lymphoreticular tumors, 434
Lymphosarcoma, 427–430
  alimentary, 428
  classification of, 427–429
  clinical signs of, 427–428
  cytologic evaluation of, 202, 204–205, 205*f*
  diagnosis of, 112*t*, 428
    with body fluid aspiration, 111
    with liver aspiration, 104, 105*f*
    with spleen aspiration, 105, 105*f*
    with thoracic mass aspiration, 107
  etiology of, 360
  gastrointestinal, 226, 431–432
    radiologic findings with, 118, 120*f*
  mediastinal (thymic), 427–428
  multicentric, 428
  prognosis for, 429–430
  pulmonary, 182, 190, 190*f*
  radiation therapy for, 430
  renal, 428–429, 435
    radiologic findings with, 122, 124*f*
  in spinal canal, radiologic findings with, 136, 136*f*
  of third eyelid, 325, 327*f*
  tracheal collapse caused by, 177, 178*f*
  treatment of, 429*t*, 429–430
Lynxacarus radovsky, 515–516, 517*f*
Lysosomal storage disease, 165
  ocular manifestations of, 346

MacEwen's Protocol, 429*t*
MacKenzie brush technique, 506, 580
Macrocytes, 64, 65*f*
Macrocytosis, 162
Macrophages, morphologic characteristics of, 201
Magnesium, dietary levels of, and feline urologic syndrome, 370
Magnesium hydroxide, 559
Magnesium sulfate
  contraindications to, 554–555
  for toxicosis, 554
Magnus neck reflex, definition of, 39
Maine Coon, 3, 15*f*, 15–16
  periodontitis in, 443
Major motor seizures. *See* Tonic-clonic seizures
Malassezia canis, 537–538
Malathion dips, for demodectic mange, 515
Malathion toxicity, 560–561
Male cats
  aggression among, 240–241
  catheterization of, 124
  characteristics of, 36
Male infertility, 467
Male reproduction, 466–467
Malocclusions, 300–303
  acquired, 301
  brachygnathic, 301, 302*f*, 302–303
  clinical signs of, 301, 301*f*
  etiology of, 301
  prognathic, 301–302
Mammary adenocarcinoma, cytologic findings with, 106*f*, 109
Mammary glands
  enlarged/swollen, differential diagnosis of, 654
  physical examination of, 35
Mammary hypertrophy, benign, caused by megestrol acetate, 51, 51*f*
Mammary tumors, 430–431
Mandibular anatomy, 290–291, 291*f*
Mandibular condylectomy, 449
Mandibular trauma, 139, 290, 448*f*, 448–449
  clinical signs of, 448
  lip avulsion with, 447
  and malocclusion, 301
  management of, 397*f*, 398, 488, 489*f*
  radiologic findings with, 139
Maneki-Neko. *See* Japanese Bobtail
Mange
  demodectic, 514–515
  notoedric, 512–513
  otodectic, 511–512
Mannitol
  contraindications to, 280
  dosage, 169
  for glaucoma, 340
  indications for, 169
  for oliguric renal failure, 280
  for toxicosis, 555
α-Mannosidosis, 346
Manx, 3, 16, 16*f*. *See also* Cymric
  nervous system disorders in, 165*t*
Manx syndrome, 416, 417*f*, 472
Marginal biopsy, 426
Marginal ear vein, blood collection from, 63
Marking behavior, 236. *See also* Spraying
  drug therapy for, 238–239
  surgical therapy for, 238
  treatment of, 238–239
Mason metasplint, 395
Masses, dermal and epidermal, 95
  cytologic findings with, 108*f*–109*f*, 108–110
Mast cells, 434
  morphologic characteristics of, 201–202
Mast cell tumors, 434
  cytologic findings with, 104–105, 106*f*, 108, 205, 206*f*
  gastrointestinal, 431–432
  histiocytic, 526, 530–531
  intestinal, 434
  originating in gastrointestinal tract, 226
  of skin, 530–531
  visceral, 434
Mastectomy, indications for, 463
Mastitis, 465–466
Mastocytoma, 434
Mastocytosis, 434
  diagnosis of, with spleen aspiration, 104–105, 106*f*
Maternal antibodies, 38
Mau. *See* Egyptian Mau
Maxilla, 290, 291*f*
Maxillary fractures, 290
  treatment of, 447
Maxillary-mandibular cerclage wire, stabilization of temporomandibular luxation or mandibular fracture with, 397*f*, 398
MCH. *See* Mean corpuscular hemoglobin
MCHC. *See* Mean corpuscular hemoglobin concentration
MCT. *See* Mast cell tumors
MCT oil, 288
MCV. *See* Mean corpuscular volume
MDB. *See* Minimum data base
Mean corpuscular hemoglobin, test for, normal value, 82
Mean corpuscular hemoglobin concentration, test for, normal value, 82
Mean corpuscular volume, 160
  test for, normal value, 82
Medial saphenous vein, catheterization, 477–478
Median lethal dose, 551
Mediastinal lymphosarcoma, 427–428
Mediastinal masses
  aspiration of, indications for, 176
  radiologic findings with, 114, 115*f*
Medication dosage charts, 631–633
  milliliters for 10-lb cat, 632
  number of pills for 10-lb cat, 633
Medications. *See* Drug(s)
Medicol. *See* Chloramphenicol
Medicut short catheter, 477
Medroxyprogesterone acetate
  dosage, 239
  for eosinophilic granuloma complex, 446
  for intermale aggression, 240
  for marking behavior, 239
  for miliary dermatitis, 532
  for sex hormone imbalance, 537
  side effects of, 239
Medullary hypertonicity, 208, 211
Medullary washout, 208
  and water deprivation test, 214–216
Megace. *See* Megestrol acetate
Megacolon, 416–419
  diagnosis of, 416
  differential diagnosis of, 416
  history and clinical signs of, 416
  pathophysiology of, 416, 417*f*
  pharmacological treatment of, 416, 418*t*–419*t*
  radiographic findings with, 121, 121*f*, 416, 417*f*
  surgical treatment of, 416, 417*f*, 480–481
  treatment of, 416
Megaesophagus, 178, 182*f*
  radiologic findings with, 114, 115*f*
Megalocornea, 339, 339*f*, 340
Megestrol acetate
  adverse effects of, 50*f*, 50–51, 51*f*
  client education about, 54
  clinical use of, guidelines for, 50–54
  contraindications to, 314, 374
  diabetes mellitus related to, 313
  dosage and administration of, 51*t*, 54, 239, 330
  for eosinophilic granuloma complex, 446
  for estrus prevention/suppression, 461
  for hyperesthesia syndrome, 400
  for idiopathic vomiting syndrome, 226
  indications for, 50, 51*t*, 330
  for intermale aggression, 240
  for marking behavior, 239
  for miliary dermatitis, 532
  physiologic effects of, 50
  for plasmacytic-lymphocytic stomatitis, 444
  for sex hormone imbalance, 537
  side effects of, 49, 207, 461
  for urge incontinence, 372
Meibomian gland, obstruction of, 322
Melanoma
  cytologic findings with, 109*f*, 109–110
  of iris, 335
Melanosarcoma, oral, 444–445
Menace reflex, definition of, 39
Mental foramina, 291*f*
Mesenchymal tumors, 530–531
Mesenteric lymph node enlargement, cytologic findings with, 107
Metabolic disease/disorder, 166
  diagnosis of, 226
  vomiting/diarrhea caused by, 226
Metacarpal fractures, management of, 395
Metamucil, 419*t*
Metarubricytes, 64, 65*f*, 159, 160*t*
Metatarsal fractures, management of, 395
Methazolamide, for glaucoma, 340
Methemoglobin, 384
Methemoglobinemia, 384–388
Methenamine, 372
  drug interactions, 52*t*–53*t*
Methimazole
  continuous management of hyperthyroidism with, 406–407
  dosage and administration of, 404–405
  indications for, 404, 498
Methioform. *See* Methionine
Methionine, 50
  contraindications to, 410, 410*t*
  Heinz body hemolytic anemia caused by, 387
  side effects of, 50
DL-Methionine, 372
Methocarbamol, 552
Methomyl, 560–561
Methotrexate
  dose, 427*t*
  route of administration, 427*t*
  toxicity, 427*t*
Methoxyflurane
  advantages and indications for, 58
  dosage, 58
  drug interactions, 53*t*
Methylene blue. *See also* New methylene blue staining
  anemia caused by, 160
  contraindications to, 387
  Heinz body hemolytic anemia caused by, 385, 386*t*
Methylene blue-containing compounds, side effects of, 372
Methyl methacrylate, 449
Methylprednisolone
  for eosinophilic granuloma complex, 446, 535
  for flea allergic dermatitis, 520
Methylprednisolone acetate
  dosage and administration of, 234*t*, 335
  for feline asthma, 234
  for inflammatory bowel disease, 414
  for miliary dermatitis, 532
  for plasmacytic-lymphocytic stomatitis, 444
Methylprednisolone sodium succinate
  dosage and administration of, 169
  indications for, 169
  for spinal cord trauma, 395
4-Methylpyrazole, 567
Metoclopramide
  dosage and administration of, 284
  indications for, 284
  for vomiting, 223
Metophane. *See* Methoxyflurane
Metritis, postpartum, 465, 465*f*
Metronidazole
  for cholangitis/cholangiohepatitis, 262
  for chronic diarrhea, 224
  dosage and administration of, 265, 410
  indications for, 265, 410, 480
  for plasmacytic-lymphocytic stomatitis, 444
  prophylactic, for inflammatory bowel disease, 414
MGK 264. *See* *N*-Octyl-bicycloheptene dicarboximide
Mibolerone
  for estrus prevention/suppression, 461
  side effects of, 461
Michel's medium, 444
Miconazole, for dermatophytosis, 507, 507*t*
Microfilaria, 379
  treatment for, 383
Microphthalmia, 317
Microscope, for reading cytologic preparations, 96
Microsporum canis, 504, 579
  macroconidia of, 506, 506*f*
Microsporum canis infection
  clinical signs of, 504–505, 505*f*
  diagnosis of, 505*f*, 505–506, 506*f*–507*f*
Microsporum gypseum, 504, 579
Milbemycin oxime, prevention of heartworm disease with, 383
Miliary dermatitis, 532–533
  clinical signs of, 532, 533*f*
  diagnosis of, 532
  differential diagnosis of, 533*t*
  etiology of, 532, 533*t*
  therapy for, 532–533
Milk of magnesia, 559
Mineral oil, 419*t*
  as cathartic, 555
  for demodectic mange, 515
  for obstipation, 416

Mini Bain Anesthesia Circuit, 58
Minimum data base
for inflammatory bowel disease, 414
for neurologic disease, 167, 168*t*
for PU/PD syndrome, 214, 214*t*
for reproductive failure, 467, 469–470
for seizure disorders, 220, 221*t*
for vomiting/diarrhea, 223
Minnesota Feline Olive Tipped Urethral Catheter, 373, 373*f*
Minocycline, drug interactions, 53*t*
Miosis, differential diagnosis of, 652
Miotic agents, topical
for glaucoma, 340
mechanism of action, 340
Mirror image artifact, in ultrasonography, 145
Mismating, 460
Misoprostol, contraindications to, 472
Missouri Rex, 16–17, 17*f*
Mitaban. *See* Amitraz
Mitotane, contraindications to, 472
Mitoxantrone, 431
Mixed pattern, cytologic interpretation of, 99*f*, 99–100
M-Mode, 145
Moderator bands
excessive, 251
clinical signs and diagnosis of, 251
treatment and prognosis for, 251
functions of, 251
Molt periosteal elevator, 298, 300
Moniliella, 509
Monocytes, test for
diseases affecting, 85–86
normal value, 82
Monoject Catheter-Tipped Syringe, 41
Mo Rex. *See* Missouri Rex
Morphine, 253
Motion mode, 145
Mouth, physical examination of, 33–34
Mouth opening, painful, differential diagnosis of, 654
MPS. *See* Mucopolysaccharidosis
Mucociliary apparatus, 231
Mucomyst. *See N*-Acetylcysteine
Mucopolysaccharidosis, 346
ocular manifestations of, 346
Mucous membranes, bluish coloration of, differential diagnosis of, 643
Multicat facilities
disease control in, 420–424
disinfection of, 423–424
prevention of upper respiratory infections in, 575
types of, 420, 422–423
Multicat household(s)
control of infectious diseases in, 423
definition of, 420
Multicentric lymphosarcoma, 428
Multisystem disseminating diseases, 344–346
Munchkin, 17, 17*f*
Mural thickening, ultrasonographic appearance of, 151
Murmur, differential diagnosis of, 655
Muscle atrophy, differential diagnosis of, 655
Muscle massage, for thromboembolic disease, 253
Musculoskeletal system, physical examination of, 35
Mutations, and evolution of cat breeds, 3
Muzzle, open front
for fractures of ramus, 448–449
for temporomandibular joint luxation, 449
Mycetoma, 509
clinical signs of, 509
diagnosis of, 509
therapy for, 509
Mycobacteria, 472
Mycoplasma
abortions caused by, 472
respiratory infection caused by, 573
Mycotic diseases, 540–550
Mydriasis
caused by glaucoma, 339
differential diagnosis of, 654–655
Myeloblastopenia, caused by feline leukemia virus, 365
Myelogram, 134–136
clinical indications for, 134
common lesions diagnosed with, 136, 136*f*
goal of, 134
materials for, 134
normal findings with, 135*f*, 136
technique for, 134*f*, 134–136
Myeloid:erythroid ratio, test for, normal value, 83
Myopathy(ies)
differential diagnosis of, 258
hypernatremic, CVF/MW complex caused by, 256
pathogenesis of, 257
Myositis, steroid-responsive, CVF/MW complex caused by, 256

Nandrolone decanoate
contraindications to, 410*t*
indications for, 284
NAPCC. *See* National Animal Poison Control Center
Nasal cavity
anatomy of, 266, 269*f*
common lesions of, radiologic findings with, 140
radiologic evaluation of, 140, 141*f*–142*f*
ventrodorsal view of, 266–267, 271*f*
Nasal discharge
chronic, 266–273, 267*f*
analysis of, 267–272
diagnosis of, 266–273
etiology of, 266, 267*t*
history of cat with, 266
medical intervention for, 272–273
prognosis for, 273
radiographic studies with, 266–267, 269*f*–271*f*
serologic studies of, 272
surgical treatment of, 273
treatment of, 272–273
differential diagnosis of, 655
Nasal flush(es)
for chronic nasal discharge, 273
for collection of discharge sample, 267–272, 272*f*
Nasal foreign bodies, 266, 267*f*
Nasal planum
black pigment depositions on, 33, 34*f*
color of, interpretation of, 157
tumor of, 433–434
Nasal polyps, benign (inflammatory), 266, 268*f*
Nasal surgical exploration, indications for, 273
Nasal tumors, 266, 268*f*, 433–434
malignant, 266, 268*f*
Nasogastric tube, 43
National Animal Poison Control Center, 551
National Cat Club, 3
National Cat Show, 3
Nausea, in CRD cats, 284
NDI. *See* Nephrogenic diabetes insipidus
NE. *See* Neurologic examination
Nebelung, 17
Neck, persistent ventroflexion of, 35
Needle punch biopsy, 425–426
Neomycin
dosage and administration of, 410
drug interactions, 52*t*–53*t*
indications for, 410
Neonatal bacterial sepsis, 466
Neonatal conjunctivitis, 321, 322*f*
Neonatal isoerythrolysis, 66–67
Neonatal kittens, 38
death of, 466
Neoplastic disease. *See* Tumor(s)
Neoplastic pattern
cytologic interpretation of, 99, 99*f*
mixed with inflammatory pattern, 99*f*, 99–100
Neo-Synephrine. *See* Phenylephrine
Nepeta cataria. *See* Catnip
Nephrectomy, 435
Nephrogenic diabetes insipidus
primary, 208
secondary, 208, 211
water deprivation testing in, 216, 216*t*
Nephrons, 274
Nephrotoxins, exposure to, prevention of, and chronic renal disease, 283
Neptazane. *See* Methazolamide
Nerve conduction testing, 194
Nervous system, radiologic evaluation of, 134–136
Nervous system anomalies, 165
Nervous tissue, traumatic injury to, therapy for, 169
Neurodermatitis. *See* Hyperesthesia syndrome
Neuroendocrine response, failure of, 469
Neurologic disease. *See* Ataxia/paresis
Neurologic examination, 164–165
with seizure disorders, 218
Neurologic parameters, of physical examination, 35
Neurologic syndrome, caused by feline leukemia virus, 365
Neuromuscular junction diseases, differential diagnosis of, 258
Neutering. *See* Castration
Neutropenia, chemotherapy-induced, 426–427
Neutrophilic lymphadenitis, 203–204, 204*f*
Neutrophils
morphologic characteristics of, 202
segmented, normal value for, 82
test for, diseases affecting, 85
values, at different ages, 83
New cat, introducing, to resident cat, 242
New methylene blue staining, 96
of Heinz bodies, 160, 162*f*
NI. *See* Neonatal isoerythrolysis
Nicotinic acid, 438
NIDDM. *See* Non–insulin-dependent diabetes mellitus
Nitrofurantoin, drug interactions, 53*t*
Nitroglycerin
for dilated cardiomyopathy, 250
for hypertrophic cardiomyopathy, 247
Nitrostat Ointment 2%. *See* Nitroglycerin
Nizoral. *See* Ketoconazole
NMB stain. *See* New methylene blue staining
Nocardia, 509
Nolvasan. *See* Chlorhexidine
Nonabsorbable cat litter, for home urine monitoring, 312, 376
Non–insulin-dependent diabetes mellitus, 306, 313
Nonliquid medications
administration of, 44–47, 45*f*–46*f*
dissolving in liquids, 47
Non-rebreathing anesthetic system, 58
Nonregenerative anemia, 159, 162
associated with chronic renal disease, 277, 283
associated with feline leukemia virus infection, 365
associated with *Hemobartonella felis*, 390–391
Nonsteroidal anti-inflammatory agents, side effects of, 49
Nonsteroidal anti-inflammatory drugs, 558–559
Nontapetum, multifocal hypopigmentation in, 344, 344*f*
Nonvisual placing response, definition of, 39
Norwegian Forest Cat, 17–18, 18*f*
Nose, physical examination of, 33
Nosebleed, differential diagnosis of, 649
Nose-to-nose transmission, of infectious diseases, 420
Notoedres cati, 512, 512*f*
Notoedric mange, 512–513
clinical signs of, 512, 513*f*
diagnosis of, 513
etiology and pathogenesis of, 512, 512*f*
therapy for, 513
Novolin L. *See* Insulin, intermediate-acting
Novolin N. *See* Insulin, intermediate-acting
Novolin R. *See* Insulin, regular
NPH. *See* Insulin, intermediate-acting
Nutrition, and gingival health, 438–439
Nutritional deficiency
neurologic manifestations of, 166
pregnancy loss caused by, 472
treatment of, 169
Nutritional needs, of anorectic cat, 40
Nutritional state, positive, maintenance of, in chronic renal disease, 284–285
Nutritional support, in chronic renal disease, 282
Nylon bands, for ligation or fracture fixation, 488–490
adverse reactions to and complications of, 490
indications for, 490, 490*f*
Nystagmus, differential diagnosis of, 655–656

Obesity
in diabetic cats, 314
extreme, dyspnea caused by, 190, 190*f*
Obstipation
caused by megacolon, 416
differential diagnosis of, 641
treatment of, 416
Ocicat, 18, 18*f*
Ocreata, 11
N-Octyl-bicycloheptene dicarboximide, 561–562
Ocular discharge, differential diagnosis of, 656
Ocular lesions, caused by *Cryptococcus neoformans*, 542
Ocular mycotic disease, 333, 333*f*, 344–345, 344*f*–345*f*
Ocular toxoplasmosis, 345
Odontomas, 445
Ojos Azules, 18–19, 19*f*
Oliguria, 280

Oliguric renal failure, 280
  diagnosis of, 280, 280*t*
  treatment of, 280
Ollulanus tricuspis, 224
Omnipaque 240. *See also* Iohexol
ONF. *See* Oronasal fistula
Onions, anemia caused by, 387
Onychectomy, 240, 490–491
  alternative to, 482–483
  surgical technique for, 490–491, 491*f*
Oocyte collection, 469
Open-mouth breathing, 172. *See also* Aerophagia
Open mouth disorders, 290
Ophthalmic antibiotics, indications for, 574
Ophthalmoscopy, direct, examination of posterior segment with, 341
Oral abscessation, 290
Oral anatomy, 290–291, 291*f*
Oral burns, 448
Oral cavity, autoimmune diseases involving, 444
Oral cellulitis, 290
Oral diseases, 438–453. *See also* Dental diseases/disorders
Oral examination, 290
Oral hygiene products, therapeutic, 296–297
Oral injury, from direct ingestion of chemicals/caustic agents, 448
Oral medications
  administration of, 44–47
  dissolving in liquids, 47
  forms of, 44–47
  hiding in food, 44–45
Oral problems. *See* Dental disease(s)
Oral trauma, 446–448
  clinical signs of, 446
Oral tumors, 431, 444–445, 445*f*
Orange cats, black pigment depositions in, 33–34, 34*f*
Orbicularis oculi muscle, 319
Orbit, anatomy of, 317
Orbital arteriography, 319
Orbital cellulitis, 318
  clinical signs of, 318–319, 319*f*
Orbital cone, 317
Orbital disease, 317–319
  clinical signs of, 317
  congenital, 317
  etiology of, 317
  inflammatory, 318–319
    clinical signs of, 318–319
    diagnosis of, 319
    drainage of, procedures for, 319
    etiology of, 318
    sequelae, 319
Orbital trauma, 317–318
Orbital tumors, 319, 325
Organ, enlarged, cytologic findings with, 106–107
Organic iodine. *See* Gastrografin
Organophosphate insecticides
  lethal doses of, 561*t*
  toxicity, 166, 472, 560–561
    treatment of, 169
Organ pattern, normal, cytologic interpretation of, 98, 98*f*
Orient, evolution of cat breeds in, 3
Oriental Longhair, 14, 14*f*
Oriental Shorthair, 19, 19*f*
Orogastric tube feeding, 41–42
  of neonatal kittens, 466
Oronasal fistula, 441
  treatment of, 441–442
Orphaned kittens, raising, 38
Orthocide. *See* Captan
Orthodontia. *See* Tooth movement
Orthodontics, interceptive, for malocclusions, 302
Orthopedic trauma, caused by high-rise fall, 395
Orthoplast splint, 478
Orthopnea, 172
  definition of, 173*t*
Osmolal gap, 566–567
Osmoreceptors, 207
Osmotic agents, for glaucoma, 340
Osmotic diuresis, 281–282
  PU/PD syndrome caused by, 207, 211
Osteochondromatosis, 433
Osteomas, ossifying, 433
Osteomyelitis, of tympanic bullae, 139
Osteosarcoma, 432–433
  nasal, 434
  parosteal, 433
Otoacariasis. *See* Otodectic mange
Otodectes cynotis, 511, 512*f*
Otodectic mange, 511–512
  clinical signs of, 511, 512*f*
  diagnosis of, 511
  etiology and pathogenesis of, 511, 512*f*
  therapy for, 511–512
Ovaban. *See* Megestrol acetate
Ovarian activity
  absence of, 467
  detection of, 467
  inhibition of, 467
Ovarian dysgenesis, unilateral, 473
Ovarian tumors, 468
Ovariohysterectomy
  for estrus prevention/suppression, 461
  indications for, 463, 465, 468–469
  in pregnant cats, use of nylon bands for, 490, 490*f*
  for pyometra, 462–463
Oviductal transport, of embryo, 460
Ovulation, 459–460
  failure of, and repeated breeding, 468–469
  hormone levels in, 460, 460*t*
  increasing likelihood of, 460
  induction of, 458
    by copulation, 458–459
    with exogenous hormones, 460
    by mechanical stimulation, 459
Owner. *See also* Children; Human(s); Pregnant women
  approach to, 28
  presence of, during euthanasia, 71
Oxalate plants, 564*t*, 564–565
Oxalic acid toxicosis, 564–565
Oxazepam
  indications for, 285
  preparations, 42*t*
  recommended dosage, 42*t*
Oxidants, anemia caused by, 160, 384–387
Oxygen administration
  for asthmatic cat, 234
  for cardiomyopathy, 247, 249
  indications for, 251
Oxygen supplementation, for toxicosis, 552
Oxymethalone
  contraindications to, 410*t*
  indications for, 284
Oxytetracycline
  drug interactions, 53*t*
  indications for, 574
  in pleurodesis, 289
Oxytocin, for uterine inertia, 464

Packed cell volume, 64
  after transfusion, 68
  in diagnosis of anemia, 157
  at different ages, 83
  diseases affecting, 84–85
  effects of blood transfusion on, 67
  normal value for, 158
Pain, treatment of, in cats with thromboembolic disease, 253
Pain relievers, human, toxicity, 558–560
Palate. *See* Hard palate
Palate defects, 449–451
  clinical signs of, 449–450, 450*f*
  congenital, 451*f*
  treatment of, 450–451
Palate lesions, 450, 451*f*
Palpebral conjunctiva, 319
Palpebral reflex, definition of, 39
2-PAM. *See* Pralidoxime chloride
Panadol. *See* Acetaminophen
Pancreas, ultrasonographic evaluation of, 147–148
Pancreatic disorders, ultrasonographic findings with, 148, 148*f*
Pancreatitis, 226
  traumatic, caused by high-rise fall, 394
  ultrasonographic signs of, 148
Pancytopenia, 162
  caused by feline leukemia virus, 365
Panleukopenia-like syndrome, caused by feline leukemia virus, 365
Panniculus reflex, definition of, 39
Panophthalmitis, caused by FHV-induced corneal ulcers, 571, 572*f*
Papillomas, oral, 445
Paragonimus kellicolli, pulmonary cysts caused by, 182, 183*f*
Paralysis. *See also* Ataxia/paresis
  differential diagnosis of, 656
  facial, 323
  posterior
    in cardiac disease, 244, 248, 250, 252
    secondary to saddle thrombus, 252–254
Paraneoplastic syndromes, 227
Parasites, intestinal, 224
Parasitic diseases
  pulmonary manifestations of, 182, 183*f*
  of skin, 511–517
Paresis. *See* Ataxia/paresis
Paresthesia, differential diagnosis of, 399
Paromomycin, drug interactions, 52*t*
Parosteal osteosarcoma, 433
Partial motor seizures, 220*t*
Parti-color Persian, 20
Parturition, 463–465
  abnormal, 464–465
  initiation of, 463
  length of, 464
  normal, 463–464
Parvovirus. *See* Feline panleukopenia
Pasteurella multocida, 479, 577
Patch testing, in diagnosis of contact allergic dermatitis, 524
PCV. *See* Packed cell volume
PD. *See* Polydipsia
Pediculosis, 515, 515*f*
Pedigrees, 4
Pelvic fracture, physical examination for, 35, 35*f*
Pemphigus vulgaris, 444
Penicillin
  in combination with aminoglycosides, for pyothorax, 456
  drug interactions, 53*t*
  indications for, 509
  for neurologic disease, 168
Penicillin G, indications for, 456
Penicillin G procaine/penicillin G benzathine combination
  for chronic nasal discharge, 273
  indications for, 574
Pennyroyal oil, 563
Pentobarbital
  antagonist, 57*t*
  for central nervous system overstimulation, 552
  concentrations, 57*t*
  contraindications to, 472
  dosage, 57*t*
    for 10-lb cat, 57*t*
  for seizure control, 220
Pentothal. *See* Sodium thiopental
Pepto Bismol. *See* Bismuth subsalicylate
Percutaneous needle biopsy. *See* Tissue aspiration
Perianal area, physical examination of, 36, 36*f*
Pericardial diaphragmatic hernias, 178, 181*f*
Perineal urethrostomy, 479, 491–496
  complications of, 492–496
  indications for, 375
  results of, 496
  surgical technique for, 491–492, 493*f*–495*f*
Perinodal fat aspirates, 206, 206*f*
Periodic acid-Schiff staining (PAS), 506
Periodontal disease, 438–442
  associated with cervical line lesions, 293–294
  clinical signs of, 439, 439*f*
  diagnosis of, 439
  home care for, 442
  pathology of, 438–439
  prophylactic treatment of, 441, 441*t*
  radiographic signs of, 440–441
  stage I, 439–440, 440*t*
  stage II, 440, 440*t*
  stage III, 440, 440*t*
  stage IV, 440, 440*t*
  staging of, 439–441, 440*t*
  treatment of, 441–442
Periodontal explorer/probe, 439
Periodontal ligament, 291, 291*f*
  inflammation of, 293–294
Periodontal pockets, depth of, in staging of disease, 439–440, 440*t*
Periodontitis, juvenile-onset, 443
Periodontium, 291, 291*f*
Periorbital cellulitis, 318
  clinical signs of, 318–319, 319*f*
Peripheral lymph nodes, physical examination of, 35
Peripheral nervous system disorders. *See* Ataxia/paresis
Peritoneal effusion, ultrasonographic findings with, 151

Peritonitis. *See also* Feline infectious peritonitis
aseptic, diagnosis of, with abdominal fluid aspiration, 99*f*, 111
septic, diagnosis of, with abdominal fluid aspiration, 111, 112*f*
ultrasonographic findings with, 151
Persians, 19–20, 20*f*
ankyloblepharon in, 321
congenital orbital disorders in, 317
corneal sequestrum in, 330
entropion in, 322, 324*f*
epiphora in, 322
eyelid diseases in, 320*t*
malocclusions in, 301–302, 302*f*
nervous system disorders in, 165*t*
periodontitis in, 442
Persistent hyperplastic primary vitreous, 338
Petit mal seizures. *See* Absence seizures
Pet Loss Support Hotline, 76
Petting, aggression related to, 243
$PGF_{2\alpha}$. *See* Prostaglandin $F_{2\alpha}$
Phaeohyphomycosis, 509
Phagolytic uveitis, 336
Pharyngeal mucoceles, 446
Pharyngostomy tube, 43
Phenacetin toxicosis, 387
Phenazopyridine
anemia caused by, 160, 387
contraindications to, 49
Phenobarbital
for central nervous system overstimulation, 552
dosage, 169
drug interactions, 53*t*
for hyperesthesia syndrome, 400
indications for, 169, 262
as maintenance anticonvulsant, 221
for psychogenic alopecia, 537
for seizure control, 220–221
side effects of, 207
Phenothiazine tranquilizers, 553
for uremia, 284
Phenoxybenzamine
indications for, 374
for urge incontinence, 372
Phenylbutazone, drug interactions, 53*t*
Phenylephrine, indications for, 322–323
Phenytoin, contraindications to, 49, 472
Phialophora, 509
pHiso-Hex. *See* Hexachlorophene
Phlebotomy, for hypertrophic cardiomyopathy, 247
Phosmet, 560–561
for demodectic mange, 515
Phosphate binders, 283
Phosphate enemas, contraindications to, 49
Phospholine Iodide. *See* Echothiophate
Phosphorus
dietary, reduction of, and chronic renal disease, 283
test for
diseases affecting, 87
normal value, 82
Photoperiod, and reproductive cycle, 458, 467
Physaloptera, 224
Physical examination, 32–36
general assessment in, 32
Physostigmine, 558
Phytonadione, 556
for hepatic lipidosis, 411*t*
Picrotoxin, 558
Piezoelectric crystals, 144–145
Pilling devices, commercial, 45–47
Pill size, effect on administration, 44
Pilocarpine
for glaucoma, 340
indications for, 322
Pinna, abnormal carriage of, 33, 34*f*
Piperazine, 558
Piperonyl butoxide, 561–562
Pitressin Tannate in Oil. *See* Vasopressin tannate in oil
Placenta, retained, 465
Plain film radiography
of cardiomyopathy, 245, 246*f*, 248, 249*f*, 250–251
of feline asthma, 232, 232*f*–233*f*
Plant(s)
cardiotoxic, 565
ingestion of, gastrointestinal irritation caused by, 565
nontoxic, 563
Plantigrade posture, 305, 306*f*
Plant oxalate, 564*t*, 564–565
Plant toxicoses, 563*t*, 563–565
Plaque
accumulation of, 438
removal of, 441
Plasma cells, morphologic characteristics of, 201
Plasmacytic-lymphocytic stomatitis, 442–444
associated with cervical line lesions, 293
clinical signs of, 443, 443*f*
diagnosis of, 443
home care for, 444
pathology of, 442–443
treatment of, 443–444
Plasma osmolality, and antidiuretic hormone secretion, 207
Plasma protein values, interpretation of, 279*t*
Platelet(s), 157
Platelet estimation, 92
normal values for, 82
Play aggression, 242
treatment of, 242
Pleural effusions. *See also* Chylothorax
with advanced hypertrophic cardiomyopathy, 245, 246*f*
in asthmatic cat, 232, 234*f*
caused by effusive feline infectious peritonitis, 354, 354*f*–355*f*
cytologic analysis of, 110–111, 111*f*
in dyspnea, 176
in feline infectious peritonitis, 356
in pyothorax, 454, 455*f*
diagnostic criteria for, 112*t*
dyspnea caused by, 172–173, 177, 190
radiographic findings with, 173, 175*f*, 287, 288*f*
Pleural expansion, loss of, 182
Pleural space
common diseases involving, 111
drainage of, for pyothorax, 456, 457*f*
ultrasonographic evaluation of, 153, 153*f*
Pleurodesis, for chylothorax, 289
Pleuroperitoneal shunt, implantation of, for chylothorax, 289
PMMA. *See* Polymethyl methacrylate bone cement
PMSG. *See* Pregnant mare serum gonadotropin
Pneumocystography, 126*f*, 126–128
Pneumonia, 182
aspiration, 182, 187*f*
bacterial, 182, 186*f*
diagnosis of, 107
systemic fungal, diagnosis of, 107
Pneumoperitoneogram, 141–143
clinical indications for, 141
complications of, 143
contraindications to, 141, 143
goal of, 141
materials for, 141
normal findings with, 141, 143*f*
technique for, 141
Pneumothorax, 182. *See also* Tension pneumothorax
caused by high-rise fall, 393, 393*f*
definition of, 173
radiographic signs of, 173–176, 176*f*
treatment of, 497
Poinsettia, 565
Pointed Persian. *See* Himalayan
Pollakiuria
definition of, 370
differential diagnosis of, 656–657
Polychromasia, of erythrocytes, 160
Polychromatophilic erythrocytes, 157, 158*f*
Polycystic renal disease
radiologic findings with, 122, 125*f*
ultrasonographic findings with, 149, 149*f*
Polydipsia, 207–217. *See also* PU/PD syndrome
causes of, 207–211
definition of, 207
in diabetes mellitus, 305–306
diagnostic approach to, 211–216
differential diagnosis of, 657
history of cat with, 211
physical examination of cat with, 211–214, 212*f*–213*f*
primary, 207, 211
treatment of, 217
water deprivation testing in, 216, 216*t*
treatment of, 216–217
verification of, 214
Polyflex. *See* Ampicillin
Polymerase chain reaction assay, detection of feline leukemia virus with, 361
Polymethyl methacrylate bone cement, for frontal sinus obliteration, 486
Polymyopathy. *See* Hypokalemic polymyopathy
Polymyositis, differential diagnosis of, 657
Polyneuritis, differential diagnosis of, 657–658
Polyneuropathies, differential diagnosis of, 258
Polyp(s)
bladder, radiologic findings with, 128, 131*f*
nasal, 266, 268*f*
Polyphagia
in diabetes mellitus, 305–306
differential diagnosis of, 658
Polypnea, definition of, 172
Polyuria, 207–217. *See also* PU/PD syndrome
causes of, 207–211
definition of, 207
in diabetes mellitus, 305–306
diagnostic approach to, 211–216
differential diagnosis of, 658
due to hyperthyroidism, 209
history of cat with, 211
physical examination of cat with, 211–214, 212*f*–213*f*
treatment of, 216–217
verification of, 214
Polyuric renal disease, nonazotemic, 214
water deprivation testing in, 216, 216*t*
Portable Omnicage, 60
Port-A-Cul Tubes, 456
Portosystemic shunt, 166
Postobstructive diuresis, PU/PD syndrome caused by, 211
Postpartum metritis, 465, 465*f*
Postpartum period, 465–466
abnormal, 465–466
normal, 465
Postprandial alkaline tide, 50
Posturethral obstruction, PU/PD syndrome caused by, 211
Potassium
for hepatic lipidosis, 411*t*
for hypokalemia, 310
serum measurements of, in hypokalemic polymyopathic cat, 258
test for
diseases affecting, 87
normal value, 82
Potassium concentration, regulation of, in diabetic cats, 309–310
Potassium gluconate
dosage and administration of, 259–260
indications for, 259
Potassium hydroxide
for diagnosis of phaeohyphomycosis, 509
in fungal stains, 506
Potassium hydroxide, dimethyl sulfoxide, and chlorazol fungal stain, recipe for, 506*t*
Potassium supplementation
for hypokalemic polymyopathy, 257–259
intense, 259
intravenous, guidelines for, 259*t*
long-term, 259–260
routine, 259
Power chains, for tooth movement, 302
Pralidoxime chloride
indications for, 169
for toxicosis, 561
Pred Forte. *See* Prednisolone acetate
Prednisolone
contraindications to, 410*t*
dosage and administration of, 234*t*, 335, 444
for eosinophilic granuloma complex, 446, 535
for feline asthma, 234
for flea allergic dermatitis, 520
for heartworm disease, 382
for hemobartonellosis, 390
for hyperesthesia syndrome, 400
indications for, 358, 444
for inflammatory bowel disease, 414
for lymphocytic cholangitis/cholangiohepatitis, 263
for plasmacytic-lymphocytic stomatitis, 444
for toxicosis, 557
Prednisolone acetate, 330, 335
Prednisolone sodium succinate
dosage and administration of, 173, 234*t*
for feline asthma, 234
indications for, 173
for shock, 393
Prednisone
for eosinophilic granuloma complex, 535

Prednisone (*continued*)
for flea allergic dermatitis, 520
for hyperesthesia syndrome, 400
indications for, 434
for inflammatory bowel disease, 414
for mast cell tumors, 531
Pregnancy, 37, 461–462. *See also* Delivery
care during, 462
confirmed, loss of, 470*f*, 470–473
in diabetic cats, 313
diagnosis of, 462
ectopic, 464–465
hormones of, 461–462
length of, 462
prevention of, with estradiol cypionate, 460
progesterone levels in, 460, 460*t*, 461–462
ultrasonographic evaluation of, 150, 151*f*
undetected, loss of, 469–470
Pregnant mare serum gonadotropin, estrus induction with, 460–461
Pregnant women, and toxoplasmosis, 581–582
Premature gonadal failure, 473
Premier RC Prep, 299
Prescription Diet Feline c/d, 372, 375, 414
Prescription Diet Feline d/d, 521
Prescription Diet Feline h/d, 250
Prescription Diet Feline k/d, 265
Prescription Diet Feline p/d, 40
deficiencies of, 41
preparation of, 40–41
Prescription Diet Feline r/d, 288, 416
canned, 308
dry, 308
Prescription Diet Feline s/d, 375
Prescription Diet Feline w/d, 288, 416
dry, 308
Primary generalized epilepsy
clinical presentation of, 219
definition of, 218
Primidone, contraindications to, 221
Primucell FIP, 358, 471
PR interval, normal value for, 84
Pro-Banthine. *See* Propantheline
Procaine, drug interactions, 53*t*
Proestrus, 458
Progestational compounds
indications for, 463
for miliary dermatitis, 532–533
Progesterone
for eosinophilic granuloma complex, 446
levels
associated with reproduction, 460, 460*t*
and ovulation, 460, 460*t*
in pregnancy, 460, 460*t*, 461–462
in pseudopregnancy, 460, 460*t*, 461
test for, normal value, 83
Progesterone in oil, for hypoluteoidism, 472
Progestins
for intermale aggression, 240
for marking behavior, 238–239
Progestogens
for sex hormone imbalance, 537
side effects of, 461
Prognathic malocclusions, 301–302
treatment of, 301–302
Prolactin production, during pregnancy, 462–463
PromAce. *See* Acetylpromazine
Propantheline
indications for, 374
for urge incontinence, 372
Propetamphos, 560–561
Propoxur, 560–561
Propranolol
contraindications to, 253
dosage and administration of, 405
indications for, 405
for intraoperative tachycardia, 498
Proprioception deficit, differential diagnosis of, 658
Proptosis. *See* Traumatic proptosis
Propylene glycol, anemia caused by, 160, 384–385
Propylthiouracil
hemolysis caused by, 162
indications for, 404
Prorubricytes, 159, 160*t*
Prostaglandin(s), 460
for pyometra, 463, 469–470
role in ocular inflammations, 335
side effects of, 463
Prostaglandin $F_{2\alpha}$
induction of abortion with, 463, 472
for pyometra, 463
Protein
produced by conceptus, 461
quantitative, normal value for, 82
serum, analysis of, in diagnosis of feline infectious peritonitis, 356–357
total, normal value for, 82–83
urinary, normal value for, 84
Protein/creatine ratio, normal value for, 82
Protein electrophoresis, normal values for, 83
Protein level, dietary, and chronic renal disease, 283
Protein Multistix, 84
Protein requirements, 283
Protein sulfosalicylic acid, urinary, normal value for, 84
Proteinuria, 276
Prothrombin consumption, normal value for, 82
Prothrombin time, normal value for, 82
Protopam. *See* Pralidoxime chloride
Protozoal infections
gastrointestinal, 225
reproductive failure caused by, 472
Protozoal parasites, 224
Pruritic alopecia, 537
Pruritis, differential diagnosis of, 399, 658–659
Pseudogenetra, 461
Pseudomonas aeruginosa, 487, 571
Pseudopregnancy, 458
physiology of, 461
progesterone levels in, 460, 460*t*
Psychogenic alopecia, 537
Psychomotor seizures, 220*t*
Psyllium, 419*t*, 555
PT. *See* Prothrombin time
Ptyalism
and administration of oral medication, 45
caused by ketamine, 60*f*, 61
differential diagnosis of, 653
PU. *See* Polyuria
Pubertal estrus
absence of, 473
failure to exhibit, 467
Puberty, 458, 466
Pulex irritans, 518
Pulmonary compression
dyspnea caused by, 177
secondary to ectopic or enlarged organs, dyspnea caused by, 178
Pulmonary diseases/disorders, dyspnea caused by, 182
Pulmonary edema, 182, 185*f*–186*f*
Pulmonary embolism, 252, 252*f*
caused by heartworm disease, 379, 380*f*
Pulmonary hemorrhage, 182, 184*f*
Pulmonary histoplasmosis, 182, 188*f*
Pulmonary injuries, caused by high-rise fall, 393, 393*f*
Pulmonary lymphosarcoma, 182, 190, 190*f*
Pulmonary metastasis, 182, 188*f*
Pulmonary radiolucency, in asthmatic cat, 232, 232*f*–233*f*
Pulmonary toxoplasmosis, 182, 189*f*
Pulmonary tumors, 434–435
primary or metastatic, 182, 188*f*
Pulpal exposure, with tooth fracture, 297, 298*f*
treatment of, 298–300
Pulp capping, 302
indications for, 302–303
Pulp cavity, 291, 291*f*
Pulpotomy, 298–299, 302
Pumpkin, canned, 419*t*
Punctate reticulocytes, 158, 159*f*, 159–160
Punishment
for clawing, 240
for urination/defecation problems, 239
PU/PD syndrome, 207
causes of, 207–211
diagnostic approach to, 211–216
frequency of diagnoses in, 208*t*
history of cat with, 211
minimum data base for cats with, 214, 214*t*
pathologic causes of, 208*t*
physical examination of cat with, 211–214, 212*f*–213*f*
treatment of, 216–217
verification of, 214
Pupillary constriction, differential diagnosis of, 654
Pupillary dilation, differential diagnosis of, 654–655
Pupillary light reflex, decreased, differential diagnosis of, 659
Pupils, unequal, differential diagnosis of, 637
P wave, normal value for, 84
PWW diet
deficiencies of, 41
preparation of, 40–41
Pyelogram, intravenous. *See* Excretory urography
Pyelonephritis
PU/PD syndrome caused by, 208
radiologic findings with, 122
Pyoderma, differential diagnosis of, 659
Pyogranulomas, multiple, caused by noneffusive feline infectious peritonitis, 355, 355*f*
Pyometra, 462–463
clinical signs of, 462, 462*f*
diagnosis of, 209, 209*t*
prevention of, 463
PU/PD syndrome caused by, 209, 209*t*
treatment of, 462–463, 463*f*
Pyothorax, 454–457
clinical presentation of, 454
common pathogens of, 455*t*
definition of, 454
diagnosis of, 112*t*, 454, 455*f*
with body fluid aspiration, 99*f*, 111
microbiology of, 455–456, 456*t*
pathogenesis of, 454
prognosis for, 456
treatment of, 456, 457*f*, 497
Pyrethin insecticides, 561–562, 562*t*
Pyrethroid insecticides, 561–562, 562*t*
Pyridium. *See* Phenazopyridine
Pyrimethamine, with sulfadiazine or triple sulfas, for toxoplasmosis, 168
Pyrogens, 191
Pythiosis, 509*f*, 509–510
Pyuria, differential diagnosis of, 659

QRS complex, normal value for, 84
QT interval, normal value for, 84
Queen. *See* Female cats
Queening box, 464
Quinolones, contraindications to, 472
QyGel, 297

Rabies
in multicat facilities, 421–423
vaccination against, 38
recommendations for, 423*t*
Radial fractures, management of, 395–396, 396*f*
Radioiodine, for hyperthyroidism, 405, 405*f*
Radiology, 114–143. *See also* Plain film radiography; Thoracic radiography
of cardiovascular system, 137–138
of digestive system, 114–121
in evaluation of chronic renal disease, 277–278
in evaluation of nasal discharge, 266–267, 269*f*–271*f*
of heartworm disease, 379, 380*f*–381*f*
identification of fluid in thoracic and abdominal cavity with, 110
indications for, 193
of inflammatory orbital disease, 319
of nervous system, 134–136
for root canal procedures, 297, 299, 299*f*–300*f*
of skull, 139–140
in staging of periodontal disease, 440–441
of tooth fractures, 297–298
of urinary system, 122–133
Ragdoll, 20–21, 21*f*
Rales, differential diagnosis of, 659–660
Ramus, fracture of, 448–449
Ranitidine
dosage and administration of, 284, 434
indications for, 284, 434, 559
Raw liver, and cervical line lesions, 294, 296
RBC. *See* Red blood cells
Rebound hyperglycemia, 311–312, 312*f*
Reception room, separation of cats and dogs in, 28
Recombinant human erythropoietin. *See* r-HuEPO
Rectal bleeding, differential diagnosis of, 660
Rectal culture
evaluation of, 225, 225*f*
indications for, 225
Red blood cell count
based on blood smear, in diagnosis of anemia, 157, 158*f*
in chronic renal disease, 277
in diagnosis of anemia, 157
at different ages, 83
diseases affecting, 84–85
normal value for, 82
Red blood cell inclusions, 157, 158*f*

Red blood cell parasites, 157, 158*f*
Red blood cell production, steps in, 159–160, 160*t*
Red blood cells
  in bone marrow, test for, normal value, 83
  effects of oxidant agents on, 384
  fragmented, 157
  nucleated, 157, 158*f*, 160
  peripheral, survival time of, 159
Redirected aggression, 242
  treatment of, 242
Reflectance meters, hand-held, 311
Regenerative anemia
  associated with hemobartonellosis, 390, 390*f*
  caused by feline leukemia virus, 365
Regenerative anemias, 159–162
  differential diagnosis of, 160
  etiology of, 159–160
  secondary to blood loss, 162
  secondary to hemolysis, 160–162
Reglan. *See* Metoclopramide
Regurgitation, differential diagnosis of, 660
Relaxin production, during pregnancy, 462–463
Renal agenesis, radiologic findings with, 122, 123*f*
Renal arteries, thrombus in, 253, 254*f*
Renal biopsy, in diagnosis of chronic renal disease, 278–279
Renal calculi, radiologic findings with, 122, 126*f*
Renal capsule, tear of, radiologic findings with, 122
Renal disease. *See also* Chronic renal disease
  associated with hyperthyroidism, 403
  end-stage, radiologic findings with, 122
  polyuric, nonazotemic, 214
    water deprivation testing in, 216, 216*t*
  progression of, 275*t*
  PU/PD syndrome caused by, 207–208, 208*t*
Renal elimination, of toxins, 555
Renal failure, 207. *See also* Chronic renal failure; Oliguric renal failure
  definition of, 274
  end-stage, definition of, 274
  polyuric and oliguric primary, biochemical similarities and differences in patients with, 280*t*
Renal function, poor, radiologic findings with, 122, 123*f*
Renal hypoperfusion, in cats with chronic renal disease, 282–283
Renal insufficiency, 207, 211
  definition of, 274
Renal lymphosarcoma, 428–429, 435
  radiologic findings with, 122, 124*f*
Renal parenchymal disease, ultrasonographic findings with, 149, 149*f*
Renal tubular necrosis, ultrasonographic findings with, 149
Renal tumors, 435
Renografin-76
  for angiocardiography, 137–138
  for celiogram, 141
  for excretory urogram, 122
  for urethrogram, 133
  for urinary cystogram, 122, 124
Reovirus, 573
Repositol progesterone, for miliary dermatitis, 532
Reproduction
  female, 458–466
  hormone levels associated with, 460, 460*t*
  male, 466–467
Reproductive cycle, cyclicity of, 458–459
Reproductive disorders, 458–476
Reproductive failure, 467–473. *See also* Infertility
Respiratory distress, in cat with high-rise syndrome, 393
Respiratory infections. *See* Upper respiratory infections
Respiratory pathogens, minor, 573
Respiratory rate, normal, 172
Respiratory sounds/patterns, terms relating to, definition of, 173*t*
Respiratory support, with toxicosis, 552, 552*t*
Respiratory tract tumors, 434–435
Respiratory viruses, vaccination against, 38
Restore FL-1, 295
Restricted-protein diet, recipe for, 285*t*
Restrictive cardiomyopathy, 250–251
Retained placenta, 465
Reticular pattern, 182
Reticulocyte(s), 64
  aggregate, 158, 159*f*, 159–160
  punctate, 158, 159*f*, 159–160
  types of, 158, 159*f*
Reticulocyte count, 92
  correction of, 92
    formula for, 158
  in diagnosis of anemia, 157–158
Reticulocyte stain, 64
Retinal changes/separation, associated with feline leukemia virus, 346, 346*f*
Retinal degeneration, 341–342
  central, 341, 342*f*–343*f*
  generalized, 342
Retinal dysplasia, 341, 342*f*
Retinal examination, indications for, 177
Retinal hemorrhage, 343, 343*f*–344*f*
Retinol-binding protein, 461
Retinopathy, 341*t*
  anemic, 343
  hypertensive, 342–343, 343*f*
Retrobulbar abscess, 318
Reverberation artifact, in ultrasonography, 144–145, 155*f*
Rex, 3. *See also* Cornish Rex; Devon Rex; Missouri Rex; Wyoming (Selkirk) Rex
Rhinitis. *See also* Nasal discharge
  chronic bacterial
    septic inflammatory pattern with, 272, 272*f*
    treatment of, 273, 500*f*, 500–502
  chronic viral, 266, 502
Rhinotracheitis. *See* Feline viral rhinotracheitis
Rhododendron species. *See* Azaleas
r-HuEPO, 283–284
  benefits of, 283
  preliminary recommendations for use of, 284*t*
  side effects of, 283
Righting response, definition of, 39
Ringer's solution, 308. *See also* Lactated Ringer's solution
Ringworm. *See* Dermatophytosis
Robert-Jones bandage, 395
Robinul-V. *See* Glycopyrrolate
Rodenticides, 555–557
Rodent ulcers, 445, 533*f*, 533–534
Romanowsky-type stains, 201
Rompun. *See* Xylazine
Root canal(s), 293, 299–300
  indications for, 295, 299, 302, 447
  materials for, 295, 300
  procedures for, 299–300
  radiographic procedures for, 297, 299, 299*f*–300*f*
Root exposure, for tooth extraction, 298
Root exposure indices, in staging of periodontal disease, 439–440, 440*t*
Rooting response, definition of, 39
Root planing, 441
Root resorption, 293
Root tips, 293
Rotenone, 562
  indications for, 515
Roto Pro burr, 304
Roundworms, 224
Rubriblasts, 159, 160*t*
Rubricytes, 159, 160*t*
Russell's viper venom time, normal value for, 82
Russian Blue, 21, 21*f*
Rx for Fleas. *See* Sodium polyborate

Sab-Duets. *See* Dermatophyte test media
Saddle thrombus, 252, 252*f*
  clinical signs of, 253
  radiographic findings with, 253, 253*f*
  treatment of, 253
Salicylates, drug interactions, 53*t*
Saliva, enzyme-linked immunosorbent assay of, 81
Salivary gland aspirates, 206, 206*f*
Salivary gland disease, 446
Salivary gland infarction, 446
Salivary gland tumors, 432, 446
Salivary mucoceles, 446
Salivation, excessive. *See* Ptyalism
Salmonella, 225, 472
Salmonellosis, 225
Saphenous vein, drug administration through, for euthanasia, 72
Sarcoma, nasal, 434
Sarcoma virus, 360
Scale, microscopic examination of, for diagnosis of ringworm, 506, 506*t*, 507*f*
Scalers, for prophylactic dental care, 441
Scan head. *See* Transducer(s)
SCC. *See* Squamous cell carcinoma
Schiotz tonometer, 339
Schroeder-Thomas splints, 395
Science Diet Feline Maintenance, 372, 414
Science Diet Feline Maintenance Light, 308
Sclera, anatomy of, 328
Scleral disease, 328
Scleral edema, differential diagnosis of, 640
Scottish Fold, 21–22, 22*f*. *See also* Longhair Scottish Fold
Scratching. *See* Clawing
Scratching post, 240
Scratch reflex, definition of, 39
Seal postural reflex, definition of, 39
Seasonality, 458–459
Seborrhea, 538
  differential diagnosis of, 660
Secondary generalized epilepsy, definition of, 218
Sector transducers, 145
Sectrol Flea Foam, 520
Seizure(s)
  behavior/activity frequently mistaken for, 220*t*
  differential diagnosis of, 641–642
  types of, 220*t*
Seizure disorder(s), 218–222. *See also* Epilepsy
  breed predilections for, 219*t*
  clinical presentation of, 219
  diagnostic plan for, 220, 221*t*
  differential diagnosis of, 219, 221*t*
  etiology of, 219*t*
  history of cat with, 218
  lesion localization with, 218–219
  maintenance therapy for, 221
    client education about, 221, 221*t*
  physical examination of cat with, 218
  signalment, 218
  therapy for, 220–221
Self-mutilation, differential diagnosis of, 649–650
Semen sample, collection of, 466
Semilente. *See* Insulin, regular
Sensitive teeth, 294
Sensors, 191
Sepsis, generalized, differential diagnosis of, 258
Serax. *See* Oxazepam
Serologic tests, in evaluation of fever, 194*t*
Serum glutamic-oxaloacetic transaminase, normal value for, 82
Serum glutamic-pyruvic transaminase
  diseases affecting, 86
  normal value for, 82
Serum osmolality, normal value for, 82
Sevin. *See* Carbaryl
Sexual development, abnormal, 473
  diagnostic evaluation of, 467
SGOT. *See* Serum glutamic-oxaloacetic transaminase
SGPT. *See* Serum glutamic-pyruvic transaminase
Shaded Persian, 20
Shag. *See* Maine Coon
Shelter(s)
  control of infectious diseases in, 422–423
  definition of, 420
Shock
  caused by high-rise fall, 393–394
  clinical signs of, 393
  treatment of, 393
Short catheters, 477
  placement of, procedure for, 478, 478*f*
Shorthair. *See* American Shorthair; British Shorthair; Colorpoint Shorthair; Exotic Shorthair; Oriental Shorthair
Siamese, 22–23, 23*f*
  corneal sequestrum in, 330
  hyperesthesia syndrome in, 399
  intestinal tumors in, 431
  mast cell tumors in, 526
  nervous system disorders in, 165*t*
  periodontitis in, 442–443
  seizure disorders in, 219*t*
Siberian Cat, 23, 23*f*
Singapura, 23–24, 24*f*
Sinuses, 266, 269*f*
Sinusitis. *See also* Nasal discharge
  chronic bacterial, septic inflammatory pattern with, 272, 272*f*
  chronic purulent, 266
  frontal, treatment of, 273
Si-Sawat. *See* Korat
Sisomicin, drug interactions, 52*t*
Skeletal deformities, 165
Skin. *See also under* Dermal
  fungal diseases of, 504–511

Skin (*continued*)
 parasitic diseases of, 511–517
 physical examination of, 32–33
 purulent. *See* Pyoderma
Skin irritation, differential diagnosis of, 399, 549
Skin tumors, 526–531, 527*t*
 examination of, 526
Skogkatt. *See* Norwegian Forest Cat
Skull
 anatomy of, 290–291, 291*f*
 lateral view of, 266–267, 269*f*
 radiologic evaluation of, 139–140
 rostral-caudal (skyline) view of, 266–267, 270*f*
Skyline view, of skull, 139, 140*f*
Slow blink reflex, definition of, 39
Small bowel, intussusception of, radiologic findings with, 118, 120*f*
Smoke inhalation, bronchial pattern caused by, 233*f*
Smoke Persian, 20
Smooth muscle relaxants, 49
Snappy Snare, 59
Sneezing
 chronic treatment of, 574–575
 differential diagnosis of, 570, 571*f*, 660
Snowshoe, 24, 24*f*
Sodium, test for
 diseases affecting, 87
 normal value, 82
Sodium bicarbonate
 for acidosis, 310–311
 contraindications to, 310
 dosage and administration of, 284, 311, 374*t*
 drug interactions, 52*t*
 indications for, 374
Sodium concentration, regulation of, in diabetic cats, 308–309
Sodium hypochlorite, as irrigant for root canal procedures, 299
Sodium iodide, for sporotrichosis, 508–509
Sodium phosphate, drug interactions, 52*t*
Sodium polyborate, 520
Sodium/potassium ratio, test for, normal value, 82
Sodium salicylate, for plasmacytic-lymphocytic stomatitis, 444
Sodium sulfate
 for acetaminophen toxicosis, 385
 for toxicosis, 554
Sodium thiopental
 advantages and indications for, 56
 concentrations, 57*t*
 disadvantages of, 56
 dosage, 56, 57*t*
Soft palate defects, 449–451
Soft palate lesions, treatment of, 451
Solid Persian, 20
Solid tissue masses, ultrasonographic characteristics of, 145
Solu-Delta-Cortef. *See* Prednisolone sodium succinate
Somali, 24*f*, 24–25
Somogyi Overswing. *See* Rebound hyperglycemia
Sorbitol, for toxicosis, 554–555
Sound, properties of, and ultrasonography, 144
Sovereign short catheter, 477
Spaying, and reduction in marking behavior, 238. *See also* Ovariohysterectomy
Spermatogenesis, determination of, in breeding soundness examination, 466
Spherocytes, 157
Sphynx, 3, 25, 25*f*
Spica splints, 395
Spinal canal, lymphosarcoma of, radiologic findings with, 136, 136*f*
Spinal cord lesions, 136, 136*f*
Spinal injuries
 caused by high-rise fall, 394–395
 treatment of, 169
Spinal needle, for myelography, 134
Spindle cell tumors, malignant, cytologic findings with, 205
Spirochetes, homogenous population of, in cat with diarrhea, 225*f*
Spleen aspiration, 104–106, 105*f*–106*f*
Splenectomy, for systemic mast cell tumors, 434
Splenomegaly, differential diagnosis of, 660–661
Splints, for intravenous catheterizations, 478, 478*f*
Sporotrichium schenkii, 508, 509*f*
Sporotrichosis, 508–509
 clinical signs of, 508, 508*f*
 diagnosis of, 508, 509*f*
 therapy for, 508–509
Spraying, 236. *See also* Marking behavior
 differential diagnosis of, 661
 versus inappropriate urination, 488
 treatment of, 488
Squamous cell carcinoma. *See also* Bowen's disease
 cytologic findings with, 108, 109*f*
 of eyelid and third eyelid, 325–326, 327*f*
 gastrointestinal, 431
 involving bone, 433
 nasal, 433–434
 oral, 431, 444–445, 445*f*
 pulmonary, 434–435
 of skin, classic form, 526–528
  biologic behavior of, 526
  clinical signs of, 526, 528*f*
  treatment of, 526–528
 on tips of pinnae, 483, 484*f*
  surgical treatment of, 483, 484*f*
Staining, 201
 for cytologic preparations, 96
Stannous fluoride, 297, 442
Stanozolol
 contraindications to, 410*t*
 indications for, 284
Staphylococcus, 465, 472, 577
Status epilepticus, treatment of, 220–221
Steatorrhea, differential diagnosis of, 661
Sterile inflammatory pattern, in FIP-induced fluid recovered from thorax or abdomen, 355, 355*f*
Sternal recumbency, in dyspneic cats, 172, 173*f*
Steroids. *See also* Anabolic steroids
 contraindications to, 314, 387, 472
 nasal flushes with, for chronic nasal discharge, 273
Stillbirth, 470*f*, 470–473
 differential diagnosis of, 635–636
Stomach. *See also under* Gastric
Stomach gas, acoustic shadowing caused by, 147–148
Stomach tumors, 432
Stomach wall masses, cytologic findings with, 106, 106*f*
Stomach worms, 224
Stomatitis. *See also* Plasmacytic-lymphocytic stomatitis
 chronic, associated with feline immunodeficiency virus, 349, 349*f*
 differential diagnosis of, 661
Stones. *See* Urolith(s)
Straining, differential diagnosis of, 662–663
Strangiuria
 definition of, 370
 differential diagnosis of, 661
Streptococcus, 465, 472, 479, 577
Streptomyces, 509
Streptomycin, drug interactions, 52*t*
Stress, minimizing, for cat with chronic renal disease, 285
Striate keratopathy, 340
String of pearls sign, 115, 116*f*
Struvite crystals, in feline urologic syndrome, 370, 370*f*
 treatment for, 372
ST segment, normal value for, 84
Stud tail, 538, 538*f*
Subarachnoid injection, preferred sites for, 134*f*, 134–136
Subconjunctival hemorrhage, 328
Sucking reflex, definition of, 39
Sucralfate, indications for, 559
Sulcus depth, measurement of, 291–292
Sulfasalazine
 for inflammatory bowel disease, 414
 side effects of, 414
 toxicity, 560
Sulfonamides
 drug interactions, 53*t*
 for eosinophilic granuloma complex, 535
 indications for, 509
Superfetation, 462
Supernumerary roots, 303, 303*f*
Supernumerary teeth, 301, 303
Superstitions, and evolution of cat breeds, 3
Suppositories, 418*t*
Suppurative cholangitis/cholangiohepatitis, 261–262
 clinical and examination findings with, 261
 diagnosis of, 261–262
 etiology of, 261
 prognosis for, 262
 radiographic and laboratory findings with, 261
 treatment of, 262
Surgical oncology, 426
Symblepharon, 328
Sympathy card, after euthanasia, 72, 73*f*
Symphyseal separation/fracture, 448, 448*f*
 classification of, 448*t*
 management of, 398
 repair of, 488
  surgical technique for, 488, 489*f*
 treatment of, 448
Synchysis scintillans, of vitreous, 338
Syncope, differential diagnosis of, 662
Synovial fluid analysis, indications for, 193–194
Syringe feeding, 42
Systemic fungal infections, 540–550
 anemia caused by, 162
 diagnosis of, 227
 differential diagnosis of, 356
 ocular manifestations of, 333, 333*f*, 344–345
 public health implications of, 548–549
 pulmonary manifestations of, 182, 188*f*–189*f*
 vomiting/diarrhea caused by, 226–227

T_3. *See* Triiodothyronine
T_4. *See* Thyroxine
Tabby Persian, 20
Tablets
 administration of, 45*f*, 45–47, 46*f*
  versus capsules, 44
 dissolving in liquids, 47
 masking taste/lubricating of, 45
Tachycardia, differential diagnosis of, 662
Tachypnea, definition of, 172
Tagamet. *See* Cimetidine
Tapazole. *See* Methimazole
Tapetum
 bullous retinal separation of, 344, 345*f*
 granulomatous lesions in, 344, 345*f*
 multifocal hyperpigmentation of, 344, 344*f*
Tapeworms, 224
 physical examination for, 36, 36*f*
Tarsal bones, comminuted fractures of, management of, 397
Tarsal glands, additional cilia emerging from, 322
Tarsorrhaphy
 permanent partial, indications for, 325
 temporary
  indications for, 318, 326
  premature removal of, 318
Tarsus, 319
Taurine deficiency
 cardiomyopathy caused by, 244, 248, 251
 during pregnancy, 462, 472
 retinal degeneration caused by, 342, 343*f*
 seizure disorders caused by, 221
Taurine supplementation
 for dilated cardiomyopathy, 250
 for hepatic lipidosis, 411*t*
 for seizure disorders, 221
Tears, enzyme-linked immunosorbent assay of, 81
Technetium-99m pertechnetate thyroid scanning
 for diagnosis of hyperthyroidism, 402–403, 403*f*, 404
 procedure for, 402
Telazol. *See* Tiletamine-zolazepam
Telogen defluxion, 537
Tempera. *See* Acetaminophen
Temperature. *See* Body temperature
Temporomandibular joint, 291*f*
 common lesions of, radiologic findings with, 139, 140*f*
 dislocation of, 290
 injuries, 449
 luxation of, 448–449, 450*f*
  management of, 397*f*, 398, 449, 450*f*
  radiologic findings with, 139, 140*f*
 normal orientation of, 449*f*
 radiologic evaluation of, 139, 139*f*
Tender Vittles, 414
Tendonectomy. *See* Deep digital flexor tendonectomy
Tenesmus, differential diagnosis of, 662–663
Tension pneumothorax, 182, 183*f*
Tenure, 298
Terbutaline
 dosage, 234*t*
 for feline asthma, 234–235

Terramycin. *See* Oxytetracycline
Territorial aggression, 240–241, 243
Testosterone
 levels, associated with reproduction, 460*t*
 for sex hormone imbalance, 537
Testosterone analogs, contraindications to, 472
Testosterone enanthate, indications for, 284
Testosterone proprionate, indications for, 284
Tetracycline
 for cholangitis/cholangiohepatitis, 262
 contraindications to, 410*t*, 472, 574
 drug interactions, 53*t*
 for hemobartonellosis, 390
 indications for, 49–50, 322
 in pleurodesis, 289
 side effects of, 50, 390
Tetracycline staining, of teeth, 304
TGEV. *See* Transmissible gastroenteritis virus
Theo-Dur. *See* Theophylline
Theophylline
 dosage, 234*t*
 for feline asthma, 235
 indications for, 262
Thermoreceptors, 191
Thiabendazole, for dermatophytosis, 507*t*
Thiacetarsamide
 dosage and administration of, 50
 for heartworm disease, 383
 for hemobartonellosis, 390
 indications for, 50
 toxicity, 50
Thiamine, dietary, for hepatic lipidosis, 411*t*
Thiamine deficiency, cervical ventroflexion caused by, 258
Thiamylal sodium
 advantages and indications for, 56
 concentrations, 57*t*
 disadvantages of, 56
 dosage, 56, 57*t*
  for 10-lb cat, 57*t*
 indications for, 50, 373, 498, 552
 tolerance, 50
Thiazide diuretics, indications for, 216–217
Thiobarbiturate, indications for, 498
Third eyelid
 bilateral protrusion of, 322
 cartilage of, eversion of, 322
 conditions affecting, 319, 320*t*
 lymphosarcoma of, 325, 327*f*
 squamous cell carcinoma of, 325–326, 327*f*
Third eyelid follicles
 hyperplasia of, 325, 325*f*
 removal of, 325
Third eyelid gland, prolapse of, 326
Third eye prolapse, 33
Thirst center, stimulation of, 207
Thomas splint, 478
Thoracentesis, for pyothorax, 456
Thoracic cavity, fluid in
 aspiration of, 110
 radiologic signs of, 110
Thoracic duct ligation, for chylothorax, 288–289
Thoracic masses, aspiration of, 107–108
 common diseases diagnosed by, 107–108
 technique for, 107
Thoracic radiography
 in cat with high-rise syndrome, 393, 393*f*
 of chylothorax, 287, 288*f*
 with lung aspiration, 107
 of pyothorax, 454, 455*f*
Thoracic trauma, caused by high-rise fall, 393, 393*f*
Thoracocentesis, 172–173, 176
 for chylothorax, 288
 for dilated cardiomyopathy, 249
 indications for, 251
 for thoracic trauma, 393
Thoracostomy tube, 497
 drainage of pleural space with, 456, 457*f*
 placement of, surgical technique for, 497, 497*f*–498*f*
Thoracotomy, 107
 indications for, 176, 456
Thread Mate System, 449
Thrombi, surgical removal of, indications for, 253, 254*f*
Thrombocytes, test for, diseases affecting, 86
Thromboembolic disease, 252–255
 and cardiomyopathy, 252
 clinical signs of, 244, 252, 252*f*
 diagnosis of, 252–253
  with blood profile, 248
 incidence of, 252
 pathophysiology of, 252
 prognosis for, 254
 radiologic findings with, 137, 137*f*
 treatment of, 253–254
Thrombosis, definition of, 252
Thrombus formation, prevention of, 253–254
Thymic atrophy, caused by feline leukemia virus, 364–365
Thymoma
 diagnosis of, with thoracic mass aspiration, 107–108, 108*f*
 dyspnea caused by, 177, 179*f*
Thyroid adenomas, 401. *See also* Hyperthyroidism
Thyroidectomy, 498–499
 anatomic considerations for, 498
 anesthetic precautions with, 498
 bilateral, 406
 complications of, 406
 for hyperthyroidism, 405–406
  precautions with, 406*t*
 modified extracapsular technique for, 499, 499*f*–500*f*
 modified intracapsular technique for, 499
 surgical options for, 498
 surgical techniques for, 499
 unilateral, 405
Thyroid gland
 anatomy of, 498
 palpation of, 402
Thyroid hormone, drug interactions, 53*t*
Thyroid hormone concentration, deregulation of, after thyroidectomy, 406
Thyroid-stimulating hormone, test for, normal value, 83
Thyroid tumors, 401. *See also* Hyperthyroidism
 metastatic, 403, 403*f*
Thyrotropin-releasing hormone stimulation test, in diagnosis of hyperthyroidism, 404
Thyroxine
 free, normal value for, 83
 test
  for diagnosis of hyperthyroidism, 402
  normal value, 83
Thyroxine supplementation, after thyroidectomy, 406
Tibial fracture, management of, 396, 396*f*
Ticked. *See* Abyssinian
Ticks, anemia caused by, 162
Tiger lily, 564
Tiletamine-zolazepam
 concentrations, 57*t*
 dosage, 57*t*
Tissue aspiration, 96, 97*f*–98*f*, 103–110. *See also specific type*
 in cancer diagnosis, 425
 in diagnosis of feline infectious peritonitis, 356
 indications for, 193
 organ-specific considerations for, 104–110
 technique for, 103–104
Tissue impression, 96–97
Tissue scraping, 97
Toenails
 blood collection from, 63
 physical examination of, 35, 35*f*–36*f*
Tom. *See* Male cats
Tom Cat Catheter, 373, 492
Tonic-clonic seizures, 220*t*
Tonic neck reflex, definition of, 39
Tonkinese, 25, 25*f*
Tonometry, 339
Tooth avulsion, 446–447
Tooth extraction, 293, 298
 indications for, 294–296, 298, 301–303, 446
 procedures for, 298
Tooth fracture(s), 297–300
 clinical signs of, 297
 diagnosis of, 297
 incidence of, 297
 pulpal exposure with, 297, 298*f*
  treatment of, 298–300
 radiographic findings with, 297
 treatment of, 298–300
 visual examination of, 297
Tooth identification, 292*f*, 292–293
Tooth movement
 indications for, 302–303
 procedures for, 302
Tooth structure, impressions of, for crown, 300
Tooth/teeth. *See also under* Dental
 bleaching of, 304
 cervical line lesions of, 293–297
 chipped, with no canal exposure (vital), treatment of, 298
 eruption times of, 292*t*
 examination of, 290
  age assessed by, 34, 34*f*
 fusion, 303
 gemination, 303, 303*f*
 improper alignment of, 139
 loss of, caused by periodontal disease, 438
 missing, 301, 303
 physical examination of, 34
 polishing of, 442
 restoration of, and cervical line lesions, 295
 retained deciduous, 301, 301*f*, 303
 root resorption of, 293
 root tips of, 293
 scaling of, 442
 sensitive, 294
 supernumerary, 301, 303
 with supernumerary roots, 303, 303*f*
 tetracycline staining of, 304
Torbugesic. *See* Butorphanol
Tourniquet, for blood collection, 62
Toxicosis, 166–167, 551–569
 client communication with, 551
 decontamination procedures for, 553*t*, 553–555
 determining exposure potential in, 551–552, 552*t*
 diagnosis of, 226, 553
  with liver aspirate, 104
 emergency stabilization with, 552*t*, 552–553
 enhancing elimination with, 555
 initial treatment of, 551–555
 prevention of reabsorption with, 555
 professional consultation with, 551
 treatment of, 169
 vomiting/diarrhea caused by, 226
Toxins, 555–567
Toxoplasma gondii, 261, 334, 345, 472, 580
Toxoplasmosis, 225, 580–582
 anterior uveitis caused by, 334, 334*f*
 diagnosis of, 345
 human disease, 581
 human infections, 580–581
 ocular manifestations of, 345
 and pregnant women, factors to consider, 581
 prevention of, recommendations for, 581
 pulmonary, 182, 189*f*
 role of cat in, 580
 treatment of, 168, 345
Tracheal collapse, 177, 178*f*–179*f*
Tracheal endoscopy, indications for, 176
Tracheal obstruction, 177, 179*f*
Tracheal rupture, 177
Tracheal strictures, 177
Tracheal wash, 93
 for feline asthma, 231–234
 indications for, 176, 194
Tranquilizer(s)
 for aggression, 242
 for asthmatic cats, 235
 before euthanasia, 71–72
 phenothiazine, for uremia, 284
Transducer(s), in ultrasonography, 145
Transducer configurations, in ultrasonography, 145
Transferrin, 461
Transient diabetes mellitus, 313
Transient hyperglycemia, 305–306
Transitional cell carcinoma, of bladder, 435
Transmissible gastroenteritis virus, porcine, 352
Transtracheal wash, 92–93
Trauma. *See also* Fracture(s); High-rise syndrome; *specific type*
 ataxia/paresis caused by, 166
 blunt, diagnosis of, with liver aspirate, 104
Traumatic cataracts, 336, 337*f*
Traumatic dental injuries. *See* Tooth fracture(s)
Traumatic injury
 to nervous tissue, therapy for, 169
 suspected, examination for, 35, 36*f*
Traumatic pancreatitis, caused by high-rise fall, 394
Traumatic proptosis, 317, 318*f*
 complications of, 318
 prognosis for, 318
 treatment of, 317–318
Trench mouth, 444
Tresaderm. *See* Thiabendazole
TRH stimulation test. *See* Thyrotropin-releasing hormone stimulation test
Triadan tooth-numbering system, 292–293

Triamcinolone
dosage, 234t
for eosinophilic granuloma complex, 446
for feline asthma, 234
for plasmacytic-lymphocytic stomatitis, 444
Trichiasis, 326
Trichogram, 93
Trichomoniasis, 225
Trichophyton mentagrophytes, 504, 579
Trifluridine, 574
indications for, 328
Triglycerides, medium-chain, supplementation with, 238
Triiodothyronine, test for, normal value, 83
Triiodothyronine suppression test, 92
in diagnosis of hyperthyroidism, 404
Trimethoprim, drug interactions, 53t
Trimethoprim-sulfa drugs
contraindications to, 410t
dosage, 168
Trombiculidiasis, 515
Tru-Cut Biopsy Needle, 425
TSH. *See* Thyroid-stimulating hormone
Tumil-K. *See* Potassium gluconate
Tumor(s), 166, 425–437. *See also specific type*
anemia caused by, 162
associated with feline immunodeficiency virus, 349
associated with feline leukemia virus, 156, 333, 333f, 363, 427
chemotherapy for, 426–427
cytologic findings with, 99f, 100, 101f–103f, 108–110, 109f–110f
diagnosis of, 425
incidence of, 425
metastatic, cytologic findings with, from lymph node aspirates, 203
nonlymphoid, cytologic evaluation of, 205, 205f–206f
surgical treatment of, 426
treatment modalities for, 426–427
ultrasonographic characteristics of, 145
Turbinate bones, 269f
Turbinectomy, 500–502
indications for, 273
results of, 502
surgical technique for, 500f, 500–502
Turkish Angora, 26, 26f
Turkish Van, 26–27, 27f
T wave, normal value for, 84
Tylenol. *See* Acetaminophen
Tympanic bullae
common lesions of, radiologic findings with, 139, 139f
radiologic evaluation of, 139, 139f

U/A. *See* Urinalysis
Ulcer(s)
corneal, differential diagnosis of, 642
dermal and epidermal, 95
cytologic findings with, 108f–109f, 108–110
eosinophilic (rodent), 445, 533f, 533–534
eyelid, geriatric-associated, 326
lip, 455, 533f, 533–535
of stomach or bowel
perforated, radiologic findings with, 117, 117f–118f
radiologic findings with, 117
Ulnar fractures, management of, 395–396, 396f
Ultralente. *See* Insulin, long-acting
Ultrasonography, 144–154
artifacts, 144–145, 147, 147f–148f, 150f–151f
of ascites, 151, 152f
of bladder, 150, 150f
clinical application of, 146–153
definition of, 144
in evaluation of chronic renal disease, 278
frequencies employed in, 144–145
of gallbladder, 146–147, 147f–148f
of gastrointestinal tract, 150–151
of heart, 152–153
image display modes in, 145
image interpretation with, 145–146
indications for, 193
of kidney, 148–149, 149f
of liver, 146, 146f–147f
of pancreas, 147–148
physics of, 144–145
of pleural space, 153, 153f
of pregnancy, 150, 151f, 462
transducer configurations in, 145
Unconsciousness, differential diagnosis of, 641
Upper gastrointestinal series. *See* Gastrointestinal series
Upper respiratory infections, 570–576
acute, treatment of, 573–574
chronic, treatment of, 574–575
diagnosis of, 573
etiologic agents of, 570
prevention of, 575
public health considerations with, 575
rates of, 570
transmission of, 570
treatment of, 573–575
viral carriers of, treatment of, 574
Urachal diverticula, 375–376, 376f
radiologic findings with, 128, 132f
Urachus, 375–376
URDs. *See* Upper respiratory infections
Urea, urinary, normal value for, 84
Ureaplasma, abortions caused by, 472
Urecholine. *See* Bethanechol
Uremia
clinical manifestations of, 274, 275, 275t
definition of, 274
serum chemistries in, 275, 275t
signs of, control of, 283–284
vomiting caused by, 284
Uremic crises, causes of, differentiating features among, 277t
changes in, after treatment of hypotension and hypovolemia, 278t
Uremic gastritis, treatment of, 284
Uremic syndrome, 274
Ureter
ectopic, radiologic findings with, 122
tear of, radiologic findings with, 122
Urethra
back flushing of, for removal of urethral obstructions, 373–374
ruptured, radiologic findings with, 127, 131f
strictured, radiologic findings with, 133, 134f
Urethral obstruction/plug
removal of, 373–375, 479, 491–496, 493f–495f. *See also* Feline urologic syndrome, obstructed form
restraint for, 372–373, 373f
that cannot be relieved, 375, 375f
versus urolith, 376
Urethral tumors, 377
Urethrogram, 133
clinical indications for, 133
common lesions diagnosed with, 133, 134f
goals of, 133
materials for, 133
normal findings with, 133, 133f
technique for, 133
Urge incontinence
caused by feline urologic syndrome, 372
treatment of, 372
Urinalysis
for feline urologic syndrome, 371
interpretation of, in chronic renal disease, 276
for PU/PD syndrome, 214
for renal disease, 403–404
Urinary acidifiers, 50, 372
drug interactions, 52t
prophylactic use of, for feline urologic syndrome, 376
Urinary bladder. *See* Bladder
Urinary collecting system, closed, 281, 281t
Urinary cystogram, 122–128
clinical indications for, 122
common lesions diagnosed with, 127–128, 129f–131f
contraindications to, 122
double contrast, 127, 128, 128f
technique for, 126
gas source for, 122, 128
general technique for, 124, 126f
goals of, 122
honeycomb appearance with, 128, 132f
materials for, 122
negative contrast. *See* Pneumocystography
positive contrast, 127, 127f, 128
technique for, 124–126
Urinary incontinence, 239
differential diagnosis of, 663
Urinary output, measurement of, during diuresis, 281, 281t
Urinary pH, 84
alkaline, and feline urologic syndrome, 370
home monitoring of, 376
Urinary system, radiologic evaluation of, 122–133
Urinary system hematoma, radiologic appearance of, 128, 133f
Urinary tract antiseptics, indications for, 372
Urinary tract infections. *See also* Feline urologic syndrome; Lower urinary tract diseases
early identification of, and chronic renal disease, 283
Urinary tract tumors, 435
Urination
difficult. *See* Strangiuria
frequent. *See* Pollakiuria
inappropriate
differential diagnosis of, 661
versus spraying, 488
increased. *See* Polyuria
painful. *See* Dysuria
Urination problems, 239
treatment of, 239
Urine
normal color of, 84
purulent. *See* Pyuria
Urine glucose monitoring
limitations of, 312
by owner, 312
Urine marking. *See* Spraying
Urine osmolality, normal value for, 84
Urine production, 207. *See also* Polyuria
Urine specific gravity, 84
in evaluation of PU/PD syndrome, 214
Urine tests, normal values for, 84
URIs. *See* Upper respiratory infections
Urobilinogen, normal value for, 84
Uro-Collect Feline Kit, 312, 376
UroEze. *See* Methionine
Uroeze. *See* Ammonium chloride
Urogram. *See* Excretory urography
Urolith(s)
radiologic findings with, 127–128, 129f–130f
urethral, 134f
versus urethral plug, 376
Urolithiasis, 376–377, 377f
after perineal urethrostomy, 496
ultrasonographic findings with, 150
Urticaria, differential diagnosis of, 663
USG. *See* Urine specific gravity
USP. *See* Calcium hydroxide
Uterine enlargement
caused by pyometra, 462f
ultrasonographic evaluation of, 150
Uterine inertia, 464
Uterine involution, 465
Uterine prolapse, 465
Uterine rupture, 464–465
and pyometra, 462, 463f
Uterine torsion, 464–465
Uvea, anatomy of, 332
Uveal tract, diseases of, 332–335
Uveitis, 332. *See also* Anterior uveitis
caused by feline infectious peritonitis, 345f, 345–346
complications of, 335
phagolytic, 336
prognosis for, 335

Vaccination(s). *See also specific type*
contraindications to, 472
of kittens, 38
in multicat facilities, 422–423
recommended program for, 423
recommendations for, 423t
Vaccine reaction granulomas, cytologic findings with, 99f, 108
VacSYN/FeLV, 366
Vagina, artificial, for breeding soundness examination, 466
Vaginal cytology, 459, 459f, 467
Vaginal discharge, differential diagnosis of, 664
Vaginal stimulation. *See also* Coital stimulation
mechanical, and induction of ovulation, 459
Valentine-shaped heart, in hypertrophic cardiomyopathy, 245, 246f
Valium. *See* Diazepam
Valproic acid, contraindications to, 221
Vasculitis. *See* Disseminated pyogranulomatous vasculitis

Vasectomy, 502
indications for, 502
surgical technique for, 501*f*, 502
Vasodilation, for dilated cardiomyopathy, 250
Vasopressin. *See* Antidiuretic hormone
Vasopressin tannate in oil
dosage and administration, 216
for PU/PD syndrome, 216
Vegetable fiber, 555
Vegetable oil, addition of, to prescription diet, 40–41
Veltrim. *See* Clotrimazole
Venipuncture
for euthanasia, 71–72
repeated, 311
Venocath long catheter, 477
placement of, procedures for, 478–479
Ventroflexion. *See* Cervical ventroflexion
Vertical ramus, 291*f*
fractures of, 449
Vertiginous signs, treatment of, 169
Vesicles, differential diagnosis of, 639
Vesicourachal diverticula, 375–376, 376*f*
Vestibular mechanism, during fall, 392
Vetalar. *See* Ketamine
Vet Alarm Respiratory Monitor, 59, 59*t*
Vetalog. *See* Triamcinolone
Vetasyl. *See* Psyllium
Vibramycin. *See* Doxycycline
Vicryl, 481
Vincent's stomatitis, 444
Vincristine
dose, 427*t*
route of administration, 427*t*
toxicity, 427*t*
Viral infections, gastrointestinal, 224
Viral rhinitis, 266
Viruses, transmission of, 420
Visual deficit, differential diagnosis of, 664
Vitamin A, 438
and pregnancy, 462, 472
Vitamin A analogs, contraindications to, 472
Vitamin B complex, with Vitamin C, drug interactions, 53*t*
Vitamin B deficiency, 438–439
Vitamin C, 372, 439, 559–560
Vitamin D_3. *See* Dihydrotachysterol
Vitamin K. *See* Phytonadione
Vitamino 4×, 47
Vitamin supplementation
for hepatic lipidosis, 411*t*
for plasmacytic-lymphocytic stomatitis, 444
Vitreous, 338
anatomy of, 338
clinical examination of, 338
congenital anomalies of, 338
pathologic conditions of, 338
primary retention of, 338
Vocalization, differential diagnosis of, 643
Vomiting/diarrhea, 223–227. *See also* Gastrointestinal disorders
caused by hyperthyroidism, 401
caused by metabolic disorders, 226
caused by nongastrointestinal disorders, 226–227
caused by primary gastrointestinal disorders, 223–226
caused by systemic fungal infections, 226–227
caused by toxic disorders, 226
chronic, and cervical line lesions, 293, 296
diagnosis of, 223
differential diagnosis of, 644–645, 647–648
induction of, for toxicosis, 554
treatment of, 223, 262
guidelines for, 223
in uremic CRD cat, 284
Vomitus hemorrhagic, differential diagnosis of, 651
V-to-Y technique, for surgical correction of ectropion, 322, 324*f*

Walchia americana, 515
Warfarin, 556
Water consumption, 207. *See also* Polydipsia
Water deprivation test, 214–216
disease differentiation based on, 216, 216*t*
indications for, 208, 214
procedure for, 215*t*
WBC count. *See* White blood cell count
WDT. *See* Water deprivation test
Weakness, episodic/intermittent, differential diagnosis of, 649
Wegie. *See* Norwegian Forest Cat
Weight loss, with diabetes mellitus, 305–306
Weight-to-body surface area, conversion table for, 629
Wheezing, differential diagnosis of, 659–660
White bile syndrome, 264–265
White blood cell count
from blood smear, 93
with chylothorax, 287
corrected, 93
from Hct tube, 93
total, diseases affecting, 85
values for
at different ages, 83
normal, 82
White blood cell pipette, 63
White petrolatum, 419*t*
Whole blood coagulation time, normal value for, 82
Wild Child, 60, 60*f*
Winstrol-V. *See* Stanozolol
Wirehair. *See* American wirehair
Wood's light examination, 506
Wool hair, 7
Wry mouth, 303
clinical signs of, 301
Wyoming (Selkirk) Rex, 16

Xenodine. *See* Iodine
XO chromosomal abnormality, 473
Xylazine
combined with ketamine, recommended dosage, 57*t*
contraindications to, 498
indications for, 71–72
for induction of emesis, 554
Xylocaine. *See* Lidocaine

Yobine. *See* Yohimbine
Yohimbine, 554
concentrations, 57*t*
dosage, 57*t*

Zantac. *See* Ranitidine
Zinc oxide, in sealer cement for root canal procedures, 300
Zinc oxide/eugenol sealer, 295
ZOE obturation, 300, 300*f*
Zoonotic diseases, 577–582, 578*t*
mode of transmission, 578*t*
Zygomatic arch, 291*f*
Zygomatic arch fractures, 447
Zygomatic salivary gland, 318

ISBN 0-397-51204-X
90000
9 780397 512041